**contexo** | media

Solutions from DecisionHealth

Draft

International Classification of Diseases
10th Revision Procedural Coding System

# ICD-10-PCS Expert for Hospitals

**DECISIONHEALTH®**

**2015 ICD-10-PCS (Draft)**

**International Classification of Diseases, 10th Revision, Procedural Coding System**

Published by DecisionHealth

9737 Washingtonian Blvd., Ste. 200
Gaithersburg, MD 20878-7364
www.codingbooks.com

Please call 800.334.5724 for questions or technical support

Printed in the United States of America

ISBN: 978-1-58383-788-7

**DISCLAIMER**

**ACKNOWLEDGEMENTS**

Tonya Nevin, *Vice President, Medical Practice Group*
Jerry M. Okabe, *Vice President, Business Development*
Gregory A. Kemp, MA, *Product Manager*
Lori Becks, RHIA, *Clinical Technical Editor*
Layne Shipley, *Database & Applications Manager*
Lori Cipro, *Production Manager*
Robyn Bernstein, *Designer*

# Table of Contents

# Introduction to ICD-10-PCS

## Development of the ICD-10 Procedure Coding System (ICD-10-PCS)

The *International Classification of Diseases 10th Revision Procedure Classification System* (ICD-10-PCS) has been developed as a replacement for Volume 3 of the *International Classification of Diseases 9th Revision* (ICD-9-CM). The development of ICD-10-PCS was funded by the U.S. Centers for Medicare and Medicaid Services (CMS).[1] ICD-10-PCS has a multiaxial seven character alphanumeric code structure that provides a unique code for all substantially different procedures, and allows new procedures to be easily incorporated as new codes. ICD-10-PCS was under development for over five years. The initial draft was formally tested and evaluated by an independent contractor; the final version was released in the Spring of 1998, with annual updates since the final release. The design, development and testing of ICD-10-PCS are discussed.

## Introduction

Volume 3 of the *International Classification of Diseases 9th Revision Clinical Modification* (ICD-9-CM) has been used in the U.S. for the reporting of inpatient procedures since 1979. The structure of Volume 3 of ICD-9-CM has not allowed new procedures associated with rapidly changing technology to be effectively incorporated as new codes. As a result, in 1992 the U.S. Centers for Medicare and Medicaid Services (CMS) funded a project to design a replacement for Volume 3 of ICD-9-CM. After a review of the preliminary design, CMS in 1995 awarded 3M Health Information Systems a three-year contract to complete development of the replacement system. The new system is the ICD-10 Procedure Coding System (ICD-10-PCS).

### Attributes Used in Development

The development of ICD-10-PCS had as its goal the incorporation of four major attributes:

#### Completeness

There should be a unique code for all substantially different procedures. In Volume 3 of ICD-9-CM, procedures on different body parts, with different approaches, or of different types are sometimes assigned to the same code.

#### Expandability

As new procedures are developed, the structure of ICD-10-PCS should allow them to be easily incorporated as unique codes.

#### Multiaxial

ICD-10-PCS codes should consist of independent characters, with each individual axis retaining its meaning across broad ranges of codes to the extent possible.

#### Standardized Terminology

ICD-10-PCS should include definitions of the terminology used. While the meaning of specific words varies in common usage, ICD-10-PCS should not include multiple meanings for the same term, and each term must be assigned a specific meaning.

If these four objectives are met, then ICD-10-PCS should enhance the ability of health information coders to construct accurate codes with minimal effort.

### General Development Principles

In the development of ICD-10-PCS, several general principles were followed:

### Diagnostic Information is Not Included in Procedure Description

When procedures are performed for specific diseases or disorders, the disease or disorder is not contained in the procedure code. There are no codes for procedures exclusive to aneurysms, cleft lip, strictures, neoplasms, hernias, etc. The diagnosis codes, not the procedure codes, specify the disease or disorder.

### Not Otherwise Specified (NOS) Options are Restricted

ICD-9-CM often provides a "not otherwise specified" code option. Certain NOS options made available in ICD-10-PCS are restricted to the uses laid out in the ICD-10-PCS draft guidelines. A minimal level of specificity is required for each component of the procedure.

### Limited Use of Not Elsewhere Classified (NEC) Option

ICD-9-CM often provides a "not elsewhere classified" code option. Because all significant components of a procedure are specified in ICD-10-PCS, there is generally no need for an NEC code option. However, limited NEC options are incorporated into ICD-10-PCS where necessary. For example, new devices are frequently developed, and therefore it is necessary to provide an "Other Device" option for use until the new device can be explicitly added to the coding system. Additional NEC options are discussed later, in the sections of the system where they occur.

### Level of Specificity

All procedures currently performed can be specified in ICD-10-PCS. The frequency with which a procedure is performed was not a consideration in the development of the system. Rather, a unique code is available for variations of a procedure that can be performed.

## ICD-10-PCS Structure

ICD-10-PCS has a seven character alphanumeric code structure. Each character contains up to 34 possible values. Each value represents a specific option for the general character definition (e.g., stomach is one of the values for the body part character). The ten digits 0-9 and the 24 letters A-H,J-N and P-Z may be used in each character. The letters O and I are not used in order to avoid confusion with the digits 0 and 1.

Procedures are divided into sections that identify the general type of procedure (e.g., medical and surgical, obstetrics, imaging). The first character of the procedure code always specifies the section. The sections are shown in Table 1.

### Table 1: ICD-10-CM Sections

| | |
|---|---|
| 0 | Medical and Surgical |
| 1 | Obstetrics |
| 2 | Placement |
| 3 | Administration |
| 4 | Measurement and Monitoring |
| 5 | Extracorporeal Assistance and Performance |
| 6 | Extracorporeal Therapies |
| 7 | Osteopathic |
| 8 | Other Procedures |
| 9 | Chiropractic |
| B | Imaging |
| C | Nuclear Medicine |
| D | Radiation Therapy |
| F | Physical Rehabilitation and Diagnostic Audiology |
| G | Mental Health |
| H | Substance Abuse Treatment |

[1] *The ICD-10-PCS is being developed with the support of the Centers for Medicare and Medicaid Services, under contract Nos. 90-1138, 91-22300, 500-95-0005, HHSM-500-2004-00011C and HHSM-500-2010-000555-C to 3M Health Information System.*

The second through seventh characters mean the same thing within each section, but may mean different things in other sections. In all sections, the third character specifies the general type of procedure performed (e.g., resection, transfusion, fluoroscopy), while the other characters give additional information such as the body part and approach. In ICD-10-PCS, the term "procedure" refers to the complete specification of the seven characters.

## ICD-10-PCS Format

The ICD-10-PCS is made up of three separate parts:

- Tables
- Index
- List of codes

The Index allows codes to be located by an alphabetic lookup. The index entry refers to a specific location in the Tables. The Tables must be used in order to construct a complete and valid code. The List of Codes provides a comprehensive listing of all valid codes, with a complete text description accompanying each code.

### Tables in ICD-10-PCS

The Tables in ICD-10-PCS are organized differently from ICD-9-CM. Each page in the Tables is composed of rows that specify the valid combinations of code values. *Table 2* is an excerpt from the ICD-10-PCS tables. In the system, the upper portion of each table specifies the values for the first three characters of the codes in that table. In the medical and surgical section, the first three characters are the section, the body system and the root operation.

In ICD-10-PCS, the values 027 specify the section Medical and Surgical (0), the body system Heart and Great Vessels (2) and the root operation Dilation (7). As shown in *Table 2*, the root operation (i.e., Dilation) is accompanied by its definition. The lower portion of the table specifies all the valid combinations of the remaining characters four through seven. The four columns in the table specify the last four characters. In the medical and surgical section they are labeled Body Part, Approach, Device and Qualifier, respectively. Each row in the table specifies the valid combination of values for characters four through seven. The Tables contain only those combinations of values that result in a valid procedure code.

*Table 2: Row from the Tables*

| 0 Medical and Surgical |
| :--- |
| **2 Heart and Great Vessels** |
| **7 Dilation: Expanding an orifice or the lumen of a tubular body part** |

| Character 4<br>Body Part | Character 5<br>Approach | Character 6<br>Device | Character 7<br>Qualifier |
| :--- | :--- | :--- | :--- |
| 0 Coronary Artery, One Site | 0 Open | 4 Drug-eluting Intraluminal Device | 6 Bifurcation |
| 1 Coronary Arteries, Two Sites | 3 Percutaneous | D Intraluminal Device | Z No Qualifier |
| 2 Coronary Arteries, Three Sites | 4 Percutaneous Endoscopic | T Radioactive Intraluminal Device | |
| 3 Coronary Arteries, Four or More Sites | | Z No Device | |

*Specifies the valid combinations of characters 4 through 7 for the medical and surgical root operation dilation of the heart and great vessels body system (027)*

The row in *Table 2* can be used to construct 96 unique procedure codes. For example, code 02703DZ specifies the procedure for dilation of one coronary artery using an intraluminal device via percutaneous approach (i.e., percutaneous transluminal coronary angioplasty with stent). *Table 3* provides code descriptions for a sample of valid codes constructed from the row shown in *Table 2*.

### List of Codes

The valid codes shown in Table 3 are constructed using the first body part value in *Table 2* (i.e., one coronary artery), combined with all the valid approaches and devices listed in the table, and the value "No Qualifier". The codes listed in *Table 3* are examples of entries in the List of Codes. Each code has a text description that is complete and easy to read. The List of Codes with complete descriptions is not included in print versions of the ICD-10-PCS due to the number procedure codes available in this coding system.

*Table 3: Code descriptions for dilation of one coronary artery (0270)*

| | |
| :--- | :--- |
| 027004Z | Dilation of Coronary Artery, One Site with Drug-eluting Intraluminal Device, Open Approach |
| 02700DZ | Dilation of Coronary Artery, One Site with Intraluminal Device, Open Approach |
| 02700TZ | Dilation of Coronary Artery, One Site with Radioactive Intraluminal Device, Open Approach |
| 02700ZZ | Dilation, Coronary Artery, One Site, Open Approach |
| 027034Z | Dilation, Coronary Artery, One Site with Drug-eluting Intraluminal Device, Percutaneous Approach |
| 02703DZ | Dilation, Coronary Artery, One Site with Intraluminal Device, Percutaneous Approach |
| 02703TZ | Dilation, Coronary Artery, One Site with Radioactive Intraluminal Device, Percutaneous Approach |
| 02703ZZ | Dilation, Coronary Artery, One Site, Percutaneous Approach |
| 027044Z | Dilation, Coronary Artery, One Site with Drug-eluting Intraluminal Device, Percutaneous Endoscopic Approach |
| 02704DZ | Dilation, Coronary Artery, One Site with Intraluminal Device, Percutaneous Endoscopic Approach |
| 02704TZ | Dilation, Coronary Artery, One Site with Radioactive Intraluminal Device, Percutaneous Endoscopic Approach |
| 02704ZZ | Dilation, Coronary Artery, One Site, Percutaneous Endoscopic Approach |

### Index

The Index allows codes to be located based on an alphabetic lookup. Codes may be found in the index based on the general type of the procedure (e.g., resection, transfusion, fluoroscopy), or a more commonly used term (e.g., appendectomy). The code for percutaneous intraluminal dilation of the coronary arteries with an intraluminal device can be found in the index under dilation, or a synonym of dilation (e.g., angioplasty).

Once the desired term is located in the index, the index specifies the first three or four values of the code (e.g., 027), or directs the user to see another term. In rare instances additional characters or the entire code is listed. Each table also identifies the first three values of the code (e.g., 027). Based on the first three values of the code obtained from the index, the corresponding table can be located. The table is then used to obtain the complete code by specifying the last four values.

## Medical and Surgical Section (0)

### Character Meanings

The seven characters for medical and surgical procedures have the following meaning:

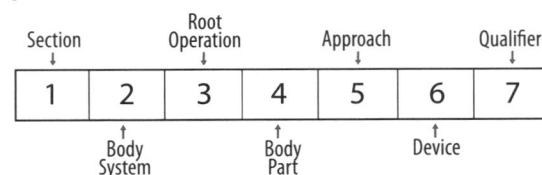

The medical and surgical section codes represent the vast majority of procedures reported in an inpatient setting. Medical and surgical procedure codes have a first character value of "0". The second character indicates the general body system (e.g., gastrointestinal). The third character indicates the root operation, or specific objective, of the procedure (e.g., excision). The fourth character indicates the specific body part on which the procedure was performed (e.g., duodenum). The fifth character indicates the approach used to reach the procedure site (e.g., open). The sixth character indicates whether any device was used and remained at the end of the procedure (e.g., synthetic substitute). The seventh character is a qualifier that may have a specific meaning for a limited range of values. For example, the qualifier can be used to identify the destination site of the root operation Bypass.

The first through fifth characters are always assigned a specific value, but the device (sixth character) and the qualifier (seventh character) are not applicable to all procedures. The value Z is used for the sixth and seventh characters to indicate that a specific device or qualifier does not apply to the procedure.

## Section (Character 1)

The first character for the Medical and Surgical Section has a value of "Ø".

## Body Systems (Character 2)

The body systems for medical and surgical section codes are specified in the second character, shown in *Table 4*. In order to provide necessary detail, some body systems are subdivided. For example, body system values K (muscles), L (tendons), M (bursae and ligaments), N (head and facial bones), P (upper bones), Q (lower bones), R (upper joints) and S (lower joints) are divisions of the musculoskeletal system.

*Table 4: Medical and Surgical Body Systems*

| | |
|---|---|
| Ø | Central Nervous System |
| 1 | Peripheral Nervous System |
| 2 | Heart and Great Vessels |
| 3 | Upper Arteries |
| 4 | Lower Arteries |
| 5 | Upper Veins |
| 6 | Lower Veins |
| 7 | Lymphatic and Hemic System |
| 8 | Eye |
| 9 | Ear, Nose, Sinus |
| B | Respiratory System |
| C | Mouth and Throat |
| D | Gastrointestinal System |
| F | Hepatobiliary System and Pancreas |
| G | Endocrine System |
| H | Skin and Breast |
| J | Subcutaneous Tissue and Fascia |
| K | Muscles |
| L | Tendons |
| M | Bursae and Ligaments |
| N | Head and Facial Bones |
| P | Upper Bones |
| Q | Lower Bones |
| R | Upper Joints |
| S | Lower Joints |
| T | Urinary System |
| U | Female Reproductive System |
| V | Male Reproductive System |
| W | Anatomical Regions, General |
| X | Anatomical Regions, Upper Extremities |
| Y | Anatomical Regions, Lower Extremities |

## Root Operation (Character 3)

The root operation is specified in the third character. In the medical and surgical section there are 31 different root operation values, as shown in *Table 5*.

*Table 5: Medical and Surgical Root Operations Definitions*

| Root Operation | Definition |
|---|---|
| Alteration | Modifying the anatomic structure of a body part without affecting the function of the body part |
| Bypass | Altering the route of passage of the contents of a tubular body part |
| Change | Taking out or off a device from a body part and putting back an identical or similar device in or on the same body part without cutting or puncturing the skin or a mucous membrane |
| Control | Stopping, or attempting to stop, postprocedural bleeding |
| Creation | Making a new genital structure that does not take over the function of a body part |
| Destruction | Physical eradication of all or a portion of a body part by the direct use of energy, force or a destructive agent |
| Detachment | Cutting off all or part of the upper or lower extremities |
| Dilation | Expanding an orifice or the lumen of a tubular body part |
| Division | Cutting into a body part without draining fluids and/or gases from the body part in order to separate or transect a body part |
| Drainage | Taking or letting out fluids and/or gases from a body part |

| Root Operation | Definition |
|---|---|
| Excision | Cutting out or off, without replacement, a portion of a body part |
| Extirpation | Taking or cutting out solid matter from a body part |
| Extraction | Pulling or stripping out or off all or a portion of a body part by the use of force |
| Fragmentation | Breaking solid matter in a body part into pieces |
| Fusion | Joining together portions of an articular body part rendering the articular body part immobile |
| Insertion | Putting in a non-biological appliance that monitors, assists, performs or prevents a physiological function but does not physically take the place of a body part |
| Inspection | Visually and/or manually exploring a body part |
| Map | Locating the route of passage of electrical impulses and/or locating functional areas in a body part |
| Occlusion | Completely closing an orifice or the lumen of a tubular body part |
| Reattachment | Putting back in or on all or a portion of a separated body part to its normal location or other suitable location |
| Release | Freeing a body part from an abnormal physical constraint by cutting or by use of force |
| Removal | Taking out or off a device from a body part |
| Repair | Restoring, to the extent possible, a body part to its normal anatomic structure and function |
| Replacement | Putting in or on biological or synthetic material that physically takes the place of all or a portion of a body part |
| Reposition | Moving to its normal location or other suitable location all or a portion of a body part |
| Resection | Cutting out or off, without replacement, all of a body part |
| Restriction | Partially closing an orifice or the lumen of a tubular body part |
| Revision | Correcting, to the extent possible, a portion of a malfunctioning device or the position of a displaced device |
| Supplement | Putting in or on biological or synthetic material that physically reinforces and/or augments the function of a portion of a body part |
| Transfer | Moving, without taking out, all or a portion of a body part to another location to take over the function of all or a portion of a body part |
| Transplantation | Putting in or on all or a portion of a living body part taken from another individual or animal to physically take the place and/or function of all or a portion of a similar body part |

The root operation identifies the objective of the procedure. Each root operation has a precise definition. For example, the root operation Insertion is used for procedures where devices are put in or on a body part. If a device is taken out but no equivalent device is put in, then the root operation Removal is used. The root operation Extirpation is used when solid matter such as a foreign body, embolus or calculus is taken out of a body part without taking out any of the body part. The root operation Excision is used when a portion of a body part is cut out, while the root operation Resection is used when all of a body part as defined by the body part value is cut out. If biological or synthetic material is put in to take the place of all or a portion of a body part, then the root operation Replacement is used. If the body part has a living body part from a donor put in its place, then the root operation Transplantation is used.

The above examples of root operation terminology illustrate the precision of the values defined in the system. There is a clear distinction between each root operation. A root operation specifies the objective of the procedure. The term "anastomosis" is not a root operation, because it is a means of joining and is always an integral part of another procedure (e.g., bypass, resection) with a specific objective. Similarly, "incision" is not a root operation, since it is always part of the objective of another procedure (e.g., division, drainage). The root operation Repair in the medical and surgical section functions as a "not elsewhere classified" option. It is used when the procedure performed is not one of the other specific root operations.

*Appendix A* provides additional explanation and representative examples of the medical and surgical root operations. *Appendix D* groups all root operations in the medical and surgical section into sub-categories and provides an example of each root operation.

## Body Part (Character 4)

The body part is specified in the fourth character. The body part indicates the specific part of the body system on which the procedure was performed (e.g., duodenum). Tubular body parts are defined in ICD-10-PCS as those hollow body parts that provide a route of passage for solids, liquids, or gases. They include the cardiovascular system, and body parts such as those contained in the gastrointestinal tract, genitourinary tract, biliary tract, and respiratory tract.

*Appendix A* contains a list of body parts included in the Medical and Surgical Section and identifies all structures included in the body part designation. For example, body part value G, Intracranial Artery, includes: anterior cerebral artery, anterior choroidal artery, anterior communicating artery, basilar artery, Circle of Willis, middle cerebral artery, posterior cerebral artery, posterior communicating artery, and posterior inferior cerebellar artery (PICA). A procedure performed on one of the listed arteries is reported with body part value G.

## Approach (Character 5)

The technique used to reach the site of the procedure is specified in the fifth character. There are seven different approaches, as shown in *Table 6*. The approach is comprised of three components: the access location, method, and type of instrumentation.

### Access Location

For procedures performed on an internal body part, the access location specifies the external site through which the site of the procedure is reached. There are two general types of access locations: skin or mucous membranes, and external orifices. Every approach value except external includes one of these two access locations. The skin or mucous membrane can be cut or punctured to reach the procedure site. All open and percutaneous approach values use this access location. The site of a procedure can also be reached through an external opening. External openings can be natural (e.g., mouth) or artificial (e.g., colostomy stoma).

### Method

For procedures performed on an internal body part, the method specifies how the external access location is entered. An open method specifies cutting through the skin or mucous membrane and any other intervening body layers necessary to expose the site of the procedure. An instrumental method specifies the entry of instrumentation through the access location to the internal procedure site. Instrumentation can be introduced by puncture or minor incision, or through an external opening. The puncture or minor incision does not constitute an open approach, because it does not expose the site of the procedure. An approach can define multiple methods. For example, the open endoscopic approach includes both the open method to expose the body part and the introduction of instrumentation into the body part to perform the procedure.

### Type of Instrumentation

For procedures performed on an internal body part, instrumentation means that specialized equipment is used to perform the procedure. Instrumentation is used in all internal approaches other than the basic open approach. Instrumentation may or may not include the capacity to visualize the procedure site. For example, the instrumentation used to perform a sigmoidoscopy permits the internal site of the procedure to be visualized, while the instrumentation used to perform a needle biopsy of the liver does not. The term "endoscopic" as used in approach values refers to instrumentation that permits a site to be visualized.

### External Approaches

Procedures performed directly on the skin or mucous membrane are identified by the external approach (e.g., skin excision). Procedures performed indirectly by the application of external force are also identified by the external approach (e.g., closed reduction of fracture).

*Table 6* contains a definition of each approach. *Appendix E* compares the components (access location, method, and type of instrumentation) of each approach, and provides an example of each approach.

### Table 6: Medical and Surgical Approach Definitions

| Approach Value | Approach Definition |
|---|---|
| Open | Cutting through the skin or mucous membrane and any other body layers necessary to expose the site of the procedure |
| Percutaneous | Entry, by puncture or minor incision, of instrumentation through the skin or mucous membrane and/or any other body layers necessary to reach the site of the procedure |
| Percutaneous Endoscopic | Entry, by puncture or minor incision, of instrumentation through the skin or mucous membrane and/or any other body layers necessary to reach and visualize the site of the procedure |
| Via Natural or Artificial Opening | Entry of instrumentation through a natural or artificial external opening to reach the site of the procedure |
| Via Natural or Artificial Opening Endoscopic | Entry of instrumentation through a natural or artificial external opening to reach and visualize the site of the procedure |
| Via Natural or Artificial Opening Endoscopic with Percutaneous Endoscopic Assistance | Entry of instrumentation through a natural or artificial external opening to reach and visualize the site of the procedure, and entry, by puncture or minor incision, of instrumentation through the skin or mucous membrane and any other body layers necessary to aid in the performance of the procedure |
| External | Procedures performed directly on the skin or mucous membrane and procedures performed indirectly by the application of external force through the skin or mucous membrane |

## Device (Character 6)

The device is specified in the sixth character and is only used to specify devices that remain after the procedure is completed. There are four general types of devices:

1. Biological or synthetic material that takes the place of all or a portion of a body part (e.g, skin graft, joint prosthesis).

2. Biological or synthetic material that assists or prevents a physiological function (e.g., IUD).

3. Therapeutic material that is not absorbed by, eliminated by, or incorporated into a body part (e.g., radioactive implant).

4. Mechanical or electronic appliances used to assist, monitor, take the place of or prevent a physiological function (e.g., cardiac pacemaker, orthopedic pin).

While all devices can be removed, some devices cannot be removed without putting in another non-biological appliance or body part substitute. Specific device values may be coded with the root operations Alteration, Bypass, Creation, Dilation, Drainage, Fusion, Occlusion, Reposition, and Restriction. Specific device values must be coded with the root operations Change, Insertion, Removal, Replacement, and Revision. Instruments used to visualize the procedure site are not specified in the device value. This information is specified in the approach value.

If the objective of the procedure is to put in the device, then the root operation is Insertion. If the device is put in to meet an objective other than insertion, then the root operation defining the underlying objective of the procedure is used, with the device specified in the device character. For example, if a procedure to replace the hip joint is performed, the root operation Replacement is coded and the prosthetic device is specified in the device character. Materials incidental to a procedure such as clips, ligatures and sutures are not specified in the device character. Because new devices can be developed, the value "Other Device" is provided as a temporary option for use until a specific device value is added to the system.

## Qualifier (Character 7)

The qualifier is specified in the seventh character. The qualifier contains unique values for individual procedures as needed. For example, the qualifier can be used to identify the destination site in a bypass.

# Medical and Surgical Section Principles

In developing the medical and surgical procedure codes, several specific principles were followed:

## Composite Terms are Not Root Operations

The only component of a procedure specified in the root operation is the objective of the procedure. Composite terms such as colonoscopy and sigmoidectomy are not root operations because they specify multiple components of a procedure. The term "colonoscopy" is a composite of information contained in the root operation value, i.e., inspection, the body part value, i.e., large intestine, and the endoscopic approach value, i.e., via natural or artificial opening endoscopic. In ICD-10-PCS, the components of a procedure are defined separately. The underlying objective of the procedure is specified by the root operation (third character), the precise part of the gastrointestinal tract inspected is specified by the body part (fourth character), and the method used to reach and visualize the procedure site is specified by the approach (fifth character). A partial sigmoidectomy is likewise a composite of information contained in the root operation value, i.e., excision, and the body part value, i.e., sigmoid colon. In ICD-10-PCS, a partial sigmoidectomy is coded as excision (cutting out or off, without replacement, a portion of a body part) of the sigmoid body part. While the terms colonoscopy and sigmoidectomy are listed in the index, they do not constitute separate root operations in the Tables, but instead refer to the correct root operation and body system in the Tables.

### Root Operation Based on the Objective of the Procedure

The root operation is based on the objective of the procedure, such as resection of transverse colon or dilation of an artery. The assignment of the root operation is based on the procedure actually performed, which may or may not have been the intended procedure. If the intended procedure is modified or discontinued (e.g., excision instead of resection is performed), the root operation is determined by the procedure actually performed. If the desired result fails to persist after completion of the procedure (i.e., the artery does not remain expanded after the dilation procedure), the root operation is still determined by the procedure actually performed.

If the procedure performed takes out a foreign body, then the procedure is coded to the Extirpation. Dilating the urethra is coded as Dilation, since the objective of the procedure is to dilate the urethra. If dilation of the urethra includes putting in an intraluminal stent, the root operation remains Dilation and not Insertion of the intraluminal device, because the underlying objective of the procedure is dilation of the urethra. The stent is identified by the intraluminal device value in the sixth character of the dilation procedure code. If the objective is solely to put a radioactive element in the urethra, then the procedure is coded to the root operation Insertion, with the radioactive element identified in the sixth character of the code. If the objective of the procedure is to correct a malfunctioning or displaced device, then the procedure is coded to the root operation Revision. In the root operation Revision, the original device being revised is identified in the device character. Revision is typically performed on mechanical appliances (e.g., pacemaker), or materials used in replacement procedures (e.g., synthetic substitute) Typical revision procedures include adjustment of pacemaker position and correction of malfunctioning knee prosthesis.

### Combination Procedures are Coded Separately

If multiple procedures as defined by distinct objectives are performed during an operative episode, then multiple codes are used. For example, obtaining the vein graft used for coronary bypass surgery is coded as a separate procedure from the bypass itself.

### Redo of Procedures are Coded to the Procedure Performed

The complete or partial redo of the original procedure is coded to the root operation that identifies the procedure performed rather than revision. For example, a complete redo of a hip replacement procedure which requires putting in a new prosthesis is coded to the root operation Replacement rather than Revision. The correction of complications arising from the original procedure other than device complications as defined in the root operation Revision are also coded to the procedure performed. For example, a procedure to control hemorrhage arising from the original procedure is coded to Control rather than Revision.

### Examples of Procedures Coded in ICD-10-PCS

The following are examples from the Medical and Surgical section:

**0HQEXZZ**    **Suture of skin laceration, left lower arm**
Medical and surgical section (0), body system skin and breast (H), root operation repair (Q), body part skin left lower arm (E), external approach (X) no device (Z) and no qualifier (Z).

**0DTJ4ZZ**    **Laparoscopic appendectomy**
Medical and surgical section (0), body system gastrointestinal (D), root operation resection (T), body part appendix (J), percutaneous endoscopic approach (4), no device (Z) and no qualifier (Z).

**0DBN8ZX**    **Sigmoidoscopy with biopsy**
Medical and surgical section (0), body system gastrointestinal (D), root operation excision (B), body part sigmoid colon (N), via natural or artificial opening endoscopic approach (8), no device (Z) and with qualifier diagnostic (X).

**0B110F4**    **Tracheostomy using tracheostomy tube**
Medical and surgical section (0), body system respiratory (B), root operation bypass (1), body part trachea (1), open approach (0), with tracheostomy device (F) and qualifier cutaneous (4).

## Obstetrics Section

The seven characters in the obstetrics section have the same meaning as in the medical and surgical section.

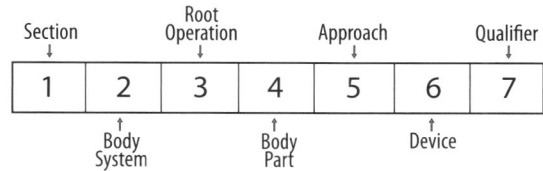

### Section (Character 1)

Obstetrics procedure codes have a first character value of "1".

### Body System (Character 2)

The second character value for body system is pregnancy.

### Root Operation (Character 3)

The root operations Change, Drainage, Extraction, Insertion, Inspection, Removal, Repair, Reposition, Resection and Transplantation are used in the obstetrics section, and have the same meaning as in the medical and surgical section. The obstetrics section also includes two additional root operations, Abortion and Delivery, defined below:

| Root Operation | Definition |
|---|---|
| *Abortion* | Artificially terminating a pregnancy |
| *Delivery* | Assisting the products of conception from the genital canal |

A cesarean section is not its own unique root operation, because the underlying objective is Extraction (i.e., pulling out all or a portion of a body part).

### Body Part (Character 4)

The body part values in the obstetrics section are:

- Products of conception
- Products of conception, retained
- Products of conception, ectopic

The obstetrics section includes procedures performed on the products of conception only; procedures on the pregnant female are coded in the medical and surgical section (e.g., episiotomy). The term "products of conception" refers to all physical components of a pregnancy, including the fetus, amnion, umbilical cord and placenta. There is no differentiation of the products of conception based on gestational age. Thus, the specification of the products of conception as a zygote, embryo or fetus, or the trimester of the pregnancy, is not part of the procedure code but can be found in the diagnosis code.

### Approach (Character 5)

The fifth character specifies approaches as defined in the medical and surgical section.

### Device (Character 6)

The sixth character is used for devices such as fetal monitoring electrodes.

### Qualifier (Character 7)

Qualifier values are specific to the root operation, and are used to specify the type of extraction (e.g., low forceps, high forceps, low cervical cesarean, etc.), the type of fluid taken out during a drainage procedure (e.g., amniotic fluid, fetal blood, etc.) or the body system of the products of conception on which a repair was performed.

## Placement Section

The seven characters in the placement section have the following meaning:

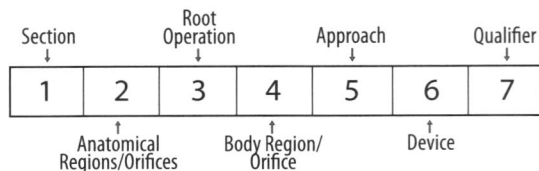

Placement section codes represent procedures for putting an externally placed device in or on a body region for the purpose of protection, immobilization, stretching, compression or packing.

### Section (Character 1)

Placement procedure codes have a first character value of "2".

### Anatomical Region/Orifices (Character 2)

The second character value for body system is either anatomical regions or anatomical orifices.

### Root Operation (Character 3)

The root operations Change and Removal are contained in the placement section, and have the same meaning as in the medical and surgical section.

The placement section also includes five additional root operations, defined as follows:

| Root Operation | Definition |
|---|---|
| Compression | Putting pressure on a body region |
| Dressing | Putting material on a body region for protection |
| Immobilization | Limiting or preventing motion of an external body region |
| Packing | Putting material in a body region or orifice |
| Traction | Exerting a pulling force on a body region in a distal direction |

### Body Region/Orifice (Character 4)

The fourth character values are either body regions (e.g., upper leg) or natural orifices (e.g., ear).

### Approach (Character 5)

Since all placement procedures are performed directly on the skin or mucous membrane, or performed indirectly by the application of external force through the skin or mucous membrane, the approach value is always External.

### Device (Character 6)

The device character is always specified (except in the case of manual traction) and indicates the device placed during the procedure (e.g., cast, splint, bandage, etc.). Except for casts for fractures and dislocations, devices in the placement section are off the shelf and do not require any extensive design, fabrication or fitting. Placement of devices that require extensive design, fabrication or fitting are coded in the rehabilitation section.

### Qualifier (Character 7)

The qualifier character is not specified in the placement section; thus the qualifier value is always No Qualifier.

## Administration Section

The seven characters in the administration section have the following meaning:

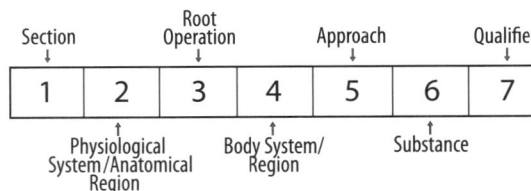

Administration section codes represent procedures for putting in or on a therapeutic, prophylactic, protective, diagnostic, nutritional or physiological substance.

### Section (Character 1)

Administration procedure codes have a first character value of "3".

### Physiological System & Anatomical Region (Character 2)

The physiological system and anatomical region character contains three values: circulatory system, indwelling device, and physiological systems and anatomical regions. The circulatory body system is used for transfusion procedures.

### Root Operation (Character 3)

There are three root operations in the administration section:

| Root Operation | Definition |
|---|---|
| Introduction | Putting in or on a therapeutic, diagnostic, nutritional, physiological or prophylactic substance except blood or blood products |
| Irrigation | Putting in or on a cleansing substance |
| Transfusion | Putting in blood or blood products |

### Body System/Region (Character 4)

The fourth character specifies the body system/region. It identifies the site where the substance is administered, not the site where the substance administered takes effect. Sites include skin and mucous membrane, subcutaneous tissue and muscle. These differentiate intradermal, subcutaneous, and intramuscular injections respectively. Other sites include eye, respiratory tract, peritoneal cavity, and epidural space.

### Approach (Character 5)

The fifth character specifies approaches as defined in the medical and surgical section. The approach for intradermal, subcutaneous and intramuscular introductions (i.e., injections) is percutaneous. If a catheter is placed to introduce a substance into an internal site within the circulatory system, then the approach is percutaneous. For example, if a catheter is advanced directly into the heart to introduce contrast for angiography, then the procedure would be coded as a percutaneous introduction of contrast into the heart.

The body systems/regions for arteries and veins are peripheral artery, central artery, peripheral vein and central vein. The peripheral artery or vein is typically used when a substance is introduced locally into an artery or vein. For example, chemotherapy is the introduction of an antineoplastic substance into a peripheral artery or vein by a percutaneous approach. In general, the substance introduced into a peripheral artery or vein has a systemic effect.

The central artery or vein is typically used when the site where the substance is introduced is distant from the point of entry into the artery or vein. For example, the introduction of a substance directly at the site of a clot within an artery or vein using a catheter is coded as an introduction of a thrombolytic substance into a central artery or vein by a percutaneous approach. In general, the substance introduced into a central artery or vein has a local effect.

### Substance (Character 6)

The sixth character specifies the substance being introduced. Broad categories of substances are defined, such as anesthetic, contrast, dialysate, and blood products such as platelets.

## Qualifier (Character 7)

The seventh character is a qualifier, and is used to indicate whether a substance transfused is autologous or nonautologous, or to further specify a substance introduced.

## Measurement and Monitoring Section

The characters in the measuring and monitoring section have the following meaning:

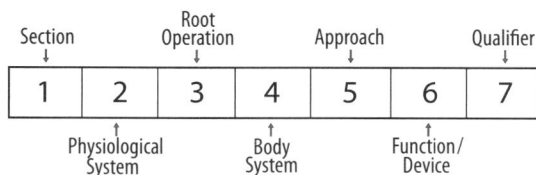

Measurement and monitoring section codes represent procedures for determining the level of a physiological or physical function.

### Section (Character 1)

Measurement and monitoring procedure codes have a first character value of "4."

### Physiological Systems (Character 2)

The second character value for body system is either physiological systems or physiological devices.

### Root Operation (Character 3)

There are two root operations in the measurement and monitoring section, as defined below:

| Root Operation | Definition |
|---|---|
| Measurement | Determining the level of a physiological or physical function at a point in time |
| Monitoring | Determining the level of a physiological or physical function repetitively over a period of time |

### Body System (Character 4)

The fourth character specifies the body system measured or monitored.

### Approach (Character 5)

The fifth character specifies approaches as defined in the medical and surgical section.

### Function (Character 6)

Instead of specifying device, the sixth character specifies the physiological or physical function being measured or monitored. Examples of physiological or physical function values are conductivity, metabolism, pulse, temperature, and volume. If a device used to perform the measurement or monitoring is inserted and left in, then insertion of the device is coded as a separate medical and surgical section procedure.

### Qualifier (Character 7)

The seventh character qualifier contains specific values as needed to further specify the body part (e.g., central, portal, pulmonary) or a variation of the procedure performed (e.g., ambulatory, stress).

Examples of typical procedures coded in this section are EKG, EEG, and cardiac catheterization. An EKG is the measurement of cardiac electrical activity, while an EEG is the measurement of electrical activity of the central nervous system. A cardiac catheterization performed to measure the pressure in the heart is coded as the measurement of cardiac pressure by percutaneous approach.

## Extracorporeal Assistance and Performance Section

The seven characters in the extracorporeal assistance and performance section have the following meaning.

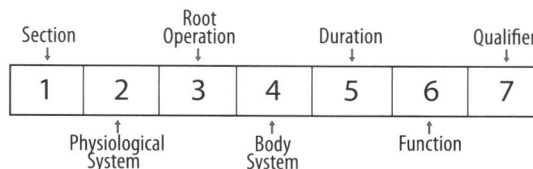

In extracorporeal assistance and performance procedures, equipment outside the body is used to assist or perform a physiological function.

### Section (Character 1)

Extracorporeal assistance and performance procedure codes have a first character value of "5".

### Physiological Systems (Character 2)

The second character value for body system is physiological systems.

### Root Operation (Character 3)

There are three root operations in the extracorporeal assistance and performance section, as defined below.

| Root Operation | Definition |
|---|---|
| Assistance | Taking over a portion of a physiological function by extracorporeal means |
| Performance | Completely taking over a physiological function by extracorporeal means |
| Restoration | Returning, or attempting to return, a physiological function to its natural state by extracorporeal means |

The root operation Restoration contains a single procedure code that identifies extracorporeal cardioversion.

### Body System (Character 4)

The fourth character specifies the body system (e.g., cardiac, respiratory) to which extracorporeal assistance or performance is applied.

### Approach (Character 5)

The fifth character specifies the duration of the procedure, i.e., single, intermittent, continuous. For respiratory ventilation assistance or performance, the duration is specified in hours, i.e., <24 hours, 24-96 hours or >96 hours.

### Function (Character 6)

The sixth character specifies the physiological function assisted or performed (e.g., oxygenation, ventilation) during the procedure.

### Qualifier (Character 7)

The seventh character qualifier specifies the type of equipment used, if any.

## Extracorporeal Therapies Section

The seven characters in the extracorporeal therapies section have the following meaning:

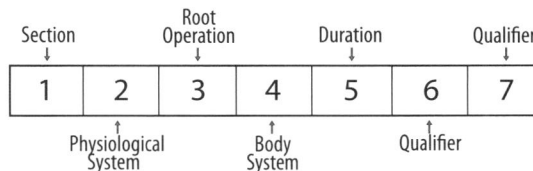

In extracorporeal therapy, equipment outside the body is used for a therapeutic purpose that does not involve the assistance or performance of a physiological function.

### Section (Character 1)

Extracorporeal therapy procedure codes have a first character value of "6".

### Physiological Systems (Character 2)

There is a single second character value of "A" for physiological systems in the extracorporeal therapies section.

## Root Operation (Character 3)

There are ten root operations in the extracorporeal therapy section, as defined below.

| Root Operation | Definition |
|---|---|
| Atmospheric Control | Extracorporeal control of atmospheric pressure and composition |
| Decompression | Extracorporeal elimination of undissolved gas from body fluids |
| Electromagnetic Therapy | Extracorporeal treatment by electromagnetic rays |
| Hyperthermia | Extracorporeal raising of body temperature |
| Hypothermia | Extracorporeal lowering of body temperature |
| Pheresis | Extracorporeal separation of blood products |
| Phototherapy | Extracorporeal treatment by light rays |
| Shock Wave Therapy | Extracorporeal treatment by shock waves |
| Ultrasound Therapy | Extracorporeal treatment by ultrasound |
| Ultraviolet Light Therapy | Extracorporeal treatment by ultraviolet light |

## Body System (Character 4)

The fourth character specifies the body system on which the extracorporeal therapy is performed (e.g., skin, circulatory).

## Duration (Character 5)

The fifth character specifies the duration of the procedure (e.g., single or intermittent).

## Qualifier (Character 6)

The sixth character is not specified for extracorporeal therapies, and always has the value No Qualifier.

## Qualifier (Character 7)

The seventh character qualifier is used in the root operation Pheresis to specify the blood component on which pheresis is performed.

## Osteopathic Section

The seven characters in the osteopathic section have the following meaning:

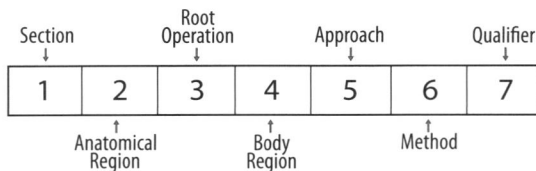

## Section (Character 1)

Osteopathic procedure codes have a first character value of "7".

## Anatomical Regions (Character 2)

There is a single second character value of "W" for anatomical regions in the osteopathic section.

## Root Operation (Character 3)

There is only one root operation in the osteopathic section.

| Root Operation | Definition |
|---|---|
| Treatment | Manual treatment to eliminate or alleviate somatic dysfunction and related disorders |

## Body Region (Character 4)

The fourth character specifies the body region on which the osteopathic manipulation is performed.

## Approach (Character 5)

The approach for osteopathic manipulations is always External.

## Method (Character 6)

The sixth character specifies the method by which the manipulation is accomplished.

## Qualifier (Character 7)

The seventh character is not specified in the osteopathic section and always has the value No Qualifier.

## Other Procedures Section

The seven characters in the other procedures section have the following meaning:

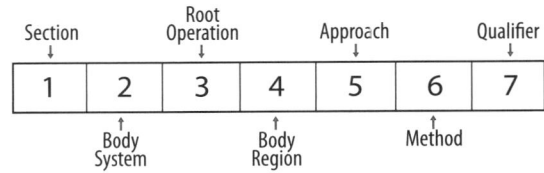

The other procedures section includes acupuncture, suture removal and in vitro fertilization.

## Section (Character 1)

Other procedures section codes have a first character value of "8".

## Body System (Character 2)

The second character value for body system represents either an indwelling device with a character value of "C" or physiological systems and anatomical regions with a character value of "E".

## Root Operation (Character 3)

The other procedures section has only one root operation, defined as follows:

| Root Operation | Definition |
|---|---|
| Other Procedures | Methodologies which attempt to remediate or cure a disorder or disease |

## Body Region (Character 4)

The fourth character contains specified body region values, and also the body region value none for extracorporeal procedures.

## Approach (Character 5)

Approaches included are percutaneous and external.

## Method (Character 6)

The sixth character specifies the method (e.g., acupuncture, robotic-assisted procedure).

## Qualifier (Character 7)

The seventh character is a qualifier, and contains specific values as needed.

## Chiropractic Section

The seven characters in the chiropractic section have the following meaning:

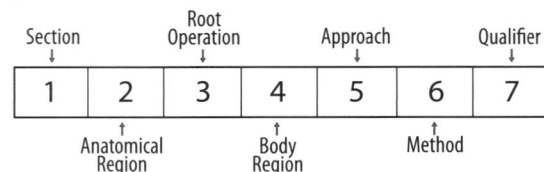

## Section (Character 1)

Chiropractic section procedure codes have a first character value of "9".

## Anatomical Regions (Character 2)

There is a single second character value of "W" for anatomical regions in the chiropractic section.

## Root Operation (Character 3)

There is only one root operation in the chiropractic section.

| Root Operation | Definition |
|---|---|
| Manipulation | Manual procedure that involves a directed thrust to move a joint past the physiological range of motion, without exceeding the anatomical limit |

## Body Region (Character 4)

The fourth character specifies the body region on which the chiropractic manipulation is performed.

## Approach (Character 5)

The approach for chiropractic manipulation is always External.

## Method (Character 6)

The sixth character is the method by which the manipulation is accomplished.

## Qualifier (Character 7)

The seventh character is not specified in the chiropractic section, and always has the value No Qualifier.

## Imaging Section

The seven characters in the imaging section have the following meaning:

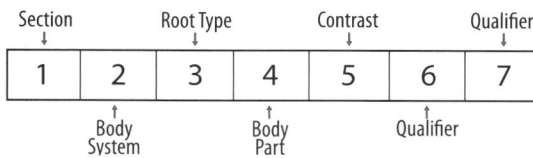

Imaging section codes represent procedures including plain radiography, fluoroscopy, CT, MRI, and ultrasound. Nuclear medicine procedure codes, including PET, uptakes, and scans, are in the nuclear medicine section. Therapeutic radiation procedure codes are in a separate radiation therapy section.

## Section (Character 1)

Imaging procedure codes have a first character value of "B".

## Body System (Character 2)

In the imaging section, the second character defines the body system.

## Root Type (Character 3)

The third character defines the root type of imaging procedure (e.g, MRI, ultrasound). There are five root types in the imaging section as defined below:

| Root Type | Definition |
| --- | --- |
| Plain Radiography | Planar display of an image developed from the capture of external ionizing radiation on photographic or photoconductive plate |
| Fluoroscopy | Single plane or bi-plane real time display of an image developed from the capture of external ionizing radiation on fluorescent screen. The image may also be stored by either digital or analog means |
| Computerized Tomography (CT Scan) | Computer-reformatted digital display of multiplanar images developed from the capture of multiple exposures of external ionizing radiation |
| Magnetic Resonance Imaging (MRI) | Computer reformatted digital display of multiplanar images developed from the capture of radio frequency signals emitted by nuclei in a body site excited within a magnetic field |
| Ultrasonography | Real time display of images of anatomy or flow information developed from the capture of reflected and attenuated high frequency sound waves |

## Body Part (Character 4)

The fourth character defines the body part.

## Contrast (Character 5)

The fifth character specifies whether the contrast material used in the imaging procedure is high or low osmolar, when applicable.

## Qualifier (Character 6)

The sixth character qualifier provides further detail as needed, such as unenhanced followed by enhanced.

## Qualifier (Character 7)

The seventh character qualifier contains specific values as needed to further specify the objective of the imaging procedure, e.g., densitometry, or the approach used, e.g., intravascular.

## Nuclear Medicine Section

The seven characters in the nuclear medicine section have the following meaning:

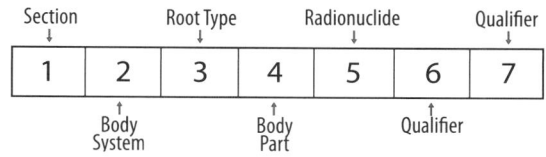

Nuclear medicine section codes represent procedures that introduce radioactive material into the body in order to create an image, to diagnose and treat pathologic conditions, or to assess metabolic functions. The nuclear medicine section does not include the introduction of encapsulated radioactive material for the treatment of cancer. These procedures are included in the radiation therapy section.

## Section (Character 1)

Nuclear medicine procedure codes have a first character value of "C".

## Body System (Character 2)

The second character specifies the body system on which the nuclear medicine procedure is performed.

## Root Type (Character 3)

The third character root type indicates the type of nuclear medicine procedure (e.g., planar imaging or non-imaging uptake). There are seven root types in the nuclear medicine section as defined below:

| Root Type | Definition |
| --- | --- |
| Nonimaging Assay | Introduction of radioactive materials into the body for the study of body fluids and blood elements, by the detection of radioactive emissions |
| Nonimaging Probe | Introduction of radioactive materials into the body for the study of distribution and fate of certain substances by the detection of radioactive emissions; or, alternatively, measurement of absorption of radioactive emissions from an external source |
| Nonimaging Uptake | Introduction of radioactive materials into the body for measurements of organ function, from the detection of radioactive emissions |
| Planar Imaging | Introduction of radioactive materials into the body for single plane display of images developed from the capture of radioactive emissions |
| Positron Emission Tomographic (PET) Imaging | Introduction of radioactive materials into the body for three dimensional display of images developed from the simultaneous capture, 180 degrees apart, of radioactive emissions |
| Systemic Therapy | Introduction of unsealed radioactive materials into the body for treatment |
| Tomographic (Tomo) Imaging | Introduction of radioactive materials into the body for three dimensional display of images developed from the capture of radioactive emissions |

## Body Part (Character 4)

The fourth character indicates the body part or body region studied. Regional (e.g., lower extremity veins) and combination (e.g., liver and spleen) body part values are used in this section.

## Radionuclide (Character 5)

The fifth character specifies the radionuclide, the radiation source. The option "Other Radionuclide" is provided in the nuclear medicine section for newly approved radionuclides until they can be added to the coding system. If more than one radiopharmaceutical is used to perform the procedure, then more than one code is used.

## Qualifier (Character 6/7)

The sixth and seventh characters are not specified in the nuclear medicine section, and always have the value None.

# Radiation Therapy Section

The seven characters in the radiation oncology section have the following meaning:

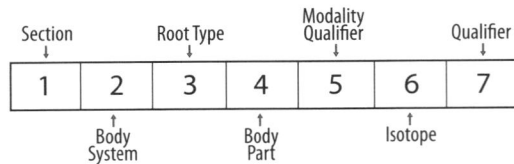

| Section | | Root Type | | Modality Qualifier | | Qualifier |
|---|---|---|---|---|---|---|
| 1 | 2 | 3 | 4 | 5 | 6 | 7 |
| | Body System | | Body Part | | Isotope | |

## Section (Character 1)

Radiation therapy procedure codes have a first character value of "D".

## Body System (Character 2)

The second character specifies the body system (e.g., central nervous system, musculoskeletal) irradiated.

## Modality (Character 3)

The third character root type specifies the general modality used (e.g., beam radiation).

## Body Part (Character 4)

The fourth character specifies the body part that is the focus of the radiation therapy.

## Modality Qualifier (Character 5)

The fifth character further specifies the radiation modality used (e.g., photons, electrons).

## Isotope (Character 6)

The sixth character specifies the isotopes introduced into the body, if applicable, or whether the beam used is a gamma beam or other photon.

## Qualifier (Character 7)

The seventh character is not specified in the radiation therapy section, and always has the value None.

# Physical Rehabilitation and Diagnostic Audiology Section

The seven characters in the physical rehabilitation and diagnostic audiology section have the following meaning:

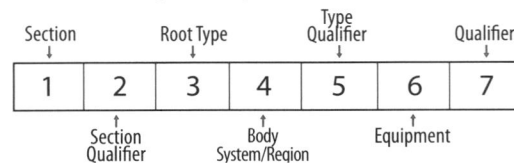

| Section | | Root Type | | Type Qualifier | | Qualifier |
|---|---|---|---|---|---|---|
| 1 | 2 | 3 | 4 | 5 | 6 | 7 |
| | Section Qualifier | | Body System/Region | | Equipment | |

Physical rehabilitation section codes represent procedures including physical therapy, occupational therapy and speech-language pathology. Osteopathic procedures and chiropractic procedures are in sections 7 and 9 respectively.

## Section (Character 1)

Physical rehabilitation and diagnostic audiology procedure codes have a first character value of "F".

## Section Qualifier (Character 2)

The section qualifier rehabilitation or diagnostic audiology is specified in the second character.

## Root Type (Character 3)

The third character specifies the root type. There are 14 different root type values, which can be classified into four basic categories of rehabilitation and diagnostic audiology procedures, defined as follows:

**Treatment:** Use of specific activities or methods to develop, improve and/or restore the performance of necessary functions, compensate for dysfunction and/or minimize debilitation.

**Assessment:** Includes a determination of the patient's diagnosis when appropriate, need for treatment, planning for treatment, periodic assessment and documentation related to these activities.

**Fitting(s):** Design, fabrication, modification, selection and/or application of splint, orthosis, prosthesis, hearing aids and/or other rehabilitation device.

**Caregiver Training:** Educating caregiver with the skills and knowledge used to interact with and assist the patient.

The root type "Treatment" includes training as well as activities which restore function.

## Body Region/System (Character 4)

The fourth character specifies the body region and/or system on which the procedure is performed.

## Type Qualifier (Character 5)

The fifth character is a type qualifier that further specifies the procedure performed. Examples include therapy to improve the range of motion and training for bathing techniques.

## Equipment (Character 6)

The sixth character specifies the equipment used. Specific equipment is not defined in the equipment value. Instead, broad categories of equipment are specified (e.g., aerobic endurance and conditioning, assistive/ adaptive/ supportive, etc.)

## Qualifier (Character 7)

The seventh character is not specified in the rehabilitation and diagnostic audiology section, and always has the value None.

# Mental Health Section

The seven characters in the mental health section have the following meaning:

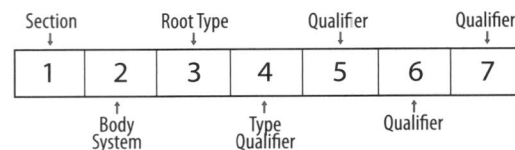

| Section | | Root Type | | Qualifier | | Qualifier |
|---|---|---|---|---|---|---|
| 1 | 2 | 3 | 4 | 5 | 6 | 7 |
| | Body System | | Type Qualifier | | Qualifier | |

## Section (Character 1)

Mental Health procedure codes have a first character value of "G".

## Body System (Character 2)

The second character is used to identify the body system elsewhere in ICD-10-PCS. Since it does not apply in this section it always has the value None.

## Root Type (Character 3)

The third character specifies the root type, such as crisis intervention or counseling.

## Type Qualifier (Character 4)

The fourth character is a type qualifier (e.g., to indicate that counseling was educational or vocational).

## Qualifier (Character 5/6/7)

The fifth, sixth and seventh characters are not specified and always have the value None.

# Substance Abuse Treatment Section

The seven characters in the substance abuse treatment section have the following meaning:

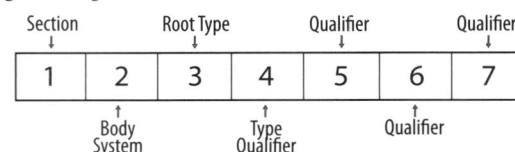

| Section | | Root Type | | Qualifier | | Qualifier |
|---|---|---|---|---|---|---|
| 1 | 2 | 3 | 4 | 5 | 6 | 7 |
| | Body System | | Type Qualifier | | Qualifier | |

## Section (Character 1)

Substance abuse treatment codes have a first character value of "H".

    2015 ICD-10-PCS Expert for Hospitals, Draft | © 2014 DecisionHealth

## Body System (Character 2)

The second character is used to identify the body system elsewhere in ICD-10-PCS. Since it does not apply in this section it always has the value None.

## Root Type (Character 3)

The third character specifies the root type. Examples include detoxification services and individual counseling.

## Type Qualifier (Character 4)

The fourth character is a type qualifier that further specifies the procedure type. The individual counseling procedure further specified in the fourth character includes the values Cognitive Behavioral, 12-step, and Interpersonal.

## Qualifier (Character 5/6/7)

The fifth, sixth and seventh characters are not specified and always have the value None.

# Modifications to ICD-10-PCS

During the development phase of ICD10-PCS, extensive input from a wide range of organizations was obtained. A Technical Advisory Panel, which included representatives from the American Health Information Management Association, American Hospital Association and the American Medical Association, provided review and comment throughout.

The initial draft of ICD-10-PCS was widely disseminated. Both a paper and electronic version of the system were made available. Copies of ICD-10-PCS were distributed to all major physician specialty societies. CMS made ICD-10-PCS available for downloading from its web site.

As a result of feedback received, the system was modified from its initial version to reflect suggestions from reviewers. The most frequent request was to add entries to the Tables to represent procedures for which there was no corresponding PCS code. A common request was to add endoscopic or percutaneous approach values for a specific procedure, to reflect the increased use of less invasive approaches. Additional root operations were specified in the medical and surgical section (e.g., fusion).

The approaches were simplified. Originally, there were 17 different approaches. The approaches that specified the access location as the lining of an orifice itself were eliminated. These approaches did not constitute a critical distinction in describing the procedure performed, and were incorporated into the remaining approaches by modifying the definitions.

Biopsy is not a separate root operation, and many reviewers suggested that it was important to distinguish biopsies from therapeutic procedures. Therefore, the qualifier diagnostic was added for use with the root operations drainage, excision, and extraction.

The issue of NOS codes was one of the most frequent issues raised. The concern was that sufficient documentation may not be present in the medical record to support the detail required by ICD-10-PCS. Originally, ICD-10-PCS did not provide NOS code options. As a result of these concerns, modifications were made to address this issue. Since ICD-10-PCS is a multiaxial system, the NOS issue was addressed separately for each character. In the Medical and Surgical section, the NOS issue primarily concerns the root operation, body part, and approach characters. The root operation value Repair is an operation of exclusion. If the objective of the procedure meets the definition of one of the other root operations, then Repair is not coded. Repair is only coded when none of the other operations apply. The ICD-10-PCS coding guidelines were modified to indicate that if the root operation cannot be determined from the documentation and the necessary information cannot be obtained from the physician, then the root operation Repair may be coded. Repair is the NOS option for the root operation character.

In order to address the issue of insufficient anatomic specificity in the medical record, the use of general body part values was expanded. General body part values were added to several body systems as needed, for use if the precise body part is not specified. For example, for procedures performed on the liver, originally the precise part of the liver excised was

required (i.e., right lobe, left lobe or caudate lobe). The general body part value Liver was added. If the documentation in the medical record does not indicate the precise part of the liver, and the detail cannot be obtained from the physician, then the coder may assign the general body part value Liver. This provides the user with a "liver NOS" option.

Three separate body systems were also added, containing fourth character body/region values for general anatomical regions, regions in the upper extremities and regions in the lower extremities. The coder may identify the broad anatomic region where the procedure was performed, when the full anatomic detail is not available in the medical record and the necessary information cannot be obtained from the physician.

There are four general approach categories: open, percutaneous, via natural or artificial opening, and external. The ICD-10-PCS coding guidelines were modified to indicate that if the full definition of the approach cannot be determined, then the general open, percutaneous or transorifice approach may be coded. The coder will still need to be able to specify whether the approach was open, percutaneous, transorifice or external. This distinction is so fundamental to the description of the procedure that any less specificity is not appropriate.

While the NOS issue primarily concerns the medical and surgical section, there were also NOS-related issues in other sections of ICD-10-PCS. The imaging, nuclear medicine and radiation therapy sections of ICD-10-PCS contain detail that may not be readily available in the medical record. Further, the level of detail provided by ICD-10-PCS in these sections, while important for research or internal management, may not be required by payers. For characters in these sections where the full detail of ICD-10-PCS may not be required, an "Other" value is provided. The sections and characters for which an "Other" value is provided are summarized as:

| Section | Character |
| --- | --- |
| *Medical and Surgical* | 6 (Device) |
| *Imaging* | 5 (Contrast) |
| *Nuclear Medicine* | 5 (Radionuclide) |
| *Radiation Therapy* | 5 (Isotope) |

The modifications made to ICD-10-PCS to address the NOS issue strike a balance between a precise description of the procedure and the realities of the current state of medical record documentation.

# Number of Codes in ICD-10-PCS

The below table summarizes the number of ICD-10-PCS codes by section.

| Section | Number of Codes |
| --- | --- |
| Medical and Surgical | 61,898 |
| Obstetrics | 300 |
| Placement | 861 |
| Administration | 1,388 |
| Measurement and Monitoring | 339 |
| Extracorporeal Assistance and Performance | 41 |
| Extracorporeal Therapies | 42 |
| Osteopathic | 100 |
| Other Procedures | 60 |
| Chiropractic | 90 |
| Imaging | 2,934 |
| Nuclear Medicine | 463 |
| Radiation Therapy | 1,939 |
| Rehabilitation and Diagnostic Audiology | 1,380 |
| Mental Health | 30 |
| Substance Abuse Treatment | 59 |
| **Total for 2013** | **71,924** |

There are a total of 71,924 codes in ICD-10-PCS. This represents a substantial increase over the number of ICD-9-CM procedure codes. The table structure of ICD-10-PCS permits the specification of a large number of codes on a single page in the Tables. The combined Tables and Index of ICD-10-PCS are approximately half the physical size of the ICD-10 diagnosis coding manual from the World Health Organization.

## Testing of ICD-10-PCS

As an informal test, in October 1996, seventy health information professionals were trained in the use of ICD-10-PCS. After the training, they coded a sample of records from their institutions using ICD-10-PCS and reported suggestions and problems to the ICD-10-PCS project staff.

CMS conducted a formal test of ICD-10-PCS in order to determine if it would be a practical replacement for the current ICD-9-CM procedures. CMS used two contractors to evaluate ICD-10-PCS: the two Clinical Data Abstraction Centers (CDACs): DynKePRO in York, PA, and FMAS in Columbia, MD.

As part of a contract awarded in 1994, the primary task of the CDACs was to collect clinical data from approximately 1.5 million medical records over a period of five years. The primary end product of the CDAC contracts was the development of accurate and reliable clinical data in quantities sufficient to support the analytical efforts of the PROs as they carry out the Health Care Quality Improvement Program. Since the CDACs had a ready supply of current medical records and extensive experience in reviewing, abstracting, and coding medical records, they were selected to test ICD-10-PCS.

Using the ICD-10-PCS training manual, the CDACs were trained for two days on the medical/surgical part of the system, and a separate one-day session was held for the remaining sections (nuclear medicine, radiation oncology osteopathic, etc.) The CDACs then spent several weeks coding with ICD-10-PCS to gain experience. Conference calls were held to answer questions prior to the start of the formal testing.

In the first phase of the test, a sample of 5000 medical records (2500 per CDAC) was selected, including cases with a wide distribution of ICD-9-CM procedure codes. The CDACs coded the cases using ICD-10-PCS, and noted any questions or concerns. Questions and concerns were forwarded to project staff, which then responded on an ongoing basis. As a result of this interaction, a list of proposed revisions to the final draft was made. This included terms that needed clarification, and omissions identified in the Tables or Index. In addition, areas where the training manual could be improved were identified.

In the second phase of the test, a subset of 100 medical records was coded blindly using both ICD-9-CM and ICD-10-PCS. The reviewers coded the initial 50 records first with ICD-9-CM, then with ICD-10-PCS. For the last 50 records the process was reversed, and ICD-10-PCS was coded first followed by ICD-9-CM. The systems were compared on issues such as ease of use, time needed to identify codes, number of codes required, problems identifying codes, strengths and weaknesses of each system, and any other issues identified by the coding personnel.

After an initial learning curve, the CDAC coders were able to use ICD-10-PCS easily, with a few challenges. Because of the added detail in ICD-10-PCS, it was occasionally necessary for the coders to consult a medical dictionary or an anatomy textbook. The coders required a greater understanding of anatomy and surgical terms to use ICD-10-PCS than is required for ICD-9-CM. As a result, more training time will be necessary for ICD-10-PCS than is currently required for ICD-9-CM. Although the initial ICD-10-PCS training manual was very useful, the CDACs felt that it needed to be enhanced with additional examples before any national training takes place. It was also suggested by the CDACs that the addition of diagrams of the body systems would be useful in the training manual.

Once the CDAC coders became proficient in ICD-10-PCS, they were able to suggest a number of improvements, such as additional index entries and modifications of body part and approach values. These suggestions have been incorporated in ongoing drafts of ICD-10-PCS. Testing demonstrated the ease with which ICD-10-PCS can be updated and expanded when issues are identified.

Another area of concern was the issue of correct code assignment in several situations: when records did not provide enough documentation to code the precise body part or procedure, or when the coders did not have enough knowledge of anatomy to select a precise code. These concerns resulted in the NOS modifications of ICD-10-PCS and the coding guidelines previously mentioned.

A side-by-side comparison of ICD-10-PCS and ICD-9-CM was performed once test coders became proficient in the new system. One CDAC reported that the staff did not detect a significant time difference using ICD-10-PCS as compared to ICD-9-CM. The other CDAC found that ICD-10-PCS coding took somewhat longer. ICD-10-PCS sometimes required more codes than ICD-9-CM. This was due in part to the fact that ICD-9-CM contains combination procedure codes, and their equivalents are coded separately in ICD-10-PCS. However, it was felt that the precision of ICD-10-PCS resulted in greater detail about the nature of the procedure and was therefore worth the possible increase in coding time. It was suggested that once coders became familiar with the greater detail and precision of ICD-10-PCS, the result would be improved accuracy and efficiency of coding.

Both CDACs pointed out that once the coders were familiar with ICD-10-PCS, they rarely used the index. The ICD-10-PCS tables were found to be so well organized and so well structured that coders could quickly find the correct section of the tables. The index was used more often for definitions of the root operations and other terms used in ICD-10-PCS. However, once coders understood ICD-10-PCS, they found it easy to code straight from the Tables.

Both CDACs found ICD-10-PCS an improvement over ICD-9-CM, because it provided greater specificity for use in research, statistical analysis, and administrative areas. A major strength of the system was its detailed structure, which allowed users to more precisely report the procedures performed.

### Comparison of ICD-10-PCS and ICD-9-CM

In 1993, the National Committee on Vital and Health Statistics (NCVHS) issued a report specifying recommendations for a new procedure classification system. NCVHS identified the essential characteristics that a procedure classification system should possess. Included in the report is a comparison of ICD-9-CM and ICD-10-PCS for each of the NCVHS characteristics. As the comparisons indicate, ICD-10-PCS meets virtually all NCVHS characteristics, while ICD-9-CM fails to meet many NCVHS characteristics. In addition to the NCVHS characteristics, there are several other attributes of a procedure coding system that should be taken into consideration when comparing systems.

### Training Effort

As the independent evaluation of ICD-10-PCS demonstrates, there is a learning curve associated with ICD-10-PCS. Since the CDAC staff consisted of trained ICD-9-CM coders, the independent evaluation could not include a formal comparison of initial training time for ICD-10-PCS and ICD-9-CM. Because of the additional specificity in ICD-10-PCS, it is likely that the training time needed to achieve a minimum level of coding proficiency is greater for ICD-10-PCS than for ICD-9-CM.

However, while it may take longer to reach a minimum level of proficiency with ICD-10-PCS, it should take less time to become highly proficient with ICD-10-PCS than with ICD-9-CM. Because ICD-9-CM lacks clear definitions, and because many substantially different procedures are coded with the same code, the identification of the correct code requires extensive knowledge of the contents of Coding Clinic and other coding guidelines. Becoming completely familiar with all the conventions associated with ICD-9-CM requires extensive effort, and as a result, the process of becoming highly proficient in ICD-9-CM can require a long learning curve.

### Completeness and Accuracy of Codes

The CDACs concluded that procedures coded in ICD-10-PCS provided a much more complete and accurate description of the procedure performed. The specification of the procedures performed not only affects payment, but is integral to internal management systems, external performance comparisons, and the assessment of quality of care. The detail and completeness of ICD-10-PCS is essential in today's healthcare environment.

### Communications with Physicians

ICD-9-CM procedure codes often provide a poor description of the precise procedure performed. Physicians reviewing or analyzing data coded in ICD-9-CM may have difficulty developing clinical pathways, evaluating the coding for possible fraud and abuse, or conducting research. The ICD-10-PCS codes provide more clinically relevant procedure descriptions that can be more readily understood and used by physicians.

## Conclusion

ICD-10-PCS has been developed as a replacement for Volume 3 of ICD-9-CM. The system has evolved during its development based on extensive input from many segments of the healthcare industry. The multiaxial structure of the system, combined with its detailed definition of terminology, permit a precise specification of procedures for use in health services research, epidemiology, statistical analysis and administrative areas. It will also enhance the ability of health information coders to determine accurate procedure codes with minimal effort.

## Changes for 2015

There were minor changes to the 2015 ICD-10-PCS. No changes were made to the tabular tables. New files were updated for the Index and Definitions addenda. The Index addenda show new, revised, and deleted index entries. The Definition addenda reports revised and deleted PCS definitions. Long and abbreviated ICD-10-PCS code titles are available.

### New Index Addenda

- New file showing new, revised and deleted index entries in response to public comment
- See list of updated files for details

### New Definitions Addenda

- New file showing new, revised and deleted PCS definitions entries (e.g. Body Part Key) in response to public comment
- See list of updated files for details

### Updated Files

#### ICD-10-PCS Tables/Index/Definitions

ICD-10-PCS Code Tables and Index
- Downloadable PDF format
- Downloadable xml format for developers, with accompanying schema

#### ICD-10-PCS Code Titles, Long and Abbreviated

- Tabular order file defines an unambiguous order for all ICD-10-CM/PCS codes
- Text file format
- Provides a unique five-digit "order number" for each ICD-10-PCS table and code
- Accompanying documentation

### ICD-10-PCS 2015 Final Addenda

- Downloadable xml format for developers
- Accompanying documentation
- Index addenda in downloadable PDF
- PCS Definitions addenda in downloadable PDF
- Index and Definitions addenda in machine readable text format for developers

### ICD-10-PCS Reference Manual

- Downloadable PDF file
- Revised in response to public comment and internal review
- Addenda to 2015 version of reference manual specifies the changes

### ICD-10-PCS Official Coding Guidelines

- Downloadable PDF format
- Revised in response to public comment and internal review

### ICD-10-PCS and ICD-9-CM General Equivalence Mappings

- Downloadable text format
- Documentation for general users and technical users
- Documentation for technical users

### ICD-10 Reimbursement Mappings

- Downloadable text format
- FY2015 version uses the FY2015 GEM files
- Accompanying documentation includes rules used in the mapping

# 2015 ICD-1Ø-PCS Official Guidelines for Coding and Reporting

The Centers for Medicare and Medicaid Services (CMS) and the National Center for Health Statistics (NCHS), two departments within the U.S. Federal Government's Department of Health and Human Services (DHHS) provide the following guidelines for coding and reporting using the *International Classification of Diseases, 10th Revision, Procedure Coding System* (ICD-10-PCS). These guidelines should be used as a companion document to the official version of the ICD-10-PCS as published on the CMS website. The ICD-10-PCS is a procedure classification published by the United States for classifying procedures performed in hospital inpatient health care settings.

These guidelines have been approved by the four organizations that make up the Cooperating Parties for the ICD-10-PCS: the American Hospital Association (AHA), the American Health Information Management Association (AHIMA), CMS, and NCHS.

These guidelines are a set of rules that have been developed to accompany and complement the official conventions and instructions provided within the ICD-10-PCS itself. The instructions and conventions of the classification take precedence over guidelines. These guidelines are based on the coding and sequencing instructions in the Tables, Index and Definitions of ICD-10-PCS, but provide additional instruction. Adherence to these guidelines when assigning ICD-10-PCS procedure codes is required under the Health Insurance Portability and Accountability Act (HIPAA). The procedure codes have been adopted under HIPAA for hospital inpatient healthcare settings. A joint effort between the healthcare provider and the coder is essential to achieve complete and accurate documentation, code assignment, and reporting of diagnoses and procedures. These guidelines have been developed to assist both the healthcare provider and the coder in identifying those procedures that are to be reported. The importance of consistent, complete documentation in the medical record cannot be overemphasized. Without such documentation accurate coding cannot be achieved.

## Conventions

**A1** ICD-10-PCS codes are composed of seven characters. Each character is an axis of classification that specifies information about the procedure performed. Within a defined code range, a character specifies the same type of information in that axis of classification.

*Example:* The fifth axis of classification specifies the approach in sections Ø through 4 and 7 through 9 of the system.

**A2** One of 34 possible values can be assigned to each axis of classification in the seven-character code: they are the numbers Ø through 9 and the alphabet (except I and O because they are easily confused with the numbers 1 and Ø). The number of unique values used in an axis of classification differs as needed.

*Example:* Where the fifth axis of classification specifies the approach, seven different approach values are currently used to specify the approach.

**A3** The valid values for an axis of classification can be added to as needed.

*Example:* If a significantly distinct type of device is used in a new procedure, a new device value can be added to the system.

**A4** As with words in their context, the meaning of any single value is a combination of its axis of classification and any preceding values on which it may be dependent.

*Example:* The meaning of a body part value in the Medical and Surgical section is always dependent on the body system value. The body part value Ø in the Central Nervous body system specifies Brain and the body part value Ø in the Peripheral Nervous body system specifies Cervical Plexus.

**A5** As the system is expanded to become increasingly detailed, over time more values will depend on preceding values for their meaning.

*Example:* In the Lower Joints body system, the device value 3 in the root operation Insertion specifies Infusion Device and the device value 3 in the root operation Fusion specifies Interbody Fusion Device.

**A6** The purpose of the alphabetic index is to locate the appropriate table that contains all information necessary to construct a procedure code. The PCS Tables should always be consulted to find the most appropriate valid code.

**A7** It is not required to consult the index first before proceeding to the tables to complete the code. A valid code may be chosen directly from the tables.

**A8** All seven characters must be specified to be a valid code. If the documentation is incomplete for coding purposes, the physician should be queried for the necessary information.

**A9** Within a PCS table, valid codes include all combinations of choices in characters 4 through 7 contained in the same row of the table. In the example below, ØJHT3VZ is a valid code, and ØJHW3VZ is *not* a valid code.

**Section:** Ø Medical and Surgical

**Body System:** J Subcutaneous Tissue and Fascia

**Operation:** H Insertion: Putting in a nonbiological appliance that monitors, assists, performs, or prevents a physiological function but does not physically take the place of a body part

| Body Part | Approach | Device | Qualifier |
|---|---|---|---|
| S Subcutaneous Tissue and Fascia, Head and Neck<br>V Subcutaneous Tissue and Fascia, Upper Extremity<br>W Subcutaneous Tissue and Fascia, Lower Extremity | Ø Open<br>3 Percutaneous | 1 Radioactive Element<br>3 Infusion Device | Z No Qualifier |
| T Subcutaneous Tissue and Fascia, Trunk | Ø Open<br>3 Percutaneous | 1 Radioactive Element<br>3 Infusion Device<br>V Infusion Pump | Z No Qualifier |

**A10** "And," when used in a code description, means "and/or."

*Example:* Lower Arm and Wrist Muscle means lower arm and/or wrist muscle.

**A11** Many of the terms used to construct PCS codes are defined within the system. It is the coder's responsibility to determine what the documentation in the medical record equates to in the PCS definitions. The physician is not expected to use the terms used in PCS code descriptions, nor is the coder required to query the physician when the correlation between the documentation and the defined PCS terms is clear.

*Example:* When the physician documents "partial resection" the coder can independently correlate "partial resection" to the root operation Excision without querying the physician for clarification.

## Medical and Surgical Section Guidelines (Section Ø)

### B2. Body system

#### General Guidelines

**B2.1a.** The procedure codes in the general anatomical regions body systems should only be used when the procedure is performed on an anatomical region rather than a specific body part (e.g., root operations Control and Detachment, Drainage of a body cavity) or on the rare occasion when no information is available to support assignment of a code to a specific body part.

*Example:* Control of postoperative hemorrhage is coded to the root operation Control found in the general anatomical regions body systems.

B2.1b Where the general body part values "upper" and "lower" are provided as an option in the Upper Arteries, Lower Arteries, Upper Veins, Lower Veins, Muscles and Tendons body systems, "upper" or "lower "specifies body parts located above or below the diaphragm respectively.

*Example:* Vein body parts above the diaphragm are found in the Upper Veins body system; vein body parts below the diaphragm are found in the Lower Veins body system.

## B3. Root Operation

### General Guidelines

B3.1a In order to determine the appropriate root operation, the full definition of the root operation as contained in the PCS Tables must be applied.

B3.1b Components of a procedure specified in the root operation definition and explanation are not coded separately. Procedural steps necessary to reach the operative site and close the operative site, including anastomosis of a tubular body part, are also not coded separately.

*Example:* Resection of a joint as part of a joint replacement procedure is included in the root operation definition of Replacement and is not coded separately. Laparotomy performed to reach the site of an open liver biopsy is not coded separately. In a resection of sigmoid colon with anastomosis of descending colon to rectum, the anastomosis is not coded separately.

### Multiple Procedures

B3.2 During the same operative episode, multiple procedures are coded if:

a. The same root operation is performed on different body parts as defined by distinct values of the body part character.

   *Example:* Diagnostic excision of liver and pancreas are coded separately.

b. The same root operation is repeated at different body sites that are included in the same body part value.

   *Example:* Excision of the sartorius muscle and excision of the gracilis muscle are both included in the upper leg muscle body part value, and multiple procedures are coded.

c. Multiple root operations with distinct objectives are performed on the same body part.

   *Example:* Destruction of sigmoid lesion and bypass of sigmoid colon are coded separately.

d. The intended root operation is attempted using one approach, but is converted to a different approach.

   *Example:* Laparoscopic cholecystectomy converted to an open cholecystectomy is coded as percutaneous endoscopic Inspection and open Resection.

### Discontinued Procedures

B3.3 If the intended procedure is discontinued, code the procedure to the root operation performed. If a procedure is discontinued before any other root operation is performed, code the root operation Inspection of the body part or anatomical region inspected.

*Example:* A planned aortic valve replacement procedure is discontinued after the initial thoracotomy and before any incision is made in the heart muscle, when the patient becomes hemodynamically unstable. This procedure is coded as an open Inspection of the mediastinum.

### Biopsy Procedures

B3.4a Biopsy procedures are coded using the root operations Excision, Extraction, or Drainage and the qualifier Diagnostic. The qualifier Diagnostic is used only for biopsies.

*Examples:* Fine needle aspiration biopsy of lung is coded to the root operation Drainage with the qualifier Diagnostic. Biopsy of bone marrow is coded to the root operation Extraction with the qualifier Diagnostic. Lymph node sampling for biopsy is coded to the root operation Excision with the qualifier Diagnostic.

### Biopsy followed by more Definitive Treatment

B3.4b If a diagnostic Excision, Extraction, or Drainage procedure (biopsy) is followed by a more definitive procedure, such as Destruction, Excision or Resection at the same procedure site, both the biopsy and the more definitive treatment are coded.

*Example*: Biopsy of breast followed by partial mastectomy at the same procedure site, both the biopsy and the partial mastectomy procedure are coded.

### Overlapping Body Layers

B3.5 If the root operations Excision, Repair or Inspection are performed on overlapping layers of the musculoskeletal system, the body part specifying the deepest layer is coded.

*Example:* Excisional debridement that includes skin and subcutaneous tissue and muscle is coded to the muscle body part.

### Bypass Procedures

B3.6a Bypass procedures are coded by identifying the body part bypassed "from" and the body part bypassed "to." The fourth character body part specifies the body part bypassed from, and the qualifier specifies the body part bypassed to.

*Example:* Bypass from stomach to jejunum, stomach is the body part and jejunum is the qualifier.

B3.6b Coronary arteries are classified by number of distinct sites treated, rather than number of coronary arteries or anatomic name of a coronary artery (e.g., left anterior descending). Coronary artery bypass procedures are coded differently than other bypass procedures as described in the previous guideline. Rather than identifying the body part bypassed from, the body part identifies the number of coronary artery sites bypassed to, and the qualifier specifies the vessel bypassed from.

*Example:* Aortocoronary artery bypass of one site on the left anterior descending coronary artery and one site on the obtuse marginal coronary artery is classified in the body part axis of classification as two coronary artery sites and the qualifier specifies the aorta as the body part bypassed from.

B3.6c If multiple coronary artery sites are bypassed, a separate procedure is coded for each coronary artery site that uses a different device and/or qualifier.

*Example:* Aortocoronary artery bypass and internal mammary coronary artery bypass are coded separately.

### Control vs. More Definitive Root Operations

B3.7 The root operation Control is defined as, "Stopping, or attempting to stop, postprocedural bleeding." If an attempt to stop postprocedural bleeding is initially unsuccessful, and to stop the bleeding requires performing any of the definitive root operations Bypass, Detachment, Excision, Extraction, Reposition, Replacement, or Resection, then that root operation is coded instead of Control.

*Example:* Resection of spleen to stop postprocedural bleeding is coded to Resection instead of Control.

### Excision vs. Resection

B3.8 PCS contains specific body parts for anatomical subdivisions of a body part, such as lobes of the lungs or liver and regions of the intestine. Resection of the specific body part is coded whenever all of the body part is cut out or off, rather than coding Excision of a less specific body part.

*Example:* Left upper lung lobectomy is coded to Resection of Upper Lung Lobe, Left rather than Excision of Lung, Left.

### Excision for Graft

B3.9  If an autograft is obtained from a different body part in order to complete the objective of the procedure, a separate procedure is coded.

*Example:* Coronary bypass with excision of saphenous vein graft, excision of saphenous vein is coded separately.

### Fusion Procedures of the Spine

B3.10a The body part coded for a spinal vertebral joint(s) rendered immobile by a spinal fusion procedure is classified by the level of the spine (e.g. thoracic). There are distinct body part values for a single vertebral joint and for multiple vertebral joints at each spinal level.

*Example:* Body part values specify Lumbar Vertebral Joint, Lumbar Vertebral Joints, 2 or More and Lumbosacral Vertebral Joint.

B3.10b If multiple vertebral joints are fused, a separate procedure is coded for each vertebral joint that uses a different device and/or qualifier.

*Example:* Fusion of lumbar vertebral joint, posterior approach, anterior column and fusion of lumbar vertebral joint, posterior approach, posterior column are coded separately.

B3.10c Combinations of devices and materials are often used on a vertebral joint to render the joint immobile. When combinations of devices are used on the same vertebral joint, the device value coded for the procedure is as follows:

- If an interbody fusion device is used to render the joint immobile (alone or containing other material like bone graft), the procedure is coded with the device value Interbody Fusion Device
- If bone graft is the only device used to render the joint immobile, the procedure is coded with the device value Nonautologous Tissue Substitute or Autologous Tissue Substitute
- If a mixture of autologous and nonautologous bone graft (with or without biological or synthetic extenders or binders) is used to render the joint immobile, code the procedure with the device value Autologous Tissue Substitute

*Examples:* Fusion of a vertebral joint using a cage style interbody fusion device containing morsellized bone graft is coded to the device Interbody Fusion Device.

Fusion of a vertebral joint using a bone dowel interbody fusion device made of cadaver bone and packed with a mixture of local morsellized bone and demineralized bone matrix is coded to the device Interbody Fusion Device.

Fusion of a vertebral joint using both autologous bone graft and bone bank bone graft is coded to the device Autologous Tissue Substitute.

### Inspection Procedures

B3.11a Inspection of a body part(s) performed in order to achieve the objective of a procedure is not coded separately.

*Example:* Fiberoptic bronchoscopy performed for irrigation of bronchus, only the irrigation procedure is coded.

B3.11b If multiple tubular body parts are inspected, the most distal body part inspected is coded. If multiple non-tubular body parts in a region are inspected, the body part that specifies the entire area inspected is coded.

*Examples:* Cystoureteroscopy with inspection of bladder and ureters is coded to the ureter body part value.

Exploratory laparotomy with general inspection of abdominal contents is coded to the peritoneal cavity body part value.

B3.11c When both an Inspection procedure and another procedure are performed on the same body part during the same episode, if the Inspection procedure is performed using a different approach than the other procedure, the Inspection procedure is coded separately.

*Example:* Endoscopic Inspection of the duodenum is coded separately when open Excision of the duodenum is performed during the same procedural episode.

### Occlusion vs. Restriction for Vessel Embolization Procedures

B3.12 If the objective of an embolization procedure is to completely close a vessel, the root operation Occlusion is coded. If the objective of an embolization procedure is to narrow the lumen of a vessel, the root operation Restriction is coded.

*Examples:* Tumor embolization is coded to the root operation Occlusion, because the objective of the procedure is to cut off the blood supply to the vessel.

Embolization of a cerebral aneurysm is coded to the root operation Restriction, because the objective of the procedure is not to close off the vessel entirely, but to narrow the lumen of the vessel at the site of the aneurysm where it is abnormally wide.

### Release Procedures

B3.13 In the root operation Release, the body part value coded is the body part being freed and not the tissue being manipulated or cut to free the body part.

*Example:* Lysis of intestinal adhesions is coded to the specific intestine body part value.

### Release vs. Division

B3.14 If the sole objective of the procedure is freeing a body part without cutting the body part, the root operation is Release. If the sole objective of the procedure is separating or transecting a body part, the root operation is Division.

*Examples:* Freeing a nerve root from surrounding scar tissue to relieve pain is coded to the root operation Release.

Severing a nerve root to relieve pain is coded to the root operation Division.

### Reposition for Fracture Treatment

B3.15 Reduction of a displaced fracture is coded to the root operation Reposition and the application of a cast or splint in conjunction with the Reposition procedure is not coded separately. Treatment of a nondisplaced fracture is coded to the procedure performed.

*Examples:* Putting a pin in a nondisplaced fracture is coded to the root operation Insertion.

Casting of a nondisplaced fracture is coded to the root operation Immobilization in the Placement section.

### Transplantation vs. Administration

B3.16 Putting in a mature and functioning living body part taken from another individual or animal is coded to the root operation Transplantation. Putting in autologous or nonautologous cells is coded to the Administration section.

*Example:* Putting in autologous or nonautologous bone marrow, pancreatic islet cells or stem cells is coded to the Administration section.

## B4. Body Part

### General Guidelines

B4.1a If a procedure is performed on a portion of a body part that does not have a separate body part value, code the body part value corresponding to the whole body part.

*Example:* A procedure performed on the alveolar process of the mandible is coded to the mandible body part.

B4.1b If the prefix "peri" is combined with a body part to identify the site of the procedure, the procedure is coded to the body part named.

*Example:* A procedure site identified as perirenal is coded to the kidney body part.

### Branches of Body Parts

B4.2 Where a specific branch of a body part does not have its own body part value in PCS, the body part is coded to the closest proximal branch that has a specific body part value.

*Example:* A procedure performed on the mandibular branch of the trigeminal nerve is coded to the trigeminal nerve body part value

## Bilateral Body Part Values

B4.3　Bilateral body part values are available for a limited number of body parts. If the identical procedure is performed on contralateral body parts, and a bilateral body part value exists for that body part, a single procedure is coded using the bilateral body part value. If no bilateral body part value exists, each procedure is coded separately using the appropriate body part value.

*Example:* The identical procedure performed on both fallopian tubes is coded once using the body part value Fallopian Tube, Bilateral. The identical procedure performed on both knee joints is coded twice using the body part values Knee Joint, Right and Knee Joint, Left.

## Coronary Arteries

B4.4　The coronary arteries are classified as a single body part that is further specified by number of sites treated and not by name or number of arteries. Separate body part values are used to specify the number of sites treated when the same procedure is performed on multiple sites in the coronary arteries.

*Examples:* Angioplasty of two distinct sites in the left anterior descending coronary artery with placement of two stents is coded as Dilation of Coronary Arteries, Two Sites, with Intraluminal Device.

Angioplasty of two distinct sites in the left anterior descending coronary artery, one with stent placed and one without, is coded separately as Dilation of Coronary Artery, One Site with Intraluminal Device, and Dilation of Coronary Artery, One Site with no device.

## Tendons, Ligaments, Bursae and Fascia Near a Joint

B4.5　Procedures performed on tendons, ligaments, bursae and fascia supporting a joint are coded to the body part in the respective body system that is the focus of the procedure. Procedures performed on joint structures themselves are coded to the body part in the joint body systems.

*Example:* Repair of the anterior cruciate ligament of the knee is coded to the knee bursae and ligament body part in the bursae and ligaments body system. Knee arthroscopy with shaving of articular cartilage is coded to the knee joint body part in the Lower Joints body system.

## Skin, Subcutaneous Tissue and Fascia Overlying a Joint

B4.6　If a procedure is performed on the skin, subcutaneous tissue or fascia overlying a joint, the procedure is coded to the following body part:

• Shoulder is coded to Upper Arm

• Elbow is coded to Lower Arm

• Wrist is coded to Lower Arm

• Hip is coded to Upper Leg

• Knee is coded to Lower Leg

• Ankle is coded to Foot

## Fingers and Toes

B4.7　If a body system does not contain a separate body part value for fingers, procedures performed on the fingers are coded to the body part value for the hand. If a body system does not contain a separate body part value for toes, procedures performed on the toes are coded to the body part value for the foot.

*Example:* Excision of finger muscle is coded to one of the hand muscle body part values in the Muscles body system.

## Upper and Lower Intestinal Tract

B4.8　In the Gastrointestinal body system, the general body part values Upper Intestinal Tract and Lower Intestinal Tract are provided as an option for the root operations Change, Inspection, Removal and Revision. Upper Intestinal Tract includes the portion of the gastrointestinal tract from the esophagus down to and including the duodenum, and Lower Intestinal Tract includes the portion of the gastrointestinal tract from the jejunum down to and including the rectum and anus.

*Example:* In the root operation Change table, change of a device in the jejunum is coded using the body part Lower Intestinal Tract.

## B5. Approach

### Open Approach with Percutaneous Endoscopic Assistance

B5.2　Procedures performed using the open approach with percutaneous endoscopic assistance are coded to the approach Open.

*Example:* Laparoscopic-assisted sigmoidectomy is coded to the approach Open.

### External Approach

B5.3a　Procedures performed within an orifice on structures that are visible without the aid of any instrumentation are coded to the approach External.

*Example:* Resection of tonsils is coded to the approach External.

B5.3b　Procedures performed indirectly by the application of external force through the intervening body layers are coded to the approach External.

*Example:* Closed reduction of fracture is coded to the approach External.

### Percutaneous Procedure via Device

B5.4　Procedures performed percutaneously via a device placed for the procedure are coded to the approach Percutaneous.

*Example:* Fragmentation of kidney stone performed via percutaneous nephrostomy is coded to the approach Percutaneous.

## B6. Device

### General Guidelines

B6.1a　A device is coded only if a device remains after the procedure is completed. If no device remains, the device value No Device is coded.

B6.1b　Materials such as sutures, ligatures, radiological markers and temporary post-operative wound drains are considered integral to the performance of a procedure and are not coded as devices.

B6.1c　Procedures performed on a device only and not on a body part are specified in the root operations Change, Irrigation, Removal and Revision, and are coded to the procedure performed.

*Example:*  Irrigation of percutaneous nephrostomy tube is coded to the root operation Irrigation of indwelling device in the Administration section.

### Drainage Device

B6.2　A separate procedure to put in a drainage device is coded to the root operation Drainage with the device value Drainage Device.

# Obstetrics Section Guidelines (Section 1)

## C. Obstetrics Sections

### Products of Conception

C1　Procedures performed on the products of conception are coded to the Obstetrics section. Procedures performed on the pregnant female other than the products of conception are coded to the appropriate root operation in the Medical and Surgical section.

*Example:* Amniocentesis is coded to the products of conception body part in the Obstetrics section. Repair of obstetric urethral laceration is coded to the urethra body part in the Medical and Surgical section.

### Procedures Following Delivery or Abortion

C2　Procedures performed following a delivery or abortion for curettage of the endometrium or evacuation of retained products of conception are all coded in the Obstetrics section, to the root operation Extraction and the body part Products of Conception, Retained. Diagnostic or therapeutic dilation and curettage performed during times other than the postpartum or post-abortion period are all coded in the Medical and Surgical section, to the root operation Extraction and the body part Endometrium.

## Selection of Principal Procedure

The following instructions should be applied in the selection of principal procedure and clarification on the importance of the relation to the principal diagnosis when more than one procedure is performed:

1. Procedure performed for definitive treatment of both principal diagnosis and secondary diagnosis

    a. Sequence procedure performed for definitive treatment most related to principal diagnosis as principal procedure.

2. Procedure performed for definitive treatment and diagnostic procedures performed for both principal diagnosis and secondary diagnosis

    a. Sequence procedure performed for definitive treatment most related to principal diagnosis as principal procedure.

3. A diagnostic procedure was performed for the principal diagnosis and a procedure is performed for definitive treatment of a secondary diagnosis.

    a. Sequence diagnostic procedure as principal procedure, since the procedure most related to the principal diagnosis takes precedence.

4. No procedures performed that are related to principal diagnosis; procedures performed for definitive treatment and diagnostic procedures were performed for secondary diagnosis

    a. Sequence procedure performed for definitive treatment of secondary diagnosis as principal procedure, since there are no procedures (definitive or nondefinitive treatment) related to principal diagnosis.

# Coding Practice

Below are descriptions of procedures for coding practice. The procedures are divided into the ICD-10-PCS section for the general type of procedure. Answers can be found in Appendix G.

## Section Ø – Medical and Surgical

| Procedure | Description | Code(s) |
|---|---|---|
| 1. | Excision of malignant melanoma from skin of right ear | |
| 2. | Laparoscopy with excision of endometrial implant from left ovary | |
| 3. | Percutaneous needle core biopsy of right kidney | |
| 4. | EGD with gastric biopsy | |
| 5. | Laparotomy with wedge resection of left lateral segment of liver | |
| 6. | Excision of basal cell carcinoma of lower lip | |
| 7. | Open excision of tail of pancreas | |
| 8. | Percutaneous biopsy of right gastrocnemius muscle | |
| 9. | Sigmoidoscopy with sigmoid polypectomy | |
| 10. | Open excision of lesion from right Achilles tendon | |
| 11. | Open resection of cecum | |
| 12. | Total excision of pituitary gland, open | |
| 13. | Explantation of left failed kidney, open | |
| 14. | Open left axillary total lymphadenectomy – Hint: RESECTION is coded for cutting out a chain of lymph nodes. | |
| 15. | Laparoscopic-assisted vaginal hysterectomy, supracervical resection | |
| 16. | Right total mastectomy, open | |
| 17. | Open resection of papillary muscle – Hint: The papillary muscle refers to the heart and is found in the HEART AND GREAT VESSELS body system. | |
| 18. | Radical retropubic prostatectomy, open | |
| 19. | Laparoscopic cholecystectomy | |
| 20. | Endoscopic bilateral total maxillary sinusectomy | |
| 21. | Amputation at right elbow level | |
| 22. | Right below-knee amputation, proximal tibia/fibula – Hint: The qualifier HIGH is used for the portion of the tib/fib closest to the knee. | |
| 23. | Fifth ray carpometacarpal joint amputation, left hand – Hint: A COMPLETE ray amputation is through the carpometacarpal joint. | |
| 24. | Right leg and hip amputation through ischium – Hint: The HINDQUARTER body part includes amputation along any part of the hip bone. | |
| 25. | DIP joint amputation of right thumb – Hint: The qualifier LOW is used for amputation through the distal interphalangeal joint. | |
| 26. | Right wrist joint amputation – Hint: Amputation at the wrist joint is actually complete amputation of the hand. | |
| 27. | Trans-metatarsal amputation of foot at left big toe – Hint: A PARTIAL amputation is through the shaft of the metatarsal bone. | |
| 28. | Mid-shaft amputation, right humerus | |
| 29. | Left fourth toe amputation, mid-proximal phalanx – Hint: The qualifier HIGH means anywhere along the proximal phalanx. | |
| 30. | Right above-knee amputation, distal femur | |
| 31. | Cryotherapy of wart on left hand | |
| 32. | Percutaneous radiofrequency ablation of right vocal cord lesion | |
| 33. | Left heart catheterization with laser destruction of arrhythmogenic focus, A-V node | |
| 34. | Cautery of nosebleed | |
| 35. | Transurethral endoscopic laser ablation of prostate | |
| 36. | Cautery of oozing varicose vein, left calf – Hint: The approach is coded PERCUTANEOUS because that is the normal route to a vein. No mention is made of approach, because likely the skin has eroded at that spot. | |
| 37. | Laparoscopy with destruction of endometriosis, bilateral ovaries | |
| 38. | Laser coagulation of right retinal vessel hemorrhage, percutaneous – Hint: The RETINAL VESSEL body part values are in the EYE body system. | |
| 39. | Thoracoscopy with mechanical abrasion and application of talc for pleurodesis | |
| 40. | Percutaneous insertion of Greenfield IVC filter | |
| 41. | Forceps total mouth extraction, upper and lower teeth | |
| 42. | Removal of left thumbnail – Hint: No separate body part value is given for thumbnail, so this is coded to FINGERNAIL. | |

| Procedure | Description | Code(s) |
|---|---|---|
| 43. | Extraction of right intraocular lens without replacement, percutaneous | |
| 44. | Laparoscopy with needle aspiration of ova for in-vitro fertilization | |
| 45. | Non-excisional debridement of skin ulcer, right foot | |
| 46. | Open stripping of abdominal fascia, right side | |
| 47. | Hysteroscopy with D&C, diagnostic | |
| 48. | Liposuction for medical purposes, left upper arm – Hint: The PERCUTANEOUS approach is inherent in the liposuction technique. | |
| 49. | Removal of tattered right ear drum fragments with tweezers | |
| 50. | Microincisional phlebectomy of spider veins, right lower leg | |
| 51. | Routine Foley catheter placement | |
| 52. | Incision and drainage of external perianal abscess | |
| 53. | Percutaneous drainage of ascites – Hint: This is drainage of the cavity and not the peritoneal membrane itself. | |
| 54. | Laparoscopy with left ovarian cystotomy and drainage | |
| 55. | Laparotomy with hepatotomy and drain placement for liver abscess, right lobe | |
| 56. | Right knee arthrotomy with drain placement | |
| 57. | Thoracentesis of left pleural effusion – Hint: This is drainage of the pleural cavity. | |
| 58. | Phlebotomy of left median cubital vein for polycythemia vera Hint: The median cubital vein is a branch of the cephalic vein. | |
| 59. | Percutaneous chest tube placement for right pneumothorax | |
| 60. | Endoscopic drainage of left ethmoid sinus | |
| 61. | Extracorporeal shock-wave lithotripsy (ESWL), bilateral ureters – Hint: The bilateral ureter body part value is not available for the root operation FRAGMENTATION, so two codes are used, one for right, one for left. | |
| 62. | Endoscopic Retrograde Cholangiopancreatography (ERCP) with lithotripsy of common bile duct stone – Hint: ERCP is performed through the mouth to the biliary system via the duodenum, so the approach value is VIA NATURAL OR ARTIFICIAL OPENING ENDOSCOPIC. | |
| 63. | Thoracotomy with crushing of pericardial calcifications | |
| 64. | Transurethral cystoscopy with fragmentation of bladder calculus | |
| 65. | Hysteroscopy with intraluminal lithotripsy of left fallopian tube calcification | |
| 66. | Division of right foot tendon, percutaneous | |
| 67. | Left heart catheterization with division of bundle of HIS | |
| 68. | Open osteotomy of capitate, left hand – Hint: The capitate is one of the carpal bones of the hand. | |
| 69. | EGD with esophagotomy of esophagogastric junction | |
| 70. | Sacral rhizotomy for pain control, percutaneous | |
| 71. | Laparotomy with exploration and adhesiolysis of right ureter | |
| 72. | Incision of scar contracture, right elbow – Hint: The skin of the elbow region is coded to the lower arm. | |
| 73. | Frenulotomy for treatment of tongue-tie syndrome – Hint: The frenulum is coded to the body part value TONGUE. | |
| 74. | Right shoulder arthroscopy with coracoacromial ligament release | |
| 75. | Mitral valvulotomy for release of fused leaflets, open approach | |
| 76. | Percutaneous left Achilles tendon release | |
| 77. | Laparoscopy with lysis of peritoneal adhesions | |
| 78. | Manual rupture of right shoulder joint adhesions under general anesthesia | |
| 79. | Open posterior tarsal tunnel release – Hint: The nerve released in the posterior tarsal tunnel is the tibial nerve. | |
| 80. | Laparoscopy with freeing of left ovary and fallopian tube | |
| 81. | Liver transplant with donor matched liver | |
| 82. | Orthotopic heart transplant using porcine heart – Hint: The donor heart comes from an animal (pig), so the qualifier value is ZOOPLASTIC. | |
| 83. | Right lung transplant, open, using organ donor match | |
| 84. | Transplant of large intestine, organ donor match | |
| 85. | Left kidney/pancreas organ bank transplant | |
| 86. | Replantation of avulsed scalp | |
| 87. | Reattachment of severed right ear | |
| 88. | Reattachment of traumatic left gastrocnemius avulsion, open | |

| Procedure | Description | Code(s) |
|---|---|---|
| 89. | Closed replantation of three avulsed teeth, lower jaw | |
| 90. | Reattachment of severed left hand | |
| 91. | Right hand open palmaris longus tendon transfer | |
| 92. | Endoscopic radial to median nerve transfer | |
| 93. | Fasciocutaneous flap closure of left thigh, open — Hint: The qualifier identifies the body layers in addition to the fascia performed as part of the procedure | |
| 94. | Transfer left index finger to left thumb position, open | |
| 95. | Percutaneous fascia transfer to fill defect, anterior neck | |
| 96. | Trigeminal to facial nerve transfer, percutaneous endoscopic | |
| 97. | Endoscopic left leg flexor hallucis longus tendon transfer | |
| 98. | Right scalp advancement flap to right temple | |
| 99. | Bilateral TRAM pedicle flap reconstruction status post mastectomy, muscle only, open — Hint: The transverse rectus abdominus muscle (TRAM) flap is coded for each flap developed. | |
| 100. | Skin transfer flap closure of complex open wound, left lower back | |
| 101. | Open fracture reduction, right tibia | |
| 102. | Laparoscopy with gastropexy for malrotation | |
| 103. | Left knee arthroscopy with reposition of anterior cruciate ligament | |
| 104. | Open transposition of ulnar nerve | |
| 105. | Closed reduction with percutaneous internal fixation of right femoral neck fracture | |
| 106. | Cervical cerclage using Shirodkar technique | |
| 107. | Thoracotomy with banding of left pulmonary artery using extraluminal device | |
| 108. | Restriction of thoracic duct with intraluminal stent, percutaneous | |
| 109. | Craniotomy with clipping of cerebral aneurysm — Hint: A clip is placed lengthwise on the outside wall of the widened portion of the vessel. | |
| 110. | Non-incisional, trans-nasal placement of restrictive stent in right lacrimal duct | |
| 111. | Percutaneous ligation of esophageal vein | |
| 112. | Percutaneous embolization of left internal carotid-cavernous fistula | |
| 113. | Laparoscopy with bilateral occlusion of fallopian tubes using Hulka extraluminal clips | |
| 114. | Open suture ligation of failed AV graft, left brachial artery | |
| 115. | Percutaneous embolization of vascular supply, intracranial meningioma | |
| 116. | ERCP with balloon dilation of common bile duct | |
| 117. | PTCA of two coronary arteries, LAD with stent placement, RCA with no stent Hint: A separate procedure is coded for each artery dilated, since the device value differs for each artery. | |
| 118. | Cystoscopy with intraluminal dilation of bladder neck stricture | |
| 119. | Open dilation of old anastomosis, left femoral artery | |
| 120. | Dilation of upper esophageal stricture, direct visualization, with Bougie sound | |
| 121. | PTA of right brachial artery stenosis | |
| 122. | Trans-nasal dilation and stent placement in right lacrimal duct | |
| 123. | Hysteroscopy with balloon dilation of bilateral fallopian tubes | |
| 124. | Tracheoscopy with intraluminal dilation of tracheal stenosis | |
| 125. | Cystoscopy with dilation of left ureteral stricture, with stent placement | |
| 126. | Open gastric bypass with Roux-en-Y limb to jejunum | |
| 127. | Right temporal artery to intracranial artery bypass using goretex graft, open | |
| 128. | Tracheostomy formation with tracheostomy tube placement, percutaneous | |
| 129. | PICVA (Percutaneous in-situ coronary venous arterialization) of single coronary artery | |
| 130. | Open left femoral-popliteal artery bypass using cadaver vein graft | |
| 131. | Shunting of intrathecal cerebrospinal fluid to peritoneal cavity using synthetic shunt | |
| 132. | Colostomy formation, open, transverse colon to abdominal wall | |
| 133. | Open urinary diversion, left ureter, using ileal conduit to skin | |
| 134. | CABG of LAD using left internal mammary artery, open off-bypass | |
| 135. | Open pleuroperitoneal shunt, right pleural cavity, using synthetic device | |
| 136. | End-of-life replacement of spinal neurostimulator generator, multiple array, in lower abdomen — Hint: Taking out the old generator is coded separately to the root operation REMOVAL. | |
| 137. | Percutaneous replacement of broken pacemaker lead in left atrium — Hint: Taking out the broken pacemaker lead is coded separately to the root operation REMOVAL. | |
| 138. | Open placement of dual chamber pacemaker generator in chest wall | |

| Procedure | Description | Code(s) |
|---|---|---|
| 139. | Percutaneous placement of venous central line in right internal jugular | |
| 140. | Open insertion of multiple channel cochlear implant, left ear | |
| 141. | Percutaneous placement of Swan-Ganz catheter in superior vena cava — Hint: The Swan-Ganz catheter is coded to the device value MONITORING DEVICE because it monitors pulmonary artery output. | |
| 142. | Bronchoscopy with insertion of brachytherapy seeds, right main bronchus | |
| 143. | Placement of intrathecal infusion pump for pain management, percutaneous — Hint: The device resides principally in the subcutaneous tissue of the back, so it is coded to body system J. | |
| 144. | Open placement of bone growth stimulator, left femoral shaft | |
| 145. | Cystoscopy with placement of brachytherapy seeds in prostate gland | |
| 146. | Full-thickness skin graft to right lower arm, autograft (do not code graft harvest for this exercise) | |
| 147. | Excision of necrosed left femoral head with bone bank bone graft to fill the defect, open | |
| 148. | Penetrating keratoplasty of right cornea with donor matched cornea, percutaneous approach | |
| 149. | Bilateral mastectomy with concomitant saline breast implants, open | |
| 150. | Excision of abdominal aorta with goretex graft replacement, open | |
| 151. | Total right knee arthroplasty with insertion of total knee prosthesis | |
| 152. | Bilateral mastectomy with free TRAM flap reconstruction | |
| 153. | Tenonectomy with graft to right ankle using cadaver graft, open | |
| 154. | Mitral valve replacement using porcine valve, open | |
| 155. | Percutaneous phacoemulsification of right eye cataract with prosthetic lens insertion | |
| 156. | Removal of foreign body, right cornea | |
| 157. | Percutaneous mechanical thrombectomy, left brachial artery | |
| 158. | Esophagogastroscopy with removal of bezoar from stomach | |
| 159. | Foreign body removal, skin of left thumb — Hint: There is no specific value for thumb skin, so the procedure is coded to the hand. | |
| 160. | Transurethral cystoscopy with removal of bladder stone | |
| 161. | Forceps removal of foreign body in right nostril — Hint: Nostril is coded to the NOSE body part value. | |
| 162. | Laparoscopy with excision of old suture from mesentery | |
| 163. | Incision and removal of right lacrimal duct stone | |
| 164. | Non-incisional removal of intraluminal foreign body from vagina — Hint: The approach may be VIA NATURAL OR ARTIFICAL OPENING or EXTERNAL depending on the exact location of the foreign body. EXTERNAL is used if the object removed was in the vaginal orifice. | |
| 165. | Right common carotid endarterectomy, open | |
| 166. | Aortic valve annuloplasty using ring, open | |
| 167. | Laparoscopic repair of left inguinal hernia with marlex plug | |
| 168. | Autograft nerve graft to right median nerve, percutaneous endoscopic (do not code graft harvest for this exercise) | |
| 169. | Exchange of liner in femoral component of previous left hip replacement, open approach — Hint: Taking out the old liner is coded separately to the root operation REMOVAL | |
| 170. | Anterior colporrhaphy with polypropylene mesh reinforcement, open approach | |
| 171. | Implantation of CorCap cardiac support device, open approach | |
| 172. | Abdominal wall herniorrhaphy, open, using synthetic mesh | |
| 173. | Tendon graft to strengthen injured left shoulder using autograft, open (do not code graft harvest for this exercise) | |
| 174. | Onlay lamellar keratoplasty of left cornea using autograft, external approach | |
| 175. | Resurfacing procedure on right femoral head, open approach | |
| 176. | Exchange of drainage tube from right hip joint | |
| 177. | Tracheostomy tube exchange | |
| 178. | Change chest tube for left pneumothorax | |
| 179. | Exchange of cerebral ventriculostomy drainage tube | |
| 180. | Foley urinary catheter exchange — Hint: This is coded to DRAINAGE DEVICE because urine is being drained. | |
| 181. | Open removal of lumbar sympathetic neurostimulator | |
| 182. | Non-incisional removal of Swan-Ganz catheter from right pulmonary artery | |
| 183. | Laparotomy with removal of pancreatic drain | |
| 184. | Extubation, endotracheal tube | |
| 185. | Non-incisional PEG tube removal | |

| Procedure | Description | Code(s) |
|---|---|---|
| 186. | Transvaginal removal of brachytherapy seeds | |
| 187. | Incision with removal of K-wire fixation, right first metatarsal | |
| 188. | Cystoscopy with retrieval of left ureteral stent | |
| 189. | Removal of nasogastric drainage tube for decompression | |
| 190. | Removal of external fixator, left radial fracture | |
| 191. | Reposition of Swan-Ganz catheter in superior vena cava | |
| 192. | Open revision of right hip replacement, with recementing of the prosthesis | |
| 193. | Adjustment of position, pacemaker lead in left ventricle, percutaneous | |
| 194. | Taking out loose screw and putting larger screw in fracture repair plate, left tibia | |
| 195. | Revision of VAD reservoir placement in chest wall, causing patient discomfort, open | |
| 196. | Thoracotomy with exploration of right pleural cavity | |
| 197. | Diagnostic laryngoscopy | |
| 198. | Exploratory arthrotomy of left knee | |
| 199. | Colposcopy with diagnostic hysteroscopy | |
| 200. | Digital rectal exam | |
| 201. | Diagnostic arthroscopy of right shoulder | |
| 202. | Endoscopy of maxillary sinus | |
| 203. | Laparotomy with palpation of liver | |
| 204. | Transurethral diagnostic cystoscopy | |
| 205. | Colonoscopy, discontinued at sigmoid colon | |
| 206. | Hysteroscopy with cautery of post-hysterectomy oozing and evacuation of clot | |
| 207. | Open exploration and ligation of post-op arterial bleeder, left forearm | |
| 208. | Control of post-operative retroperitoneal bleeding via laparotomy | |
| 209. | Reopening of thoracotomy site with drainage and control of post-op hemopericardium | |
| 210. | Arthroscopy with drainage of hemarthrosis at previous operative site, right knee | |
| 211. | Suture repair of left radial nerve laceration – Hint: The approach value is OPEN, though the surgical exposure may have been created by the wound itself. | |
| 212. | Laparotomy with suture repair of blunt force duodenal laceration | |
| 213. | Perineoplasty with repair of old obstetric laceration, open | |
| 214. | Suture repair of right biceps tendon laceration, open | |
| 215. | Closure of abdominal wall stab wound | |
| 216. | Percutaneous mapping of basal ganglia | |
| 217. | Heart catheterization with cardiac mapping | |
| 218. | Intraoperative whole brain mapping via craniotomy | |
| 219. | Mapping of left cerebral hemisphere, percutaneous endoscopic | |
| 220. | Intraoperative cardiac mapping during open heart surgery | |
| 221. | Radiocarpal fusion of left hand with internal fixation, open | |
| 222. | Posterior spinal fusion at L1-L3 level with BAK cage interbody fusion device, open | |
| 223. | Intercarpal fusion of right hand with bone bank bone graft, open | |
| 224. | Sacrococcygeal fusion with bone graft from same operative site, open | |
| 225. | Interphalangeal fusion of left great toe, percutaneous pin fixation | |
| 226. | Cosmetic face lift, open, no other information available | |
| 227. | Bilateral breast augmentation with silicone implants, open | |
| 228. | Cosmetic rhinoplasty with septal reduction and tip elevation using local tissue graft, open | |
| 229. | Abdominoplasty (tummy tuck), open | |
| 230. | Liposuction of bilateral thighs | |
| 231. | Creation of penis in female patient using tissue bank donor graft | |
| 232. | Creation of vagina in male patient using synthetic material | |

## Section 1 – Obstetrics

| Procedure | Description | Code(s) |
|---|---|---|
| 1. | Abortion by dilation and evacuation following laminaria insertion | |
| 2. | Manually assisted spontaneous abortion – Hint: Since the pregnancy was not artificially terminated, this is coded to DELIVERY, because it captures the procedure objective. The fact that it was an abortion will be identified in the diagnosis code. | |
| 3. | Abortion by abortifacient insertion | |
| 4. | Bimanual pregnancy examination | |
| 5. | Extraperitoneal c-section, low transverse incision | |

| Procedure | Description | Code(s) |
|---|---|---|
| 6. | Fetal spinal tap, percutaneous | |
| 7. | Fetal kidney transplant, laparoscopic | |
| 8. | Open in utero repair of congenital diaphragmatic hernia – Hint: Diaphragm is classified to the RESPIRATORY body system in the MEDICAL AND SURGICAL section. | |
| 9. | Laparoscopy with total excision of tubal pregnancy | |
| 10. | Transvaginal removal of fetal monitoring electrode | |

## Section 2 – Placement

| Procedure | Description | Code(s) |
|---|---|---|
| 1. | Placement of packing material, right ear | |
| 2. | Mechanical traction of entire left leg | |
| 3. | Removal of splint, right shoulder | |
| 4. | Placement of neck brace | |
| 5. | Change of vaginal packing | |
| 6. | Packing of wound, chest wall | |
| 7. | Sterile dressing placement to left groin region | |
| 8. | Removal of packing material from pharynx | |
| 9. | Placement of intermittent pneumatic compression device, covering entire right arm | |
| 10. | Exchange of pressure dressing to left thigh | |

## Section 3 – Administration

| Procedure | Description | Code(s) |
|---|---|---|
| 1. | Peritoneal dialysis via indwelling catheter | |
| 2. | Transvaginal artificial insemination | |
| 3. | Infusion of total parenteral nutrition via central venous catheter | |
| 4. | Esophagogastroscopy with botox injection into esophageal sphincter – Hint: Botulinum toxin is a paralyzing agent with temporary effects; it does not sclerose or destroy the nerve. | |
| 5. | Percutaneous irrigation of knee joint | |
| 6. | Epidural injection of mixed steroid and local anesthetic for pain control – Hint: This is coded to the substance value ANTI-INFLAMMATORY. The anesthetic is only added to lessen the pain of the injection. | |
| 7. | Transfusion of antihemophilic factor, (nonautologous) via arterial central line | |
| 8. | Transabdominal in-vitro fertilization, implantation of donor ovum | |
| 9. | Autologous bone marrow transplant via central venous line | |
| 10. | Implantation antimicrobial envelope with cardiac defibrillator placement, open | |

## Section 4 – Measurement and Monitoring

| Procedure | Description | Code(s) |
|---|---|---|
| 1. | Cardiac stress test, single measurement | |
| 2. | EGD with biliary flow measurement | |
| 3. | Right and left heart cardiac catheterization with bilateral sampling and pressure measurements | |
| 4. | Peripheral venous pulse, external, single measurement | |
| 5. | Holter monitoring | |
| 6. | Respiratory rate, external, single measurement | |
| 7. | Fetal heart rate monitoring, transvaginal | |
| 8. | Visual mobility test, single measurement | |
| 9. | Left ventricular cardiac output monitoring from pulmonary artery wedge (Swan-Ganz catheter) | |
| 10. | Olfactory acuity test, single measurement | |

## Section 5 – Extracorporeal Assistance and Performance

| Procedure | Description | Code(s) |
|---|---|---|
| 1. | Intermittent mechanical ventilation, 16 hours | |
| 2. | Liver dialysis, single encounter | |
| 3. | Cardiac countershock with successful conversion to sinus rhythm | |
| 4. | IPPB (intermittent positive pressure breathing) for mobilization of secretions, 22 hours | |
| 5. | Renal dialysis, series of encounters | |
| 6. | IABP (intra-aortic balloon pump) continuous | |
| 7. | Intra-operative cardiac pacing, continuous – Hint: The procedure to insert the balloon pump is coded to the root operation INSERTION in the MEDICAL AND SURGICAL section. | |
| 8. | ECMO (extracorporeal membrane oxygenation), continuous | |
| 9. | Controlled mechanical ventilation (CMV), 45 hours – Hint: The endotracheal tube associated with the mechanical ventilation procedure is considered a component of the equipment used in performing the procedure and is not coded separately. | |

| Procedure | Description | Code(s) |
|---|---|---|
| 10. | Pulsatile compression boot with intermittent inflation — Hint: This is coded to the function value CARDIAC OUTPUT, because the purpose of such compression devices is to return blood to the heart faster.. | |

## Section 6 — Extracorporeal Therapies

| Procedure | Description | Code(s) |
|---|---|---|
| 1. | Donor thrombocytapheresis, single encounter | |
| 2. | Bili-lite UV phototherapy, series treatment | |
| 3. | Whole body hypothermia, single treatment | |
| 4. | Circulatory phototherapy, single encounter | |
| 5. | Shock wave therapy of plantar fascia, single treatment | |
| 6. | Antigen-free air conditioning, series treatment | |
| 7. | TMS (transcranial magnetic stimulation), series treatment | |
| 8. | Therapeutic ultrasound of peripheral vessels, single treatment | |
| 9. | Plasmapheresis, series treatment | |
| 10. | Extracorporeal electromagnetic stimulation (EMS) for urinary incontinence, single treatment | |

## Section 7 — Osteopathic

| Procedures | Description | Code(s) |
|---|---|---|
| 1. | Isotonic muscle energy treatment of right leg | |
| 2. | Low velocity-high amplitude osteopathic treatment of head | |
| 3. | Lymphatic pump osteopathic treatment of left axilla | |
| 4. | Indirect osteopathic treatment of sacrum | |
| 5. | Articulatory osteopathic treatment of cervical region | |

## Section 8 — Other Procedures

| Procedure | Description | Code(s) |
|---|---|---|
| 1. | Near infrared spectroscopy of leg vessels | |
| 2. | CT computer assisted sinus surgery — Hint: The sinus surgery is the primary procedure and is coded separately, but there is not enough information to code the sinus procedure here. | |
| 3. | Suture removal, abdominal wall | |
| 4. | Isolation after infectious disease exposure | |
| 5. | Robotic assisted open prostatectomy — Hint: The prostatectomy is the primary procedure and is coded separately. Code only the robotic assistance for this coding practice. | |

## Section 9 — Chiropractics

| Procedure | Description | Code(s) |
|---|---|---|
| 1. | Chiropractic treatment of lumbar region using long lever specific contact | |
| 2. | Chiropractic manipulation of abdominal region, indirect visceral | |
| 3. | Chiropractic extra-articular treatment of hip region | |
| 4. | Chiropractic treatment of sacrum using long and short lever specific contact | |
| 5. | Mechanically-assisted chiropractic manipulation of head | |

## Section B — Imaging

| Procedure | Description | Code(s) |
|---|---|---|
| 1. | Non-contrast CT of abdomen and pelvis | |
| 2. | Intravascular ultrasound, left subclavian artery | |
| 3. | Fluoroscopic guidance for insertion of central venous catheter in SVC, low osmolar contrast | |
| 4. | Endoluminal ultrasound of gallbladder and bile ducts | |
| 5. | Left ventriculography using low osmolar contrast | |
| 6. | Esophageal videofluoroscopy study with oral barium contrast | |
| 7. | Portable X-ray study of right radius/ulna shaft, standard series | |
| 8. | Routine fetal ultrasound, second trimester twin gestation | |
| 9. | CT scan of bilateral lungs, high osmolar contrast with densitometry | |
| 10. | Fluoroscopic guidance for percutaneous transluminal angioplasty (PTA) of left common femoral artery, low osmolar contrast | |

## Section C — Nuclear Medicine

| Procedure | Description | Code(s) |
|---|---|---|
| 1. | Tomo scan of right and left heart, unspecified radiopharmaceutical, qualitative gated rest | |
| 2. | Technetium pentetate assay of kidneys, ureters, and bladder | |
| 3. | Uniplanar scan of spine using technetium oxidronate, with first pass study | |
| 4. | Thallous chloride tomographic scan of bilateral breasts | |
| 5. | PET scan of myocardium using rubidium | |
| 6. | Gallium citrate scan of head and neck, single plane imaging | |
| 7. | Xenon gas nonimaging probe of brain | |
| 8. | Upper GI scan, radiopharmaceutical unspecified, for gastric emptying | |
| 9. | Carbon 11 PET scan of brain with quantification | |
| 10. | Iodinated albumin nuclear medicine assay, blood plasma volume study | |

## Section D — Radiation Therapy

| Procedure | Description | Code(s) |
|---|---|---|
| 1. | Plaque radiation of left eye, single port | |
| 2. | 8 MeV photon beam radiation to brain | |
| 3. | IORT of colon, 3 ports | |
| 4. | HDR Brachytherapy of prostate using Palladium 103 | |
| 5. | Electron radiation treatment of right breast, custom device | |
| 6. | Hyperthermia oncology treatment of pelvic region | |
| 7. | Contact radiation of tongue | |
| 8. | Heavy particle radiation treatment of pancreas, four risk sites | |
| 9. | LDR brachytherapy to spinal cord using iodine | |
| 10. | Whole body Phosphorus 32 administration with risk to hematopoetic system | |

## Section F — Physical Rehabilitation and Diagnostic Audiology

| Procedure | Description | Code(s) |
|---|---|---|
| 1. | Bekesy assessment using audiometer | |
| 2. | Individual fitting of left eye prosthesis | |
| 3. | Physical therapy for range of motion and mobility, patient right hip, no special equipment | |
| 4. | Bedside swallow assessment using assessment kit | |
| 5. | Caregiver training in airway clearance techniques | |
| 6. | Application of short arm cast in rehabilitation setting — Hint: Inhibitory cast is listed in the equipment reference table under ORTHOSIS. | |
| 7. | Verbal assessment of patient's pain level | |
| 8. | Caregiver training in communication skills using manual communication board — Hint: Manual communication board is listed in the equipment reference table under AUGMENTATIVE/ALTERNATIVE COMMUNICATION. | |
| 9. | Group musculoskeletal balance training exercises, whole body, no special equipment — Hint: Balance training is included in the MOTOR TREATMENT reference table under THERAPEUTIC EXERCISE. | |
| 10. | Individual therapy for auditory processing using tape recorder — Hint: Tape recorder is listed in the equipment reference table under AUDIOVISUAL EQUIPMENT. | |

## Section G — Mental Health

| Procedure | Description | Code(s) |
|---|---|---|
| 1. | Cognitive-behavioral psychotherapy, individual | |
| 2. | Narcosynthesis | |
| 3. | Light therapy | |
| 4. | ECT (Electroconvulsive therapy), unilateral, multiple seizure | |
| 5. | Crisis intervention | |
| 6. | Neuropsychological testing | |
| 7. | Hypnosis | |
| 8. | Developmental testing | |
| 9. | Vocational counseling | |
| 10. | Family psychotherapy | |

## Section H — Substance Abuse Treatment

| Procedure | Description | Code(s) |
|---|---|---|
| 1. | Naltrexone treatment for drug dependency | |
| 2. | Substance abuse treatment family counseling | |
| 3. | Medication monitoring of patient on methadone maintenance | |
| 4. | Individual interpersonal psychotherapy for drug abuse | |
| 5. | Patient in for alcohol detoxification treatment | |
| 6. | Group motivational counseling | |
| 7. | Individual 12-step psychotherapy for substance abuse | |
| 8. | Post-test infectious disease counseling for IV drug abuser | |
| 9. | Psychodynamic psychotherapy for drug dependent patient | |
| 10. | Group cognitive-behavioral counseling for substance abuse | |

# 2015 ICD-10-PCS Code Changes

## New Index Entries

Absolute Pro Vascular (OTW) Self-Expanding Stent System – use Intraluminal

Acculink (RX) Carotid Stent System – use Intraluminal Device

Advisa (MRI) – use Pacemaker, Dual Chamber in 0JH

AIGISRx Antibacterial Envelope – use Anti-Infective Envelope

Antimicrobial envelope – use Anti-Infective Envelope

Ascenda Intrathecal Catheter – use Infusion Device

Baroreflex Activation Therapy® (BAT®)
 – use Stimulator Generator in Subcutaneous Tissue and Fascia

Bedside swallow F00ZJWZ

Bone morphogenetic protein 2 (BMP 2) – use Recombinant Bone Morphogenetic Protein

Clolar – use Clofarabine

Evera (XT)(S)(DR/VR) – use Defibrillator Generator in 0JH

Hemilaminotomy
 – see Excision, Upper Bones 0PB
 – see Excision, Lower Bones 0QB
 – see Release, Central Nervous System 00N
 – see Release, Peripheral Nervous System 01N
 – see Drainage, Upper Bones 0P9
 – see Release, Upper Bones 0PN
 – see Drainage, Lower Bones 0Q9
 – see Release, Lower Bones 0QN

Herculink (RX) Elite Renal Stent System – use Intraluminal Device

Infusion Device, Pump
 Insertion of device in
 Abdomen 0JH8
 Back 0JH7
 Chest 0JH6
 Lower Arm
 Left 0JHH
 Right 0JHG
 Lower Leg
 Left 0JHP
 Right 0JHN
 Trunk 0JHT
 Upper Arm
 Left 0JHF
 Right 0JHD
 Upper Leg
 Left 0JHM
 Right 0JHL
 Removal of device from
 Lower Extremity 0JPW
 Trunk 0JPT
 Upper Extremity 0JPV
 Revision of device in
 Lower Extremity 0JWW
 Trunk 0JWT
 Upper Extremity 0JWV

Kcentra – use 4-Factor Prothrombin Complex Concentrate

Laminotomy
 – see Drainage, Upper Bones 0P9
 – see Drainage, Lower Bones 0Q9
 – see Release, Upper Bones 0PN
 – see Release, Lower Bones 0QN
 – see Excision, Upper Bones 0PB
 – see Excision, Lower Bones 0QB

Monitoring Device, Hemodynamic
 Abdomen 0JH8
 Chest 0JH6

Mosaic Bioprosthesis (aortic) (mitral) valve – use Zooplastic Tissue in Heart and Great Vessels

MULTI-LINK (VISION)(MINI-VISION)(ULTRA) Coronary Stent System – use Intraluminal Device

Nesiritide – use Human B-type Natriuretic Peptide

Omnilink Elite Vascular Balloon Expandable Stent System – use Intraluminal Device

Open Pivot (mechanical) valve – use Synthetic Substitute

Open Pivot Aortic Valve Graft (AVG) – use Synthetic Substitute

Pharmacotherapy, for substance abuse
 Antabuse HZ93ZZZ
 Bupropion HZ97ZZZ
 Clonidine HZ96ZZZ
 Levo-alpha-acetyl-methadol (LAAM) HZ92ZZZ
 Methadone Maintenance HZ91ZZZ
 Naloxone HZ95ZZZ
 Naltrexone HZ94ZZZ
 Nicotine Replacement HZ90ZZZ
 Psychiatric Medication HZ98ZZZ
 Replacement Medication, Other HZ99ZZZ

PrimeAdvanced neurostimulator (SureScan)(MRI Safe) – use Stimulator Generator, Multiple Array in 0JH

RestoreAdvanced neurostimulator (SureScan)(MRI Safe) – use Stimulator Generator, Multiple Array Rechargeable in 0JH

RestoreSensor neurostimulator (SureScan)(MRI Safe) – use Stimulator Generator, Multiple Array Rechargeable in 0JH

RestoreUltra neurostimulator (SureScan)(MRI Safe) – use Stimulator Generator, Multiple Array Rechargeable in 0JH

rhBMP-2 – use Recombinant Bone Morphogenetic Protein

Seprafilm – use Adhesion Barrier

Stent, intraluminal (cardiovascular)(gastrointestinal)(hepatobiliary) (urinary) – use Intraluminal Device

SynchroMed pump – use Infusion Device, Pump in Subcutaneous Tissue and Fascia

Tissue Plasminogen Activator (tPA)(r-tPA) – use Thrombolytic, Other

Viva (XT)(S) – use Cardiac Resynchronization Defibrillator Pulse Generator in 0JH

Voraxaze – use Glucarpidase

Xact Carotid Stent System – use Intraluminal Device

XIENCE Everolimus Eluting Coronary Stent System – use Intraluminal Device, Drug-eluting in Heart and Great Vessels

Zyvox – use Oxazolidinones

## Revised Index Entries

Banding
 – see Restriction
 – see Occlusion

Centrimag® Blood Pump – use External Heart Assist System in Heart and Great Vessels

Costotransverse joint – use Joint, Thoracic Vertebral

Costovertebral joint – use Joint, Thoracic Vertebral

Lumbar facet joint – use Joint, Lumbar Vertebral

Extracorporeal membrane (ECMO) – see Performance, Circulatory 5A15

Rheos® System device – use Stimulator Generator in Subcutaneous Tissue and Fascia

Thoracic facet joint – use Joint, Thoracic Vertebral

TURP (transurethral resection of prostate)
 – see Excision, Prostate 0VB0
 – see Resection, Prostate 0VT0

## Deleted Index Entries

Baroreflex Activation Therapy® (BAT®)
 – use Cardiac Rhythm Related Device in Subcutaneous Tissue and Fascia

Costotransverse joint
 – use Joint, Thoracic Vertebral
 – use Joint, Thoracic Vertebral, 2 to 7
 – use Joint, Thoracic Vertebral, 8 or more

Costovertebral joint
 – use Joint, Thoracic Vertebral, 8 or more
 – use Joint, Thoracic Vertebral, 2 to 7
 – use Joint, Thoracic Vertebral

Impella® (2.5)(5.0)(LD) cardiac assist device – use Intraluminal Device

Infusion Device
   Insertion of device in
      Abdomen 0JH8
      Back 0JH7
      Chest 0JH6
      Lower Arm
         Left 0JHH
         Right 0JHG
      Lower Leg
         Left 0JHP
         Right 0JHN
      Trunk 0JHT
      Upper Arm
         Left 0JHF
         Right 0JHD
      Upper Leg
         Left 0JHM
         Right 0JHL
   Removal of device from
      Lower Extremity 0JPW
      Trunk 0JPT
      Upper Extremity 0JPV
   Revision of device in
      Lower Extremity 0JWW
      Trunk 0JWT
      Upper Extremity 0JWV
Kinetra® neurostimulator – use Stimulator Generator, Multiple Array in 0JH
Laminotomy
   – see Drainage, Upper Joints 0R9
   – see Drainage, Lower Joints 0S9
   – see Release, Upper Joints 0RN
   – see Release, Lower Joints 0SN

Lumbar facet joint
   – use Joint, Lumbar Vertebral, 2 or more
   – use Joint, Lumbar Vertebral
Monitoring Device
   Abdomen 0JH8
   Chest 0JH6
Pharmacotherapy
   Antabuse HZ93ZZZ
   Bupropion HZ97ZZZ
   Clonidine HZ96ZZZ
   Levo-alpha-acetyl-methadol (LAAM) HZ92ZZZ
   Methadone Maintenance HZ91ZZZ
   Naloxone HZ95ZZZ
   Naltrexone HZ94ZZZ
   Nicotine Replacement HZ90ZZZ
   Psychiatric Medication HZ98ZZZ
   Replacement Medication, Other HZ99ZZZ
PrimeAdvanced neurostimulator – use Stimulator Generator, Multiple Array in 0JH
RestoreAdvanced neurostimulator – use Stimulator Generator, Multiple Array Rechargeable in 0JH
RestoreSensor neurostimulator – use Stimulator Generator, Multiple Array Rechargeable in 0JH
RestoreUltra neurostimulator – use Stimulator Generator, Multiple Array Rechargeable in 0JH
Soletra® neurostimulator – use Stimulator Generator, Single Array in 0JH
Stent (angioplasty)(embolization) – use Intraluminal Device
Thoracic facet joint
   – use Joint, Thoracic Vertebral, 2 to 7
   – use Joint, Thoracic Vertebral, 8 or more
   – use Joint, Thoracic Vertebral

# 3

**3f** (Aortic) **Bioprosthesis valve** – *use* Zooplastic Tissue in Heart and Great Vessels

# A

**Abdominal aortic plexus** – *use* Nerve, Abdominal Sympathetic
**Abdominal esophagus** – *use* Esophagus, Lower
**Abdominohysterectomy**
  – *see* Excision, Uterus ØUB9
  – *see* Resection, Uterus ØUT9
**Abdominoplasty**
  – *see* Alteration, Abdominal Wall ØWØF
  – *see* Repair, Abdominal Wall ØWQF
  – *see* Supplement, Abdominal Wall ØWUF
**Abductor hallucis muscle**
  – *use* Muscle, Foot, Right
  – *use* Muscle, Foot, Left
**AbioCor® Total Replacement Heart** – *use* Synthetic Substitute
**Ablation** – *see* Destruction
**Abortion**
  Products of Conception 1ØAØ
  Abortifacient 1ØAØ7ZX
  Laminaria 1ØAØ7ZW
  Vacuum 1ØAØ7Z6
**Abrasion** – *see* Extraction
**Absolute Pro Vascular (OTW) Self-Expanding Stent System** – *use* Intraluminal Device
**Accessory cephalic vein**
  – *use* Vein, Cephalic, Right
  – *use* Vein, Cephalic, Left
**Accessory obturator nerve** – *use* Nerve, Lumbar Plexus
**Accessory phrenic nerve** – *use* Nerve, Phrenic
**Accessory spleen** – *use* Spleen
**Acculink (RX) Carotid Stent System** – *use* Intraluminal Device
**Acellular Hydrated Dermis** – *use* Nonautologous Tissue Substitute
**Acetabulectomy**
  – *see* Excision, Lower Bones ØQB
  – *see* Resection, Lower Bones ØQT
**Acetabulofemoral joint**
  – *use* Joint, Hip, Right
  – *use* Joint, Hip, Left
**Acetabuloplasty**
  – *see* Repair, Lower Bones ØQQ
  – *see* Replacement, Lower Bones ØQR
  – *see* Supplement, Lower Bones ØQU
**Achilles tendon**
  – *use* Tendon, Lower Leg, Left
  – *use* Tendon, Lower Leg, Right
**Achillorrhaphy** – *see* Repair, Tendons ØLQ
**Achillotenotomy, achillotomy**
  – *see* Division, Tendons ØL8
  – *see* Drainage, Tendons ØL9
**Acromioclavicular ligament**
  – *use* Bursa and Ligament, Shoulder, Right
  – *use* Bursa and Ligament, Shoulder, Left
**Acromion** (process)
  – *use* Scapula, Left
  – *use* Scapula, Right
**Acromionectomy**
  – *see* Excision, Upper Joints ØRB
  – *see* Resection, Upper Joints ØRT
**Acromioplasty**
  – *see* Repair, Upper Joints ØRQ
  – *see* Replacement, Upper Joints ØRR
  – *see* Supplement, Upper Joints ØRU
**Activa PC neurostimulator** – *use* Stimulator Generator, Multiple Array in ØJH
**Activa RC neurostimulator** – *use* Stimulator Generator, Multiple Array Rechargeable in ØJH
**Activa SC neurostimulator** – *use* Stimulator Generator, Single Array in ØJH
**Activities of Daily Living Assessment** FØ2
**Activities of Daily Living Treatment** FØ8
**ACUITY™ Steerable Lead**
  – *use* Cardiac Lead, Defibrillator in Ø2H
  – *use* Cardiac Lead, Pacemaker in Ø2H
**Acupuncture**
  Breast
    Anesthesia 8EØH3ØØ
    No Qualifier 8EØH3ØZ

**Acupuncture** – *continued*
  Integumentary System
    Anesthesia 8EØH3ØØ
    No Qualifier 8EØH3ØZ
**Adductor brevis muscle**
  – *use* Muscle, Upper Leg, Left
  – *use* Muscle, Upper Leg, Right
**Adductor hallucis muscle**
  – *use* Muscle, Foot, Left
  – *use* Muscle, Foot, Right
**Adductor longus muscle**
  – *use* Muscle, Upper Leg, Right
  – *use* Muscle, Upper Leg, Left
**Adductor magnus muscle**
  – *use* Muscle, Upper Leg, Right
  – *use* Muscle, Upper Leg, Left
**Adenohypophysis** – *use* Gland, Pituitary
**Adenoidectomy**
  – *see* Excision, Adenoids ØCBQ
  – *see* Resection, Adenoids ØCTQ
**Adenoidotomy** – *see* Drainage, Adenoids ØC9Q
**Adhesiolysis** – *see* Release
**Administration**
  Blood products – *see* Transfusion
  Other substance – *see* Introduction of substance in or on
**Adrenalectomy**
  – *see* Excision, Endocrine System ØGB
  – *see* Resection, Endocrine System ØGT
**Adrenalorrhaphy** – *see* Repair, Endocrine System ØGQ
**Adrenalotomy** – *see* Drainage, Endocrine System ØG9
**Advancement**
  – *see* Reposition
  – *see* Transfer
**Advisa (MRI)** – *use* Pacemaker, Dual Chamber in ØJH
**AIGISRx Antibacterial Envelope** – *use* Anti-Infective Envelope
**Alar ligament of axis** – *use* Bursa and Ligament, Head and Neck
**Alimentation** – *see* Introduction of substance in or on
**Alteration**
  Abdominal Wall ØWØF
  Ankle Region
    Left ØYØL
    Right ØYØK
  Arm
    Lower
      Left ØXØF
      Right ØXØD
    Upper
      Left ØXØ9
      Right ØXØ8
  Axilla
    Left ØXØ5
    Right ØXØ4
  Back
    Lower ØWØL
    Upper ØWØK
  Breast
    Bilateral ØHØV
    Left ØHØU
    Right ØHØT
  Buttock
    Left ØYØ1
    Right ØYØØ
  Chest Wall ØWØ8
  Ear
    Bilateral Ø9Ø2
    Left Ø9Ø1
    Right Ø9ØØ
  Elbow Region
    Left ØXØC
    Right ØXØB
  Extremity
    Lower
      Left ØYØB
      Right ØYØ9
    Upper
      Left ØXØ7
      Right ØXØ6
  Eyelid
    Lower
      Left Ø8ØR
      Right Ø8ØQ
    Upper
      Left Ø8ØP
      Right Ø8ØN
  Face ØWØ2
  Head ØWØØ

**Alteration** – *continued*
  Jaw
    Lower ØWØ5
    Upper ØWØ4
  Knee Region
    Left ØYØG
    Right ØYØF
  Leg
    Lower
      Left ØYØJ
      Right ØYØH
    Upper
      Left ØYØD
      Right ØYØC
  Lip
    Lower ØCØ1X
    Upper ØCØØX
  Neck ØWØ6
  Nose Ø9ØK
  Perineum
    Female ØWØN
    Male ØWØM
  Shoulder Region
    Left ØXØ3
    Right ØXØ2
  Subcutaneous Tissue and Fascia
    Abdomen ØJØ8
    Back ØJØ7
    Buttock ØJØ9
    Chest ØJØ6
    Face ØJØ1
    Lower Arm
      Left ØJØH
      Right ØJØG
    Lower Leg
      Left ØJØP
      Right ØJØN
    Neck
      Anterior ØJØ4
      Posterior ØJØ5
    Upper Arm
      Left ØJØF
      Right ØJØD
    Upper Leg
      Left ØJØM
      Right ØJØL
  Wrist Region
    Left ØXØH
    Right ØXØG
**Alveolar process of mandible**
  – *use* Mandible, Left
  – *use* Mandible, Right
**Alveolar process of maxilla**
  – *use* Maxilla, Right
  – *use* Maxilla, Left
**Alveolectomy**
  – *see* Excision, Head and Facial Bones ØNB
  – *see* Resection, Head and Facial Bones ØNT
**Alveoloplasty**
  – *see* Repair, Head and Facial Bones ØNQ
  – *see* Replacement, Head and Facial Bones ØNR
  – *see* Supplement, Head and Facial Bones ØNU
**Alveolotomy**
  – *see* Division, Head and Facial Bones ØN8
  – *see* Drainage, Head and Facial Bones ØN9
**Ambulatory cardiac monitoring** 4A12X45
**Amniocentesis** – *see* Drainage, Products of Conception 1Ø9Ø
**Amnioinfusion** – *see* Introduction of substance in or on, Products of Conception 3EØE
**Amnioscopy** 1ØJØ8ZZ
**Amniotomy** – *see* Drainage, Products of Conception 1Ø9Ø
**AMPLATZER® Muscular VSD Occluder** – *use* Synthetic Substitute
**Amputation** – *see* Detachment
**AMS 800® Urinary Control System** – *use* Artificial Sphincter in Urinary System
**Anal orifice** – *use* Anus
**Analog radiography** – *see* Plain Radiography
**Analog radiology** – *see* Plain Radiography
**Anastomosis** – *see* Bypass
**Anatomical snuffbox**
  – *use* Muscle, Lower Arm and Wrist, Left
  – *use* Muscle, Lower Arm and Wrist, Right
**AneuRx® AAA Advantage®** – *use* Intraluminal Device
**Angiectomy**
  – *see* Excision, Heart and Great Vessels Ø2B
  – *see* Excision, Upper Arteries Ø3B
  – *see* Excision, Lower Arteries Ø4B
  – *see* Excision, Upper Veins Ø5B
  – *see* Excision, Lower Veins Ø6B

**Angiocardiography**
Combined right and left heart – *see* Fluoroscopy, Heart, Right and Left Heart B216
Left Heart – *see* Fluoroscopy, Heart, Left B215
Right Heart – *see* Fluoroscopy, Heart, Right B214
SPY – *see* Fluoroscopy, Heart B21

**Angiography**
– *see* Plain Radiography, Heart B20
– *see* Fluoroscopy, Heart B21

**Angioplasty**
– *see* Dilation, Heart and Great Vessels 027
– *see* Repair, Heart and Great Vessels 02Q
– *see* Replacement, Heart and Great Vessels 02R
– *see* Dilation, Upper Arteries 037
– *see* Repair, Upper Arteries 03Q
– *see* Replacement, Upper Arteries 03R
– *see* Dilation, Lower Arteries 047
– *see* Repair, Lower Arteries 04Q
– *see* Replacement, Lower Arteries 04R
– *see* Supplement, Heart and Great Vessels 02U
– *see* Supplement, Upper Arteries 03U
– *see* Supplement, Lower Arteries 04U

**Angiorrhaphy**
– *see* Repair, Heart and Great Vessels 02Q
– *see* Repair, Upper Arteries 03Q
– *see* Repair, Lower Arteries 04Q

**Angioscopy**
02JY4ZZ
03JY4ZZ
04JY4ZZ

**Angiotripsy**
– *see* Occlusion, Upper Arteries 03L
– *see* Occlusion, Lower Arteries 04L

**Angular artery** – *use* Artery, Face

**Angular vein**
– *use* Vein, Face, Left
– *use* Vein, Face, Right

**Annular ligament**
– *use* Bursa and Ligament, Elbow, Left
– *use* Bursa and Ligament, Elbow, Right

**Annuloplasty**
– *see* Repair, Heart and Great Vessels 02Q
– *see* Supplement, Heart and Great Vessels 02U

**Annuloplasty ring** – *use* Synthetic Substitute

**Anoplasty**
– *see* Repair, Anus 0DQQ
– *see* Supplement, Anus 0DUQ

**Anorectal junction** – *use* Rectum

**Anoscopy** 0DJD8ZZ

**Ansa cervicalis** – *use* Nerve, Cervical Plexus

**Antabuse therapy** HZ93ZZZ

**Antebrachial fascia**
– *use* Subcutaneous Tissue and Fascia, Lower Arm, Left
– *use* Subcutaneous Tissue and Fascia, Lower Arm, Right

**Anterior** (pectoral) **lymph node**
– *use* Lymphatic, Axillary, Right
– *use* Lymphatic, Axillary, Left

**Anterior cerebral artery** – *use* Artery, Intracranial
**Anterior cerebral vein** – *use* Vein, Intracranial
**Anterior choroidal artery** – *use* Artery, Intracranial
**Anterior circumflex humeral artery**
– *use* Artery, Axillary, Left
– *use* Artery, Axillary, Right

**Anterior communicating artery** – *use* Artery, Intracranial

**Anterior cruciate ligament (ACL)**
– *use* Bursa and Ligament, Knee, Left
– *use* Bursa and Ligament, Knee, Right

**Anterior crural nerve** – *use* Nerve, Femoral

**Anterior facial vein**
– *use* Vein, Face, Left
– *use* Vein, Face, Right

**Anterior intercostal artery**
– *use* Artery, Internal Mammary, Right
– *use* Artery, Internal Mammary, Left

**Anterior interosseous nerve** – *use* Nerve, Median

**Anterior lateral malleolar artery**
– *use* Artery, Anterior Tibial, Right
– *use* Artery, Anterior Tibial, Left

**Anterior lingual gland** – *use* Gland, Minor Salivary

**Anterior medial malleolar artery**
– *use* Artery, Anterior Tibial, Right
– *use* Artery, Anterior Tibial, Left

**Anterior spinal artery**
– *use* Artery, Vertebral, Right
– *use* Artery, Vertebral, Left

**Anterior tibial recurrent artery**
– *use* Artery, Anterior Tibial, Right
– *use* Artery, Anterior Tibial, Left

**Anterior ulnar recurrent artery**
– *use* Artery, Ulnar, Right
– *use* Artery, Ulnar, Left

**Anterior vagal trunk** – *use* Nerve, Vagus

**Anterior vertebral muscle**
– *use* Muscle, Neck, Left
– *use* Muscle, Neck, Right

**Antihelix**
– *use* Ear, External, Right
– *use* Ear, External, Left
– *use* Ear, External, Bilateral

**Antimicrobial envelope** – *use* Anti-Infective Envelope

**Antitragus**
– *use* Ear, External, Bilateral
– *use* Ear, External, Right
– *use* Ear, External, Left

**Antrostomy** – *see* Drainage, Ear, Nose, Sinus 099
**Antrotomy** – *see* Drainage, Ear, Nose, Sinus 099

**Antrum of Highmore**
– *use* Sinus, Maxillary, Left
– *use* Sinus, Maxillary, Right

**Aortic annulus** – *use* Valve, Aortic
**Aortic arch** – *use* Aorta, Thoracic
**Aortic intercostal artery** – *use* Aorta, Thoracic

**Aortography**
– *see* Plain Radiography, Upper Arteries B30
– *see* Fluoroscopy, Upper Arteries B31
– *see* Plain Radiography, Lower Arteries B40
– *see* Fluoroscopy, Lower Arteries B41

**Aortoplasty**
– *see* Repair, Aorta, Thoracic 02QW
– *see* Replacement, Aorta, Thoracic 02RW
– *see* Supplement, Aorta, Thoracic 02UW
– *see* Repair, Aorta, Abdominal 04Q0
– *see* Replacement, Aorta, Abdominal 04R0
– *see* Supplement, Aorta, Abdominal 04U0

**Apical** (subclavicular) **lymph node**
– *use* Lymphatic, Axillary, Left
– *use* Lymphatic, Axillary, Right

**Apneustic center** – *use* Pons

**Appendectomy**
– *see* Excision, Appendix 0DBJ
– *see* Resection, Appendix 0DTJ

**Appendicolysis** – *see* Release, Appendix 0DNJ

**Appendicotomy** – *see* Drainage, Appendix 0D9J

**Application** – *see* Introduction of substance in or on

**Aquapheresis** 6A550Z3

**Aqueduct of Sylvius** – *use* Cerebral Ventricle

**Aqueous humour**
– *use* Anterior Chamber, Right
– *use* Anterior Chamber, Left

**Arachnoid mater**
– *use* Spinal Meninges
– *use* Cerebral Meninges

**Arcuate artery**
– *use* Artery, Foot, Left
– *use* Artery, Foot, Right

**Areola**
– *use* Nipple, Left
– *use* Nipple, Right

**AROM (artificial rupture of membranes)** 10907ZC

**Arterial canal** (duct) – *use* Artery, Pulmonary, Left

**Arterial pulse tracing** – *see* Measurement, Arterial 4A03

**Arteriectomy**
– *see* Excision, Heart and Great Vessels 02B
– *see* Excision, Upper Arteries 03B
– *see* Excision, Lower Arteries 04B

**Arteriography**
– *see* Plain Radiography, Heart B20
– *see* Fluoroscopy, Heart B21
– *see* Plain Radiography, Upper Arteries B30
– *see* Fluoroscopy, Upper Arteries B31
– *see* Plain Radiography, Lower Arteries B40
– *see* Fluoroscopy, Lower Arteries B41

**Arterioplasty**
– *see* Repair, Heart and Great Vessels 02Q
– *see* Replacement, Heart and Great Vessels 02R
– *see* Repair, Upper Arteries 03Q
– *see* Replacement, Upper Arteries 03R
– *see* Repair, Lower Arteries 04Q
– *see* Replacement, Lower Arteries 04R
– *see* Supplement, Upper Arteries 03U
– *see* Supplement, Lower Arteries 04U
– *see* Supplement, Heart and Great Vessels 02U

**Arteriorrhaphy**
– *see* Repair, Heart and Great Vessels 02Q
– *see* Repair, Upper Arteries 03Q
– *see* Repair, Lower Arteries 04Q

**Arterioscopy**
02JY4ZZ
03JY4ZZ
04JY4ZZ

**Arthrectomy**
– *see* Excision, Upper Joints 0RB
– *see* Resection, Upper Joints 0RT
– *see* Excision, Lower Joints 0SB
– *see* Resection, Lower Joints 0ST

**Arthrocentesis**
– *see* Drainage, Upper Joints 0R9
– *see* Drainage, Lower Joints 0S9

**Arthrodesis**
– *see* Fusion, Upper Joints 0RG
– *see* Fusion, Lower Joints 0SG

**Arthrography**
– *see* Plain Radiography, Skull and Facial Bones BN0
– *see* Plain Radiography, Non–Axial Upper Bones BP0
– *see* Plain Radiography, Non–Axial Lower Bones BQ0

**Arthrolysis**
– *see* Release, Upper Joints 0RN
– *see* Release, Lower Joints 0SN

**Arthropexy**
– *see* Repair, Upper Joints 0RQ
– *see* Reposition, Upper Joints 0RS
– *see* Repair, Lower Joints 0SQ
– *see* Reposition, Lower Joints 0SS

**Arthroplasty**
– *see* Repair, Upper Joints 0RQ
– *see* Replacement, Upper Joints 0RR
– *see* Repair, Lower Joints 0SQ
– *see* Replacement, Lower Joints 0SR
– *see* Supplement, Lower Joints 0SU
– *see* Supplement, Upper Joints 0RU

**Arthroscopy**
– *see* Inspection, Upper Joints 0RJ
– *see* Inspection, Lower Joints 0SJ

**Arthrotomy**
– *see* Drainage, Upper Joints 0R9
– *see* Drainage, Lower Joints 0S9

**Artificial anal sphincter (AAS)** – *use* Artificial Sphincter in Gastrointestinal System

**Artificial bowel sphincter** (neosphincter) – *use* Artificial Sphincter in Gastrointestinal System

**Artificial Sphincter**
Insertion of device in
Anus 0DHQ
Bladder 0THB
Bladder Neck 0THC
Urethra 0THD
Removal of device from
Anus 0DPQ
Bladder 0TPB
Urethra 0TPD
Revision of device in
Anus 0DWQ
Bladder 0TWB
Urethra 0TWD

**Artificial urinary sphincter (AUS)** – *use* Artificial Sphincter in Urinary System

**Aryepiglottic fold** – *use* Larynx
**Arytenoid cartilage** – *use* Larynx

**Arytenoid muscle**
– *use* Muscle, Neck, Left
– *use* Muscle, Neck, Right

**Arytenoidectomy** – *see* Excision, Larynx 0CBS
**Arytenoidopexy** – *see* Repair, Larynx 0CQS

**Ascenda Intrathecal Catheter** – *use* Infusion Device

**Ascending aorta** – *use* Aorta, Thoracic

**Ascending palatine artery** – *use* Artery, Face

**Ascending pharyngeal artery**
– *use* Artery, External Carotid, Left
– *use* Artery, External Carotid, Right

**Aspiration** – *see* Drainage

**Assessment**
Activities of daily living – *see* Activities of Daily Living Assessment, Rehabilitation F02
Hearing – *see* Hearing Assessment, Diagnostic Audiology F13
Hearing aid – *see* Hearing Aid Assessment, Diagnostic Audiology F14
Motor function – *see* Motor Function Assessment, Rehabilitation F01
Nerve function – *see* Motor Function Assessment, Rehabilitation F01

**Assessment** – *continued*
Speech – *see* Speech Assessment, Rehabilitation F00
Vestibular – *see* Vestibular Assessment, Diagnostic Audiology F15
Vocational – *see* Activities of Daily Living Treatment, Rehabilitation F08

**Assistance**
Cardiac
Continuous
Balloon Pump 5A02210
Impeller Pump 5A0221D
Other Pump 5A02216
Pulsatile Compression 5A02215
Intermittent
Balloon Pump 5A02110
Impeller Pump 5A0211D
Other Pump 5A02116
Pulsatile Compression 5A02115
Circulatory
Continuous
Hyperbaric 5A05221
Supersaturated 5A0522C
Intermittent
Hyperbaric 5A05121
Supersaturated 5A0512C
Respiratory
24–96 Consecutive Hours
Continuous Negative Airway Pressure 5A09459
Continuous Positive Airway Pressure 5A09457
Intermittent Negative Airway Pressure 5A0945B
Intermittent Positive Airway Pressure 5A09458
No Qualifier 5A0945Z
Greater than 96 Consecutive Hours
Continuous Negative Airway Pressure 5A09559
Continuous Positive Airway Pressure 5A09557
Intermittent Negative Airway Pressure 5A0955B
Intermittent Positive Airway Pressure 5A09558
No Qualifier 5A0955Z
Less than 24 Consecutive Hours
Continuous Negative Airway Pressure 5A09359
Continuous Positive Airway Pressure 5A09357
Intermittent Negative Airway Pressure 5A0935B
Intermittent Positive Airway Pressure 5A09358
No Qualifier 5A0935Z

**Assurant** (Cobalt) **stent** – *use* Intraluminal Device
**Atherectomy**
– *see* Extirpation, Heart and Great Vessels 02C
– *see* Extirpation, Upper Arteries 03C
– *see* Extirpation, Lower Arteries 04C
**Atlantoaxial joint** – *use* Joint, Cervical Vertebral
**Atmospheric Control** 6A0Z
**Atrioseptoplasty**
– *see* Repair, Heart and Great Vessels 02Q
– *see* Replacement, Heart and Great Vessels 02R
– *see* Supplement, Heart and Great Vessels 02U
**Atrioventricular node** – *use* Conduction Mechanism
**Atrium dextrum cordis** – *use* Atrium, Right
**Atrium pulmonale** – *use* Atrium, Left
**Attain Ability® lead**
– *use* Cardiac Lead, Pacemaker in 02H
– *use* Cardiac Lead, Defibrillator in 02H
**Attain StarFix® (OTW) lead**
– *use* Cardiac Lead, Defibrillator in 02H
– *use* Cardiac Lead, Pacemaker in 02H
**Audiology, diagnostic**
– *see* Hearing Assessment, Diagnostic Audiology F13
– *see* Hearing Aid Assessment, Diagnostic Audiology F14
– *see* Vestibular Assessment, Diagnostic Audiology F15
**Audiometry** – *see* Hearing Assessment, Diagnostic Audiology F13
**Auditory tube**
– *use* Eustachian Tube, Right
– *use* Eustachian Tube, Left
**Auerbach's** (myenteric) **plexus** – *use* Nerve, Abdominal Sympathetic
**Auricle**
– *use* Ear, External, Left
– *use* Ear, External, Bilateral
– *use* Ear, External, Right
**Auricularis muscle** – *use* Muscle, Head
**Autograft** – *use* Autologous Tissue Substitute
**Autologous artery graft**
– *use* Autologous Arterial Tissue in Lower Arteries
– *use* Autologous Arterial Tissue in Upper Veins
– *use* Autologous Arterial Tissue in Lower Veins
– *use* Autologous Arterial Tissue in Heart and Great Vessels
– *use* Autologous Arterial Tissue in Upper Arteries

**Autologous vein graft**
– *use* Autologous Venous Tissue in Lower Arteries
– *use* Autologous Venous Tissue in Upper Veins
– *use* Autologous Venous Tissue in Lower Veins
– *use* Autologous Venous Tissue in Heart and Great Vessels
– *use* Autologous Venous Tissue in Upper Arteries
**Autotransfusion** – *see* Transfusion
**Autotransplant**
Adrenal tissue – *see* Reposition, Endocrine System 0GS
Kidney – *see* Reposition, Urinary System 0TS
Pancreatic tissue – *see* Reposition, Pancreas 0FSG
Parathyroid tissue – *see* Reposition, Endocrine System 0GS
Thyroid tissue – *see* Reposition, Endocrine System 0GS
Tooth – *see* Reattachment, Mouth and Throat 0CM
**Avulsion** – *see* Extraction
**Axial Lumbar Interbody Fusion System** – *use* Interbody Fusion Device in Lower Joints
**AxiaLIF® System** – *use* Interbody Fusion Device in Lower Joints
**Axillary fascia**
– *use* Subcutaneous Tissue and Fascia, Upper Arm, Left
– *use* Subcutaneous Tissue and Fascia, Upper Arm, Right
**Axillary nerve** – *use* Nerve, Brachial Plexus

# B

**BAK/C® Interbody Cervical Fusion System** – *use* Interbody Fusion Device in Upper Joints
**BAL (bronchial alveolar lavage), diagnostic** – *see* Drainage, Respiratory System 0B9
**Balanoplasty**
– *see* Repair, Penis 0VQS
– *see* Supplement, Penis 0VUS
**Balloon Pump**
Continuous, Output 5A02210
Intermittent, Output 5A02110
**Bandage, Elastic** – *see* Compression
**Banding**
– *see* Restriction
– *see* Occlusion
**Bard® Composix®** (E/X)(LP) **mesh** – *use* Synthetic Substitute
**Bard® Composix® Kugel® patch** – *use* Synthetic Substitute
**Bard® Dulex™ mesh** – *use* Synthetic Substitute
**Bard® Ventralex™ hernia patch** – *use* Synthetic Substitute
**Barium swallow** – *see* Fluoroscopy, Gastrointestinal System BD1
**Baroreflex Activation Therapy® (BAT®)**
– *use* Stimulator Generator in Subcutaneous Tissue and Fascia
– *use* Stimulator Lead in Upper Arteries
**Bartholin's** (greater vestibular) **gland** – *use* Gland, Vestibular
**Basal** (internal) **cerebral vein** – *use* Vein, Intracranial
**Basal metabolic rate (BMR)** – *see* Measurement, Physiological Systems 4A0Z
**Basal nuclei** – *use* Basal Ganglia
**Basilar artery** – *use* Artery, Intracranial
**Basis pontis** – *use* Pons
**Beam Radiation**
Abdomen DW03
Intraoperative DW033Z0
Adrenal Gland DG02
Intraoperative DG023Z0
Bile Ducts DF02
Intraoperative DF023Z0
Bladder DT02
Intraoperative DT023Z0
Bone
Other DP0C
Intraoperative DP0C3Z0
Bone Marrow D700
Intraoperative D7003Z0
Brain D000
Intraoperative D0003Z0
Brain Stem D001
Intraoperative D0013Z0
Breast
Left DM00
Intraoperative DM003Z0
Right DM01
Intraoperative DM013Z0
Bronchus DB01
Intraoperative DB013Z0

**Beam Radiation** – *continued*
Cervix DU01
Intraoperative DU013Z0
Chest DW02
Intraoperative DW023Z0
Chest Wall DB07
Intraoperative DB073Z0
Colon DD05
Intraoperative DD053Z0
Diaphragm DB08
Intraoperative DB083Z0
Duodenum DD02
Intraoperative DD023Z0
Ear D900
Intraoperative D9003Z0
Esophagus DD00
Intraoperative DD003Z0
Eye D800
Intraoperative D8003Z0
Femur DP09
Intraoperative DP093Z0
Fibula DP0B
Intraoperative DP0B3Z0
Gallbladder DF01
Intraoperative DF013Z0
Gland
Adrenal DG02
Intraoperative DG023Z0
Parathyroid DG04
Intraoperative DG043Z0
Pituitary DG00
Intraoperative DG003Z0
Thyroid DG05
Intraoperative DG053Z0
Glands
Salivary D906
Intraoperative D9063Z0
Head and Neck DW01
Intraoperative DW013Z0
Hemibody DW04
Intraoperative DW043Z0
Humerus DP06
Intraoperative DP063Z0
Hypopharynx D903
Intraoperative D9033Z0
Ileum DD04
Intraoperative DD043Z0
Jejunum DD03
Intraoperative DD033Z0
Kidney DT00
Intraoperative DT003Z0
Larynx D90B
Intraoperative D90B3Z0
Liver DF00
Intraoperative DF003Z0
Lung DB02
Intraoperative DB023Z0
Lymphatics
Abdomen D706
Intraoperative D7063Z0
Axillary D704
Intraoperative D7043Z0
Inguinal D708
Intraoperative D7083Z0
Neck D703
Intraoperative D7033Z0
Pelvis D707
Intraoperative D7073Z0
Thorax D705
Intraoperative D7053Z0
Mandible DP03
Intraoperative DP033Z0
Maxilla DP02
Intraoperative DP023Z0
Mediastinum DB06
Intraoperative DB063Z0
Mouth D904
Intraoperative D9043Z0
Nasopharynx D90D
Intraoperative D90D3Z0
Neck and Head DW01
Intraoperative DW013Z0
Nerve
Peripheral D007
Intraoperative D0073Z0
Nose D901
Intraoperative D9013Z0
Oropharynx D90F
Intraoperative D90F3Z0
Ovary DU00
Intraoperative DU003Z0

**Beam Radiation** – *continued*
  Palate
    Hard D908
      Intraoperative D9083Z0
    Soft D909
      Intraoperative D9093Z0
  Pancreas DF03
    Intraoperative DF033Z0
  Parathyroid Gland DG04
    Intraoperative DG043Z0
  Pelvic Bones DP08
    Intraoperative DP083Z0
  Pelvic Region DW06
    Intraoperative DW063Z0
  Pineal Body DG01
    Intraoperative DG013Z0
  Pituitary Gland DG00
    Intraoperative DG003Z0
  Pleura DB05
    Intraoperative DB053Z0
  Prostate DV00
    Intraoperative DV003Z0
  Radius DP07
    Intraoperative DP073Z0
  Rectum DD07
    Intraoperative DD073Z0
  Rib DP05
    Intraoperative DP053Z0
  Sinuses D907
    Intraoperative D9073Z0
  Skin
    Abdomen DH08
      Intraoperative DH083Z0
    Arm DH04
      Intraoperative DH043Z0
    Back DH07
      Intraoperative DH073Z0
    Buttock DH09
      Intraoperative DH093Z0
    Chest DH06
      Intraoperative DH063Z0
    Face DH02
      Intraoperative DH023Z0
    Leg DH0B
      Intraoperative DH0B3Z0
    Neck DH03
      Intraoperative DH033Z0
  Skull DP00
    Intraoperative DP003Z0
  Spinal Cord D006
    Intraoperative D0063Z0
  Spleen D702
    Intraoperative D7023Z0
  Sternum DP04
    Intraoperative DP043Z0
  Stomach DD01
    Intraoperative DD013Z0
  Testis DV01
    Intraoperative DV013Z0
  Thymus D701
    Intraoperative D7013Z0
  Thyroid Gland DG05
    Intraoperative DG053Z0
  Tibia DP0B
    Intraoperative DP0B3Z0
  Tongue D905
    Intraoperative D9053Z0
  Trachea DB00
    Intraoperative DB003Z0
  Ulna DP07
    Intraoperative DP073Z0
  Ureter DT01
    Intraoperative DT013Z0
  Urethra DT03
    Intraoperative DT033Z0
  Uterus DU02
    Intraoperative DU023Z0
  Whole Body DW05
    Intraoperative DW053Z0
**Bedside swallow** F00ZJWZ
**Berlin Heart Ventricular Assist Device** – *use* Implantable Heart Assist System in Heart and Great Vessels
**Biceps brachii muscle**
  – *use* Muscle, Upper Arm, Right
  – *use* Muscle, Upper Arm, Left
**Biceps femoris muscle**
  – *use* Muscle, Upper Leg, Right
  – *use* Muscle, Upper Leg, Left
**Bicipital aponeurosis**
  – *use* Subcutaneous Tissue and Fascia, Lower Arm, Left
  – *use* Subcutaneous Tissue and Fascia, Lower Arm, Right

**Bicuspid valve** – *use* Valve, Mitral
**Bililite therapy** – *see* Ultraviolet Light Therapy, Skin 6A80
**Bioactive embolization coil(s)** – *use* Intraluminal Device, Bioactive in Upper Arteries
**Biofeedback** GZC9ZZZ
**Biopsy**
  – *see* Drainage with qualifier Diagnostic
  – *see* Excision with qualifier Diagnostic
  Bone Marrow – *see* Extraction with qualifier Diagnostic
**BiPAP** – *see* Assistance, Respiratory 5A09
**Bisection** – *see* Division
**Biventricular external heart assist system** – *use* External Heart Assist System in Heart and Great Vessels
**Blepharectomy**
  – *see* Excision, Eye 08B
  – *see* Resection, Eye 08T
**Blepharoplasty**
  – *see* Repair, Eye 08Q
  – *see* Replacement, Eye 08R
  – *see* Supplement, Eye 08U
  – *see* Reposition, Eye 08S
**Blepharorrhaphy** – *see* Repair, Eye 08Q
**Blepharotomy** – *see* Drainage, Eye 089
**Block, Nerve, anesthetic injection** 3E0T3CZ
**Blood glucose monitoring system** – *use* Monitoring Device
**Blood pressure** – *see* Measurement, Arterial 4A03
**BMR (basal metabolic rate)** – *see* Measurement, Physiological Systems 4A0Z
**Body of femur**
  – *use* Femoral Shaft, Right
  – *use* Femoral Shaft, Left
**Body of fibula**
  – *use* Fibula, Right
  – *use* Fibula, Left
**Bone anchored hearing device**
  – *use* Hearing Device, Bone Conduction in 09H
  – *use* Hearing Device in Head and Facial Bones
**Bone bank bone graft** – *use* Nonautologous Tissue Substitute
**Bone Growth Stimulator**
  Insertion of device in
    Bone
      Facial 0NHW
      Lower 0QHY
      Nasal 0NHB
      Upper 0PHY
    Skull 0NH0
  Removal of device from
    Bone
      Facial 0NPW
      Lower 0QPY
      Nasal 0NPB
      Upper 0PPY
    Skull 0NP0
  Revision of device in
    Bone
      Facial 0NWW
      Lower 0QWY
      Nasal 0NWB
      Upper 0PWY
    Skull 0NW0
**Bone marrow transplant** – *see* Transfusion
**Bone morphogenetic protein 2 (BMP 2)** – *use* Recombinant Bone Morphogenetic Protein
**Bone screw** (interlocking)(lag)(pedicle)(recessed)
  – *use* Internal Fixation Device in Head and Facial Bones
  – *use* Internal Fixation Device in Upper Bones
  – *use* Internal Fixation Device in Lower Bones
**Bony labyrinth**
  – *use* Ear, Inner, Left
  – *use* Ear, Inner, Right
**Bony orbit**
  – *use* Orbit, Right
  – *use* Orbit, Left
**Bony vestibule**
  – *use* Ear, Inner, Right
  – *use* Ear, Inner, Left
**Botallo's duct** – *use* Artery, Pulmonary, Left
**Bovine pericardial valve** – *use* Zooplastic Tissue in Heart and Great Vessels
**Bovine pericardium graft** – *use* Zooplastic Tissue in Heart and Great Vessels
**BP (blood pressure)** – *see* Measurement, Arterial 4A03
**Brachial (lateral) lymph node**
  – *use* Lymphatic, Axillary, Left
  – *use* Lymphatic, Axillary, Right

**Brachialis muscle**
  – *use* Muscle, Upper Arm, Right
  – *use* Muscle, Upper Arm, Left
**Brachiocephalic artery** – *use* Artery, Innominate
**Brachiocephalic trunk** – *use* Artery, Innominate
**Brachiocephalic vein**
  – *use* Vein, Innominate, Right
  – *use* Vein, Innominate, Left
**Brachioradialis muscle**
  – *use* Muscle, Lower Arm and Wrist, Right
  – *use* Muscle, Lower Arm and Wrist, Left
**Brachytherapy**
  Abdomen DW13
  Adrenal Gland DG12
  Bile Ducts DF12
  Bladder DT12
  Bone Marrow D710
  Brain D010
  Brain Stem D011
  Breast
    Left DM10
    Right DM11
  Bronchus DB11
  Cervix DU11
  Chest DW12
  Chest Wall DB17
  Colon DD15
  Diaphragm DB18
  Duodenum DD12
  Ear D910
  Esophagus DD10
  Eye D810
  Gallbladder DF11
  Gland
    Adrenal DG12
    Parathyroid DG14
    Pituitary DG10
    Thyroid DG15
  Glands, Salivary D916
  Head and Neck DW11
  Hypopharynx D913
  Ileum DD14
  Jejunum DD13
  Kidney DT10
  Larynx D91B
  Liver DF10
  Lung DB12
  Lymphatics
    Abdomen D716
    Axillary D714
    Inguinal D718
    Neck D713
    Pelvis D717
    Thorax D715
  Mediastinum DB16
  Mouth D914
  Nasopharynx D91D
  Neck and Head DW11
  Nerve, Peripheral D017
  Nose D911
  Oropharynx D91F
  Ovary DU10
  Palate
    Hard D918
    Soft D919
  Pancreas DF13
  Parathyroid Gland DG14
  Pelvic Region DW16
  Pineal Body DG11
  Pituitary Gland DG10
  Pleura DB15
  Prostate DV10
  Rectum DD17
  Sinuses D917
  Spinal Cord D016
  Spleen D712
  Stomach DD11
  Testis DV11
  Thymus D711
  Thyroid Gland DG15
  Tongue D915
  Trachea DB10
  Ureter DT11
  Urethra DT13
  Uterus DU12
**Brachytherapy seeds** – *use* Radioactive Element
**Broad ligament** – *use* Uterine Supporting Structure
**Bronchial artery** – *use* Aorta, Thoracic
**Bronchography**
  – *see* Plain Radiography, Respiratory System BB0
  – *see* Fluoroscopy, Respiratory System BB1

**Bronchoplasty**
– see Repair, Respiratory System ØBQ
– see Supplement, Respiratory System ØBU

**Bronchorrhaphy** – see Repair, Respiratory System ØBQ

**Bronchoscopy** ØBJØ8ZZ

**Bronchotomy** – see Drainage, Respiratory System ØB9

**BRYAN® Cervical Disc System** – use Synthetic Substitute

**Buccal gland** – use Buccal Mucosa

**Buccinator lymph node** – use Lymphatic, Head

**Buccinator muscle** – use Muscle, Facial

**Buckling, scleral with implant** – see Supplement, Eye Ø8U

**Bulbospongiosus muscle** – use Muscle, Perineum

**Bulbourethral (Cowper's) gland** – use Urethra

**Bundle of His** – use Conduction Mechanism

**Bundle of Kent** – use Conduction Mechanism

**Bunionectomy** – see Excision, Lower Bones ØQB

**Bursectomy**
– see Excision, Bursae and Ligaments ØMB
– see Resection, Bursae and Ligaments ØMT

**Bursocentesis** – see Drainage, Bursae and Ligaments ØM9

**Bursography**
– see Plain Radiography, Non–Axial Upper Bones BPØ
– see Plain Radiography, Non–Axial Lower Bones BQØ

**Bursotomy**
– see Division, Bursae and Ligaments ØM8
– see Drainage, Bursae and Ligaments ØM9

**BVS 5000 Ventricular Assist Device** – use External Heart Assist System in Heart and Great Vessels

**Bypass**
Anterior Chamber
Left Ø8133
Right Ø8123
Aorta
Abdominal Ø41Ø
Thoracic Ø21W
Artery
Axillary
Left Ø316Ø
Right Ø315Ø
Brachial
Left Ø318Ø
Right Ø317Ø
Common Carotid
Left Ø31JØ
Right Ø31HØ
Common Iliac
Left Ø41D
Right Ø41C
Coronary
Four or More Sites Ø213
One Site Ø210
Three Sites Ø212
Two Sites Ø211
External Carotid
Left Ø31NØ
Right Ø31MØ
External Iliac
Left Ø41J
Right Ø41H
Femoral
Left Ø41L
Right Ø41K
Innominate Ø312Ø
Internal Carotid
Left Ø31LØ
Right Ø31KØ
Internal Iliac
Left Ø41F
Right Ø41E
Intracranial Ø31GØ
Popliteal
Left Ø41N
Right Ø41M
Radial
Left Ø31CØ
Right Ø31BØ
Splenic Ø414
Subclavian
Left Ø314Ø
Right Ø313Ø
Temporal
Left Ø31TØ
Right Ø31SØ
Ulnar
Left Ø31AØ
Right Ø319Ø
Atrium
Left Ø217
Right Ø216

**Bypass** – continued
Bladder ØT1B
Cavity, Cranial ØW11ØJ
Cecum ØD1H
Cerebral Ventricle ØØ16
Colon
Ascending ØD1K
Descending ØD1M
Sigmoid ØD1N
Transverse ØD1L
Duct
Common Bile ØF19
Cystic ØF18
Hepatic
Left ØF16
Right ØF15
Lacrimal
Left Ø81Y
Right Ø81X
Pancreatic ØF1D
Accessory ØF1F
Duodenum ØD19
Ear
Left Ø91EØ
Right Ø91DØ
Esophagus ØD15
Lower ØD13
Middle ØD12
Upper ØD11
Fallopian Tube
Left ØU16
Right ØU15
Gallbladder ØF14
Ileum ØD1B
Jejunum ØD1A
Kidney Pelvis
Left ØT14
Right ØT13
Pancreas ØF1G
Pelvic Cavity ØW1J
Peritoneal Cavity ØW1G
Pleural Cavity
Left ØW1B
Right ØW19
Spinal Canal ØØ1U
Stomach ØD16
Trachea ØB11
Ureter
Left ØT17
Right ØT16
Ureters, Bilateral ØT18
Vas Deferens
Bilateral ØV1Q
Left ØV1P
Right ØV1N
Vein
Axillary
Left Ø518
Right Ø517
Azygos Ø510
Basilic
Left Ø51C
Right Ø51B
Brachial
Left Ø51A
Right Ø519
Cephalic
Left Ø51F
Right Ø51D
Colic Ø617
Common Iliac
Left Ø61D
Right Ø61C
Esophageal Ø613
External Iliac
Left Ø61G
Right Ø61F
External Jugular
Left Ø51Q
Right Ø51P
Face
Left Ø51V
Right Ø51T
Femoral
Left Ø61N
Right Ø61M
Foot
Left Ø61V
Right Ø61T
Gastric Ø612
Greater Saphenous
Left Ø61Q
Right Ø61P

**Bypass** – continued
Vein – continued
Hand
Left Ø51H
Right Ø51G
Hemiazygos Ø511
Hepatic Ø614
Hypogastric
Left Ø61J
Right Ø61H
Inferior Mesenteric Ø616
Innominate
Left Ø514
Right Ø513
Internal Jugular
Left Ø51N
Right Ø51M
Intracranial Ø51L
Lesser Saphenous
Left Ø61S
Right Ø61R
Portal Ø618
Renal
Left Ø61B
Right Ø619
Splenic Ø611
Subclavian
Left Ø516
Right Ø515
Superior Mesenteric Ø615
Vertebral
Left Ø51S
Right Ø51R
Vena Cava
Inferior Ø61Ø
Superior Ø21V
Ventricle
Left Ø21L
Right Ø21K

**Bypass, cardiopulmonary** 5A1221Z

# C

**Caesarean section** – see Extraction, Products of Conception 10DØ

**Calcaneocuboid joint**
– use Joint, Tarsal, Left
– use Joint, Tarsal, Right

**Calcaneocuboid ligament**
– use Bursa and Ligament, Foot, Right
– use Bursa and Ligament, Foot, Left

**Calcaneofibular ligament**
– use Bursa and Ligament, Ankle, Left
– use Bursa and Ligament, Ankle, Right

**Calcaneus**
– use Tarsal, Right
– use Tarsal, Left

**Cannulation**
– see Bypass
– see Dilation
– see Drainage
– see Irrigation

**Canthorrhaphy** – see Repair, Eye Ø8Q

**Canthotomy** – see Release, Eye Ø8N

**Capitate bone**
– use Carpal, Left
– use Carpal, Right

**Capsulectomy, lens** – see Excision, Eye Ø8B

**Capsulorrhaphy, joint**
– see Repair, Upper Joints ØRQ
– see Repair, Lower Joints ØSQ

**Cardia** – use Esophagogastric Junction

**Cardiac contractility modulation lead** – use Cardiac Lead in Heart and Great Vessels

**Cardiac event recorder** – use Monitoring Device

**Cardiac Lead**
Defibrillator
Atrium
Left Ø2H7
Right Ø2H6
Pericardium Ø2HN
Vein, Coronary Ø2H4
Ventricle
Left Ø2HL
Right Ø2HK
Insertion of device in
Atrium
Left Ø2H7
Right Ø2H6

**Cardiac Lead** – *continued*
  Insertion of device in – *continued*
    Pericardium Ø2HN
    Vein, Coronary Ø2H4
    Ventricle
      Left Ø2HL
      Right Ø2HK
  Pacemaker
    Atrium
      Left Ø2H7
      Right Ø2H6
    Pericardium Ø2HN
    Vein, Coronary Ø2H4
    Ventricle
      Left Ø2HL
      Right Ø2HK
  Removal of device from, Heart Ø2PA
  Revision of device in, Heart Ø2WA
**Cardiac plexus** – *use* Nerve, Thoracic Sympathetic
**Cardiac Resynchronization Defibrillator Pulse Generator**
  Abdomen ØJH8
  Chest ØJH6
**Cardiac Resynchronization Pacemaker Pulse Generator**
  Abdomen ØJH8
  Chest ØJH6
**Cardiac resynchronization therapy (CRT) lead**
  – *use* Cardiac Lead, Pacemaker in Ø2H
  – *use* Cardiac Lead, Defibrillator in Ø2H
**Cardiac Rhythm Related Device**
  Insertion of device in
    Abdomen ØJH8
    Chest ØJH6
  Removal of device from, Subcutaneous Tissue and Fascia, Trunk ØJPT
  Revision of device in, Subcutaneous Tissue and Fascia, Trunk ØJWT
**Cardiocentesis** – *see* Drainage, Pericardial Cavity ØW9D
**Cardioesophageal junction** – *use* Esophagogastric Junction
**Cardiolysis** – *see* Release, Heart and Great Vessels Ø2N
**CardioMEMS® pressure sensor** – *use* Monitoring Device, Pressure Sensor in Ø2H
**Cardiomyotomy** – *see* Division, Esophagogastric Junction ØD84
**Cardioplegia** – *see* Introduction of substance in or on, Heart 3EØ8
**Cardiorrhaphy** – *see* Repair, Heart and Great Vessels Ø2Q
**Cardioversion** 5A2204Z
**Caregiver Training** FØFZ
**Caroticotympanic artery**
  – *use* Artery, Internal Carotid, Right
  – *use* Artery, Internal Carotid, Left
**Carotid (artery) sinus (baroreceptor) lead** – *use* Stimulator Lead in Upper Arteries
**Carotid glomus**
  – *use* Carotid Bodies, Bilateral
  – *use* Carotid Body, Right
  – *use* Carotid Body, Left
**Carotid sinus**
  – *use* Artery, Internal Carotid, Left
  – *use* Artery, Internal Carotid, Right
**Carotid sinus nerve** – *use* Nerve, Glossopharyngeal
**Carotid WALLSTENT® Monorail® Endoprosthesis** – *use* Intraluminal Device
**Carpectomy**
  – *see* Excision, Upper Bones ØPB
  – *see* Resection, Upper Bones ØPT
**Carpometacarpal (CMC) joint**
  – *use* Joint, Metacarpocarpal, Left
  – *use* Joint, Metacarpocarpal, Right
**Carpometacarpal ligament**
  – *use* Bursa and Ligament, Hand, Left
  – *use* Bursa and Ligament, Hand, Right
**Casting** – *see* Immobilization
**CAT scan** – *see* Computerized Tomography (CT Scan)
**Catheterization**
  – *see* Dilation
  – *see* Drainage
  – *see* Irrigation
  – *see* Insertion of device in
  Heart – *see* Measurement, Cardiac 4AØ2
  Umbilical vein, for infusion Ø6HØ33T
**Cauda equina** – *use* Spinal Cord, Lumbar
**Cauterization**
  – *see* Destruction
  – *see* Repair

**Cavernous plexus** – *use* Nerve, Head and Neck Sympathetic
**Cecectomy**
  – *see* Excision, Cecum ØDBH
  – *see* Resection, Cecum ØDTH
**Cecocolostomy**
  – *see* Bypass, Gastrointestinal System ØD1
  – *see* Drainage, Gastrointestinal System ØD9
**Cecopexy**
  – *see* Repair, Cecum ØDQH
  – *see* Reposition, Cecum ØDSH
**Cecoplication** – *see* Restriction, Cecum ØDVH
**Cecorrhaphy** – *see* Repair, Cecum ØDQH
**Cecostomy**
  – *see* Bypass, Cecum ØD1H
  – *see* Drainage, Cecum ØD9H
**Cecotomy** – *see* Drainage, Cecum ØD9H
**Celiac (solar) plexus** – *use* Nerve, Abdominal Sympathetic
**Celiac ganglion** – *use* Nerve, Abdominal Sympathetic
**Celiac lymph node** – *use* Lymphatic, Aortic
**Celiac trunk** – *use* Artery, Celiac
**Central axillary lymph node**
  – *use* Lymphatic, Axillary, Left
  – *use* Lymphatic, Axillary, Right
**Central venous pressure** – *see* Measurement, Venous 4AØ4
**Centrimag® Blood Pump** – *use* External Heart Assist System in Heart and Great Vessels
**Cephalogram** BNØØZZZ
**Cerclage** – *see* Restriction
**Cerebral aqueduct** (Sylvius) – *use* Cerebral Ventricle
**Cerebrum** – *use* Brain
**Cervical esophagus** – *use* Esophagus, Upper
**Cervical facet joint**
  – *use* Joint, Cervical Vertebral
  – *use* Joint, Cervical Vertebral, 2 or more
**Cervical ganglion** – *use* Nerve, Head and Neck Sympathetic
**Cervical interspinous ligament** – *use* Bursa and Ligament, Head and Neck
**Cervical intertransverse ligament** – *use* Bursa and Ligament, Head and Neck
**Cervical ligamentum flavum** – *use* Bursa and Ligament, Head and Neck
**Cervical lymph node**
  – *use* Lymphatic, Neck, Right
  – *use* Lymphatic, Neck, Left
**Cervicectomy**
  – *see* Excision, Cervix ØUBC
  – *see* Resection, Cervix ØUTC
**Cervicothoracic facet joint** – *use* Joint, Cervicothoracic Vertebral
**Cesarean section** – *see* Extraction, Products of Conception 1ØDØ
**Change device in**
  Abdominal Wall ØW2FX
  Back
    Lower ØW2LX
    Upper ØW2KX
  Bladder ØT2BX
  Bone
    Facial ØN2WX
    Lower ØQ2YX
    Nasal ØN2BX
    Upper ØP2YX
  Bone Marrow Ø72TX
  Brain ØØ2ØX
  Breast
    Left ØH2UX
    Right ØH2TX
  Bursa and Ligament
    Lower ØM2YX
    Upper ØM2XX
  Cavity, Cranial ØW21X
  Chest Wall ØW28X
  Cisterna Chyli Ø72LX
  Diaphragm ØB2TX
  Duct
    Hepatobiliary ØF2BX
    Pancreatic ØF2DX
  Ear
    Left Ø92JX
    Right Ø92HX
  Epididymis and Spermatic Cord ØV2MX
  Extremity
    Lower
      Left ØY2BX
      Right ØY29X

**Change device in** – *continued*
  Extremity – *continued*
    Upper
      Left ØX27X
      Right ØX26X
  Eye
    Left Ø821X
    Right Ø82ØX
  Face ØW22X
  Fallopian Tube ØU28X
  Gallbladder ØF24X
  Gland
    Adrenal ØG25X
    Endocrine ØG2SX
    Pituitary ØG2ØX
    Salivary ØC2AX
  Head ØW2ØX
  Intestinal Tract
    Lower ØD2DXUZ
    Upper ØD2ØXUZ
  Jaw
    Lower ØW25X
    Upper ØW24X
  Joint
    Lower ØS2YX
    Upper ØR2YX
  Kidney ØT25X
  Larynx ØC2SX
  Liver ØF2ØX
  Lung
    Left ØB2LX
    Right ØB2KX
  Lymphatic Ø72NX
    Thoracic Duct Ø72KX
  Mediastinum ØW2CX
  Mesentery ØD2VX
  Mouth and Throat ØC2YX
  Muscle
    Lower ØK2YX
    Upper ØK2XX
  Neck ØW26X
  Nerve
    Cranial ØØ2EX
    Peripheral Ø12YX
  Nose Ø92KX
  Omentum ØD2UX
  Ovary ØU23X
  Pancreas ØF2GX
  Parathyroid Gland ØG2RX
  Pelvic Cavity ØW2JX
  Penis ØV2SX
  Pericardial Cavity ØW2DX
  Perineum
    Female ØW2NX
    Male ØW2MX
  Peritoneal Cavity ØW2GX
  Peritoneum ØD2WX
  Pineal Body ØG21X
  Pleura ØB2QX
  Pleural Cavity
    Left ØW2BX
    Right ØW29X
  Products of Conception 1Ø2Ø7
  Prostate and Seminal Vesicles ØV24X
  Retroperitoneum ØW2HX
  Scrotum and Tunica Vaginalis ØV28X
  Sinus Ø92YX
  Skin ØH2PX
  Skull ØN2ØX
  Spinal Canal ØØ2UX
  Spleen Ø72PX
  Subcutaneous Tissue and Fascia
    Head and Neck ØJ2SX
    Lower Extremity ØJ2WX
    Trunk ØJ2TX
    Upper Extremity ØJ2VX
  Tendon
    Lower ØL2YX
    Upper ØL2XX
  Testis ØV2DX
  Thymus Ø72MX
  Thyroid Gland ØG2KX
  Trachea ØB21
  Tracheobronchial Tree ØB2ØX
  Ureter ØT29X
  Urethra ØT2DX
  Uterus and Cervix ØU2DXHZ
  Vagina and Cul-de-sac ØU2HXGZ
  Vas Deferens ØV2RX
  Vulva ØU2MX
**Change device in or on**
  Abdominal Wall 2WØ3X
  Anorectal 2YØ3X5Z

**Change device in or on** – *continued*
  Arm
    Lower
      Left 2W0DX
      Right 2W0CX
    Upper
      Left 2W0BX
      Right 2W0AX
  Back 2W05X
  Chest Wall 2W04X
  Ear 2Y02X5Z
  Extremity
    Lower
      Left 2W0MX
      Right 2W0LX
    Upper
      Left 2W09X
      Right 2W08X
  Face 2W01X
  Finger
    Left 2W0KX
    Right 2W0JX
  Foot
    Left 2W0TX
    Right 2W0SX
  Genital Tract, Female 2Y04X5Z
  Hand
    Left 2W0FX
    Right 2W0EX
  Head 2W00X
  Inguinal Region
    Left 2W07X
    Right 2W06X
  Leg
    Lower
      Left 2W0RX
      Right 2W0QX
    Upper
      Left 2W0PX
      Right 2W0NX
  Mouth and Pharynx 2Y00X5Z
  Nasal 2Y01X5Z
  Neck 2W02X
  Thumb
    Left 2W0HX
    Right 2W0GX
  Toe
    Left 2W0VX
    Right 2W0UX
  Urethra 2Y05X5Z
**Chemoembolization** – *see* Introduction of substance in or on
**Chemosurgery, Skin** 3E00XTZ
**Chemothalamectomy** – *see* Destruction, Thalamus 0059
**Chemotherapy, Infusion for cancer** – *see* Introduction of substance in or on
**Chest x-ray** – *see* Plain Radiography, Chest BW03
**Chiropractic Manipulation**
  Abdomen 9WB9X
  Cervical 9WB1X
  Extremities
    Lower 9WB6X
    Upper 9WB7X
  Head 9WB0X
  Lumbar 9WB3X
  Pelvis 9WB5X
  Rib Cage 9WB8X
  Sacrum 9WB4X
  Thoracic 9WB2X
**Choana** – *use* Nasopharynx
**Cholangiogram**
  – *see* Plain Radiography, Hepatobiliary System and Pancreas BF0
  – *see* Fluoroscopy, Hepatobiliary System and Pancreas BF1
**Cholecystectomy**
  – *see* Excision, Gallbladder 0FB4
  – *see* Resection, Gallbladder 0FT4
**Cholecystojejunostomy**
  – *see* Bypass, Hepatobiliary System and Pancreas 0F1
  – *see* Drainage, Hepatobiliary System and Pancreas 0F9
**Cholecystopexy**
  – *see* Repair, Gallbladder 0FQ4
  – *see* Reposition, Gallbladder 0FS4
**Cholecystoscopy** 0FJ44ZZ
**Cholecystostomy**
  – *see* Drainage, Gallbladder 0F94
  – *see* Bypass, Gallbladder 0F14
**Cholecystotomy** – *see* Drainage, Gallbladder 0F94

**Choledochectomy**
  – *see* Excision, Hepatobiliary System and Pancreas 0FB
  – *see* Resection, Hepatobiliary System and Pancreas 0FT
**Choledocholithotomy** – *see* Extirpation, Duct, Common Bile 0FC9
**Choledochoplasty**
  – *see* Repair, Hepatobiliary System and Pancreas 0FQ
  – *see* Replacement, Hepatobiliary System and Pancreas 0FR
  – *see* Supplement, Hepatobiliary System and Pancreas 0FU
**Choledochoscopy** 0FJB8ZZ
**Choledochotomy** – *see* Drainage, Hepatobiliary System and Pancreas 0F9
**Cholelithotomy** – *see* Extirpation, Hepatobiliary System and Pancreas 0FC
**Chondrectomy**
  – *see* Excision, Upper Joints 0RB
  – *see* Excision, Lower Joints 0SB
  Knee – *see* Excision, Lower Joints 0SB
  Semilunar cartilage – *see* Excision, Lower Joints 0SB
**Chondroglossus muscle** – *use* Muscle, Tongue, Palate, Pharynx
**Chorda tympani** – *use* Nerve, Facial
**Chordotomy** – *see* Division, Central Nervous System 008
**Choroid plexus** – *use* Cerebral Ventricle
**Choroidectomy**
  – *see* Excision, Eye 08B
  – *see* Resection, Eye 08T
**Ciliary body**
  – *use* Eye, Right
  – *use* Eye, Left
**Ciliary ganglion** – *use* Nerve, Head and Neck Sympathetic
**Circle of Willis** – *use* Artery, Intracranial
**Circumflex iliac artery**
  – *use* Artery, Femoral, Right
  – *use* Artery, Femoral, Left
**Clamp and rod internal fixation system (CRIF)**
  – *use* Internal Fixation Device in Upper Bones
  – *use* Internal Fixation Device in Lower Bones
**Clamping** – *see* Occlusion
**Claustrum** – *use* Basal Ganglia
**Claviculectomy**
  – *see* Excision, Upper Bones 0PB
  – *see* Resection, Upper Bones 0PT
**Claviculotomy**
  – *see* Division, Upper Bones 0P8
  – *see* Drainage, Upper Bones 0P9
**Clipping, aneurysm** – *see* Restriction using Extraluminal Device
**Clitorectomy, clitoridectomy**
  – *see* Excision, Clitoris 0UBJ
  – *see* Resection, Clitoris 0UTJ
**Clolar** – *use* Clofarabine
**Closure**
  – *see* Occlusion
  – *see* Repair
**Clysis** – *see* Introduction of substance in or on
**Coagulation** – *see* Destruction
**CoAxia NeuroFlo catheter** – *use* Intraluminal Device
**Cobalt/chromium head and polyethylene socket** – *use* Synthetic Substitute, Metal on Polyethylene in 0SR
**Cobalt/chromium head and socket** – *use* Synthetic Substitute, Metal in 0SR
**Coccygeal body** – *use* Coccygeal Glomus
**Coccygeus muscle**
  – *use* Muscle, Trunk, Left
  – *use* Muscle, Trunk, Right
**Cochlea**
  – *use* Ear, Inner, Left
  – *use* Ear, Inner, Right
**Cochlear implant (CI), multiple channel** (electrode)
  – *use* Hearing Device, Multiple Channel Cochlear Prosthesis in 09H
**Cochlear implant (CI), single channel** (electrode) – *use* Hearing Device, Single Channel Cochlear Prosthesis in 09H
**Cochlear Implant Treatment**
**Cochlear nerve** – *use* Nerve, Acoustic
**COGNIS® CRT-D** – *use* Cardiac Resynchronization Defibrillator Pulse Generator in 0JH
**Colectomy**
  – *see* Excision, Gastrointestinal System 0DB
  – *see* Resection, Gastrointestinal System 0DT
**Collapse** – *see* Occlusion

**Collection from**
  Breast, Breast Milk 8E0HX62
  Indwelling Device
    Circulatory System
      Blood 8C02X6K
      Other Fluid 8C02X6L
    Nervous System
      Cerebrospinal Fluid 8C01X6J
      Other Fluid 8C01X6L
  Integumentary System, Breast Milk 8E0HX62
  Reproductive System, Male, Sperm 8E0VX63
**Colocentesis** – *see* Drainage, Gastrointestinal System 0D9
**Colofixation**
  – *see* Repair, Gastrointestinal System 0DQ
  – *see* Reposition, Gastrointestinal System 0DS
**Cololysis** – *see* Release, Gastrointestinal System 0DN
**Colonic Z-Stent®** – *use* Intraluminal Device
**Colonoscopy** 0DJD8ZZ
**Colopexy**
  – *see* Repair, Gastrointestinal System 0DQ
  – *see* Reposition, Gastrointestinal System 0DS
**Coloplication** – *see* Restriction, Gastrointestinal System 0DV
**Coloproctectomy**
  – *see* Excision, Gastrointestinal System 0DB
  – *see* Resection, Gastrointestinal System 0DT
**Coloproctostomy**
  – *see* Bypass, Gastrointestinal System 0D1
  – *see* Drainage, Gastrointestinal System 0D9
**Colopuncture** – *see* Drainage, Gastrointestinal System 0D9
**Colorrhaphy** – *see* Repair, Gastrointestinal System 0DQ
**Colostomy**
  – *see* Bypass, Gastrointestinal System 0D1
  – *see* Drainage, Gastrointestinal System 0D9
**Colpectomy**
  – *see* Excision, Vagina 0UBG
  – *see* Resection, Vagina 0UTG
**Colpocentesis** – *see* Drainage, Vagina 0U9G
**Colpopexy**
  – *see* Repair, Vagina 0UQG
  – *see* Reposition, Vagina 0USG
**Colpoplasty**
  – *see* Repair, Vagina 0UQG
  – *see* Supplement, Vagina 0UUG
**Colporrhaphy** – *see* Repair, Vagina 0UQG
**Colposcopy** 0UJH8ZZ
**Columella** – *use* Nose
**Common digital vein**
  – *use* Vein, Foot, Right
  – *use* Vein, Foot, Left
**Common facial vein**
  – *use* Vein, Face, Left
  – *use* Vein, Face, Right
**Common fibular nerve** – *use* Nerve, Peroneal
**Common hepatic artery** – *use* Artery, Hepatic
**Common iliac** (subaortic) **lymph node** – *use* Lymphatic, Pelvis
**Common interosseous artery**
  – *use* Artery, Ulnar, Left
  – *use* Artery, Ulnar, Right
**Common peroneal nerve** – *use* Nerve, Peroneal
**Complete** (SE) **stent** – *use* Intraluminal Device
**Compression**
  – *see* Restriction
  Abdominal Wall 2W13X
  Arm
    Lower
      Left 2W1DX
      Right 2W1CX
    Upper
      Left 2W1BX
      Right 2W1AX
  Back 2W15X
  Chest Wall 2W14X
  Extremity
    Lower
      Left 2W1MX
      Right 2W1LX
    Upper
      Left 2W19X
      Right 2W18X
  Face 2W11X
  Finger
    Left 2W1KX
    Right 2W1JX
  Foot
    Left 2W1TX
    Right 2W1SX

**Compression** – *continued*
  Hand
    Left 2W1FX
    Right 2W1EX
  Head 2W10X
  Inguinal Region
    Left 2W17X
    Right 2W16X
  Leg
    Lower
      Left 2W1RX
      Right 2W1QX
    Upper
      Left 2W1PX
      Right 2W1NX
  Neck 2W12X
  Thumb
    Left 2W1HX
    Right 2W1GX
  Toe
    Left 2W1VX
    Right 2W1UX

**Computer Assisted Procedure**
  Extremity
    Lower
      No Qualifier 8E0YXBZ
      With Computerized Tomography 8E0YXBG
      With Fluoroscopy 8E0YXBF
      With Magnetic Resonance Imaging 8E0YXBH
    Upper
      No Qualifier 8E0XXBZ
      With Computerized Tomography 8E0XXBG
      With Fluoroscopy 8E0XXBF
      With Magnetic Resonance Imaging 8E0XXBH
  Head and Neck Region
    No Qualifier 8E09XBZ
    With Computerized Tomography 8E09XBG
    With Fluoroscopy 8E09XBF
    With Magnetic Resonance Imaging 8E09XBH
  Trunk Region
    No Qualifier 8E0WXBZ
    With Computerized Tomography 8E0WXBG
    With Fluoroscopy 8E0WXBF
    With Magnetic Resonance Imaging 8E0WXBH

**Computerized Tomography (CT Scan)**
  Abdomen BW20
    Chest and Pelvis BW25
  Abdomen and Chest BW24
  Abdomen and Pelvis BW21
  Airway, Trachea BB2F
  Ankle
    Left BQ2H
    Right BQ2G
  Aorta
    Abdominal B420
      Intravascular Optical Coherence B420Z2Z
    Thoracic B320
      Intravascular Optical Coherence B320Z2Z
  Arm
    Left BP2F
    Right BP2E
  Artery
    Celiac B421
      Intravascular Optical Coherence B421Z2Z
    Common Carotid
      Bilateral B325
      Intravascular Optical Coherence B325Z2Z
    Coronary
      Bypass Graft
        Multiple B223
          Intravascular Optical Coherence B223Z2Z
        Multiple B221
          Intravascular Optical Coherence B221Z2Z
    Internal Carotid
      Bilateral B328
      Intravascular Optical Coherence B328Z2Z
    Intracranial B32R
      Intravascular Optical Coherence B32RZ2Z
    Lower Extremity
      Bilateral B42H
        Intravascular Optical Coherence B42HZ2Z
      Left B42G
        Intravascular Optical Coherence B42GZ2Z
      Right B42F
        Intravascular Optical Coherence B42FZ2Z
    Pelvic B42C
      Intravascular Optical Coherence B42CZ2Z
    Pulmonary
      Left B32T
        Intravascular Optical Coherence B32TZ2Z
      Right B32S
        Intravascular Optical Coherence B32SZ2Z

**Computerized Tomography (CT Scan)** – *continued*
  Artery – *continued*
    Renal
      Bilateral B428
        Intravascular Optical Coherence B428Z2Z
      Transplant B42M
        Intravascular Optical Coherence B42MZ2Z
    Superior Mesenteric B424
      Intravascular Optical Coherence B424Z2Z
    Vertebral
      Bilateral B32G
        Intravascular Optical Coherence B32GZ2Z
  Bladder BT20
  Bone
    Facial BN25
    Temporal BN2F
  Brain B020
  Calcaneus
    Left BQ2K
    Right BQ2J
  Cerebral Ventricle B028
  Chest, Abdomen and Pelvis BW25
  Chest and Abdomen BW24
  Cisterna B027
  Clavicle
    Left BP25
    Right BP24
  Coccyx BR2F
  Colon BD24
  Ear B920
  Elbow
    Left BP2H
    Right BP2G
  Extremity
    Lower
      Left BQ2S
      Right BQ2R
    Upper
      Bilateral BP2V
      Left BP2U
      Right BP2T
  Eye
    Bilateral B827
    Left B826
    Right B825
  Femur
    Left BQ24
    Right BQ23
  Fibula
    Left BQ2C
    Right BQ2B
  Finger
    Left BP2S
    Right BP2R
  Foot
    Left BQ2M
    Right BQ2L
  Forearm
    Left BP2K
    Right BP2J
  Gland
    Adrenal, Bilateral BG22
    Parathyroid BG23
    Parotid, Bilateral B926
    Salivary, Bilateral B92D
    Submandibular, Bilateral B929
    Thyroid BG24
  Hand
    Left BP2P
    Right BP2N
  Hands and Wrists, Bilateral BP2Q
  Head BW28
  Head and Neck BW29
  Heart
    Right and Left B226
      Intravascular Optical Coherence B226Z2Z
  Hepatobiliary System, All BF2C
  Hip
    Left BQ21
    Right BQ20
  Humerus
    Left BP2B
    Right BP2A
  Intracranial Sinus B522
    Intravascular Optical Coherence B522Z2Z
  Joint
    Acromioclavicular, Bilateral BP23
    Finger
      Left BP2DZZZ
      Right BP2CZZZ
    Foot
      Left BQ2Y
      Right BQ2X

**Computerized Tomography (CT Scan)** – *continued*
  Joint – *continued*
    Hand
      Left BP2DZZZ
      Right BP2CZZZ
    Sacroiliac BR2D
    Sternoclavicular
      Bilateral BP22
      Left BP21
      Right BP20
    Temporomandibular, Bilateral BN29
    Toe
      Left BQ2Y
      Right BQ2X
  Kidney
    Bilateral BT23
    Left BT22
    Right BT21
    Transplant BT29
  Knee
    Left BQ28
    Right BQ27
  Larynx B92J
  Leg
    Left BQ2F
    Right BQ2D
  Liver BF25
  Liver and Spleen BF26
  Lung, Bilateral BB24
  Mandible BN26
  Nasopharynx B92F
  Neck BW2F
  Neck and Head BW29
  Orbit, Bilateral BN23
  Oropharynx B92F
  Pancreas BF27
  Patella
    Left BQ2W
    Right BQ2V
  Pelvic Region BW2G
  Pelvis BR2C
    Chest and Abdomen BW25
  Pelvis and Abdomen BW21
  Pituitary Gland B029
  Prostate BV23
  Ribs
    Left BP2Y
    Right BP2X
  Sacrum BR2F
  Scapula
    Left BP27
    Right BP26
  Sella Turcica B029
  Shoulder
    Left BP29
    Right BP28
  Sinus
    Intracranial B522
      Intravascular Optical Coherence B522Z2Z
    Paranasal B922
  Skull BN20
  Spinal Cord B02B
  Spine
    Cervical BR20
    Lumbar BR29
    Thoracic BR27
  Spleen and Liver BF26
  Thorax BP2W
  Tibia
    Left BQ2C
    Right BQ2B
  Toe
    Left BQ2Q
    Right BQ2P
  Trachea BB2F
  Tracheobronchial Tree
    Bilateral BB29
    Left BB28
    Right BB27
  Vein
    Pelvic (Iliac)
      Left B52G
        Intravascular Optical Coherence B52GZ2Z
      Right B52F
        Intravascular Optical Coherence B52FZ2Z
    Pelvic (Iliac) Bilateral B52H
      Intravascular Optical Coherence B52HZ2Z
    Portal B52T
      Intravascular Optical Coherence B52TZ2Z
    Pulmonary
      Bilateral B52S
        Intravascular Optical Coherence B52SZ2Z

**Computerized Tomography (CT Scan)** – *continued*
  Vein – *continued*
    Pulmonary – *continued*
      Left B52R
        Intravascular Optical Coherence B52RZ2Z
      Right B52Q
        Intravascular Optical Coherence B52QZ2Z
    Renal
      Bilateral B52L
        Intravascular Optical Coherence B52LZ2Z
      Left B52K
        Intravascular Optical Coherence B52KZ2Z
      Right B52J
        Intravascular Optical Coherence B52JZ2Z
    Spanchnic B52T
      Intravascular Optical Coherence B52TZ2Z
    Vena Cava
      Inferior B529
        Intravascular Optical Coherence B529Z2Z
      Superior B528
        Intravascular Optical Coherence B528Z2Z
    Ventricle, Cerebral B028
    Wrist
      Left BP2M
      Right BP2L
**Concerto II CRT-D** – *use* Cardiac Resynchronization Defibrillator Pulse Generator in 0JH
**Condylectomy**
  – *see* Excision, Head and Facial Bones 0NB
  – *see* Excision, Upper Bones 0PB
  – *see* Excision, Lower Bones 0QB
**Condyloid process**
  – *use* Mandible, Left
  – *use* Mandible, Right
**Condylotomy**
  – *see* Division, Head and Facial Bones 0N8
  – *see* Drainage, Head and Facial Bones 0N9
  – *see* Division, Upper Bones 0P8
  – *see* Drainage, Upper Bones 0P9
  – *see* Division, Lower Bones 0Q8
  – *see* Drainage, Lower Bones 0Q9
**Condylysis**
  – *see* Release, Head and Facial Bones 0NN
  – *see* Release, Upper Bones 0PN
  – *see* Release, Lower Bones 0QN
**Conization, cervix** – *see* Excision, Uterus 0UB9
**Conjunctivoplasty**
  – *see* Repair, Eye 08Q
  – *see* Replacement, Eye 08R
**CONSERVE® PLUS Total Resurfacing Hip System** – *use* Resurfacing Device in Lower Joints
**Construction**
  Auricle, ear – *see* Replacement, Ear, Nose, Sinus 09R
  Ileal conduit – *see* Bypass, Urinary System 0T1
**Consulta CRT-D** – *use* Cardiac Resynchronization Defibrillator Pulse Generator in 0JH
**Consulta CRT-P** – *use* Cardiac Resynchronization Pacemaker Pulse Generator in 0JH
**Contact Radiation**
  Abdomen DWY37ZZ
  Adrenal Gland DGY27ZZ
  Bile Ducts DFY27ZZ
  Bladder DTY27ZZ
  Bone, Other DPYC7ZZ
  Brain D0Y07ZZ
  Brain Stem D0Y17ZZ
  Breast
    Left DMY07ZZ
    Right DMY17ZZ
  Bronchus DBY17ZZ
  Cervix DUY17ZZ
  Chest DWY27ZZ
  Chest Wall DBY77ZZ
  Colon DDY57ZZ
  Diaphragm DBY87ZZ
  Duodenum DDY27ZZ
  Ear D9Y07ZZ
  Esophagus DDY07ZZ
  Eye D8Y07ZZ
  Femur DPY97ZZ
  Fibula DPYB7ZZ
  Gallbladder DFY17ZZ
  Gland
    Adrenal DGY27ZZ
    Parathyroid DGY47ZZ
    Pituitary DGY07ZZ
    Thyroid DGY57ZZ
  Glands, Salivary D9Y67ZZ
  Head and Neck DWY17ZZ
  Hemibody DWY47ZZ
  Humerus DPY67ZZ

**Contact Radiation** – *continued*
  Hypopharynx D9Y37ZZ
  Ileum DDY47ZZ
  Jejunum DDY37ZZ
  Kidney DTY07ZZ
  Larynx D9YB7ZZ
  Liver DFY07ZZ
  Lung DBY27ZZ
  Mandible DPY37ZZ
  Maxilla DPY27ZZ
  Mediastinum DBY67ZZ
  Mouth D9Y47ZZ
  Nasopharynx D9YD7ZZ
  Neck and Head DWY17ZZ
  Nerve, Peripheral D0Y77ZZ
  Nose D9Y17ZZ
  Oropharynx D9YF7ZZ
  Ovary DUY07ZZ
  Palate
    Hard D9Y87ZZ
    Soft D9Y97ZZ
  Pancreas DFY37ZZ
  Parathyroid Gland DGY47ZZ
  Pelvic Bones DPY87ZZ
  Pelvic Region DWY67ZZ
  Pineal Body DGY17ZZ
  Pituitary Gland DGY07ZZ
  Pleura DBY57ZZ
  Prostate DVY07ZZ
  Radius DPY77ZZ
  Rectum DDY77ZZ
  Rib DPY57ZZ
  Sinuses D9Y77ZZ
  Skin
    Abdomen DHY87ZZ
    Arm DHY47ZZ
    Back DHY77ZZ
    Buttock DHY97ZZ
    Chest DHY67ZZ
    Face DHY27ZZ
    Leg DHYB7ZZ
    Neck DHY37ZZ
  Skull DPY07ZZ
  Spinal Cord D0Y67ZZ
  Sternum DPY47ZZ
  Stomach DDY17ZZ
  Testis DVY17ZZ
  Thyroid Gland DGY57ZZ
  Tibia DPYB7ZZ
  Tongue D9Y57ZZ
  Trachea DBY07ZZ
  Ulna DPY77ZZ
  Ureter DTY17ZZ
  Urethra DTY37ZZ
  Uterus DUY27ZZ
  Whole Body DWY57ZZ

**CONTAK RENEWAL® 3 RF** (HE) **CRT-D** – *use* Cardiac Resynchronization Defibrillator Pulse Generator in 0JH
**Contegra Pulmonary Valved Conduit** – *use* Zooplastic Tissue in Heart and Great Vessels
**Continuous Glucose Monitoring (CGM) device** – *use* Monitoring Device
**Continuous Negative Airway Pressure**
  24–96 Consecutive Hours, Ventilation 5A09459
  Greater than 96 Consecutive Hours, Ventilation 5A09559
  Less than 24 Consecutive Hours, Ventilation 5A09359
**Continuous Positive Airway Pressure**
  24–96 Consecutive Hours, Ventilation 5A09457
  Greater than 96 Consecutive Hours, Ventilation 5A09557
  Less than 24 Consecutive Hours, Ventilation 5A09357
**Contraceptive Device**
  Change device in, Uterus and Cervix 0U2DXHZ
  Insertion of device in
    Cervix 0UHC
    Subcutaneous Tissue and Fascia
      Abdomen 0JH8
      Chest 0JH6
      Lower Arm
        Left 0JHH
        Right 0JHG
      Lower Leg
        Left 0JHP
        Right 0JHN
      Upper Arm
        Left 0JHF
        Right 0JHD
      Upper Leg
        Left 0JHM
        Right 0JHL

**Contraceptive Device** – *continued*
    Insertion of device in – *continued*
      Uterus 0UH9
  Removal of device from
    Subcutaneous Tissue and Fascia
      Lower Extremity 0JPW
      Trunk 0JPT
      Upper Extremity 0JPV
    Uterus and Cervix 0UPD
  Revision of device in
    Subcutaneous Tissue and Fascia
      Lower Extremity 0JWW
      Trunk 0JWT
      Upper Extremity 0JWV
    Uterus and Cervix 0UWD
**Contractility Modulation Device**
  Abdomen 0JH8
  Chest 0JH6
**Control postprocedural bleeding in**
  Abdominal Wall 0W3F
  Ankle Region
    Left 0Y3L
    Right 0Y3K
  Arm
    Lower
      Left 0X3F
      Right 0X3D
    Upper
      Left 0X39
      Right 0X38
  Axilla
    Left 0X35
    Right 0X34
  Back
    Lower 0W3L
    Upper 0W3K
  Buttock
    Left 0Y31
    Right 0Y30
  Cavity, Cranial 0W31
  Chest Wall 0W38
  Elbow Region
    Left 0X3C
    Right 0X3B
  Extremity
    Lower
      Left 0Y3B
      Right 0Y39
    Upper
      Left 0X37
      Right 0X36
  Face 0W32
  Femoral Region
    Left 0Y38
    Right 0Y37
  Foot
    Left 0Y3N
    Right 0Y3M
  Gastrointestinal Tract 0W3P
  Genitourinary Tract 0W3R
  Hand
    Left 0X3K
    Right 0X3J
  Head 0W30
  Inguinal Region
    Left 0Y36
    Right 0Y35
  Jaw
    Lower 0W35
    Upper 0W34
  Knee Region
    Left 0Y3G
    Right 0Y3F
  Leg
    Lower
      Left 0Y3J
      Right 0Y3H
    Upper
      Left 0Y3D
      Right 0Y3C
  Mediastinum 0W3C
  Neck 0W36
  Oral Cavity and Throat 0W33
  Pelvic Cavity 0W3J
  Pericardial Cavity 0W3D
  Perineum
    Female 0W3N
    Male 0W3M
  Peritoneal Cavity 0W3G
  Pleural Cavity
    Left 0W3B
    Right 0W39
  Respiratory Tract 0W3Q

**Control postprocedural bleeding in** – *continued*
  Retroperitoneum ØW3H
  Shoulder Region
    Left ØX33
    Right ØX32
  Wrist Region
    Left ØX3H
    Right ØX3G
**Conus arteriosus** – *use* Ventricle, Right
**Conus medullaris** – *use* Spinal Cord, Lumbar
**Conversion**
  Cardiac rhythm 5A2204Z
  Gastrostomy to jejunostomy feeding device – *see* Insertion of device in, Jejunum ØDHA
**Coracoacromial ligament**
  – *use* Bursa and Ligament, Shoulder, Right
  – *use* Bursa and Ligament, Shoulder, Left
**Coracobrachialis muscle**
  – *use* Muscle, Upper Arm, Left
  – *use* Muscle, Upper Arm, Right
**Coracoclavicular ligament**
  – *use* Bursa and Ligament, Shoulder, Left
  – *use* Bursa and Ligament, Shoulder, Right
**Coracohumeral ligament**
  – *use* Bursa and Ligament, Shoulder, Left
  – *use* Bursa and Ligament, Shoulder, Right
**Coracoid process**
  – *use* Scapula, Right
  – *use* Scapula, Left
**Cordotomy** – *see* Division, Central Nervous System ØØ8
**Core needle biopsy** – *see* Excision with qualifier Diagnostic
**CoreValve transcatheter aortic valve** – *use* Zooplastic Tissue in Heart and Great Vessels
**Cormet Hip Resurfacing System** – *use* Resurfacing Device in Lower Joints
**Corniculate cartilage** – *use* Larynx
**CoRoent® XL** – *use* Interbody Fusion Device in Lower Joints
**Coronary arteriography**
  – *see* Plain Radiography, Heart B2Ø
  – *see* Fluoroscopy, Heart B21
**Corox (OTW) Bipolar Lead**
  – *use* Cardiac Lead, Pacemaker in Ø2H
  – *use* Cardiac Lead, Defibrillator in Ø2H
**Corpus callosum** – *use* Brain
**Corpus cavernosum** – *use* Penis
**Corpus spongiosum** – *use* Penis
**Corpus striatum** – *use* Basal Ganglia
**Corrugator supercilii muscle** – *use* Muscle, Facial
**Cortical strip neurostimulator lead** – *use* Neurostimulator Lead in Central Nervous System
**Costatectomy**
  – *see* Excision, Upper Bones ØPB
  – *see* Resection, Upper Bones ØPT
**Costectomy**
  – *see* Excision, Upper Bones ØPB
  – *see* Resection, Upper Bones ØPT
**Costocervical trunk**
  – *use* Artery, Subclavian, Left
  – *use* Artery, Subclavian, Right
**Costochondrectomy**
  – *see* Excision, Upper Bones ØPB
  – *see* Resection, Upper Bones ØPT
**Costoclavicular ligament**
  – *use* Bursa and Ligament, Shoulder, Left
  – *use* Bursa and Ligament, Shoulder, Right
**Costosternoplasty**
  – *see* Repair, Upper Bones ØPQ
  – *see* Replacement, Upper Bones ØPR
  – *see* Supplement, Upper Bones ØPU
**Costotomy**
  – *see* Division, Upper Bones ØP8
  – *see* Drainage, Upper Bones ØP9
**Costotransverse joint** – *use* Joint, Thoracic Vertebral
**Costotransverse ligament**
  – *use* Bursa and Ligament, Thorax, Right
  – *use* Bursa and Ligament, Thorax, Left
**Costovertebral joint** – *use* Joint, Thoracic Vertebral
**Costoxiphoid ligament**
  – *use* Bursa and Ligament, Thorax, Right
  – *use* Bursa and Ligament, Thorax, Left
**Counseling**
  Family, for substance abuse, Other Family Counseling HZ63ZZZ
  Group
    12-Step HZ43ZZZ
    Behavioral HZ41ZZZ

**Counseling** – *continued*
  Group – *continued*
    Cognitive HZ4ØZZZ
    Cognitive-Behavioral HZ42ZZZ
    Confrontational HZ48ZZZ
    Continuing Care HZ49ZZZ
    Infectious Disease
      Post-Test HZ4CZZZ
      Pre-Test HZ4CZZZ
    Interpersonal HZ44ZZZ
    Motivational Enhancement HZ47ZZZ
    Psychoeducation HZ46ZZZ
    Spiritual HZ4BZZZ
    Vocational HZ45ZZZ
  Individual
    12-Step HZ33ZZZ
    Behavioral HZ31ZZZ
    Cognitive HZ3ØZZZ
    Cognitive-Behavioral HZ32ZZZ
    Confrontational HZ38ZZZ
    Continuing Care HZ39ZZZ
    Infectious Disease
      Post-Test HZ3CZZZ
      Pre-Test HZ3CZZZ
    Interpersonal HZ34ZZZ
    Motivational Enhancement HZ37ZZZ
    Psychoeducation HZ36ZZZ
    Spiritual HZ3BZZZ
    Vocational HZ35ZZZ
  Mental Health Services
    Educational GZ6ØZZZ
    Other Counseling GZ63ZZZ
    Vocational GZ61ZZZ
**Countershock, cardiac** 5A2204Z
**Cowper's (bulbourethral) gland** – *use* Urethra
**CPAP (continuous positive airway pressure)** – *see* Assistance, Respiratory 5AØ9
**Cranial dura mater** – *use* Dura Mater
**Cranial epidural space** – *use* Epidural Space
**Cranial subarachnoid space** – *use* Subarachnoid Space
**Cranial subdural space** – *use* Subdural Space
**Craniectomy**
  – *see* Excision, Head and Facial Bones ØNB
  – *see* Resection, Head and Facial Bones ØNT
**Cranioplasty**
  – *see* Repair, Head and Facial Bones ØNQ
  – *see* Replacement, Head and Facial Bones ØNR
  – *see* Supplement, Head and Facial Bones ØNU
**Craniotomy**
  – *see* Drainage, Central Nervous System ØØ9
  – *see* Division, Head and Facial Bones ØN8
  – *see* Drainage, Head and Facial Bones ØN9
**Creation**
  Female ØW4NØ
  Male ØW4MØ
**Cremaster muscle** – *use* Muscle, Perineum
**Cribriform plate**
  – *use* Bone, Ethmoid, Left
  – *use* Bone, Ethmoid, Right
**Cricoid cartilage** – *use* Larynx
**Cricoidectomy** – *see* Excision, Larynx ØCBS
**Cricothyroid artery**
  – *use* Artery, Thyroid, Left
  – *use* Artery, Thyroid, Right
**Cricothyroid muscle**
  – *use* Muscle, Neck, Right
  – *use* Muscle, Neck, Left
**Crisis Intervention** GZ2ZZZZ
**Crural fascia**
  – *use* Subcutaneous Tissue and Fascia, Upper Leg, Right
  – *use* Subcutaneous Tissue and Fascia, Upper Leg, Left
**Crushing, nerve**
  Cranial – *see* Destruction, Central Nervous System ØØ5
  Peripheral – *see* Destruction, Peripheral Nervous System Ø15
**Cryoablation** – *see* Destruction
**Cryotherapy** – *see* Destruction
**Cryptorchidectomy**
  – *see* Excision, Male Reproductive System ØVB
  – *see* Resection, Male Reproductive System ØVT
**Cryptorchiectomy**
  – *see* Excision, Male Reproductive System ØVB
  – *see* Resection, Male Reproductive System ØVT
**Cryptotomy**
  – *see* Division, Gastrointestinal System ØD8
  – *see* Drainage, Gastrointestinal System ØD9
**CT scan** – *see* Computerized Tomography (CT Scan)

**CT sialogram** – *see* Computerized Tomography (CT Scan), Ear, Nose, Mouth and Throat B92
**Cubital lymph node**
  – *use* Lymphatic, Upper Extremity, Left
  – *use* Lymphatic, Upper Extremity, Right
**Cubital nerve** – *use* Nerve, Ulnar
**Cuboid bone**
  – *use* Tarsal, Left
  – *use* Tarsal, Right
**Cuboideonavicular joint**
  – *use* Joint, Tarsal, Right
  – *use* Joint, Tarsal, Left
**Culdocentesis** – *see* Drainage, Cul-de-sac ØU9F
**Culdoplasty**
  – *see* Repair, Cul-de-sac ØUQF
  – *see* Supplement, Cul-de-sac ØUUF
**Culdoscopy** ØUJH8ZZ
**Culdotomy** – *see* Drainage, Cul-de-sac ØU9F
**Culmen** – *use* Cerebellum
**Cultured epidermal cell autograft** – *use* Autologous Tissue Substitute
**Cuneiform cartilage** – *use* Larynx
**Cuneonavicular joint**
  – *use* Joint, Tarsal, Left
  – *use* Joint, Tarsal, Right
**Cuneonavicular ligament**
  – *use* Bursa and Ligament, Foot, Left
  – *use* Bursa and Ligament, Foot, Right
**Curettage**
  – *see* Excision
  – *see* Extraction
**Cutaneous (transverse) cervical nerve** – *use* Nerve, Cervical Plexus
**CVP (central venous pressure)** – *see* Measurement, Venous 4AØ4
**Cyclodiathermy** – *see* Destruction, Eye Ø85
**Cyclophotocoagulation** – *see* Destruction, Eye Ø85
**CYPHER® Stent** – *use* Intraluminal Device, Drug-eluting in Heart and Great Vessels
**Cystectomy**
  – *see* Excision, Bladder ØTBB
  – *see* Resection, Bladder ØTTB
**Cystocele repair** – *see* Repair, Subcutaneous Tissue and Fascia, Pelvic Region ØJQC
**Cystography**
  – *see* Plain Radiography, Urinary System BTØ
  – *see* Fluoroscopy, Urinary System BT1
**Cystolithotomy** – *see* Extirpation, Bladder ØTCB
**Cystopexy**
  – *see* Repair, Bladder ØTQB
  – *see* Reposition, Bladder ØTSB
**Cystoplasty**
  – *see* Repair, Bladder ØTQB
  – *see* Replacement, Bladder ØTRB
  – *see* Supplement, Bladder ØTUB
**Cystorrhaphy** – *see* Repair, Bladder ØTQB
**Cystoscopy** ØTJB8ZZ
**Cystostomy** – *see* Bypass, Bladder ØT1B
**Cystostomy tube** – *use* Drainage Device
**Cystotomy** – *see* Drainage, Bladder ØT9B
**Cystourethrography**
  – *see* Plain Radiography, Urinary System BTØ
  – *see* Fluoroscopy, Urinary System BT1
**Cystourethroplasty**
  – *see* Repair, Urinary System ØTQ
  – *see* Replacement, Urinary System ØTR
  – *see* Supplement, Urinary System ØTU

# D

**DBS lead** – *use* Neurostimulator Lead in Central Nervous System
**DeBakey Left Ventricular Assist Device** – *use* Implantable Heart Assist System in Heart and Great Vessels
**Debridement**
  Excisional – *see* Excision
  Non-excisional – *see* Extraction
**Decompression, Circulatory** 6A15
**Decortication, lung** – *see* Extraction, Respiratory System ØBD
**Deep brain neurostimulator lead** – *use* Neurostimulator Lead in Central Nervous System
**Deep cervical fascia** – *use* Subcutaneous Tissue and Fascia, Neck, Anterior

**Deep cervical vein**
– *use* Vein, Vertebral, Left
– *use* Vein, Vertebral, Right
**Deep circumflex iliac artery**
– *use* Artery, External Iliac, Left
– *use* Artery, External Iliac, Right
**Deep facial vein**
– *use* Vein, Face, Left
– *use* Vein, Face, Right
**Deep femoral (profunda femoris) vein**
– *use* Vein, Femoral, Left
– *use* Vein, Femoral, Right
**Deep femoral artery**
– *use* Artery, Femoral, Right
– *use* Artery, Femoral, Left
**Deep Inferior Epigastric Artery Perforator Flap**
Bilateral ØHRVØ77
Left ØHRUØ77
Right ØHRTØ77
**Deep palmar arch**
– *use* Artery, Hand, Left
– *use* Artery, Hand, Right
**Deep transverse perineal muscle** – *use* Muscle, Perineum
**Deferential artery**
– *use* Artery, Internal Iliac, Right
– *use* Artery, Internal Iliac, Left
**Defibrillator Generator**
Abdomen ØJH8
Chest ØJH6
**Delivery**
Cesarean – *see* Extraction, Products of Conception 10DØ
Forceps – *see* Extraction, Products of Conception 10DØ
Manually assisted 10EØXZZ
Products of Conception 10EØXZZ
Vacuum assisted – *see* Extraction, Products of Conception 10DØ
**Delta frame external fixator**
– *use* External Fixation Device, Hybrid in ØPH
– *use* External Fixation Device, Hybrid in ØPS
– *use* External Fixation Device, Hybrid in ØQH
– *use* External Fixation Device, Hybrid in ØQS
**Delta III Reverse shoulder prosthesis** – *use* Synthetic Substitute, Reverse Ball and Socket in ØRR
**Deltoid fascia**
– *use* Subcutaneous Tissue and Fascia, Upper Arm, Right
– *use* Subcutaneous Tissue and Fascia, Upper Arm, Left
**Deltoid ligament**
– *use* Bursa and Ligament, Ankle, Left
– *use* Bursa and Ligament, Ankle, Right
**Deltoid muscle**
– *use* Muscle, Shoulder, Left
– *use* Muscle, Shoulder, Right
**Deltopectoral (infraclavicular) lymph node**
– *use* Lymphatic, Upper Extremity, Right
– *use* Lymphatic, Upper Extremity, Left
**Denervation**
Cranial nerve – *see* Destruction, Central Nervous System 005
Peripheral nerve – *see* Destruction, Peripheral Nervous System 015
**Densitometry**
Plain Radiography
Femur
Left BQ04ZZ1
Right BQ03ZZ1
Hip
Left BQ01ZZ1
Right BQ00ZZ1
Spine
Cervical BR00ZZ1
Lumbar BR09ZZ1
Thoracic BR07ZZ1
Whole BR0GZZ1
Ultrasonography
Elbow
Left BP4HZZ1
Right BP4GZZ1
Hand
Left BP4PZZ1
Right BP4NZZ1
Shoulder
Left BP49ZZ1
Right BP48ZZ1
Wrist
Left BP4MZZ1
Right BP4LZZ1

**Dentate ligament** – *use* Dura Mater
**Denticulate ligament** – *use* Spinal Meninges
**Depressor anguli oris muscle** – *use* Muscle, Facial
**Depressor labii inferioris muscle** – *use* Muscle, Facial
**Depressor septi nasi muscle** – *use* Muscle, Facial
**Depressor supercilii muscle** – *use* Muscle, Facial
**Dermabrasion** – *see* Extraction, Skin and Breast ØHD
**Dermis** – *use* Skin
**Descending genicular artery**
– *use* Artery, Femoral, Right
– *use* Artery, Femoral, Left
**Destruction**
Acetabulum
Left ØQ55
Right ØQ54
Adenoids ØC5Q
Ampulla of Vater ØF5C
Anal Sphincter ØD5R
Anterior Chamber
Left Ø8533ZZ
Right Ø8523ZZ
Anus ØD5Q
Aorta
Abdominal Ø45Ø
Thoracic Ø25W
Aortic Body ØG5D
Appendix ØD5J
Artery
Anterior Tibial
Left Ø45Q
Right Ø45P
Axillary
Left Ø356
Right Ø355
Brachial
Left Ø358
Right Ø357
Celiac Ø451
Colic
Left Ø457
Middle Ø458
Right Ø456
Common Carotid
Left Ø35J
Right Ø35H
Common Iliac
Left Ø45D
Right Ø45C
External Carotid
Left Ø35N
Right Ø35M
External Iliac
Left Ø45J
Right Ø45H
Face Ø35R
Femoral
Left Ø45L
Right Ø45K
Foot
Left Ø45W
Right Ø45V
Gastric Ø452
Hand
Left Ø35F
Right Ø35D
Hepatic Ø453
Inferior Mesenteric Ø45B
Innominate Ø352
Internal Carotid
Left Ø35L
Right Ø35K
Internal Iliac
Left Ø45F
Right Ø45E
Internal Mammary
Left Ø351
Right Ø35Ø
Intracranial Ø35G
Lower Ø45Y
Peroneal
Left Ø45U
Right Ø45T
Popliteal
Left Ø45N
Right Ø45M
Posterior Tibial
Left Ø45S
Right Ø45R
Pulmonary
Left Ø25R
Right Ø25Q
Pulmonary Trunk Ø25P

**Destruction** – *continued*
Artery – *continued*
Radial
Left Ø35C
Right Ø35B
Renal
Left Ø45A
Right Ø459
Splenic Ø454
Subclavian
Left Ø354
Right Ø353
Superior Mesenteric Ø455
Temporal
Left Ø35T
Right Ø35S
Thyroid
Left Ø35V
Right Ø35U
Ulnar
Left Ø35A
Right Ø359
Upper Ø35Y
Vertebral
Left Ø35Q
Right Ø35P
Atrium
Left Ø257
Right Ø256
Auditory Ossicle
Left Ø95AØZZ
Right Ø959ØZZ
Basal Ganglia ØØ58
Bladder ØT5B
Bladder Neck ØT5C
Bone
Ethmoid
Left ØN5G
Right ØN5F
Frontal
Left ØN52
Right ØN51
Hyoid ØN5X
Lacrimal
Left ØN5J
Right ØN5H
Nasal ØN5B
Occipital
Left ØN58
Right ØN57
Palatine
Left ØN5L
Right ØN5K
Parietal
Left ØN54
Right ØN53
Pelvic
Left ØQ53
Right ØQ52
Sphenoid
Left ØN5D
Right ØN5C
Temporal
Left ØN56
Right ØN55
Zygomatic
Left ØN5N
Right ØN5M
Brain ØØ5Ø
Breast
Bilateral ØH5V
Left ØH5U
Right ØH5T
Bronchus
Lingula ØB59
Lower Lobe
Left ØB5B
Right ØB56
Main
Left ØB57
Right ØB53
Middle Lobe, Right ØB55
Upper Lobe
Left ØB58
Right ØB54
Buccal Mucosa ØC54
Bursa and Ligament
Abdomen
Left ØM5J
Right ØM5H
Ankle
Left ØM5R
Right ØM5Q

**Destruction** – *continued*
Bursa and Ligament – *continued*
  Elbow
    Left ØM54
    Right ØM53
  Foot
    Left ØM5T
    Right ØM5S
  Hand
    Left ØM58
    Right ØM57
  Head and Neck ØM50
  Hip
    Left ØM5M
    Right ØM5L
  Knee
    Left ØM5P
    Right ØM5N
  Lower Extremity
    Left ØM5W
    Right ØM5V
  Perineum ØM5K
  Shoulder
    Left ØM52
    Right ØM51
  Thorax
    Left ØM5G
    Right ØM5F
  Trunk
    Left ØM5D
    Right ØM5C
  Upper Extremity
    Left ØM5B
    Right ØM59
  Wrist
    Left ØM56
    Right ØM55
Carina ØB52
Carotid Bodies, Bilateral ØG58
Carotid Body
  Left ØG56
  Right ØG57
Carpal
  Left ØP5N
  Right ØP5M
Cecum ØD5H
Cerebellum ØØ5C
Cerebral Hemisphere ØØ57
Cerebral Meninges ØØ51
Cerebral Ventricle ØØ56
Cervix ØU5C
Chordae Tendineae Ø259
Choroid
  Left Ø85B
  Right Ø85A
Cisterna Chyli Ø75L
Clavicle
  Left ØP5B
  Right ØP59
Clitoris ØU5J
Coccygeal Glomus ØG5B
Coccyx ØQ5S
Colon
  Ascending ØD5K
  Descending ØD5M
  Sigmoid ØD5N
  Transverse ØD5L
Conduction Mechanism Ø258
Conjunctiva
  Left Ø85TXZZ
  Right Ø85SXZZ
Cord
  Bilateral ØV5H
  Left ØV5G
  Right ØV5F
Cornea
  Left Ø859XZZ
  Right Ø858XZZ
Cul-de-sac ØU5F
Diaphragm
  Left ØB5S
  Right ØB5R
Disc
  Cervical Vertebral ØR53
  Cervicothoracic Vertebral ØR55
  Lumbar Vertebral ØS52
  Lumbosacral ØS54
  Thoracic Vertebral ØR59
  Thoracolumbar Vertebral ØR5B
Duct
  Common Bile ØF59
  Cystic ØF58

**Destruction** – *continued*
Duct – *continued*
  Hepatic
    Left ØF56
    Right ØF55
  Lacrimal
    Left Ø85Y
    Right Ø85X
  Pancreatic ØF5D
    Accessory ØF5F
  Parotid
    Left ØC5C
    Right ØC5B
Duodenum ØD59
Dura Mater ØØ52
Ear
  External
    Left Ø951
    Right Ø950
  External Auditory Canal
    Left Ø954
    Right Ø953
  Inner
    Left Ø95EØZZ
    Right Ø95DØZZ
  Middle
    Left Ø956ØZZ
    Right Ø955ØZZ
Endometrium ØU5B
Epididymis
  Bilateral ØV5L
  Left ØV5K
  Right ØV5J
Epiglottis ØC5R
Esophagogastric Junction ØD54
Esophagus ØD55
  Lower ØD53
  Middle ØD52
  Upper ØD51
Eustachian Tube
  Left Ø95G
  Right Ø95F
Eye
  Left Ø851XZZ
  Right Ø850XZZ
Eyelid
  Lower
    Left Ø85R
    Right Ø85Q
  Upper
    Left Ø85P
    Right Ø85N
Fallopian Tube
  Left ØU56
  Right ØU55
Fallopian Tubes, Bilateral ØU57
Femoral Shaft
  Left ØQ59
  Right ØQ58
Femur
  Lower
    Left ØQ5C
    Right ØQ5B
  Upper
    Left ØQ57
    Right ØQ56
Fibula
  Left ØQ5K
  Right ØQ5J
Finger Nail ØH5QXZZ
Gallbladder ØF54
Gingiva
  Lower ØC56
  Upper ØC55
Gland
  Adrenal
    Bilateral ØG54
    Left ØG52
    Right ØG53
  Lacrimal
    Left Ø85W
    Right Ø85V
  Minor Salivary ØC5J
  Parotid
    Left ØC59
    Right ØC58
  Pituitary ØG5Ø
  Sublingual
    Left ØC5F
    Right ØC5D
  Submaxillary
    Left ØC5H
    Right ØC5G

**Destruction** – *continued*
Gland – *continued*
  Vestibular ØU5L
Glenoid Cavity
  Left ØP58
  Right ØP57
Glomus Jugulare ØG5C
Humeral Head
  Left ØP5D
  Right ØP5C
Humeral Shaft
  Left ØP5G
  Right ØP5F
Hymen ØU5K
Hypothalamus ØØ5A
Ileocecal Valve ØD5C
Ileum ØD5B
Intestine
  Large ØD5E
    Left ØD5G
    Right ØD5F
  Small ØD58
Iris
  Left Ø85D3ZZ
  Right Ø85C3ZZ
Jejunum ØD5A
Joint
  Acromioclavicular
    Left ØR5H
    Right ØR5G
  Ankle
    Left ØS5G
    Right ØS5F
  Carpal
    Left ØR5R
    Right ØR5Q
  Cervical Vertebral ØR51
  Cervicothoracic Vertebral ØR54
  Coccygeal ØS56
  Elbow
    Left ØR5M
    Right ØR5L
  Finger Phalangeal
    Left ØR5X
    Right ØR5W
  Hip
    Left ØS5B
    Right ØS59
  Knee
    Left ØS5D
    Right ØS5C
  Lumbar Vertebral ØS5Ø
  Lumbosacral ØS53
  Metacarpocarpal
    Left ØR5T
    Right ØR5S
  Metacarpophalangeal
    Left ØR5V
    Right ØR5U
  Metatarsal–Phalangeal
    Left ØS5N
    Right ØS5M
  Metatarsal–Tarsal
    Left ØS5L
    Right ØS5K
  Occipital–cervical ØR5Ø
  Sacrococcygeal ØS55
  Sacroiliac
    Left ØS58
    Right ØS57
  Shoulder
    Left ØR5K
    Right ØR5J
  Sternoclavicular
    Left ØR5F
    Right ØR5E
  Tarsal
    Left ØS5J
    Right ØS5H
  Temporomandibular
    Left ØR5D
    Right ØR5C
  Thoracic Vertebral ØR56
  Thoracolumbar Vertebral ØR5A
  Toe Phalangeal
    Left ØS5Q
    Right ØS5P
  Wrist
    Left ØR5P
    Right ØR5N
Kidney
  Left ØT51
  Right ØT5Ø

**Destruction** – continued
  Kidney Pelvis
    Left ØT54
    Right ØT53
  Larynx ØC5S
  Lens
    Left Ø85K3ZZ
    Right Ø85J3ZZ
  Lip
    Lower ØC51
    Upper ØC5Ø
  Liver ØF5Ø
    Left Lobe ØF52
    Right Lobe ØF51
  Lung
    Bilateral ØB5M
    Left ØB5L
    Lower Lobe
      Left ØB5J
      Right ØB5F
    Middle Lobe, Right ØB5D
    Right ØB5K
    Upper Lobe
      Left ØB5G
      Right ØB5C
  Lung Lingula ØB5H
  Lymphatic
    Aortic Ø75D
    Axillary
      Left Ø756
      Right Ø755
    Head Ø75Ø
    Inguinal
      Left Ø75J
      Right Ø75H
    Internal Mammary
      Left Ø759
      Right Ø758
    Lower Extremity
      Left Ø75G
      Right Ø75F
    Mesenteric Ø75B
    Neck
      Left Ø752
      Right Ø751
    Pelvis Ø75C
    Thoracic Duct Ø75K
    Thorax Ø757
    Upper Extremity
      Left Ø754
      Right Ø753
  Mandible
    Left ØN5V
    Right ØN5T
  Maxilla
    Left ØN5S
    Right ØN5R
  Medulla Oblongata ØØ5D
  Mesentery ØD5V
  Metacarpal
    Left ØP5Q
    Right ØP5P
  Metatarsal
    Left ØQ5P
    Right ØQ5N
  Muscle
    Abdomen
      Left ØK5L
      Right ØK5K
    Extraocular
      Left Ø85M
      Right Ø85L
    Facial ØK51
    Foot
      Left ØK5W
      Right ØK5V
    Hand
      Left ØK5D
      Right ØK5C
    Head ØK5Ø
    Hip
      Left ØK5P
      Right ØK5N
    Lower Arm and Wrist
      Left ØK5B
      Right ØK59
    Lower Leg
      Left ØK5T
      Right ØK5S
    Neck
      Left ØK53
      Right ØK52
    Papillary Ø25D

**Destruction** – continued
  Muscle – continued
    Perineum ØK5M
    Shoulder
      Left ØK56
      Right ØK55
    Thorax
      Left ØK5J
      Right ØK5H
    Tongue, Palate, Pharynx ØK54
    Trunk
      Left ØK5G
      Right ØK5F
    Upper Arm
      Left ØK58
      Right ØK57
    Upper Leg
      Left ØK5R
      Right ØK5Q
  Nasopharynx Ø95N
  Nerve
    Abdominal Sympathetic Ø15M
    Abducens ØØ5L
    Accessory ØØ5R
    Acoustic ØØ5N
    Brachial Plexus Ø153
    Cervical Ø151
    Cervical Plexus Ø15Ø
    Facial ØØ5M
    Femoral Ø15D
    Glossopharyngeal ØØ5P
    Head and Neck Sympathetic Ø15K
    Hypoglossal ØØ5S
    Lumbar Ø15B
    Lumbar Plexus Ø159
    Lumbar Sympathetic Ø15N
    Lumbosacral Plexus Ø15A
    Median Ø155
    Oculomotor ØØ5H
    Olfactory ØØ5F
    Optic ØØ5G
    Peroneal Ø15H
    Phrenic Ø152
    Pudendal Ø15C
    Radial Ø156
    Sacral Ø15R
    Sacral Plexus Ø15Q
    Sacral Sympathetic Ø15P
    Sciatic Ø15F
    Thoracic Ø158
    Thoracic Sympathetic Ø15L
    Tibial Ø15G
    Trigeminal ØØ5K
    Trochlear ØØ5J
    Ulnar Ø154
    Vagus ØØ5Q
  Nipple
    Left ØH5X
    Right ØH5W
  Nose Ø95K
  Omentum
    Greater ØD5S
    Lesser ØD5T
  Orbit
    Left ØN5Q
    Right ØN5P
  Ovary
    Bilateral ØU52
    Left ØU51
    Right ØU5Ø
  Palate
    Hard ØC52
    Soft ØC53
  Pancreas ØF5G
  Para–aortic Body ØG59
  Paraganglion Extremity ØG5F
  Parathyroid Gland ØG5R
    Inferior
      Left ØG5P
      Right ØG5N
    Multiple ØG5Q
    Superior
      Left ØG5M
      Right ØG5L
  Patella
    Left ØQ5F
    Right ØQ5D
  Penis ØV5S
  Pericardium Ø25N
  Peritoneum ØD5W
  Phalanx
    Finger
      Left ØP5V

**Destruction** – continued
  Phalanx– continued
    Finger– continued
      Right ØP5T
    Thumb
      Left ØP5S
      Right ØP5R
    Toe
      Left ØQ5R
      Right ØQ5Q
  Pharynx ØC5M
  Pineal Body ØG51
  Pleura
    Left ØB5P
    Right ØB5N
  Pons ØØ5B
  Prepuce ØV5T
  Prostate ØV5Ø
  Radius
    Left ØP5J
    Right ØP5H
  Rectum ØD5P
  Retina
    Left Ø85F3ZZ
    Right Ø85E3ZZ
  Retinal Vessel
    Left Ø85H3ZZ
    Right Ø85G3ZZ
  Rib
    Left ØP52
    Right ØP51
  Sacrum ØQ51
  Scapula
    Left ØP56
    Right ØP55
  Sclera
    Left Ø857XZZ
    Right Ø856XZZ
  Scrotum ØV55
  Septum
    Atrial Ø255
    Nasal Ø95M
    Ventricular Ø25M
  Sinus
    Accessory Ø95P
    Ethmoid
      Left Ø95V
      Right Ø95U
    Frontal
      Left Ø95T
      Right Ø95S
    Mastoid
      Left Ø95C
      Right Ø95B
    Maxillary
      Left Ø95R
      Right Ø95Q
    Sphenoid
      Left Ø95X
      Right Ø95W
  Skin
    Abdomen ØH57XZ
    Back ØH56XZ
    Buttock ØH58XZ
    Chest ØH55XZ
    Ear
      Left ØH53XZ
      Right ØH52XZ
    Face ØH51XZ
    Foot
      Left ØH5NXZ
      Right ØH5MXZ
    Genitalia ØH5AXZ
    Hand
      Left ØH5GXZ
      Right ØH5FXZ
    Lower Arm
      Left ØH5EXZ
      Right ØH5DXZ
    Lower Leg
      Left ØH5LXZ
      Right ØH5KXZ
    Neck ØH54XZ
    Perineum ØH59XZ
    Scalp ØH5ØXZ
    Upper Arm
      Left ØH5CXZ
      Right ØH5BXZ
    Upper Leg
      Left ØH5JXZ
      Right ØH5HXZ
  Skull ØN5Ø

**Destruction** – *continued*
Spinal Cord
  Cervical 005W
  Lumbar 005Y
  Thoracic 005X
Spinal Meninges 005T
Spleen 075P
Sternum 0P50
Stomach 0D56
  Pylorus 0D57
Subcutaneous Tissue and Fascia
  Abdomen 0J58
  Back 0J57
  Buttock 0J59
  Chest 0J56
  Face 0J51
  Foot
    Left 0J5R
    Right 0J5Q
  Hand
    Left 0J5K
    Right 0J5J
  Lower Arm
    Left 0J5H
    Right 0J5G
  Lower Leg
    Left 0J5P
    Right 0J5N
  Neck
    Anterior 0J54
    Posterior 0J55
  Pelvic Region 0J5C
  Perineum 0J5B
  Scalp 0J50
  Upper Arm
    Left 0J5F
    Right 0J5D
  Upper Leg
    Left 0J5M
    Right 0J5L
Tarsal
  Left 0Q5M
  Right 0Q5L
Tendon
  Abdomen
    Left 0L5G
    Right 0L5F
  Ankle
    Left 0L5T
    Right 0L5S
  Foot
    Left 0L5W
    Right 0L5V
  Hand
    Left 0L58
    Right 0L57
  Head and Neck 0L50
  Hip
    Left 0L5K
    Right 0L5J
  Knee
    Left 0L5R
    Right 0L5Q
  Lower Arm and Wrist
    Left 0L56
    Right 0L55
  Lower Leg
    Left 0L5P
    Right 0L5N
  Perineum 0L5H
  Shoulder
    Left 0L52
    Right 0L51
  Thorax
    Left 0L5D
    Right 0L5C
  Trunk
    Left 0L5B
    Right 0L59
  Upper Arm
    Left 0L54
    Right 0L53
  Upper Leg
    Left 0L5M
    Right 0L5L
Testis
  Bilateral 0V5C
  Left 0V5B
  Right 0V59
Thalamus 0059
Thymus 075M
Thyroid Gland 0G5K
  Left Lobe 0G5G

**Destruction** – *continued*
Thyroid Gland – *continued*
  Right Lobe 0G5H
Tibia
  Left 0Q5H
  Right 0Q5G
Toe Nail 0H5RXZZ
Tongue 0C57
Tonsils 0C5P
Tooth
  Lower 0C5X
  Upper 0C5W
Trachea 0B51
Tunica Vaginalis
  Left 0V57
  Right 0V56
Turbinate, Nasal 095L
Tympanic Membrane
  Left 0958
  Right 0957
Ulna
  Left 0P5L
  Right 0P5K
Ureter
  Left 0T57
  Right 0T56
Urethra 0T5D
Uterine Supporting Structure 0U54
Uterus 0U59
Uvula 0C5N
Vagina 0U5G
Valve
  Aortic 025F
  Mitral 025G
  Pulmonary 025H
  Tricuspid 025J
Vas Deferens
  Bilateral 0V5Q
  Left 0V5P
  Right 0V5N
Vein
  Axillary
    Left 0558
    Right 0557
  Azygos 0550
  Basilic
    Left 055C
    Right 055B
  Brachial
    Left 055A
    Right 0559
  Cephalic
    Left 055F
    Right 055D
  Colic 0657
  Common Iliac
    Left 065D
    Right 065C
  Coronary 0254
  Esophageal 0653
  External Iliac
    Left 065G
    Right 065F
  External Jugular
    Left 055Q
    Right 055P
  Face
    Left 055V
    Right 055T
  Femoral
    Left 065N
    Right 065M
  Foot
    Left 065V
    Right 065T
  Gastric 0652
  Greater Saphenous
    Left 065Q
    Right 065P
  Hand
    Left 055H
    Right 055G
  Hemiazygos 0551
  Hepatic 0654
  Hypogastric
    Left 065J
    Right 065H
  Inferior Mesenteric 0656
  Innominate
    Left 0554
    Right 0553
  Internal Jugular
    Left 055N

**Destruction** – *continued*
Vein – *continued*
  Internal Jugular – *continued*
    Right 055M
  Intracranial 055L
  Lesser Saphenous
    Left 065S
    Right 065R
  Lower 065Y
  Portal 0658
  Pulmonary
    Left 025T
    Right 025S
  Renal
    Left 065B
    Right 0659
  Splenic 0651
  Subclavian
    Left 0556
    Right 0555
  Superior Mesenteric 0655
  Upper 055Y
  Vertebral
    Left 055S
    Right 055R
Vena Cava
  Inferior 0650
  Superior 025V
Ventricle
  Left 025L
  Right 025K
Vertebra
  Cervical 0P53
  Lumbar 0Q50
  Thoracic 0P54
Vesicle
  Bilateral 0V53
  Left 0V52
  Right 0V51
Vitreous
  Left 08553ZZ
  Right 08543ZZ
Vocal Cord
  Left 0C5V
  Right 0C5T
Vulva 0U5M
**Detachment**
Arm
  Lower
    Left 0X6F0Z
    Right 0X6D0Z
  Upper
    Left 0X690Z
    Right 0X680Z
Elbow Region
  Left 0X6C0ZZ
  Right 0X6B0ZZ
Femoral Region
  Left 0Y680ZZ
  Right 0Y670ZZ
Finger
  Index
    Left 0X6P0Z
    Right 0X6N0Z
  Little
    Left 0X6W0Z
    Right 0X6V0Z
  Middle
    Left 0X6R0Z
    Right 0X6Q0Z
  Ring
    Left 0X6T0Z
    Right 0X6S0Z
Foot
  Left 0Y6N0Z
  Right 0Y6M0Z
Forequarter
  Left 0X610ZZ
  Right 0X600ZZ
Hand
  Left 0X6K0Z
  Right 0X6J0Z
Hindquarter
  Bilateral 0Y640ZZ
  Left 0Y630ZZ
  Right 0Y620ZZ
Knee Region
  Left 0Y6G0ZZ
  Right 0Y6F0ZZ
Leg
  Lower
    Left 0Y6J0Z
    Right 0Y6H0Z

**Detachment** – *continued*
Leg – *continued*
Upper
Left ØY6DØZ
Right ØY6CØZ
Shoulder Region
Left ØX63ØZZ
Right ØX62ØZZ
Thumb
Left ØX6MØZ
Right ØX6LØZ
Toe
1st
Left ØY6QØZ
Right ØY6PØZ
2nd
Left ØY6SØZ
Right ØY6RØZ
3rd
Left ØY6UØZ
Right ØY6TØZ
4th
Left ØY6WØZ
Right ØY6VØZ
5th
Left ØY6YØZ
Right ØY6XØZ
**Determination, Mental status** GZ14ZZZ
**Detorsion**
 – *see* Release
 – *see* Reposition
**Detoxification Services, for substance abuse** HZ2ZZZZ
**Device Fitting** FØDZ
**Diagnostic Audiology** – *see* Audiology, Diagnostic
**Diagnostic imaging** – *see* Imaging, Diagnostic
**Diagnostic radiology** – *see* Imaging, Diagnostic
**Dialysis**
Hemodialysis 5A1DØØZ
Peritoneal 3E1M39Z
**Diaphragma sellae** – *use* Dura Mater
**Diaphragmatic pacemaker generator** – *use* Stimulator
Generator in Subcutaneous Tissue and Fascia
**Diaphragmatic Pacemaker Lead**
Insertion of device in
Left ØBHS
Right ØBHR
Removal of device from, Diaphragm ØBPT
Revision of device in, Diaphragm ØBWT
**Digital radiography, plain** – *see* Plain Radiography
**Dilation**
Ampulla of Vater ØF7C
Anus ØD7Q
Aorta
Abdominal Ø47Ø
Thoracic Ø27W
Artery
Anterior Tibial
Left Ø47Q
Right Ø47P
Axillary
Left Ø376
Right Ø375
Brachial
Left Ø378
Right Ø377
Celiac Ø471
Colic
Left Ø477
Middle Ø478
Right Ø476
Common Carotid
Left Ø37J
Right Ø37H
Common Iliac
Left Ø47D
Right Ø47C
Coronary
Four or More Sites Ø273
One Site Ø27Ø
Three Sites Ø272
Two Sites Ø271
External Carotid
Left Ø37N
Right Ø37M
External Iliac
Left Ø47J
Right Ø47H
Face Ø37R
Femoral
Left Ø47L
Right Ø47K

**Dilation** – *continued*
Artery – *continued*
Foot
Left Ø47W
Right Ø47V
Gastric Ø472
Hand
Left Ø37F
Right Ø37D
Hepatic Ø473
Inferior Mesenteric Ø47B
Innominate Ø372
Internal Carotid
Left Ø37L
Right Ø37K
Internal Iliac
Left Ø47F
Right Ø47E
Internal Mammary
Left Ø371
Right Ø37Ø
Intracranial Ø37G
Lower Ø47Y
Peroneal
Left Ø47U
Right Ø47T
Popliteal
Left Ø47N
Right Ø47M
Posterior Tibial
Left Ø47S
Right Ø47R
Pulmonary
Left Ø27R
Right Ø27Q
Pulmonary Trunk Ø27P
Radial
Left Ø37C
Right Ø37B
Renal
Left Ø47A
Right Ø479
Splenic Ø474
Subclavian
Left Ø374
Right Ø373
Superior Mesenteric Ø475
Temporal
Left Ø37T
Right Ø37S
Thyroid
Left Ø37V
Right Ø37U
Ulnar
Left Ø37A
Right Ø379
Upper Ø37Y
Vertebral
Left Ø37Q
Right Ø37P
Bladder ØT7B
Bladder Neck ØT7C
Bronchus
Lingula ØB79
Lower Lobe
Left ØB7B
Right ØB76
Main
Left ØB77
Right ØB73
Middle Lobe, Right ØB75
Upper Lobe
Left ØB78
Right ØB74
Carina ØB72
Cecum ØD7H
Cervix ØU7C
Colon
Ascending ØD7K
Descending ØD7M
Sigmoid ØD7N
Transverse ØD7L
Duct
Common Bile ØF79
Cystic ØF78
Hepatic
Left ØF76
Right ØF75
Lacrimal
Left Ø87Y
Right Ø87X
Pancreatic ØF7D
Accessory ØF7F

**Dilation** – *continued*
Duct – *continued*
Parotid
Left ØC7C
Right ØC7B
Duodenum ØD79
Esophagogastric Junction ØD74
Esophagus ØD75
Lower ØD73
Middle ØD72
Upper ØD71
Eustachian Tube
Left Ø97G
Right Ø97F
Fallopian Tube
Left ØU76
Right ØU75
Fallopian Tubes, Bilateral ØU77
Hymen ØU7K
Ileocecal Valve ØD7C
Ileum ØD7B
Intestine
Large ØD7E
Left ØD7G
Right ØD7F
Small ØD78
Jejunum ØD7A
Kidney Pelvis
Left ØT74
Right ØT73
Larynx ØC7S
Pharynx ØC7M
Rectum ØD7P
Stomach ØD76
Pylorus ØD77
Trachea ØB71
Ureter
Left ØT77
Right ØT76
Ureters, Bilateral ØT78
Urethra ØT7D
Uterus ØU79
Vagina ØU7G
Valve
Aortic Ø27F
Mitral Ø27G
Pulmonary Ø27H
Tricuspid Ø27J
Vas Deferens
Bilateral ØV7Q
Left ØV7P
Right ØV7N
Vein
Axillary
Left Ø578
Right Ø577
Azygos Ø57Ø
Basilic
Left Ø57C
Right Ø57B
Brachial
Left Ø57A
Right Ø579
Cephalic
Left Ø57F
Right Ø57D
Colic Ø677
Common Iliac
Left Ø67D
Right Ø67C
Esophageal Ø673
External Iliac
Left Ø67G
Right Ø67F
External Jugular
Left Ø57Q
Right Ø57P
Face
Left Ø57V
Right Ø57T
Femoral
Left Ø67N
Right Ø67M
Foot
Left Ø67V
Right Ø67T
Gastric Ø672
Greater Saphenous
Left Ø67Q
Right Ø67P
Hand
Left Ø57H
Right Ø57G

**Dilation** – *continued*
Vein – *continued*
Hemiazygos 0571
Hepatic 0674
Hypogastric
Left 067J
Right 067H
Inferior Mesenteric 0676
Innominate
Left 0574
Right 0573
Internal Jugular
Left 057N
Right 057M
Intracranial 057L
Lesser Saphenous
Left 067S
Right 067R
Lower 067Y
Portal 0678
Pulmonary
Left 027T
Right 027S
Renal
Left 067B
Right 0679
Splenic 0671
Subclavian
Left 0576
Right 0575
Superior Mesenteric 0675
Upper 057Y
Vertebral
Left 057S
Right 057R
Vena Cava
Inferior 0670
Superior 027V
Ventricle, Right 027K
**Direct Lateral Interbody Fusion (DLIF) device** – *use*
Interbody Fusion Device in Lower Joints
**Disarticulation** – *see* Detachment
**Discectomy, diskectomy**
– *see* Excision, Lower Joints 0SB
– *see* Excision, Upper Joints 0RB
– *see* Resection, Lower Joints 0ST
– *see* Resection, Upper Joints 0RT
**Discography**
– *see* Fluoroscopy, Axial Skeleton, Except Skull and Facial Bones BR1
– *see* Plain Radiography, Axial Skeleton, Except Skull and Facial Bones BR0
**Distal humerus**
– *use* Humeral Shaft, Right
– *use* Humeral Shaft, Left
**Distal humerus, involving joint**
– *use* Joint, Elbow, Right
– *use* Joint, Elbow, Left
**Distal radioulnar joint**
– *use* Joint, Wrist, Right
– *use* Joint, Wrist, Left
**Diversion** – *see* Bypass
**Diverticulectomy** – *see* Excision, Gastrointestinal System 0DB
**Division**
Acetabulum
Left 0Q85
Right 0Q84
Anal Sphincter 0D8R
Basal Ganglia 0088
Bladder Neck 0T8C
Bone
Ethmoid
Left 0N8G
Right 0N8F
Frontal
Left 0N82
Right 0N81
Hyoid 0N8X
Lacrimal
Left 0N8J
Right 0N8H
Nasal 0N8B
Occipital
Left 0N88
Right 0N87
Palatine
Left 0N8L
Right 0N8K
Parietal
Left 0N84
Right 0N83

**Division** – *continued*
Bone – *continued*
Pelvic
Left 0Q83
Right 0Q82
Sphenoid
Left 0N8D
Right 0N8C
Temporal
Left 0N86
Right 0N85
Zygomatic
Left 0N8N
Right 0N8M
Brain 0080
Bursa and Ligament
Abdomen
Left 0M8J
Right 0M8H
Ankle
Left 0M8R
Right 0M8Q
Elbow
Left 0M84
Right 0M83
Foot
Left 0M8T
Right 0M8S
Hand
Left 0M88
Right 0M87
Head and Neck 0M80
Hip
Left 0M8M
Right 0M8L
Knee
Left 0M8P
Right 0M8N
Lower Extremity
Left 0M8W
Right 0M8V
Perineum 0M8K
Shoulder
Left 0M82
Right 0M81
Thorax
Left 0M8G
Right 0M8F
Trunk
Left 0M8D
Right 0M8C
Upper Extremity
Left 0M8B
Right 0M89
Wrist
Left 0M86
Right 0M85
Carpal
Left 0P8N
Right 0P8M
Cerebral Hemisphere 0087
Chordae Tendineae 0289
Clavicle
Left 0P8B
Right 0P89
Coccyx 0Q8S
Conduction Mechanism 0288
Esophagogastric Junction 0D84
Femoral Shaft
Left 0Q89
Right 0Q88
Femur
Lower
Left 0Q8C
Right 0Q8B
Upper
Left 0Q87
Right 0Q86
Fibula
Left 0Q8K
Right 0Q8J
Gland, Pituitary 0G80
Glenoid Cavity
Left 0P88
Right 0P87
Humeral Head
Left 0P8D
Right 0P8C
Humeral Shaft
Left 0P8G
Right 0P8F
Hymen 0U8K
Kidneys, Bilateral 0T82

**Division** – *continued*
Mandible
Left 0N8V
Right 0N8T
Maxilla
Left 0N8S
Right 0N8R
Metacarpal
Left 0P8Q
Right 0P8P
Metatarsal
Left 0Q8P
Right 0Q8N
Muscle
Abdomen
Left 0K8L
Right 0K8K
Facial 0K81
Foot
Left 0K8W
Right 0K8V
Hand
Left 0K8D
Right 0K8C
Head 0K80
Hip
Left 0K8P
Right 0K8N
Lower Arm and Wrist
Left 0K8B
Right 0K89
Lower Leg
Left 0K8T
Right 0K8S
Neck
Left 0K83
Right 0K82
Papillary 028D
Perineum 0K8M
Shoulder
Left 0K86
Right 0K85
Thorax
Left 0K8J
Right 0K8H
Tongue, Palate, Pharynx 0K84
Trunk
Left 0K8G
Right 0K8F
Upper Arm
Left 0K88
Right 0K87
Upper Leg
Left 0K8R
Right 0K8Q
Nerve
Abdominal Sympathetic 018M
Abducens 008L
Accessory 008R
Acoustic 008N
Brachial Plexus 0183
Cervical 0181
Cervical Plexus 0180
Facial 008M
Femoral 018D
Glossopharyngeal 008P
Head and Neck Sympathetic 018K
Hypoglossal 008S
Lumbar 018B
Lumbar Plexus 0189
Lumbar Sympathetic 018N
Lumbosacral Plexus 018A
Median 0185
Oculomotor 008H
Olfactory 008F
Optic 008G
Peroneal 018H
Phrenic 0182
Pudendal 018C
Radial 0186
Sacral 018R
Sacral Plexus 018Q
Sacral Sympathetic 018P
Sciatic 018F
Thoracic 0188
Thoracic Sympathetic 018L
Tibial 018G
Trigeminal 008K
Trochlear 008J
Ulnar 0184
Vagus 008Q
Orbit
Left 0N8Q

## Division – continued

Orbit – continued
Right ØN8P
Ovary
Bilateral ØU82
Left ØU81
Right ØU80
Pancreas ØF8G
Patella
Left ØQ8F
Right ØQ8D
Perineum, Female ØW8NXZZ
Phalanx
Finger
Left ØP8V
Right ØP8T
Thumb
Left ØP8S
Right ØP8R
Toe
Left ØQ8R
Right ØQ8Q
Radius
Left ØP8J
Right ØP8H
Rib
Left ØP82
Right ØP81
Sacrum ØQ81
Scapula
Left ØP86
Right ØP85
Skin
Abdomen ØH87XZZ
Back ØH86XZZ
Buttock ØH88XZZ
Chest ØH85XZZ
Ear
Left ØH83XZZ
Right ØH82XZZ
Face ØH81XZZ
Foot
Left ØH8NXZZ
Right ØH8MXZZ
Genitalia ØH8AXZZ
Hand
Left ØH8GXZZ
Right ØH8FXZZ
Lower Arm
Left ØH8EXZZ
Right ØH8DXZZ
Lower Leg
Left ØH8LXZZ
Right ØH8KXZZ
Neck ØH84XZZ
Perineum ØH89XZZ
Scalp ØH80XZZ
Upper Arm
Left ØH8CXZZ
Right ØH8BXZZ
Upper Leg
Left ØH8JXZZ
Right ØH8HXZZ
Skull ØN8Ø
Spinal Cord
Cervical ØØ8W
Lumbar ØØ8Y
Thoracic ØØ8X
Sternum ØP8Ø
Stomach, Pylorus ØD87
Subcutaneous Tissue and Fascia
Abdomen ØJ88
Back ØJ87
Buttock ØJ89
Chest ØJ86
Face ØJ81
Foot
Left ØJ8R
Right ØJ8Q
Hand
Left ØJ8K
Right ØJ8J
Head and Neck ØJ8S
Lower Arm
Left ØJ8H
Right ØJ8G
Lower Extremity ØJ8W
Lower Leg
Left ØJ8P
Right ØJ8N
Neck
Anterior ØJ84
Posterior ØJ85

## Division – continued

Subcutaneous Tissue and Fascia – continued
Pelvic Region ØJ8C
Perineum ØJ8B
Scalp ØJ8Ø
Trunk ØJ8T
Upper Arm
Left ØJ8F
Right ØJ8D
Upper Extremity ØJ8V
Upper Leg
Left ØJ8M
Right ØJ8L
Tarsal
Left ØQ8M
Right ØQ8L
Tendon
Abdomen
Left ØL8G
Right ØL8F
Ankle
Left ØL8T
Right ØL8S
Foot
Left ØL8W
Right ØL8V
Hand
Left ØL88
Right ØL87
Head and Neck ØL8Ø
Hip
Left ØL8K
Right ØL8J
Knee
Left ØL8R
Right ØL8Q
Lower Arm and Wrist
Left ØL86
Right ØL85
Lower Leg
Left ØL8P
Right ØL8N
Perineum ØL8H
Shoulder
Left ØL82
Right ØL81
Thorax
Left ØL8D
Right ØL8C
Trunk
Left ØL8B
Right ØL89
Upper Arm
Left ØL84
Right ØL83
Upper Leg
Left ØL8M
Right ØL8L
Thyroid Gland Isthmus ØG8J
Tibia
Left ØQ8H
Right ØQ8G
Turbinate, Nasal Ø98L
Ulna
Left ØP8L
Right ØP8K
Uterine Supporting Structure ØU84
Vertebra
Cervical ØP83
Lumbar ØQ8Ø
Thoracic ØP84

**Doppler study** – *see* Ultrasonography
**Dorsal digital nerve** – *use* Nerve, Radial
**Dorsal metacarpal vein**
– *use* Vein, Hand, Left
– *use* Vein, Hand, Right
**Dorsal metatarsal artery**
– *use* Artery, Foot, Left
– *use* Artery, Foot, Right
**Dorsal metatarsal vein**
– *use* Vein, Foot, Right
– *use* Vein, Foot, Left
**Dorsal scapular artery**
– *use* Artery, Subclavian, Right
– *use* Artery, Subclavian, Left
**Dorsal scapular nerve** – *use* Nerve, Brachial Plexus
**Dorsal venous arch**
– *use* Vein, Foot, Right
– *use* Vein, Foot, Left
**Dorsalis pedis artery**
– *use* Artery, Anterior Tibial, Right
– *use* Artery, Anterior Tibial, Left

## Drainage

Abdominal Wall ØW9F
Acetabulum
Left ØQ95
Right ØQ94
Adenoids ØC9Q
Ampulla of Vater ØF9C
Anal Sphincter ØD9R
Ankle Region
Left ØY9L
Right ØY9K
Anterior Chamber
Left Ø893
Right Ø892
Anus ØD9Q
Aorta, Abdominal Ø49Ø
Aortic Body ØG9D
Appendix ØD9J
Arm
Lower
Left ØX9F
Right ØX9D
Upper
Left ØX99
Right ØX98
Artery
Anterior Tibial
Left Ø49Q
Right Ø49P
Axillary
Left Ø396
Right Ø395
Brachial
Left Ø398
Right Ø397
Celiac Ø491
Colic
Left Ø497
Middle Ø498
Right Ø496
Common Carotid
Left Ø39J
Right Ø39H
Common Iliac
Left Ø49D
Right Ø49C
External Carotid
Left Ø39N
Right Ø39M
External Iliac
Left Ø49J
Right Ø49H
Face Ø39R
Femoral
Left Ø49L
Right Ø49K
Foot
Left Ø49W
Right Ø49V
Gastric Ø492
Hand
Left Ø39F
Right Ø39D
Hepatic Ø493
Inferior Mesenteric Ø49B
Innominate Ø392
Internal Carotid
Left Ø39L
Right Ø39K
Internal Iliac
Left Ø49F
Right Ø49E
Internal Mammary
Left Ø391
Right Ø39Ø
Intracranial Ø39G
Lower Ø49Y
Peroneal
Left Ø49U
Right Ø49T
Popliteal
Left Ø49N
Right Ø49M
Posterior Tibial
Left Ø49S
Right Ø49R
Radial
Left Ø39C
Right Ø39B
Renal
Left Ø49A
Right Ø499
Splenic Ø494

**Drainage** – *continued*
  Artery – *continued*
    Subclavian
      Left Ø394
      Right Ø393
    Superior Mesenteric Ø495
    Temporal
      Left Ø39T
      Right Ø39S
    Thyroid
      Left Ø39V
      Right Ø39U
    Ulnar
      Left Ø39A
      Right Ø399
    Upper Ø39Y
    Vertebral
      Left Ø39Q
      Right Ø39P
  Auditory Ossicle
    Left Ø99A
    Right Ø999
  Axilla
    Left ØX95
    Right ØX94
  Back
    Lower ØW9L
    Upper ØW9K
  Basal Ganglia ØØ98
  Bladder ØT9B
  Bladder Neck ØT9C
  Bone
    Ethmoid
      Left ØN9G
      Right ØN9F
    Frontal
      Left ØN92
      Right ØN91
    Hyoid ØN9X
    Lacrimal
      Left ØN9J
      Right ØN9H
    Nasal ØN9B
    Occipital
      Left ØN98
      Right ØN97
    Palatine
      Left ØN9L
      Right ØN9K
    Parietal
      Left ØN94
      Right ØN93
    Pelvic
      Left ØQ93
      Right ØQ92
    Sphenoid
      Left ØN9D
      Right ØN9C
    Temporal
      Left ØN96
      Right ØN95
    Zygomatic
      Left ØN9N
      Right ØN9M
  Bone Marrow Ø79T
  Brain ØØ9Ø
  Breast
    Bilateral ØH9V
    Left ØH9U
    Right ØH9T
  Bronchus
    Lingula ØB99
    Lower Lobe
      Left ØB9B
      Right ØB96
    Main
      Left ØB97
      Right ØB93
    Middle Lobe, Right ØB95
    Upper Lobe
      Left ØB98
      Right ØB94
  Buccal Mucosa ØC94
  Bursa and Ligament
    Abdomen
      Left ØM9J
      Right ØM9H
    Ankle
      Left ØM9R
      Right ØM9Q
    Elbow
      Left ØM94
      Right ØM93

**Drainage** – *continued*
  Bursa and Ligament – *continued*
    Foot
      Left ØM9T
      Right ØM9S
    Hand
      Left ØM98
      Right ØM97
    Head and Neck ØM9Ø
    Hip
      Left ØM9M
      Right ØM9L
    Knee
      Left ØM9P
      Right ØM9N
    Lower Extremity
      Left ØM9W
      Right ØM9V
    Perineum ØM9K
    Shoulder
      Left ØM92
      Right ØM91
    Thorax
      Left ØM9G
      Right ØM9F
    Trunk
      Left ØM9D
      Right ØM9C
    Upper Extremity
      Left ØM9B
      Right ØM99
    Wrist
      Left ØM96
      Right ØM95
  Buttock
    Left ØY91
    Right ØY9Ø
  Carina ØB92
  Carotid Bodies, Bilateral ØG98
  Carotid Body
    Left ØG96
    Right ØG97
  Carpal
    Left ØP9N
    Right ØP9M
  Cavity, Cranial ØW91
  Cecum ØD9H
  Cerebellum ØØ9C
  Cerebral Hemisphere ØØ97
  Cerebral Meninges ØØ91
  Cerebral Ventricle ØØ96
  Cervix ØU9C
  Chest Wall ØW98
  Choroid
    Left Ø89B
    Right Ø89A
  Cisterna Chyli Ø79L
  Clavicle
    Left ØP9B
    Right ØP99
  Clitoris ØU9J
  Coccygeal Glomus ØG9B
  Coccyx ØQ9S
  Colon
    Ascending ØD9K
    Descending ØD9M
    Sigmoid ØD9N
    Transverse ØD9L
  Conjunctiva
    Left Ø89T
    Right Ø89S
  Cord
    Bilateral ØV9H
    Left ØV9G
    Right ØV9F
  Cornea
    Left Ø899
    Right Ø898
  Cul-de-sac ØU9F
  Diaphragm
    Left ØB9S
    Right ØB9R
  Disc
    Cervical Vertebral ØR93
    Cervicothoracic Vertebral ØR95
    Lumbar Vertebral ØS92
    Lumbosacral ØS94
    Thoracic Vertebral ØR99
    Thoracolumbar Vertebral ØR9B
  Duct
    Common Bile ØF99
    Cystic ØF98
    Hepatic
      Left ØF96

**Drainage** – *continued*
  Duct – *continued*
    Hepatic – *continued*
      Right ØF95
    Lacrimal
      Left Ø89Y
      Right Ø89X
    Pancreatic ØF9D
      Accessory ØF9F
    Parotid
      Left ØC9C
      Right ØC9B
  Duodenum ØD99
  Dura Mater ØØ92
  Ear
    External
      Left Ø991
      Right Ø990
    External Auditory Canal
      Left Ø994
      Right Ø993
    Inner
      Left Ø99E
      Right Ø99D
    Middle
      Left Ø996
      Right Ø995
  Elbow Region
    Left ØX9C
    Right ØX9B
  Epididymis
    Bilateral ØV9L
    Left ØV9K
    Right ØV9J
  Epidural Space ØØ93
  Epiglottis ØC9R
  Esophagogastric Junction ØD94
  Esophagus ØD95
    Lower ØD93
    Middle ØD92
    Upper ØD91
  Eustachian Tube
    Left Ø99G
    Right Ø99F
  Extremity
    Lower
      Left ØY9B
      Right ØY99
    Upper
      Left ØX97
      Right ØX96
  Eye
    Left Ø891
    Right Ø890
  Eyelid
    Lower
      Left Ø89R
      Right Ø89Q
    Upper
      Left Ø89P
      Right Ø89N
  Face ØW92
  Fallopian Tube
    Left ØU96
    Right ØU95
  Fallopian Tubes, Bilateral ØU97
  Femoral Region
    Left ØY98
    Right ØY97
  Femoral Shaft
    Left ØQ99
    Right ØQ98
  Femur
    Lower
      Left ØQ9C
      Right ØQ9B
    Upper
      Left ØQ97
      Right ØQ96
  Fibula
    Left ØQ9K
    Right ØQ9J
  Finger Nail ØH9Q
  Foot
    Left ØY9N
    Right ØY9M
  Gallbladder ØF94
  Gingiva
    Lower ØC96
    Upper ØC95
  Gland
    Adrenal
      Bilateral ØG94
      Left ØG92

**Drainage** – *continued*
  Gland – *continued*
    Adrenal – *continued*
      Right ØG93
    Lacrimal
      Left Ø89W
      Right Ø89V
    Minor Salivary ØC9J
    Parotid
      Left ØC99
      Right ØC98
    Pituitary ØG90
    Sublingual
      Left ØC9F
      Right ØC9D
    Submaxillary
      Left ØC9H
      Right ØC9G
    Vestibular ØU9L
  Glenoid Cavity
    Left ØP98
    Right ØP97
  Glomus Jugulare ØG9C
  Hand
    Left ØX9K
    Right ØX9J
  Head ØW90
  Humeral Head
    Left ØP9D
    Right ØP9C
  Humeral Shaft
    Left ØP9G
    Right ØP9F
  Hymen ØU9K
  Hypothalamus ØØ9A
  Ileocecal Valve ØD9C
  Ileum ØD9B
  Inguinal Region
    Left ØY96
    Right ØY95
  Intestine
    Large ØD9E
      Left ØD9G
      Right ØD9F
    Small ØD98
  Iris
    Left Ø89D
    Right Ø89C
  Jaw
    Lower ØW95
    Upper ØW94
  Jejunum ØD9A
  Joint
    Acromioclavicular
      Left ØR9H
      Right ØR9G
    Ankle
      Left ØS9G
      Right ØS9F
    Carpal
      Left ØR9R
      Right ØR9Q
    Cervical Vertebral ØR91
    Cervicothoracic Vertebral ØR94
    Coccygeal ØS96
    Elbow
      Left ØR9M
      Right ØR9L
    Finger Phalangeal
      Left ØR9X
      Right ØR9W
    Hip
      Left ØS9B
      Right ØS99
    Knee
      Left ØS9D
      Right ØS9C
    Lumbar Vertebral ØS90
    Lumbosacral ØS93
    Metacarpocarpal
      Left ØR9T
      Right ØR9S
    Metacarpophalangeal
      Left ØR9V
      Right ØR9U
    Metatarsal-Phalangeal
      Left ØS9N
      Right ØS9M
    Metatarsal-Tarsal
      Left ØS9L
      Right ØS9K
    Occipital-cervical ØR90
    Sacrococcygeal ØS95

**Drainage** – *continued*
  Joint – *continued*
    Sacroiliac
      Left ØS98
      Right ØS97
    Shoulder
      Left ØR9K
      Right ØR9J
    Sternoclavicular
      Left ØR9F
      Right ØR9E
    Tarsal
      Left ØS9J
      Right ØS9H
    Temporomandibular
      Left ØR9D
      Right ØR9C
    Thoracic Vertebral ØR96
    Thoracolumbar Vertebral ØR9A
    Toe Phalangeal
      Left ØS9Q
      Right ØS9P
    Wrist
      Left ØR9P
      Right ØR9N
  Kidney
    Left ØT91
    Right ØT90
  Kidney Pelvis
    Left ØT94
    Right ØT93
  Knee Region
    Left ØY9G
    Right ØY9F
  Larynx ØC9S
  Leg
    Lower
      Left ØY9J
      Right ØY9H
    Upper
      Left ØY9D
      Right ØY9C
  Lens
    Left Ø89K
    Right Ø89J
  Lip
    Lower ØC91
    Upper ØC90
  Liver ØF90
    Left Lobe ØF92
    Right Lobe ØF91
  Lung
    Bilateral ØB9M
    Left ØB9L
    Lower Lobe
      Left ØB9J
      Right ØB9F
    Middle Lobe, Right ØB9D
    Right ØB9K
    Upper Lobe
      Left ØB9G
      Right ØB9C
  Lung Lingula ØB9H
  Lymphatic
    Aortic Ø79D
    Axillary
      Left Ø796
      Right Ø795
    Head Ø790
    Inguinal
      Left Ø79J
      Right Ø79H
    Internal Mammary
      Left Ø799
      Right Ø798
    Lower Extremity
      Left Ø79G
      Right Ø79F
    Mesenteric Ø79B
    Neck
      Left Ø792
      Right Ø791
    Pelvis Ø79C
    Thoracic Duct Ø79K
    Thorax Ø797
    Upper Extremity
      Left Ø794
      Right Ø793
  Mandible
    Left ØN9V
    Right ØN9T
  Maxilla
    Left ØN9S

**Drainage** – *continued*
  Maxilla – *continued*
    Right ØN9R
  Mediastinum ØW9C
  Medulla Oblongata ØØ9D
  Mesentery ØD9V
  Metacarpal
    Left ØP9Q
    Right ØP9P
  Metatarsal
    Left ØQ9P
    Right ØQ9N
  Muscle
    Abdomen
      Left ØK9L
      Right ØK9K
    Extraocular
      Left Ø89M
      Right Ø89L
    Facial ØK91
    Foot
      Left ØK9W
      Right ØK9V
    Hand
      Left ØK9D
      Right ØK9C
    Head ØK90
    Hip
      Left ØK9P
      Right ØK9N
    Lower Arm and Wrist
      Left ØK9B
      Right ØK99
    Lower Leg
      Left ØK9T
      Right ØK9S
    Neck
      Left ØK93
      Right ØK92
    Perineum ØK9M
    Shoulder
      Left ØK96
      Right ØK95
    Thorax
      Left ØK9J
      Right ØK9H
    Tongue, Palate, Pharynx ØK94
    Trunk
      Left ØK9G
      Right ØK9F
    Upper Arm
      Left ØK98
      Right ØK97
    Upper Leg
      Left ØK9R
      Right ØK9Q
  Nasopharynx Ø99N
  Neck ØW96
  Nerve
    Abdominal Sympathetic Ø19M
    Abducens ØØ9L
    Accessory ØØ9R
    Acoustic ØØ9N
    Brachial Plexus Ø193
    Cervical Ø191
    Cervical Plexus Ø190
    Facial ØØ9M
    Femoral Ø19D
    Glossopharyngeal ØØ9P
    Head and Neck Sympathetic Ø19K
    Hypoglossal ØØ9S
    Lumbar Ø19B
    Lumbar Plexus Ø199
    Lumbar Sympathetic Ø19N
    Lumbosacral Plexus Ø19A
    Median Ø195
    Oculomotor ØØ9H
    Olfactory ØØ9F
    Optic ØØ9G
    Peroneal Ø19H
    Phrenic Ø192
    Pudendal Ø19C
    Radial Ø196
    Sacral Ø19R
    Sacral Plexus Ø19Q
    Sacral Sympathetic Ø19P
    Sciatic Ø19F
    Thoracic Ø198
    Thoracic Sympathetic Ø19L
    Tibial Ø19G
    Trigeminal ØØ9K
    Trochlear ØØ9J
    Ulnar Ø194

**Drainage** – *continued*
Nerve – *continued*
Vagus 009Q
Nipple
Left 0H9X
Right 0H9W
Nose 099K
Omentum
Greater 0D9S
Lesser 0D9T
Oral Cavity and Throat 0W93
Orbit
Left 0N9Q
Right 0N9P
Ovary
Bilateral 0U92
Left 0U91
Right 0U90
Palate
Hard 0C92
Soft 0C93
Pancreas 0F9G
Para-aortic Body 0G99
Paraganglion Extremity 0G9F
Parathyroid Gland 0G9R
Inferior
Left 0G9P
Right 0G9N
Multiple 0G9Q
Superior
Left 0G9M
Right 0G9L
Patella
Left 0Q9F
Right 0Q9D
Pelvic Cavity 0W9J
Penis 0V9S
Pericardial Cavity 0W9D
Perineum
Female 0W9N
Male 0W9M
Peritoneal Cavity 0W9G
Peritoneum 0D9W
Phalanx
Finger
Left 0P9V
Right 0P9T
Thumb
Left 0P9S
Right 0P9R
Toe
Left 0Q9R
Right 0Q9Q
Pharynx 0C9M
Pineal Body 0G91
Pleura
Left 0B9P
Right 0B9N
Pleural Cavity
Left 0W9B
Right 0W99
Pons 009B
Prepuce 0V9T
Products of Conception
Amniotic Fluid
Diagnostic 1090
Therapeutic 1090
Fetal Blood 1090
Fetal Cerebrospinal Fluid 1090
Fetal Fluid, Other 1090
Fluid, Other 1090
Prostate 0V90
Radius
Left 0P9J
Right 0P9H
Rectum 0D9P
Retina
Left 089F
Right 089E
Retinal Vessel
Left 089H
Right 089G
Retroperitoneum 0W9H
Rib
Left 0P92
Right 0P91
Sacrum 0Q91
Scapula
Left 0P96
Right 0P95
Sclera
Left 0897
Right 0896

**Drainage** – *continued*
Scrotum 0V95
Septum, Nasal 099M
Shoulder Region
Left 0X93
Right 0X92
Sinus
Accessory 099P
Ethmoid
Left 099V
Right 099U
Frontal
Left 099T
Right 099S
Mastoid
Left 099C
Right 099B
Maxillary
Left 099R
Right 099Q
Sphenoid
Left 099X
Right 099W
Skin
Abdomen 0H97
Back 0H96
Buttock 0H98
Chest 0H95
Ear
Left 0H93
Right 0H92
Face 0H91
Foot
Left 0H9N
Right 0H9M
Genitalia 0H9A
Hand
Left 0H9G
Right 0H9F
Lower Arm
Left 0H9E
Right 0H9D
Lower Leg
Left 0H9L
Right 0H9K
Neck 0H94
Perineum 0H99
Scalp 0H90
Upper Arm
Left 0H9C
Right 0H9B
Upper Leg
Left 0H9J
Right 0H9H
Skull 0N90
Spinal Canal 009U
Spinal Cord
Cervical 009W
Lumbar 009Y
Thoracic 009X
Spinal Meninges 009T
Spleen 079P
Sternum 0P90
Stomach 0D96
Pylorus 0D97
Subarachnoid Space 0095
Subcutaneous Tissue and Fascia
Abdomen 0J98
Back 0J97
Buttock 0J99
Chest 0J96
Face 0J91
Foot
Left 0J9R
Right 0J9Q
Hand
Left 0J9K
Right 0J9J
Lower Arm
Left 0J9H
Right 0J9G
Lower Leg
Left 0J9P
Right 0J9N
Neck
Anterior 0J94
Posterior 0J95
Pelvic Region 0J9C
Perineum 0J9B
Scalp 0J90
Upper Arm
Left 0J9F
Right 0J9D

**Drainage** – *continued*
Subcutaneous Tissue and Fascia – *continued*
Upper Leg
Left 0J9M
Right 0J9L
Subdural Space 0094
Tarsal
Left 0Q9M
Right 0Q9L
Tendon
Abdomen
Left 0L9G
Right 0L9F
Ankle
Left 0L9T
Right 0L9S
Foot
Left 0L9W
Right 0L9V
Hand
Left 0L98
Right 0L97
Head and Neck 0L90
Hip
Left 0L9K
Right 0L9J
Knee
Left 0L9R
Right 0L9Q
Lower Arm and Wrist
Left 0L96
Right 0L95
Lower Leg
Left 0L9P
Right 0L9N
Perineum 0L9H
Shoulder
Left 0L92
Right 0L91
Thorax
Left 0L9D
Right 0L9C
Trunk
Left 0L9B
Right 0L99
Upper Arm
Left 0L94
Right 0L93
Upper Leg
Left 0L9M
Right 0L9L
Testis
Bilateral 0V9C
Left 0V9B
Right 0V99
Thalamus 0099
Thymus 079M
Thyroid Gland 0G9K
Left Lobe 0G9G
Right Lobe 0G9H
Tibia
Left 0Q9H
Right 0Q9G
Toe Nail 0H9R
Tongue 0C97
Tonsils 0C9P
Tooth
Lower 0C9X
Upper 0C9W
Trachea 0B91
Tunica Vaginalis
Left 0V97
Right 0V96
Turbinate, Nasal 099L
Tympanic Membrane
Left 0998
Right 0997
Ulna
Left 0P9L
Right 0P9K
Ureter
Left 0T97
Right 0T96
Ureters, Bilateral 0T98
Urethra 0T9D
Uterine Supporting Structure 0U94
Uterus 0U99
Uvula 0C9N
Vagina 0U9G
Vas Deferens
Bilateral 0V9Q
Left 0V9P
Right 0V9N

**Drainage** – *continued*
Vein
Axillary
Left 0598
Right 0597
Azygos 0590
Basilic
Left 059C
Right 059B
Brachial
Left 059A
Right 0599
Cephalic
Left 059F
Right 059D
Colic 0697
Common Iliac
Left 069D
Right 069C
Esophageal 0693
External Iliac
Left 069G
Right 069F
External Jugular
Left 059Q
Right 059P
Face
Left 059V
Right 059T
Femoral
Left 069N
Right 069M
Foot
Left 069V
Right 069T
Gastric 0692
Greater Saphenous
Left 069Q
Right 069P
Hand
Left 059H
Right 059G
Hemiazygos 0591
Hepatic 0694
Hypogastric
Left 069J
Right 069H
Inferior Mesenteric 0696
Innominate
Left 0594
Right 0593
Internal Jugular
Left 059N
Right 059M
Intracranial 059L
Lesser Saphenous
Left 069S
Right 069R
Lower 069Y
Portal 0698
Renal
Left 069B
Right 0699
Splenic 0691
Subclavian
Left 0596
Right 0595
Superior Mesenteric 0695
Upper 059Y
Vertebral
Left 059S
Right 059R
Vena Cava, Inferior 0690
Vertebra
Cervical 0P93
Lumbar 0Q90
Thoracic 0P94
Vesicle
Bilateral 0V93
Left 0V92
Right 0V91
Vitreous
Left 0895
Right 0894
Vocal Cord
Left 0C9V
Right 0C9T
Vulva 0U9M
Wrist Region
Left 0X9H
Right 0X9G

**Dressing**
Abdominal Wall 2W23X4Z
Arm
Lower
Left 2W2DX4Z
Right 2W2CX4Z
Upper
Left 2W2BX4Z
Right 2W2AX4Z
Back 2W25X4Z
Chest Wall 2W24X4Z
Extremity
Lower
Left 2W2MX4Z
Right 2W2LX4Z
Upper
Left 2W29X4Z
Right 2W28X4Z
Face 2W21X4Z
Finger
Left 2W2KX4Z
Right 2W2JX4Z
Foot
Left 2W2TX4Z
Right 2W2SX4Z
Hand
Left 2W2FX4Z
Right 2W2EX4Z
Head 2W20X4Z
Inguinal Region
Left 2W27X4Z
Right 2W26X4Z
Leg
Lower
Left 2W2RX4Z
Right 2W2QX4Z
Upper
Left 2W2PX4Z
Right 2W2NX4Z
Neck 2W22X4Z
Thumb
Left 2W2HX4Z
Right 2W2GX4Z
Toe
Left 2W2VX4Z
Right 2W2UX4Z
**Driver stent** (RX) (OTW) – *use* Intraluminal Device
**Drotrecogin alfa** – *see* Introduction of Recombinant Human–activated Protein C
**Duct of Santorini** – *use* Duct, Pancreatic, Accessory
**Duct of Wirsung** – *use* Duct, Pancreatic
**Ductogram, mammary** – *see* Plain Radiography, Skin, Subcutaneous Tissue and Breast BH0
**Ductography, mammary** – *see* Plain Radiography, Skin, Subcutaneous Tissue and Breast BH0
**Ductus deferens**
– *use* Vas Deferens, Left
– *use* Vas Deferens, Right
– *use* Vas Deferens, Bilateral
**Duodenal ampulla** – *use* Ampulla of Vater
**Duodenectomy**
– *see* Excision, Duodenum 0DB9
– *see* Resection, Duodenum 0DT9
**Duodenocholedochotomy** – *see* Drainage, Gallbladder 0F94
**Duodenocystostomy**
– *see* Bypass, Gallbladder 0F14
– *see* Drainage, Gallbladder 0F94
**Duodenoenterostomy**
– *see* Bypass, Gastrointestinal System 0D1
– *see* Drainage, Gastrointestinal System 0D9
**Duodenojejunal flexure** – *use* Jejunum
**Duodenolysis** – *see* Release, Duodenum 0DN9
**Duodenorrhaphy** – *see* Repair, Duodenum 0DQ9
**Duodenostomy**
– *see* Bypass, Duodenum 0D19
– *see* Drainage, Duodenum 0D99
**Duodenotomy** – *see* Drainage, Duodenum 0D99
**DuraHeart Left Ventricular Assist System** – *use* Implantable Heart Assist System in Heart and Great Vessels
**Dural venous sinus** – *use* Vein, Intracranial
**Durata® Defibrillation Lead** – *use* Cardiac Lead, Defibrillator in 02H
**Dynesys® Dynamic Stabilization System**
– *use* Spinal Stabilization Device, Pedicle–Based in 0RH
– *use* Spinal Stabilization Device, Pedicle–Based in 0SH

# E

**E-Luminexx™** (Biliary)(Vascular) **Stent** – *use* Intraluminal Device
**Earlobe**
– *use* Ear, External, Left
– *use* Ear, External, Bilateral
– *use* Ear, External, Right
**Echocardiogram** – *see* Ultrasonography, Heart B24
**Echography** – *see* Ultrasonography
**ECMO** – *see* Performance, Circulatory 5A15
**EEG (electroencephalogram)** – *see* Measurement, Central Nervous 4A00
**EGD (esophagogastroduodenscopy)** 0DJ08ZZ
**Eighth cranial nerve** – *use* Nerve, Acoustic
**Ejaculatory duct**
– *use* Vas Deferens, Bilateral
– *use* Vas Deferens, Left
– *use* Vas Deferens, Right
**EKG (electrocardiogram)** – *see* Measurement, Cardiac 4A02
**Electrical bone growth stimulator (EBGS)**
– *use* Bone Growth Stimulator in Head and Facial Bones
– *use* Bone Growth Stimulator in Upper Bones
– *use* Bone Growth Stimulator in Lower Bones
**Electrical muscle stimulation (EMS) lead** – *use* Stimulator Lead in Muscles
**Electrocautery**
Destruction – *see* Destruction
Repair – *see* Repair
**Electroconvulsive Therapy**
Bilateral-Multiple Seizure GZB3ZZZ
Bilateral-Single Seizure GZB2ZZZ
Electroconvulsive Therapy, Other GZB4ZZZ
Unilateral-Multiple Seizure GZB1ZZZ
Unilateral-Single Seizure GZB0ZZZ
**Electroencephalogram (EEG)** – *see* Measurement, Central Nervous 4A00
**Electromagnetic Therapy**
Central Nervous 6A22
Urinary 6A21
**Electronic muscle stimulator lead** – *use* Stimulator Lead in Muscles
**Electrophysiologic stimulation (EPS)** – *see* Measurement, Cardiac 4A02
**Electroshock therapy** – *see* Electroconvulsive Therapy
**Elevation, bone fragments, skull** – *see* Reposition, Head and Facial Bones 0NS
**Eleventh cranial nerve** – *use* Nerve, Accessory
**Embolectomy** – *see* Extirpation
**Embolization**
– *see* Occlusion
– *see* Restriction
**Embolization coil(s)** – *use* Intraluminal Device
**EMG (electromyogram)** – *see* Measurement, Musculoskeletal 4A0F
**Encephalon** – *use* Brain
**Endarterectomy**
– *see* Extirpation, Upper Arteries 03C
– *see* Extirpation, Lower Arteries 04C
**Endeavor®** (III)(IV) (Sprint) **Zotarolimus-eluting Coronary Stent System** – *use* Intraluminal Device, Drug-eluting in Heart and Great Vessels
**EndoSure® sensor** – *use* Monitoring Device, Pressure Sensor in 02H
**ENDOTAK RELIANCE®** (G) **Defibrillation Lead** – *use* Cardiac Lead, Defibrillator in 02H
**Endotracheal tube** (cuffed)(double-lumen) – *use* Intraluminal Device, Endotracheal Airway in Respiratory System
**Endurant® Endovascular Stent Graft** – *use* Intraluminal Device
**Enlargement**
– *see* Dilation
– *see* Repair
**EnRhythm** – *use* Pacemaker, Dual Chamber in 0JH
**Enterorrhaphy** – *see* Repair, Gastrointestinal System 0DQ
**Enterra gastric neurostimulator** – *use* Stimulator Generator, Multiple Array in 0JH
**Enucleation**
Eyeball – *see* Resection, Eye 08T
Eyeball with prosthetic implant – *see* Replacement, Eye 08R
**Ependyma** – *use* Cerebral Ventricle
**Epicel® cultured epidermal autograft** – *use* Autologous Tissue Substitute

**Epic™ Stented Tissue Valve** (aortic) – use Zooplastic Tissue in Heart and Great Vessels

**Epidermis** – use Skin

**Epididymectomy**
– see Excision, Male Reproductive System ØVB
– see Resection, Male Reproductive System ØVT

**Epididymoplasty**
– see Repair, Male Reproductive System ØVQ
– see Supplement, Male Reproductive System ØVU

**Epididymorrhaphy** – see Repair, Male Reproductive System ØVQ

**Epididymotomy** – see Drainage, Male Reproductive System ØV9

**Epiphysiodesis**
– see Fusion, Upper Joints ØRG
– see Fusion, Lower Joints ØSG

**Epiploic foramen** – use Peritoneum

**Epiretinal Visual Prosthesis**
– use Epiretinal Visual Prosthesis in Eye
Insertion of device in
Left Ø8H1Ø5Z
Right Ø8HØØ5Z

**Episiorrhaphy** – see Repair, Perineum, Female ØWQN

**Episiotomy** – see Division, Perineum, Female ØW8N

**Epithalamus** – use Thalamus

**Epitrochlear lymph node**
– use Lymphatic, Upper Extremity, Left
– use Lymphatic, Upper Extremity, Right

**EPS (electrophysiologic stimulation)** – see Measurement, Cardiac 4AØ2

**Eptifibatide, infusion** – see Introduction of Platelet Inhibitor

**ERCP (endoscopic retrograde cholangiopancreatography)**
– see Fluoroscopy, Hepatobiliary System and Pancreas BF1

**Erector spinae muscle**
– use Muscle, Trunk, Left
– use Muscle, Trunk, Right

**Esophageal artery** – use Aorta, Thoracic

**Esophageal obturator airway (EOA)** – use Intraluminal Device, Airway in Gastrointestinal System

**Esophageal plexus** – use Nerve, Thoracic Sympathetic

**Esophagectomy**
– see Excision, Gastrointestinal System ØDB
– see Resection, Gastrointestinal System ØDT

**Esophagocoloplasty**
– see Repair, Gastrointestinal System ØDQ
– see Supplement, Gastrointestinal System ØDU

**Esophagoenterostomy**
– see Bypass, Gastrointestinal System ØD1
– see Drainage, Gastrointestinal System ØD9

**Esophagoesophagostomy**
– see Bypass, Gastrointestinal System ØD1
– see Drainage, Gastrointestinal System ØD9

**Esophagogastrectomy**
– see Excision, Gastrointestinal System ØDB
– see Resection, Gastrointestinal System ØDT

**Esophagogastroduodenscopy (EGD)** ØDJØ8ZZ

**Esophagogastroplasty**
– see Repair, Gastrointestinal System ØDQ
– see Supplement, Gastrointestinal System ØDU

**Esophagogastroscopy** ØDJ68ZZ

**Esophagogastrostomy**
– see Bypass, Gastrointestinal System ØD1
– see Drainage, Gastrointestinal System ØD9

**Esophagojejunoplasty** – see Supplement, Gastrointestinal System ØDU

**Esophagojejunostomy**
– see Drainage, Gastrointestinal System ØD9
– see Bypass, Gastrointestinal System ØD1

**Esophagomyotomy** – see Division, Esophagogastric Junction ØD84

**Esophagoplasty**
– see Repair, Gastrointestinal System ØDQ
– see Replacement, Esophagus ØDR5
– see Supplement, Gastrointestinal System ØDU

**Esophagoplication** – see Restriction, Gastrointestinal System ØDV

**Esophagorrhaphy** – see Repair, Gastrointestinal System ØDQ

**Esophagoscopy** ØDJØ8ZZ

**Esophagotomy** – see Drainage, Gastrointestinal System ØD9

**Esteem® implantable hearing system** – use Hearing Device in Ear, Nose, Sinus

**ESWL (extracorporeal shock wave lithotripsy)** – see Fragmentation

**Ethmoidal air cell**
– use Sinus, Ethmoid, Left
– use Sinus, Ethmoid, Right

**Ethmoidectomy**
– see Excision, Ear, Nose, Sinus Ø9B
– see Resection, Ear, Nose, Sinus Ø9T
– see Excision, Head and Facial Bones ØNB
– see Resection, Head and Facial Bones ØNT

**Ethmoidotomy** – see Drainage, Ear, Nose, Sinus Ø99

**Evacuation**
Hematoma – see Extirpation
Other Fluid – see Drainage

**Evera (XT)(S)(DR/VR)** – use Defibrillator Generator in ØJH

**Everolimus-eluting coronary stent** – use Intraluminal Device, Drug-eluting in Heart and Great Vessels

**Evisceration**
Eyeball – see Resection, Eye Ø8T
Eyeball with prosthetic implant – see Replacement, Eye Ø8R

**Ex-PRESS™ mini glaucoma shunt** – use Synthetic Substitute

**Examination** – see Inspection

**Exchange** – see Change device in

**Excision**
Abdominal Wall ØWBF
Acetabulum
Left ØQB5
Right ØQB4
Adenoids ØCBQ
Ampulla of Vater ØFBC
Anal Sphincter ØDBR
Ankle Region
Left ØYBL
Right ØYBK
Anus ØDBQ
Aorta
Abdominal Ø4BØ
Thoracic Ø2BW
Aortic Body ØGBD
Appendix ØDBJ
Arm
Lower
Left ØXBF
Right ØXBD
Upper
Left ØXB9
Right ØXB8
Artery
Anterior Tibial
Left Ø4BQ
Right Ø4BP
Axillary
Left Ø3B6
Right Ø3B5
Brachial
Left Ø3B8
Right Ø3B7
Celiac Ø4B1
Colic
Left Ø4B7
Middle Ø4B8
Right Ø4B6
Common Carotid
Left Ø3BJ
Right Ø3BH
Common Iliac
Left Ø4BD
Right Ø4BC
External Carotid
Left Ø3BN
Right Ø3BM
External Iliac
Left Ø4BJ
Right Ø4BH
Face Ø3BR
Femoral
Left Ø4BL
Right Ø4BK
Foot
Left Ø4BW
Right Ø4BV
Gastric Ø4B2
Hand
Left Ø3BF
Right Ø3BD
Hepatic Ø4B3
Inferior Mesenteric Ø4BB
Innominate Ø3B2
Internal Carotid
Left Ø3BL
Right Ø3BK

**Excision** – continued
Artery – continued
Internal Iliac
Left Ø4BF
Right Ø4BE
Internal Mammary
Left Ø3B1
Right Ø3BØ
Intracranial Ø3BG
Lower Ø4BY
Peroneal
Left Ø4BU
Right Ø4BT
Popliteal
Left Ø4BN
Right Ø4BM
Posterior Tibial
Left Ø4BS
Right Ø4BR
Pulmonary
Left Ø2BR
Right Ø2BQ
Pulmonary Trunk Ø2BP
Radial
Left Ø3BC
Right Ø3BB
Renal
Left Ø4BA
Right Ø4B9
Splenic Ø4B4
Subclavian
Left Ø3B4
Right Ø3B3
Superior Mesenteric Ø4B5
Temporal
Left Ø3BT
Right Ø3BS
Thyroid
Left Ø3BV
Right Ø3BU
Ulnar
Left Ø3BA
Right Ø3B9
Upper Ø3BY
Vertebral
Left Ø3BQ
Right Ø3BP
Atrium
Left Ø2B7
Right Ø2B6
Auditory Ossicle
Left Ø9BAØZ
Right Ø9B9ØZ
Axilla
Left ØXB5
Right ØXB4
Back
Lower ØWBL
Upper ØWBK
Basal Ganglia ØØB8
Bladder ØTBB
Bladder Neck ØTBC
Bone
Ethmoid
Left ØNBG
Right ØNBF
Frontal
Left ØNB2
Right ØNB1
Hyoid ØNBX
Lacrimal
Left ØNBJ
Right ØNBH
Nasal ØNBB
Occipital
Left ØNB8
Right ØNB7
Palatine
Left ØNBL
Right ØNBK
Parietal
Left ØNB4
Right ØNB3
Pelvic
Left ØQB3
Right ØQB2
Sphenoid
Left ØNBD
Right ØNBC
Temporal
Left ØNB6
Right ØNB5

**Excision** – *continued*
  Bone – *continued*
    Zygomatic
      Left ØNBN
      Right ØNBM
  Brain ØØBØ
  Breast
    Bilateral ØHBV
    Left ØHBU
    Right ØHBT
    Supernumerary ØHBY
  Bronchus
    Lingula ØBB9
    Lower Lobe
      Left ØBBB
      Right ØBB6
    Main
      Left ØBB7
      Right ØBB3
    Middle Lobe, Right ØBB5
    Upper Lobe
      Left ØBB8
      Right ØBB4
  Buccal Mucosa ØCB4
  Bursa and Ligament
    Abdomen
      Left ØMBJ
      Right ØMBH
    Ankle
      Left ØMBR
      Right ØMBQ
    Elbow
      Left ØMB4
      Right ØMB3
    Foot
      Left ØMBT
      Right ØMBS
    Hand
      Left ØMB8
      Right ØMB7
    Head and Neck ØMBØ
    Hip
      Left ØMBM
      Right ØMBL
    Knee
      Left ØMBP
      Right ØMBN
    Lower Extremity
      Left ØMBW
      Right ØMBV
    Perineum ØMBK
    Shoulder
      Left ØMB2
      Right ØMB1
    Thorax
      Left ØMBG
      Right ØMBF
    Trunk
      Left ØMBD
      Right ØMBC
    Upper Extremity
      Left ØMBB
      Right ØMB9
    Wrist
      Left ØMB6
      Right ØMB5
  Buttock
    Left ØYB1
    Right ØYBØ
  Carina ØBB2
  Carotid Bodies, Bilateral ØGB8
  Carotid Body
    Left ØGB6
    Right ØGB7
  Carpal
    Left ØPBN
    Right ØPBM
  Cecum ØDBH
  Cerebellum ØØBC
  Cerebral Hemisphere ØØB7
  Cerebral Meninges ØØB1
  Cerebral Ventricle ØØB6
  Cervix ØUBC
  Chest Wall ØWB8
  Chordae Tendineae Ø2B9
  Choroid
    Left Ø8BB
    Right Ø8BA
  Cisterna Chyli Ø7BL
  Clavicle
    Left ØPBB
    Right ØPB9
  Clitoris ØUBJ
  Coccygeal Glomus ØGBB

**Excision** – *continued*
  Coccyx ØQBS
  Colon
    Ascending ØDBK
    Descending ØDBM
    Sigmoid ØDBN
    Transverse ØDBL
  Conduction Mechanism Ø2B8
  Conjunctiva
    Left Ø8BTXZ
    Right Ø8BSXZ
  Cord
    Bilateral ØVBH
    Left ØVBG
    Right ØVBF
  Cornea
    Left Ø8B9XZ
    Right Ø8B8XZ
  Cul-de-sac ØUBF
  Diaphragm
    Left ØBBS
    Right ØBBR
  Disc
    Cervical Vertebral ØRB3
    Cervicothoracic Vertebral ØRB5
    Lumbar Vertebral ØSB2
    Lumbosacral ØSB4
    Thoracic Vertebral ØRB9
    Thoracolumbar Vertebral ØRBB
  Duct
    Common Bile ØFB9
    Cystic ØFB8
    Hepatic
      Left ØFB6
      Right ØFB5
    Lacrimal
      Left Ø8BY
      Right Ø8BX
    Pancreatic ØFBD
      Accessory ØFBF
    Parotid
      Left ØCBC
      Right ØCBB
  Duodenum ØDB9
  Dura Mater ØØB2
  Ear
    External
      Left Ø9B1
      Right Ø9BØ
    External Auditory Canal
      Left Ø9B4
      Right Ø9B3
    Inner
      Left Ø9BEØZ
      Right Ø9BDØZ
    Middle
      Left Ø9B6ØZ
      Right Ø9B5ØZ
  Elbow Region
    Left ØXBC
    Right ØXBB
  Epididymis
    Bilateral ØVBL
    Left ØVBK
    Right ØVBJ
  Epiglottis ØCBR
  Esophagogastric Junction ØDB4
  Esophagus ØDB5
    Lower ØDB3
    Middle ØDB2
    Upper ØDB1
  Eustachian Tube
    Left Ø9BG
    Right Ø9BF
  Extremity
    Lower
      Left ØYBB
      Right ØYB9
    Upper
      Left ØXB7
      Right ØXB6
  Eye
    Left Ø8B1
    Right Ø8BØ
  Eyelid
    Lower
      Left Ø8BR
      Right Ø8BQ
    Upper
      Left Ø8BP
      Right Ø8BN
  Face ØWB2
  Fallopian Tube
    Left ØUB6

**Excision** – *continued*
  Fallopian Tube – *continued*
    Right ØUB5
  Fallopian Tubes, Bilateral ØUB7
  Femoral Region
    Left ØYB8
    Right ØYB7
  Femoral Shaft
    Left ØQB9
    Right ØQB8
  Femur
    Lower
      Left ØQBC
      Right ØQBB
    Upper
      Left ØQB7
      Right ØQB6
  Fibula
    Left ØQBK
    Right ØQBJ
  Finger Nail ØHBQXZ
  Foot
    Left ØYBN
    Right ØYBM
  Gallbladder ØFB4
  Gingiva
    Lower ØCB6
    Upper ØCB5
  Gland
    Adrenal
      Bilateral ØGB4
      Left ØGB2
      Right ØGB3
    Lacrimal
      Left Ø8BW
      Right Ø8BV
    Minor Salivary ØCBJ
    Parotid
      Left ØCB9
      Right ØCB8
    Pituitary ØGBØ
    Sublingual
      Left ØCBF
      Right ØCBD
    Submaxillary
      Left ØCBH
      Right ØCBG
    Vestibular ØUBL
  Glenoid Cavity
    Left ØPB8
    Right ØPB7
  Glomus Jugulare ØGBC
  Hand
    Left ØXBK
    Right ØXBJ
  Head ØWBØ
  Humeral Head
    Left ØPBD
    Right ØPBC
  Humeral Shaft
    Left ØPBG
    Right ØPBF
  Hymen ØUBK
  Hypothalamus ØØBA
  Ileocecal Valve ØDBC
  Ileum ØDBB
  Inguinal Region
    Left ØYB6
    Right ØYB5
  Intestine
    Large ØDBE
      Left ØDBG
      Right ØDBF
    Small ØDB8
  Iris
    Left Ø8BD3Z
    Right Ø8BC3Z
  Jaw
    Lower ØWB5
    Upper ØWB4
  Jejunum ØDBA
  Joint
    Acromioclavicular
      Left ØRBH
      Right ØRBG
    Ankle
      Left ØSBG
      Right ØSBF
    Carpal
      Left ØRBR
      Right ØRBQ
    Cervical Vertebral ØRB1
    Cervicothoracic Vertebral ØRB4
    Coccygeal ØSB6

**Excision** – *continued*
  Joint – *continued*
    Elbow
      Left ØRBM
      Right ØRBL
    Finger Phalangeal
      Left ØRBX
      Right ØRBW
    Hip
      Left ØSBB
      Right ØSB9
    Knee
      Left ØSBD
      Right ØSBC
    Lumbar Vertebral ØSBØ
    Lumbosacral ØSB3
    Metacarpocarpal
      Left ØRBT
      Right ØRBS
    Metacarpophalangeal
      Left ØRBV
      Right ØRBU
    Metatarsal–Phalangeal
      Left ØSBN
      Right ØSBM
    Metatarsal–Tarsal
      Left ØSBL
      Right ØSBK
    Occipital–cervical ØRBØ
    Sacrococcygeal ØSB5
    Sacroiliac
      Left ØSB8
      Right ØSB7
    Shoulder
      Left ØRBK
      Right ØRBJ
    Sternoclavicular
      Left ØRBF
      Right ØRBE
    Tarsal
      Left ØSBJ
      Right ØSBH
    Temporomandibular
      Left ØRBD
      Right ØRBC
    Thoracic Vertebral ØRB6
    Thoracolumbar Vertebral ØRBA
    Toe Phalangeal
      Left ØSBQ
      Right ØSBP
    Wrist
      Left ØRBP
      Right ØRBN
  Kidney
    Left ØTB1
    Right ØTBØ
  Kidney Pelvis
    Left ØTB4
    Right ØTB3
  Knee Region
    Left ØYBG
    Right ØYBF
  Larynx ØCBS
  Leg
    Lower
      Left ØYBJ
      Right ØYBH
    Upper
      Left ØYBD
      Right ØYBC
  Lens
    Left Ø8BK3Z
    Right Ø8BJ3Z
  Lip
    Lower ØCB1
    Upper ØCBØ
  Liver ØFBØ
    Left Lobe ØFB2
    Right Lobe ØFB1
  Lung
    Bilateral ØBBM
    Left ØBBL
    Lower Lobe
      Left ØBBJ
      Right ØBBF
    Middle Lobe, Right ØBBD
    Right ØBBK
    Upper Lobe
      Left ØBBG
      Right ØBBC
  Lung Lingula ØBBH
  Lymphatic
    Aortic Ø7BD

**Excision** – *continued*
  Lymphatic – *continued*
    Axillary
      Left Ø7B6
      Right Ø7B5
    Head Ø7BØ
    Inguinal
      Left Ø7BJ
      Right Ø7BH
    Internal Mammary
      Left Ø7B9
      Right Ø7B8
    Lower Extremity
      Left Ø7BG
      Right Ø7BF
    Mesenteric Ø7BB
    Neck
      Left Ø7B2
      Right Ø7B1
    Pelvis Ø7BC
    Thoracic Duct Ø7BK
    Thorax Ø7B7
    Upper Extremity
      Left Ø7B4
      Right Ø7B3
  Mandible
    Left ØNBV
    Right ØNBT
  Maxilla
    Left ØNBS
    Right ØNBR
  Mediastinum ØWBC
  Medulla Oblongata ØØBD
  Mesentery ØDBV
  Metacarpal
    Left ØPBQ
    Right ØPBP
  Metatarsal
    Left ØQBP
    Right ØQBN
  Muscle
    Abdomen
      Left ØKBL
      Right ØKBK
    Extraocular
      Left Ø8BM
      Right Ø8BL
    Facial ØKB1
    Foot
      Left ØKBW
      Right ØKBV
    Hand
      Left ØKBD
      Right ØKBC
    Head ØKBØ
    Hip
      Left ØKBP
      Right ØKBN
    Lower Arm and Wrist
      Left ØKBB
      Right ØKB9
    Lower Leg
      Left ØKBT
      Right ØKBS
    Neck
      Left ØKB3
      Right ØKB2
    Papillary Ø2BD
    Perineum ØKBM
    Shoulder
      Left ØKB6
      Right ØKB5
    Thorax
      Left ØKBJ
      Right ØKBH
    Tongue, Palate, Pharynx ØKB4
    Trunk
      Left ØKBG
      Right ØKBF
    Upper Arm
      Left ØKB8
      Right ØKB7
    Upper Leg
      Left ØKBR
      Right ØKBQ
  Nasopharynx Ø9BN
  Neck ØWB6
  Nerve
    Abdominal Sympathetic Ø1BM
    Abducens ØØBL
    Accessory ØØBR
    Acoustic ØØBN
    Brachial Plexus Ø1B3

**Excision** – *continued*
  Nerve – *continued*
    Cervical Ø1B1
    Cervical Plexus Ø1BØ
    Facial ØØBM
    Femoral Ø1BD
    Glossopharyngeal ØØBP
    Head and Neck Sympathetic Ø1BK
    Hypoglossal ØØBS
    Lumbar Ø1BB
    Lumbar Plexus Ø1B9
    Lumbar Sympathetic Ø1BN
    Lumbosacral Plexus Ø1BA
    Median Ø1B5
    Oculomotor ØØBH
    Olfactory ØØBF
    Optic ØØBG
    Peroneal Ø1BH
    Phrenic Ø1B2
    Pudendal Ø1BC
    Radial Ø1B6
    Sacral Ø1BR
    Sacral Plexus Ø1BQ
    Sacral Sympathetic Ø1BP
    Sciatic Ø1BF
    Thoracic Ø1B8
    Thoracic Sympathetic Ø1BL
    Tibial Ø1BG
    Trigeminal ØØBK
    Trochlear ØØBJ
    Ulnar Ø1B4
    Vagus ØØBQ
  Nipple
    Left ØHBX
    Right ØHBW
  Nose Ø9BK
  Omentum
    Greater ØDBS
    Lesser ØDBT
  Orbit
    Left ØNBQ
    Right ØNBP
  Ovary
    Bilateral ØUB2
    Left ØUB1
    Right ØUBØ
  Palate
    Hard ØCB2
    Soft ØCB3
  Pancreas ØFBG
  Para–aortic Body ØGB9
  Paraganglion Extremity ØGBF
  Parathyroid Gland ØGBR
    Inferior
      Left ØGBP
      Right ØGBN
    Multiple ØGBQ
    Superior
      Left ØGBM
      Right ØGBL
  Patella
    Left ØQBF
    Right ØQBD
  Penis ØVBS
  Pericardium Ø2BN
  Perineum
    Female ØWBN
    Male ØWBM
  Peritoneum ØDBW
  Phalanx
    Finger
      Left ØPBV
      Right ØPBT
    Thumb
      Left ØPBS
      Right ØPBR
    Toe
      Left ØQBR
      Right ØQBQ
  Pharynx ØCBM
  Pineal Body ØGB1
  Pleura
    Left ØBBP
    Right ØBBN
  Pons ØØBB
  Prepuce ØVBT
  Prostate ØVBØ
  Radius
    Left ØPBJ
    Right ØPBH
  Rectum ØDBP
  Retina
    Left Ø8BF3Z
    Right Ø8BE3Z

**Excision** – *continued*
  Retroperitoneum ØWBH
  Rib
    Left ØPB2
    Right ØPB1
  Sacrum ØQB1
  Scapula
    Left ØPB6
    Right ØPB5
  Sclera
    Left Ø8B7XZ
    Right Ø8B6XZ
  Scrotum ØVB5
  Septum
    Atrial Ø2B5
    Nasal Ø9BM
    Ventricular Ø2BM
  Shoulder Region
    Left ØXB3
    Right ØXB2
  Sinus
    Accessory Ø9BP
    Ethmoid
      Left Ø9BV
      Right Ø9BU
    Frontal
      Left Ø9BT
      Right Ø9BS
    Mastoid
      Left Ø9BC
      Right Ø9BB
    Maxillary
      Left Ø9BR
      Right Ø9BQ
    Sphenoid
      Left Ø9BX
      Right Ø9BW
  Skin
    Abdomen ØHB7XZ
    Back ØHB6XZ
    Buttock ØHB8XZ
    Chest ØHB5XZ
    Ear
      Left ØHB3XZ
      Right ØHB2XZ
    Face ØHB1XZ
    Foot
      Left ØHBNXZ
      Right ØHBMXZ
    Genitalia ØHBAXZ
    Hand
      Left ØHBGXZ
      Right ØHBFXZ
    Lower Arm
      Left ØHBEXZ
      Right ØHBDXZ
    Lower Leg
      Left ØHBLXZ
      Right ØHBKXZ
    Neck ØHB4XZ
    Perineum ØHB9XZ
    Scalp ØHBØXZ
    Upper Arm
      Left ØHBCXZ
      Right ØHBBXZ
    Upper Leg
      Left ØHBJXZ
      Right ØHBHXZ
  Skull ØNBØ
  Spinal Cord
    Cervical ØØBW
    Lumbar ØØBY
    Thoracic ØØBX
  Spinal Meninges ØØBT
  Spleen Ø7BP
  Sternum ØPBØ
  Stomach ØDB6
    Pylorus ØDB7
  Subcutaneous Tissue and Fascia
    Abdomen ØJB8
    Back ØJB7
    Buttock ØJB9
    Chest ØJB6
    Face ØJB1
    Foot
      Left ØJBR
      Right ØJBQ
    Hand
      Left ØJBK
      Right ØJBJ
    Lower Arm
      Left ØJBH
      Right ØJBG

**Excision** – *continued*
  Subcutaneous Tissue and Fascia – *continued*
    Lower Leg
      Left ØJBP
      Right ØJBN
    Neck
      Anterior ØJB4
      Posterior ØJB5
    Pelvic Region ØJBC
    Perineum ØJBB
    Scalp ØJBØ
    Upper Arm
      Left ØJBF
      Right ØJBD
    Upper Leg
      Left ØJBM
      Right ØJBL
  Tarsal
    Left ØQBM
    Right ØQBL
  Tendon
    Abdomen
      Left ØLBG
      Right ØLBF
    Ankle
      Left ØLBT
      Right ØLBS
    Foot
      Left ØLBW
      Right ØLBV
    Hand
      Left ØLB8
      Right ØLB7
    Head and Neck ØLBØ
    Hip
      Left ØLBK
      Right ØLBJ
    Knee
      Left ØLBR
      Right ØLBQ
    Lower Arm and Wrist
      Left ØLB6
      Right ØLB5
    Lower Leg
      Left ØLBP
      Right ØLBN
    Perineum ØLBH
    Shoulder
      Left ØLB2
      Right ØLB1
    Thorax
      Left ØLBD
      Right ØLBC
    Trunk
      Left ØLBB
      Right ØLB9
    Upper Arm
      Left ØLB4
      Right ØLB3
    Upper Leg
      Left ØLBM
      Right ØLBL
  Testis
    Bilateral ØVBC
    Left ØVBB
    Right ØVB9
  Thalamus ØØB9
  Thymus Ø7BM
  Thyroid Gland
    Left Lobe ØGBG
    Right Lobe ØGBH
  Tibia
    Left ØQBH
    Right ØQBG
  Toe Nail ØHBRXZ
  Tongue ØCB7
  Tonsils ØCBP
  Tooth
    Lower ØCBX
    Upper ØCBW
  Trachea ØBB1
  Tunica Vaginalis
    Left ØVB7
    Right ØVB6
  Turbinate, Nasal Ø9BL
  Tympanic Membrane
    Left Ø9B8
    Right Ø9B7
  Ulna
    Left ØPBL
    Right ØPBK
  Ureter
    Left ØTB7

**Excision** – *continued*
  Ureter – *continued*
    Right ØTB6
  Urethra ØTBD
  Uterine Supporting Structure ØUB4
  Uterus ØUB9
  Uvula ØCBN
  Vagina ØUBG
  Valve
    Aortic Ø2BF
    Mitral Ø2BG
    Pulmonary Ø2BH
    Tricuspid Ø2BJ
  Vas Deferens
    Bilateral ØVBQ
    Left ØVBP
    Right ØVBN
  Vein
    Axillary
      Left Ø5B8
      Right Ø5B7
    Azygos Ø5BØ
    Basilic
      Left Ø5BC
      Right Ø5BB
    Brachial
      Left Ø5BA
      Right Ø5B9
    Cephalic
      Left Ø5BF
      Right Ø5BD
    Colic Ø6B7
    Common Iliac
      Left Ø6BD
      Right Ø6BC
    Coronary Ø2B4
    Esophageal Ø6B3
    External Iliac
      Left Ø6BG
      Right Ø6BF
    External Jugular
      Left Ø5BQ
      Right Ø5BP
    Face
      Left Ø5BV
      Right Ø5BT
    Femoral
      Left Ø6BN
      Right Ø6BM
    Foot
      Left Ø6BV
      Right Ø6BT
    Gastric Ø6B2
    Greater Saphenous
      Left Ø6BQ
      Right Ø6BP
    Hand
      Left Ø5BH
      Right Ø5BG
    Hemiazygos Ø5B1
    Hepatic Ø6B4
    Hypogastric
      Left Ø6BJ
      Right Ø6BH
    Inferior Mesenteric Ø6B6
    Innominate
      Left Ø5B4
      Right Ø5B3
    Internal Jugular
      Left Ø5BN
      Right Ø5BM
    Intracranial Ø5BL
    Lesser Saphenous
      Left Ø6BS
      Right Ø6BR
    Lower Ø6BY
    Portal Ø6B8
    Pulmonary
      Left Ø2BT
      Right Ø2BS
    Renal
      Left Ø6BB
      Right Ø6B9
    Splenic Ø6B1
    Subclavian
      Left Ø5B6
      Right Ø5B5
    Superior Mesenteric Ø6B5
    Upper Ø5BY
    Vertebral
      Left Ø5BS
      Right Ø5BR

**Excision** – *continued*
  Vena Cava
    Inferior 06B0
    Superior 02BV
  Ventricle
    Left 02BL
    Right 02BK
  Vertebra
    Cervical 0PB3
    Lumbar 0QB0
    Thoracic 0PB4
  Vesicle
    Bilateral 0VB3
    Left 0VB2
    Right 0VB1
  Vitreous
    Left 08B53Z
    Right 08B43Z
  Vocal Cord
    Left 0CBV
    Right 0CBT
  Vulva 0UBM
  Wrist Region
    Left 0XBH
    Right 0XBG
**Exclusion, Left atrial appendage (LAA)** – *see* Occlusion, Atrium, Left 02L7
**Exercise, rehabilitation** – *see* Motor Treatment, Rehabilitation F07
**Exploration** – *see* Inspection
**Express®** (LD) **Premounted Stent System** – *use* Intraluminal Device
**Express® Biliary SD Monorail® Premounted Stent System** – *use* Intraluminal Device
**Express® SD Renal Monorail® Premounted Stent System** – *use* Intraluminal Device
**Extensor carpi radialis muscle**
  – *use* Muscle, Lower Arm and Wrist, Left
  – *use* Muscle, Lower Arm and Wrist, Right
**Extensor carpi ulnaris muscle**
  – *use* Muscle, Lower Arm and Wrist, Left
  – *use* Muscle, Lower Arm and Wrist, Right
**Extensor digitorum brevis muscle**
  – *use* Muscle, Foot, Right
  – *use* Muscle, Foot, Left
**Extensor digitorum longus muscle**
  – *use* Muscle, Lower Leg, Left
  – *use* Muscle, Lower Leg, Right
**Extensor hallucis brevis muscle**
  – *use* Muscle, Foot, Right
  – *use* Muscle, Foot, Left
**Extensor hallucis longus muscle**
  – *use* Muscle, Lower Leg, Right
  – *use* Muscle, Lower Leg, Left
**External anal sphincter** – *use* Anal Sphincter
**External auditory meatus**
  – *use* Ear, External Auditory Canal, Left
  – *use* Ear, External Auditory Canal, Right
**External fixator**
  – *use* External Fixation Device in Head and Facial Bones
  – *use* External Fixation Device in Upper Bones
  – *use* External Fixation Device in Lower Bones
  – *use* External Fixation Device in Upper Joints
  – *use* External Fixation Device in Lower Joints
**External maxillary artery** – *use* Artery, Face
**External naris** – *use* Nose
**External oblique aponeurosis** – *use* Subcutaneous Tissue and Fascia, Trunk
**External oblique muscle**
  – *use* Muscle, Abdomen, Left
  – *use* Muscle, Abdomen, Right
**External popliteal nerve** – *use* Nerve, Peroneal
**External pudendal artery**
  – *use* Artery, Femoral, Right
  – *use* Artery, Femoral, Left
**External pudendal vein**
  – *use* Vein, Greater Saphenous, Right
  – *use* Vein, Greater Saphenous, Left
**External urethral sphincter** – *use* Urethra
**Extirpation**
  Acetabulum
    Left 0QC5
    Right 0QC4
  Adenoids 0CCQ
  Ampulla of Vater 0FCC
  Anal Sphincter 0DCR
  Anterior Chamber
    Left 08C3
    Right 08C2

**Extirpation** – *continued*
  Anus 0DCQ
  Aorta
    Abdominal 04C0
    Thoracic 02CW
  Aortic Body 0GCD
  Appendix 0DCJ
  Artery
    Anterior Tibial
      Left 04CQ
      Right 04CP
    Axillary
      Left 03C6
      Right 03C5
    Brachial
      Left 03C8
      Right 03C7
    Celiac 04C1
    Colic
      Left 04C7
      Middle 04C8
      Right 04C6
    Common Carotid
      Left 03CJ
      Right 03CH
    Common Iliac
      Left 04CD
      Right 04CC
    Coronary
      Four or More Sites 02C3
      One Site 02C0
      Three Sites 02C2
      Two Sites 02C1
    External Carotid
      Left 03CN
      Right 03CM
    External Iliac
      Left 04CJ
      Right 04CH
    Face 03CR
    Femoral
      Left 04CL
      Right 04CK
    Foot
      Left 04CW
      Right 04CV
    Gastric 04C2
    Hand
      Left 03CF
      Right 03CD
    Hepatic 04C3
    Inferior Mesenteric 04CB
    Innominate 03C2
    Internal Carotid
      Left 03CL
      Right 03CK
    Internal Iliac
      Left 04CF
      Right 04CE
    Internal Mammary
      Left 03C1
      Right 03C0
    Intracranial 03CG
    Lower 04CY
    Peroneal
      Left 04CU
      Right 04CT
    Popliteal
      Left 04CN
      Right 04CM
    Posterior Tibial
      Left 04CS
      Right 04CR
    Pulmonary
      Left 02CR
      Right 02CQ
    Pulmonary Trunk 02CP
    Radial
      Left 03CC
      Right 03CB
    Renal
      Left 04CA
      Right 04C9
    Splenic 04C4
    Subclavian
      Left 03C4
      Right 03C3
    Superior Mesenteric 04C5
    Temporal
      Left 03CT
      Right 03CS
    Thyroid
      Left 03CV

**Extirpation** – *continued*
  Artery – *continued*
    Thyroid – *continued*
      Right 03CU
    Ulnar
      Left 03CA
      Right 03C9
    Upper 03CY
    Vertebral
      Left 03CQ
      Right 03CP
  Atrium
    Left 02C7
    Right 02C6
  Auditory Ossicle
    Left 09CA0ZZ
    Right 09C90ZZ
  Basal Ganglia 00C8
  Bladder 0TCB
  Bladder Neck 0TCC
  Bone
    Ethmoid
      Left 0NCG
      Right 0NCF
    Frontal
      Left 0NC2
      Right 0NC1
    Hyoid 0NCX
    Lacrimal
      Left 0NCJ
      Right 0NCH
    Nasal 0NCB
    Occipital
      Left 0NC8
      Right 0NC7
    Palatine
      Left 0NCL
      Right 0NCK
    Parietal
      Left 0NC4
      Right 0NC3
    Pelvic
      Left 0QC3
      Right 0QC2
    Sphenoid
      Left 0NCD
      Right 0NCC
    Temporal
      Left 0NC6
      Right 0NC5
    Zygomatic
      Left 0NCN
      Right 0NCM
  Brain 00C0
  Breast
    Bilateral 0HCV
    Left 0HCU
    Right 0HCT
  Bronchus
    Lingula 0BC9
    Lower Lobe
      Left 0BCB
      Right 0BC6
    Main
      Left 0BC7
      Right 0BC3
    Middle Lobe, Right 0BC5
    Upper Lobe
      Left 0BC8
      Right 0BC4
  Buccal Mucosa 0CC4
  Bursa and Ligament
    Abdomen
      Left 0MCJ
      Right 0MCH
    Ankle
      Left 0MCR
      Right 0MCQ
    Elbow
      Left 0MC4
      Right 0MC3
    Foot
      Left 0MCT
      Right 0MCS
    Hand
      Left 0MC8
      Right 0MC7
    Head and Neck 0MC0
    Hip
      Left 0MCM
      Right 0MCL
    Knee
      Left 0MCP

**Extirpation** – *continued*
  Bursa and Ligament – *continued*
    Knee – *continued*
      Right ØMCN
    Lower Extremity
      Left ØMCW
      Right ØMCV
    Perineum ØMCK
    Shoulder
      Left ØMC2
      Right ØMC1
    Thorax
      Left ØMCG
      Right ØMCF
    Trunk
      Left ØMCD
      Right ØMCC
    Upper Extremity
      Left ØMCB
      Right ØMC9
    Wrist
      Left ØMC6
      Right ØMC5
  Carina ØBC2
  Carotid Bodies, Bilateral ØGC8
  Carotid Body
    Left ØGC6
    Right ØGC7
  Carpal
    Left ØPCN
    Right ØPCM
  Cavity, Cranial ØWC1
  Cecum ØDCH
  Cerebellum ØØCC
  Cerebral Hemisphere ØØC7
  Cerebral Meninges ØØC1
  Cerebral Ventricle ØØC6
  Cervix ØUCC
  Chordae Tendineae Ø2C9
  Choroid
    Left Ø8CB
    Right Ø8CA
  Cisterna Chyli Ø7CL
  Clavicle
    Left ØPCB
    Right ØPC9
  Clitoris ØUCJ
  Coccygeal Glomus ØGCB
  Coccyx ØQCS
  Colon
    Ascending ØDCK
    Descending ØDCM
    Sigmoid ØDCN
    Transverse ØDCL
  Conduction Mechanism Ø2C8
  Conjunctiva
    Left Ø8CTXZZ
    Right Ø8CSXZZ
  Cord
    Bilateral ØVCH
    Left ØVCG
    Right ØVCF
  Cornea
    Left Ø8C9XZZ
    Right Ø8C8XZZ
  Cul-de-sac ØUCF
  Diaphragm
    Left ØBCS
    Right ØBCR
  Disc
    Cervical Vertebral ØRC3
    Cervicothoracic Vertebral ØRC5
    Lumbar Vertebral ØSC2
    Lumbosacral ØSC4
    Thoracic Vertebral ØRC9
    Thoracolumbar Vertebral ØRCB
  Duct
    Common Bile ØFC9
    Cystic ØFC8
    Hepatic
      Left ØFC6
      Right ØFC5
    Lacrimal
      Left Ø8CY
      Right Ø8CX
    Pancreatic ØFCD
      Accessory ØFCF
    Parotid
      Left ØCCC
      Right ØCCB
  Duodenum ØDC9
  Dura Mater ØØC2

**Extirpation** – *continued*
  Ear
    External
      Left Ø9C1
      Right Ø9CØ
    External Auditory Canal
      Left Ø9C4
      Right Ø9C3
    Inner
      Left Ø9CEØZZ
      Right Ø9CDØZZ
    Middle
      Left Ø9C6ØZZ
      Right Ø9C5ØZZ
  Endometrium ØUCB
  Epididymis
    Bilateral ØVCL
    Left ØVCK
    Right ØVCJ
  Epidural Space ØØC3
  Epiglottis ØCCR
  Esophagogastric Junction ØDC4
  Esophagus ØDC5
    Lower ØDC3
    Middle ØDC2
    Upper ØDC1
  Eustachian Tube
    Left Ø9CG
    Right Ø9CF
  Eye
    Left Ø8C1XZZ
    Right Ø8CØXZZ
  Eyelid
    Lower
      Left Ø8CR
      Right Ø8CQ
    Upper
      Left Ø8CP
      Right Ø8CN
  Fallopian Tube
    Left ØUC6
    Right ØUC5
  Fallopian Tubes, Bilateral ØUC7
  Femoral Shaft
    Left ØQC9
    Right ØQC8
  Femur
    Lower
      Left ØQCC
      Right ØQCB
    Upper
      Left ØQC7
      Right ØQC6
  Fibula
    Left ØQCK
    Right ØQCJ
  Finger Nail ØHCQXZZ
  Gallbladder ØFC4
  Gastrointestinal Tract ØWCP
  Genitourinary Tract ØWCR
  Gingiva
    Lower ØCC6
    Upper ØCC5
  Gland
    Adrenal
      Bilateral ØGC4
      Left ØGC2
      Right ØGC3
    Lacrimal
      Left Ø8CW
      Right Ø8CV
    Minor Salivary ØCCJ
    Parotid
      Left ØCC9
      Right ØCC8
    Pituitary ØGCØ
    Sublingual
      Left ØCCF
      Right ØCCD
    Submaxillary
      Left ØCCH
      Right ØCCG
    Vestibular ØUCL
  Glenoid Cavity
    Left ØPC8
    Right ØPC7
  Glomus Jugulare ØGCC
  Humeral Head
    Left ØPCD
    Right ØPCC
  Humeral Shaft
    Left ØPCG
    Right ØPCF

**Extirpation** – *continued*
  Hymen ØUCK
  Hypothalamus ØØCA
  Ileocecal Valve ØDCC
  Ileum ØDCB
  Intestine
    Large ØDCE
      Left ØDCG
      Right ØDCF
    Small ØDC8
  Iris
    Left Ø8CD
    Right Ø8CC
  Jejunum ØDCA
  Joint
    Acromioclavicular
      Left ØRCH
      Right ØRCG
    Ankle
      Left ØSCG
      Right ØSCF
    Carpal
      Left ØRCR
      Right ØRCQ
    Cervical Vertebral ØRC1
    Cervicothoracic Vertebral ØRC4
    Coccygeal ØSC6
    Elbow
      Left ØRCM
      Right ØRCL
    Finger Phalangeal
      Left ØRCX
      Right ØRCW
    Hip
      Left ØSCB
      Right ØSC9
    Knee
      Left ØSCD
      Right ØSCC
    Lumbar Vertebral ØSCØ
    Lumbosacral ØSC3
    Metacarpocarpal
      Left ØRCT
      Right ØRCS
    Metacarpophalangeal
      Left ØRCV
      Right ØRCU
    Metatarsal–Phalangeal
      Left ØSCN
      Right ØSCM
    Metatarsal–Tarsal
      Left ØSCL
      Right ØSCK
    Occipital–cervical ØRCØ
    Sacrococcygeal ØSC5
    Sacroiliac
      Left ØSC8
      Right ØSC7
    Shoulder
      Left ØRCK
      Right ØRCJ
    Sternoclavicular
      Left ØRCF
      Right ØRCE
    Tarsal
      Left ØSCJ
      Right ØSCH
    Temporomandibular
      Left ØRCD
      Right ØRCC
    Thoracic Vertebral ØRC6
    Thoracolumbar Vertebral ØRCA
    Toe Phalangeal
      Left ØSCQ
      Right ØSCP
    Wrist
      Left ØRCP
      Right ØRCN
  Kidney
    Left ØTC1
    Right ØTCØ
  Kidney Pelvis
    Left ØTC4
    Right ØTC3
  Larynx ØCCS
  Lens
    Left Ø8CK
    Right Ø8CJ
  Lip
    Lower ØCC1
    Upper ØCCØ
  Liver ØFCØ
    Left Lobe ØFC2

**Extirpation** – *continued*
Liver – *continued*
Right Lobe ØFC1
Lung
Bilateral ØBCM
Left ØBCL
Lower Lobe
Left ØBCJ
Right ØBCF
Middle Lobe, Right ØBCD
Right ØBCK
Upper Lobe
Left ØBCG
Right ØBCC
Lung Lingula ØBCH
Lymphatic
Aortic Ø7CD
Axillary
Left Ø7C6
Right Ø7C5
Head Ø7CØ
Inguinal
Left Ø7CJ
Right Ø7CH
Internal Mammary
Left Ø7C9
Right Ø7C8
Lower Extremity
Left Ø7CG
Right Ø7CF
Mesenteric Ø7CB
Neck
Left Ø7C2
Right Ø7C1
Pelvis Ø7CC
Thoracic Duct Ø7CK
Thorax Ø7C7
Upper Extremity
Left Ø7C4
Right Ø7C3
Mandible
Left ØNCV
Right ØNCT
Maxilla
Left ØNCS
Right ØNCR
Mediastinum ØWCC
Medulla Oblongata ØØCD
Mesentery ØDCV
Metacarpal
Left ØPCQ
Right ØPCP
Metatarsal
Left ØQCP
Right ØQCN
Muscle
Abdomen
Left ØKCL
Right ØKCK
Extraocular
Left Ø8CM
Right Ø8CL
Facial ØKC1
Foot
Left ØKCW
Right ØKCV
Hand
Left ØKCD
Right ØKCC
Head ØKCØ
Hip
Left ØKCP
Right ØKCN
Lower Arm and Wrist
Left ØKCB
Right ØKC9
Lower Leg
Left ØKCT
Right ØKCS
Neck
Left ØKC3
Right ØKC2
Papillary Ø2CD
Perineum ØKCM
Shoulder
Left ØKC6
Right ØKC5
Thorax
Left ØKCJ
Right ØKCH
Tongue, Palate, Pharynx ØKC4
Trunk
Left ØKCG

**Extirpation** – *continued*
Muscle – *continued*
Trunk – *continued*
Right ØKCF
Upper Arm
Left ØKC8
Right ØKC7
Upper Leg
Left ØKCR
Right ØKCQ
Nasopharynx Ø9CN
Nerve
Abdominal Sympathetic Ø1CM
Abducens ØØCL
Accessory ØØCR
Acoustic ØØCN
Brachial Plexus Ø1C3
Cervical Ø1C1
Cervical Plexus Ø1CØ
Facial ØØCM
Femoral Ø1CD
Glossopharyngeal ØØCP
Head and Neck Sympathetic Ø1CK
Hypoglossal ØØCS
Lumbar Ø1CB
Lumbar Plexus Ø1C9
Lumbar Sympathetic Ø1CN
Lumbosacral Plexus Ø1CA
Median Ø1C5
Oculomotor ØØCH
Olfactory ØØCF
Optic ØØCG
Peroneal Ø1CH
Phrenic Ø1C2
Pudendal Ø1CC
Radial Ø1C6
Sacral Ø1CR
Sacral Plexus Ø1CQ
Sacral Sympathetic Ø1CP
Sciatic Ø1CF
Thoracic Ø1C8
Thoracic Sympathetic Ø1CL
Tibial Ø1CG
Trigeminal ØØCK
Trochlear ØØCJ
Ulnar Ø1C4
Vagus ØØCQ
Nipple
Left ØHCX
Right ØHCW
Nose Ø9CK
Omentum
Greater ØDCS
Lesser ØDCT
Oral Cavity and Throat ØWC3
Orbit
Left ØNCQ
Right ØNCP
Ovary
Bilateral ØUC2
Left ØUC1
Right ØUCØ
Palate
Hard ØCC2
Soft ØCC3
Pancreas ØFCG
Para–aortic Body ØGC9
Paraganglion Extremity ØGCF
Parathyroid Gland ØGCR
Inferior
Left ØGCP
Right ØGCN
Multiple ØGCQ
Superior
Left ØGCM
Right ØGCL
Patella
Left ØQCF
Right ØQCD
Pelvic Cavity ØWCJ
Penis ØVCS
Pericardial Cavity ØWCD
Pericardium Ø2CN
Peritoneal Cavity ØWCG
Peritoneum ØDCW
Phalanx
Finger
Left ØPCV
Right ØPCT
Thumb
Left ØPCS
Right ØPCR

**Extirpation** – *continued*
Phalanx – *continued*
Toe
Left ØQCR
Right ØQCQ
Pharynx ØCCM
Pineal Body ØGC1
Pleura
Left ØBCP
Right ØBCN
Pleural Cavity
Left ØWCB
Right ØWC9
Pons ØØCB
Prepuce ØVCT
Prostate ØVCØ
Radius
Left ØPCJ
Right ØPCH
Rectum ØDCP
Respiratory Tract ØWCQ
Retina
Left Ø8CF
Right Ø8CE
Retinal Vessel
Left Ø8CH
Right Ø8CG
Rib
Left ØPC2
Right ØPC1
Sacrum ØQC1
Scapula
Left ØPC6
Right ØPC5
Sclera
Left Ø8C7XZZ
Right Ø8C6XZZ
Scrotum ØVC5
Septum
Atrial Ø2C5
Nasal Ø9CM
Ventricular Ø2CM
Sinus
Accessory Ø9CP
Ethmoid
Left Ø9CV
Right Ø9CU
Frontal
Left Ø9CT
Right Ø9CS
Mastoid
Left Ø9CC
Right Ø9CB
Maxillary
Left Ø9CR
Right Ø9CQ
Sphenoid
Left Ø9CX
Right Ø9CW
Skin
Abdomen ØHC7XZZ
Back ØHC6XZZ
Buttock ØHC8XZZ
Chest ØHC5XZZ
Ear
Left ØHC3XZZ
Right ØHC2XZZ
Face ØHC1XZZ
Foot
Left ØHCNXZZ
Right ØHCMXZZ
Genitalia ØHCAXZZ
Hand
Left ØHCGXZZ
Right ØHCFXZZ
Lower Arm
Left ØHCEXZZ
Right ØHCDXZZ
Lower Leg
Left ØHCLXZZ
Right ØHCKXZZ
Neck ØHC4XZZ
Perineum ØHC9XZZ
Scalp ØHCØXZZ
Upper Arm
Left ØHCCXZZ
Right ØHCBXZZ
Upper Leg
Left ØHCJXZZ
Right ØHCHXZZ
Spinal Cord
Cervical ØØCW
Lumbar ØØCY

**Extirpation** – *continued*
  Spinal Cord – *continued*
    Thoracic 00CX
  Spinal Meninges 00CT
  Spleen 07CP
  Sternum 0PC0
  Stomach 0DC6
    Pylorus 0DC7
  Subarachnoid Space 00C5
  Subcutaneous Tissue and Fascia
    Abdomen 0JC8
    Back 0JC7
    Buttock 0JC9
    Chest 0JC6
    Face 0JC1
    Foot
      Left 0JCR
      Right 0JCQ
    Hand
      Left 0JCK
      Right 0JCJ
    Lower Arm
      Left 0JCH
      Right 0JCG
    Lower Leg
      Left 0JCP
      Right 0JCN
    Neck
      Anterior 0JC4
      Posterior 0JC5
    Pelvic Region 0JCC
    Perineum 0JCB
    Scalp 0JC0
    Upper Arm
      Left 0JCF
      Right 0JCD
    Upper Leg
      Left 0JCM
      Right 0JCL
  Subdural Space 00C4
  Tarsal
    Left 0QCM
    Right 0QCL
  Tendon
    Abdomen
      Left 0LCG
      Right 0LCF
    Ankle
      Left 0LCT
      Right 0LCS
    Foot
      Left 0LCW
      Right 0LCV
    Hand
      Left 0LC8
      Right 0LC7
    Head and Neck 0LC0
    Hip
      Left 0LCK
      Right 0LCJ
    Knee
      Left 0LCR
      Right 0LCQ
    Lower Arm and Wrist
      Left 0LC6
      Right 0LC5
    Lower Leg
      Left 0LCP
      Right 0LCN
    Perineum 0LCH
    Shoulder
      Left 0LC2
      Right 0LC1
    Thorax
      Left 0LCD
      Right 0LCC
    Trunk
      Left 0LCB
      Right 0LC9
    Upper Arm
      Left 0LC4
      Right 0LC3
    Upper Leg
      Left 0LCM
      Right 0LCL
  Testis
    Bilateral 0VCC
    Left 0VCB
    Right 0VC9
  Thalamus 00C9
  Thymus 07CM
  Thyroid Gland 0GCK
    Left Lobe 0GCG

**Extirpation** – *continued*
  Thyroid Gland – *continued*
    Right Lobe 0GCH
  Tibia
    Left 0QCH
    Right 0QCG
  Toe Nail 0HCRXZZ
  Tongue 0CC7
  Tonsils 0CCP
  Tooth
    Lower 0CCX
    Upper 0CCW
  Trachea 0BC1
  Tunica Vaginalis
    Left 0VC7
    Right 0VC6
  Turbinate, Nasal 09CL
  Tympanic Membrane
    Left 09C8
    Right 09C7
  Ulna
    Left 0PCL
    Right 0PCK
  Ureter
    Left 0TC7
    Right 0TC6
  Urethra 0TCD
  Uterine Supporting Structure 0UC4
  Uterus 0UC9
  Uvula 0CCN
  Vagina 0UCG
  Valve
    Aortic 02CF
    Mitral 02CG
    Pulmonary 02CH
    Tricuspid 02CJ
  Vas Deferens
    Bilateral 0VCQ
    Left 0VCP
    Right 0VCN
  Vein
    Axillary
      Left 05C8
      Right 05C7
    Azygos 05C0
    Basilic
      Left 05CC
      Right 05CB
    Brachial
      Left 05CA
      Right 05C9
    Cephalic
      Left 05CF
      Right 05CD
    Colic 06C7
    Common Iliac
      Left 06CD
      Right 06CC
    Coronary 02C4
    Esophageal 06C3
    External Iliac
      Left 06CG
      Right 06CF
    External Jugular
      Left 05CQ
      Right 05CP
    Face
      Left 05CV
      Right 05CT
    Femoral
      Left 06CN
      Right 06CM
    Foot
      Left 06CV
      Right 06CT
    Gastric 06C2
    Greater Saphenous
      Left 06CQ
      Right 06CP
    Hand
      Left 05CH
      Right 05CG
    Hemiazygos 05C1
    Hepatic 06C4
    Hypogastric
      Left 06CJ
      Right 06CH
    Inferior Mesenteric 06C6
    Innominate
      Left 05C4
      Right 05C3
    Internal Jugular
      Left 05CN

**Extirpation** – *continued*
  Vein – *continued*
    Internal Jugular – *continued*
      Right 05CM
    Intracranial 05CL
    Lesser Saphenous
      Left 06CS
      Right 06CR
    Lower 06CY
    Portal 06C8
    Pulmonary
      Left 02CT
      Right 02CS
    Renal
      Left 06CB
      Right 06C9
    Splenic 06C1
    Subclavian
      Left 05C6
      Right 05C5
    Superior Mesenteric 06C5
    Upper 05CY
    Vertebral
      Left 05CS
      Right 05CR
  Vena Cava
    Inferior 06C0
    Superior 02CV
  Ventricle
    Left 02CL
    Right 02CK
  Vertebra
    Cervical 0PC3
    Lumbar 0QC0
    Thoracic 0PC4
  Vesicle
    Bilateral 0VC3
    Left 0VC2
    Right 0VC1
  Vitreous
    Left 08C5
    Right 08C4
  Vocal Cord
    Left 0CCV
    Right 0CCT
  Vulva 0UCM
**Extracorporeal shock wave lithotripsy** – *see*
  Fragmentation
**Extracranial-intracranial bypass** (EC-IC) – *see* Bypass,
  Upper Arteries 031
**Extraction**
  Auditory Ossicle
    Left 09DA0ZZ
    Right 09D90ZZ
  Bone Marrow
    Iliac 07DR
    Sternum 07DQ
    Vertebral 07DS
  Bursa and Ligament
    Abdomen
      Left 0MDJ
      Right 0MDH
    Ankle
      Left 0MDR
      Right 0MDQ
    Elbow
      Left 0MD4
      Right 0MD3
    Foot
      Left 0MDT
      Right 0MDS
    Hand
      Left 0MD8
      Right 0MD7
    Head and Neck 0MD0
    Hip
      Left 0MDM
      Right 0MDL
    Knee
      Left 0MDP
      Right 0MDN
    Lower Extremity
      Left 0MDW
      Right 0MDV
    Perineum 0MDK
    Shoulder
      Left 0MD2
      Right 0MD1
    Thorax
      Left 0MDG
      Right 0MDF
    Trunk
      Left 0MDD

**Extraction** – *continued*
  Bursa and Ligament – *continued*
    Trunk – *continued*
      Right 0MDC
    Upper Extremity
      Left 0MDB
      Right 0MD9
    Wrist
      Left 0MD6
      Right 0MD5
  Cerebral Meninges 00D1
  Cornea
    Left 08D9XZ
    Right 08D8XZ
  Dura Mater 00D2
  Endometrium 0UDB
  Finger Nail 0HDQXZZ
  Hair 0HDSXZZ
  Kidney
    Left 0TD1
    Right 0TD0
  Lens
    Left 08DK3ZZ
    Right 08DJ3ZZ
  Nerve
    Abdominal Sympathetic 01DM
    Abducens 00DL
    Accessory 00DR
    Acoustic 00DN
    Brachial Plexus 01D3
    Cervical 01D1
    Cervical Plexus 01D0
    Facial 00DM
    Femoral 01DD
    Glossopharyngeal 00DP
    Head and Neck Sympathetic 01DK
    Hypoglossal 00DS
    Lumbar 01DB
    Lumbar Plexus 01D9
    Lumbar Sympathetic 01DN
    Lumbosacral Plexus 01DA
    Median 01D5
    Oculomotor 00DH
    Olfactory 00DF
    Optic 00DG
    Peroneal 01DH
    Phrenic 01D2
    Pudendal 01DC
    Radial 01D6
    Sacral 01DR
    Sacral Plexus 01DQ
    Sacral Sympathetic 01DP
    Sciatic 01DF
    Thoracic 01D8
    Thoracic Sympathetic 01DL
    Tibial 01DG
    Trigeminal 00DK
    Trochlear 00DJ
    Ulnar 01D4
    Vagus 00DQ
  Ova 0UDN
  Pleura
    Left 0BDP
    Right 0BDN
  Products of Conception
    Classical 10D00Z0
    Ectopic 10D2
    Extraperitoneal 10D00Z2
    High Forceps 10D07Z5
    Internal Version 10D07Z7
    Low Cervical 10D00Z1
    Low Forceps 10D07Z3
    Mid Forceps 10D07Z4
    Other 10D07Z8
    Retained 10D1
    Vacuum 10D07Z6
  Septum, Nasal 09DM
  Sinus
    Accessory 09DP
    Ethmoid
      Left 09DV
      Right 09DU
    Frontal
      Left 09DT
      Right 09DS
    Mastoid
      Left 09DC
      Right 09DB
    Maxillary
      Left 09DR
      Right 09DQ
    Sphenoid
      Left 09DX

**Extraction** – *continued*
  Sinus – *continued*
    Sphenoid – *continued*
      Right 09DW
  Skin
    Abdomen 0HD7XZZ
    Back 0HD6XZZ
    Buttock 0HD8XZZ
    Chest 0HD5XZZ
    Ear
      Left 0HD3XZZ
      Right 0HD2XZZ
    Face 0HD1XZZ
    Foot
      Left 0HDNXZZ
      Right 0HDMXZZ
    Genitalia 0HDAXZZ
    Hand
      Left 0HDGXZZ
      Right 0HDFXZZ
    Lower Arm
      Left 0HDEXZZ
      Right 0HDDXZZ
    Lower Leg
      Left 0HDLXZZ
      Right 0HDKXZZ
    Neck 0HD4XZZ
    Perineum 0HD9XZZ
    Scalp 0HD0XZZ
    Upper Arm
      Left 0HDCXZZ
      Right 0HDBXZZ
    Upper Leg
      Left 0HDJXZZ
      Right 0HDHXZZ
  Spinal Meninges 00DT
  Subcutaneous Tissue and Fascia
    Abdomen 0JD8
    Back 0JD7
    Buttock 0JD9
    Chest 0JD6
    Face 0JD1
    Foot
      Left 0JDR
      Right 0JDQ
    Hand
      Left 0JDK
      Right 0JDJ
    Lower Arm
      Left 0JDH
      Right 0JDG
    Lower Leg
      Left 0JDP
      Right 0JDN
    Neck
      Anterior 0JD4
      Posterior 0JD5
    Pelvic Region 0JDC
    Perineum 0JDB
    Scalp 0JD0
    Upper Arm
      Left 0JDF
      Right 0JDD
    Upper Leg
      Left 0JDM
      Right 0JDL
  Toe Nail 0HDRXZZ
  Tooth
    Lower 0CDXXZ
    Upper 0CDWXZ
  Turbinate, Nasal 09DL
  Tympanic Membrane
    Left 09D8
    Right 09D7
  Vein
    Basilic
      Left 05DC
      Right 05DB
    Brachial
      Left 05DA
      Right 05D9
    Cephalic
      Left 05DF
      Right 05DD
    Femoral
      Left 06DN
      Right 06DM
    Foot
      Left 06DV
      Right 06DT
    Greater Saphenous
      Left 06DQ
      Right 06DP

**Extraction** – *continued*
  Vein – *continued*
    Hand
      Left 05DH
      Right 05DG
    Lesser Saphenous
      Left 06DS
      Right 06DR
    Lower 06DY
    Upper 05DY
  Vocal Cord
    Left 0CDV
    Right 0CDT
**Extradural space** – *use* Epidural Space
**EXtreme Lateral Interbody Fusion (XLIF) device** – *use*
  Interbody Fusion Device in Lower Joints

# F

**Face lift** – *see* Alteration, Face 0W02
**Facet replacement spinal stabilization device**
  – *use* Spinal Stabilization Device, Facet Replacement
    in 0RH
  – *use* Spinal Stabilization Device, Facet Replacement
    in 0SH
**Facial artery** – *use* Artery, Face
**False vocal cord** – *use* Larynx
**Falx cerebri** – *use* Dura Mater
**Fascia lata**
  – *use* Subcutaneous Tissue and Fascia, Upper Leg,
    Left
  – *use* Subcutaneous Tissue and Fascia, Upper Leg,
    Right
**Fasciaplasty, fascioplasty**
  – *see* Repair, Subcutaneous Tissue and Fascia 0JQ
  – *see* Replacement, Subcutaneous Tissue and
    Fascia 0JR
**Fasciectomy** – *see* Excision, Subcutaneous Tissue and
  Fascia 0JB
**Fasciorrhaphy** – *see* Repair, Subcutaneous Tissue and
  Fascia 0JQ
**Fasciotomy**
  – *see* Division, Subcutaneous Tissue and Fascia 0J8
  – *see* Drainage, Subcutaneous Tissue and Fascia 0J9
**Feeding Device**
  Change device in
    Lower 0D2DXUZ
    Upper 0D20XUZ
  Insertion of device in
    Duodenum 0DH9
    Esophagus 0DH5
    Ileum 0DHB
    Intestine, Small 0DH8
    Jejunum 0DHA
    Stomach 0DH6
  Removal of device from
    Esophagus 0DP5
    Intestinal Tract
      Lower 0DPD
      Upper 0DP0
    Stomach 0DP6
  Revision of device in
    Intestinal Tract
      Lower 0DWD
      Upper 0DW0
    Stomach 0DW6
**Femoral head**
  – *use* Femur, Upper, Right
  – *use* Femur, Upper, Left
**Femoral lymph node**
  – *use* Lymphatic, Lower Extremity, Left
  – *use* Lymphatic, Lower Extremity, Right
**Femoropatellar joint**
  – *use* Joint, Knee, Right
  – *use* Joint, Knee, Left
  – *use* Joint, Knee, Right, Femoral Surface
  – *use* Joint, Knee, Left, Femoral Surface
**Femorotibial joint**
  – *use* Joint, Knee, Right
  – *use* Joint, Knee, Left
  – *use* Joint, Knee, Right, Tibial Surface
  – *use* Joint, Knee, Left, Tibial Surface
**Fibular artery**
  – *use* Artery, Peroneal, Right
  – *use* Artery, Peroneal, Left
**Fibularis brevis muscle**
  – *use* Muscle, Lower Leg, Left
  – *use* Muscle, Lower Leg, Right

**Fibularis longus muscle**
 – *use* Muscle, Lower Leg, Left
 – *use* Muscle, Lower Leg, Right
**Fifth cranial nerve** – *use* Nerve, Trigeminal
**Fimbriectomy**
 – *see* Excision, Female Reproductive System ØUB
 – *see* Resection, Female Reproductive System ØUT
**First cranial nerve** – *use* Nerve, Olfactory
**First intercostal nerve** – *use* Nerve, Brachial Plexus
**Fistulization**
 – *see* Bypass
 – *see* Drainage
 – *see* Repair
**Fitting**
 Arch bars, for fracture reduction – *see* Reposition,
  Mouth and Throat ØCS
 Arch bars, for immobilization – *see* Immobilization,
  Face 2W31
 Artificial limb – *see* Device Fitting, Rehabilitation FØD
 Hearing aid – *see* Device Fitting, Rehabilitation FØD
 Ocular prosthesis FØDZ8UZ
 Prosthesis, limb – *see* Device Fitting,
  Rehabilitation FØD
 Prosthesis, ocular FØDZ8UZ
**Fixation, bone**
 External, with fracture reduction – *see* Reposition
 External, without fracture reduction – *see* Insertion
 Internal, with fracture reduction – *see* Reposition
 Internal, without fracture reduction – *see* Insertion
**FLAIR® Endovascular Stent Graft** – *use* Intraluminal
  Device
**Flexible Composite Mesh** – *use* Synthetic Substitute
**Flexor carpi radialis muscle**
 – *use* Muscle, Lower Arm and Wrist, Right
 – *use* Muscle, Lower Arm and Wrist, Left
**Flexor carpi ulnaris muscle**
 – *use* Muscle, Lower Arm and Wrist, Right
 – *use* Muscle, Lower Arm and Wrist, Left
**Flexor digitorum brevis muscle**
 – *use* Muscle, Foot, Left
 – *use* Muscle, Foot, Right
**Flexor digitorum longus muscle**
 – *use* Muscle, Lower Leg, Left
 – *use* Muscle, Lower Leg, Right
**Flexor hallucis brevis muscle**
 – *use* Muscle, Foot, Left
 – *use* Muscle, Foot, Right
**Flexor hallucis longus muscle**
 – *use* Muscle, Lower Leg, Right
 – *use* Muscle, Lower Leg, Left
**Flexor pollicis longus muscle**
 – *use* Muscle, Lower Arm and Wrist, Left
 – *use* Muscle, Lower Arm and Wrist, Right
**Fluoroscopy**
 Abdomen and Pelvis BW11
 Airway, Upper BB1DZZZ
 Ankle
  Left BQ1H
  Right BQ1G
 Aorta
  Abdominal B41Ø
   Laser, Intraoperative B41Ø
  Thoracic B31Ø
   Laser, Intraoperative B31Ø
  Thoraco–Abdominal B31P
   Laser, Intraoperative B31P
 Aorta and Bilateral Lower Extremity Arteries B41D
  Laser, Intraoperative B41D
 Arm
  Left BP1FZZZ
  Right BP1EZZZ
 Artery
  Brachiocephalic–Subclavian
   Right B311
    Laser, Intraoperative B311
  Bronchial B31L
   Laser, Intraoperative B31L
  Bypass Graft, Other B21F
  Cervico–Cerebral Arch B31Q
   Laser, Intraoperative B31Q
  Common Carotid
   Bilateral B315
    Laser, Intraoperative B315
   Left B314
    Laser, Intraoperative B314
   Right B313
    Laser, Intraoperative B313
  Coronary
   Bypass Graft
    Multiple B213
     Laser, Intraoperative B213

**Fluoroscopy** – *continued*
 Artery – *continued*
  Coronary – *continued*
   Bypass Graft – *continued*
    Single B212
     Laser, Intraoperative B212
   Multiple B211
    Laser, Intraoperative B211
   Single B210
    Laser, Intraoperative B210
  External Carotid
   Bilateral B31C
    Laser, Intraoperative B31C
   Left B31B
    Laser, Intraoperative B31B
   Right B319
    Laser, Intraoperative B319
  Hepatic B412
   Laser, Intraoperative B412
  Inferior Mesenteric B415
   Laser, Intraoperative B415
  Intercostal B31L
   Laser, Intraoperative B31L
  Internal Carotid
   Bilateral B318
    Laser, Intraoperative B318
   Left B317
    Laser, Intraoperative B317
   Right B316
    Laser, Intraoperative B316
  Internal Mammary Bypass Graft
   Left B218
   Right B217
  Intra–Abdominal
   Other B41B
   Laser, Intraoperative B41B
  Intracranial B31R
   Laser, Intraoperative B31R
  Lower
   Other B41J
   Laser, Intraoperative B41J
  Lower Extremity
   Bilateral and Aorta B41D
    Laser, Intraoperative B41D
   Left B41G
    Laser, Intraoperative B41G
   Right B41F
    Laser, Intraoperative B41F
  Lumbar B419
   Laser, Intraoperative B419
  Pelvic B41C
   Laser, Intraoperative B41C
  Pulmonary
   Left B31T
    Laser, Intraoperative B31T
   Right B31S
    Laser, Intraoperative B31S
  Renal
   Bilateral B418
    Laser, Intraoperative B418
   Left B417
    Laser, Intraoperative B417
   Right B416
    Laser, Intraoperative B416
  Spinal B31M
   Laser, Intraoperative B31M
  Splenic B413
   Laser, Intraoperative B413
  Subclavian
   Left B312
    Laser, Intraoperative B312
  Superior Mesenteric B414
   Laser, Intraoperative B414
  Upper
   Other B31N
   Laser, Intraoperative B31N
  Upper Extremity
   Bilateral B31K
    Laser, Intraoperative B31K
   Left B31J
    Laser, Intraoperative B31J
   Right B31H
    Laser, Intraoperative B31H
  Vertebral
   Bilateral B31G
    Laser, Intraoperative B31G
   Left B31F
    Laser, Intraoperative B31F
   Right B31D
    Laser, Intraoperative B31D
 Bile Duct BF1Ø
  Pancreatic Duct and Gallbladder BF14
 Bile Duct and Gallbladder BF13

**Fluoroscopy** – *continued*
 Biliary Duct BF11
 Bladder BT1Ø
  Kidney and Ureter BT14
  Left BT1F
  Right BT1D
 Bladder and Urethra BT1B
 Bowel, Small BD1
 Calcaneus
  Left BQ1KZZZ
  Right BQ1JZZZ
 Clavicle
  Left BP15ZZZ
  Right BP14ZZZ
 Coccyx BR1F
 Colon BD14
 Corpora Cavernosa BV1Ø
 Dialysis Fistula B51W
 Dialysis Shunt B51W
 Diaphragm BB16ZZZ
 Disc
  Cervical BR11
  Lumbar BR13
  Thoracic BR12
 Duodenum BD19
 Elbow
  Left BP1H
  Right BP1G
 Epiglottis B91G
 Esophagus BD11
 Extremity
  Lower BW1C
  Upper BW1J
 Facet Joint
  Cervical BR14
  Lumbar BR16
  Thoracic BR15
 Fallopian Tube
  Bilateral BU12
  Left BU11
  Right BU1Ø
 Fallopian Tube and Uterus BU18
 Femur
  Left BQ14ZZZ
  Right BQ13ZZZ
 Finger
  Left BP1SZZZ
  Right BP1RZZZ
 Foot
  Left BQ1MZZZ
  Right BQ1LZZZ
 Forearm
  Left BP1KZZZ
  Right BP1JZZZ
 Gallbladder BF12
  Bile Duct and Pancreatic Duct BF14
 Gallbladder and Bile Duct BF13
 Gastrointestinal, Upper BD1
 Hand
  Left BP1PZZZ
  Right BP1NZZZ
 Head and Neck BW19
 Heart
  Left B215
  Right B214
  Right and Left B216
 Hip
  Left BQ11
  Right BQ1Ø
 Humerus
  Left BP1BZZZ
  Right BP1AZZZ
 Ileal Diversion Loop BT1C
 Ileal Loop, Ureters and Kidney BT1G
 Intracranial Sinus B512
 Joint
  Acromioclavicular, Bilateral BP13ZZZ
  Finger
   Left BP1D
   Right BP1C
  Foot
   Left BQ1Y
   Right BQ1X
  Hand
   Left BP1D
   Right BP1C
  Lumbosacral BR1B
  Sacroiliac BR1D
  Sternoclavicular
   Bilateral BP12ZZZ
   Left BP11ZZZ
   Right BP1ØZZZ

**Fluoroscopy** – *continued*
Joint – *continued*
Temporomandibular
Bilateral BN19
Left BN18
Right BN17
Thoracolumbar BR18
Toe
Left BQ1Y
Right BQ1X
Kidney
Bilateral BT13
Ileal Loop and Ureter BT1G
Left BT12
Right BT11
Ureter and Bladder BT14
Left BT1F
Right BT1D
Knee
Left BQ18
Right BQ17
Larynx B91J
Leg
Left BQ1FZZZ
Right BQ1DZZZ
Lung
Bilateral BB14ZZZ
Left BB13ZZZ
Right BB12ZZZ
Mediastinum BB1CZZZ
Mouth BD1B
Neck and Head BW19
Oropharynx BD1B
Pancreatic Duct BF1
Gallbladder and Bile Buct BF14
Patella
Left BQ1WZZZ
Right BQ1VZZZ
Pelvis BR1C
Pelvis and Abdomen BW11
Pharynx B91G
Ribs
Left BP1YZZZ
Right BP1XZZZ
Sacrum BR1F
Scapula
Left BP17ZZZ
Right BP16ZZZ
Shoulder
Left BP19
Right BP18
Sinus, Intracranial B512
Spinal Cord B01B
Spine
Cervical BR10
Lumbar BR19
Thoracic BR17
Whole BR1G
Sternum BR1H
Stomach BD12
Toe
Left BQ1QZZZ
Right BQ1PZZZ
Tracheobronchial Tree
Bilateral BB19YZZ
Left BB18YZZ
Right BB17YZZ
Ureter
Ileal Loop and Kidney BT1G
Kidney and Bladder BT14
Left BT1F
Right BT1D
Left BT17
Right BT16
Urethra BT15
Urethra and Bladder BT1B
Uterus BU16
Uterus and Fallopian Tube BU18
Vagina BU19
Vasa Vasorum BV18
Vein
Cerebellar B511
Cerebral B511
Epidural B510
Jugular
Bilateral B515
Left B514
Right B513
Lower Extremity
Bilateral B51D
Left B51C
Right B51B
Other B51V

**Fluoroscopy** – *continued*
Vein – *continued*
Pelvic (Iliac)
Left B51G
Right B51F
Pelvic (Iliac) Bilateral B51H
Portal B51T
Pulmonary
Bilateral B51S
Left B51R
Right B51Q
Renal
Bilateral B51L
Left B51K
Right B51J
Spanchnic B51T
Subclavian
Left B517
Right B516
Upper Extremity
Bilateral B51P
Left B51N
Right B51M
Vena Cava
Inferior B519
Superior B518
Wrist
Left BP1M
Right BP1L
**Flushing** – *see* Irrigation
**Foley catheter** – *use* Drainage Device
**Foramen magnum**
– *use* Bone, Occipital, Right
– *use* Bone, Occipital, Left
**Foramen of Monro** (intraventricular) – *use* Cerebral Ventricle
**Foreskin** – *use* Prepuce
**Formula™ Balloon-Expandable Renal Stent System** – *use* Intraluminal Device
**Fossa of Rosenmuller** – *use* Nasopharynx
**Fourth cranial nerve** – *use* Nerve, Trochlear
**Fourth ventricle** – *use* Cerebral Ventricle
**Fovea**
– *use* Retina, Right
– *use* Retina, Left
**Fragmentation**
Ampulla of Vater 0FFC
Anus 0DFQ
Appendix 0DFJ
Bladder 0TFB
Bladder Neck 0TFC
Bronchus
Lingula 0BF9
Lower Lobe
Left 0BFB
Right 0BF6
Main
Left 0BF7
Right 0BF3
Middle Lobe, Right 0BF5
Upper Lobe
Left 0BF8
Right 0BF4
Carina 0BF2
Cavity, Cranial 0WF1
Cecum 0DFH
Cerebral Ventricle 00F6
Colon
Ascending 0DFK
Descending 0DFM
Sigmoid 0DFN
Transverse 0DFL
Duct
Common Bile 0FF9
Cystic 0FF8
Hepatic
Left 0FF6
Right 0FF5
Pancreatic 0FFD
Accessory 0FFF
Parotid
Left 0CFC
Right 0CFB
Duodenum 0DF9
Epidural Space 00F3
Esophagus 0DF5
Fallopian Tube
Left 0UF6
Right 0UF5
Fallopian Tubes, Bilateral 0UF7
Gallbladder 0FF4
Gastrointestinal Tract 0WFP

**Fragmentation** – *continued*
Genitourinary Tract 0WFR
Ileum 0DFB
Intestine
Large 0DFE
Left 0DFG
Right 0DFF
Small 0DF8
Jejunum 0DFA
Kidney Pelvis
Left 0TF4
Right 0TF3
Mediastinum 0WFC
Oral Cavity and Throat 0WF3
Pelvic Cavity 0WFJ
Pericardial Cavity 0WFD
Pericardium 02FN
Peritoneal Cavity 0WFG
Pleural Cavity
Left 0WFB
Right 0WF9
Rectum 0DFP
Respiratory Tract 0WFQ
Spinal Canal 00FU
Stomach 0DF6
Subarachnoid Space 00F5
Subdural Space 00F4
Trachea 0BF1
Ureter
Left 0TF7
Right 0TF6
Urethra 0TFD
Uterus 0UF9
Vitreous
Left 08F5
Right 08F4
**Freestyle** (Stentless) **Aortic Root Bioprosthesis** – *use* Zooplastic Tissue in Heart and Great Vessels
**Frenectomy**
– *see* Excision, Mouth and Throat 0CB
– *see* Resection, Mouth and Throat 0CT
**Frenoplasty, frenuloplasty**
– *see* Repair, Mouth and Throat 0CQ
– *see* Replacement, Mouth and Throat 0CR
– *see* Supplement, Mouth and Throat 0CU
**Frenotomy**
– *see* Drainage, Mouth and Throat 0C9
– *see* Release, Mouth and Throat 0CN
**Frenulotomy**
– *see* Drainage, Mouth and Throat 0C9
– *see* Release, Mouth and Throat 0CN
**Frenulum labii inferioris** – *use* Lip, Lower
**Frenulum labii superioris** – *use* Lip, Upper
**Frenulum linguae** – *use* Tongue
**Frenulumectomy**
– *see* Excision, Mouth and Throat 0CB
– *see* Resection, Mouth and Throat 0CT
**Frontal lobe** – *use* Cerebral Hemisphere
**Frontal vein**
– *use* Vein, Face, Right
– *use* Vein, Face, Left
**Fulguration** – *see* Destruction
**Fundoplication, gastroesophageal** – *see* Restriction, Esophagogastric Junction 0DV4
**Fundus uteri** – *use* Uterus
**Fusion**
Acromioclavicular
Left 0RGH
Right 0RGG
Ankle
Left 0SGG
Right 0SGF
Carpal
Left 0RGR
Right 0RGQ
Cervical Vertebral 0RG1
2 or more 0RG2
Cervicothoracic Vertebral 0RG4
Coccygeal 0SG6
Elbow
Left 0RGM
Right 0RGL
Finger Phalangeal
Left 0RGX
Right 0RGW
Hip
Left 0SGB
Right 0SG9
Knee
Left 0SGD
Right 0SGC

**Fusion** – continued
  Lumbar Vertebral ØSGØ
    2 or more ØSG1
  Lumbosacral ØSG3
  Metacarpocarpal
    Left ØRGT
    Right ØRGS
  Metacarpophalangeal
    Left ØRGV
    Right ØRGU
  Metatarsal–Phalangeal
    Left ØSGN
    Right ØSGM
  Metatarsal–Tarsal
    Left ØSGL
    Right ØSGK
  Occipital–cervical ØRGØ
  Sacrococcygeal ØSG5
  Sacroiliac
    Left ØSG8
    Right ØSG7
  Shoulder
    Left ØRGK
    Right ØRGJ
  Sternoclavicular
    Left ØRGF
    Right ØRGE
  Tarsal
    Left ØSGJ
    Right ØSGH
  Temporomandibular
    Left ØRGD
    Right ØRGC
  Thoracic Vertebral ØRG6
    2 to 7 ØRG7
    8 or more ØRG8
  Thoracolumbar Vertebral ØRGA
  Toe Phalangeal
    Left ØSGQ
    Right ØSGP
  Wrist
    Left ØRGP
    Right ØRGN
**Fusion screw** (compression)(lag)(locking)
  – *use* Internal Fixation Device in Upper Joints
  – *use* Internal Fixation Device in Lower Joints

# G

**Gait training** – *see* Motor Treatment, Rehabilitation FØ7
**Galea aponeurotica** – *use* Subcutaneous Tissue and Fascia, Scalp
**Ganglion impar** (ganglion of Walther) – *use* Nerve, Sacral Sympathetic
**Ganglionectomy**
  Destruction of lesion – *see* Destruction
  Excision of lesion – *see* Excision
**Gasserian ganglion** – *use* Nerve, Trigeminal
**Gastrectomy**
  Partial – *see* Excision, Stomach ØDB6
  Total – *see* Resection, Stomach ØDT6
  Vertical (sleeve) – *see* Excision, Stomach ØDB6
**Gastric electrical stimulation (GES) lead** – *use* Stimulator Lead in Gastrointestinal System
**Gastric lymph node** – *use* Lymphatic, Aortic
**Gastric pacemaker lead** – *use* Stimulator Lead in Gastrointestinal System
**Gastric plexus** – *use* Nerve, Abdominal Sympathetic
**Gastrocnemius muscle**
  – *use* Muscle, Lower Leg, Left
  – *use* Muscle, Lower Leg, Right
**Gastrocolic ligament** – *use* Omentum, Greater
**Gastrocolic omentum** – *use* Omentum, Greater
**Gastrocolostomy**
  – *see* Bypass, Gastrointestinal System ØD1
  – *see* Drainage, Gastrointestinal System ØD9
**Gastroduodenal artery** – *use* Artery, Hepatic
**Gastroduodenectomy**
  – *see* Excision, Gastrointestinal System ØDB
  – *see* Resection, Gastrointestinal System ØDT
**Gastroduodenoscopy** ØDJ08ZZ
**Gastroenteroplasty**
  – *see* Repair, Gastrointestinal System ØDQ
  – *see* Supplement, Gastrointestinal System ØDU
**Gastroenterostomy**
  – *see* Bypass, Gastrointestinal System ØD1
  – *see* Drainage, Gastrointestinal System ØD9
**Gastroesophageal (GE) junction** – *use* Esophagogastric Junction

**Gastrogastrostomy**
  – *see* Bypass, Stomach ØD16
  – *see* Drainage, Stomach ØD96
**Gastrohepatic omentum** – *use* Omentum, Lesser
**Gastrojejunostomy**
  – *see* Bypass, Stomach ØD16
  – *see* Drainage, Stomach ØD96
**Gastrolysis** – *see* Release, Stomach ØDN6
**Gastropexy**
  – *see* Repair, Stomach ØDQ6
  – *see* Reposition, Stomach ØDS6
**Gastrophrenic ligament** – *use* Omentum, Greater
**Gastroplasty**
  – *see* Repair, Stomach ØDQ6
  – *see* Supplement, Stomach ØDU6
**Gastroplication** – *see* Restriction, Stomach ØDV6
**Gastropylorectomy** – *see* Excision, Gastrointestinal System ØDB
**Gastrorrhaphy** – *see* Repair, Stomach ØDQ6
**Gastroscopy** ØDJ68ZZ
**Gastrosplenic ligament** – *use* Omentum, Greater
**Gastrostomy**
  – *see* Bypass, Stomach ØD16
  – *see* Drainage, Stomach ØD96
**Gastrotomy** – *see* Drainage, Stomach ØD96
**Gemellus muscle**
  – *use* Muscle, Hip, Left
  – *use* Muscle, Hip, Right
**Geniculate ganglion** – *use* Nerve, Facial
**Geniculate nucleus** – *use* Thalamus
**Genioglossus muscle** – *use* Muscle, Tongue, Palate, Pharynx
**Genioplasty** – *see* Alteration, Jaw, Lower ØWØ5
**Genitofemoral nerve** – *use* Nerve, Lumbar Plexus
**Gingivectomy** – *see* Excision, Mouth and Throat ØCB
**Gingivoplasty**
  – *see* Repair, Mouth and Throat ØCQ
  – *see* Replacement, Mouth and Throat ØCR
  – *see* Supplement, Mouth and Throat ØCU
**Glans penis** – *use* Prepuce
**Glenohumeral joint**
  – *use* Joint, Shoulder, Left
  – *use* Joint, Shoulder, Right
**Glenohumeral ligament**
  – *use* Bursa and Ligament, Shoulder, Right
  – *use* Bursa and Ligament, Shoulder, Left
**Glenoid fossa** (of scapula)
  – *use* Glenoid Cavity, Left
  – *use* Glenoid Cavity, Right
**Glenoid ligament** (labrum)
  – *use* Bursa and Ligament, Shoulder, Right
  – *use* Bursa and Ligament, Shoulder, Left
**Globus pallidus** – *use* Basal Ganglia
**Glomectomy**
  – *see* Excision, Endocrine System ØGB
  – *see* Resection, Endocrine System ØGT
**Glossectomy**
  – *see* Excision, Tongue ØCB7
  – *see* Resection, Tongue ØCT7
**Glossoepiglottic fold** – *use* Epiglottis
**Glossopexy**
  – *see* Repair, Tongue ØCQ7
  – *see* Reposition, Tongue ØCS7
**Glossoplasty**
  – *see* Repair, Tongue ØCQ7
  – *see* Replacement, Tongue ØCR7
  – *see* Supplement, Tongue ØCU7
**Glossorrhaphy** – *see* Repair, Tongue ØCQ7
**Glossotomy** – *see* Drainage, Tongue ØC97
**Glottis** – *use* Larynx
**Gluteal Artery Perforator Flap**
  Bilateral ØHRVØ79
  Left ØHRUØ79
  Right ØHRTØ79
**Gluteal lymph node** – *use* Lymphatic, Pelvis
**Gluteal vein**
  – *use* Vein, Hypogastric, Right
  – *use* Vein, Hypogastric, Left
**Gluteus maximus muscle**
  – *use* Muscle, Hip, Right
  – *use* Muscle, Hip, Left
**Gluteus medius muscle**
  – *use* Muscle, Hip, Right
  – *use* Muscle, Hip, Left
**Gluteus minimus muscle**
  – *use* Muscle, Hip, Left
  – *use* Muscle, Hip, Right

**GORE® DUALMESH®** – *use* Synthetic Substitute
**Gracilis muscle**
  – *use* Muscle, Upper Leg, Left
  – *use* Muscle, Upper Leg, Right
**Graft**
  – *see* Replacement
  – *see* Supplement
**Great auricular nerve** – *use* Nerve, Cervical Plexus
**Great cerebral vein** – *use* Vein, Intracranial
**Great saphenous vein**
  – *use* Vein, Greater Saphenous, Left
  – *use* Vein, Greater Saphenous, Right
**Greater alar cartilage** – *use* Nose
**Greater occipital nerve** – *use* Nerve, Cervical
**Greater splanchnic nerve** – *use* Nerve, Thoracic Sympathetic
**Greater superficial petrosal nerve** – *use* Nerve, Facial
**Greater trochanter**
  – *use* Femur, Upper, Left
  – *use* Femur, Upper, Right
**Greater tuberosity**
  – *use* Humeral Head, Right
  – *use* Humeral Head, Left
**Greater vestibular** (Bartholin's) **gland** – *use* Gland, Vestibular
**Greater wing**
  – *use* Bone, Sphenoid, Left
  – *use* Bone, Sphenoid, Right
**Guedel airway** – *use* Intraluminal Device, Airway in Mouth and Throat
**Guidance, catheter placement**
  EKG – *see* Measurement, Physiological Systems 4AØ
  Fluoroscopy – *see* Fluoroscopy, Veins B51
  Ultrasound – *see* Ultrasonography, Veins B54

# H

**Hallux**
  – *use* Toe, 1st, Right
  – *use* Toe, 1st, Left
**Hamate bone**
  – *use* Carpal, Right
  – *use* Carpal, Left
**Hancock Bioprosthesis** (aortic) (mitral) **valve** – *use* Zooplastic Tissue in Heart and Great Vessels
**Hancock Bioprosthetic Valved Conduit** – *use* Zooplastic Tissue in Heart and Great Vessels
**Harvesting, stem cells** – *see* Pheresis, Circulatory 6A55
**Head of fibula**
  – *use* Fibula, Right
  – *use* Fibula, Left
**Hearing Aid Assessment** F14Z
**Hearing Assessment** F13Z
**Hearing Device**
  Bone Conduction
    Left 09HE
    Right 09HD
  Insertion of device in
    Left ØNH6
    Right ØNH5
  Multiple Channel Cochlear Prosthesis
    Left 09HE
    Right 09HD
  Removal of device from, Skull ØNPØ
  Revision of device in, Skull ØNWØ
  Single Channel Cochlear Prosthesis
    Left 09HE
    Right 09HD
**Hearing Treatment** FØ9Z
**Heart Assist System**
  External
    Insertion of device in, Heart 02HA
    Removal of device from, Heart 02PA
    Revision of device in, Heart 02WA
  Implantable
    Insertion of device in, Heart 02HA
    Removal of device from, Heart 02PA
    Revision of device in, Heart 02WA
**HeartMate II® Left Ventricular Assist Device (LVAD)** – *use* Implantable Heart Assist System in Heart and Great Vessels
**HeartMate XVE® Left Ventricular Assist Device (LVAD)** – *use* Implantable Heart Assist System in Heart and Great Vessels
**HeartMate® implantable heart assist system** – *see* Insertion of device in, Heart 02HA

**Helix**
– *use* Ear, External, Bilateral
– *use* Ear, External, Left
– *use* Ear, External, Right
**Hemicolectomy** – *see* Resection, Gastrointestinal System ØDT
**Hemicystectomy** – *see* Excision, Urinary System ØTB
**Hemigastrectomy** – *see* Excision, Gastrointestinal System ØDB
**Hemiglossectomy** – *see* Excision, Mouth and Throat ØCB
**Hemilaminectomy**
– *see* Excision, Lower Bones ØQB
– *see* Excision, Upper Bones ØPB
**Hemilaminotomy**
– *see* Drainage, Lower Bones ØQ9
– *see* Drainage, Upper Bones ØP9
– *see* Excision, Lower Bones ØQB
– *see* Excision, Upper Bones ØPB
– *see* Release, Central Nervous System ØØN
– *see* Release, Lower Bones ØQN
– *see* Release, Peripheral Nervous System Ø1N
– *see* Release, Upper Bones ØPN
**Hemilaryngectomy** – *see* Excision, Larynx ØCBS
**Hemimandibulectomy** – *see* Excision, Head and Facial Bones ØNB
**Hemimaxillectomy** – *see* Excision, Head and Facial Bones ØNB
**Hemipylorectomy** – *see* Excision, Gastrointestinal System ØDB
**Hemispherectomy**
– *see* Excision, Central Nervous System ØØB
– *see* Resection, Central Nervous System ØØT
**Hemithyroidectomy**
– *see* Excision, Endocrine System ØGB
– *see* Resection, Endocrine System ØGT
**Hemodialysis** 5A1DØØZ
**Hepatectomy**
– *see* Excision, Hepatobiliary System and Pancreas ØFB
– *see* Resection, Hepatobiliary System and Pancreas ØFT
**Hepatic artery proper** – *use* Artery, Hepatic
**Hepatic flexure** – *use* Colon, Ascending
**Hepatic lymph node** – *use* Lymphatic, Aortic
**Hepatic plexus** – *use* Nerve, Abdominal Sympathetic
**Hepatic portal vein** – *use* Vein, Portal
**Hepaticoduodenostomy**
– *see* Bypass, Hepatobiliary System and Pancreas ØF1
– *see* Drainage, Hepatobiliary System and Pancreas ØF9
**Hepaticotomy** – *see* Drainage, Hepatobiliary System and Pancreas ØF9
**Hepatocholedochostomy** – *see* Drainage, Duct, Common Bile ØF99
**Hepatogastric ligament** – *use* Omentum, Lesser
**Hepatopancreatic ampulla** – *use* Ampulla of Vater
**Hepatopexy**
– *see* Repair, Hepatobiliary System and Pancreas ØFQ
– *see* Reposition, Hepatobiliary System and Pancreas ØFS
**Hepatorrhaphy** – *see* Repair, Hepatobiliary System and Pancreas ØFQ
**Hepatotomy** – *see* Drainage, Hepatobiliary System and Pancreas ØF9
**Herculink (RX) Elite Renal Stent System** – *use* Intraluminal Device
**Herniorrhaphy**
– *see* Repair, Anatomical Regions, General ØWQ
– *see* Repair, Anatomical Regions, Lower Extremities ØYQ
with synthetic substitute
– *see* Supplement, Anatomical Regions, General ØWU
– *see* Supplement, Anatomical Regions, Lower Extremities ØYU
**Hip** (joint) **liner** – *use* Liner in Lower Joints
**Holter monitoring** 4A12X45
**Holter valve ventricular shunt** – *use* Synthetic Substitute
**Humeroradial joint**
– *use* Joint, Elbow, Right
– *use* Joint, Elbow, Left
**Humeroulnar joint**
– *use* Joint, Elbow, Left
– *use* Joint, Elbow, Right
**Humerus, distal**
– *use* Humeral Shaft, Right
– *use* Humeral Shaft, Left

**Hydrocelectomy** – *see* Excision, Male Reproductive System ØVB
**Hydrotherapy**
Assisted exercise in pool – *see* Motor Treatment, Rehabilitation FØ7
Whirlpool – *see* Activities of Daily Living Treatment, Rehabilitation FØ8
**Hymenectomy**
– *see* Excision, Hymen ØUBK
– *see* Resection, Hymen ØUTK
**Hymenoplasty**
– *see* Repair, Hymen ØUQK
– *see* Supplement, Hymen ØUUK
**Hymenorrhaphy** – *see* Repair, Hymen ØUQK
**Hymenotomy**
– *see* Division, Hymen ØU8K
– *see* Drainage, Hymen ØU9K
**Hyoglossus muscle** – *use* Muscle, Tongue, Palate, Pharynx
**Hyoid artery**
– *use* Artery, Thyroid, Right
– *use* Artery, Thyroid, Left
**Hyperalimentation** – *see* Introduction of substance in or on
**Hyperbaric oxygenation**
Decompression sickness treatment – *see* Decompression, Circulatory 6A15
Wound treatment – *see* Assistance, Circulatory 5AØ5
**Hyperthermia**
Radiation Therapy
Abdomen DWY38ZZ
Adrenal Gland DGY28ZZ
Bile Ducts DFY28ZZ
Bladder DTY28ZZ
Bone, Other DPYC8ZZ
Bone Marrow D7YØ8ZZ
Brain DØYØ8ZZ
Brain Stem DØY18ZZ
Breast
Left DMYØ8ZZ
Right DMY18ZZ
Bronchus DBY18ZZ
Cervix DUY18ZZ
Chest DWY28ZZ
Chest Wall DBY78ZZ
Colon DDY58ZZ
Diaphragm DBY88ZZ
Duodenum DDY28ZZ
Ear D9YØ8ZZ
Esophagus DDYØ8ZZ
Eye D8YØ8ZZ
Femur DPY98ZZ
Fibula DPYB8ZZ
Gallbladder DFY18ZZ
Gland
Adrenal DGY28ZZ
Parathyroid DGY48ZZ
Pituitary DGYØ8ZZ
Thyroid DGY58ZZ
Glands, Salivary D9Y68ZZ
Head and Neck DWY18ZZ
Hemibody DWY48ZZ
Humerus DPY68ZZ
Hypopharynx D9Y38ZZ
Ileum DDY48ZZ
Jejunum DDY38ZZ
Kidney DTYØ8ZZ
Larynx D9YB8ZZ
Liver DFYØ8ZZ
Lung DBY28ZZ
Lymphatics
Abdomen D7Y68ZZ
Axillary D7Y48ZZ
Inguinal D7Y88ZZ
Neck D7Y38ZZ
Pelvis D7Y78ZZ
Thorax D7Y58ZZ
Mandible DPY38ZZ
Maxilla DPY28ZZ
Mediastinum DBY68ZZ
Mouth D9Y48ZZ
Nasopharynx D9YD8ZZ
Neck and Head DWY18ZZ
Nerve, Peripheral DØY78ZZ
Nose D9Y18ZZ
Oropharynx D9YF8ZZ
Ovary DUYØ8ZZ
Palate
Hard D9Y88ZZ
Soft D9Y98ZZ
Pancreas DFY38ZZ
Parathyroid Gland DGY48ZZ

**Hyperthermia** – *continued*
Radiation Therapy – *continued*
Pelvic Bones DPY88ZZ
Pelvic Region DWY68ZZ
Pineal Body DGY18ZZ
Pituitary Gland DGYØ8ZZ
Pleura DBY58ZZ
Prostate DVYØ8ZZ
Radius DPY78ZZ
Rectum DDY78ZZ
Rib DPY58ZZ
Sinuses D9Y78ZZ
Skin
Abdomen DHY88ZZ
Arm DHY48ZZ
Back DHY78ZZ
Buttock DHY98ZZ
Chest DHY68ZZ
Face DHY28ZZ
Leg DHYB8ZZ
Neck DHY38ZZ
Skull DPYØ8ZZ
Spinal Cord DØY68ZZ
Spleen D7Y28ZZ
Sternum DPY48ZZ
Stomach DDY18ZZ
Testis DVY18ZZ
Thymus D7Y18ZZ
Thyroid Gland DGY58ZZ
Tibia DPYB8ZZ
Tongue D9Y58ZZ
Trachea DBYØ8ZZ
Ulna DPY78ZZ
Ureter DTY18ZZ
Urethra DTY38ZZ
Uterus DUY28ZZ
Whole Body DWY58ZZ
Whole Body 6A3Z
**Hypnosis** GZFZZZZ
**Hypogastric artery**
– *use* Artery, Internal Iliac, Right
– *use* Artery, Internal Iliac, Left
**Hypopharynx** – *use* Pharynx
**Hypophysectomy**
– *see* Excision, Gland, Pituitary ØGBØ
– *see* Resection, Gland, Pituitary ØGTØ
**Hypophysis** – *use* Gland, Pituitary
**Hypothalamotomy** – *see* Destruction, Thalamus ØØ59
**Hypothenar muscle**
– *use* Muscle, Hand, Right
– *use* Muscle, Hand, Left
**Hypothermia, Whole Body** 6A4Z
**Hysterectomy**
– *see* Excision, Uterus ØUB9
– *see* Resection, Uterus ØUT9
**Hysterolysis** – *see* Release, Uterus ØUN9
**Hysteropexy**
– *see* Repair, Uterus ØUQ9
– *see* Reposition, Uterus ØUS9
**Hysteroplasty** – *see* Repair, Uterus ØUQ9
**Hysterorrhaphy** – *see* Repair, Uterus ØUQ9
**Hysteroscopy** ØUJD8ZZ
**Hysterotomy** – *see* Drainage, Uterus ØU99
**Hysterotrachelectomy** – *see* Resection, Uterus ØUT9
**Hysterotracheloplasty** – *see* Repair, Uterus ØUQ9
**Hysterotrachelorrhaphy** – *see* Repair, Uterus ØUQ9

# I

**IABP (Intra-aortic balloon pump)** – *see* Assistance, Cardiac 5AØ2
**IAEMT (Intraoperative anesthetic effect monitoring and titration)** – *see* Monitoring, Central Nervous 4A1Ø
**Ileal artery** – *use* Artery, Superior Mesenteric
**Ileectomy**
– *see* Excision, Ileum ØDBB
– *see* Resection, Ileum ØDTB
**Ileocolic artery** – *use* Artery, Superior Mesenteric
**Ileocolic vein** – *use* Vein, Colic
**Ileopexy**
– *see* Repair, Ileum ØDQB
– *see* Reposition, Ileum ØDSB
**Ileorrhaphy** – *see* Repair, Ileum ØDQB
**Ileoscopy** ØDJD8ZZ
**Ileostomy**
– *see* Bypass, Ileum ØD1B
– *see* Drainage, Ileum ØD9B

**Ileotomy** – *see* Drainage, Ileum ØD9B
**Ileoureterostomy** – *see* Bypass, Urinary System ØT1
**Iliac crest**
 – *use* Bone, Pelvic, Left
 – *use* Bone, Pelvic, Right
**Iliac fascia**
 – *use* Subcutaneous Tissue and Fascia, Upper Leg, Left
 – *use* Subcutaneous Tissue and Fascia, Upper Leg, Right
**Iliac lymph node** – *use* Lymphatic, Pelvis
**Iliacus muscle**
 – *use* Muscle, Hip, Right
 – *use* Muscle, Hip, Left
**Iliofemoral ligament**
 – *use* Bursa and Ligament, Hip, Left
 – *use* Bursa and Ligament, Hip, Right
**Iliohypogastric nerve** – *use* Nerve, Lumbar Plexus
**Ilioinguinal nerve** – *use* Nerve, Lumbar Plexus
**Iliolumbar artery**
 – *use* Artery, Internal Iliac, Left
 – *use* Artery, Internal Iliac, Right
**Iliolumbar ligament**
 – *use* Bursa and Ligament, Trunk, Left
 – *use* Bursa and Ligament, Trunk, Right
**Iliotibial tract** (band)
 – *use* Subcutaneous Tissue and Fascia, Upper Leg, Right
 – *use* Subcutaneous Tissue and Fascia, Upper Leg, Left
**Ilium**
 – *use* Bone, Pelvic, Left
 – *use* Bone, Pelvic, Right
**Ilizarov external fixator**
 – *use* External Fixation Device, Ring in ØPH
 – *use* External Fixation Device, Ring in ØPS
 – *use* External Fixation Device, Ring in ØQH
 – *use* External Fixation Device, Ring in ØQS
**Ilizarov-Vecklich device**
 – *use* External Fixation Device, Limb Lengthening in ØPH
 – *use* External Fixation Device, Limb Lengthening in ØQH
**Imaging, diagnostic**
 – *see* Plain Radiography
 – *see* Fluoroscopy
 – *see* Computerized Tomography (CT Scan)
 – *see* Magnetic Resonance Imaging (MRI)
 – *see* Ultrasonography
**Immobilization**
 Abdominal Wall 2W33X
 Arm
  Lower
   Left 2W3DX
   Right 2W3CX
  Upper
   Left 2W3BX
   Right 2W3AX
 Back 2W35X
 Chest Wall 2W34X
 Extremity
  Lower
   Left 2W3MX
   Right 2W3LX
  Upper
   Left 2W39X
   Right 2W38X
 Face 2W31X
 Finger
  Left 2W3KX
  Right 2W3JX
 Foot
  Left 2W3TX
  Right 2W3SX
 Hand
  Left 2W3FX
  Right 2W3EX
 Head 2W30X
 Inguinal Region
  Left 2W37X
  Right 2W36X
 Leg
  Lower
   Left 2W3RX
   Right 2W3QX
  Upper
   Left 2W3PX
   Right 2W3NX
 Neck 2W32X
 Thumb
  Left 2W3HX

**Immobilization** – *continued*
 Thumb – *continued*
  Right 2W3GX
 Toe
  Left 2W3VX
  Right 2W3UX
**Immunization** – *see* Introduction of Serum, Toxoid, and Vaccine
**Immunotherapy** – *see* Introduction of Immunotherapeutic Substance
**Immunotherapy, antineoplastic**
 Interferon – *see* Introduction of Low-dose Interleukin-2
 Interleukin-2, high-dose – *see* Introduction of High-dose Interleukin-2
 Interleukin-2, low–dose – *see* Introduction of Low-dose Interleukin-2
 Monoclonal antibody – *see* Introduction of Monoclonal Antibody
 Proleukin, high–dose – *see* Introduction of High-dose Interleukin-2
 Proleukin, low–dose – *see* Introduction of Low-dose Interleukin-2
**Impeller Pump**
 Continuous, Output 5A0221D
 Intermittent, Output 5A0211D
**Implantable cardioverter-defibrillator (ICD)** – *use* Defibrillator Generator in ØJH
**Implantable drug infusion pump** (anti-spasmodic) (chemotherapy)(pain) – *use* Infusion Device, Pump in Subcutaneous Tissue and Fascia
**Implantable glucose monitoring device** – *use* Monitoring Device
**Implantable hemodynamic monitor (IHM)** – *use* Monitoring Device, Hemodynamic in ØJH
**Implantable hemodynamic monitoring system (IHMS)** – *use* Monitoring Device, Hemodynamic in ØJH
**Implantable Miniature Telescope™ (IMT)** – *use* Synthetic Substitute, Intraocular Telescope in Ø8R
**Implantation**
 – *see* Insertion
 – *see* Replacement
**Implanted** (venous)(access) **port** – *use* Vascular Access Device, Reservoir in Subcutaneous Tissue and Fascia
**IMV (intermittent mandatory ventilation)** – *see* Assistance, Respiratory 5A09
**In Vitro Fertilization** 8E0ZXY1
**Incision, abscess** – *see* Drainage
**Incudectomy**
 – *see* Excision, Ear, Nose, Sinus Ø9B
 – *see* Resection, Ear, Nose, Sinus Ø9T
**Incudopexy**
 – *see* Reposition, Ear, Nose, Sinus Ø9S
 – *see* Repair, Ear, Nose, Sinus Ø9Q
**Incus**
 – *use* Auditory Ossicle, Left
 – *use* Auditory Ossicle, Right
**Induction of labor**
 Artificial rupture of membranes – *see* Drainage, Pregnancy 1Ø9
 Oxytocin – *see* Introduction of Hormone
**InDura, intrathecal catheter** (1P) (spinal) – *use* Infusion Device
**Inferior cardiac nerve** – *use* Nerve, Thoracic Sympathetic
**Inferior cerebellar vein** – *use* Vein, Intracranial
**Inferior cerebral vein** – *use* Vein, Intracranial
**Inferior epigastric artery**
 – *use* Artery, External Iliac, Right
 – *use* Artery, External Iliac, Left
**Inferior epigastric lymph node** – *use* Lymphatic, Pelvis
**Inferior genicular artery**
 – *use* Artery, Popliteal, Left
 – *use* Artery, Popliteal, Right
**Inferior gluteal artery**
 – *use* Artery, Internal Iliac, Right
 – *use* Artery, Internal Iliac, Left
**Inferior gluteal nerve** – *use* Nerve, Sacral Plexus
**Inferior hypogastric plexus** – *use* Nerve, Abdominal Sympathetic
**Inferior labial artery** – *use* Artery, Face
**Inferior longitudinal muscle** – *use* Muscle, Tongue, Palate, Pharynx
**Inferior mesenteric ganglion** – *use* Nerve, Abdominal Sympathetic

**Inferior mesenteric lymph node** – *use* Lymphatic, Mesenteric
**Inferior mesenteric plexus** – *use* Nerve, Abdominal Sympathetic
**Inferior oblique muscle**
 – *use* Muscle, Extraocular, Right
 – *use* Muscle, Extraocular, Left
**Inferior pancreaticoduodenal artery** – *use* Artery, Superior Mesenteric
**Inferior phrenic artery** – *use* Aorta, Abdominal
**Inferior rectus muscle**
 – *use* Muscle, Extraocular, Right
 – *use* Muscle, Extraocular, Left
**Inferior suprarenal artery**
 – *use* Artery, Renal, Left
 – *use* Artery, Renal, Right
**Inferior tarsal plate**
 – *use* Eyelid, Lower, Right
 – *use* Eyelid, Lower, Left
**Inferior thyroid vein**
 – *use* Vein, Innominate, Left
 – *use* Vein, Innominate, Right
**Inferior tibiofibular joint**
 – *use* Joint, Ankle, Right
 – *use* Joint, Ankle, Left
**Inferior turbinate** – *use* Turbinate, Nasal
**Inferior ulnar collateral artery**
 – *use* Artery, Brachial, Right
 – *use* Artery, Brachial, Left
**Inferior vesical artery**
 – *use* Artery, Internal Iliac, Right
 – *use* Artery, Internal Iliac, Left
**Infraauricular lymph node** – *use* Lymphatic, Head
**Infraclavicular** (deltopectoral) **lymph node**
 – *use* Lymphatic, Upper Extremity, Left
 – *use* Lymphatic, Upper Extremity, Right
**Infrahyoid muscle**
 – *use* Muscle, Neck, Left
 – *use* Muscle, Neck, Right
**Infraparotid lymph node** – *use* Lymphatic, Head
**Infraspinatus fascia**
 – *use* Subcutaneous Tissue and Fascia, Upper Arm, Right
 – *use* Subcutaneous Tissue and Fascia, Upper Arm, Left
**Infraspinatus muscle**
 – *use* Muscle, Shoulder, Right
 – *use* Muscle, Shoulder, Left
**Infundibulopelvic ligament** – *use* Uterine Supporting Structure
**Infusion** – *see* Introduction of substance in or on
**Infusion device, pump**
 Insertion of device in
  Abdomen ØJH8
  Back ØJH7
  Chest ØJH6
  Lower Arm
   Left ØJHH
   Right ØJHG
  Lower Leg
   Left ØJHP
   Right ØJHN
  Trunk ØJHT
  Upper Arm
   Left ØJHF
   Right ØJHD
  Upper Leg
   Left ØJHM
   Right ØJHL
 Removal of device from
  Lower Extremity ØJPW
  Trunk ØJPT
  Upper Extremity ØJPV
 Revision of device in
  Lower Extremity ØJWW
  Trunk ØJWT
  Upper Extremity ØJWV
**Infusion, glucarpidase**
 Central vein 3E043GQ
 Peripheral vein 3E033GQ
**Inguinal canal**
 – *use* Inguinal Region, Right
 – *use* Inguinal Region, Left
 – *use* Inguinal Region, Bilateral
**Inguinal triangle**
 – *use* Inguinal Region, Right
 – *use* Inguinal Region, Bilateral
 – *use* Inguinal Region, Left
**Injection** – *see* Introduction of substance in or on

**Injection reservoir, port** – *use* Vascular Access Device, Reservoir in Subcutaneous Tissue and Fascia

**Injection reservoir, pump** – *use* Infusion Device, Pump in Subcutaneous Tissue and Fascia

**Insemination, artificial** 3E0P7LZ

**Insertion**
Antimicrobial envelope – *see* Introduction of Anti-infective
Aqueous drainage shunt
– *see* Bypass, Eye 081
– *see* Drainage, Eye 089
Products of Conception 10H0
Spinal Stabilization Device
– *see* Insertion of device in, Upper Joints 0RH
– *see* Insertion of device in, Lower Joints 0SH

**Insertion of device in**
Abdominal Wall 0WHF
Acetabulum
Left 0QH5
Right 0QH4
Anal Sphincter 0DHR
Ankle Region
Left 0YHL
Right 0YHK
Anus 0DHQ
Aorta
Abdominal 04H0
Thoracic 02HW
Arm
Lower
Left 0XHF
Right 0XHD
Upper
Left 0XH9
Right 0XH8
Artery
Anterior Tibial
Left 04HQ
Right 04HP
Axillary
Left 03H6
Right 03H5
Brachial
Left 03H8
Right 03H7
Celiac 04H1
Colic
Left 04H7
Middle 04H8
Right 04H6
Common Carotid
Left 03HJ
Right 03HH
Common Iliac
Left 04HD
Right 04HC
External Carotid
Left 03HN
Right 03HM
External Iliac
Left 04HJ
Right 04HH
Face 03HR
Femoral
Left 04HL
Right 04HK
Foot
Left 04HW
Right 04HV
Gastric 04H2
Hand
Left 03HF
Right 03HD
Hepatic 04H3
Inferior Mesenteric 04HB
Innominate 03H2
Internal Carotid
Left 03HL
Right 03HK
Internal Iliac
Left 04HF
Right 04HE
Internal Mammary
Left 03H1
Right 03H0
Intracranial 03HG
Lower 04HY
Peroneal
Left 04HU
Right 04HT
Popliteal
Left 04HN
Right 04HM

**Insertion of device in** – *continued*
Artery – *continued*
Posterior Tibial
Left 04HS
Right 04HR
Pulmonary
Left 02HR
Right 02HQ
Pulmonary Trunk 02HP
Radial
Left 03HC
Right 03HB
Renal
Left 04HA
Right 04H9
Splenic 04H4
Subclavian
Left 03H4
Right 03H3
Superior Mesenteric 04H5
Temporal
Left 03HT
Right 03HS
Thyroid
Left 03HV
Right 03HU
Ulnar
Left 03HA
Right 03H9
Upper 03HY
Vertebral
Left 03HQ
Right 03HP
Atrium
Left 02H7
Right 02H6
Axilla
Left 0XH5
Right 0XH4
Back
Lower 0WHL
Upper 0WHK
Bladder 0THB
Bladder Neck 0THC
Bone
Ethmoid
Left 0NHG
Right 0NHF
Facial 0NHW
Frontal
Left 0NH2
Right 0NH1
Hyoid 0NHX
Lacrimal
Left 0NHJ
Right 0NHH
Lower 0QHY
Nasal 0NHB
Occipital
Left 0NH8
Right 0NH7
Palatine
Left 0NHL
Right 0NHK
Parietal
Left 0NH4
Right 0NH3
Pelvic
Left 0QH3
Right 0QH2
Sphenoid
Left 0NHD
Right 0NHC
Temporal
Left 0NH6
Right 0NH5
Upper 0PHY
Zygomatic
Left 0NHN
Right 0NHM
Brain 00H0
Breast
Bilateral 0HHV
Left 0HHU
Right 0HHT
Bronchus
Lingula 0BH9
Lower Lobe
Left 0BHB
Right 0BH6
Main
Left 0BH7
Right 0BH3

**Insertion of device in** – *continued*
Bronchus – *continued*
Middle Lobe, Right 0BH5
Upper Lobe
Left 0BH8
Right 0BH4
Buttock
Left 0YH1
Right 0YH0
Carpal
Left 0PHN
Right 0PHM
Cavity, Cranial 0WH1
Cerebral Ventricle 00H6
Cervix 0UHC
Chest Wall 0WH8
Cisterna Chyli 07HL
Clavicle
Left 0PHB
Right 0PH9
Coccyx 0QHS
Cul-de-sac 0UHF
Diaphragm
Left 0BHS
Right 0BHR
Disc
Cervical Vertebral 0RH3
Cervicothoracic Vertebral 0RH5
Lumbar Vertebral 0SH2
Lumbosacral 0SH4
Thoracic Vertebral 0RH9
Thoracolumbar Vertebral 0RHB
Duct
Hepatobiliary 0FHB
Pancreatic 0FHD
Duodenum 0DH9
Ear
Left 09HE
Right 09HD
Elbow Region
Left 0XHC
Right 0XHB
Epididymis and Spermatic Cord 0VHM
Esophagus 0DH5
Extremity
Lower
Left 0YHB
Right 0YH9
Upper
Left 0XH7
Right 0XH6
Eye
Left 08H1
Right 08H0
Face 0WH2
Fallopian Tube 0UH8
Femoral Region
Left 0YH8
Right 0YH7
Femoral Shaft
Left 0QH9
Right 0QH8
Femur
Lower
Left 0QHC
Right 0QHB
Upper
Left 0QH7
Right 0QH6
Fibula
Left 0QHK
Right 0QHJ
Foot
Left 0YHN
Right 0YHM
Gallbladder 0FH4
Gastrointestinal Tract 0WHP
Genitourinary Tract 0WHR
Gland, Endocrine 0GHS
Glenoid Cavity
Left 0PH8
Right 0PH7
Hand
Left 0XHK
Right 0XHJ
Head 0WH0
Heart 02HA
Humeral Head
Left 0PHD
Right 0PHC
Humeral Shaft
Left 0PHG
Right 0PHF

## Insertion of device in – *continued*

Ileum ØDHB
Inguinal Region
   Left ØYH6
   Right ØYH5
Intestine
   Large ØDHE
   Small ØDH8
Jaw
   Lower ØWH5
   Upper ØWH4
Jejunum ØDHA
Joint
   Acromioclavicular
      Left ØRHH
      Right ØRHG
   Ankle
      Left ØSHG
      Right ØSHF
   Carpal
      Left ØRHR
      Right ØRHQ
   Cervical Vertebral ØRH1
   Cervicothoracic Vertebral ØRH4
   Coccygeal ØSH6
   Elbow
      Left ØRHM
      Right ØRHL
   Finger Phalangeal
      Left ØRHX
      Right ØRHW
   Hip
      Left ØSHB
      Right ØSH9
   Knee
      Left ØSHD
      Right ØSHC
   Lumbar Vertebral ØSHØ
   Lumbosacral ØSH3
   Metacarpocarpal
      Left ØRHT
      Right ØRHS
   Metacarpophalangeal
      Left ØRHV
      Right ØRHU
   Metatarsal–Phalangeal
      Left ØSHN
      Right ØSHM
   Metatarsal–Tarsal
      Left ØSHL
      Right ØSHK
   Occipital–cervical ØRHØ
   Sacrococcygeal ØSH5
   Sacroiliac
      Left ØSH8
      Right ØSH7
   Shoulder
      Left ØRHK
      Right ØRHJ
   Sternoclavicular
      Left ØRHF
      Right ØRHE
   Tarsal
      Left ØSHJ
      Right ØSHH
   Temporomandibular
      Left ØRHD
      Right ØRHC
   Thoracic Vertebral ØRH6
   Thoracolumbar Vertebral ØRHA
   Toe Phalangeal
      Left ØSHQ
      Right ØSHP
   Wrist
      Left ØRHP
      Right ØRHN
Kidney ØTH5
Knee Region
   Left ØYHG
   Right ØYHF
Leg
   Lower
      Left ØYHJ
      Right ØYHH
   Upper
      Left ØYHD
      Right ØYHC
Liver ØFHØ
   Left Lobe ØFH2
   Right Lobe ØFH1
Lung
   Left ØBHL
   Right ØBHK

## Insertion of device in – *continued*

Lymphatic Ø7HN
   Thoracic Duct Ø7HK
Mandible
   Left ØNHV
   Right ØNHT
Maxilla
   Left ØNHS
   Right ØNHR
Mediastinum ØWHC
Metacarpal
   Left ØPHQ
   Right ØPHP
Metatarsal
   Left ØQHP
   Right ØQHN
Mouth and Throat ØCHY
Muscle
   Lower ØKHY
   Upper ØKHX
Nasopharynx Ø9HN
Neck ØWH6
Nerve
   Cranial ØØHE
   Peripheral Ø1HY
Nipple
   Left ØHHX
   Right ØHHW
Oral Cavity and Throat ØWH3
Orbit
   Left ØNHQ
   Right ØNHP
Ovary ØUH3
Pancreas ØFHG
Patella
   Left ØQHF
   Right ØQHD
Pelvic Cavity ØWHJ
Penis ØVHS
Pericardial Cavity ØWHD
Pericardium Ø2HN
Perineum
   Female ØWHN
   Male ØWHM
Peritoneal Cavity ØWHG
Phalanx
   Finger
      Left ØPHV
      Right ØPHT
   Thumb
      Left ØPHS
      Right ØPHR
   Toe
      Left ØQHR
      Right ØQHQ
Pleural Cavity
   Left ØWHB
   Right ØWH9
Prostate ØVHØ
Prostate and Seminal Vesicles ØVH4
Radius
   Left ØPHJ
   Right ØPHH
Rectum ØDHP
Respiratory Tract ØWHQ
Retroperitoneum ØWHH
Rib
   Left ØPH2
   Right ØPH1
Sacrum ØQH1
Scapula
   Left ØPH6
   Right ØPH5
Scrotum and Tunica Vaginalis ØVH8
Shoulder Region
   Left ØXH3
   Right ØXH2
Skull ØNHØ
Spinal Canal ØØHU
Spinal Cord ØØHV
Spleen Ø7HP
Sternum ØPHØ
Stomach ØDH6
Subcutaneous Tissue and Fascia
   Abdomen ØJH8
   Back ØJH7
   Buttock ØJH9
   Chest ØJH6
   Face ØJH1
   Foot
      Left ØJHR
      Right ØJHQ

## Insertion of device in – *continued*

Subcutaneous Tissue and Fascia – *continued*
   Hand
      Left ØJHK
      Right ØJHJ
   Head and Neck ØJHS
   Lower Arm
      Left ØJHH
      Right ØJHG
   Lower Extremity ØJHW
   Lower Leg
      Left ØJHP
      Right ØJHN
   Neck
      Anterior ØJH4
      Posterior ØJH5
   Pelvic Region ØJHC
   Perineum ØJHB
   Scalp ØJHØ
   Trunk ØJHT
   Upper Arm
      Left ØJHF
      Right ØJHD
   Upper Extremity ØJHV
   Upper Leg
      Left ØJHM
      Right ØJHL
Tarsal
   Left ØQHM
   Right ØQHL
Testis ØVHD
Thymus Ø7HM
Tibia
   Left ØQHH
   Right ØQHG
Tongue ØCH7
Trachea ØBH1
Tracheobronchial Tree ØBHØ
Ulna
   Left ØPHL
   Right ØPHK
Ureter ØTH9
Urethra ØTHD
Uterus ØUH9
Uterus and Cervix ØUHD
Vagina ØUHG
Vagina and Cul-de-sac ØUHH
Vas Deferens ØVHR
Vein
   Axillary
      Left Ø5H8
      Right Ø5H7
   Azygos Ø5HØ
   Basilic
      Left Ø5HC
      Right Ø5HB
   Brachial
      Left Ø5HA
      Right Ø5H9
   Cephalic
      Left Ø5HF
      Right Ø5HD
   Colic Ø6H7
   Common Iliac
      Left Ø6HD
      Right Ø6HC
   Coronary Ø2H4
   Esophageal Ø6H3
   External Iliac
      Left Ø6HG
      Right Ø6HF
   External Jugular
      Left Ø5HQ
      Right Ø5HP
   Face
      Left Ø5HV
      Right Ø5HT
   Femoral
      Left Ø6HN
      Right Ø6HM
   Foot
      Left Ø6HV
      Right Ø6HT
   Gastric Ø6H2
   Greater Saphenous
      Left Ø6HQ
      Right Ø6HP
   Hand
      Left Ø5HH
      Right Ø5HG
   Hemiazygos Ø5H1
   Hepatic Ø6H4

**Insertion of device in** – *continued*
  Vein – *continued*
    Hypogastric
      Left 06HJ
      Right 06HH
    Inferior Mesenteric 06H6
    Innominate
      Left 05H4
      Right 05H3
    Internal Jugular
      Left 05HN
      Right 05HM
    Intracranial 05HL
    Lesser Saphenous
      Left 06HS
      Right 06HR
    Lower 06HY
    Portal 06H8
    Pulmonary
      Left 02HT
      Right 02HS
    Renal
      Left 06HB
      Right 06H9
    Splenic 06H1
    Subclavian
      Left 05H6
      Right 05H5
    Superior Mesenteric 06H5
    Upper 05HY
    Vertebral
      Left 05HS
      Right 05HR
  Vena Cava
    Inferior 06H0
    Superior 02HV
  Ventricle
    Left 02HL
    Right 02HK
  Vertebra
    Cervical 0PH3
    Lumbar 0QH0
    Thoracic 0PH4
  Wrist Region
    Left 0XHH
    Right 0XHG

**Inspection**
  Abdominal Wall 0WJF
  Ankle Region
    Left 0YJL
    Right 0YJK
  Arm
    Lower
      Left 0XJF
      Right 0XJD
    Upper
      Left 0XJ9
      Right 0XJ8
  Artery
    Lower 04JY
    Upper 03JY
  Axilla
    Left 0XJ5
    Right 0XJ4
  Back
    Lower 0WJL
    Upper 0WJK
  Bladder 0TJB
  Bone
    Facial 0NJW
    Lower 0QJY
    Nasal 0NJB
    Upper 0PJY
  Bone Marrow 07JT
  Brain 00J0
  Breast
    Left 0HJU
    Right 0HJT
  Bursa and Ligament
    Lower 0MJY
    Upper 0MJX
  Buttock
    Left 0YJ1
    Right 0YJ0
  Cavity, Cranial 0WJ1
  Chest Wall 0WJ8
  Cisterna Chyli 07JL
  Diaphragm 0BJT
  Disc
    Cervical Vertebral 0RJ3
    Cervicothoracic Vertebral 0RJ5
    Lumbar Vertebral 0SJ2
    Lumbosacral 0SJ4

**Inspection** – *continued*
  Disc – *continued*
    Thoracic Vertebral 0RJ9
    Thoracolumbar Vertebral 0RJB
  Duct
    Hepatobiliary 0FJB
    Pancreatic 0FJD
  Ear
    Inner
      Left 09JE
      Right 09JD
    Left 09JJ
    Right 09JH
  Elbow Region
    Left 0XJC
    Right 0XJB
  Epididymis and Spermatic Cord 0VJM
  Extremity
    Lower
      Left 0YJB
      Right 0YJ9
    Upper
      Left 0XJ7
      Right 0XJ6
  Eye
    Left 08J1XZZ
    Right 08J0XZZ
  Face 0WJ2
  Fallopian Tube 0UJ8
  Femoral Region
    Bilateral 0YJE
    Left 0YJ8
    Right 0YJ7
  Finger Nail 0HJQXZZ
  Foot
    Left 0YJN
    Right 0YJM
  Gallbladder 0FJ4
  Gastrointestinal Tract 0WJP
  Genitourinary Tract 0WJR
  Gland
    Adrenal 0GJ5
    Endocrine 0GJS
    Pituitary 0GJ0
    Salivary 0CJA
  Great Vessel 02JY
  Hand
    Left 0XJK
    Right 0XJJ
  Head 0WJ0
  Heart 02JA
  Inguinal Region
    Bilateral 0YJA
    Left 0YJ6
    Right 0YJ5
  Intestinal Tract
    Lower 0DJD
    Upper 0DJ0
  Jaw
    Lower 0WJ5
    Upper 0WJ4
  Joint
    Acromioclavicular
      Left 0RJH
      Right 0RJG
    Ankle
      Left 0SJG
      Right 0SJF
    Carpal
      Left 0RJR
      Right 0RJQ
    Cervical Vertebral 0RJ1
    Cervicothoracic Vertebral 0RJ4
    Coccygeal 0SJ6
    Elbow
      Left 0RJM
      Right 0RJL
    Finger Phalangeal
      Left 0RJX
      Right 0RJW
    Hip
      Left 0SJB
      Right 0SJ9
    Knee
      Left 0SJD
      Right 0SJC
    Lumbar Vertebral 0SJ0
    Lumbosacral 0SJ3
    Metacarpocarpal
      Left 0RJT
      Right 0RJS
    Metacarpophalangeal
      Left 0RJV

**Inspection** – *continued*
  Joint – *continued*
    Metacarpophalangeal – *continued*
      Right 0RJU
    Metatarsal–Phalangeal
      Left 0SJN
      Right 0SJM
    Metatarsal–Tarsal
      Left 0SJL
      Right 0SJK
    Occipital–cervical 0RJ0
    Sacrococcygeal 0SJ5
    Sacroiliac
      Left 0SJ8
      Right 0SJ7
    Shoulder
      Left 0RJK
      Right 0RJJ
    Sternoclavicular
      Left 0RJF
      Right 0RJE
    Tarsal
      Left 0SJJ
      Right 0SJH
    Temporomandibular
      Left 0RJD
      Right 0RJC
    Thoracic Vertebral 0RJ6
    Thoracolumbar Vertebral 0RJA
    Toe Phalangeal
      Left 0SJQ
      Right 0SJP
    Wrist
      Left 0RJP
      Right 0RJN
  Kidney 0TJ5
  Knee Region
    Left 0YJG
    Right 0YJF
  Larynx 0CJS
  Leg
    Lower
      Left 0YJJ
      Right 0YJH
    Upper
      Left 0YJD
      Right 0YJC
  Lens
    Left 08JKXZZ
    Right 08JJXZZ
  Liver 0FJ0
  Lung
    Left 0BJL
    Right 0BJK
  Lymphatic 07JN
    Thoracic Duct 07JK
  Mediastinum 0WJC
  Mesentery 0DJV
  Mouth and Throat 0CJY
  Muscle
    Extraocular
      Left 08JM
      Right 08JL
    Lower 0KJY
    Upper 0KJX
  Neck 0WJ6
  Nerve
    Cranial 00JE
    Peripheral 01JY
  Nose 09JK
  Omentum 0DJU
  Oral Cavity and Throat 0WJ3
  Ovary 0UJ3
  Pancreas 0FJG
  Parathyroid Gland 0GJR
  Pelvic Cavity 0WJJ
  Penis 0VJS
  Pericardial Cavity 0WJD
  Perineum
    Female 0WJN
    Male 0WJM
  Peritoneal Cavity 0WJG
  Peritoneum 0DJW
  Pineal Body 0GJ1
  Pleura 0BJQ
  Pleural Cavity
    Left 0WJB
    Right 0WJ9
  Products of Conception 10J0
    Ectopic 10J2
    Retained 10J1
  Prostate and Seminal Vesicles 0VJ4
  Respiratory Tract 0WJQ

**Inspection** – *continued*
  Retroperitoneum ØWJH
  Scrotum and Tunica Vaginalis ØVJ8
  Shoulder Region
    Left ØXJ3
    Right ØXJ2
  Sinus Ø9JY
  Skin ØHJPXZZ
  Skull ØNJØ
  Spinal Canal ØØJU
  Spinal Cord ØØJV
  Spleen Ø7JP
  Stomach ØDJ6
  Subcutaneous Tissue and Fascia
    Head and Neck ØJJS
    Lower Extremity ØJJW
    Trunk ØJJT
    Upper Extremity ØJJV
  Tendon
    Lower ØLJY
    Upper ØLJX
  Testis ØVJD
  Thymus Ø7JM
  Thyroid Gland ØGJK
  Toe Nail ØHJRXZZ
  Trachea ØBJ1
  Tracheobronchial Tree ØBJØ
  Tympanic Membrane
    Left Ø9J8
    Right Ø9J7
  Ureter ØTJ9
  Urethra ØTJD
  Uterus and Cervix ØUJD
  Vagina and Cul-de-sac ØUJH
  Vas Deferens ØVJR
  Vein
    Lower Ø6JY
    Upper Ø5JY
  Vulva ØUJM
  Wrist Region
    Left ØXJH
    Right ØXJG
**Instillation** – *see* Introduction of substance in or on
**Insufflation** – *see* Introduction of substance in or on
**Interatrial septum** – *use* Septum, Atrial
**Interbody fusion** (spine) **cage**
  – *use* Interbody Fusion Device in Upper Joints
  – *use* Interbody Fusion Device in Lower Joints
**Intercarpal joint**
  – *use* Joint, Carpal, Right
  – *use* Joint, Carpal, Left
**Intercarpal ligament**
  – *use* Bursa and Ligament, Hand, Right
  – *use* Bursa and Ligament, Hand, Left
**Interclavicular ligament**
  – *use* Bursa and Ligament, Shoulder, Right
  – *use* Bursa and Ligament, Shoulder, Left
**Intercostal lymph node** – *use* Lymphatic, Thorax
**Intercostal muscle**
  – *use* Muscle, Thorax, Right
  – *use* Muscle, Thorax, Left
**Intercostal nerve** – *use* Nerve, Thoracic
**Intercostobrachial nerve** – *use* Nerve, Thoracic
**Intercuneiform joint**
  – *use* Joint, Tarsal, Right
  – *use* Joint, Tarsal, Left
**Intercuneiform ligament**
  – *use* Bursa and Ligament, Foot, Left
  – *use* Bursa and Ligament, Foot, Right
**Intermediate cuneiform bone**
  – *use* Tarsal, Right
  – *use* Tarsal, Left
**Intermittent mandatory ventilation** – *see* Assistance, Respiratory 5AØ9
**Intermittent Negative Airway Pressure**
  24–96 Consecutive Hours, Ventilation 5AØ945B
  Greater than 96 Consecutive Hours, Ventilation 5AØ955B
  Less than 24 Consecutive Hours, Ventilation 5AØ935B
**Intermittent Positive Airway Pressure**
  24–96 Consecutive Hours, Ventilation 5AØ9458
  Greater than 96 Consecutive Hours, Ventilation 5AØ9558
  Less than 24 Consecutive Hours, Ventilation 5AØ9358
**Intermittent positive pressure breathing** – *see* Assistance, Respiratory 5AØ9
**Internal** (basal) **cerebral vein** – *use* Vein, Intracranial
**Internal anal sphincter** – *use* Anal Sphincter
**Internal carotid plexus** – *use* Nerve, Head and Neck Sympathetic

**Internal iliac vein**
  – *use* Vein, Hypogastric, Right
  – *use* Vein, Hypogastric, Left
**Internal maxillary artery**
  – *use* Artery, External Carotid, Left
  – *use* Artery, External Carotid, Right
**Internal naris** – *use* Nose
**Internal oblique muscle**
  – *use* Muscle, Abdomen, Right
  – *use* Muscle, Abdomen, Left
**Internal pudendal artery**
  – *use* Artery, Internal Iliac, Right
  – *use* Artery, Internal Iliac, Left
**Internal pudendal vein**
  – *use* Vein, Hypogastric, Right
  – *use* Vein, Hypogastric, Left
**Internal thoracic artery**
  – *use* Artery, Subclavian, Right
  – *use* Artery, Subclavian, Left
  – *use* Artery, Internal Mammary, Left
  – *use* Artery, Internal Mammary, Right
**Internal urethral sphincter** – *use* Urethra
**Interphalangeal (IP) joint**
  – *use* Joint, Finger Phalangeal, Left
  – *use* Joint, Toe Phalangeal, Right
  – *use* Joint, Toe Phalangeal, Left
  – *use* Joint, Finger Phalangeal, Right
**Interphalangeal ligament**
  – *use* Bursa and Ligament, Hand, Left
  – *use* Bursa and Ligament, Hand, Right
  – *use* Bursa and Ligament, Foot, Right
  – *use* Bursa and Ligament, Foot, Left
**Interrogation, cardiac rhythm related device**
  Interrogation only – *see* Measurement, Cardiac 4BØ2
  With cardiac function testing – *see* Measurement, Cardiac 4AØ2
**Interruption** – *see* Occlusion
**Interspinalis muscle**
  – *use* Muscle, Trunk, Right
  – *use* Muscle, Trunk, Left
**Interspinous ligament**
  – *use* Bursa and Ligament, Trunk, Right
  – *use* Bursa and Ligament, Trunk, Left
**Interspinous process spinal stabilization device**
  – *use* Spinal Stabilization Device, Interspinous Process in ØRH
  – *use* Spinal Stabilization Device, Interspinous Process in ØSH
**InterStim® Therapy lead** – *use* Neurostimulator Lead in Peripheral Nervous System
**InterStim® Therapy neurostimulator** – *use* Stimulator Generator, Single Array in ØJH
**Intertransversarius muscle**
  – *use* Muscle, Trunk, Left
  – *use* Muscle, Trunk, Right
**Intertransverse ligament**
  – *use* Bursa and Ligament, Trunk, Right
  – *use* Bursa and Ligament, Trunk, Left
**Interventricular foramen** (Monro) – *use* Cerebral Ventricle
**Interventricular septum** – *use* Septum, Ventricular
**Intestinal lymphatic trunk** – *use* Cisterna Chyli
**Intraluminal Device**
  Airway
    Esophagus ØDH5
    Mouth and Throat ØCHY
    Nasopharynx Ø9HN
  Bioactive
    Occlusion
      Common Carotid
        Left Ø3LJ
        Right Ø3LH
      External Carotid
        Left Ø3LN
        Right Ø3LM
      Internal Carotid
        Left Ø3LL
        Right Ø3LK
      Intracranial Ø3LG
      Vertebral
        Left Ø3LQ
        Right Ø3LP
    Restriction
      Common Carotid
        Left Ø3VJ
        Right Ø3VH
      External Carotid
        Left Ø3VN
        Right Ø3VM

**Intraluminal Device** – *continued*
  Bioactive – *continued*
    Restriction – *continued*
      Internal Carotid
        Left Ø3VL
        Right Ø3VK
      Intracranial Ø3VG
      Vertebral
        Left Ø3VQ
        Right Ø3VP
  Endobronchial Valve
    Lingula ØBH9
    Lower Lobe
      Left ØBHB
      Right ØBH6
    Main
      Left ØBH7
      Right ØBH3
    Middle Lobe, Right ØBH5
    Upper Lobe
      Left ØBH8
      Right ØBH4
  Endotracheal Airway
    Change device in, Trachea ØB21XEZ
    Insertion of device in, Trachea ØBH1
  Pessary
    Change device in, Vagina and Cul-de-sac ØU2HXGZ
    Insertion of device in
      Cul-de-sac ØUHF
      Vagina ØUHG
**Intramedullary (IM) rod** (nail)
  – *use* Internal Fixation Device, Intramedullary in Upper Bones
  – *use* Internal Fixation Device, Intramedullary in Lower Bones
**Intramedullary skeletal kinetic distractor (ISKD)**
  – *use* Internal Fixation Device, Intramedullary in Upper Bones
  – *use* Internal Fixation Device, Intramedullary in Lower Bones
**Intraocular Telescope**
  Left Ø8RK3ØZ
  Right Ø8RJ3ØZ
**Intraoperative Radiation Therapy (IORT)**
  Anus DDY8CZZ
  Bile Ducts DFY2CZZ
  Bladder DTY2CZZ
  Cervix DUY1CZZ
  Colon DDY5CZZ
  Duodenum DDY2CZZ
  Gallbladder DFY1CZZ
  Ileum DDY4CZZ
  Jejunum DDY3CZZ
  Kidney DTY0CZZ
  Larynx D9YBCZZ
  Liver DFY0CZZ
  Mouth D9Y4CZZ
  Nasopharynx D9YDCZZ
  Ovary DUY0CZZ
  Pancreas DFY3CZZ
  Pharynx D9YCCZZ
  Prostate DVY0CZZ
  Rectum DDY7CZZ
  Stomach DDY1CZZ
  Ureter DTY1CZZ
  Urethra DTY3CZZ
  Uterus DUY2CZZ
**Intrauterine device (IUD)** – *use* Contraceptive Device in Female Reproductive System
**Introduction of substance in or on**
  Artery
    Central 3EØ6
      Analgesics 3EØ6
      Anesthetic, Intracirculatory 3EØ6
      Anti-infective 3EØ6
      Anti-inflammatory 3EØ6
      Antiarrhythmic 3EØ6
      Antineoplastic 3EØ6
      Destructive Agent 3EØ6
      Diagnostic Substance, Other 3EØ6
      Electrolytic Substance 3EØ6
      Hormone 3EØ6
      Hypnotics 3EØ6
      Immunotherapeutic 3EØ6
      Nutritional Substance 3EØ6
      Platelet Inhibitor 3EØ6
      Radioactive Substance 3EØ6
      Sedatives 3EØ6
      Serum 3EØ6
      Thrombolytic 3EØ6
      Toxoid 3EØ6

**Introduction of substance in or on** – *continued*
- Artery – *continued*
  - Central – *continued*
    - Vaccine 3E06
    - Vasopressor 3E06
    - Water Balance Substance 3E06
  - Coronary 3E07
    - Diagnostic Substance, Other 3E07
    - Platelet Inhibitor 3E07
    - Thrombolytic 3E07
  - Peripheral 3E05
    - Analgesics 3E05
    - Anesthetic, Intracirculatory 3E05
    - Anti-infective 3E05
    - Anti-inflammatory 3E05
    - Antiarrhythmic 3E05
    - Antineoplastic 3E05
    - Destructive Agent 3E05
    - Diagnostic Substance, Other 3E05
    - Electrolytic Substance 3E05
    - Hormone 3E05
    - Hypnotics 3E05
    - Immunotherapeutic 3E05
    - Nutritional Substance 3E05
    - Platelet Inhibitor 3E05
    - Radioactive Substance 3E05
    - Sedatives 3E05
    - Serum 3E05
    - Thrombolytic 3E05
    - Toxoid 3E05
    - Vaccine 3E05
    - Vasopressor 3E05
    - Water Balance Substance 3E05
- Biliary Tract 3E0J
  - Analgesics 3E0J
  - Anesthetic, Local 3E0J
  - Anti-infective 3E0J
  - Anti-inflammatory 3E0J
  - Antineoplastic 3E0J
  - Destructive Agent 3E0J
  - Diagnostic Substance, Other 3E0J
  - Electrolytic Substance 3E0J
  - Gas 3E0J
  - Hypnotics 3E0J
  - Islet Cells, Pancreatic 3E0J
  - Nutritional Substance 3E0J
  - Radioactive Substance 3E0J
  - Sedatives 3E0J
  - Water Balance Substance 3E0J
- Bone 3E0V
  - Analgesics 3E0V3NZ
  - Anesthetic, Local 3E0V3BZ
  - Anti-infective 3E0V32
  - Anti-inflammatory 3E0V33Z
  - Antineoplastic 3E0V30
  - Destructive Agent 3E0V3TZ
  - Diagnostic Substance, Other 3E0V3KZ
  - Electrolytic Substance 3E0V37Z
  - Hypnotics 3E0V3NZ
  - Nutritional Substance 3E0V36Z
  - Radioactive Substance 3E0V3HZ
  - Sedatives 3E0V3NZ
  - Water Balance Substance 3E0V37Z
- Bone Marrow 3E0A3GC
  - Antineoplastic 3E0A30
- Brain 3E0Q3GC
  - Analgesics 3E0Q3NZ
  - Anesthetic, Local 3E0Q3BZ
  - Anti-infective 3E0Q32
  - Anti-inflammatory 3E0Q33Z
  - Antineoplastic 3E0Q
  - Destructive Agent 3E0Q3TZ
  - Diagnostic Substance, Other 3E0Q3KZ
  - Electrolytic Substance 3E0Q37Z
  - Gas 3E0Q
  - Hypnotics 3E0Q3NZ
  - Nutritional Substance 3E0Q36Z
  - Radioactive Substance 3E0Q3HZ
  - Sedatives 3E0Q3NZ
  - Stem Cells
    - Embryonic 3E0Q
    - Somatic 3E0Q
  - Water Balance Substance 3E0Q37Z
- Cranial Cavity 3E0Q3GC
  - Analgesics 3E0Q3NZ
  - Anesthetic, Local 3E0Q3BZ
  - Anti-infective 3E0Q32
  - Anti-inflammatory 3E0Q33Z
  - Antineoplastic 3E0Q
  - Destructive Agent 3E0Q3TZ
  - Diagnostic Substance, Other 3E0Q3KZ
  - Electrolytic Substance 3E0Q37Z
  - Gas 3E0Q

**Introduction of substance in or on** – *continued*
- Cranial Cavity – *continued*
  - Hypnotics 3E0Q3NZ
  - Nutritional Substance 3E0Q36Z
  - Radioactive Substance 3E0Q3HZ
  - Sedatives 3E0Q3NZ
  - Stem Cells
    - Embryonic 3E0Q
    - Somatic 3E0Q
  - Water Balance Substance 3E0Q37Z
- Ear 3E0B
  - Analgesics 3E0B
  - Anesthetic, Local 3E0B
  - Anti-infective 3E0B
  - Anti-inflammatory 3E0B
  - Antineoplastic 3E0B
  - Destructive Agent 3E0B
  - Diagnostic Substance, Other 3E0B
  - Hypnotics 3E0B
  - Radioactive Substance 3E0B
  - Sedatives 3E0B
- Epidural Space 3E0S3GC
  - Analgesics 3E0S3NZ
  - Anesthetic
    - Local 3E0S3BZ
    - Regional 3E0S3CZ
  - Anti-infective 3E0S32
  - Anti-inflammatory 3E0S33Z
  - Antineoplastic 3E0S30
  - Destructive Agent 3E0S3TZ
  - Diagnostic Substance, Other 3E0S3KZ
  - Electrolytic Substance 3E0S37Z
  - Gas 3E0S
  - Hypnotics 3E0S3NZ
  - Nutritional Substance 3E0S36Z
  - Radioactive Substance 3E0S3HZ
  - Sedatives 3E0S3NZ
  - Water Balance Substance 3E0S37Z
- Eye 3E0C
  - Analgesics 3E0C
  - Anesthetic, Local 3E0C
  - Anti-infective 3E0C
  - Anti-inflammatory 3E0C
  - Antineoplastic 3E0C
  - Destructive Agent 3E0C
  - Diagnostic Substance, Other 3E0C
  - Gas 3E0C
  - Hypnotics 3E0C
  - Pigment 3E0C
  - Radioactive Substance 3E0C
  - Sedatives 3E0C
- Gastrointestinal Tract
  - Lower 3E0H
    - Analgesics 3E0H
    - Anesthetic, Local 3E0H
    - Anti-infective 3E0H
    - Anti-inflammatory 3E0H
    - Antineoplastic 3E0H
    - Destructive Agent 3E0H
    - Diagnostic Substance, Other 3E0H
    - Electrolytic Substance 3E0H
    - Gas 3E0H
    - Hypnotics 3E0H
    - Nutritional Substance 3E0H
    - Radioactive Substance 3E0H
    - Sedatives 3E0H
    - Water Balance Substance 3E0H
  - Upper 3E0G
    - Analgesics 3E0G
    - Anesthetic, Local 3E0G
    - Anti-infective 3E0G
    - Anti-inflammatory 3E0G
    - Antineoplastic 3E0G
    - Destructive Agent 3E0G
    - Diagnostic Substance, Other 3E0G
    - Electrolytic Substance 3E0G
    - Gas 3E0G
    - Hypnotics 3E0G
    - Nutritional Substance 3E0G
    - Radioactive Substance 3E0G
    - Sedatives 3E0G
    - Water Balance Substance 3E0G
- Genitourinary Tract 3E0K
  - Analgesics 3E0K
  - Anesthetic, Local 3E0K
  - Anti-infective 3E0K
  - Anti-inflammatory 3E0K
  - Antineoplastic 3E0K
  - Destructive Agent 3E0K
  - Diagnostic Substance, Other 3E0K
  - Electrolytic Substance 3E0K
  - Gas 3E0K
  - Hypnotics 3E0K

**Introduction of substance in or on** – *continued*
- Genitourinary Tract – *continued*
  - Nutritional Substance 3E0K
  - Radioactive Substance 3E0K
  - Sedatives 3E0K
  - Water Balance Substance 3E0K
- Heart 3E08
  - Diagnostic Substance, Other 3E08
  - Platelet Inhibitor 3E08
  - Thrombolytic 3E08
- Joint 3E0U
  - Analgesics 3E0U3NZ
  - Anesthetic, Local 3E0U3BZ
  - Anti-infective 3E0U
  - Anti-inflammatory 3E0U33Z
  - Antineoplastic 3E0U30
  - Destructive Agent 3E0U3TZ
  - Diagnostic Substance, Other 3E0U3KZ
  - Electrolytic Substance 3E0U37Z
  - Gas 3E0U3SF
  - Hypnotics 3E0U3NZ
  - Nutritional Substance 3E0U36Z
  - Radioactive Substance 3E0U3HZ
  - Sedatives 3E0U3NZ
  - Water Balance Substance 3E0U37Z
- Lymphatic 3E0W3GC
  - Analgesics 3E0W3NZ
  - Anesthetic, Local 3E0W3BZ
  - Anti-infective 3E0W32
  - Anti-inflammatory 3E0W33Z
  - Antineoplastic 3E0W30
  - Destructive Agent 3E0W3TZ
  - Diagnostic Substance, Other 3E0W3KZ
  - Electrolytic Substance 3E0W37Z
  - Hypnotics 3E0W3NZ
  - Nutritional Substance 3E0W36Z
  - Radioactive Substance 3E0W3HZ
  - Sedatives 3E0W3NZ
  - Water Balance Substance 3E0W37Z
- Mouth 3E0D
  - Analgesics 3E0D
  - Anesthetic, Local 3E0D
  - Anti-infective 3E0D
  - Anti-inflammatory 3E0D
  - Antiarrhythmic 3E0D
  - Antineoplastic 3E0D
  - Destructive Agent 3E0D
  - Diagnostic Substance, Other 3E0D
  - Electrolytic Substance 3E0D
  - Hypnotics 3E0D
  - Nutritional Substance 3E0D
  - Radioactive Substance 3E0D
  - Sedatives 3E0D
  - Serum 3E0D
  - Toxoid 3E0D
  - Vaccine 3E0D
  - Water Balance Substance 3E0D
- Mucous Membrane 3E00XGC
  - Analgesics 3E00XNZ
  - Anesthetic, Local 3E00XBZ
  - Anti-infective 3E00X2
  - Anti-inflammatory 3E00X3Z
  - Antineoplastic 3E00X0
  - Destructive Agent 3E00XTZ
  - Diagnostic Substance, Other 3E00XKZ
  - Hypnotics 3E00XNZ
  - Pigment 3E00XMZ
  - Sedatives 3E00XNZ
  - Serum 3E00X4Z
  - Toxoid 3E00X4Z
  - Vaccine 3E00X4Z
- Muscle 3E023GC
  - Analgesics 3E023NZ
  - Anesthetic, Local 3E023BZ
  - Anti-infective 3E0232
  - Anti-inflammatory 3E0233Z
  - Antineoplastic 3E0230
  - Destructive Agent 3E023TZ
  - Diagnostic Substance, Other 3E023KZ
  - Electrolytic Substance 3E0237Z
  - Hypnotics 3E023NZ
  - Nutritional Substance 3E0236Z
  - Radioactive Substance 3E023HZ
  - Sedatives 3E023NZ
  - Serum 3E0234Z
  - Toxoid 3E0234Z
  - Vaccine 3E0234Z
  - Water Balance Substance 3E0237Z
- Nerve
  - Cranial 3E0X3GC
    - Anesthetic
      - Local 3E0X3BZ
      - Regional 3E0X3CZ

**Introduction of substance in or on** – *continued*
　Nerve – *continued*
　　Cranial – *continued*
　　　Anti-inflammatory 3E0X33Z
　　　Destructive Agent 3E0X3TZ
　　Peripheral 3E0T3GC
　　　Anesthetic
　　　　Local 3E0T3BZ
　　　　Regional 3E0T3CZ
　　　Anti-inflammatory 3E0T33Z
　　　Destructive Agent 3E0T3TZ
　　Plexus 3E0T3GC
　　　Anesthetic
　　　　Local 3E0T3BZ
　　　　Regional 3E0T3CZ
　　　Anti-inflammatory 3E0T33Z
　　　Destructive Agent 3E0T3TZ
　Nose 3E09
　　Analgesics 3E09
　　Anesthetic, Local 3E09
　　Anti-infective 3E09
　　Anti-inflammatory 3E09
　　Antineoplastic 3E09
　　Destructive Agent 3E09
　　Diagnostic Substance, Other 3E09
　　Hypnotics 3E09
　　Radioactive Substance 3E09
　　Sedatives 3E09
　　Serum 3E09
　　Toxoid 3E09
　　Vaccine 3E09
　Pancreatic Tract 3E0J
　　Analgesics 3E0J
　　Anesthetic, Local 3E0J
　　Anti-infective 3E0J
　　Anti-inflammatory 3E0J
　　Antineoplastic 3E0J
　　Destructive Agent 3E0J
　　Diagnostic Substance, Other 3E0J
　　Electrolytic Substance 3E0J
　　Gas 3E0J
　　Hypnotics 3E0J
　　Islet Cells, Pancreatic 3E0J
　　Nutritional Substance 3E0J
　　Radioactive Substance 3E0J
　　Sedatives 3E0J
　　Water Balance Substance 3E0J
　Pericardial Cavity 3E0Y3GC
　　Analgesics 3E0Y3NZ
　　Anesthetic, Local 3E0Y3BZ
　　Anti-infective 3E0Y32
　　Anti-inflammatory 3E0Y33Z
　　Antineoplastic 3E0Y
　　Destructive Agent 3E0Y3TZ
　　Diagnostic Substance, Other 3E0Y3KZ
　　Electrolytic Substance 3E0Y37Z
　　Gas 3E0Y
　　Hypnotics 3E0Y3NZ
　　Nutritional Substance 3E0Y36Z
　　Radioactive Substance 3E0Y3HZ
　　Sedatives 3E0Y3NZ
　　Water Balance Substance 3E0Y37Z
　Peritoneal Cavity 3E0M3GC
　　Adhesion Barrier 3E0M05Z
　　Analgesics 3E0M3NZ
　　Anesthetic, Local 3E0M3BZ
　　Anti-infective 3E0M32
　　Anti-inflammatory 3E0M33Z
　　Antineoplastic 3E0M
　　Destructive Agent 3E0M3TZ
　　Diagnostic Substance, Other 3E0M3KZ
　　Electrolytic Substance 3E0M37Z
　　Gas 3E0M
　　Hypnotics 3E0M3NZ
　　Nutritional Substance 3E0M36Z
　　Radioactive Substance 3E0M3HZ
　　Sedatives 3E0M3NZ
　　Water Balance Substance 3E0M37Z
　Pharynx 3E0D
　　Analgesics 3E0D
　　Anesthetic, Local 3E0D
　　Anti-infective 3E0D
　　Anti-inflammatory 3E0D
　　Antiarrhythmic 3E0D
　　Antineoplastic 3E0D
　　Destructive Agent 3E0D
　　Diagnostic Substance, Other 3E0D
　　Electrolytic Substance 3E0D
　　Hypnotics 3E0D
　　Nutritional Substance 3E0D
　　Radioactive Substance 3E0D
　　Sedatives 3E0D
　　Serum 3E0D

**Introduction of substance in or on** – *continued*
　Pharynx – *continued*
　　Toxoid 3E0D
　　Vaccine 3E0D
　　Water Balance Substance 3E0D
　Pleural Cavity 3E0L3GC
　　Adhesion Barrier 3E0L05Z
　　Analgesics 3E0L3NZ
　　Anesthetic, Local 3E0L3BZ
　　Anti-infective 3E0L32
　　Anti-inflammatory 3E0L33Z
　　Antineoplastic 3E0L
　　Destructive Agent 3E0L3TZ
　　Diagnostic Substance, Other 3E0L3KZ
　　Electrolytic Substance 3E0L37Z
　　Gas 3E0L
　　Hypnotics 3E0L3NZ
　　Nutritional Substance 3E0L36Z
　　Radioactive Substance 3E0L3HZ
　　Sedatives 3E0L3NZ
　　Water Balance Substance 3E0L37Z
　Products of Conception 3E0E
　　Analgesics 3E0E
　　Anesthetic, Local 3E0E
　　Anti-infective 3E0E
　　Anti-inflammatory 3E0E
　　Antineoplastic 3E0E
　　Destructive Agent 3E0E
　　Diagnostic Substance, Other 3E0E
　　Electrolytic Substance 3E0E
　　Gas 3E0E
　　Hypnotics 3E0E
　　Nutritional Substance 3E0E
　　Radioactive Substance 3E0E
　　Sedatives 3E0E
　　Water Balance Substance 3E0E
　Reproductive
　　Female 3E0P
　　　Adhesion Barrier 3E0P05Z
　　　Analgesics 3E0P
　　　Anesthetic, Local 3E0P
　　　Anti-infective 3E0P
　　　Anti-inflammatory 3E0P
　　　Antineoplastic 3E0P
　　　Destructive Agent 3E0P
　　　Diagnostic Substance, Other 3E0P
　　　Electrolytic Substance 3E0P
　　　Gas 3E0P
　　　Hypnotics 3E0P
　　　Nutritional Substance 3E0P
　　　Ovum, Fertilized 3E0P
　　　Radioactive Substance 3E0P
　　　Sedatives 3E0P
　　　Sperm 3E0P
　　　Water Balance Substance 3E0P
　　Male 3E0N
　　　Analgesics 3E0N
　　　Anesthetic, Local 3E0N
　　　Anti-infective 3E0N
　　　Anti-inflammatory 3E0N
　　　Antineoplastic 3E0N
　　　Destructive Agent 3E0N
　　　Diagnostic Substance, Other 3E0N
　　　Electrolytic Substance 3E0N
　　　Gas 3E0N
　　　Hypnotics 3E0N
　　　Nutritional Substance 3E0N
　　　Radioactive Substance 3E0N
　　　Sedatives 3E0N
　　　Water Balance Substance 3E0N
　Respiratory Tract 3E0F
　　Analgesics 3E0F
　　Anesthetic
　　　Inhalation 3E0F
　　　Local 3E0F
　　Anti-infective 3E0F
　　Anti-inflammatory 3E0F
　　Antineoplastic 3E0F
　　Destructive Agent 3E0F
　　Diagnostic Substance, Other 3E0F
　　Electrolytic Substance 3E0F
　　Gas 3E0F
　　Hypnotics 3E0F
　　Nutritional Substance 3E0F
　　Radioactive Substance 3E0F
　　Sedatives 3E0F
　　Water Balance Substance 3E0F
　Skin 3E00XGC
　　Analgesics 3E00XNZ
　　Anesthetic, Local 3E00XBZ
　　Anti-infective 3E00X2
　　Anti-inflammatory 3E00X3Z
　　Antineoplastic 3E00X0

**Introduction of substance in or on** – *continued*
　Skin – *continued*
　　Destructive Agent 3E00XTZ
　　Diagnostic Substance, Other 3E00XKZ
　　Hypnotics 3E00XNZ
　　Pigment 3E00XMZ
　　Sedatives 3E00XNZ
　　Serum 3E00X4Z
　　Toxoid 3E00X4Z
　　Vaccine 3E00X4Z
　Spinal Canal 3E0R3GC
　　Analgesics 3E0R3NZ
　　Anesthetic
　　　Local 3E0R3BZ
　　　Regional 3E0R3CZ
　　Anti-infective 3E0R32
　　Anti-inflammatory 3E0R33Z
　　Antineoplastic 3E0R30
　　Destructive Agent 3E0R3TZ
　　Diagnostic Substance, Other 3E0R3KZ
　　Electrolytic Substance 3E0R37Z
　　Gas 3E0R
　　Hypnotics 3E0R3NZ
　　Nutritional Substance 3E0R36Z
　　Radioactive Substance 3E0R3HZ
　　Sedatives 3E0R3NZ
　　Stem Cells
　　　Embryonic 3E0R
　　　Somatic 3E0R
　　Water Balance Substance 3E0R37Z
　Subcutaneous Tissue 3E013GC
　　Analgesics 3E013NZ
　　Anesthetic, Local 3E013BZ
　　Anti-infective 3E01
　　Anti-inflammatory 3E0133Z
　　Antineoplastic 3E0130
　　Destructive Agent 3E013TZ
　　Diagnostic Substance, Other 3E013KZ
　　Electrolytic Substance 3E0137Z
　　Hormone 3E013V
　　Hypnotics 3E013NZ
　　Nutritional Substance 3E0136Z
　　Radioactive Substance 3E013HZ
　　Sedatives 3E013NZ
　　Serum 3E0134Z
　　Toxoid 3E0134Z
　　Vaccine 3E0134Z
　　Water Balance Substance 3E0137Z
　Vein
　　Central 3E04
　　　Analgesics 3E04
　　　Anesthetic, Intracirculatory 3E04
　　　Anti-infective 3E04
　　　Anti-inflammatory 3E04
　　　Antiarrhythmic 3E04
　　　Antineoplastic 3E04
　　　Destructive Agent 3E04
　　　Diagnostic Substance, Other 3E04
　　　Electrolytic Substance 3E04
　　　Hormone 3E04
　　　Hypnotics 3E04
　　　Immunotherapeutic 3E04
　　　Nutritional Substance 3E04
　　　Platelet Inhibitor 3E04
　　　Radioactive Substance 3E04
　　　Sedatives 3E04
　　　Serum 3E04
　　　Thrombolytic 3E04
　　　Toxoid 3E04
　　　Vaccine 3E04
　　　Vasopressor 3E04
　　　Water Balance Substance 3E04
　　Peripheral 3E03
　　　Analgesics 3E03
　　　Anesthetic, Intracirculatory 3E03
　　　Anti-infective 3E03
　　　Anti-inflammatory 3E03
　　　Antiarrhythmic 3E03
　　　Antineoplastic 3E03
　　　Destructive Agent 3E03
　　　Diagnostic Substance, Other 3E03
　　　Electrolytic Substance 3E03
　　　Hormone 3E03
　　　Hypnotics 3E03
　　　Immunotherapeutic 3E03
　　　Islet Cells, Pancreatic 3E03
　　　Nutritional Substance 3E03
　　　Platelet Inhibitor 3E03
　　　Radioactive Substance 3E03
　　　Sedatives 3E03
　　　Serum 3E03
　　　Thrombolytic 3E03
　　　Toxoid 3E03

**Introduction of substance in or on** – *continued*
Vein – *continued*
Peripheral – *continued*
Vaccine 3E03
Vasopressor 3E03
Water Balance Substance 3E03
**Intubation**
Airway
– *see* Insertion of device in, Trachea ØBH1
– *see* Insertion of device in, Mouth and Throat ØCHY
– *see* Insertion of device in, Esophagus ØDH5
Drainage device – *see* Drainage
Feeding Device – *see* Insertion of device in, Gastrointestinal System ØDH
**IPPB (intermittent positive pressure breathing)** – *see* Assistance, Respiratory 5A09
**Iridectomy**
– *see* Excision, Eye Ø8B
– *see* Resection, Eye Ø8T
**Iridoplasty**
– *see* Repair, Eye Ø8Q
– *see* Replacement, Eye Ø8R
– *see* Supplement, Eye Ø8U
**Iridotomy** – *see* Drainage, Eye Ø89
**Irrigation**
Biliary Tract, Irrigating Substance 3E1J
Brain, Irrigating Substance 3E1Q38Z
Cranial Cavity, Irrigating Substance 3E1Q38Z
Ear, Irrigating Substance 3E1B
Epidural Space, Irrigating Substance 3E1S38Z
Eye, Irrigating Substance 3E1C
Gastrointestinal Tract
Lower, Irrigating Substance 3E1H
Upper, Irrigating Substance 3E1G
Genitourinary Tract, Irrigating Substance 3E1K
Irrigating Substance 3C1ZX8Z
Joint, Irrigating Substance 3E1U38Z
Mucous Membrane, Irrigating Substance 3E10
Nose, Irrigating Substance 3E19
Pancreatic Tract, Irrigating Substance 3E1J
Pericardial Cavity, Irrigating Substance 3E1Y38Z
Peritoneal Cavity
Dialysate 3E1M39Z
Irrigating Substance 3E1M38Z
Pleural Cavity, Irrigating Substance 3E1L38Z
Reproductive
Female, Irrigating Substance 3E1P
Male, Irrigating Substance 3E1N
Respiratory Tract, Irrigating Substance 3E1F
Skin, Irrigating Substance 3E10
Spinal Canal, Irrigating Substance 3E1R38Z
**Ischiatic nerve** – *use* Nerve, Sciatic
**Ischiocavernosus muscle** – *use* Muscle, Perineum
**Ischiofemoral ligament**
– *use* Bursa and Ligament, Hip, Left
– *use* Bursa and Ligament, Hip, Right
**Ischium**
– *use* Bone, Pelvic, Right
– *use* Bone, Pelvic, Left
**Isolation** 8E0ZXY6
**Isotope Administration, Whole Body** DWY5G
**Itrel (3)(4) neurostimulator** – *use* Stimulator Generator, Single Array in ØJH

## J

**Jejunal artery** – *use* Artery, Superior Mesenteric
**Jejunectomy**
– *see* Excision, Jejunum ØDBA
– *see* Resection, Jejunum ØDTA
**Jejunocolostomy**
– *see* Bypass, Gastrointestinal System ØD1
– *see* Drainage, Gastrointestinal System ØD9
**Jejunopexy**
– *see* Repair, Jejunum ØDQA
– *see* Reposition, Jejunum ØDSA
**Jejunostomy**
– *see* Bypass, Jejunum ØD1A
– *see* Drainage, Jejunum ØD9A
**Jejunotomy** – *see* Drainage, Jejunum ØD9A
**Joint fixation plate**
– *use* Internal Fixation Device in Upper Joints
– *use* Internal Fixation Device in Lower Joints
**Joint liner (insert)** – *use* Liner in Lower Joints
**Joint spacer (antibiotic)**
– *use* Spacer in Upper Joints
– *use* Spacer in Lower Joints
**Jugular body** – *use* Glomus Jugulare

**Jugular lymph node**
– *use* Lymphatic, Neck, Left
– *use* Lymphatic, Neck, Right

## K

**Kappa** – *use* Pacemaker, Dual Chamber in ØJH
**Kcentra** – *use* 4-Factor Prothrombin Complex Concentrate
**Keratectomy, kerectomy**
– *see* Excision, Eye Ø8B
– *see* Resection, Eye Ø8T
**Keratocentesis** – *see* Drainage, Eye Ø89
**Keratoplasty**
– *see* Repair, Eye Ø8Q
– *see* Replacement, Eye Ø8R
– *see* Supplement, Eye Ø8U
**Keratotomy**
– *see* Drainage, Eye Ø89
– *see* Repair, Eye Ø8Q
**Kirschner wire** (K-wire)
– *use* Internal Fixation Device in Head and Facial Bones
– *use* Internal Fixation Device in Lower Bones
– *use* Internal Fixation Device in Upper Bones
– *use* Internal Fixation Device in Lower Joints
– *use* Internal Fixation Device in Upper Joints
**Knee** (implant) **insert** – *use* Liner in Lower Joints
**KUB x-ray** – *see* Plain Radiography, Kidney, Ureter and Bladder BT04
**Kuntscher nail**
– *use* Internal Fixation Device, Intramedullary in Upper Bones
– *use* Internal Fixation Device, Intramedullary in Lower Bones

## L

**Labia majora** – *use* Vulva
**Labia minora** – *use* Vulva
**Labial gland**
– *use* Lip, Lower
– *use* Lip, Upper
**Labiectomy**
– *see* Excision, Female Reproductive System ØUB
– *see* Resection, Female Reproductive System ØUT
**Lacrimal canaliculus**
– *use* Duct, Lacrimal, Left
– *use* Duct, Lacrimal, Right
**Lacrimal punctum**
– *use* Duct, Lacrimal, Left
– *use* Duct, Lacrimal, Right
**Lacrimal sac**
– *use* Duct, Lacrimal, Left
– *use* Duct, Lacrimal, Right
**Laminectomy**
– *see* Excision, Lower Bones ØQB
– *see* Excision, Upper Bones ØPB
**Laminotomy**
– *see* Drainage, Lower Bones ØQ9
– *see* Drainage, Upper Bones ØP9
– *see* Excision, Lower Bones ØQB
– *see* Excision, Upper Bones ØPB
– *see* Release, Central Nervous System 00N
– *see* Release, Lower Bones ØQN
– *see* Release, Peripheral Nervous System 01N
– *see* Release, Upper Bones ØPN
**LAP-BAND® adjustable gastric banding system** – *use* Extraluminal Device
**Laparoscopy** – *see* Inspection
**Laparotomy**
Drainage – *see* Drainage, Peritoneal Cavity ØW9G
Exploratory – *see* Inspection, Peritoneal Cavity ØWJG
**Laryngectomy**
– *see* Excision, Larynx ØCBS
– *see* Resection, Larynx ØCTS
**Laryngocentesis** – *see* Drainage, Larynx ØC9S
**Laryngogram** – *see* Fluoroscopy, Larynx B91J
**Laryngopexy** – *see* Repair, Larynx ØCQS
**Laryngopharynx** – *use* Pharynx
**Laryngoplasty**
– *see* Repair, Larynx ØCQS
– *see* Replacement, Larynx ØCRS
– *see* Supplement, Larynx ØCUS
**Laryngorrhaphy** – *see* Repair, Larynx ØCQS
**Laryngoscopy** ØCJS8ZZ
**Laryngotomy** – *see* Drainage, Larynx ØC9S

**Laser Interstitial Thermal Therapy**
Adrenal Gland DGY2KZZ
Anus DDY8KZZ
Bile Ducts DFY2KZZ
Brain D0Y0KZZ
Brain Stem D0Y1KZZ
Breast
Left DMY0KZZ
Right DMY1KZZ
Bronchus DBY1KZZ
Chest Wall DBY7KZZ
Colon DDY5KZZ
Diaphragm DBY8KZZ
Duodenum DDY2KZZ
Esophagus DDY0KZZ
Gallbladder DFY1KZZ
Gland
Adrenal DGY2KZZ
Parathyroid DGY4KZZ
Pituitary DGY0KZZ
Thyroid DGY5KZZ
Ileum DDY4KZZ
Jejunum DDY3KZZ
Liver DFY0KZZ
Lung DBY2KZZ
Mediastinum DBY6KZZ
Nerve, Peripheral D0Y7KZZ
Pancreas DFY3KZZ
Parathyroid Gland DGY4KZZ
Pineal Body DGY1KZZ
Pituitary Gland DGY0KZZ
Pleura DBY5KZZ
Prostate DVY0KZZ
Rectum DDY7KZZ
Spinal Cord D0Y6KZZ
Stomach DDY1KZZ
Thyroid Gland DGY5KZZ
Trachea DBY0KZZ
**Lateral** (brachial) **lymph node**
– *use* Lymphatic, Axillary, Left
– *use* Lymphatic, Axillary, Right
**Lateral canthus**
– *use* Eyelid, Upper, Right
– *use* Eyelid, Upper, Left
**Lateral collateral ligament (LCL)**
– *use* Bursa and Ligament, Knee, Right
– *use* Bursa and Ligament, Knee, Left
**Lateral condyle of femur**
– *use* Femur, Lower, Right
– *use* Femur, Lower, Left
**Lateral condyle of tibia**
– *use* Tibia, Left
– *use* Tibia, Right
**Lateral cuneiform bone**
– *use* Tarsal, Right
– *use* Tarsal, Left
**Lateral epicondyle of femur**
– *use* Femur, Lower, Left
– *use* Femur, Lower, Right
**Lateral epicondyle of humerus**
– *use* Humeral Shaft, Right
– *use* Humeral Shaft, Left
**Lateral femoral cutaneous nerve** – *use* Nerve, Lumbar Plexus
**Lateral malleolus**
– *use* Fibula, Right
– *use* Fibula, Left
**Lateral meniscus**
– *use* Joint, Knee, Left
– *use* Joint, Knee, Right
**Lateral nasal cartilage** – *use* Nose
**Lateral plantar artery**
– *use* Artery, Foot, Left
– *use* Artery, Foot, Right
**Lateral plantar nerve** – *use* Nerve, Tibial
**Lateral rectus muscle**
– *use* Muscle, Extraocular, Left
– *use* Muscle, Extraocular, Right
**Lateral sacral artery**
– *use* Artery, Internal Iliac, Left
– *use* Artery, Internal Iliac, Right
**Lateral sacral vein**
– *use* Vein, Hypogastric, Left
– *use* Vein, Hypogastric, Right
**Lateral sural cutaneous nerve** – *use* Nerve, Peroneal
**Lateral tarsal artery**
– *use* Artery, Foot, Right
– *use* Artery, Foot, Left
**Lateral temporomandibular ligament** – *use* Bursa and Ligament, Head and Neck

**Lateral thoracic artery**
- *use* Artery, Axillary, Left
- *use* Artery, Axillary, Right

**Latissimus dorsi muscle**
- *use* Muscle, Trunk, Left
- *use* Muscle, Trunk, Right

**Latissimus Dorsi Myocutaneous Flap**
Bilateral ØHRVØ75
Left ØHRUØ75
Right ØHRTØ75

**Lavage**
- *see* Irrigation~ bronchial alveolar, diagnostic – *see* Drainage, Respiratory System ØB9

**Least splanchnic nerve** – *use* Nerve, Thoracic Sympathetic

**Left ascending lumbar vein** – *use* Vein, Hemiazygos

**Left atrioventricular valve** – *use* Valve, Mitral

**Left auricular appendix** – *use* Atrium, Left

**Left colic vein** – *use* Vein, Colic

**Left coronary sulcus** – *use* Heart, Left

**Left gastric artery** – *use* Artery, Gastric

**Left gastroepiploic artery** – *use* Artery, Splenic

**Left gastroepiploic vein** – *use* Vein, Splenic

**Left inferior phrenic vein** – *use* Vein, Renal, Left

**Left inferior pulmonary vein** – *use* Vein, Pulmonary, Left

**Left jugular trunk** – *use* Lymphatic, Thoracic Duct

**Left lateral ventricle** – *use* Cerebral Ventricle

**Left ovarian vein** – *use* Vein, Renal, Left

**Left second lumbar vein** – *use* Vein, Renal, Left

**Left subclavian trunk** – *use* Lymphatic, Thoracic Duct

**Left subcostal vein** – *use* Vein, Hemiazygos

**Left superior pulmonary vein** – *use* Vein, Pulmonary, Left

**Left suprarenal vein** – *use* Vein, Renal, Left

**Left testicular vein** – *use* Vein, Renal, Left

**Lengthening**
Bone, with device – *see* Insertion of Limb Lengthening Device
Muscle, by incision – *see* Division, Muscles ØK8
Tendon, by incision – *see* Division, Tendons ØL8

**Leptomeninges**
- *use* Cerebral Meninges
- *use* Spinal Meninges

**Lesser alar cartilage** – *use* Nose

**Lesser occipital nerve** – *use* Nerve, Cervical Plexus

**Lesser splanchnic nerve** – *use* Nerve, Thoracic Sympathetic

**Lesser trochanter**
- *use* Femur, Upper, Right
- *use* Femur, Upper, Left

**Lesser tuberosity**
- *use* Humeral Head, Left
- *use* Humeral Head, Right

**Lesser wing**
- *use* Bone, Sphenoid, Right
- *use* Bone, Sphenoid, Left

**Leukopheresis, therapeutic** – *see* Pheresis, Circulatory 6A55

**Levator anguli oris muscle** – *use* Muscle, Facial

**Levator ani muscle**
- *use* Muscle, Trunk, Left
- *use* Muscle, Trunk, Right

**Levator labii superioris alaeque nasi muscle** – *use* Muscle, Facial

**Levator labii superioris muscle** – *use* Muscle, Facial

**Levator palpebrae superioris muscle**
- *use* Eyelid, Upper, Left
- *use* Eyelid, Upper, Right

**Levator scapulae muscle**
- *use* Muscle, Neck, Left
- *use* Muscle, Neck, Right

**Levator veli palatini muscle** – *use* Muscle, Tongue, Palate, Pharynx

**Levatores costarum muscle**
- *use* Muscle, Thorax, Left
- *use* Muscle, Thorax, Right

**LifeStent®** (Flexstar)(XL) **Vascular Stent System** – *use* Intraluminal Device

**Ligament of head of fibula**
- *use* Bursa and Ligament, Knee, Right
- *use* Bursa and Ligament, Knee, Left

**Ligament of the lateral malleolus**
- *use* Bursa and Ligament, Ankle, Left
- *use* Bursa and Ligament, Ankle, Right

**Ligamentum flavum**
- *use* Bursa and Ligament, Trunk, Left
- *use* Bursa and Ligament, Trunk, Right

**Ligation** – *see* Occlusion

**Ligation, hemorrhoid** – *see* Occlusion, Lower Veins, Hemorrhoidal Plexus

**Light Therapy** GZJZZZZ

**Liner**
Removal of device from
Hip
Left ØSPBØ9Z
Right ØSP9Ø9Z
Knee
Left ØSPDØ9Z
Right ØSPCØ9Z
Revision of device in
Hip
Left ØSWBØ9Z
Right ØSW9Ø9Z
Knee
Left ØSWDØ9Z
Right ØSWCØ9Z
Supplement
Hip
Left ØSUBØ9Z
Acetabular Surface ØSUEØ9Z
Femoral Surface ØSUSØ9Z
Right ØSU9Ø9Z
Acetabular Surface ØSUAØ9Z
Femoral Surface ØSURØ9Z
Knee
Left ØSUDØ9
Femoral Surface ØSUUØ9Z
Tibial Surface ØSUWØ9Z
Right ØSUCØ9
Femoral Surface ØSUTØ9Z
Tibial Surface ØSUVØ9Z

**Lingual artery**
- *use* Artery, External Carotid, Right
- *use* Artery, External Carotid, Left

**Lingual tonsil** – *use* Tongue

**Lingulectomy, lung**
- *see* Excision, Lung Lingula ØBBH
- *see* Resection, Lung Lingula ØBTH

**Lithotripsy**
- *see* Fragmentation
with removal of fragments – *see* Extirpation

**LIVIAN™ CRT-D** – *use* Cardiac Resynchronization Defibrillator Pulse Generator in ØJH

**Lobectomy**
- *see* Excision, Central Nervous System ØØB
- *see* Excision, Respiratory System ØBB
- *see* Resection, Respiratory System ØBT
- *see* Excision, Hepatobiliary System and Pancreas ØFB
- *see* Resection, Hepatobiliary System and Pancreas ØFT
- *see* Excision, Endocrine System ØGB
- *see* Resection, Endocrine System ØGT

**Lobotomy** – *see* Division, Brain ØØ8Ø

**Localization**
- *see* Map
- *see* Imaging

**Locus ceruleus** – *use* Pons

**Long thoracic nerve** – *use* Nerve, Brachial Plexus

**Loop ileostomy** – *see* Bypass, Ileum ØD1B

**Loop recorder, implantable** – *use* Monitoring Device

**Lower GI series** – *see* Fluoroscopy, Colon BD14

**Lumbar artery** – *use* Aorta, Abdominal

**Lumbar facet joint** – *use* Joint, Lumbar Vertebral

**Lumbar ganglion** – *use* Nerve, Lumbar Sympathetic

**Lumbar lymph node** – *use* Lymphatic, Aortic

**Lumbar lymphatic trunk** – *use* Cisterna Chyli

**Lumbar splanchnic nerve** – *use* Nerve, Lumbar Sympathetic

**Lumbosacral facet joint** – *use* Joint, Lumbosacral

**Lumbosacral trunk** – *use* Nerve, Lumbar

**Lumpectomy** – *see* Excision

**Lunate bone**
- *use* Carpal, Left
- *use* Carpal, Right

**Lunotriquetral ligament**
- *use* Bursa and Ligament, Hand, Left
- *use* Bursa and Ligament, Hand, Right

**Lymphadenectomy**
- *see* Excision, Lymphatic and Hemic Systems Ø7B
- *see* Resection, Lymphatic and Hemic Systems Ø7T

**Lymphadenotomy** – *see* Drainage, Lymphatic and Hemic Systems Ø79

**Lymphangiectomy**
- *see* Excision, Lymphatic and Hemic Systems Ø7B
- *see* Resection, Lymphatic and Hemic Systems Ø7T

**Lymphangiogram** – *see* Plain Radiography, Lymphatic System B7Ø

**Lymphangioplasty**
- *see* Repair, Lymphatic and Hemic Systems Ø7Q
- *see* Supplement, Lymphatic and Hemic Systems Ø7U

**Lymphangiorrhaphy** – *see* Repair, Lymphatic and Hemic Systems Ø7Q

**Lymphangiotomy** – *see* Drainage, Lymphatic and Hemic Systems Ø79

**Lysis** – *see* Release

# M

**Macula**
- *use* Retina, Right
- *use* Retina, Left

**Magnet extraction, ocular foreign body** – *see* Extirpation, Eye Ø8C

**Magnetic Resonance Imaging (MRI)**
Abdomen BW3Ø
Ankle
Left BQ3H
Right BQ3G
Aorta
Abdominal B43Ø
Thoracic B33Ø
Arm
Left BP3F
Right BP3E
Artery
Celiac B431
Cervico–Cerebral Arch B33Q
Common Carotid, Bilateral B335
Coronary
Bypass Graft, Multiple B233
Multiple B231
Internal Carotid, Bilateral B338
Intracranial B33R
Lower Extremity
Bilateral B43H
Left B43G
Right B43F
Pelvic B43C
Renal, Bilateral B438
Spinal B33M
Superior Mesenteric B434
Upper Extremity
Bilateral B33K
Left B33J
Right B33H
Vertebral, Bilateral B33G
Bladder BT3Ø
Brachial Plexus BW3P
Brain BØ3Ø
Breast
Bilateral BH32
Left BH31
Right BH3Ø
Calcaneus
Left BQ3K
Right BQ3J
Chest BW33Y
Coccyx BR3F
Connective Tissue
Lower Extremity BL31
Upper Extremity BL32
Corpora Cavernosa BV3Ø
Disc
Cervical BR31
Lumbar BR33
Thoracic BR32
Ear B93Ø
Elbow
Left BP3H
Right BP3G
Eye
Bilateral B837
Left B836
Right B835
Femur
Left BQ34
Right BQ33
Fetal Abdomen BY33
Fetal Extremity BY35
Fetal Head BY3Ø
Fetal Heart BY31
Fetal Spine BY34
Fetal Thorax BY32

**Magnetic Resonance Imaging (MRI)** – *continued*
  Fetus, Whole BY36
  Foot
    Left BQ3M
    Right BQ3L
  Forearm
    Left BP3K
    Right BP3J
  Gland
    Adrenal, Bilateral BG32
    Parathyroid BG33
    Parotid, Bilateral B936
    Salivary, Bilateral B93D
    Submandibular, Bilateral B939
    Thyroid BG34
  Head BW38
  Heart, Right and Left B236
  Hip
    Left BQ31
    Right BQ30
  Intracranial Sinus B532
  Joint
    Finger
      Left BP3D
      Right BP3C
    Hand
      Left BP3D
      Right BP3C
    Temporomandibular, Bilateral BN39
  Kidney
    Bilateral BT33
    Left BT32
    Right BT31
    Transplant BT39
  Knee
    Left BQ38
    Right BQ37
  Larynx B93J
  Leg
    Left BQ3F
    Right BQ3D
  Liver BF35
  Liver and Spleen BF36
  Lung Apices BB3G
  Nasopharynx B93F
  Neck BW3F
  Nerve
    Acoustic B03C
    Brachial Plexus BW3P
  Oropharynx B93F
  Ovary
    Bilateral BU35
    Left BU34
    Right BU33
  Ovary and Uterus BU3C
  Pancreas BF37
  Patella
    Left BQ3W
    Right BQ3V
  Pelvic Region BW3G
  Pelvis BR3C
  Pituitary Gland B039
  Plexus, Brachial BW3P
  Prostate BV33
  Retroperitoneum BW3H
  Sacrum BR3F
  Scrotum BV34
  Sella Turcica B039
  Shoulder
    Left BP39
    Right BP38
  Sinus
    Intracranial B532
    Paranasal B932
  Spinal Cord B03B
  Spine
    Cervical BR30
    Lumbar BR39
    Thoracic BR37
  Spleen and Liver BF36
  Subcutaneous Tissue
    Abdomen BH3H
    Extremity
      Lower BH3J
      Upper BH3F
    Head BH3D
    Neck BH3D
    Pelvis BH3H
    Thorax BH3G
  Tendon
    Lower Extremity BL33
    Upper Extremity BL32

**Magnetic Resonance Imaging (MRI)** – *continued*
  Testicle
    Bilateral BV37
    Left BV36
    Right BV35
  Toe
    Left BQ3Q
    Right BQ3P
  Uterus BU36
    Pregnant BU3B
  Uterus and Ovary BU3C
  Vagina BU39
  Vein
    Cerebellar B531
    Cerebral B531
    Jugular, Bilateral B535
    Lower Extremity
      Bilateral B53D
      Left B53C
      Right B53B
    Other B53V
    Pelvic (Iliac) Bilateral B53H
    Portal B53T
    Pulmonary, Bilateral B53S
    Renal, Bilateral B53L
    Spanchnic B53T
    Upper Extremity
      Bilateral B53P
      Left B53N
      Right B53M
  Vena Cava
    Inferior B539
    Superior B538
  Wrist
    Left BP3M
    Right BP3L
**Malleotomy** – *see* Drainage, Ear, Nose, Sinus 099
**Malleus**
  – *use* Auditory Ossicle, Right
  – *use* Auditory Ossicle, Left
**Mammaplasty, mammoplasty**
  – *see* Alteration, Skin and Breast 0H0
  – *see* Repair, Skin and Breast 0HQ
  – *see* Replacement, Skin and Breast 0HR
  – *see* Supplement, Skin and Breast 0HU
**Mammary duct**
  – *use* Breast, Bilateral
  – *use* Breast, Right
  – *use* Breast, Left
**Mammary gland**
  – *use* Breast, Bilateral
  – *use* Breast, Right
  – *use* Breast, Left
**Mammectomy**
  – *see* Excision, Skin and Breast 0HB
  – *see* Resection, Skin and Breast 0HT
**Mammillary body** – *use* Hypothalamus
**Mammography** – *see* Plain Radiography, Skin,
    Subcutaneous Tissue and Breast BH0
**Mammotomy** – *see* Drainage, Skin and Breast 0H9
**Mandibular nerve** – *use* Nerve, Trigeminal
**Mandibular notch**
  – *use* Mandible, Right
  – *use* Mandible, Left
**Mandibulectomy**
  – *see* Excision, Head and Facial Bones 0NB
  – *see* Resection, Head and Facial Bones 0NT
**Manipulation**
  Adhesions – *see* Release
  Chiropractic – *see* Chiropractic Manipulation
**Manubrium** – *use* Sternum
**Map**
  Basal Ganglia 00K8
  Brain 00K0
  Cerebellum 00KC
  Cerebral Hemisphere 00K7
  Conduction Mechanism 02K8
  Hypothalamus 00KA
  Medulla Oblongata 00KD
  Pons 00KB
  Thalamus 00K9
**Mapping**
  Doppler ultrasound – *see* Ultrasonography
  Electrocardiogram only – *see* Measurement,
    Cardiac 4A02
**Mark IV Breathing Pacemaker System** – *use* Stimulator
    Generator in Subcutaneous Tissue and Fascia
**Marsupialization**
  – *see* Drainage
  – *see* Excision

**Massage, cardiac**
  External 5A12012
  Open 02QA0ZZ
**Masseter muscle** – *use* Muscle, Head
**Masseteric fascia** – *use* Subcutaneous Tissue and Fascia,
    Face
**Mastectomy**
  – *see* Excision, Skin and Breast 0HB
  – *see* Resection, Skin and Breast 0HT
**Mastoid (postauricular) lymph node**
  – *use* Lymphatic, Neck, Left
  – *use* Lymphatic, Neck, Right
**Mastoid air cells**
  – *use* Sinus, Mastoid, Left
  – *use* Sinus, Mastoid, Right
**Mastoid process**
  – *use* Bone, Temporal, Right
  – *use* Bone, Temporal, Left
**Mastoidectomy**
  – *see* Excision, Ear, Nose, Sinus 09B
  – *see* Resection, Ear, Nose, Sinus 09T
**Mastoidotomy** – *see* Drainage, Ear, Nose, Sinus 099
**Mastopexy**
  – *see* Reposition, Skin and Breast 0HS
  – *see* Repair, Skin and Breast 0HQ
**Mastorrhaphy** – *see* Repair, Skin and Breast 0HQ
**Mastotomy** – *see* Drainage, Skin and Breast 0H9
**Maxillary artery**
  – *use* Artery, External Carotid, Right
  – *use* Artery, External Carotid, Left
**Maxillary nerve** – *use* Nerve, Trigeminal
**Maximo II DR** (VR) – *use* Defibrillator Generator in 0JH
**Maximo II DR CRT-D** – *use* Cardiac Resynchronization
    Defibrillator Pulse Generator in 0JH
**Measurement**
  Arterial
    Flow
      Coronary 4A03
      Peripheral 4A03
      Pulmonary 4A03
    Pressure
      Coronary 4A03
      Peripheral 4A03
      Pulmonary 4A03
      Thoracic, Other 4A03
    Pulse
      Coronary 4A03
      Peripheral 4A03
      Pulmonary 4A03
    Saturation, Peripheral 4A03
    Sound, Peripheral 4A03
  Biliary
    Flow 4A0C
    Pressure 4A0C
  Cardiac
    Action Currents 4A02
    Defibrillator 4B02XTZ
    Electrical Activity 4A02
      Guidance 4A02X4A
      No Qualifier 4A02X4Z
    Output 4A02
    Pacemaker 4B02XSZ
    Rate 4A02
    Rhythm 4A02
    Sampling and Pressure
      Bilateral 4A02
      Left Heart 4A02
      Right Heart 4A02
    Sound 4A02
    Total Activity, Stress 4A02XM4
  Central Nervous
    Conductivity 4A00
    Electrical Activity 4A00
    Pressure 4A000BZ
      Intracranial 4A00
    Saturation, Intracranial 4A00
    Stimulator 4B00XVZ
    Temperature, Intracranial 4A00
  Circulatory, Volume 4A05XLZ
  Gastrointestinal
    Motility 4A0B
    Pressure 4A0B
    Secretion 4A0B
  Lymphatic
    Flow 4A06
    Pressure 4A06
  Metabolism 4A0Z
  Musculoskeletal
    Contractility 4A0F
    Stimulator 4B0FXVZ
  Olfactory, Acuity 4A08X0Z

**Measurement** – *continued*
  Peripheral Nervous
    Conductivity
      Motor 4A01
      Sensory 4A01
    Electrical Activity 4A01
    Stimulator 4B01XVZ
  Products of Conception
    Cardiac
      Electrical Activity 4A0H
      Rate 4A0H
      Rhythm 4A0H
      Sound 4A0H
    Nervous
      Conductivity 4A0J
      Electrical Activity 4A0J
      Pressure 4A0J
  Respiratory
    Capacity 4A09
    Flow 4A09
    Pacemaker 4B09XSZ
    Rate 4A09
    Resistance 4A09
    Total Activity 4A09
    Volume 4A09
  Sleep 4A0ZXQZ
  Temperature 4A0Z
  Urinary
    Contractility 4A0D73Z
    Flow 4A0D75Z
    Pressure 4A0D7BZ
    Resistance 4A0D7DZ
    Volume 4A0D7LZ
  Venous
    Flow
      Central 4A04
      Peripheral 4A04
      Portal 4A04
      Pulmonary 4A04
    Pressure
      Central 4A04
      Peripheral 4A04
      Portal 4A04
      Pulmonary 4A04
    Pulse
      Central 4A04
      Peripheral 4A04
      Portal 4A04
      Pulmonary 4A04
    Saturation, Peripheral 4A04
  Visual
    Acuity 4A07X0Z
    Mobility 4A07X7Z
    Pressure 4A07XBZ
**Meatoplasty, urethra** – *see* Repair, Urethra 0TQD
**Meatotomy** – *see* Drainage, Urinary System 0T9
**Mechanical ventilation** – *see* Performance, Respiratory 5A19
**Medial canthus**
  – *use* Eyelid, Lower, Left
  – *use* Eyelid, Lower, Right
**Medial collateral ligament (MCL)**
  – *use* Bursa and Ligament, Knee, Left
  – *use* Bursa and Ligament, Knee, Right
**Medial condyle of femur**
  – *use* Femur, Lower, Right
  – *use* Femur, Lower, Left
**Medial condyle of tibia**
  – *use* Tibia, Left
  – *use* Tibia, Right
**Medial cuneiform bone**
  – *use* Tarsal, Right
  – *use* Tarsal, Left
**Medial epicondyle of femur**
  – *use* Femur, Lower, Right
  – *use* Femur, Lower, Left
**Medial epicondyle of humerus**
  – *use* Humeral Shaft, Left
  – *use* Humeral Shaft, Right
**Medial malleolus**
  – *use* Tibia, Right
  – *use* Tibia, Left
**Medial meniscus**
  – *use* Joint, Knee, Right
  – *use* Joint, Knee, Left
**Medial plantar artery**
  – *use* Artery, Foot, Right
  – *use* Artery, Foot, Left
**Medial plantar nerve** – *use* Nerve, Tibial
**Medial popliteal nerve** – *use* Nerve, Tibial

**Medial rectus muscle**
  – *use* Muscle, Extraocular, Right
  – *use* Muscle, Extraocular, Left
**Medial sural cutaneous nerve** – *use* Nerve, Tibial
**Median antebrachial vein**
  – *use* Vein, Basilic, Left
  – *use* Vein, Basilic, Right
**Median cubital vein**
  – *use* Vein, Basilic, Left
  – *use* Vein, Basilic, Right
**Median sacral artery** – *use* Aorta, Abdominal
**Mediastinal lymph node** – *use* Lymphatic, Thorax
**Mediastinoscopy** 0WJC4ZZ
**Medication Management** GZ3ZZZZ
  for substance abuse
    Antabuse HZ83ZZZ
    Bupropion HZ87ZZZ
    Clonidine HZ86ZZZ
    Levo–alpha–acetyl–methadol (LAAM) HZ82ZZZ
    Methadone Maintenance HZ81ZZZ
    Naloxone HZ85ZZZ
    Naltrexone HZ84ZZZ
    Nicotine Replacement HZ80ZZZ
    Other Replacement Medication HZ89ZZZ
    Psychiatric Medication HZ88ZZZ
**Meditation** 8E0ZXY5
**Meissner's** (submucous) **plexus** – *use* Nerve, Abdominal Sympathetic
**Melody® transcatheter pulmonary valve** – *use* Zooplastic Tissue in Heart and Great Vessels
**Membranous urethra** – *use* Urethra
**Meningeorrhaphy**
  – *see* Repair, Cerebral Meninges 00Q1
  – *see* Repair, Spinal Meninges 00QT
**Meniscectomy**
  – *see* Excision, Lower Joints 0SB
  – *see* Resection, Lower Joints 0ST
**Mental foramen**
  – *use* Mandible, Left
  – *use* Mandible, Right
**Mentalis muscle** – *use* Muscle, Facial
**Mentoplasty** – *see* Alteration, Jaw, Lower 0W05
**Mesenterectomy** – *see* Excision, Mesentery 0DBV
**Mesenteriorrhaphy, mesenterorrhaphy** – *see* Repair, Mesentery 0DQV
**Mesenteriplication** – *see* Repair, Mesentery 0DQV
**Mesoappendix** – *use* Mesentery
**Mesocolon** – *use* Mesentery
**Metacarpal ligament**
  – *use* Bursa and Ligament, Hand, Left
  – *use* Bursa and Ligament, Hand, Right
**Metacarpophalangeal ligament**
  – *use* Bursa and Ligament, Hand, Right
  – *use* Bursa and Ligament, Hand, Left
**Metatarsal ligament**
  – *use* Bursa and Ligament, Foot, Right
  – *use* Bursa and Ligament, Foot, Left
**Metatarsectomy**
  – *see* Excision, Lower Bones 0QB
  – *see* Resection, Lower Bones 0QT
**Metatarsophalangeal (MTP) joint**
  – *use* Joint, Metatarsal–Phalangeal, Left
  – *use* Joint, Metatarsal–Phalangeal, Right
**Metatarsophalangeal ligament**
  – *use* Bursa and Ligament, Foot, Right
  – *use* Bursa and Ligament, Foot, Left
**Metathalamus** – *use* Thalamus
**Micro-Driver stent** (RX) (OTW) – *use* Intraluminal Device
**MicroMed HeartAssist** – *use* Implantable Heart Assist System in Heart and Great Vessels
**Micrus CERECYTE microcoil** – *use* Intraluminal Device, Bioactive in Upper Arteries
**Midcarpal joint**
  – *use* Joint, Carpal, Right
  – *use* Joint, Carpal, Left
**Middle cardiac nerve** – *use* Nerve, Thoracic Sympathetic
**Middle cerebral artery** – *use* Artery, Intracranial
**Middle cerebral vein** – *use* Vein, Intracranial
**Middle colic vein** – *use* Vein, Colic
**Middle genicular artery**
  – *use* Artery, Popliteal, Left
  – *use* Artery, Popliteal, Right
**Middle hemorrhoidal vein**
  – *use* Vein, Hypogastric, Left
  – *use* Vein, Hypogastric, Right

**Middle rectal artery**
  – *use* Artery, Internal Iliac, Right
  – *use* Artery, Internal Iliac, Left
**Middle suprarenal artery** – *use* Aorta, Abdominal
**Middle temporal artery**
  – *use* Artery, Temporal, Left
  – *use* Artery, Temporal, Right
**Middle turbinate** – *use* Turbinate, Nasal
**MitraClip valve repair system** – *use* Synthetic Substitute
**Mitral annulus** – *use* Valve, Mitral
**Mitroflow® Aortic Pericardial Heart Valve** – *use* Zooplastic Tissue in Heart and Great Vessels
**Mobilization, adhesions** – *see* Release
**Molar gland** – *use* Buccal Mucosa
**Monitoring**
  Arterial
    Flow
      Coronary 4A13
      Peripheral 4A13
      Pulmonary 4A13
    Pressure
      Coronary 4A13
      Peripheral 4A13
      Pulmonary 4A13
    Pulse
      Coronary 4A13
      Peripheral 4A13
      Pulmonary 4A13
    Saturation, Peripheral 4A13
    Sound, Peripheral 4A13
  Cardiac
    Electrical Activity 4A12
      Ambulatory 4A12X45
      No Qualifier 4A12X4Z
    Output 4A12
    Rate 4A12
    Rhythm 4A12
    Sound 4A12
    Total Activity, Stress 4A12XM4
  Central Nervous
    Conductivity 4A10
    Electrical Activity
      Intraoperative 4A10
      No Qualifier 4A10
    Pressure 4A100BZ
      Intracranial 4A10
    Saturation, Intracranial 4A10
    Temperature, Intracranial 4A10
  Gastrointestinal
    Motility 4A1B
    Pressure 4A1B
    Secretion 4A1B
  Lymphatic
    Flow 4A16
    Pressure 4A16
  Peripheral Nervous
    Conductivity
      Motor 4A11
      Sensory 4A11
    Electrical Activity
      Intraoperative 4A11
      No Qualifier 4A11
  Products of Conception
    Cardiac
      Electrical Activity 4A1H
      Rate 4A1H
      Rhythm 4A1H
      Sound 4A1H
    Nervous
      Conductivity 4A1J
      Electrical Activity 4A1J
      Pressure 4A1J
  Respiratory
    Capacity 4A19
    Flow 4A19
    Rate 4A19
    Resistance 4A19
    Volume 4A19
  Sleep 4A1ZXQZ
  Temperature 4A1Z
  Urinary
    Contractility 4A1D73Z
    Flow 4A1D75Z
    Pressure 4A1D7BZ
    Resistance 4A1D7DZ
    Volume 4A1D7LZ
  Venous
    Flow
      Central 4A14
      Peripheral 4A14
      Portal 4A14
      Pulmonary 4A14

**Monitoring** – *continued*
  Venous – *continued*
    Pressure
      Central 4A14
      Peripheral 4A14
      Portal 4A14
      Pulmonary 4A14
    Pulse
      Central 4A14
      Peripheral 4A14
      Portal 4A14
      Pulmonary 4A14
    Saturation
      Central 4A14
      Portal 4A14
      Pulmonary 4A14

**Monitoring Device, Hemodynamic**
  Abdomen ØJH8
  Chest ØJH6

**Mosaic Bioprosthesis (aortic) (mitral) valve** – *use* Zooplastic Tissue in Heart and Great Vessels

**Motor Function Assessment** FØ1

**Motor Treatment** FØ7

**MR Angiography**
  – *see* Magnetic Resonance Imaging (MRI), Heart B23
  – *see* Magnetic Resonance Imaging (MRI), Upper Arteries B33
  – *see* Magnetic Resonance Imaging (MRI), Lower Arteries B43

**MULTI-LINK (VISION)(MINI-VISION)(ULTRA) Coronary Stent System** – *use* Intraluminal Device

**Multiple sleep latency test** 4AØZXQZ

**Musculocutaneous nerve** – *use* Nerve, Brachial Plexus

**Musculopexy**
  – *see* Repair, Muscles ØKQ
  – *see* Reposition, Muscles ØKS

**Musculophrenic artery**
  – *use* Artery, Internal Mammary, Left
  – *use* Artery, Internal Mammary, Right

**Musculoplasty**
  – *see* Repair, Muscles ØKQ
  – *see* Supplement, Muscles ØKU

**Musculorrhaphy** – *see* Repair, Muscles ØKQ

**Musculospiral nerve** – *use* Nerve, Radial

**Myectomy**
  – *see* Excision, Muscles ØKB
  – *see* Resection, Muscles ØKT

**Myelencephalon** – *use* Medulla Oblongata

**Myelogram**
  CT – *see* Computerized Tomography (CT Scan), Central Nervous System BØ2
  MRI – *see* Magnetic Resonance Imaging (MRI), Central Nervous System BØ3

**Myenteric (Auerbach's) plexus** – *use* Nerve, Abdominal Sympathetic

**Myomectomy** – *see* Excision, Female Reproductive System ØUB

**Myometrium** – *use* Uterus

**Myopexy**
  – *see* Repair, Muscles ØKQ
  – *see* Reposition, Muscles ØKS

**Myoplasty**
  – *see* Repair, Muscles ØKQ
  – *see* Supplement, Muscles ØKU

**Myorrhaphy** – *see* Repair, Muscles ØKQ

**Myoscopy** – *see* Inspection, Muscles ØKJ

**Myotomy**
  – *see* Division, Muscles ØK8
  – *see* Drainage, Muscles ØK9

**Myringectomy**
  – *see* Excision, Ear, Nose, Sinus Ø9B
  – *see* Resection, Ear, Nose, Sinus Ø9T

**Myringoplasty**
  – *see* Repair, Ear, Nose, Sinus Ø9Q
  – *see* Replacement, Ear, Nose, Sinus Ø9R
  – *see* Supplement, Ear, Nose, Sinus Ø9U

**Myringostomy** – *see* Drainage, Ear, Nose, Sinus Ø99

**Myringotomy** – *see* Drainage, Ear, Nose, Sinus Ø99

# N

**Nail bed**
  – *use* Finger Nail
  – *use* Toe Nail

**Nail plate**
  – *use* Finger Nail
  – *use* Toe Nail

**Narcosynthesis** GZGZZZZ

**Nasal cavity** – *use* Nose

**Nasal concha** – *use* Turbinate, Nasal

**Nasalis muscle** – *use* Muscle, Facial

**Nasolacrimal duct**
  – *use* Duct, Lacrimal, Right
  – *use* Duct, Lacrimal, Left

**Nasopharyngeal airway (NPA)** – *use* Intraluminal Device, Airway in Ear, Nose, Sinus

**Navicular bone**
  – *use* Tarsal, Left
  – *use* Tarsal, Right

**Near Infrared Spectroscopy, Circulatory System** 8E023DZ

**Neck of femur**
  – *use* Femur, Upper, Right
  – *use* Femur, Upper, Left

**Neck of humerus** (anatomical)(surgical)
  – *use* Humeral Head, Right
  – *use* Humeral Head, Left

**Nephrectomy**
  – *see* Excision, Urinary System ØTB
  – *see* Resection, Urinary System ØTT

**Nephrolithotomy** – *see* Extirpation, Urinary System ØTC

**Nephrolysis** – *see* Release, Urinary System ØTN

**Nephropexy**
  – *see* Repair, Urinary System ØTQ
  – *see* Reposition, Urinary System ØTS

**Nephroplasty**
  – *see* Repair, Urinary System ØTQ
  – *see* Supplement, Urinary System ØTU

**Nephropyeloureterostomy**
  – *see* Bypass, Urinary System ØT1
  – *see* Drainage, Urinary System ØT9

**Nephrorrhaphy** – *see* Repair, Urinary System ØTQ

**Nephroscopy, transurethral** ØTJ58ZZ

**Nephrostomy**
  – *see* Bypass, Urinary System ØT1
  – *see* Drainage, Urinary System ØT9

**Nephrotomography**
  – *see* Plain Radiography, Urinary System BTØ
  – *see* Fluoroscopy, Urinary System BT1

**Nephrotomy**
  – *see* Drainage, Urinary System ØT9
  – *see* Division, Urinary System ØT8

**Nerve conduction study**
  – *see* Measurement, Central Nervous 4A00
  – *see* Measurement, Peripheral Nervous 4A01

**Nerve Function Assessment** FØ1

**Nerve to the stapedius** – *use* Nerve, Facial

**Nesiritide** – *use* Human B-type Natriuretic Peptide

**Neurectomy**
  – *see* Excision, Central Nervous System ØØB
  – *see* Excision, Peripheral Nervous System Ø1B

**Neurexeresis**
  – *see* Extraction, Central Nervous System ØØD
  – *see* Extraction, Peripheral Nervous System Ø1D

**Neurohypophysis** – *use* Gland, Pituitary

**Neurolysis**
  – *see* Release, Central Nervous System ØØN
  – *see* Release, Peripheral Nervous System Ø1N

**Neuromuscular electrical stimulation (NEMS) lead** – *use* Stimulator Lead in Muscles

**Neurophysiologic monitoring** – *see* Monitoring, Central Nervous 4A10

**Neuroplasty**
  – *see* Repair, Central Nervous System ØØQ
  – *see* Repair, Peripheral Nervous System Ø1Q
  – *see* Supplement, Central Nervous System ØØU
  – *see* Supplement, Peripheral Nervous System Ø1U

**Neurorrhaphy**
  – *see* Repair, Central Nervous System ØØQ
  – *see* Repair, Peripheral Nervous System Ø1Q

**Neurostimulator Generator**
  Insertion of device in, Skull ØNHØØNZ
  Removal of device from, Skull ØNPØØNZ
  Revision of device in, Skull ØNWØØNZ

**Neurostimulator generator, multiple channel** – *use* Stimulator Generator, Multiple Array in ØJH

**Neurostimulator generator, multiple channel rechargeable** – *use* Stimulator Generator, Multiple Array Rechargeable in ØJH

**Neurostimulator generator, single channel** – *use* Stimulator Generator, Single Array in ØJH

**Neurostimulator generator, single channel rechargeable** – *use* Stimulator Generator, Single Array Rechargeable in ØJH

**Neurostimulator Lead**
  Insertion of device in
    Brain ØØHØ
    Cerebral Ventricle ØØH6
    Nerve
      Cranial ØØHE
      Peripheral Ø1HY
    Spinal Canal ØØHU
    Spinal Cord ØØHV
  Removal of device from
    Brain ØØPØ
    Cerebral Ventricle ØØP6
    Nerve
      Cranial ØØPE
      Peripheral Ø1PY
    Spinal Canal ØØPU
    Spinal Cord ØØPV
  Revision of device in
    Brain ØØWØ
    Cerebral Ventricle ØØW6
    Nerve
      Cranial ØØWE
      Peripheral Ø1WY
    Spinal Canal ØØWU
    Spinal Cord ØØWV

**Neurotomy**
  – *see* Division, Central Nervous System ØØ8
  – *see* Division, Peripheral Nervous System Ø18

**Neurotripsy**
  – *see* Destruction, Central Nervous System ØØ5
  – *see* Destruction, Peripheral Nervous System Ø15

**Neutralization plate**
  – *use* Internal Fixation Device in Head and Facial Bones
  – *use* Internal Fixation Device in Upper Bones
  – *use* Internal Fixation Device in Lower Bones

**Ninth cranial nerve** – *use* Nerve, Glossopharyngeal

**Nitinol framed polymer mesh** – *use* Synthetic Substitute

**Non-tunneled central venous catheter** – *use* Infusion Device

**Nonimaging Nuclear Medicine Assay**
  Bladder, Kidneys and Ureters CT63
  Blood C763
  Kidneys, Ureters and Bladder CT63
  Lymphatics and Hematologic System C76YYZZ
  Ureters, Kidneys and Bladder CT63
  Urinary System CT6YYZZ

**Nonimaging Nuclear Medicine Probe** CP5YYZZ
  Abdomen CW50
  Abdomen and Chest CW54
  Abdomen and Pelvis CW51
  Brain C050
  Central Nervous System C05YYZZ
  Chest CW53
  Chest and Abdomen CW54
  Chest and Neck CW56
  Extremity
    Lower CP5
    Upper CP5
  Head and Neck CW5B
  Heart C25YYZZ
    Right and Left C256
  Lymphatics
    Head C75J
    Head and Neck C755
    Lower Extremity C75P
    Neck C75K
    Pelvic C75D
    Trunk C75M
    Upper Chest C75L
    Upper Extremity C75N
  Lymphatics and Hematologic System C75YYZZ
  Neck and Chest CW56
  Neck and Head CW5B
  Pelvic Region CW5J
  Pelvis and Abdomen CW51
  Spine CP55ZZZ

**Nonimaging Nuclear Medicine Uptake**
  Endocrine System CG4YYZZ
  Gland, Thyroid CG42

**Nostril** – *use* Nose

**Novacor Left Ventricular Assist Device** – *use* Implantable Heart Assist System in Heart and Great Vessels

**Novation® Ceramic AHS® (Articulation Hip System)** – *use* Synthetic Substitute, Ceramic in ØSR

**Nuclear medicine**
  – *see* Nonimaging Nuclear Medicine Assay
  – *see* Nonimaging Nuclear Medicine Probe
  – *see* Nonimaging Nuclear Medicine Uptake

**Nuclear medicine** – *continued*
 – *see* Planar Nuclear Medicine Imaging
 – *see* Positron Emission Tomographic (PET) Imaging
 – *see* Systemic Nuclear Medicine Therapy
 – *see* Tomographic (Tomo) Nuclear Medicine Imaging
**Nuclear scintigraphy** – *see* Nuclear Medicine
**Nutrition, concentrated substances**
 Enteral infusion 3E0G36Z
 Parenteral (peripheral) infusion – *see* Introduction of
  Nutritional Substance

# O

**Obliteration** – *see* Destruction
**Obturator artery**
 – *use* Artery, Internal Iliac, Left
 – *use* Artery, Internal Iliac, Right
**Obturator lymph node** – *use* Lymphatic, Pelvis
**Obturator muscle**
 – *use* Muscle, Hip, Left
 – *use* Muscle, Hip, Right
**Obturator nerve** – *use* Nerve, Lumbar Plexus
**Obturator vein**
 – *use* Vein, Hypogastric, Right
 – *use* Vein, Hypogastric, Left
**Obtuse margin** – *use* Heart, Left
**Occipital artery**
 – *use* Artery, External Carotid, Right
 – *use* Artery, External Carotid, Left
**Occipital lobe** – *use* Cerebral Hemisphere
**Occipital lymph node**
 – *use* Lymphatic, Neck, Left
 – *use* Lymphatic, Neck, Right
**Occipitofrontalis muscle** – *use* Muscle, Facial
**Occlusion**
 Ampulla of Vater 0FLC
 Anus 0DLQ
 Aorta, Abdominal 04L0
 Artery
  Anterior Tibial
   Left 04LQ
   Right 04LP
  Axillary
   Left 03L6
   Right 03L5
  Brachial
   Left 03L8
   Right 03L7
  Celiac 04L1
  Colic
   Left 04L7
   Middle 04L8
   Right 04L6
  Common Carotid
   Left 03LJ
   Right 03LH
  Common Iliac
   Left 04LD
   Right 04LC
  External Carotid
   Left 03LN
   Right 03LM
  External Iliac
   Left 04LJ
   Right 04LH
  Face 03LR
  Femoral
   Left 04LL
   Right 04LK
  Foot
   Left 04LW
   Right 04LV
  Gastric 04L2
  Hand
   Left 03LF
   Right 03LD
  Hepatic 04L3
  Inferior Mesenteric 04LB
  Innominate 03L2
  Internal Carotid
   Left 03LL
   Right 03LK
  Internal Iliac
   Left, Uterine Artery, Left 04LF
   Right, Uterine Artery, Right 04LE
  Internal Mammary
   Left 03L1
   Right 03L0
  Intracranial 03LG
  Lower 04LY

**Occlusion** – *continued*
 Artery – *continued*
  Peroneal
   Left 04LU
   Right 04LT
  Popliteal
   Left 04LN
   Right 04LM
  Posterior Tibial
   Left 04LS
   Right 04LR
  Pulmonary, Left 02LR
  Radial
   Left 03LC
   Right 03LB
  Renal
   Left 04LA
   Right 04L9
  Splenic 04L4
  Subclavian
   Left 03L4
   Right 03L3
  Superior Mesenteric 04L5
  Temporal
   Left 03LT
   Right 03LS
  Thyroid
   Left 03LV
   Right 03LU
  Ulnar
   Left 03LA
   Right 03L9
  Upper 03LY
  Vertebral
   Left 03LQ
   Right 03LP
 Atrium, Left 02L7
 Bladder 0TLB
 Bladder Neck 0TLC
 Bronchus
  Lingula 0BL9
  Lower Lobe
   Left 0BLB
   Right 0BL6
  Main
   Left 0BL7
   Right 0BL3
  Middle Lobe, Right 0BL5
  Upper Lobe
   Left 0BL8
   Right 0BL4
 Carina 0BL2
 Cecum 0DLH
 Cisterna Chyli 07LL
 Colon
  Ascending 0DLK
  Descending 0DLM
  Sigmoid 0DLN
  Transverse 0DLL
 Cord
  Bilateral 0VLH
  Left 0VLG
  Right 0VLF
 Cul-de-sac 0ULF
 Duct
  Common Bile 0FL9
  Cystic 0FL8
  Hepatic
   Left 0FL6
   Right 0FL5
  Lacrimal
   Left 08LY
   Right 08LX
  Pancreatic 0FLD
   Accessory 0FLF
  Parotid
   Left 0CLC
   Right 0CLB
 Duodenum 0DL9
 Esophagogastric Junction 0DL4
 Esophagus 0DL5
  Lower 0DL3
  Middle 0DL2
  Upper 0DL1
 Fallopian Tube
  Left 0UL6
  Right 0UL5
 Fallopian Tubes, Bilateral 0UL7
 Ileocecal Valve 0DLC
 Ileum 0DLB
 Intestine
  Large 0DLE
   Left 0DLG

**Occlusion** – *continued*
 Intestine – *continued*
  Large – *continued*
   Right 0DLF
  Small 0DL8
 Jejunum 0DLA
 Kidney Pelvis
  Left 0TL4
  Right 0TL3
 Left atrial appendage (LAA) – *see* Occlusion, Atrium,
  Left 02L7
 Lymphatic
  Aortic 07LD
  Axillary
   Left 07L6
   Right 07L5
  Head 07L0
  Inguinal
   Left 07LJ
   Right 07LH
  Internal Mammary
   Left 07L9
   Right 07L8
  Lower Extremity
   Left 07LG
   Right 07LF
  Mesenteric 07LB
  Neck
   Left 07L2
   Right 07L1
  Pelvis 07LC
  Thoracic Duct 07LK
  Thorax 07L7
  Upper Extremity
   Left 07L4
   Right 07L3
 Rectum 0DLP
 Stomach 0DL6
  Pylorus 0DL7
 Trachea 0BL1
 Ureter
  Left 0TL7
  Right 0TL6
 Urethra 0TLD
 Vagina 0ULG
 Vas Deferens
  Bilateral 0VLQ
  Left 0VLP
  Right 0VLN
 Vein
  Axillary
   Left 05L8
   Right 05L7
  Azygos 05L0
  Basilic
   Left 05LC
   Right 05LB
  Brachial
   Left 05LA
   Right 05L9
  Cephalic
   Left 05LF
   Right 05LD
  Colic 06L7
  Common Iliac
   Left 06LD
   Right 06LC
  Esophageal 06L3
  External Iliac
   Left 06LG
   Right 06LF
  External Jugular
   Left 05LQ
   Right 05LP
  Face
   Left 05LV
   Right 05LT
  Femoral
   Left 06LN
   Right 06LM
  Foot
   Left 06LV
   Right 06LT
  Gastric 06L2
  Greater Saphenous
   Left 06LQ
   Right 06LP
  Hand
   Left 05LH
   Right 05LG
  Hemiazygos 05L1
  Hepatic 06L4

**Occlusion** – *continued*
  Vein – *continued*
    Hypogastric
      Left Ø6LJ
      Right Ø6LH
    Inferior Mesenteric Ø6L6
    Innominate
      Left Ø5L4
      Right Ø5L3
    Internal Jugular
      Left Ø5LN
      Right Ø5LM
    Intracranial Ø5LL
    Lesser Saphenous
      Left Ø6LS
      Right Ø6LR
    Lower Ø6LY
    Portal Ø6L8
    Pulmonary
      Left Ø2LT
      Right Ø2LS
    Renal
      Left Ø6LB
      Right Ø6L9
    Splenic Ø6L1
    Subclavian
      Left Ø5L6
      Right Ø5L5
    Superior Mesenteric Ø6L5
    Upper Ø5LY
    Vertebral
      Left Ø5LS
      Right Ø5LR
  Vena Cava
    Inferior Ø6LØ
    Superior Ø2LV
**Occupational therapy** – *see* Activities of Daily Living Treatment, Rehabilitation FØ8
**Odentectomy**
– *see* Excision, Mouth and Throat ØCB
– *see* Resection, Mouth and Throat ØCT
**Olecranon bursa**
– *use* Bursa and Ligament, Elbow, Left
– *use* Bursa and Ligament, Elbow, Right
**Olecranon process**
– *use* Ulna, Left
– *use* Ulna, Right
**Olfactory bulb** – *use* Nerve, Olfactory
**Omentectomy, omentumectomy**
– *see* Excision, Gastrointestinal System ØDB
– *see* Resection, Gastrointestinal System ØDT
**Omentofixation** – *see* Repair, Gastrointestinal System ØDQ
**Omentoplasty**
– *see* Repair, Gastrointestinal System ØDQ
– *see* Replacement, Gastrointestinal System ØDR
– *see* Supplement, Gastrointestinal System ØDU
**Omentorrhaphy** – *see* Repair, Gastrointestinal System ØDQ
**Omentotomy** – *see* Drainage, Gastrointestinal System ØD9
**Omnilink Elite Vascular Balloon Expandable Stent System** – *use* Intraluminal Device
**Onychectomy**
– *see* Excision, Skin and Breast ØHB
– *see* Resection, Skin and Breast ØHT
**Onychoplasty**
– *see* Repair, Skin and Breast ØHQ
– *see* Replacement, Skin and Breast ØHR
**Onychotomy** – *see* Drainage, Skin and Breast ØH9
**Oophorectomy**
– *see* Excision, Female Reproductive System ØUB
– *see* Resection, Female Reproductive System ØUT
**Oophoropexy**
– *see* Repair, Female Reproductive System ØUQ
– *see* Reposition, Female Reproductive System ØUS
**Oophoroplasty**
– *see* Repair, Female Reproductive System ØUQ
– *see* Supplement, Female Reproductive System ØUU
**Oophororrhaphy** – *see* Repair, Female Reproductive System ØUQ
**Oophorostomy** – *see* Drainage, Female Reproductive System ØU9
**Oophorotomy**
– *see* Drainage, Female Reproductive System ØU9
– *see* Division, Female Reproductive System ØU8
**Oophorrhaphy** – *see* Repair, Female Reproductive System ØUQ
**Open Pivot (mechanical) valve** – *use* Synthetic Substitute
**Open Pivot Aortic Valve Graft (AVG)** – *use* Synthetic Substitute

**Ophthalmic artery**
– *use* Artery, Internal Carotid, Right
– *use* Artery, Internal Carotid, Left
**Ophthalmic nerve** – *use* Nerve, Trigeminal
**Ophthalmic vein** – *use* Vein, Intracranial
**Opponensplasty**
  Tendon replacement – *see* Replacement, Tendons ØLR
  Tendon transfer – *see* Transfer, Tendons ØLX
**Optic chiasma** – *use* Nerve, Optic
**Optic disc**
– *use* Retina, Left
– *use* Retina, Right
**Optic foramen**
– *use* Bone, Sphenoid, Right
– *use* Bone, Sphenoid, Left
**Optical coherence tomography, intravascular** – *see* Computerized Tomography (CT Scan)
**Optimizer™ III implantable pulse generator** – *use* Contractility Modulation Device in ØJH
**Orbicularis oculi muscle**
– *use* Eyelid, Upper, Left
– *use* Eyelid, Upper, Right
**Orbicularis oris muscle** – *use* Muscle, Facial
**Orbital fascia** – *use* Subcutaneous Tissue and Fascia, Face
**Orbital portion of ethmoid bone**
– *use* Orbit, Left
– *use* Orbit, Right
**Orbital portion of frontal bone**
– *use* Orbit, Right
– *use* Orbit, Left
**Orbital portion of lacrimal bone**
– *use* Orbit, Left
– *use* Orbit, Right
**Orbital portion of maxilla**
– *use* Orbit, Left
– *use* Orbit, Right
**Orbital portion of palatine bone**
– *use* Orbit, Right
– *use* Orbit, Left
**Orbital portion of sphenoid bone**
– *use* Orbit, Right
– *use* Orbit, Left
**Orbital portion of zygomatic bone**
– *use* Orbit, Left
– *use* Orbit, Right
**Orchectomy, orchidectomy, orchiectomy**
– *see* Excision, Male Reproductive System ØVB
– *see* Resection, Male Reproductive System ØVT
**Orchidoplasty, orchioplasty**
– *see* Repair, Male Reproductive System ØVQ
– *see* Replacement, Male Reproductive System ØVR
– *see* Supplement, Male Reproductive System ØVU
**Orchidorrhaphy, orchiorrhaphy** – *see* Repair, Male Reproductive System ØVQ
**Orchidotomy, orchiotomy, orchotomy** – *see* Drainage, Male Reproductive System ØV9
**Orchiopexy**
– *see* Repair, Male Reproductive System ØVQ
– *see* Reposition, Male Reproductive System ØVS
**Oropharyngeal airway (OPA)** – *use* Intraluminal Device, Airway in Mouth and Throat
**Oropharynx** – *use* Pharynx
**Ossicular chain**
– *use* Auditory Ossicle, Left
– *use* Auditory Ossicle, Right
**Ossiculectomy**
– *see* Excision, Ear, Nose, Sinus Ø9B
– *see* Resection, Ear, Nose, Sinus Ø9T
**Ossiculotomy** – *see* Drainage, Ear, Nose, Sinus Ø99
**Ostectomy**
– *see* Excision, Head and Facial Bones ØNB
– *see* Resection, Head and Facial Bones ØNT
– *see* Excision, Upper Bones ØPB
– *see* Resection, Upper Bones ØPT
– *see* Excision, Lower Bones ØQB
– *see* Resection, Lower Bones ØQT
**Osteoclasis**
– *see* Division, Head and Facial Bones ØN8
– *see* Division, Upper Bones ØP8
– *see* Division, Lower Bones ØQ8
**Osteolysis**
– *see* Release, Head and Facial Bones ØNN
– *see* Release, Upper Bones ØPN
– *see* Release, Lower Bones ØQN
**Osteopathic Treatment**
  Abdomen 7WØ9X
  Cervical 7WØ1X

**Osteopathic Treatment** – *continued*
  Extremity
    Lower 7WØ6X
    Upper 7WØ7X
  Head 7WØØX
  Lumbar 7WØ3X
  Pelvis 7WØ5X
  Rib Cage 7WØ8X
  Sacrum 7WØ4X
  Thoracic 7WØ2X
**Osteopexy**
– *see* Repair, Head and Facial Bones ØNQ
– *see* Reposition, Head and Facial Bones ØNS
– *see* Repair, Upper Bones ØPQ
– *see* Reposition, Upper Bones ØPS
– *see* Repair, Lower Bones ØQQ
– *see* Reposition, Lower Bones ØQS
**Osteoplasty**
– *see* Repair, Head and Facial Bones ØNQ
– *see* Replacement, Head and Facial Bones ØNR
– *see* Repair, Upper Bones ØPQ
– *see* Replacement, Upper Bones ØPR
– *see* Repair, Lower Bones ØQQ
– *see* Replacement, Lower Bones ØQR
– *see* Supplement, Lower Bones ØQU
– *see* Supplement, Head and Facial Bones ØNU
– *see* Supplement, Upper Bones ØPU
**Osteorrhaphy**
– *see* Repair, Head and Facial Bones ØNQ
– *see* Repair, Upper Bones ØPQ
– *see* Repair, Lower Bones ØQQ
**Osteotomy, ostotomy**
– *see* Division, Head and Facial Bones ØN8
– *see* Drainage, Head and Facial Bones ØN9
– *see* Division, Upper Bones ØP8
– *see* Drainage, Upper Bones ØP9
– *see* Division, Lower Bones ØQ8
– *see* Drainage, Lower Bones ØQ9
**Otic ganglion** – *use* Nerve, Head and Neck Sympathetic
**Otoplasty**
– *see* Repair, Ear, Nose, Sinus Ø9Q
– *see* Replacement, Ear, Nose, Sinus Ø9R
– *see* Supplement, Ear, Nose, Sinus Ø9U
**Otoscopy** – *see* Inspection, Ear, Nose, Sinus Ø9J
**Oval window**
– *use* Ear, Middle, Left
– *use* Ear, Middle, Right
**Ovarian artery** – *use* Aorta, Abdominal
**Ovarian ligament** – *use* Uterine Supporting Structure
**Ovariectomy**
– *see* Excision, Female Reproductive System ØUB
– *see* Resection, Female Reproductive System ØUT
**Ovariocentesis** – *see* Drainage, Female Reproductive System ØU9
**Ovariopexy**
– *see* Repair, Female Reproductive System ØUQ
– *see* Reposition, Female Reproductive System ØUS
**Ovariotomy**
– *see* Drainage, Female Reproductive System ØU9
– *see* Division, Female Reproductive System ØU8
**Ovatio™ CRT-D** – *use* Cardiac Resynchronization Defibrillator Pulse Generator in ØJH
**Oversewing**
  Gastrointestinal ulcer – *see* Repair, Gastrointestinal System ØDQ
  Pleural bleb – *see* Repair, Respiratory System ØBQ
**Oviduct**
– *use* Fallopian Tube, Right
– *use* Fallopian Tube, Left
**Oxidized zirconium ceramic hip bearing surface** – *use* Synthetic Substitute, Ceramic on Polyethylene in ØSR
**Oximetry, Fetal pulse** 1ØH073Z
**Oxygenation**
  Extracorporeal membrane (ECMO) – *see* Performance, Circulatory 5A15
  Hyperbaric – *see* Assistance, Circulatory 5AØ5
  Supersaturated – *see* Assistance, Circulatory 5AØ5

# P

**Pacemaker**
  Dual Chamber
    Abdomen ØJH8
    Chest ØJH6
  Single Chamber
    Abdomen ØJH8
    Chest ØJH6
  Single Chamber Rate Responsive
    Abdomen ØJH8
    Chest ØJH6

**Packing**
- Abdominal Wall 2W43X5Z
- Anorectal 2Y43X5Z
- Arm
    - Lower
        - Left 2W4DX5Z
        - Right 2W4CX5Z
    - Upper
        - Left 2W4BX5Z
        - Right 2W4AX5Z
- Back 2W45X5Z
- Chest Wall 2W44X5Z
- Ear 2Y42X5Z
- Extremity
    - Lower
        - Left 2W4MX5Z
        - Right 2W4LX5Z
    - Upper
        - Left 2W49X5Z
        - Right 2W48X5Z
- Face 2W41X5Z
- Finger
    - Left 2W4KX5Z
    - Right 2W4JX5Z
- Foot
    - Left 2W4TX5Z
    - Right 2W4SX5Z
- Genital Tract, Female 2Y44X5Z
- Hand
    - Left 2W4FX5Z
    - Right 2W4EX5Z
- Head 2W40X5Z
- Inguinal Region
    - Left 2W47X5Z
    - Right 2W46X5Z
- Leg
    - Lower
        - Left 2W4RX5Z
        - Right 2W4QX5Z
    - Upper
        - Left 2W4PX5Z
        - Right 2W4NX5Z
- Mouth and Pharynx 2Y40X5Z
- Nasal 2Y41X5Z
- Neck 2W42X5Z
- Thumb
    - Left 2W4HX5Z
    - Right 2W4GX5Z
- Toe
    - Left 2W4VX5Z
    - Right 2W4UX5Z
- Urethra 2Y45X5Z

**Paclitaxel-eluting coronary stent** – *use* Intraluminal Device, Drug-eluting in Heart and Great Vessels

**Paclitaxel-eluting peripheral stent**
- *use* Intraluminal Device, Drug-eluting in Upper Arteries
- *use* Intraluminal Device, Drug-eluting in Lower Arteries

**Palatine gland** – *use* Buccal Mucosa

**Palatine tonsil** – *use* Tonsils

**Palatine uvula** – *use* Uvula

**Palatoglossal muscle** – *use* Muscle, Tongue, Palate, Pharynx

**Palatopharyngeal muscle** – *use* Muscle, Tongue, Palate, Pharynx

**Palatoplasty**
- *see* Repair, Mouth and Throat 0CQ
- *see* Replacement, Mouth and Throat 0CR
- *see* Supplement, Mouth and Throat 0CU

**Palatorrhaphy** – *see* Repair, Mouth and Throat 0CQ

**Palmar** (volar) **digital vein**
- *use* Vein, Hand, Right
- *use* Vein, Hand, Left

**Palmar** (volar) **metacarpal vein**
- *use* Vein, Hand, Left
- *use* Vein, Hand, Right

**Palmar cutaneous nerve**
- *use* Nerve, Radial
- *use* Nerve, Median

**Palmar fascia** (aponeurosis)
- *use* Subcutaneous Tissue and Fascia, Hand, Left
- *use* Subcutaneous Tissue and Fascia, Hand, Right

**Palmar interosseous muscle**
- *use* Muscle, Hand, Left
- *use* Muscle, Hand, Right

**Palmar ulnocarpal ligament**
- *use* Bursa and Ligament, Wrist, Right
- *use* Bursa and Ligament, Wrist, Left

**Palmaris longus muscle**
- *use* Muscle, Lower Arm and Wrist, Left
- *use* Muscle, Lower Arm and Wrist, Right

**Pancreatectomy**
- *see* Excision, Pancreas 0FBG
- *see* Resection, Pancreas 0FTG

**Pancreatic artery** – *use* Artery, Splenic

**Pancreatic plexus** – *use* Nerve, Abdominal Sympathetic

**Pancreatic vein** – *use* Vein, Splenic

**Pancreaticoduodenostomy** – *see* Bypass, Hepatobiliary System and Pancreas 0F1

**Pancreaticosplenic lymph node** – *use* Lymphatic, Aortic

**Pancreatogram, endoscopic retrograde** – *see* Fluoroscopy, Pancreatic Duct BF18

**Pancreatolithotomy** – *see* Extirpation, Pancreas 0FCG

**Pancreatotomy**
- *see* Drainage, Pancreas 0F9G
- *see* Division, Pancreas 0F8G

**Panniculectomy**
- *see* Excision, Skin, Abdomen 0HB7
- *see* Excision, Abdominal Wall 0WBF

**Paraaortic lymph node** – *use* Lymphatic, Aortic

**Paracentesis**
- Eye – *see* Drainage, Eye 089
- Peritoneal Cavity – *see* Drainage, Peritoneal Cavity 0W9G
- Tympanum – *see* Drainage, Ear, Nose, Sinus 099

**Pararectal lymph node** – *use* Lymphatic, Mesenteric

**Parasternal lymph node** – *use* Lymphatic, Thorax

**Parathyroidectomy**
- *see* Excision, Endocrine System 0GB
- *see* Resection, Endocrine System 0GT

**Paratracheal lymph node** – *use* Lymphatic, Thorax

**Paraurethral** (Skene's) **gland** – *use* Gland, Vestibular

**Parenteral nutrition, total** – *see* Introduction of Nutritional Substance

**Parietal lobe** – *use* Cerebral Hemisphere

**Parotid lymph node** – *use* Lymphatic, Head

**Parotid plexus** – *use* Nerve, Facial

**Parotidectomy**
- *see* Excision, Mouth and Throat 0CB
- *see* Resection, Mouth and Throat 0CT

**Pars flaccida**
- *use* Tympanic Membrane, Right
- *use* Tympanic Membrane, Left

**Partial joint replacement**
- Hip – *see* Replacement, Lower Joints 0SR
- Knee – *see* Replacement, Lower Joints 0SR
- Shoulder – *see* Replacement, Upper Joints 0RR

**Partially absorbable mesh** – *use* Synthetic Substitute

**Patch, blood, spinal** 3E0S3GC

**Patellapexy**
- *see* Repair, Lower Bones 0QQ
- *see* Reposition, Lower Bones 0QS

**Patellaplasty**
- *see* Repair, Lower Bones 0QQ
- *see* Replacement, Lower Bones 0QR
- *see* Supplement, Lower Bones 0QU

**Patellar ligament**
- *use* Bursa and Ligament, Knee, Right
- *use* Bursa and Ligament, Knee, Left

**Patellar tendon**
- *use* Tendon, Knee, Left
- *use* Tendon, Knee, Right

**Patellectomy**
- *see* Excision, Lower Bones 0QB
- *see* Resection, Lower Bones 0QT

**Patellofemoral joint**
- *use* Joint, Knee, Right
- *use* Joint, Knee, Left
- *use* Joint, Knee, Right, Femoral Surface
- *use* Joint, Knee, Left, Femoral Surface

**Pectineus muscle**
- *use* Muscle, Upper Leg, Left
- *use* Muscle, Upper Leg, Right

**Pectoral (anterior) lymph node**
- *use* Lymphatic, Axillary, Right
- *use* Lymphatic, Axillary, Left

**Pectoral fascia** – *use* Subcutaneous Tissue and Fascia, Chest

**Pectoralis major muscle**
- *use* Muscle, Thorax, Left
- *use* Muscle, Thorax, Right

**Pectoralis minor muscle**
- *use* Muscle, Thorax, Right
- *use* Muscle, Thorax, Left

**Pedicle-based dynamic stabilization device**
- *use* Spinal Stabilization Device, Pedicle–Based in 0RH
- *use* Spinal Stabilization Device, Pedicle–Based in 0SH

**PEEP (positive end expiratory pressure)** – *see* Assistance, Respiratory 5A09

**PEG (percutaneous endoscopic gastrostomy)** 0DH64UZ

**PEJ (percutaneous endoscopic jejunostomy)** 0DHA4UZ

**Pelvic splanchnic nerve**
- *use* Nerve, Abdominal Sympathetic
- *use* Nerve, Sacral Sympathetic

**Penectomy**
- *see* Excision, Male Reproductive System 0VB
- *see* Resection, Male Reproductive System 0VT

**Penile urethra** – *use* Urethra

**Percutaneous endoscopic gastrojejunostomy (PEG/J) tube** – *use* Feeding Device in Gastrointestinal System

**Percutaneous endoscopic gastrostomy (PEG) tube** – *use* Feeding Device in Gastrointestinal System

**Percutaneous nephrostomy catheter** – *use* Drainage Device

**Percutaneous transluminal coronary angioplasty (PTCA)** – *see* Dilation, Heart and Great Vessels 027

**Performance**
- Biliary
    - Multiple, Filtration 5A1C60Z
    - Single, Filtration 5A1C00Z
- Cardiac
    - Continuous
        - Output 5A1221Z
        - Pacing 5A1223Z
    - Intermittent, Pacing 5A1213Z
    - Single, Output, Manual 5A12012
- Circulatory, Continuous, Oxygenation, Membrane 5A15223
- Respiratory
    - 24–96 Consecutive Hours, Ventilation 5A1945Z
    - Greater than 96 Consecutive Hours, Ventilation 5A1955Z
    - Less than 24 Consecutive Hours, Ventilation 5A1935Z
    - Single, Ventilation, Nonmechanical 5A19054
- Urinary
    - Multiple, Filtration 5A1D60Z
    - Single, Filtration 5A1D00Z

**Perfusion** – *see* Introduction of substance in or on

**Pericardiectomy**
- *see* Excision, Pericardium 02BN
- *see* Resection, Pericardium 02TN

**Pericardiocentesis** – *see* Drainage, Pericardial Cavity 0W9D

**Pericardiolysis** – *see* Release, Pericardium 02NN

**Pericardiophrenic artery**
- *use* Artery, Internal Mammary, Left
- *use* Artery, Internal Mammary, Right

**Pericardioplasty**
- *see* Repair, Pericardium 02QN
- *see* Replacement, Pericardium 02RN
- *see* Supplement, Pericardium 02UN

**Pericardiorrhaphy** – *see* Repair, Pericardium 02QN

**Pericardiostomy** – *see* Drainage, Pericardial Cavity 0W9D

**Pericardiotomy** – *see* Drainage, Pericardial Cavity 0W9D

**Perimetrium** – *use* Uterus

**Peripheral parenteral nutrition** – *see* Introduction of Nutritional Substance

**Peripherally inserted central catheter (PICC)** – *use* Infusion Device

**Peritoneal dialysis** 3E1M39Z

**Peritoneocentesis**
- *see* Drainage, Peritoneum 0D9W
- *see* Drainage, Peritoneal Cavity 0W9G

**Peritoneoplasty**
- *see* Repair, Peritoneum 0DQW
- *see* Replacement, Peritoneum 0DRW
- *see* Supplement, Peritoneum 0DUW

**Peritoneoscopy** 0DJW4ZZ

**Peritoneotomy** – *see* Drainage, Peritoneum 0D9W

**Peritoneumectomy** – *see* Excision, Peritoneum 0DBW

**Peroneus brevis muscle**
- *use* Muscle, Lower Leg, Left
- *use* Muscle, Lower Leg, Right

**Peroneus longus muscle**
- *use* Muscle, Lower Leg, Right
- *use* Muscle, Lower Leg, Left

**Pessary ring** – *use* Intraluminal Device, Pessary in Female Reproductive System

**PET scan** – *see* Positron Emission Tomographic (PET) Imaging

**Petrous part of temporal bone**
– *use* Bone, Temporal, Right
– *use* Bone, Temporal, Left

**Phacoemulsification, lens**
With IOL implant – *see* Replacement, Eye 08R
Without IOL implant – *see* Extraction, Eye 08D

**Phalangectomy**
– *see* Excision, Upper Bones 0PB
– *see* Resection, Upper Bones 0PT
– *see* Excision, Lower Bones 0QB
– *see* Resection, Lower Bones 0QT

**Phallectomy**
– *see* Excision, Penis 0VBS
– *see* Resection, Penis 0VTS

**Phalloplasty**
– *see* Repair, Penis 0VQS
– *see* Supplement, Penis 0VUS

**Phallotomy** – *see* Drainage, Penis 0V9S

**Pharmocotherapy, for substance abuse**
Antabuse HZ93ZZZ
Bupropion HZ97ZZZ
Clonidine HZ96ZZZ
Levo-alpha-acetyl-methadol (LAAM) HZ92ZZZ
Methadone Maintenance HZ91ZZZ
Naloxone HZ95ZZZ
Naltrexone HZ94ZZZ
Nicotine Replacement HZ90ZZZ
Psychiatric Medication HZ98ZZZ
Replacement Medication, Other HZ99ZZZ

**Pharyngeal constrictor muscle** – *use* Muscle, Tongue, Palate, Pharynx

**Pharyngeal plexus** – *use* Nerve, Vagus

**Pharyngeal recess** – *use* Nasopharynx

**Pharyngeal tonsil** – *use* Adenoids

**Pharyngogram** – *see* Fluoroscopy, Pharynx B91G

**Pharyngoplasty**
– *see* Repair, Mouth and Throat 0CQ
– *see* Replacement, Mouth and Throat 0CR
– *see* Supplement, Mouth and Throat 0CU

**Pharyngorrhaphy** – *see* Repair, Mouth and Throat 0CQ

**Pharyngotomy** – *see* Drainage, Mouth and Throat 0C9

**Pharyngotympanic tube**
– *use* Eustachian Tube, Right
– *use* Eustachian Tube, Left

**Pheresis**
Erythrocytes 6A55
Leukocytes 6A55
Plasma 6A55
Platelets 6A55
Stem Cells
Cord Blood 6A55
Hematopoietic 6A55

**Phlebectomy**
– *see* Excision, Upper Veins 05B
– *see* Extraction, Upper Veins 05D
– *see* Excision, Lower Veins 06B
– *see* Extraction, Lower Veins 06D

**Phlebography**
– *see* Plain Radiography, Veins B50
Impedance 4A04X51

**Phleborrhaphy**
– *see* Repair, Upper Veins 05Q
– *see* Repair, Lower Veins 06Q

**Phlebotomy**
– *see* Drainage, Upper Veins 059
– *see* Drainage, Lower Veins 069

**Photocoagulation**
for Destruction – *see* Destruction
for Repair – *see* Repair

**Photopheresis, therapeutic** – *see* Phototherapy, Circulatory 6A65

**Phototherapy**
Circulatory 6A65
Skin 6A60

**Phrenectomy, phrenoneurectomy** – *see* Excision, Nerve, Phrenic 01B2

**Phrenemphraxis** – *see* Destruction, Nerve, Phrenic 0152

**Phrenic nerve stimulator generator** – *use* Stimulator Generator in Subcutaneous Tissue and Fascia

**Phrenic nerve stimulator lead** – *use* Diaphragmatic Pacemaker Lead in Respiratory System

**Phreniclasis** – *see* Destruction, Nerve, Phrenic 0152

**Phrenicoexeresis** – *see* Extraction, Nerve, Phrenic 01D2

**Phrenicotomy** – *see* Division, Nerve, Phrenic 0182

**Phrenicotripsy** – *see* Destruction, Nerve, Phrenic 0152

**Phrenoplasty**
– *see* Repair, Respiratory System 0BQ
– *see* Supplement, Respiratory System 0BU

**Phrenotomy** – *see* Drainage, Respiratory System 0B9

**Physiatry** – *see* Motor Treatment, Rehabilitation F07

**Physical medicine** – *see* Motor Treatment, Rehabilitation F07

**Physical therapy** – *see* Motor Treatment, Rehabilitation F07

**PHYSIOMESH™ Flexible Composite Mesh** – *use* Synthetic Substitute

**Pia mater**
– *use* Spinal Meninges
– *use* Cerebral Meninges

**Pinealectomy**
– *see* Excision, Pineal Body 0GB1
– *see* Resection, Pineal Body 0GT1

**Pinealoscopy** 0GJ14ZZ

**Pinealotomy** – *see* Drainage, Pineal Body 0G91

**Pinna**
– *use* Ear, External, Left
– *use* Ear, External, Bilateral
– *use* Ear, External, Right

**Pipeline™ Embolization device (PED)** – *use* Intraluminal Device

**Piriform recess** (sinus) – *use* Pharynx

**Piriformis muscle**
– *use* Muscle, Hip, Left
– *use* Muscle, Hip, Right

**Pisiform bone**
– *use* Carpal, Left
– *use* Carpal, Right

**Pisohamate ligament**
– *use* Bursa and Ligament, Hand, Right
– *use* Bursa and Ligament, Hand, Left

**Pisometacarpal ligament**
– *use* Bursa and Ligament, Hand, Left
– *use* Bursa and Ligament, Hand, Right

**Pituitectomy**
– *see* Excision, Gland, Pituitary 0GB0
– *see* Resection, Gland, Pituitary 0GT0

**Plain film radiology** – *see* Plain Radiography

**Plain Radiography**
Abdomen BW00ZZZ
Abdomen and Pelvis BW01ZZZ
Abdominal Lymphatic
Bilateral B701
Unilateral B700
Airway, Upper BB0DZZZ
Ankle
Left BQ0H
Right BQ0G
Aorta
Abdominal B400
Thoracic B300
Thoraco-Abdominal B30P
Aorta and Bilateral Lower Extremity Arteries B40D
Arch
Bilateral BN0DZZZ
Left BN0CZZZ
Right BN0BZZZ
Arm
Left BP0FZZZ
Right BP0EZZZ
Artery
Brachiocephalic-Subclavian, Right B301
Bronchial B30L
Bypass Graft, Other B20F
Cervico-Cerebral Arch B30Q
Common Carotid
Bilateral B305
Left B304
Right B303
Coronary
Bypass Graft
Multiple B203
Single B202
Multiple B201
Single B200
External Carotid
Bilateral B30C
Left B30B
Right B309
Hepatic B402
Inferior Mesenteric B405
Intercostal B30L
Internal Carotid
Bilateral B308
Left B307
Right B306
Internal Mammary Bypass Graft
Left B208
Right B207
Intra-Abdominal, Other B40B

**Plain Radiography** – *continued*
Artery – *continued*
Intracranial B30R
Lower, Other B40J
Lower Extremity
Bilateral and Aorta B40D
Left B40G
Right B40F
Lumbar B409
Pelvic B40C
Pulmonary
Left B30T
Right B30S
Renal
Bilateral B408
Left B407
Right B406
Transplant B40M
Spinal B30M
Splenic B403
Subclavian, Left B302
Superior Mesenteric B404
Upper, Other B30N
Upper Extremity
Bilateral B30K
Left B30J
Right B30H
Vertebral
Bilateral B30G
Left B30F
Right B30D
Bile Duct BF00
Bile Duct and Gallbladder BF03
Bladder BT00
Kidney and Ureter BT04
Bladder and Urethra BT0B
Bone
Facial BN05ZZZ
Nasal BN04ZZZ
Bones, Long, All BW0BZZZ
Breast
Bilateral BH02ZZZ
Left BH01ZZZ
Right BH00ZZZ
Calcaneus
Left BQ0KZZZ
Right BQ0JZZZ
Chest BW03ZZZ
Clavicle
Left BP05ZZZ
Right BP04ZZZ
Coccyx BR0FZZZ
Corpora Cavernosa BV00
Dialysis Fistula B50W
Dialysis Shunt B50W
Disc
Cervical BR01
Lumbar BR03
Thoracic BR02
Duct
Lacrimal
Bilateral B802
Left B801
Right B800
Mammary
Multiple
Left BH06
Right BH05
Single
Left BH04
Right BH03
Elbow
Left BP0H
Right BP0G
Epididymis
Left BV02
Right BV01
Extremity
Lower BW0CZZZ
Upper BW0JZZZ
Eye
Bilateral B807ZZZ
Left B806ZZZ
Right B805ZZZ
Facet Joint
Cervical BR04
Lumbar BR06
Thoracic BR05
Fallopian Tube
Bilateral BU02
Left BU01
Right BU00
Fallopian Tube and Uterus BU08

**Plain Radiography** – *continued*
  Femur
    Left, Densitometry BQ04ZZ1
    Right, Densitometry BQ03ZZ1
  Finger
    Left BP0SZZZ
    Right BP0RZZZ
  Foot
    Left BQ0MZZZ
    Right BQ0LZZZ
  Forearm
    Left BP0KZZZ
    Right BP0JZZZ
  Gallbladder and Bile Duct BF03
  Gland
    Parotid
      Bilateral B906
      Left B905
      Right B904
    Salivary
      Bilateral B90D
      Left B90C
      Right B90B
    Submandibular
      Bilateral B909
      Left B908
      Right B907
  Hand
    Left BP0PZZZ
    Right BP0NZZZ
  Heart
    Left B205
    Right B204
    Right and Left B206
  Hepatobiliary System, All BF0C
  Hip
    Left BQ01
      Densitometry BQ01ZZ1
    Right BQ00
      Densitometry BQ00ZZ1
  Humerus
    Left BP0BZZZ
    Right BP0AZZZ
  Ileal Diversion Loop BT0C
  Intracranial Sinus B502
  Joint
    Acromioclavicular, Bilateral BP03ZZZ
    Finger
      Left BP0D
      Right BP0C
    Foot
      Left BQ0Y
      Right BQ0X
    Hand
      Left BP0D
      Right BP0C
    Lumbosacral BR0BZZZ
    Sacroiliac BR0D
    Sternoclavicular
      Bilateral BP02ZZZ
      Left BP01ZZZ
      Right BP00ZZZ
    Temporomandibular
      Bilateral BN09
      Left BN08
      Right BN07
    Thoracolumbar BR08ZZZ
    Toe
      Left BQ0Y
      Right BQ0X
  Kidney
    Bilateral BT03
    Left BT02
    Right BT01
    Ureter and Bladder BT04
  Knee
    Left BQ08
    Right BQ07
  Leg
    Left BQ0FZZZ
    Right BQ0DZZZ
  Lymphatic
    Head B704
    Lower Extremity
      Bilateral B70B
      Left B709
      Right B708
    Neck B704
    Pelvic B70C
    Upper Extremity
      Bilateral B707
      Left B706
      Right B705

**Plain Radiography** – *continued*
  Mandible BN06ZZZ
  Mastoid B90HZZZ
  Nasopharynx B90FZZZ
  Optic Foramina
    Left B804ZZZ
    Right B803ZZZ
  Orbit
    Bilateral BN03ZZZ
    Left BN02ZZZ
    Right BN01ZZZ
  Oropharynx B90FZZZ
  Patella
    Left BQ0WZZZ
    Right BQ0VZZZ
  Pelvis BR0CZZZ
  Pelvis and Abdomen BW01ZZZ
  Prostate BV03
  Retroperitoneal Lymphatic
    Bilateral B701
    Unilateral B700
  Ribs
    Left BP0YZZZ
    Right BP0XZZZ
  Sacrum BR0FZZZ
  Scapula
    Left BP07ZZZ
    Right BP06ZZZ
  Shoulder
    Left BP09
    Right BP08
  Sinus
    Intracranial B502
    Paranasal B902ZZZ
  Skull BN00ZZZ
  Spinal Cord B00B
  Spine
    Cervical, Densitometry BR00ZZ1
    Lumbar, Densitometry BR09ZZ1
    Thoracic, Densitometry BR07ZZ1
    Whole, Densitometry BR0GZZ1
  Sternum BR0HZZZ
  Teeth
    All BN0JZZZ
    Multiple BN0HZZZ
  Testicle
    Left BV06
    Right BV05
  Toe
    Left BQ0QZZZ
    Right BQ0PZZZ
  Tooth, Single BN0GZZZ
  Tracheobronchial Tree
    Bilateral BB09YZZ
    Left BB08YZZ
    Right BB07YZZ
  Ureter
    Bilateral BT08
    Kidney and Bladder BT04
    Left BT07
    Right BT06
  Urethra BT05
  Urethra and Bladder BT0B
  Uterus BU06
  Uterus and Fallopian Tube BU08
  Vagina BU09
  Vasa Vasorum BV08
  Vein
    Cerebellar B501
    Cerebral B501
    Epidural B500
    Jugular
      Bilateral B505
      Left B504
      Right B503
    Lower Extremity
      Bilateral B50D
      Left B50C
      Right B50B
    Other B50V
    Pelvic (Iliac)
      Left B50G
      Right B50F
    Pelvic (Iliac) Bilateral B50H
    Portal B50T
    Pulmonary
      Bilateral B50S
      Left B50R
      Right B50Q
    Renal
      Bilateral B50L
      Left B50K
      Right B50J

**Plain Radiography** – *continued*
  Vein – *continued*
    Spanchnic B50T
    Subclavian
      Left B507
      Right B506
    Upper Extremity
      Bilateral B50P
      Left B50N
      Right B50M
  Vena Cava
    Inferior B509
    Superior B508
  Whole Body BW0KZZZ
    Infant BW0MZZZ
  Whole Skeleton BW0LZZZ
  Wrist
    Left BP0M
    Right BP0L

**Planar Nuclear Medicine Imaging** CP1
  Abdomen CW10
  Abdomen and Chest CW14
  Abdomen and Pelvis CW11
  Anatomical Regions, Multiple CW1YYZZ
  Bladder, Kidneys and Ureters CT13
  Bladder and Ureters CT1H
  Blood C713
  Bone Marrow C710
  Brain C010
  Breast CH1YYZZ
    Bilateral CH12
    Left CH11
    Right CH10
  Bronchi and Lungs CB12
  Central Nervous System C01YYZZ
  Cerebrospinal Fluid C015
  Chest CW13
  Chest and Abdomen CW14
  Chest and Neck CW16
  Digestive System CD1YYZZ
  Ducts, Lacrimal, Bilateral C819
  Ear, Nose, Mouth and Throat C91YYZZ
  Endocrine System CG1YYZZ
  Extremity
    Lower CW1D
      Bilateral CP1F
      Left CP1D
      Right CP1C
    Upper CW1M
      Bilateral CP1B
      Left CP19
      Right CP18
  Eye C81YYZZ
  Gallbladder CF14
  Gastrointestinal Tract CD17
    Upper CD15
  Gland
    Adrenal, Bilateral CG14
    Parathyroid CG11
    Thyroid CG12
  Glands, Salivary, Bilateral C91B
  Head and Neck CW1B
  Heart C21YYZZ
    Right and Left C216
  Hepatobiliary System, All CF1C
  Hepatobiliary System and Pancreas CF1YYZZ
  Kidneys, Ureters and Bladder CT13
  Liver CF15
  Liver and Spleen CF16
  Lungs and Bronchi CB12
  Lymphatics
    Head C71J
    Head and Neck C715
    Lower Extremity C71P
    Neck C71K
    Pelvic C71D
    Trunk C71M
    Upper Chest C71L
    Upper Extremity C71N
  Lymphatics and Hematologic System C71YYZZ
  Musculoskeletal System, All CP1Z
  Myocardium C21G
  Neck and Chest CW16
  Neck and Head CW1B
  Pancreas and Hepatobiliary System CF1YYZZ
  Pelvic Region CW1J
  Pelvis CP16
  Pelvis and Abdomen CW11
  Pelvis and Spine CP17
  Reproductive System, Male CV1YYZZ
  Respiratory System CB1YYZZ
  Skin CH1YYZZ
  Skull CP11

**Planar Nuclear Medicine Imaging** – *continued*
Spine CP15
Spine and Pelvis CP17
Spleen C712
Spleen and Liver CF16
Subcutaneous Tissue CH1YYZZ
Testicles, Bilateral CV19
Thorax CP14
Ureters, Kidneys and Bladder CT13
Ureters and Bladder CT1H
Urinary System CT1YYZZ
Veins C51YYZZ
  Central C51R
  Lower Extremity
    Bilateral C51D
    Left C51C
    Right C51B
  Upper Extremity
    Bilateral C51Q
    Left C51P
    Right C51N
Whole Body CW1N
**Plantar digital vein**
  – *use* Vein, Foot, Right
  – *use* Vein, Foot, Left
**Plantar fascia** (aponeurosis)
  – *use* Subcutaneous Tissue and Fascia, Foot, Right
  – *use* Subcutaneous Tissue and Fascia, Foot, Left
**Plantar metatarsal vein**
  – *use* Vein, Foot, Right
  – *use* Vein, Foot, Left
**Plantar venous arch**
  – *use* Vein, Foot, Right
  – *use* Vein, Foot, Left
**Plaque Radiation**
Abdomen DWY3FZZ
Adrenal Gland DGY2FZZ
Anus DDY8FZZ
Bile Ducts DFY2FZZ
Bladder DTY2FZZ
Bone, Other DPYCFZZ
Bone Marrow D7Y0FZZ
Brain D0Y0FZZ
Brain Stem D0Y1FZZ
Breast
  Left DMY0FZZ
  Right DMY1FZZ
Bronchus DBY1FZZ
Cervix DUY1FZZ
Chest DWY2FZZ
Chest Wall DBY7FZZ
Colon DDY5FZZ
Diaphragm DBY8FZZ
Duodenum DDY2FZZ
Ear D9Y0FZZ
Esophagus DDY0FZZ
Eye D8Y0FZZ
Femur DPY9FZZ
Fibula DPYBFZZ
Gallbladder DFY1FZZ
Gland
  Adrenal DGY2FZZ
  Parathyroid DGY4FZZ
  Pituitary DGY0FZZ
  Thyroid DGY5FZZ
Glands, Salivary D9Y6FZZ
Head and Neck DWY1FZZ
Hemibody DWY4FZZ
Humerus DPY6FZZ
Ileum DDY4FZZ
Jejunum DDY3FZZ
Kidney DTY0FZZ
Larynx D9YBFZZ
Liver DFY0FZZ
Lung DBY2FZZ
Lymphatics
  Abdomen D7Y6FZZ
  Axillary D7Y4FZZ
  Inguinal D7Y8FZZ
  Neck D7Y3FZZ
  Pelvis D7Y7FZZ
  Thorax D7Y5FZZ
Mandible DPY3FZZ
Maxilla DPY2FZZ
Mediastinum DBY6FZZ
Mouth D9Y4FZZ
Nasopharynx D9YDFZZ
Neck and Head DWY1FZZ
Nerve, Peripheral D0Y7FZZ
Nose D9Y1FZZ
Ovary DUY0FZZ
Palate
  Hard D9Y8FZZ

**Plaque Radiation** – *continued*
Palate – *continued*
  Soft D9Y9FZZ
Pancreas DFY3FZZ
Parathyroid Gland DGY4FZZ
Pelvic Bones DPY8FZZ
Pelvic Region DWY6FZZ
Pharynx D9YCFZZ
Pineal Body DGY1FZZ
Pituitary Gland DGY0FZZ
Pleura DBY5FZZ
Prostate DVY0FZZ
Radius DPY7FZZ
Rectum DDY7FZZ
Rib DPY5FZZ
Sinuses D9Y7FZZ
Skin
  Abdomen DHY8FZZ
  Arm DHY4FZZ
  Back DHY7FZZ
  Buttock DHY9FZZ
  Chest DHY6FZZ
  Face DHY2FZZ
  Foot DHYCFZZ
  Hand DHY5FZZ
  Leg DHYBFZZ
  Neck DHY3FZZ
Skull DPY0FZZ
Spinal Cord D0Y6FZZ
Spleen D7Y2FZZ
Sternum DPY4FZZ
Stomach DDY1FZZ
Testis DVY1FZZ
Thymus D7Y1FZZ
Thyroid Gland DGY5FZZ
Tibia DPYBFZZ
Tongue D9Y5FZZ
Trachea DBY0FZZ
Ulna DPY7FZZ
Ureter DTY1FZZ
Urethra DTY3FZZ
Uterus DUY2FZZ
Whole Body DWY5FZZ
**Plasmapheresis, therapeutic** 6A550Z3
**Plateletpheresis, therapeutic** 6A550Z2
**Platysma muscle**
  – *use* Muscle, Neck, Left
  – *use* Muscle, Neck, Right
**Pleurectomy**
  – *see* Excision, Respiratory System 0BB
  – *see* Resection, Respiratory System 0BT
**Pleurocentesis** – *see* Drainage, Anatomical Regions, General 0W9
**Pleurodesis, pleurosclerosis**
  Chemical injection – *see* Introduction of substance in or on, Pleural Cavity 3E0L
  Surgical – *see* Destruction, Respiratory System 0B5
**Pleurolysis** – *see* Release, Respiratory System 0BN
**Pleuroscopy** 0BJQ4ZZ
**Pleurotomy** – *see* Drainage, Respiratory System 0B9
**Plica semilunaris**
  – *use* Conjunctiva, Left
  – *use* Conjunctiva, Right
**Plication** – *see* Restriction
**Pneumectomy**
  – *see* Excision, Respiratory System 0BB
  – *see* Resection, Respiratory System 0BT
**Pneumocentesis** – *see* Drainage, Respiratory System 0B9
**Pneumogastric nerve** – *use* Nerve, Vagus
**Pneumolysis** – *see* Release, Respiratory System 0BN
**Pneumonectomy** – *see* Resection, Respiratory System 0BT
**Pneumonolysis** – *see* Release, Respiratory System 0BN
**Pneumonopexy**
  – *see* Repair, Respiratory System 0BQ
  – *see* Reposition, Respiratory System 0BS
**Pneumonorrhaphy** – *see* Repair, Respiratory System 0BQ
**Pneumonotomy** – *see* Drainage, Respiratory System 0B9
**Pneumotaxic center** – *use* Pons
**Pneumotomy** – *see* Drainage, Respiratory System 0B9
**Pollicization** – *see* Transfer, Anatomical Regions, Upper Extremities 0XX
**Polyethylene socket** – *use* Synthetic Substitute, Polyethylene in 0SR
**Polymethylmethacrylate (PMMA)** – *use* Synthetic Substitute
**Polypectomy, gastrointestinal** – *see* Excision, Gastrointestinal System 0DB
**Polypropylene mesh** – *use* Synthetic Substitute
**Polysomnogram** 4A1ZXQZ

**Pontine tegmentum** – *use* Pons
**Popliteal ligament**
  – *use* Bursa and Ligament, Knee, Right
  – *use* Bursa and Ligament, Knee, Left
**Popliteal lymph node**
  – *use* Lymphatic, Lower Extremity, Right
  – *use* Lymphatic, Lower Extremity, Left
**Popliteal vein**
  – *use* Vein, Femoral, Right
  – *use* Vein, Femoral, Left
**Popliteus muscle**
  – *use* Muscle, Lower Leg, Right
  – *use* Muscle, Lower Leg, Left
**Porcine** (bioprosthetic) **valve** – *use* Zooplastic Tissue in Heart and Great Vessels
**Positive end expiratory pressure** – *see* Performance, Respiratory 5A19
**Positron Emission Tomographic (PET) Imaging**
Brain C030
Bronchi and Lungs CB32
Central Nervous System C03YYZZ
Heart C23YYZZ
Lungs and Bronchi CB32
Myocardium C23G
Respiratory System CB3YYZZ
Whole Body CW3NYZZ
**Positron emission tomography** – *see* Positron Emission Tomographic (PET) Imaging
**Postauricular (mastoid) lymph node**
  – *use* Lymphatic, Neck, Right
  – *use* Lymphatic, Neck, Left
**Postcava** – *use* Vena Cava, Inferior
**Posterior (subscapular) lymph node**
  – *use* Lymphatic, Axillary, Left
  – *use* Lymphatic, Axillary, Right
**Posterior auricular artery**
  – *use* Artery, External Carotid, Right
  – *use* Artery, External Carotid, Left
**Posterior auricular nerve** – *use* Nerve, Facial
**Posterior auricular vein**
  – *use* Vein, External Jugular, Left
  – *use* Vein, External Jugular, Right
**Posterior cerebral artery** – *use* Artery, Intracranial
**Posterior chamber**
  – *use* Eye, Right
  – *use* Eye, Left
**Posterior circumflex humeral artery**
  – *use* Artery, Axillary, Right
  – *use* Artery, Axillary, Left
**Posterior communicating artery** – *use* Artery, Intracranial
**Posterior cruciate ligament (PCL)**
  – *use* Bursa and Ligament, Knee, Right
  – *use* Bursa and Ligament, Knee, Left
**Posterior facial** (retromandibular) **vein**
  – *use* Vein, Face, Right
  – *use* Vein, Face, Left
**Posterior femoral cutaneous nerve** – *use* Nerve, Sacral Plexus
**Posterior inferior cerebellar artery (PICA)** – *use* Artery, Intracranial
**Posterior interosseous nerve** – *use* Nerve, Radial
**Posterior labial nerve** – *use* Nerve, Pudendal
**Posterior scrotal nerve** – *use* Nerve, Pudendal
**Posterior spinal artery**
  – *use* Artery, Vertebral, Left
  – *use* Artery, Vertebral, Right
**Posterior tibial recurrent artery**
  – *use* Artery, Anterior Tibial, Right
  – *use* Artery, Anterior Tibial, Left
**Posterior ulnar recurrent artery**
  – *use* Artery, Ulnar, Left
  – *use* Artery, Ulnar, Right
**Posterior vagal trunk** – *use* Nerve, Vagus
**PPN (peripheral parenteral nutrition)** – *see* Introduction of Nutritional Substance
**Preauricular lymph node** – *use* Lymphatic, Head
**Precava** – *use* Vena Cava, Superior
**Prepatellar bursa**
  – *use* Bursa and Ligament, Knee, Right
  – *use* Bursa and Ligament, Knee, Left
**Preputiotomy** – *see* Drainage, Male Reproductive System 0V9
**Pressure support ventilation** – *see* Performance, Respiratory 5A19
**PRESTIGE® Cervical Disc** – *use* Synthetic Substitute

**Pretracheal fascia** – *use* Subcutaneous Tissue and Fascia, Neck, Anterior
**Prevertebral fascia** – *use* Subcutaneous Tissue and Fascia, Neck, Posterior
**PrimeAdvanced neurostimulator (SureScan)(MRI Safe)** – *use* Stimulator Generator, Multiple Array in ØJH
**Princeps pollicis artery**
   – *use* Artery, Hand, Left
   – *use* Artery, Hand, Right
**Probing, duct**
   Diagnostic – *see* Inspection
   Dilation – *see* Dilation
**PROCEED™ Ventral Patch** – *use* Synthetic Substitute
**Procerus muscle** – *use* Muscle, Facial
**Proctectomy**
   – *see* Excision, Rectum ØDBP
   – *see* Resection, Rectum ØDTP
**Proctoclysis** – *see* Introduction of substance in or on, Gastrointestinal Tract, Lower 3EØH
**Proctocolectomy**
   – *see* Excision, Gastrointestinal System ØDB
   – *see* Resection, Gastrointestinal System ØDT
**Proctocolpoplasty**
   – *see* Repair, Gastrointestinal System ØDQ
   – *see* Supplement, Gastrointestinal System ØDU
**Proctoperineoplasty**
   – *see* Repair, Gastrointestinal System ØDQ
   – *see* Supplement, Gastrointestinal System ØDU
**Proctoperineorrhaphy** – *see* Repair, Gastrointestinal System ØDQ
**Proctopexy**
   – *see* Repair, Rectum ØDQP
   – *see* Reposition, Rectum ØDSP
**Proctoplasty**
   – *see* Repair, Rectum ØDQP
   – *see* Supplement, Rectum ØDUP
**Proctorrhaphy** – *see* Repair, Rectum ØDQP
**Proctoscopy** ØDJD8ZZ
**Proctosigmoidectomy**
   – *see* Excision, Gastrointestinal System ØDB
   – *see* Resection, Gastrointestinal System ØDT
**Proctosigmoidoscopy** ØDJD8ZZ
**Proctostomy** – *see* Drainage, Rectum ØD9P
**Proctotomy** – *see* Drainage, Rectum ØD9P
**Prodisc-C** – *use* Synthetic Substitute
**Prodisc-L** – *use* Synthetic Substitute
**Production, atrial septal defect** – *see* Excision, Septum, Atrial Ø2B5
**Profunda brachii**
   – *use* Artery, Brachial, Right
   – *use* Artery, Brachial, Left
**Profunda femoris (deep femoral) vein**
   – *use* Vein, Femoral, Right
   – *use* Vein, Femoral, Left
**PROLENE Polypropylene Hernia System (PHS)** – *use* Synthetic Substitute
**Pronator quadratus muscle**
   – *use* Muscle, Lower Arm and Wrist, Left
   – *use* Muscle, Lower Arm and Wrist, Right
**Pronator teres muscle**
   – *use* Muscle, Lower Arm and Wrist, Right
   – *use* Muscle, Lower Arm and Wrist, Left
**Prostatectomy**
   – *see* Excision, Prostate ØVBØ
   – *see* Resection, Prostate ØVTØ
**Prostatic urethra** – *use* Urethra
**Prostatomy, prostatotomy** – *see* Drainage, Prostate ØV9Ø
**Protecta XT CRT-D** – *use* Cardiac Resynchronization Defibrillator Pulse Generator in ØJH
**Protecta XT DR** (XT VR) – *use* Defibrillator Generator in ØJH
**Protégé® RX Carotid Stent System** – *use* Intraluminal Device
**Proximal radioulnar joint**
   – *use* Joint, Elbow, Left
   – *use* Joint, Elbow, Right
**Psoas muscle**
   – *use* Muscle, Hip, Right
   – *use* Muscle, Hip, Left
**PSV (pressure support ventilation)** – *see* Performance, Respiratory 5A19
**Psychoanalysis** GZ54ZZZ
**Psychological Tests**
   Cognitive Status GZ14ZZZ
   Developmental GZ1ØZZZ
   Intellectual and Psychoeducational GZ12ZZZ

**Psychological Tests** – *continued*
   Neurobehavioral Status GZ14ZZZ
   Neuropsychological GZ13ZZZ
   Personality and Behavioral GZ11ZZZ
**Psychotherapy**
   Family, Mental Health Services GZ72ZZZ
   Group GZHZZZZ
      Mental Health Services GZHZZZZ
   Individual
      – *see* Psychotherapy, Individual, Mental Health Services
   for substance abuse
      12–Step HZ53ZZZ
      Behavioral HZ51ZZZ
      Cognitive HZ5ØZZZ
      Cognitive–Behavioral HZ52ZZZ
      Confrontational HZ58ZZZ
      Interactive HZ55ZZZ
      Interpersonal HZ54ZZZ
      Motivational Enhancement HZ57ZZZ
      Psychoanalysis HZ5BZZZ
      Psychodynamic HZ5CZZZ
      Psychoeducation HZ56ZZZ
      Psychophysiological HZ5DZZZ
      Supportive HZ59ZZZ
   Mental Health Services
      Behavioral GZ51ZZZ
      Cognitive GZ52ZZZ
      Cognitive–Behavioral GZ58ZZZ
      Interactive GZ5ØZZZ
      Interpersonal GZ53ZZZ
      Psychoanalysis GZ54ZZZ
      Psychodynamic GZ55ZZZ
      Psychophysiological GZ59ZZZ
      Supportive GZ56ZZZ
**PTCA (percutaneous transluminal coronary angioplasty)** – *see* Dilation, Heart and Great Vessels Ø27
**Pterygoid muscle** – *use* Muscle, Head
**Pterygoid process**
   – *use* Bone, Sphenoid, Right
   – *use* Bone, Sphenoid, Left
**Pterygopalatine** (sphenopalatine) **ganglion** – *use* Nerve, Head and Neck Sympathetic
**Pubic ligament**
   – *use* Bursa and Ligament, Trunk, Right
   – *use* Bursa and Ligament, Trunk, Left
**Pubis**
   – *use* Bone, Pelvic, Right
   – *use* Bone, Pelvic, Left
**Pubofemoral ligament**
   – *use* Bursa and Ligament, Hip, Left
   – *use* Bursa and Ligament, Hip, Right
**Pudendal nerve** – *use* Nerve, Sacral Plexus
**Pull-through, rectal** – *see* Resection, Rectum ØDTP
**Pulmoaortic canal** – *use* Artery, Pulmonary, Left
**Pulmonary annulus** – *use* Valve, Pulmonary
**Pulmonary artery wedge monitoring** – *see* Monitoring, Arterial 4A13
**Pulmonary plexus**
   – *use* Nerve, Vagus
   – *use* Nerve, Thoracic Sympathetic
**Pulmonic valve** – *use* Valve, Pulmonary
**Pulpectomy** – *see* Excision, Mouth and Throat ØCB
**Pulverization** – *see* Fragmentation
**Pulvinar** – *use* Thalamus
**Pump reservoir** – *use* Infusion Device, Pump in Subcutaneous Tissue and Fascia
**Punch biopsy** – *see* Excision with qualifier Diagnostic
**Puncture** – *see* Drainage
**Puncture, lumbar** – *see* Drainage, Spinal Canal ØØ9U
**Pyelography**
   – *see* Plain Radiography, Urinary System BTØ
   – *see* Fluoroscopy, Urinary System BT1
**Pyeloileostomy, urinary diversion** – *see* Bypass, Urinary System ØT1
**Pyeloplasty**
   – *see* Repair, Urinary System ØTQ
   – *see* Replacement, Urinary System ØTR
   – *see* Supplement, Urinary System ØTU
**Pyelorrhaphy** – *see* Repair, Urinary System ØTQ
**Pyeloscopy** ØTJ58ZZ
**Pyelostomy**
   – *see* Drainage, Urinary System ØT9
   – *see* Bypass, Urinary System ØT1
**Pyelotomy** – *see* Drainage, Urinary System ØT9
**Pylorectomy**
   – *see* Excision, Stomach, Pylorus ØDB7
   – *see* Resection, Stomach, Pylorus ØDT7

**Pyloric antrum** – *use* Stomach, Pylorus
**Pyloric canal** – *use* Stomach, Pylorus
**Pyloric sphincter** – *use* Stomach, Pylorus
**Pylorodiosis** – *see* Dilation, Stomach, Pylorus ØD77
**Pylorogastrectomy**
   – *see* Excision, Gastrointestinal System ØDB
   – *see* Resection, Gastrointestinal System ØDT
**Pyloroplasty**
   – *see* Repair, Stomach, Pylorus ØDQ7
   – *see* Supplement, Stomach, Pylorus ØDU7
**Pyloroscopy** ØDJ68ZZ
**Pylorotomy** – *see* Drainage, Stomach, Pylorus ØD97
**Pyramidalis muscle**
   – *use* Muscle, Abdomen, Left
   – *use* Muscle, Abdomen, Right

# Q

**Quadrangular cartilage** – *use* Septum, Nasal
**Quadrant resection of breast** – *see* Excision, Skin and Breast ØHB
**Quadrate lobe** – *use* Liver
**Quadratus femoris muscle**
   – *use* Muscle, Hip, Left
   – *use* Muscle, Hip, Right
**Quadratus lumborum muscle**
   – *use* Muscle, Trunk, Left
   – *use* Muscle, Trunk, Right
**Quadratus plantae muscle**
   – *use* Muscle, Foot, Left
   – *use* Muscle, Foot, Right
**Quadriceps (femoris)**
   – *use* Muscle, Upper Leg, Left
   – *use* Muscle, Upper Leg, Right
**Quarantine** 8EØZXY6

# R

**Radial collateral carpal ligament**
   – *use* Bursa and Ligament, Wrist, Right
   – *use* Bursa and Ligament, Wrist, Left
**Radial collateral ligament**
   – *use* Bursa and Ligament, Elbow, Left
   – *use* Bursa and Ligament, Elbow, Right
**Radial notch**
   – *use* Ulna, Left
   – *use* Ulna, Right
**Radial recurrent artery**
   – *use* Artery, Radial, Right
   – *use* Artery, Radial, Left
**Radial vein**
   – *use* Vein, Brachial, Right
   – *use* Vein, Brachial, Left
**Radialis indicis**
   – *use* Artery, Hand, Right
   – *use* Artery, Hand, Left
**Radiation Therapy**
   – *see* Beam Radiation
   – *see* Brachytherapy
**Radiation treatment** – *see* Radiation Oncology
**Radiocarpal joint**
   – *use* Joint, Wrist, Left
   – *use* Joint, Wrist, Right
**Radiocarpal ligament**
   – *use* Bursa and Ligament, Wrist, Left
   – *use* Bursa and Ligament, Wrist, Right
**Radiography** – *see* Plain Radiography
**Radiology, analog** – *see* Plain Radiography
**Radiology, diagnostic** – *see* Imaging, Diagnostic
**Radioulnar ligament**
   – *use* Bursa and Ligament, Wrist, Right
   – *use* Bursa and Ligament, Wrist, Left
**Range of motion testing** – *see* Motor Function Assessment, Rehabilitation FØ1
**REALIZE® Adjustable Gastric Band** – *use* Extraluminal Device
**Reattachment**
   Abdominal Wall ØWMFØZZ
   Ampulla of Vater ØFMC
   Ankle Region
      Left ØYMLØZZ
      Right ØYMKØZZ
   Arm
      Lower
         Left ØXMFØZZ
         Right ØXMDØZZ

**Reattachment** – *continued*
Arm – *continued*
  Upper
    Left ØXM9ØZZ
    Right ØXM8ØZZ
  Axilla
    Left ØXM5ØZZ
    Right ØXM4ØZZ
  Back
    Lower ØWMLØZZ
    Upper ØWMKØZZ
  Bladder ØTMB
  Bladder Neck ØTMC
  Breast
    Bilateral ØHMVXZZ
    Left ØHMUXZZ
    Right ØHMTXZZ
  Bronchus
    Lingula ØBM9ØZZ
    Lower Lobe
      Left ØBMBØZZ
      Right ØBM6ØZZ
    Main
      Left ØBM7ØZZ
      Right ØBM3ØZZ
    Middle Lobe, Right ØBM5ØZZ
    Upper Lobe
      Left ØBM8ØZZ
      Right ØBM4ØZZ
  Bursa and Ligament
    Abdomen
      Left ØMMJ
      Right ØMMH
    Ankle
      Left ØMMR
      Right ØMMQ
    Elbow
      Left ØMM4
      Right ØMM3
    Foot
      Left ØMMT
      Right ØMMS
    Hand
      Left ØMM8
      Right ØMM7
    Head and Neck ØMMØ
    Hip
      Left ØMMM
      Right ØMML
    Knee
      Left ØMMP
      Right ØMMN
    Lower Extremity
      Left ØMMW
      Right ØMMV
    Perineum ØMMK
    Shoulder
      Left ØMM2
      Right ØMM1
    Thorax
      Left ØMMG
      Right ØMMF
    Trunk
      Left ØMMD
      Right ØMMC
    Upper Extremity
      Left ØMMB
      Right ØMM9
    Wrist
      Left ØMM6
      Right ØMM5
  Buttock
    Left ØYM1ØZZ
    Right ØYMØØZZ
  Carina ØBM2ØZZ
  Cecum ØDMH
  Cervix ØUMC
  Chest Wall ØWM8ØZZ
  Clitoris ØUMJXZZ
  Colon
    Ascending ØDMK
    Descending ØDMM
    Sigmoid ØDMN
    Transverse ØDML
  Cord
    Bilateral ØVMH
    Left ØVMG
    Right ØVMF
  Cul-de-sac ØUMF
  Diaphragm
    Left ØBMSØZZ
    Right ØBMRØZZ

**Reattachment** – *continued*
Duct
  Common Bile ØFM9
  Cystic ØFM8
  Hepatic
    Left ØFM6
    Right ØFM5
  Pancreatic ØFMD
    Accessory ØFMF
Duodenum ØDM9
Ear
  Left Ø9M1XZZ
  Right Ø9MØXZZ
Elbow Region
  Left ØXMCØZZ
  Right ØXMBØZZ
Esophagus ØDM5
Extremity
  Lower
    Left ØYMBØZZ
    Right ØYM9ØZZ
  Upper
    Left ØXM7ØZZ
    Right ØXM6ØZZ
Eyelid
  Lower
    Left Ø8MRXZZ
    Right Ø8MQXZZ
  Upper
    Left Ø8MPXZZ
    Right Ø8MNXZZ
Face ØWM2ØZZ
Fallopian Tube
  Left ØUM6
  Right ØUM5
Fallopian Tubes, Bilateral ØUM7
Femoral Region
  Left ØYM8ØZZ
  Right ØYM7ØZZ
Finger
  Index
    Left ØXMPØZZ
    Right ØXMNØZZ
  Little
    Left ØXMWØZZ
    Right ØXMVØZZ
  Middle
    Left ØXMRØZZ
    Right ØXMQØZZ
  Ring
    Left ØXMTØZZ
    Right ØXMSØZZ
Foot
  Left ØYMNØZZ
  Right ØYMMØZZ
Forequarter
  Left ØXM1ØZZ
  Right ØXMØØZZ
Gallbladder ØFM4
Gland
  Left ØGM2
  Right ØGM3
Hand
  Left ØXMKØZZ
  Right ØXMJØZZ
Hindquarter
  Bilateral ØYM4ØZZ
  Left ØYM3ØZZ
  Right ØYM2ØZZ
Hymen ØUMK
Ileum ØDMB
Inguinal Region
  Left ØYM6ØZZ
  Right ØYM5ØZZ
Intestine
  Large ØDME
    Left ØDMG
    Right ØDMF
  Small ØDM8
Jaw
  Lower ØWM5ØZZ
  Upper ØWM4ØZZ
Jejunum ØDMA
Kidney
  Left ØTM1
  Right ØTMØ
Kidney Pelvis
  Left ØTM4
  Right ØTM3
Kidneys, Bilateral ØTM2
Knee Region
  Left ØYMGØZZ
  Right ØYMFØZZ

**Reattachment** – *continued*
Leg
  Lower
    Left ØYMJØZZ
    Right ØYMHØZZ
  Upper
    Left ØYMDØZZ
    Right ØYMCØZZ
Lip
  Lower ØCM1ØZZ
  Upper ØCMØØZZ
Liver ØFMØ
  Left Lobe ØFM2
  Right Lobe ØFM1
Lung
  Left ØBMLØZZ
  Lower Lobe
    Left ØBMJØZZ
    Right ØBMFØZZ
  Middle Lobe, Right ØBMDØZZ
  Right ØBMKØZZ
  Upper Lobe
    Left ØBMGØZZ
    Right ØBMCØZZ
Lung Lingula ØBMHØZZ
Muscle
  Abdomen
    Left ØKML
    Right ØKMK
  Facial ØKM1
  Foot
    Left ØKMW
    Right ØKMV
  Hand
    Left ØKMD
    Right ØKMC
  Head ØKMØ
  Hip
    Left ØKMP
    Right ØKMN
  Lower Arm and Wrist
    Left ØKMB
    Right ØKM9
  Lower Leg
    Left ØKMT
    Right ØKMS
  Neck
    Left ØKM3
    Right ØKM2
  Perineum ØKMM
  Shoulder
    Left ØKM6
    Right ØKM5
  Thorax
    Left ØKMJ
    Right ØKMH
  Tongue, Palate, Pharynx ØKM4
  Trunk
    Left ØKMG
    Right ØKMF
  Upper Arm
    Left ØKM8
    Right ØKM7
  Upper Leg
    Left ØKMR
    Right ØKMQ
Neck ØWM6ØZZ
Nipple
  Left ØHMXXZZ
  Right ØHMWXZZ
Nose Ø9MKXZZ
Ovary
  Bilateral ØUM2
  Left ØUM1
  Right ØUMØ
Palate, Soft ØCM3ØZZ
Pancreas ØFMG
Parathyroid Gland ØGMR
  Inferior
    Left ØGMP
    Right ØGMN
  Multiple ØGMQ
  Superior
    Left ØGMM
    Right ØGML
Penis ØVMSXZZ
Perineum
  Female ØWMNØZZ
  Male ØWMMØZZ
Rectum ØDMP
Scrotum ØVM5XZZ
Shoulder Region
  Left ØXM3ØZZ

**Reattachment** – *continued*
  Shoulder Region – *continued*
    Right ØXM2ØZZ
  Skin
    Abdomen ØHM7XZZ
    Back ØHM6XZZ
    Buttock ØHM8XZZ
    Chest ØHM5XZZ
    Ear
      Left ØHM3XZZ
      Right ØHM2XZZ
    Face ØHM1XZZ
    Foot
      Left ØHMNXZZ
      Right ØHMMXZZ
    Genitalia ØHMAXZZ
    Hand
      Left ØHMGXZZ
      Right ØHMFXZZ
    Lower Arm
      Left ØHMEXZZ
      Right ØHMDXZZ
    Lower Leg
      Left ØHMLXZZ
      Right ØHMKXZZ
    Neck ØHM4XZZ
    Perineum ØHM9XZZ
    Scalp ØHMØXZZ
    Upper Arm
      Left ØHMCXZZ
      Right ØHMBXZZ
    Upper Leg
      Left ØHMJXZZ
      Right ØHMHXZZ
  Stomach ØDM6
  Tendon
    Abdomen
      Left ØLMG
      Right ØLMF
    Ankle
      Left ØLMT
      Right ØLMS
    Foot
      Left ØLMW
      Right ØLMV
    Hand
      Left ØLM8
      Right ØLM7
    Head and Neck ØLMØ
    Hip
      Left ØLMK
      Right ØLMJ
    Knee
      Left ØLMR
      Right ØLMQ
    Lower Arm and Wrist
      Left ØLM6
      Right ØLM5
    Lower Leg
      Left ØLMP
      Right ØLMN
    Perineum ØLMH
    Shoulder
      Left ØLM2
      Right ØLM1
    Thorax
      Left ØLMD
      Right ØLMC
    Trunk
      Left ØLMB
      Right ØLM9
    Upper Arm
      Left ØLM4
      Right ØLM3
    Upper Leg
      Left ØLMM
      Right ØLML
  Testis
    Bilateral ØVMC
    Left ØVMB
    Right ØVM9
  Thumb
    Left ØXMMØZZ
    Right ØXMLØZZ
  Thyroid Gland
    Left Lobe ØGMG
    Right Lobe ØGMH
  Toe
    1st
      Left ØYMQØZZ
      Right ØYMPØZZ
    2nd
      Left ØYMSØZZ

**Reattachment** – *continued*
  Toe – *continued*
    2nd – *continued*
      Right ØYMRØZZ
    3rd
      Left ØYMUØZZ
      Right ØYMTØZZ
    4th
      Left ØYMWØZZ
      Right ØYMVØZZ
    5th
      Left ØYMYØZZ
      Right ØYMXØZZ
  Tongue ØCM7ØZZ
  Tooth
    Lower ØCMX
    Upper ØCMW
  Trachea ØBM1ØZZ
  Tunica Vaginalis
    Left ØVM7
    Right ØVM6
  Ureter
    Left ØTM7
    Right ØTM6
  Ureters, Bilateral ØTM8
  Urethra ØTMD
  Uterine Supporting Structure ØUM4
  Uterus ØUM9
  Uvula ØCMNØZZ
  Vagina ØUMG
  Vulva ØUMMXZZ
  Wrist Region
    Left ØXMHØZZ
    Right ØXMGØZZ
**Rebound HRD® (Hernia Repair Device)** – *use* Synthetic Substitute
**Recession**
  – *see* Repair
  – *see* Reposition
**Reclosure, disrupted abdominal wall** ØWQFXZZ
**Reconstruction**
  – *see* Repair
  – *see* Replacement
  – *see* Supplement
**Rectectomy**
  – *see* Excision, Rectum ØDBP
  – *see* Resection, Rectum ØDTP
**Rectocele repair** – *see* Repair, Subcutaneous Tissue and Fascia, Pelvic Region ØJQC
**Rectopexy**
  – *see* Repair, Gastrointestinal System ØDQ
  – *see* Reposition, Gastrointestinal System ØDS
**Rectoplasty**
  – *see* Repair, Gastrointestinal System ØDQ
  – *see* Supplement, Gastrointestinal System ØDU
**Rectorrhaphy** – *see* Repair, Gastrointestinal System ØDQ
**Rectoscopy** ØDJD8ZZ
**Rectosigmoid junction** – *use* Colon, Sigmoid
**Rectosigmoidectomy**
  – *see* Excision, Gastrointestinal System ØDB
  – *see* Resection, Gastrointestinal System ØDT
**Rectostomy** – *see* Drainage, Rectum ØD9P
**Rectotomy** – *see* Drainage, Rectum ØD9P
**Rectus abdominis muscle**
  – *use* Muscle, Abdomen, Left
  – *use* Muscle, Abdomen, Right
**Rectus femoris muscle**
  – *use* Muscle, Upper Leg, Left
  – *use* Muscle, Upper Leg, Right
**Recurrent laryngeal nerve** – *use* Nerve, Vagus
**Reduction**
  Dislocation – *see* Reposition
  Fracture – *see* Reposition
  Intussusception, intestinal – *see* Reposition, Gastrointestinal System ØDS
  Mammoplasty – *see* Excision, Skin and Breast ØHB
  Prolapse – *see* Reposition
  Torsion – *see* Reposition
  Volvulus, gastrointestinal – *see* Reposition, Gastrointestinal System ØDS
**Refusion** – *see* Fusion
**Reimplantation**
  – *see* Reposition
  – *see* Transfer
  – *see* Reattachment
**Reinforcement**
  – *see* Repair
  – *see* Supplement
**Relaxation, scar tissue** – *see* Release

**Release**
  Acetabulum
    Left ØQN5
    Right ØQN4
  Adenoids ØCNQ
  Ampulla of Vater ØFNC
  Anal Sphincter ØDNR
  Anterior Chamber
    Left Ø8N33ZZ
    Right Ø8N23ZZ
  Anus ØDNQ
  Aorta
    Abdominal Ø4NØ
    Thoracic Ø2NW
  Aortic Body ØGND
  Appendix ØDNJ
  Artery
    Anterior Tibial
      Left Ø4NQ
      Right Ø4NP
    Axillary
      Left Ø3N6
      Right Ø3N5
    Brachial
      Left Ø3N8
      Right Ø3N7
    Celiac Ø4N1
    Colic
      Left Ø4N7
      Middle Ø4N8
      Right Ø4N6
    Common Carotid
      Left Ø3NJ
      Right Ø3NH
    Common Iliac
      Left Ø4ND
      Right Ø4NC
    External Carotid
      Left Ø3NN
      Right Ø3NM
    External Iliac
      Left Ø4NJ
      Right Ø4NH
    Face Ø3NR
    Femoral
      Left Ø4NL
      Right Ø4NK
    Foot
      Left Ø4NW
      Right Ø4NV
    Gastric Ø4N2
    Hand
      Left Ø3NF
      Right Ø3ND
    Hepatic Ø4N3
    Inferior Mesenteric Ø4NB
    Innominate Ø3N2
    Internal Carotid
      Left Ø3NL
      Right Ø3NK
    Internal Iliac
      Left Ø4NF
      Right Ø4NE
    Internal Mammary
      Left Ø3N1
      Right Ø3NØ
    Intracranial Ø3NG
    Lower Ø4NY
    Peroneal
      Left Ø4NU
      Right Ø4NT
    Popliteal
      Left Ø4NN
      Right Ø4NM
    Posterior Tibial
      Left Ø4NS
      Right Ø4NR
    Pulmonary
      Left Ø2NR
      Right Ø2NQ
    Pulmonary Trunk Ø2NP
    Radial
      Left Ø3NC
      Right Ø3NB
    Renal
      Left Ø4NA
      Right Ø4N9
    Splenic Ø4N4
    Subclavian
      Left Ø3N4
      Right Ø3N3
    Superior Mesenteric Ø4N5

**Release** – continued
Artery – continued
Temporal
Left 03NT
Right 03NS
Thyroid
Left 03NV
Right 03NU
Ulnar
Left 03NA
Right 03N9
Upper 03NY
Vertebral
Left 03NQ
Right 03NP
Atrium
Left 02N7
Right 02N6
Auditory Ossicle
Left 09NA0ZZ
Right 09N90ZZ
Basal Ganglia 00N8
Bladder 0TNB
Bladder Neck 0TNC
Bone
Ethmoid
Left 0NNG
Right 0NNF
Frontal
Left 0NN2
Right 0NN1
Hyoid 0NNX
Lacrimal
Left 0NNJ
Right 0NNH
Nasal 0NNB
Occipital
Left 0NN8
Right 0NN7
Palatine
Left 0NNL
Right 0NNK
Parietal
Left 0NN4
Right 0NN3
Pelvic
Left 0QN3
Right 0QN2
Sphenoid
Left 0NND
Right 0NNC
Temporal
Left 0NN6
Right 0NN5
Zygomatic
Left 0NNN
Right 0NNM
Brain 00N0
Breast
Bilateral 0HNV
Left 0HNU
Right 0HNT
Bronchus
Lingula 0BN9
Lower Lobe
Left 0BNB
Right 0BN6
Main
Left 0BN7
Right 0BN3
Middle Lobe, Right 0BN5
Upper Lobe
Left 0BN8
Right 0BN4
Buccal Mucosa 0CN4
Abdomen
Left 0MNJ
Right 0MNH
Ankle
Left 0MNR
Right 0MNQ
Elbow
Left 0MN4
Right 0MN3
Foot
Left 0MNT
Right 0MNS
Hand
Left 0MN8
Right 0MN7
Head and Neck 0MN0
Hip
Left 0MNM

**Release** – continued
Buccal Mucosa – continued
Hip – continued
Right 0MNL
Knee
Left 0MNP
Right 0MNN
Lower Extremity
Left 0MNW
Right 0MNV
Perineum 0MNK
Shoulder
Left 0MN2
Right 0MN1
Thorax
Left 0MNG
Right 0MNF
Trunk
Left 0MND
Right 0MNC
Upper Extremity
Left 0MNB
Right 0MN9
Wrist
Left 0MN6
Right 0MN5
Carina 0BN2
Carotid Bodies, Bilateral 0GN8
Carotid Body
Left 0GN6
Right 0GN7
Carpal
Left 0PNN
Right 0PNM
Cecum 0DNH
Cerebellum 00NC
Cerebral Hemisphere 00N7
Cerebral Meninges 00N1
Cerebral Ventricle 00N6
Cervix 0UNC
Chordae Tendineae 02N9
Choroid
Left 08NB
Right 08NA
Cisterna Chyli 07NL
Clavicle
Left 0PNB
Right 0PN9
Clitoris 0UNJ
Coccygeal Glomus 0GNB
Coccyx 0QNS
Colon
Ascending 0DNK
Descending 0DNM
Sigmoid 0DNN
Transverse 0DNL
Conduction Mechanism 02N8
Conjunctiva
Left 08NTXZZ
Right 08NSXZZ
Cord
Bilateral 0VNH
Left 0VNG
Right 0VNF
Cornea
Left 08N9XZZ
Right 08N8XZZ
Cul-de-sac 0UNF
Diaphragm
Left 0BNS
Right 0BNR
Disc
Cervical Vertebral 0RN3
Cervicothoracic Vertebral 0RN5
Lumbar Vertebral 0SN2
Lumbosacral 0SN4
Thoracic Vertebral 0RN9
Thoracolumbar Vertebral 0RNB
Duct
Common Bile 0FN9
Cystic 0FN8
Hepatic
Left 0FN6
Right 0FN5
Lacrimal
Left 08NY
Right 08NX
Pancreatic 0FND
Accessory 0FNF
Parotid
Left 0CNC
Right 0CNB
Duodenum 0DN9

**Release** – continued
Dura Mater 00N2
Ear
External
Left 09N1
Right 09N0
External Auditory Canal
Left 09N4
Right 09N3
Inner
Left 09NE0ZZ
Right 09ND0ZZ
Middle
Left 09N60ZZ
Right 09N50ZZ
Epididymis
Bilateral 0VNL
Left 0VNK
Right 0VNJ
Epiglottis 0CNR
Esophagogastric Junction 0DN4
Esophagus 0DN5
Lower 0DN3
Middle 0DN2
Upper 0DN1
Eustachian Tube
Left 09NG
Right 09NF
Eye
Left 08N1XZZ
Right 08N0XZZ
Eyelid
Lower
Left 08NR
Right 08NQ
Upper
Left 08NP
Right 08NN
Fallopian Tube
Left 0UN6
Right 0UN5
Fallopian Tubes, Bilateral 0UN7
Femoral Shaft
Left 0QN9
Right 0QN8
Femur
Lower
Left 0QNC
Right 0QNB
Upper
Left 0QN7
Right 0QN6
Fibula
Left 0QNK
Right 0QNJ
Finger Nail 0HNQXZZ
Gallbladder 0FN4
Gingiva
Lower 0CN6
Upper 0CN5
Gland
Adrenal
Bilateral 0GN4
Left 0GN2
Right 0GN3
Lacrimal
Left 08NW
Right 08NV
Minor Salivary 0CNJ
Parotid
Left 0CN9
Right 0CN8
Pituitary 0GN0
Sublingual
Left 0CNF
Right 0CND
Submaxillary
Left 0CNH
Right 0CNG
Vestibular 0UNL
Glenoid Cavity
Left 0PN8
Right 0PN7
Glomus Jugulare 0GNC
Humeral Head
Left 0PND
Right 0PNC
Humeral Shaft
Left 0PNG
Right 0PNF
Hymen 0UNK
Hypothalamus 00NA
Ileocecal Valve 0DNC

**Release** – *continued*
Ileum ØDNB
Intestine
  Large ØDNE
    Left ØDNG
    Right ØDNF
  Small ØDN8
Iris
  Left 08ND3ZZ
  Right 08NC3ZZ
Jejunum ØDNA
Joint
  Acromioclavicular
    Left ØRNH
    Right ØRNG
  Ankle
    Left ØSNG
    Right ØSNF
  Carpal
    Left ØRNR
    Right ØRNQ
  Cervical Vertebral ØRN1
  Cervicothoracic Vertebral ØRN4
  Coccygeal ØSN6
  Elbow
    Left ØRNM
    Right ØRNL
  Finger Phalangeal
    Left ØRNX
    Right ØRNW
  Hip
    Left ØSNB
    Right ØSN9
  Knee
    Left ØSND
    Right ØSNC
  Lumbar Vertebral ØSNØ
  Lumbosacral ØSN3
  Metacarpocarpal
    Left ØRNT
    Right ØRNS
  Metacarpophalangeal
    Left ØRNV
    Right ØRNU
  Metatarsal–Phalangeal
    Left ØSNN
    Right ØSNM
  Metatarsal–Tarsal
    Left ØSNL
    Right ØSNK
  Occipital–cervical ØRNØ
  Sacrococcygeal ØSN5
  Sacroiliac
    Left ØSN8
    Right ØSN7
  Shoulder
    Left ØRNK
    Right ØRNJ
  Sternoclavicular
    Left ØRNF
    Right ØRNE
  Tarsal
    Left ØSNJ
    Right ØSNH
  Temporomandibular
    Left ØRND
    Right ØRNC
  Thoracic Vertebral ØRN6
  Thoracolumbar Vertebral ØRNA
  Toe Phalangeal
    Left ØSNQ
    Right ØSNP
  Wrist
    Left ØRNP
    Right ØRNN
Kidney
  Left ØTN1
  Right ØTNØ
Kidney Pelvis
  Left ØTN4
  Right ØTN3
Larynx ØCNS
Lens
  Left 08NK3ZZ
  Right 08NJ3ZZ
Lip
  Lower ØCN1
  Upper ØCNØ
Liver ØFNØ
  Left Lobe ØFN2
  Right Lobe ØFN1
Lung
  Bilateral ØBNM

**Release** – *continued*
Lung – *continued*
  Left ØBNL
  Lower Lobe
    Left ØBNJ
    Right ØBNF
  Middle Lobe, Right ØBND
  Right ØBNK
  Upper Lobe
    Left ØBNG
    Right ØBNC
Lung Lingula ØBNH
Lymphatic
  Aortic Ø7ND
  Axillary
    Left Ø7N6
    Right Ø7N5
  Head Ø7NØ
  Inguinal
    Left Ø7NJ
    Right Ø7NH
  Internal Mammary
    Left Ø7N9
    Right Ø7N8
  Lower Extremity
    Left Ø7NG
    Right Ø7NF
  Mesenteric Ø7NB
  Neck
    Left Ø7N2
    Right Ø7N1
  Pelvis Ø7NC
  Thoracic Duct Ø7NK
  Thorax Ø7N7
  Upper Extremity
    Left Ø7N4
    Right Ø7N3
Mandible
  Left ØNNV
  Right ØNNT
Maxilla
  Left ØNNS
  Right ØNNR
Medulla Oblongata ØØND
Mesentery ØDNV
Metacarpal
  Left ØPNQ
  Right ØPNP
Metatarsal
  Left ØQNP
  Right ØQNN
Muscle
  Abdomen
    Left ØKNL
    Right ØKNK
  Extraocular
    Left 08NM
    Right 08NL
  Facial ØKN1
  Foot
    Left ØKNW
    Right ØKNV
  Hand
    Left ØKND
    Right ØKNC
  Head ØKNØ
  Hip
    Left ØKNP
    Right ØKNN
  Lower Arm and Wrist
    Left ØKNB
    Right ØKN9
  Lower Leg
    Left ØKNT
    Right ØKNS
  Neck
    Left ØKN3
    Right ØKN2
  Papillary 02ND
  Perineum ØKNM
  Shoulder
    Left ØKN6
    Right ØKN5
  Thorax
    Left ØKNJ
    Right ØKNH
  Tongue, Palate, Pharynx ØKN4
  Trunk
    Left ØKNG
    Right ØKNF
  Upper Arm
    Left ØKN8
    Right ØKN7

**Release** – *continued*
Muscle – *continued*
  Upper Leg
    Left ØKNR
    Right ØKNQ
Nasopharynx Ø9NN
Nerve
  Abdominal Sympathetic Ø1NM
  Abducens ØØNL
  Accessory ØØNR
  Acoustic ØØNN
  Brachial Plexus Ø1N3
  Cervical Ø1N1
  Cervical Plexus Ø1NØ
  Facial ØØNM
  Femoral Ø1ND
  Glossopharyngeal ØØNP
  Head and Neck Sympathetic Ø1NK
  Hypoglossal ØØNS
  Lumbar Ø1NB
  Lumbar Plexus Ø1N9
  Lumbar Sympathetic Ø1NN
  Lumbosacral Plexus Ø1NA
  Median Ø1N5
  Oculomotor ØØNH
  Olfactory ØØNF
  Optic ØØNG
  Peroneal Ø1NH
  Phrenic Ø1N2
  Pudendal Ø1NC
  Radial Ø1N6
  Sacral Ø1NR
  Sacral Plexus Ø1NQ
  Sacral Sympathetic Ø1NP
  Sciatic Ø1NF
  Thoracic Ø1N8
  Thoracic Sympathetic Ø1NL
  Tibial Ø1NG
  Trigeminal ØØNK
  Trochlear ØØNJ
  Ulnar Ø1N4
  Vagus ØØNQ
Nipple
  Left ØHNX
  Right ØHNW
Nose Ø9NK
Omentum
  Greater ØDNS
  Lesser ØDNT
Orbit
  Left ØNNQ
  Right ØNNP
Ovary
  Bilateral ØUN2
  Left ØUN1
  Right ØUNØ
Palate
  Hard ØCN2
  Soft ØCN3
Pancreas ØFNG
Para–aortic Body ØGN9
Paraganglion Extremity ØGNF
Parathyroid Gland ØGNR
  Inferior
    Left ØGNP
    Right ØGNN
  Multiple ØGNQ
  Superior
    Left ØGNM
    Right ØGNL
Patella
  Left ØQNF
  Right ØQND
Penis ØVNS
Pericardium 02NN
Peritoneum ØDNW
Phalanx
  Finger
    Left ØPNV
    Right ØPNT
  Thumb
    Left ØPNS
    Right ØPNR
  Toe
    Left ØQNR
    Right ØQNQ
Pharynx ØCNM
Pineal Body ØGN1
Pleura
  Left ØBNP
  Right ØBNN
Pons ØØNB
Prepuce ØVNT

**Release** – *continued*
Prostate ØVNØ
Radius
    Left ØPNJ
    Right ØPNH
Rectum ØDNP
Retina
    Left Ø8NF3ZZ
    Right Ø8NE3ZZ
Retinal Vessel
    Left Ø8NH3ZZ
    Right Ø8NG3ZZ
Rib
    Left ØPN2
    Right ØPN1
Sacrum ØQN1
Scapula
    Left ØPN6
    Right ØPN5
Sclera
    Left Ø8N7XZZ
    Right Ø8N6XZZ
Scrotum ØVN5
Septum
    Atrial Ø2N5
    Nasal Ø9NM
    Ventricular Ø2NM
Sinus
    Accessory Ø9NP
    Ethmoid
        Left Ø9NV
        Right Ø9NU
    Frontal
        Left Ø9NT
        Right Ø9NS
    Mastoid
        Left Ø9NC
        Right Ø9NB
    Maxillary
        Left Ø9NR
        Right Ø9NQ
    Sphenoid
        Left Ø9NX
        Right Ø9NW
Skin
    Abdomen ØHN7XZZ
    Back ØHN6XZZ
    Buttock ØHN8XZZ
    Chest ØHN5XZZ
    Ear
        Left ØHN3XZZ
        Right ØHN2XZZ
    Face ØHN1XZZ
    Foot
        Left ØHNNXZZ
        Right ØHNMXZZ
    Genitalia ØHNAXZZ
    Hand
        Left ØHNGXZZ
        Right ØHNFXZZ
    Lower Arm
        Left ØHNEXZZ
        Right ØHNDXZZ
    Lower Leg
        Left ØHNLXZZ
        Right ØHNKXZZ
    Neck ØHN4XZZ
    Perineum ØHN9XZZ
    Scalp ØHNØXZZ
    Upper Arm
        Left ØHNCXZZ
        Right ØHNBXZZ
    Upper Leg
        Left ØHNJXZZ
        Right ØHNHXZZ
Spinal Cord
    Cervical ØØNW
    Lumbar ØØNY
    Thoracic ØØNX
Spinal Meninges ØØNT
Spleen Ø7NP
Sternum ØPNØ
Stomach ØDN6
    Pylorus ØDN7
Subcutaneous Tissue and Fascia
    Abdomen ØJN8
    Back ØJN7
    Buttock ØJN9
    Chest ØJN6
    Face ØJN1
    Foot
        Left ØJNR
        Right ØJNQ

**Release** – *continued*
Subcutaneous Tissue and Fascia – *continued*
    Hand
        Left ØJNK
        Right ØJNJ
    Lower Arm
        Left ØJNH
        Right ØJNG
    Lower Leg
        Left ØJNP
        Right ØJNN
    Neck
        Anterior ØJN4
        Posterior ØJN5
    Pelvic Region ØJNC
    Perineum ØJNB
    Scalp ØJNØ
    Upper Arm
        Left ØJNF
        Right ØJND
    Upper Leg
        Left ØJNM
        Right ØJNL
Tarsal
    Left ØQNM
    Right ØQNL
Tendon
    Abdomen
        Left ØLNG
        Right ØLNF
    Ankle
        Left ØLNT
        Right ØLNS
    Foot
        Left ØLNW
        Right ØLNV
    Hand
        Left ØLN8
        Right ØLN7
    Head and Neck ØLNØ
    Hip
        Left ØLNK
        Right ØLNJ
    Knee
        Left ØLNR
        Right ØLNQ
    Lower Arm and Wrist
        Left ØLN6
        Right ØLN5
    Lower Leg
        Left ØLNP
        Right ØLNN
    Perineum ØLNH
    Shoulder
        Left ØLN2
        Right ØLN1
    Thorax
        Left ØLND
        Right ØLNC
    Trunk
        Left ØLNB
        Right ØLN9
    Upper Arm
        Left ØLN4
        Right ØLN3
    Upper Leg
        Left ØLNM
        Right ØLNL
Testis
    Bilateral ØVNC
    Left ØVNB
    Right ØVN9
Thalamus ØØN9
Thymus Ø7NM
Thyroid Gland ØGNK
    Left Lobe ØGNG
    Right Lobe ØGNH
Tibia
    Left ØQNH
    Right ØQNG
Toe Nail ØHNRXZZ
Tongue ØCN7
Tonsils ØCNP
Tooth
    Lower ØCNX
    Upper ØCNW
Trachea ØBN1
Tunica Vaginalis
    Left ØVN7
    Right ØVN6
Turbinate, Nasal Ø9NL
Tympanic Membrane
    Left Ø9N8

**Release** – *continued*
Tympanic Membrane – *continued*
    Right Ø9N7
Ulna
    Left ØPNL
    Right ØPNK
Ureter
    Left ØTN7
    Right ØTN6
Urethra ØTND
Uterine Supporting Structure ØUN4
Uterus ØUN9
Uvula ØCNN
Vagina ØUNG
Valve
    Aortic Ø2NF
    Mitral Ø2NG
    Pulmonary Ø2NH
    Tricuspid Ø2NJ
Vas Deferens
    Bilateral ØVNQ
    Left ØVNP
    Right ØVNN
Vein
    Axillary
        Left Ø5N8
        Right Ø5N7
    Azygos Ø5NØ
    Basilic
        Left Ø5NC
        Right Ø5NB
    Brachial
        Left Ø5NA
        Right Ø5N9
    Cephalic
        Left Ø5NF
        Right Ø5ND
    Colic Ø6N7
    Common Iliac
        Left Ø6ND
        Right Ø6NC
    Coronary Ø2N4
    Esophageal Ø6N3
    External Iliac
        Left Ø6NG
        Right Ø6NF
    External Jugular
        Left Ø5NQ
        Right Ø5NP
    Face
        Left Ø5NV
        Right Ø5NT
    Femoral
        Left Ø6NN
        Right Ø6NM
    Foot
        Left Ø6NV
        Right Ø6NT
    Gastric Ø6N2
    Greater Saphenous
        Left Ø6NQ
        Right Ø6NP
    Hand
        Left Ø5NH
        Right Ø5NG
    Hemiazygos Ø5N1
    Hepatic Ø6N4
    Hypogastric
        Left Ø6NJ
        Right Ø6NH
    Inferior Mesenteric Ø6N6
    Innominate
        Left Ø5N4
        Right Ø5N3
    Internal Jugular
        Left Ø5NN
        Right Ø5NM
    Intracranial Ø5NL
    Lesser Saphenous
        Left Ø6NS
        Right Ø6NR
    Lower Ø6NY
    Portal Ø6N8
    Pulmonary
        Left Ø2NT
        Right Ø2NS
    Renal
        Left Ø6NB
        Right Ø6N9
    Splenic Ø6N1
    Subclavian
        Left Ø5N6
        Right Ø5N5

**Release** – *continued*
Vein – *continued*
Superior Mesenteric 06N5
Upper 05NY
Vertebral
Left 05NS
Right 05NR
Vena Cava
Inferior 06N0
Superior 02NV
Ventricle
Left 02NL
Right 02NK
Vertebra
Cervical 0PN3
Lumbar 0QN0
Thoracic 0PN4
Vesicle
Bilateral 0VN3
Left 0VN2
Right 0VN1
Vitreous
Left 08N53ZZ
Right 08N43ZZ
Vocal Cord
Left 0CNV
Right 0CNT
Vulva 0UNM
**Relocation** – *see* Reposition
**Removal**
Abdominal Wall 2W53X
Anorectal 2Y53X5Z
Arm
Lower
Left 2W5DX
Right 2W5CX
Upper
Left 2W5BX
Right 2W5AX
Back 2W55X
Chest Wall 2W54X
Ear 2Y52X5Z
Extremity
Lower
Left 2W5MX
Right 2W5LX
Upper
Left 2W59X
Right 2W58X
Face 2W51X
Finger
Left 2W5KX
Right 2W5JX
Foot
Left 2W5TX
Right 2W5SX
Genital Tract, Female 2Y54X5Z
Hand
Left 2W5FX
Right 2W5EX
Head 2W50X
Inguinal Region
Left 2W57X
Right 2W56X
Leg
Lower
Left 2W5RX
Right 2W5QX
Upper
Left 2W5PX
Right 2W5NX
Mouth and Pharynx 2Y50X5Z
Nasal 2Y51X5Z
Neck 2W52X
Thumb
Left 2W5HX
Right 2W5GX
Toe
Left 2W5VX
Right 2W5UX
Urethra 2Y55X5Z
**Removal of device from**
Abdominal Wall 0WPF
Acetabulum
Left 0QP5
Right 0QP4
Anal Sphincter 0DPR
Anus 0DPQ
Artery
Lower 04PY
Upper 03PY
Back
Lower 0WPL

**Removal of device from** – *continued*
Back – *continued*
Upper 0WPK
Bladder 0TPB
Bone
Facial 0NPW
Lower 0QPY
Nasal 0NPB
Pelvic
Left 0QP3
Right 0QP2
Upper 0PPY
Bone Marrow 07PT
Brain 00P0
Breast
Left 0HPU
Right 0HPT
Bursa and Ligament
Lower 0MPY
Upper 0MPX
Carpal
Left 0PPN
Right 0PPM
Cavity, Cranial 0WP1
Cerebral Ventricle 00P6
Chest Wall 0WP8
Cisterna Chyli 07PL
Clavicle
Left 0PPB
Right 0PP9
Coccyx 0QPS
Diaphragm 0BPT
Disc
Cervical Vertebral 0RP3
Cervicothoracic Vertebral 0RP5
Lumbar Vertebral 0SP2
Lumbosacral 0SP4
Thoracic Vertebral 0RP9
Thoracolumbar Vertebral 0RPB
Duct
Hepatobiliary 0FPB
Pancreatic 0FPD
Ear
Inner
Left 09PE
Right 09PD
Left 09PJ
Right 09PH
Epididymis and Spermatic Cord 0VPM
Esophagus 0DP5
Extremity
Lower
Left 0YPB
Right 0YP9
Upper
Left 0XP7
Right 0XP6
Eye
Left 08P1
Right 08P0
Face 0WP2
Fallopian Tube 0UP8
Femoral Shaft
Left 0QP9
Right 0QP8
Femur
Lower
Left 0QPC
Right 0QPB
Upper
Left 0QP7
Right 0QP6
Fibula
Left 0QPK
Right 0QPJ
Finger Nail 0HPQX
Gallbladder 0FP4
Gastrointestinal Tract 0WPP
Genitourinary Tract 0WPR
Gland
Adrenal 0GP5
Endocrine 0GPS
Pituitary 0GP0
Salivary 0CPA
Glenoid Cavity
Left 0PP8
Right 0PP7
Great Vessel 02PY
Hair 0HPSX
Head 0WP0
Heart 02PA
Humeral Head
Left 0PPD
Right 0PPC

**Removal of device from** – *continued*
Humeral Shaft
Left 0PPG
Right 0PPF
Intestinal Tract
Lower 0DPD
Upper 0DP0
Jaw
Lower 0WP5
Upper 0WP4
Joint
Acromioclavicular
Left 0RPH
Right 0RPG
Ankle
Left 0SPG
Right 0SPF
Carpal
Left 0RPR
Right 0RPQ
Cervical Vertebral 0RP1
Cervicothoracic Vertebral 0RP4
Coccygeal 0SP6
Elbow
Left 0RPM
Right 0RPL
Finger Phalangeal
Left 0RPX
Right 0RPW
Hip
Left 0SPB
Right 0SP9
Knee
Left 0SPD
Right 0SPC
Lumbar Vertebral 0SP0
Lumbosacral 0SP3
Metacarpocarpal
Left 0RPT
Right 0RPS
Metacarpophalangeal
Left 0RPV
Right 0RPU
Metatarsal–Phalangeal
Left 0SPN
Right 0SPM
Metatarsal–Tarsal
Left 0SPL
Right 0SPK
Occipital–cervical 0RP0
Sacrococcygeal 0SP5
Sacroiliac
Left 0SP8
Right 0SP7
Shoulder
Left 0RPK
Right 0RPJ
Sternoclavicular
Left 0RPF
Right 0RPE
Tarsal
Left 0SPJ
Right 0SPH
Temporomandibular
Left 0RPD
Right 0RPC
Thoracic Vertebral 0RP6
Thoracolumbar Vertebral 0RPA
Toe Phalangeal
Left 0SPQ
Right 0SPP
Wrist
Left 0RPP
Right 0RPN
Kidney 0TP5
Larynx 0CPS
Lens
Left 08PK3JZ
Right 08PJ3JZ
Liver 0FP0
Lung
Left 0BPL
Right 0BPK
Lymphatic 07PN
Thoracic Duct 07PK
Mediastinum 0WPC
Mesentery 0DPV
Metacarpal
Left 0PPQ
Right 0PPP
Metatarsal
Left 0QPP
Right 0QPN
Mouth and Throat 0CPY

**Removal of device from** – *continued*
Muscle
Extraocular
Left 08PM
Right 08PL
Lower 0KPY
Upper 0KPX
Neck 0WP6
Nerve
Cranial 00PE
Peripheral 01PY
Nose 09PK
Omentum 0DPU
Ovary 0UP3
Pancreas 0FPG
Parathyroid Gland 0GPR
Patella
Left 0QPF
Right 0QPD
Pelvic Cavity 0WPJ
Penis 0VPS
Pericardial Cavity 0WPD
Perineum
Female 0WPN
Male 0WPM
Peritoneal Cavity 0WPG
Peritoneum 0DPW
Phalanx
Finger
Left 0PPV
Right 0PPT
Thumb
Left 0PPS
Right 0PPR
Toe
Left 0QPR
Right 0QPQ
Pineal Body 0GP1
Pleura 0BPQ
Pleural Cavity
Left 0WPB
Right 0WP9
Products of Conception 10P0
Prostate and Seminal Vesicles 0VP4
Radius
Left 0PPJ
Right 0PPH
Rectum 0DPP
Respiratory Tract 0WPQ
Retroperitoneum 0WPH
Rib
Left 0PP2
Right 0PP1
Sacrum 0QP1
Scapula
Left 0PP6
Right 0PP5
Scrotum and Tunica Vaginalis 0VP8
Sinus 09PY
Skin 0HPPX
Skull 0NP0
Spinal Canal 00PU
Spinal Cord 00PV
Spleen 07PP
Sternum 0PP0
Stomach 0DP6
Subcutaneous Tissue and Fascia
Head and Neck 0JPS
Lower Extremity 0JPW
Trunk 0JPT
Upper Extremity 0JPV
Tarsal
Left 0QPM
Right 0QPL
Tendon
Lower 0LPY
Upper 0LPX
Testis 0VPD
Thymus 07PM
Thyroid Gland 0GPK
Tibia
Left 0QPH
Right 0QPG
Toe Nail 0HPRX
Trachea 0BP1
Tracheobronchial Tree 0BP0
Tympanic Membrane
Left 09P8
Right 09P7
Ulna
Left 0PPL
Right 0PPK
Ureter 0TP9

**Removal of device from** – *continued*
Urethra 0TPD
Uterus and Cervix 0UPD
Vagina and Cul-de-sac 0UPH
Vas Deferens 0VPR
Vein
Lower 06PY
Upper 05PY
Vertebra
Cervical 0PP3
Lumbar 0QP0
Thoracic 0PP4
Vulva 0UPM
**Renal calyx**
– *use* Kidney
– *use* Kidneys, Bilateral
– *use* Kidney, Left
– *use* Kidney, Right
**Renal capsule**
– *use* Kidney, Left
– *use* Kidney
– *use* Kidney, Right
– *use* Kidneys, Bilateral
**Renal cortex**
– *use* Kidneys, Bilateral
– *use* Kidney, Left
– *use* Kidney, Right
– *use* Kidney
**Renal dialysis** – *see* Performance, Urinary 5A1D
**Renal plexus** – *use* Nerve, Abdominal Sympathetic
**Renal segment**
– *use* Kidney
– *use* Kidney, Left
– *use* Kidney, Right
– *use* Kidneys, Bilateral
**Renal segmental artery**
– *use* Artery, Renal, Left
– *use* Artery, Renal, Right
**Reopening, operative site**
Control of bleeding – *see* Control postprocedural bleeding in
Inspection only – *see* Inspection
**Repair**
Abdominal Wall 0WQF
Acetabulum
Left 0QQ5
Right 0QQ4
Adenoids 0CQQ
Ampulla of Vater 0FQC
Anal Sphincter 0DQR
Ankle Region
Left 0YQL
Right 0YQK
Anterior Chamber
Left 08Q33ZZ
Right 08Q23ZZ
Anus 0DQQ
Aorta
Abdominal 04Q0
Thoracic 02QW
Aortic Body 0GQD
Appendix 0DQJ
Arm
Lower
Left 0XQF
Right 0XQD
Upper
Left 0XQ9
Right 0XQ8
Artery
Anterior Tibial
Left 04QQ
Right 04QP
Axillary
Left 03Q6
Right 03Q5
Brachial
Left 03Q8
Right 03Q7
Celiac 04Q1
Colic
Left 04Q7
Middle 04Q8
Right 04Q6
Common Carotid
Left 03QJ
Right 03QH
Common Iliac
Left 04QD
Right 04QC
Coronary
Four or More Sites 02Q3

**Repair** – *continued*
Artery – *continued*
Coronary – *continued*
One Site 02Q0
Three Sites 02Q2
Two Sites 02Q1
External Carotid
Left 03QN
Right 03QM
External Iliac
Left 04QJ
Right 04QH
Face 03QR
Femoral
Left 04QL
Right 04QK
Foot
Left 04QW
Right 04QV
Gastric 04Q2
Hand
Left 03QF
Right 03QD
Hepatic 04Q3
Inferior Mesenteric 04QB
Innominate 03Q2
Internal Carotid
Left 03QL
Right 03QK
Internal Iliac
Left 04QF
Right 04QE
Internal Mammary
Left 03Q1
Right 03Q0
Intracranial 03QG
Lower 04QY
Peroneal
Left 04QU
Right 04QT
Popliteal
Left 04QN
Right 04QM
Posterior Tibial
Left 04QS
Right 04QR
Pulmonary
Left 02QR
Right 02QQ
Pulmonary Trunk 02QP
Radial
Left 03QC
Right 03QB
Renal
Left 04QA
Right 04Q9
Splenic 04Q4
Subclavian
Left 03Q4
Right 03Q3
Superior Mesenteric 04Q5
Temporal
Left 03QT
Right 03QS
Thyroid
Left 03QV
Right 03QU
Ulnar
Left 03QA
Right 03Q9
Upper 03QY
Vertebral
Left 03QQ
Right 03QP
Atrium
Left 02Q7
Right 02Q6
Auditory Ossicle
Left 09QA0ZZ
Right 09Q90ZZ
Axilla
Left 0XQ5
Right 0XQ4
Back
Lower 0WQL
Upper 0WQK
Basal Ganglia 00Q8
Bladder 0TQB
Bladder Neck 0TQC
Bone
Ethmoid
Left 0NQG
Right 0NQF

**Repair** – continued
  Bone – continued
    Frontal
      Left ØNQ2
      Right ØNQ1
    Hyoid ØNQX
    Lacrimal
      Left ØNQJ
      Right ØNQH
    Nasal ØNQB
    Occipital
      Left ØNQ8
      Right ØNQ7
    Palatine
      Left ØNQL
      Right ØNQK
    Parietal
      Left ØNQ4
      Right ØNQ3
    Pelvic
      Left ØQQ3
      Right ØQQ2
    Sphenoid
      Left ØNQD
      Right ØNQC
    Temporal
      Left ØNQ6
      Right ØNQ5
    Zygomatic
      Left ØNQN
      Right ØNQM
  Brain ØØQ0
  Breast
    Bilateral ØHQV
    Left ØHQU
    Right ØHQT
    Supernumerary ØHQY
  Bronchus
    Lingula ØBQ9
    Lower Lobe
      Left ØBQB
      Right ØBQ6
    Main
      Left ØBQ7
      Right ØBQ3
    Middle Lobe, Right ØBQ5
    Upper Lobe
      Left ØBQ8
      Right ØBQ4
  Buccal Mucosa ØCQ4
  Bursa and Ligament
    Abdomen
      Left ØMQJ
      Right ØMQH
    Ankle
      Left ØMQR
      Right ØMQQ
    Elbow
      Left ØMQ4
      Right ØMQ3
    Foot
      Left ØMQT
      Right ØMQS
    Hand
      Left ØMQ8
      Right ØMQ7
    Head and Neck ØMQ0
    Hip
      Left ØMQM
      Right ØMQL
    Knee
      Left ØMQP
      Right ØMQN
    Lower Extremity
      Left ØMQW
      Right ØMQV
    Perineum ØMQK
    Shoulder
      Left ØMQ2
      Right ØMQ1
    Thorax
      Left ØMQG
      Right ØMQF
    Trunk
      Left ØMQD
      Right ØMQC
    Upper Extremity
      Left ØMQB
      Right ØMQ9
    Wrist
      Left ØMQ6
      Right ØMQ5

**Repair** – continued
  Buttock
    Left ØYQ1
    Right ØYQ0
  Carina ØBQ2
  Carotid Bodies, Bilateral ØGQ8
  Carotid Body
    Left ØGQ6
    Right ØGQ7
  Carpal
    Left ØPQN
    Right ØPQM
  Cecum ØDQH
  Cerebellum ØØQC
  Cerebral Hemisphere ØØQ7
  Cerebral Meninges ØØQ1
  Cerebral Ventricle ØØQ6
  Cervix ØUQC
  Chest Wall ØWQ8
  Chordae Tendineae Ø2Q9
  Choroid
    Left Ø8QB
    Right Ø8QA
  Cisterna Chyli Ø7QL
  Clavicle
    Left ØPQB
    Right ØPQ9
  Clitoris ØUQJ
  Coccygeal Glomus ØGQB
  Coccyx ØQQS
  Colon
    Ascending ØDQK
    Descending ØDQM
    Sigmoid ØDQN
    Transverse ØDQL
  Conduction Mechanism Ø2Q8
  Conjunctiva
    Left Ø8QTXZZ
    Right Ø8QSXZZ
  Cord
    Bilateral ØVQH
    Left ØVQG
    Right ØVQF
  Cornea
    Left Ø8Q9XZZ
    Right Ø8Q8XZZ
  Cul-de-sac ØUQF
  Diaphragm
    Left ØBQS
    Right ØBQR
  Disc
    Cervical Vertebral ØRQ3
    Cervicothoracic Vertebral ØRQ5
    Lumbar Vertebral ØSQ2
    Lumbosacral ØSQ4
    Thoracic Vertebral ØRQ9
    Thoracolumbar Vertebral ØRQB
  Duct
    Common Bile ØFQ9
    Cystic ØFQ8
    Hepatic
      Left ØFQ6
      Right ØFQ5
    Lacrimal
      Left Ø8QY
      Right Ø8QX
    Pancreatic ØFQD
      Accessory ØFQF
    Parotid
      Left ØCQC
      Right ØCQB
  Duodenum ØDQ9
  Dura Mater ØØQ2
  Ear
    External
      Bilateral Ø9Q2
      Left Ø9Q1
      Right Ø9Q0
    External Auditory Canal
      Left Ø9Q4
      Right Ø9Q3
    Inner
      Left Ø9QEØZZ
      Right Ø9QDØZZ
    Middle
      Left Ø9Q6ØZZ
      Right Ø9Q5ØZZ
  Elbow Region
    Left ØXQC
    Right ØXQB
  Epididymis
    Bilateral ØVQL
    Left ØVQK

**Repair** – continued
  Epididymis – continued
    Right ØVQJ
  Epiglottis ØCQR
  Esophagogastric Junction ØDQ4
  Esophagus ØDQ5
    Lower ØDQ3
    Middle ØDQ2
    Upper ØDQ1
  Eustachian Tube
    Left Ø9QG
    Right Ø9QF
  Extremity
    Lower
      Left ØYQB
      Right ØYQ9
    Upper
      Left ØXQ7
      Right ØXQ6
  Eye
    Left Ø8Q1XZZ
    Right Ø8Q0XZZ
  Eyelid
    Lower
      Left Ø8QR
      Right Ø8QQ
    Upper
      Left Ø8QP
      Right Ø8QN
  Face ØWQ2
  Fallopian Tube
    Left ØUQ6
    Right ØUQ5
  Fallopian Tubes, Bilateral ØUQ7
  Femoral Region
    Bilateral ØYQE
    Left ØYQ8
    Right ØYQ7
  Femoral Shaft
    Left ØQQ9
    Right ØQQ8
  Femur
    Lower
      Left ØQQC
      Right ØQQB
    Upper
      Left ØQQ7
      Right ØQQ6
  Fibula
    Left ØQQK
    Right ØQQJ
  Finger
    Index
      Left ØXQP
      Right ØXQN
    Little
      Left ØXQW
      Right ØXQV
    Middle
      Left ØXQR
      Right ØXQQ
    Ring
      Left ØXQT
      Right ØXQS
  Finger Nail ØHQQXZZ
  Foot
    Left ØYQN
    Right ØYQM
  Gallbladder ØFQ4
  Gingiva
    Lower ØCQ6
    Upper ØCQ5
  Gland
    Adrenal
      Bilateral ØGQ4
      Left ØGQ2
      Right ØGQ3
    Lacrimal
      Left Ø8QW
      Right Ø8QV
    Minor Salivary ØCQJ
    Parotid
      Left ØCQ9
      Right ØCQ8
    Pituitary ØGQ0
    Sublingual
      Left ØCQF
      Right ØCQD
    Submaxillary
      Left ØCQH
      Right ØCQG
    Vestibular ØUQL

**Repair** – *continued*
  Glenoid Cavity
    Left ØPQ8
    Right ØPQ7
  Glomus Jugulare ØGQC
  Hand
    Left ØXQK
    Right ØXQJ
  Head ØWQØ
  Heart Ø2QA
    Left Ø2QC
    Right Ø2QB
  Humeral Head
    Left ØPQD
    Right ØPQC
  Humeral Shaft
    Left ØPQG
    Right ØPQF
  Hymen ØUQK
  Hypothalamus ØØQA
  Ileocecal Valve ØDQC
  Ileum ØDQB
  Inguinal Region
    Bilateral ØYQA
    Left ØYQ6
    Right ØYQ5
  Intestine
    Large ØDQE
      Left ØDQG
      Right ØDQF
    Small ØDQ8
  Iris
    Left Ø8QD3ZZ
    Right Ø8QC3ZZ
  Jaw
    Lower ØWQ5
    Upper ØWQ4
  Jejunum ØDQA
  Joint
    Acromioclavicular
      Left ØRQH
      Right ØRQG
    Ankle
      Left ØSQG
      Right ØSQF
    Carpal
      Left ØRQR
      Right ØRQQ
    Cervical Vertebral ØRQ1
    Cervicothoracic Vertebral ØRQ4
    Coccygeal ØSQ6
    Elbow
      Left ØRQM
      Right ØRQL
    Finger Phalangeal
      Left ØRQX
      Right ØRQW
    Hip
      Left ØSQB
      Right ØSQ9
    Knee
      Left ØSQD
      Right ØSQC
    Lumbar Vertebral ØSQØ
    Lumbosacral ØSQ3
    Metacarpocarpal
      Left ØRQT
      Right ØRQS
    Metacarpophalangeal
      Left ØRQV
      Right ØRQU
    Metatarsal–Phalangeal
      Left ØSQN
      Right ØSQM
    Metatarsal–Tarsal
      Left ØSQL
      Right ØSQK
    Occipital–cervical ØRQØ
    Sacrococcygeal ØSQ5
    Sacroiliac
      Left ØSQ8
      Right ØSQ7
    Shoulder
      Left ØRQK
      Right ØRQJ
    Sternoclavicular
      Left ØRQF
      Right ØRQE
    Tarsal
      Left ØSQJ
      Right ØSQH
    Temporomandibular
      Left ØRQD

**Repair** – *continued*
  Joint – *continued*
    Temporomandibular – *continued*
      Right ØRQC
    Thoracic Vertebral ØRQ6
    Thoracolumbar Vertebral ØRQA
    Toe Phalangeal
      Left ØSQQ
      Right ØSQP
    Wrist
      Left ØRQP
      Right ØRQN
  Kidney
    Left ØTQ1
    Right ØTQØ
  Kidney Pelvis
    Left ØTQ4
    Right ØTQ3
  Knee Region
    Left ØYQG
    Right ØYQF
  Larynx ØCQS
  Leg
    Lower
      Left ØYQJ
      Right ØYQH
    Upper
      Left ØYQD
      Right ØYQC
  Lens
    Left Ø8QK3ZZ
    Right Ø8QJ3ZZ
  Lip
    Lower ØCQ1
    Upper ØCQØ
  Liver ØFQØ
    Left Lobe ØFQ2
    Right Lobe ØFQ1
  Lung
    Bilateral ØBQM
    Left ØBQL
    Lower Lobe
      Left ØBQJ
      Right ØBQF
    Middle Lobe, Right ØBQD
    Right ØBQK
    Upper Lobe
      Left ØBQG
      Right ØBQC
  Lung Lingula ØBQH
  Lymphatic
    Aortic Ø7QD
    Axillary
      Left Ø7Q6
      Right Ø7Q5
    Head Ø7QØ
    Inguinal
      Left Ø7QJ
      Right Ø7QH
    Internal Mammary
      Left Ø7Q9
      Right Ø7Q8
    Lower Extremity
      Left Ø7QG
      Right Ø7QF
    Mesenteric Ø7QB
    Neck
      Left Ø7Q2
      Right Ø7Q1
    Pelvis Ø7QC
    Thoracic Duct Ø7QK
    Thorax Ø7Q7
    Upper Extremity
      Left Ø7Q4
      Right Ø7Q3
  Mandible
    Left ØNQV
    Right ØNQT
  Maxilla
    Left ØNQS
    Right ØNQR
  Mediastinum ØWQC
  Medulla Oblongata ØØQD
  Mesentery ØDQV
  Metacarpal
    Left ØPQQ
    Right ØPQP
  Metatarsal
    Left ØQQP
    Right ØQQN
  Muscle
    Abdomen
      Left ØKQL

**Repair** – *continued*
  Muscle – *continued*
    Abdomen – *continued*
      Right ØKQK
    Extraocular
      Left Ø8QM
      Right Ø8QL
    Facial ØKQ1
    Foot
      Left ØKQW
      Right ØKQV
    Hand
      Left ØKQD
      Right ØKQC
    Head ØKQØ
    Hip
      Left ØKQP
      Right ØKQN
    Lower Arm and Wrist
      Left ØKQB
      Right ØKQ9
    Lower Leg
      Left ØKQT
      Right ØKQS
    Neck
      Left ØKQ3
      Right ØKQ2
    Papillary Ø2QD
    Perineum ØKQM
    Shoulder
      Left ØKQ6
      Right ØKQ5
    Thorax
      Left ØKQJ
      Right ØKQH
    Tongue, Palate, Pharynx ØKQ4
    Trunk
      Left ØKQG
      Right ØKQF
    Upper Arm
      Left ØKQ8
      Right ØKQ7
    Upper Leg
      Left ØKQR
      Right ØKQQ
  Nasopharynx Ø9QN
  Neck ØWQ6
  Nerve
    Abdominal Sympathetic Ø1QM
    Abducens ØØQL
    Accessory ØØQR
    Acoustic ØØQN
    Brachial Plexus Ø1Q3
    Cervical Ø1Q1
    Cervical Plexus Ø1QØ
    Facial ØØQM
    Femoral Ø1QD
    Glossopharyngeal ØØQP
    Head and Neck Sympathetic Ø1QK
    Hypoglossal ØØQS
    Lumbar Ø1QB
    Lumbar Plexus Ø1Q9
    Lumbar Sympathetic Ø1QN
    Lumbosacral Plexus Ø1QA
    Median Ø1Q5
    Oculomotor ØØQH
    Olfactory ØØQF
    Optic ØØQG
    Peroneal Ø1QH
    Phrenic Ø1Q2
    Pudendal Ø1QC
    Radial Ø1Q6
    Sacral Ø1QR
    Sacral Plexus Ø1QQ
    Sacral Sympathetic Ø1QP
    Sciatic Ø1QF
    Thoracic Ø1Q8
    Thoracic Sympathetic Ø1QL
    Tibial Ø1QG
    Trigeminal ØØQK
    Trochlear ØØQJ
    Ulnar Ø1Q4
    Vagus ØØQQ
  Nipple
    Left ØHQX
    Right ØHQW
  Nose Ø9QK
  Omentum
    Greater ØDQS
    Lesser ØDQT
  Orbit
    Left ØNQQ
    Right ØNQP

**Repair** – continued
Ovary
Bilateral 0UQ2
Left 0UQ1
Right 0UQ0
Palate
Hard 0CQ2
Soft 0CQ3
Pancreas 0FQG
Para–aortic Body 0GQ9
Paraganglion Extremity 0GQF
Parathyroid Gland 0GQR
Inferior
Left 0GQP
Right 0GQN
Multiple 0GQQ
Superior
Left 0GQM
Right 0GQL
Patella
Left 0QQF
Right 0QQD
Penis 0VQS
Pericardium 02QN
Perineum
Female 0WQN
Male 0WQM
Peritoneum 0DQW
Phalanx
Finger
Left 0PQV
Right 0PQT
Thumb
Left 0PQS
Right 0PQR
Toe
Left 0QQR
Right 0QQQ
Pharynx 0CQM
Pineal Body 0GQ1
Pleura
Left 0BQP
Right 0BQN
Pons 00QB
Prepuce 0VQT
Products of Conception 10Q0
Prostate 0VQ0
Radius
Left 0PQJ
Right 0PQH
Rectum 0DQP
Retina
Left 08QF3ZZ
Right 08QE3ZZ
Retinal Vessel
Left 08QH3ZZ
Right 08QG3ZZ
Rib
Left 0PQ2
Right 0PQ1
Sacrum 0QQ1
Scapula
Left 0PQ6
Right 0PQ5
Sclera
Left 08Q7XZZ
Right 08Q6XZZ
Scrotum 0VQ5
Septum
Atrial 02Q5
Nasal 09QM
Ventricular 02QM
Shoulder Region
Left 0XQ3
Right 0XQ2
Sinus
Accessory 09QP
Ethmoid
Left 09QV
Right 09QU
Frontal
Left 09QT
Right 09QS
Mastoid
Left 09QC
Right 09QB
Maxillary
Left 09QR
Right 09QQ
Sphenoid
Left 09QX
Right 09QW

**Repair** – continued
Skin
Abdomen 0HQ7XZZ
Back 0HQ6XZZ
Buttock 0HQ8XZZ
Chest 0HQ5XZZ
Ear
Left 0HQ3XZZ
Right 0HQ2XZZ
Face 0HQ1XZZ
Foot
Left 0HQNXZZ
Right 0HQMXZZ
Genitalia 0HQAXZZ
Hand
Left 0HQGXZZ
Right 0HQFXZZ
Lower Arm
Left 0HQEXZZ
Right 0HQDXZZ
Lower Leg
Left 0HQLXZZ
Right 0HQKXZZ
Neck 0HQ4XZZ
Perineum 0HQ9XZZ
Scalp 0HQ0XZZ
Upper Arm
Left 0HQCXZZ
Right 0HQBXZZ
Upper Leg
Left 0HQJXZZ
Right 0HQHXZZ
Skull 0NQ0
Spinal Cord
Cervical 00QW
Lumbar 00QY
Thoracic 00QX
Spinal Meninges 00QT
Spleen 07QP
Sternum 0PQ0
Stomach 0DQ6
Pylorus 0DQ7
Subcutaneous Tissue and Fascia
Abdomen 0JQ8
Back 0JQ7
Buttock 0JQ9
Chest 0JQ6
Face 0JQ1
Foot
Left 0JQR
Right 0JQQ
Hand
Left 0JQK
Right 0JQJ
Lower Arm
Left 0JQH
Right 0JQG
Lower Leg
Left 0JQP
Right 0JQN
Neck
Anterior 0JQ4
Posterior 0JQ5
Pelvic Region 0JQC
Perineum 0JQB
Scalp 0JQ0
Upper Arm
Left 0JQF
Right 0JQD
Upper Leg
Left 0JQM
Right 0JQL
Tarsal
Left 0QQM
Right 0QQL
Tendon
Abdomen
Left 0LQG
Right 0LQF
Ankle
Left 0LQT
Right 0LQS
Foot
Left 0LQW
Right 0LQV
Hand
Left 0LQ8
Right 0LQ7
Head and Neck 0LQ0
Hip
Left 0LQK
Right 0LQJ

**Repair** – continued
Tendon – continued
Knee
Left 0LQR
Right 0LQQ
Lower Arm and Wrist
Left 0LQ6
Right 0LQ5
Lower Leg
Left 0LQP
Right 0LQN
Perineum 0LQH
Shoulder
Left 0LQ2
Right 0LQ1
Thorax
Left 0LQD
Right 0LQC
Trunk
Left 0LQB
Right 0LQ9
Upper Arm
Left 0LQ4
Right 0LQ3
Upper Leg
Left 0LQM
Right 0LQL
Testis
Bilateral 0VQC
Left 0VQB
Right 0VQ9
Thalamus 00Q9
Thumb
Left 0XQM
Right 0XQL
Thymus 07QM
Thyroid Gland 0GQK
Left Lobe 0GQG
Right Lobe 0GQH
Thyroid Gland Isthmus 0GQJ
Tibia
Left 0QQH
Right 0QQG
Toe
1st
Left 0YQQ
Right 0YQP
2nd
Left 0YQS
Right 0YQR
3rd
Left 0YQU
Right 0YQT
4th
Left 0YQW
Right 0YQV
5th
Left 0YQY
Right 0YQX
Toe Nail 0HQRXZZ
Tongue 0CQ7
Tonsils 0CQP
Tooth
Lower 0CQX
Upper 0CQW
Trachea 0BQ1
Tunica Vaginalis
Left 0VQ7
Right 0VQ6
Turbinate, Nasal 09QL
Tympanic Membrane
Left 09Q8
Right 09Q7
Ulna
Left 0PQL
Right 0PQK
Ureter
Left 0TQ7
Right 0TQ6
Urethra 0TQD
Uterine Supporting Structure 0UQ4
Uterus 0UQ9
Uvula 0CQN
Vagina 0UQG
Valve
Aortic 02QF
Mitral 02QG
Pulmonary 02QH
Tricuspid 02QJ
Vas Deferens
Bilateral 0VQQ
Left 0VQP
Right 0VQN

**Repair** – *continued*
Vein
  Axillary
    Left 05Q8
    Right 05Q7
  Azygos 05Q0
  Basilic
    Left 05QC
    Right 05QB
  Brachial
    Left 05QA
    Right 05Q9
  Cephalic
    Left 05QF
    Right 05QD
  Colic 06Q7
  Common Iliac
    Left 06QD
    Right 06QC
  Coronary 02Q4
  Esophageal 06Q3
  External Iliac
    Left 06QG
    Right 06QF
  External Jugular
    Left 05QQ
    Right 05QP
  Face
    Left 05QV
    Right 05QT
  Femoral
    Left 06QN
    Right 06QM
  Foot
    Left 06QV
    Right 06QT
  Gastric 06Q2
  Greater Saphenous
    Left 06QQ
    Right 06QP
  Hand
    Left 05QH
    Right 05QG
  Hemiazygos 05Q1
  Hepatic 06Q4
  Hypogastric
    Left 06QJ
    Right 06QH
  Inferior Mesenteric 06Q6
  Innominate
    Left 05Q4
    Right 05Q3
  Internal Jugular
    Left 05QN
    Right 05QM
  Intracranial 05QL
  Lesser Saphenous
    Left 06QS
    Right 06QR
  Lower 06QY
  Portal 06Q8
  Pulmonary
    Left 02QT
    Right 02QS
  Renal
    Left 06QB
    Right 06Q9
  Splenic 06Q1
  Subclavian
    Left 05Q6
    Right 05Q5
  Superior Mesenteric 06Q5
  Upper 05QY
  Vertebral
    Left 05QS
    Right 05QR
Vena Cava
  Inferior 06Q0
  Superior 02QV
Ventricle
  Left 02QL
  Right 02QK
Vertebra
  Cervical 0PQ3
  Lumbar 0QQ0
  Thoracic 0PQ4
Vesicle
  Bilateral 0VQ3
  Left 0VQ2
  Right 0VQ1
Vitreous
  Left 08Q53ZZ
  Right 08Q43ZZ

**Repair** – *continued*
Vocal Cord
  Left 0CQV
  Right 0CQT
Vulva 0UQM
Wrist Region
  Left 0XQH
  Right 0XQG
**Replacement**
Acetabulum
  Left 0QR5
  Right 0QR4
Ampulla of Vater 0FRC
Anal Sphincter 0DRR
Aorta
  Abdominal 04R0
  Thoracic 02RW
Artery
  Anterior Tibial
    Left 04RQ
    Right 04RP
  Axillary
    Left 03R6
    Right 03R5
  Brachial
    Left 03R8
    Right 03R7
  Celiac 04R1
  Colic
    Left 04R7
    Middle 04R8
    Right 04R6
  Common Carotid
    Left 03RJ
    Right 03RH
  Common Iliac
    Left 04RD
    Right 04RC
  External Carotid
    Left 03RN
    Right 03RM
  External Iliac
    Left 04RJ
    Right 04RH
  Face 03RR
  Femoral
    Left 04RL
    Right 04RK
  Foot
    Left 04RW
    Right 04RV
  Gastric 04R2
  Hand
    Left 03RF
    Right 03RD
  Hepatic 04R3
  Inferior Mesenteric 04RB
  Innominate 03R2
  Internal Carotid
    Left 03RL
    Right 03RK
  Internal Iliac
    Left 04RF
    Right 04RE
  Internal Mammary
    Left 03R1
    Right 03R0
  Intracranial 03RG
  Lower 04RY
  Peroneal
    Left 04RU
    Right 04RT
  Popliteal
    Left 04RN
    Right 04RM
  Posterior Tibial
    Left 04RS
    Right 04RR
  Pulmonary
    Left 02RR
    Right 02RQ
  Pulmonary Trunk 02RP
  Radial
    Left 03RC
    Right 03RB
  Renal
    Left 04RA
    Right 04R9
  Splenic 04R4
  Subclavian
    Left 03R4
    Right 03R3
  Superior Mesenteric 04R5

**Replacement** – *continued*
Artery – *continued*
  Temporal
    Left 03RT
    Right 03RS
  Thyroid
    Left 03RV
    Right 03RU
  Ulnar
    Left 03RA
    Right 03R9
  Upper 03RY
  Vertebral
    Left 03RQ
    Right 03RP
Atrium
  Left 02R7
  Right 02R6
Auditory Ossicle
  Left 09RA0
  Right 09R90
Bladder 0TRB
Bladder Neck 0TRC
Bone
  Ethmoid
    Left 0NRG
    Right 0NRF
  Frontal
    Left 0NR2
    Right 0NR1
  Hyoid 0NRX
  Lacrimal
    Left 0NRJ
    Right 0NRH
  Nasal 0NRB
  Occipital
    Left 0NR8
    Right 0NR7
  Palatine
    Left 0NRL
    Right 0NRK
  Parietal
    Left 0NR4
    Right 0NR3
  Pelvic
    Left 0QR3
    Right 0QR2
  Sphenoid
    Left 0NRD
    Right 0NRC
  Temporal
    Left 0NR6
    Right 0NR5
  Zygomatic
    Left 0NRN
    Right 0NRM
Breast
  Bilateral 0HRV
  Left 0HRU
  Right 0HRT
Buccal Mucosa 0CR4
Carpal
  Left 0PRN
  Right 0PRM
Chordae Tendineae 02R9
Choroid
  Left 08RB
  Right 08RA
Clavicle
  Left 0PRB
  Right 0PR9
Coccyx 0QRS
Conjunctiva
  Left 08RTX
  Right 08RSX
Cornea
  Left 08R9
  Right 08R8
Disc
  Cervical Vertebral 0RR30
  Cervicothoracic Vertebral 0RR50
  Lumbar Vertebral 0SR20
  Lumbosacral 0SR40
  Thoracic Vertebral 0RR90
  Thoracolumbar Vertebral 0RRB0
Duct
  Common Bile 0FR9
  Cystic 0FR8
  Hepatic
    Left 0FR6
    Right 0FR5
  Lacrimal
    Left 08RY
    Right 08RX

**Replacement** – *continued*
  Duct – *continued*
    Pancreatic ØFRD
      Accessory ØFRF
    Parotid
      Left ØCRC
      Right ØCRB
  Ear
    External
      Bilateral Ø9R2
      Left Ø9R1
      Right Ø9RØ
    Inner
      Left Ø9REØ
      Right Ø9RDØ
    Middle
      Left Ø9R6Ø
      Right Ø9R5Ø
  Epiglottis ØCRR
  Esophagus ØDR5
  Eye
    Left Ø8R1
    Right Ø8RØ
  Eyelid
    Lower
      Left Ø8RR
      Right Ø8RQ
    Upper
      Left Ø8RP
      Right Ø8RN
  Femoral Shaft
    Left ØQR9
    Right ØQR8
  Femur
    Lower
      Left ØQRC
      Right ØQRB
    Upper
      Left ØQR7
      Right ØQR6
  Fibula
    Left ØQRK
    Right ØQRJ
  Finger Nail ØHRQX
  Gingiva
    Lower ØCR6
    Upper ØCR5
  Glenoid Cavity
    Left ØPR8
    Right ØPR7
  Hair ØHRSX
  Humeral Head
    Left ØPRD
    Right ØPRC
  Humeral Shaft
    Left ØPRG
    Right ØPRF
  Iris
    Left Ø8RD3
    Right Ø8RC3
  Joint
    Acromioclavicular
      Left ØRRHØ
      Right ØRRGØ
    Ankle
      Left ØSRG
      Right ØSRF
    Carpal
      Left ØRRRØ
      Right ØRRQØ
    Cervical Vertebral ØRR1Ø
    Cervicothoracic Vertebral ØRR4Ø
    Coccygeal ØSR6Ø
    Elbow
      Left ØRRMØ
      Right ØRRLØ
    Finger Phalangeal
      Left ØRRXØ
      Right ØRRWØ
    Hip
      Left ØSRB
        Acetabular Surface ØSRE
        Femoral Surface ØSRS
      Right ØSR9
        Acetabular Surface ØSRA
        Femoral Surface ØSRR
    Knee
      Left ØSRD
        Femoral Surface ØSRU
        Tibial Surface ØSRW
      Right ØSRC
        Femoral Surface ØSRT
        Tibial Surface ØSRV
    Lumbar Vertebral ØSRØØ

**Replacement** – *continued*
  Joint – *continued*
    Lumbosacral ØSR3Ø
    Metacarpocarpal
      Left ØRRTØ
      Right ØRRSØ
    Metacarpophalangeal
      Left ØRRVØ
      Right ØRRUØ
    Metatarsal–Phalangeal
      Left ØSRNØ
      Right ØSRMØ
    Metatarsal–Tarsal
      Left ØSRLØ
      Right ØSRKØ
    Occipital–cervical ØRRØØ
    Sacrococcygeal ØSR5Ø
    Sacroiliac
      Left ØSR8Ø
      Right ØSR7Ø
    Shoulder
      Left ØRRK
      Right ØRRJ
    Sternoclavicular
      Left ØRRFØ
      Right ØRREØ
    Tarsal
      Left ØSRJØ
      Right ØSRHØ
    Temporomandibular
      Left ØRRDØ
      Right ØRRCØ
    Thoracic Vertebral ØRR6Ø
    Thoracolumbar Vertebral ØRRAØ
    Toe Phalangeal
      Left ØSRQØ
      Right ØSRPØ
    Wrist
      Left ØRRPØ
      Right ØRRNØ
  Kidney Pelvis
    Left ØTR4
    Right ØTR3
  Larynx ØCRS
  Lens
    Left Ø8RK3ØZ
    Right Ø8RJ3ØZ
  Lip
    Lower ØCR1
    Upper ØCRØ
  Mandible
    Left ØNRV
    Right ØNRT
  Maxilla
    Left ØNRS
    Right ØNRR
  Mesentery ØDRV
  Metacarpal
    Left ØPRQ
    Right ØPRP
  Metatarsal
    Left ØQRP
    Right ØQRN
  Muscle, Papillary Ø2RD
  Nasopharynx Ø9RN
  Nipple
    Left ØHRX
    Right ØHRW
  Nose Ø9RK
  Omentum
    Greater ØDRS
    Lesser ØDRT
  Orbit
    Left ØNRQ
    Right ØNRP
  Palate
    Hard ØCR2
    Soft ØCR3
  Patella
    Left ØQRF
    Right ØQRD
  Pericardium Ø2RN
  Peritoneum ØDRW
  Phalanx
    Finger
      Left ØPRV
      Right ØPRT
    Thumb
      Left ØPRS
      Right ØPRR
    Toe
      Left ØQRR
      Right ØQRQ
  Pharynx ØCRM

**Replacement** – *continued*
  Radius
    Left ØPRJ
    Right ØPRH
  Retinal Vessel
    Left Ø8RH3
    Right Ø8RG3
  Rib
    Left ØPR2
    Right ØPR1
  Sacrum ØQR1
  Scapula
    Left ØPR6
    Right ØPR5
  Sclera
    Left Ø8R7X
    Right Ø8R6X
  Septum
    Atrial Ø2R5
    Nasal Ø9RM
    Ventricular Ø2RM
  Skin
    Abdomen ØHR7
    Back ØHR6
    Buttock ØHR8
    Chest ØHR5
    Ear
      Left ØHR3
      Right ØHR2
    Face ØHR1
    Foot
      Left ØHRN
      Right ØHRM
    Genitalia ØHRA
    Hand
      Left ØHRG
      Right ØHRF
    Lower Arm
      Left ØHRE
      Right ØHRD
    Lower Leg
      Left ØHRL
      Right ØHRK
    Neck ØHR4
    Perineum ØHR9
    Scalp ØHRØ
    Upper Arm
      Left ØHRC
      Right ØHRB
    Upper Leg
      Left ØHRJ
      Right ØHRH
  Skull ØNRØ
  Sternum ØPRØ
  Subcutaneous Tissue and Fascia
    Abdomen ØJR8
    Back ØJR7
    Buttock ØJR9
    Chest ØJR6
    Face ØJR1
    Foot
      Left ØJRR
      Right ØJRQ
    Hand
      Left ØJRK
      Right ØJRJ
    Lower Arm
      Left ØJRH
      Right ØJRG
    Lower Leg
      Left ØJRP
      Right ØJRN
    Neck
      Anterior ØJR4
      Posterior ØJR5
    Pelvic Region ØJRC
    Perineum ØJRB
    Scalp ØJRØ
    Upper Arm
      Left ØJRF
      Right ØJRD
    Upper Leg
      Left ØJRM
      Right ØJRL
  Tarsal
    Left ØQRM
    Right ØQRL
  Tendon
    Abdomen
      Left ØLRG
      Right ØLRF
    Ankle
      Left ØLRT
      Right ØLRS

**Alphabetic Index to Procedures**

**Replacement – Reposition**

**Replacement** – *continued*
  Tendon – *continued*
    Foot
      Left 0LRW
      Right 0LRV
    Hand
      Left 0LR8
      Right 0LR7
    Head and Neck 0LR0
    Hip
      Left 0LRK
      Right 0LRJ
    Knee
      Left 0LRR
      Right 0LRQ
    Lower Arm and Wrist
      Left 0LR6
      Right 0LR5
    Lower Leg
      Left 0LRP
      Right 0LRN
    Perineum 0LRH
    Shoulder
      Left 0LR2
      Right 0LR1
    Thorax
      Left 0LRD
      Right 0LRC
    Trunk
      Left 0LRB
      Right 0LR9
    Upper Arm
      Left 0LR4
      Right 0LR3
    Upper Leg
      Left 0LRM
      Right 0LRL
  Testis
    Bilateral 0VRC0JZ
    Left 0VRB0JZ
    Right 0VR90JZ
  Thumb
    Left 0XRM
    Right 0XRL
  Tibia
    Left 0QRH
    Right 0QRG
  Toe Nail 0HRRX
  Tongue 0CR7
  Tooth
    Lower 0CRX
    Upper 0CRW
  Turbinate, Nasal 09RL
  Tympanic Membrane
    Left 09R8
    Right 09R7
  Ulna
    Left 0PRL
    Right 0PRK
  Ureter
    Left 0TR7
    Right 0TR6
  Urethra 0TRD
  Uvula 0CRN
  Valve
    Aortic 02RF
    Mitral 02RG
    Pulmonary 02RH
    Tricuspid 02RJ
  Vein
    Axillary
      Left 05R8
      Right 05R7
    Azygos 05R0
    Basilic
      Left 05RC
      Right 05RB
    Brachial
      Left 05RA
      Right 05R9
    Cephalic
      Left 05RF
      Right 05RD
    Colic 06R7
    Common Iliac
      Left 06RD
      Right 06RC
    Esophageal 06R3
    External Iliac
      Left 06RG
      Right 06RF
    External Jugular
      Left 05RQ

**Replacement** – *continued*
  Vein – *continued*
    External Jugular – *continued*
      Right 05RP
    Face
      Left 05RV
      Right 05RT
    Femoral
      Left 06RN
      Right 06RM
    Foot
      Left 06RV
      Right 06RT
    Gastric 06R2
    Greater Saphenous
      Left 06RQ
      Right 06RP
    Hand
      Left 05RH
      Right 05RG
    Hemiazygos 05R1
    Hepatic 06R4
    Hypogastric
      Left 06RJ
      Right 06RH
    Inferior Mesenteric 06R6
    Innominate
      Left 05R4
      Right 05R3
    Internal Jugular
      Left 05RN
      Right 05RM
    Intracranial 05RL
    Lesser Saphenous
      Left 06RS
      Right 06RR
    Lower 06RY
    Portal 06R8
    Pulmonary
      Left 02RT
      Right 02RS
    Renal
      Left 06RB
      Right 06R9
    Splenic 06R1
    Subclavian
      Left 05R6
      Right 05R5
    Superior Mesenteric 06R5
    Upper 05RY
    Vertebral
      Left 05RS
      Right 05RR
  Vena Cava
    Inferior 06R0
    Superior 02RV
  Ventricle
    Left 02RL
    Right 02RK
  Vertebra
    Cervical 0PR3
    Lumbar 0QR0
    Thoracic 0PR4
  Vitreous
    Left 08R53
    Right 08R43
  Vocal Cord
    Left 0CRV
    Right 0CRT

**Replantation** – *see* Reposition

**Replantation, scalp** – *see* Reattachment, Skin, Scalp 0HM0

**Reposition**
  Acetabulum
    Left 0QS5
    Right 0QS4
  Ampulla of Vater 0FSC
  Anus 0DSQ
  Aorta
    Abdominal 04S0
    Thoracic 02SW0ZZ
  Artery
    Anterior Tibial
      Left 04SQ
      Right 04SP
    Axillary
      Left 03S6
      Right 03S5
    Brachial
      Left 03S8
      Right 03S7
    Celiac 04S1
    Colic
      Left 04S7

**Reposition** – *continued*
  Artery – *continued*
    Colic – *continued*
      Middle 04S8
      Right 04S6
    Common Carotid
      Left 03SJ
      Right 03SH
    Common Iliac
      Left 04SD
      Right 04SC
    External Carotid
      Left 03SN
      Right 03SM
    External Iliac
      Left 04SJ
      Right 04SH
    Face 03SR
    Femoral
      Left 04SL
      Right 04SK
    Foot
      Left 04SW
      Right 04SV
    Gastric 04S2
    Hand
      Left 03SF
      Right 03SD
    Hepatic 04S3
    Inferior Mesenteric 04SB
    Innominate 03S2
    Internal Carotid
      Left 03SL
      Right 03SK
    Internal Iliac
      Left 04SF
      Right 04SE
    Internal Mammary
      Left 03S1
      Right 03S0
    Intracranial 03SG
    Lower 04SY
    Peroneal
      Left 04SU
      Right 04ST
    Popliteal
      Left 04SN
      Right 04SM
    Posterior Tibial
      Left 04SS
      Right 04SR
    Pulmonary
      Left 02SR0ZZ
      Right 02SQ0ZZ
    Pulmonary Trunk 02SP0ZZ
    Radial
      Left 03SC
      Right 03SB
    Renal
      Left 04SA
      Right 04S9
    Splenic 04S4
    Subclavian
      Left 03S4
      Right 03S3
    Superior Mesenteric 04S5
    Temporal
      Left 03ST
      Right 03SS
    Thyroid
      Left 03SV
      Right 03SU
    Ulnar
      Left 03SA
      Right 03S9
    Upper 03SY
    Vertebral
      Left 03SQ
      Right 03SP
  Auditory Ossicle
    Left 09SA
    Right 09S9
  Bladder 0TSB
  Bladder Neck 0TSC
  Bone
    Ethmoid
      Left 0NSG
      Right 0NSF
    Frontal
      Left 0NS2
      Right 0NS1
    Hyoid 0NSX

**Reposition** – *continued*
  Bone – *continued*
    Lacrimal
      Left ØNSJ
      Right ØNSH
    Nasal ØNSB
    Occipital
      Left ØNS8
      Right ØNS7
    Palatine
      Left ØNSL
      Right ØNSK
    Parietal
      Left ØNS4
      Right ØNS3
    Pelvic
      Left ØQS3
      Right ØQS2
    Sphenoid
      Left ØNSD
      Right ØNSC
    Temporal
      Left ØNS6
      Right ØNS5
    Zygomatic
      Left ØNSN
      Right ØNSM
  Breast
    Bilateral ØHSVØZZ
    Left ØHSUØZZ
    Right ØHSTØZZ
  Bronchus
    Lingula ØBS9ØZZ
    Lower Lobe
      Left ØBSBØZZ
      Right ØBS6ØZZ
    Main
      Left ØBS7ØZZ
      Right ØBS3ØZZ
    Middle Lobe, Right ØBS5ØZZ
    Upper Lobe
      Left ØBS8ØZZ
      Right ØBS4ØZZ
  Bursa and Ligament
    Abdomen
      Left ØMSJ
      Right ØMSH
    Ankle
      Left ØMSR
      Right ØMSQ
    Elbow
      Left ØMS4
      Right ØMS3
    Foot
      Left ØMST
      Right ØMSS
    Hand
      Left ØMS8
      Right ØMS7
    Head and Neck ØMSØ
    Hip
      Left ØMSM
      Right ØMSL
    Knee
      Left ØMSP
      Right ØMSN
    Lower Extremity
      Left ØMSW
      Right ØMSV
    Perineum ØMSK
    Shoulder
      Left ØMS2
      Right ØMS1
    Thorax
      Left ØMSG
      Right ØMSF
    Trunk
      Left ØMSD
      Right ØMSC
    Upper Extremity
      Left ØMSB
      Right ØMS9
    Wrist
      Left ØMS6
      Right ØMS5
  Carina ØBS2ØZZ
  Carpal
    Left ØPSN
    Right ØPSM
  Cecum ØDSH
  Cervix ØUSC
  Clavicle
    Left ØPSB

**Reposition** – *continued*
  Clavicle – *continued*
    Right ØPS9
  Coccyx ØQSS
  Colon
    Ascending ØDSK
    Descending ØDSM
    Sigmoid ØDSN
    Transverse ØDSL
  Cord
    Bilateral ØVSH
    Left ØVSG
    Right ØVSF
  Cul-de-sac ØUSF
  Diaphragm
    Left ØBSSØZZ
    Right ØBSRØZZ
  Duct
    Common Bile ØFS9
    Cystic ØFS8
    Hepatic
      Left ØFS6
      Right ØFS5
    Lacrimal
      Left Ø8SY
      Right Ø8SX
    Pancreatic ØFSD
      Accessory ØFSF
    Parotid
      Left ØCSC
      Right ØCSB
  Duodenum ØDS9
  Ear
    Bilateral Ø9S2
    Left Ø9S1
    Right Ø9SØ
  Epiglottis ØCSR
  Esophagus ØDS5
  Eustachian Tube
    Left Ø9SG
    Right Ø9SF
  Eyelid
    Lower
      Left Ø8SR
      Right Ø8SQ
    Upper
      Left Ø8SP
      Right Ø8SN
  Fallopian Tube
    Left ØUS6
    Right ØUS5
  Fallopian Tubes, Bilateral ØUS7
  Femoral Shaft
    Left ØQS9
    Right ØQS8
  Femur
    Lower
      Left ØQSC
      Right ØQSB
    Upper
      Left ØQS7
      Right ØQS6
  Fibula
    Left ØQSK
    Right ØQSJ
  Gallbladder ØFS4
  Gland
    Adrenal
      Left ØGS2
      Right ØGS3
    Lacrimal
      Left Ø8SW
      Right Ø8SV
  Glenoid Cavity
    Left ØPS8
    Right ØPS7
  Hair ØHSSXZZ
  Humeral Head
    Left ØPSD
    Right ØPSC
  Humeral Shaft
    Left ØPSG
    Right ØPSF
  Ileum ØDSB
  Iris
    Left Ø8SD3ZZ
    Right Ø8SC3ZZ
  Jejunum ØDSA
  Joint
    Acromioclavicular
      Left ØRSH
      Right ØRSG

**Reposition** – *continued*
  Joint – *continued*
    Ankle
      Left ØSSG
      Right ØSSF
    Carpal
      Left ØRSR
      Right ØRSQ
    Cervical Vertebral ØRS1
    Cervicothoracic Vertebral ØRS4
    Coccygeal ØSS6
    Elbow
      Left ØRSM
      Right ØRSL
    Finger Phalangeal
      Left ØRSX
      Right ØRSW
    Hip
      Left ØSSB
      Right ØSS9
    Knee
      Left ØSSD
      Right ØSSC
    Lumbar Vertebral ØSSØ
    Lumbosacral ØSS3
    Metacarpocarpal
      Left ØRST
      Right ØRSS
    Metacarpophalangeal
      Left ØRSV
      Right ØRSU
    Metatarsal–Phalangeal
      Left ØSSN
      Right ØSSM
    Metatarsal–Tarsal
      Left ØSSL
      Right ØSSK
    Occipital–cervical ØRSØ
    Sacrococcygeal ØSS5
    Sacroiliac
      Left ØSS8
      Right ØSS7
    Shoulder
      Left ØRSK
      Right ØRSJ
    Sternoclavicular
      Left ØRSF
      Right ØRSE
    Tarsal
      Left ØSSJ
      Right ØSSH
    Temporomandibular
      Left ØRSD
      Right ØRSC
    Thoracic Vertebral ØRS6
    Thoracolumbar Vertebral ØRSA
    Toe Phalangeal
      Left ØSSQ
      Right ØSSP
    Wrist
      Left ØRSP
      Right ØRSN
  Kidney
    Left ØTS1
    Right ØTSØ
  Kidney Pelvis
    Left ØTS4
    Right ØTS3
  Kidneys, Bilateral ØTS2
  Lens
    Left Ø8SK3ZZ
    Right Ø8SJ3ZZ
  Lip
    Lower ØCS1
    Upper ØCSØ
  Liver ØFSØ
  Lung
    Left ØBSLØZZ
    Lower Lobe
      Left ØBSJØZZ
      Right ØBSFØZZ
    Middle Lobe, Right ØBSDØZZ
      Right ØBSKØZZ
    Upper Lobe
      Left ØBSGØZZ
      Right ØBSCØZZ
  Lung Lingula ØBSHØZZ
  Mandible
    Left ØNSV
    Right ØNST
  Maxilla
    Left ØNSS
    Right ØNSR

**Reposition** – *continued*
- Metacarpal
  - Left ØPSQ
  - Right ØPSP
- Metatarsal
  - Left ØQSP
  - Right ØQSN
- Muscle
  - Abdomen
    - Left ØKSL
    - Right ØKSK
  - Extraocular
    - Left Ø8SM
    - Right Ø8SL
  - Facial ØKS1
  - Foot
    - Left ØKSW
    - Right ØKSV
  - Hand
    - Left ØKSD
    - Right ØKSC
  - Head ØKSØ
  - Hip
    - Left ØKSP
    - Right ØKSN
  - Lower Arm and Wrist
    - Left ØKSB
    - Right ØKS9
  - Lower Leg
    - Left ØKST
    - Right ØKSS
  - Neck
    - Left ØKS3
    - Right ØKS2
  - Perineum ØKSM
  - Shoulder
    - Left ØKS6
    - Right ØKS5
  - Thorax
    - Left ØKSJ
    - Right ØKSH
  - Tongue, Palate, Pharynx ØKS4
  - Trunk
    - Left ØKSG
    - Right ØKSF
  - Upper Arm
    - Left ØKS8
    - Right ØKS7
  - Upper Leg
    - Left ØKSR
    - Right ØKSQ
- Nerve
  - Abducens ØØSL
  - Accessory ØØSR
  - Acoustic ØØSN
  - Brachial Plexus Ø1S3
  - Cervical Ø1S1
  - Cervical Plexus Ø1SØ
  - Facial ØØSM
  - Femoral Ø1SD
  - Glossopharyngeal ØØSP
  - Hypoglossal ØØSS
  - Lumbar Ø1SB
  - Lumbar Plexus Ø1S9
  - Lumbosacral Plexus Ø1SA
  - Median Ø1S5
  - Oculomotor ØØSH
  - Olfactory ØØSF
  - Optic ØØSG
  - Peroneal Ø1SH
  - Phrenic Ø1S2
  - Pudendal Ø1SC
  - Radial Ø1S6
  - Sacral Ø1SR
  - Sacral Plexus Ø1SQ
  - Sciatic Ø1SF
  - Thoracic Ø1S8
  - Tibial Ø1SG
  - Trigeminal ØØSK
  - Trochlear ØØSJ
  - Ulnar Ø1S4
  - Vagus ØØSQ
- Nipple
  - Left ØHSXXZZ
  - Right ØHSWXZZ
- Nose Ø9SK
- Orbit
  - Left ØNSQ
  - Right ØNSP
- Ovary
  - Bilateral ØUS2
  - Left ØUS1
  - Right ØUSØ

**Reposition** – *continued*
- Palate
  - Hard ØCS2
  - Soft ØCS3
- Pancreas ØFSG
- Parathyroid Gland ØGSR
  - Inferior
    - Left ØGSP
    - Right ØGSN
  - Multiple ØGSQ
  - Superior
    - Left ØGSM
    - Right ØGSL
- Patella
  - Left ØQSF
  - Right ØQSD
- Phalanx
  - Finger
    - Left ØPSV
    - Right ØPST
  - Thumb
    - Left ØPSS
    - Right ØPSR
  - Toe
    - Left ØQSR
    - Right ØQSQ
- Products of Conception 10SØ
  - Ectopic 10S2
- Radius
  - Left ØPSJ
  - Right ØPSH
- Rectum ØDSP
- Retinal Vessel
  - Left Ø8SH3ZZ
  - Right Ø8SG3ZZ
- Rib
  - Left ØPS2
  - Right ØPS1
- Sacrum ØQS1
- Scapula
  - Left ØPS6
  - Right ØPS5
- Septum, Nasal Ø9SM
- Skull ØNSØ
- Spinal Cord
  - Cervical ØØSW
  - Lumbar ØØSY
  - Thoracic ØØSX
- Spleen Ø7SPØZZ
- Sternum ØPSØ
- Stomach ØDS6
- Tarsal
  - Left ØQSM
  - Right ØQSL
- Tendon
  - Abdomen
    - Left ØLSG
    - Right ØLSF
  - Ankle
    - Left ØLST
    - Right ØLSS
  - Foot
    - Left ØLSW
    - Right ØLSV
  - Hand
    - Left ØLS8
    - Right ØLS7
  - Head and Neck ØLSØ
  - Hip
    - Left ØLSK
    - Right ØLSJ
  - Knee
    - Left ØLSR
    - Right ØLSQ
  - Lower Arm and Wrist
    - Left ØLS6
    - Right ØLS5
  - Lower Leg
    - Left ØLSP
    - Right ØLSN
  - Perineum ØLSH
  - Shoulder
    - Left ØLS2
    - Right ØLS1
  - Thorax
    - Left ØLSD
    - Right ØLSC
  - Trunk
    - Left ØLSB
    - Right ØLS9
  - Upper Arm
    - Left ØLS4
    - Right ØLS3

**Reposition** – *continued*
- Tendon – *continued*
  - Upper Leg
    - Left ØLSM
    - Right ØLSL
- Testis
  - Bilateral ØVSC
  - Left ØVSB
  - Right ØVS9
- Thymus Ø7SMØZZ
- Thyroid Gland
  - Left Lobe ØGSG
  - Right Lobe ØGSH
- Tibia
  - Left ØQSH
  - Right ØQSG
- Tongue ØCS7
- Tooth
  - Lower ØCSX
  - Upper ØCSW
- Trachea ØBS10ZZ
- Turbinate, Nasal Ø9SL
- Tympanic Membrane
  - Left Ø9S8
  - Right Ø9S7
- Ulna
  - Left ØPSL
  - Right ØPSK
- Ureter
  - Left ØTS7
  - Right ØTS6
- Ureters, Bilateral ØTS8
- Urethra ØTSD
- Uterine Supporting Structure ØUS4
- Uterus ØUS9
- Uvula ØCSN
- Vagina ØUSG
- Vein
  - Axillary
    - Left Ø5S8
    - Right Ø5S7
  - Azygos Ø5SØ
  - Basilic
    - Left Ø5SC
    - Right Ø5SB
  - Brachial
    - Left Ø5SA
    - Right Ø5S9
  - Cephalic
    - Left Ø5SF
    - Right Ø5SD
  - Colic Ø6S7
  - Common Iliac
    - Left Ø6SD
    - Right Ø6SC
  - Esophageal Ø6S3
  - External Iliac
    - Left Ø6SG
    - Right Ø6SF
  - External Jugular
    - Left Ø5SQ
    - Right Ø5SP
  - Face
    - Left Ø5SV
    - Right Ø5ST
  - Femoral
    - Left Ø6SN
    - Right Ø6SM
  - Foot
    - Left Ø6SV
    - Right Ø6ST
  - Gastric Ø6S2
  - Greater Saphenous
    - Left Ø6SQ
    - Right Ø6SP
  - Hand
    - Left Ø5SH
    - Right Ø5SG
  - Hemiazygos Ø5S1
  - Hepatic Ø6S4
  - Hypogastric
    - Left Ø6SJ
    - Right Ø6SH
  - Inferior Mesenteric Ø6S6
  - Innominate
    - Left Ø5S4
    - Right Ø5S3
  - Internal Jugular
    - Left Ø5SN
    - Right Ø5SM
  - Intracranial Ø5SL
  - Lesser Saphenous
    - Left Ø6SS

**Reposition** – *continued*
  Vein – *continued*
    Lesser Saphenous – *continued*
      Right 06SR
    Lower 06SY
    Portal 06S8
    Pulmonary
      Left 02ST0ZZ
      Right 02SS0ZZ
    Renal
      Left 06SB
      Right 06S9
    Splenic 06S1
    Subclavian
      Left 05S6
      Right 05S5
    Superior Mesenteric 06S5
    Upper 05SY
    Vertebral
      Left 05SS
      Right 05SR
  Vena Cava
    Inferior 06S0
    Superior 02SV0ZZ
  Vertebra
    Cervical 0PS3
    Lumbar 0QS0
    Thoracic 0PS4
  Vocal Cord
    Left 0CSV
    Right 0CST

**Resection**
  Acetabulum
    Left 0QT50ZZ
    Right 0QT40ZZ
  Adenoids 0CTQ
  Ampulla of Vater 0FTC
  Anal Sphincter 0DTR
  Anus 0DTQ
  Aortic Body 0GTD
  Appendix 0DTJ
  Auditory Ossicle
    Left 09TA0ZZ
    Right 09T90ZZ
  Bladder 0TTB
  Bladder Neck 0TTC
  Bone
    Ethmoid
      Left 0NTG0ZZ
      Right 0NTF0ZZ
    Frontal
      Left 0NT20ZZ
      Right 0NT10ZZ
    Hyoid 0NTX0ZZ
    Lacrimal
      Left 0NTJ0ZZ
      Right 0NTH0ZZ
    Nasal 0NTB0ZZ
    Occipital
      Left 0NT80ZZ
      Right 0NT70ZZ
    Palatine
      Left 0NTL0ZZ
      Right 0NTK0ZZ
    Parietal
      Left 0NT40ZZ
      Right 0NT30ZZ
    Pelvic
      Left 0QT30ZZ
      Right 0QT20ZZ
    Sphenoid
      Left 0NTD0ZZ
      Right 0NTC0ZZ
    Temporal
      Left 0NT60ZZ
      Right 0NT50ZZ
    Zygomatic
      Left 0NTN0ZZ
      Right 0NTM0ZZ
  Breast
    Bilateral 0HTV0ZZ
    Left 0HTU0ZZ
    Right 0HTT0ZZ
    Supernumerary 0HTY0ZZ
  Bronchus
    Lingula 0BT9
    Lower Lobe
      Left 0BTB
      Right 0BT6
    Main
      Left 0BT7
      Right 0BT3
    Middle Lobe, Right 0BT5

**Resection** – *continued*
  Bronchus – *continued*
    Upper Lobe
      Left 0BT8
      Right 0BT4
  Bursa and Ligament
    Abdomen
      Left 0MTJ
      Right 0MTH
    Ankle
      Left 0MTR
      Right 0MTQ
    Elbow
      Left 0MT4
      Right 0MT3
    Foot
      Left 0MTT
      Right 0MTS
    Hand
      Left 0MT8
      Right 0MT7
    Head and Neck 0MT0
    Hip
      Left 0MTM
      Right 0MTL
    Knee
      Left 0MTP
      Right 0MTN
    Lower Extremity
      Left 0MTW
      Right 0MTV
    Perineum 0MTK
    Shoulder
      Left 0MT2
      Right 0MT1
    Thorax
      Left 0MTG
      Right 0MTF
    Trunk
      Left 0MTD
      Right 0MTC
    Upper Extremity
      Left 0MTB
      Right 0MT9
    Wrist
      Left 0MT6
      Right 0MT5
  Carina 0BT2
  Carotid Bodies, Bilateral 0GT8
  Carotid Body
    Left 0GT6
    Right 0GT7
  Carpal
    Left 0PTN0ZZ
    Right 0PTM0ZZ
  Cecum 0DTH
  Cerebral Hemisphere 00T7
  Cervix 0UTC
  Chordae Tendineae 02T9
  Cisterna Chyli 07TL
  Clavicle
    Left 0PTB0ZZ
    Right 0PT90ZZ
  Clitoris 0UTJ
  Coccygeal Glomus 0GTB
  Coccyx 0QTS0ZZ
  Colon
    Ascending 0DTK
    Descending 0DTM
    Sigmoid 0DTN
    Transverse 0DTL
  Conduction Mechanism 02T8
  Cord
    Bilateral 0VTH
    Left 0VTG
    Right 0VTF
  Cornea
    Left 08T9XZZ
    Right 08T8XZZ
  Cul-de-sac 0UTF
  Diaphragm
    Left 0BTS
    Right 0BTR
  Disc
    Cervical Vertebral 0RT30ZZ
    Cervicothoracic Vertebral 0RT50ZZ
    Lumbar Vertebral 0ST20ZZ
    Lumbosacral 0ST40ZZ
    Thoracic Vertebral 0RT90ZZ
    Thoracolumbar Vertebral 0RTB0ZZ
  Duct
    Common Bile 0FT9
    Cystic 0FT8

**Resection** – *continued*
  Duct – *continued*
    Hepatic
      Left 0FT6
      Right 0FT5
    Lacrimal
      Left 08TY
      Right 08TX
    Pancreatic 0FTD
      Accessory 0FTF
    Parotid
      Left 0CTC0ZZ
      Right 0CTB0ZZ
  Duodenum 0DT9
  Ear
    External
      Left 09T1
      Right 09T0
    Inner
      Left 09TE0ZZ
      Right 09TD0ZZ
    Middle
      Left 09T60ZZ
      Right 09T50ZZ
  Epididymis
    Bilateral 0VTL
    Left 0VTK
    Right 0VTJ
  Epiglottis 0CTR
  Esophagogastric Junction 0DT4
  Esophagus 0DT5
    Lower 0DT3
    Middle 0DT2
    Upper 0DT1
  Eustachian Tube
    Left 09TG
    Right 09TF
  Eye
    Left 08T1XZZ
    Right 08T0XZZ
  Eyelid
    Lower
      Left 08TR
      Right 08TQ
    Upper
      Left 08TP
      Right 08TN
  Fallopian Tube
    Left 0UT6
    Right 0UT5
  Fallopian Tubes, Bilateral 0UT7
  Femoral Shaft
    Left 0QT90ZZ
    Right 0QT80ZZ
  Femur
    Lower
      Left 0QTC0ZZ
      Right 0QTB0ZZ
    Upper
      Left 0QT70ZZ
      Right 0QT60ZZ
  Fibula
    Left 0QTK0ZZ
    Right 0QTJ0ZZ
  Finger Nail 0HTQXZZ
  Gallbladder 0FT4
  Gland
    Adrenal
      Bilateral 0GT4
      Left 0GT2
      Right 0GT3
    Lacrimal
      Left 08TW
      Right 08TV
    Minor Salivary 0CTJ0ZZ
    Parotid
      Left 0CT90ZZ
      Right 0CT80ZZ
    Pituitary 0GT0
    Sublingual
      Left 0CTF0ZZ
      Right 0CTD0ZZ
    Submaxillary
      Left 0CTH0ZZ
      Right 0CTG0ZZ
    Vestibular 0UTL
  Glenoid Cavity
    Left 0PT80ZZ
    Right 0PT70ZZ
  Glomus Jugulare 0GTC
  Humeral Head
    Left 0PTD0ZZ
    Right 0PTC0ZZ

**Resection** – *continued*
Humeral Shaft
   Left ØPTGØZZ
   Right ØPTFØZZ
Hymen ØUTK
Ileocecal Valve ØDTC
Ileum ØDTB
Intestine
   Large ØDTE
      Left ØDTG
      Right ØDTF
   Small ØDT8
Iris
   Left Ø8TD3ZZ
   Right Ø8TC3ZZ
Jejunum ØDTA
Joint
   Acromioclavicular
      Left ØRTHØZZ
      Right ØRTGØZZ
   Ankle
      Left ØSTGØZZ
      Right ØSTFØZZ
   Carpal
      Left ØRTRØZZ
      Right ØRTQØZZ
   Cervicothoracic Vertebral ØRT4ØZZ
   Coccygeal ØST6ØZZ
   Elbow
      Left ØRTMØZZ
      Right ØRTLØZZ
   Finger Phalangeal
      Left ØRTXØZZ
      Right ØRTWØZZ
   Hip
      Left ØSTBØZZ
      Right ØST9ØZZ
   Knee
      Left ØSTDØZZ
      Right ØSTCØZZ
   Metacarpocarpal
      Left ØRTTØZZ
      Right ØRTSØZZ
   Metacarpophalangeal
      Left ØRTVØZZ
      Right ØRTUØZZ
   Metatarsal–Phalangeal
      Left ØSTNØZZ
      Right ØSTMØZZ
   Metatarsal–Tarsal
      Left ØSTLØZZ
      Right ØSTKØZZ
   Sacrococcygeal ØST5ØZZ
   Sacroiliac
      Left ØST8ØZZ
      Right ØST7ØZZ
   Shoulder
      Left ØRTKØZZ
      Right ØRTJØZZ
   Sternoclavicular
      Left ØRTFØZZ
      Right ØRTEØZZ
   Tarsal
      Left ØSTJØZZ
      Right ØSTHØZZ
   Temporomandibular
      Left ØRTDØZZ
      Right ØRTCØZZ
   Toe Phalangeal
      Left ØSTQØZZ
      Right ØSTPØZZ
   Wrist
      Left ØRTPØZZ
      Right ØRTNØZZ
Kidney
   Left ØTT1
   Right ØTTØ
Kidney Pelvis
   Left ØTT4
   Right ØTT3
Kidneys, Bilateral ØTT2
Larynx ØCTS
Lens
   Left Ø8TK3ZZ
   Right Ø8TJ3ZZ
Lip
   Lower ØCT1
   Upper ØCTØ
Liver ØFTØ
   Left Lobe ØFT2
   Right Lobe ØFT1

**Resection** – *continued*
Lung
   Bilateral ØBTM
   Left ØBTL
   Lower Lobe
      Left ØBTJ
      Right ØBTF
   Middle Lobe, Right ØBTD
   Right ØBTK
   Upper Lobe
      Left ØBTG
      Right ØBTC
Lung Lingula ØBTH
Lymphatic
   Aortic Ø7TD
   Axillary
      Left Ø7T6
      Right Ø7T5
   Head Ø7TØ
   Inguinal
      Left Ø7TJ
      Right Ø7TH
   Internal Mammary
      Left Ø7T9
      Right Ø7T8
   Lower Extremity
      Left Ø7TG
      Right Ø7TF
   Mesenteric Ø7TB
   Neck
      Left Ø7T2
      Right Ø7T1
   Pelvis Ø7TC
   Thoracic Duct Ø7TK
   Thorax Ø7T7
   Upper Extremity
      Left Ø7T4
      Right Ø7T3
Mandible
   Left ØNTVØZZ
   Right ØNTTØZZ
Maxilla
   Left ØNTSØZZ
   Right ØNTRØZZ
Metacarpal
   Left ØPTQØZZ
   Right ØPTPØZZ
Metatarsal
   Left ØQTPØZZ
   Right ØQTNØZZ
Muscle
   Abdomen
      Left ØKTL
      Right ØKTK
   Extraocular
      Left Ø8TM
      Right Ø8TL
   Facial ØKT1
   Foot
      Left ØKTW
      Right ØKTV
   Hand
      Left ØKTD
      Right ØKTC
   Head ØKTØ
   Hip
      Left ØKTP
      Right ØKTN
   Lower Arm and Wrist
      Left ØKTB
      Right ØKT9
   Lower Leg
      Left ØKTT
      Right ØKTS
   Neck
      Left ØKT3
      Right ØKT2
   Papillary Ø2TD
   Perineum ØKTM
   Shoulder
      Left ØKT6
      Right ØKT5
   Thorax
      Left ØKTJ
      Right ØKTH
   Tongue, Palate, Pharynx ØKT4
   Trunk
      Left ØKTG
      Right ØKTF
   Upper Arm
      Left ØKT8
      Right ØKT7

**Resection** – *continued*
Muscle – *continued*
   Upper Leg
      Left ØKTR
      Right ØKTQ
Nasopharynx Ø9TN
Nipple
   Left ØHTXXZZ
   Right ØHTWXZZ
Nose Ø9TK
Omentum
   Greater ØDTS
   Lesser ØDTT
Orbit
   Left ØNTQØZZ
   Right ØNTPØZZ
Ovary
   Bilateral ØUT2
   Left ØUT1
   Right ØUTØ
Palate
   Hard ØCT2
   Soft ØCT3
Pancreas ØFTG
Para-aortic Body ØGT9
Paraganglion Extremity ØGTF
Parathyroid Gland ØGTR
   Inferior
      Left ØGTP
      Right ØGTN
   Multiple ØGTQ
   Superior
      Left ØGTM
      Right ØGTL
Patella
   Left ØQTFØZZ
   Right ØQTDØZZ
Penis ØVTS
Pericardium Ø2TN
Phalanx
   Finger
      Left ØPTVØZZ
      Right ØPTTØZZ
   Thumb
      Left ØPTSØZZ
      Right ØPTRØZZ
   Toe
      Left ØQTRØZZ
      Right ØQTQØZZ
Pharynx ØCTM
Pineal Body ØGT1
Prepuce ØVTT
Products of Conception, Ectopic 1ØT2
Prostate ØVTØ
Radius
   Left ØPTJØZZ
   Right ØPTHØZZ
Rectum ØDTP
Rib
   Left ØPT2ØZZ
   Right ØPT1ØZZ
Scapula
   Left ØPT6ØZZ
   Right ØPT5ØZZ
Scrotum ØVT5
Septum
   Atrial Ø2T5
   Nasal Ø9TM
   Ventricular Ø2TM
Sinus
   Accessory Ø9TP
   Ethmoid
      Left Ø9TV
      Right Ø9TU
   Frontal
      Left Ø9TT
      Right Ø9TS
   Mastoid
      Left Ø9TC
      Right Ø9TB
   Maxillary
      Left Ø9TR
      Right Ø9TQ
   Sphenoid
      Left Ø9TX
      Right Ø9TW
Spleen Ø7TP
Sternum ØPTØØZZ
Stomach ØDT6
   Pylorus ØDT7
Tarsal
   Left ØQTMØZZ
   Right ØQTLØZZ

**Resection** – *continued*
  Tendon
    Abdomen
      Left ØLTG
      Right ØLTF
    Ankle
      Left ØLTT
      Right ØLTS
    Foot
      Left ØLTW
      Right ØLTV
    Hand
      Left ØLT8
      Right ØLT7
    Head and Neck ØLTØ
    Hip
      Left ØLTK
      Right ØLTJ
    Knee
      Left ØLTR
      Right ØLTQ
    Lower Arm and Wrist
      Left ØLT6
      Right ØLT5
    Lower Leg
      Left ØLTP
      Right ØLTN
    Perineum ØLTH
    Shoulder
      Left ØLT2
      Right ØLT1
    Thorax
      Left ØLTD
      Right ØLTC
    Trunk
      Left ØLTB
      Right ØLT9
    Upper Arm
      Left ØLT4
      Right ØLT3
    Upper Leg
      Left ØLTM
      Right ØLTL
  Testis
    Bilateral ØVTC
    Left ØVTB
    Right ØVT9
  Thymus Ø7TM
  Thyroid Gland ØGTK
    Left Lobe ØGTG
    Right Lobe ØGTH
  Tibia
    Left ØQTHØZZ
    Right ØQTGØZZ
  Toe Nail ØHTRXZZ
  Tongue ØCT7
  Tonsils ØCTP
  Tooth
    Lower ØCTXØZ
    Upper ØCTWØZ
  Trachea ØBT1
  Tunica Vaginalis
    Left ØVT7
    Right ØVT6
  Turbinate, Nasal Ø9TL
  Tympanic Membrane
    Left Ø9T8
    Right Ø9T7
  Ulna
    Left ØPTLØZZ
    Right ØPTKØZZ
  Ureter
    Left ØTT7
    Right ØTT6
  Urethra ØTTD
  Uterine Supporting Structure ØUT4
  Uterus ØUT9
  Uvula ØCTN
  Vagina ØUTG
  Valve, Pulmonary Ø2TH
  Vas Deferens
    Bilateral ØVTQ
    Left ØVTP
    Right ØVTN
  Vesicle
    Bilateral ØVT3
    Left ØVT2
    Right ØVT1
  Vitreous
    Left Ø8T53ZZ
    Right Ø8T43ZZ
  Vocal Cord
    Left ØCTV

**Resection** – *continued*
  Vocal Cord – *continued*
    Right ØCTT
  Vulva ØUTM
**Restoration, Cardiac, Single, Rhythm** 5A22Ø4Z
**RestoreAdvanced neurostimulator (SureScan)(MRI Safe)** – *use* Stimulator Generator, Multiple Array Rechargeable in ØJH
**RestoreSensor neurostimulator (SureScan)(MRI Safe)** – *use* Stimulator Generator, Multiple Array Rechargeable in ØJH
**RestoreUltra neurostimulator (SureScan)(MRI Safe)** – *use* Stimulator Generator, Multiple Array Rechargeable in ØJH
**Restriction**
  Ampulla of Vater ØFVC
  Anus ØDVQ
  Aorta
    Abdominal Ø4VØ
    Thoracic Ø2VW
  Artery
    Anterior Tibial
      Left Ø4VQ
      Right Ø4VP
    Axillary
      Left Ø3V6
      Right Ø3V5
    Brachial
      Left Ø3V8
      Right Ø3V7
    Celiac Ø4V1
    Colic
      Left Ø4V7
      Middle Ø4V8
      Right Ø4V6
    Common Carotid
      Left Ø3VJ
      Right Ø3VH
    Common Iliac
      Left Ø4VD
      Right Ø4VC
    External Carotid
      Left Ø3VN
      Right Ø3VM
    External Iliac
      Left Ø4VJ
      Right Ø4VH
    Face Ø3VR
    Femoral
      Left Ø4VL
      Right Ø4VK
    Foot
      Left Ø4VW
      Right Ø4VV
    Gastric Ø4V2
    Hand
      Left Ø3VF
      Right Ø3VD
    Hepatic Ø4V3
    Inferior Mesenteric Ø4VB
    Innominate Ø3V2
    Internal Carotid
      Left Ø3VL
      Right Ø3VK
    Internal Iliac
      Left Ø4VF
      Right Ø4VE
    Internal Mammary
      Left Ø3V1
      Right Ø3VØ
    Intracranial Ø3VG
    Lower Ø4VY
    Peroneal
      Left Ø4VU
      Right Ø4VT
    Popliteal
      Left Ø4VN
      Right Ø4VM
    Posterior Tibial
      Left Ø4VS
      Right Ø4VR
    Pulmonary
      Left Ø2VR
      Right Ø2VQ
    Pulmonary Trunk Ø2VP
    Radial
      Left Ø3VC
      Right Ø3VB
    Renal
      Left Ø4VA
      Right Ø4V9
    Splenic Ø4V4

**Restriction** – *continued*
  Artery – *continued*
    Subclavian
      Left Ø3V4
      Right Ø3V3
    Superior Mesenteric Ø4V5
    Temporal
      Left Ø3VT
      Right Ø3VS
    Thyroid
      Left Ø3VV
      Right Ø3VU
    Ulnar
      Left Ø3VA
      Right Ø3V9
    Upper Ø3VY
    Vertebral
      Left Ø3VQ
      Right Ø3VP
  Bladder ØTVB
  Bladder Neck ØTVC
  Bronchus
    Lingula ØBV9
    Lower Lobe
      Left ØBVB
      Right ØBV6
    Main
      Left ØBV7
      Right ØBV3
    Middle Lobe, Right ØBV5
    Upper Lobe
      Left ØBV8
      Right ØBV4
  Carina ØBV2
  Cecum ØDVH
  Cervix ØUVC
  Cisterna Chyli Ø7VL
  Colon
    Ascending ØDVK
    Descending ØDVM
    Sigmoid ØDVN
    Transverse ØDVL
  Duct
    Common Bile ØFV9
    Cystic ØFV8
    Hepatic
      Left ØFV6
      Right ØFV5
    Lacrimal
      Left Ø8VY
      Right Ø8VX
    Pancreatic ØFVD
      Accessory ØFVF
    Parotid
      Left ØCVC
      Right ØCVB
  Duodenum ØDV9
  Esophagogastric Junction ØDV4
  Esophagus ØDV5
    Lower ØDV3
    Middle ØDV2
    Upper ØDV1
  Heart Ø2VA
  Ileocecal Valve ØDVC
  Ileum ØDVB
  Intestine
    Large ØDVE
      Left ØDVG
      Right ØDVF
    Small ØDV8
  Jejunum ØDVA
  Kidney Pelvis
    Left ØTV4
    Right ØTV3
  Lymphatic
    Aortic Ø7VD
    Axillary
      Left Ø7V6
      Right Ø7V5
    Head Ø7VØ
    Inguinal
      Left Ø7VJ
      Right Ø7VH
    Internal Mammary
      Left Ø7V9
      Right Ø7V8
    Lower Extremity
      Left Ø7VG
      Right Ø7VF
    Mesenteric Ø7VB
    Neck
      Left Ø7V2
      Right Ø7V1

**Restriction** – *continued*
  Lymphatic – *continued*
    Pelvis 07VC
    Thoracic Duct 07VK
    Thorax 07V7
    Upper Extremity
      Left 07V4
      Right 07V3
  Rectum 0DVP
  Stomach 0DV6
    Pylorus 0DV7
  Trachea 0BV1
  Ureter
    Left 0TV7
    Right 0TV6
  Urethra 0TVD
  Vein
    Axillary
      Left 05V8
      Right 05V7
    Azygos 05V0
    Basilic
      Left 05VC
      Right 05VB
    Brachial
      Left 05VA
      Right 05V9
    Cephalic
      Left 05VF
      Right 05VD
    Colic 06V7
    Common Iliac
      Left 06VD
      Right 06VC
    Esophageal 06V3
    External Iliac
      Left 06VG
      Right 06VF
    External Jugular
      Left 05VQ
      Right 05VP
    Face
      Left 05VV
      Right 05VT
    Femoral
      Left 06VN
      Right 06VM
    Foot
      Left 06VV
      Right 06VT
    Gastric 06V2
    Greater Saphenous
      Left 06VQ
      Right 06VP
    Hand
      Left 05VH
      Right 05VG
    Hemiazygos 05V1
    Hepatic 06V4
    Hypogastric
      Left 06VJ
      Right 06VH
    Inferior Mesenteric 06V6
    Innominate
      Left 05V4
      Right 05V3
    Internal Jugular
      Left 05VN
      Right 05VM
    Intracranial 05VL
    Lesser Saphenous
      Left 06VS
      Right 06VR
    Lower 06VY
    Portal 06V8
    Pulmonary
      Left 02VT
      Right 02VS
    Renal
      Left 06VB
      Right 06V9
    Splenic 06V1
    Subclavian
      Left 05V6
      Right 05V5
    Superior Mesenteric 06V5
    Upper 05VY
    Vertebral
      Left 05VS
      Right 05VR
  Vena Cava
    Inferior 06V0
    Superior 02VV

**Resurfacing Device**
  Removal of device from
    Left 0SPB0BZ
    Right 0SP90BZ
  Revision of device in
    Left 0SWB0BZ
    Right 0SW90BZ
  Supplement
    Left 0SUB0BZ
      Acetabular Surface 0SUE0BZ
      Femoral Surface 0SUS0BZ
    Right 0SU90BZ
      Acetabular Surface 0SUA0BZ
      Femoral Surface 0SUR0BZ

**Resuscitation**
  Cardiopulmonary – *see* Assistance, Cardiac 5A02
  Cardioversion 5A2204Z
  Defibrillation 5A2204Z
  Endotracheal intubation – *see* Insertion of device in, Trachea 0BH1
  External chest compression 5A12012
  Pulmonary 5A19054

**Resuture, Heart valve prosthesis** – *see* Revision of device in, Heart and Great Vessels 02W

**Retraining**
  Cardiac – *see* Motor Treatment, Rehabilitation F07
  Vocational – *see* Activities of Daily Living Treatment, Rehabilitation F08

**Retrogasserian rhizotomy** – *see* Division, Nerve, Trigeminal 008K

**Retroperitoneal lymph node** – *use* Lymphatic, Aortic

**Retroperitoneal space** – *use* Retroperitoneum

**Retropharyngeal lymph node**
  – *use* Lymphatic, Neck, Left
  – *use* Lymphatic, Neck, Right

**Retropubic space** – *use* Pelvic Cavity

**Reveal** (DX)(XT) – *use* Monitoring Device

**Reverse total shoulder replacement** – *see* Replacement, Upper Joints 0RR

**Reverse® Shoulder Prosthesis** – *use* Synthetic Substitute, Reverse Ball and Socket in 0RR

**Revision of device in**
  Abdominal Wall 0WWF
  Acetabulum
    Left 0QW5
    Right 0QW4
  Anal Sphincter 0DWR
  Anus 0DWQ
  Artery
    Lower 04WY
    Upper 03WY
  Auditory Ossicle
    Left 09WA
    Right 09W9
  Back
    Lower 0WWL
    Upper 0WWK
  Bladder 0TWB
  Bone
    Facial 0NWW
    Lower 0QWY
    Nasal 0NWB
    Pelvic
      Left 0QW3
      Right 0QW2
    Upper 0PWY
  Bone Marrow 07WT
  Brain 00W0
  Breast
    Left 0HWU
    Right 0HWT
  Bursa and Ligament
    Lower 0MWY
    Upper 0MWX
  Carpal
    Left 0PWN
    Right 0PWM
  Cavity, Cranial 0WW1
  Cerebral Ventricle 00W6
  Chest Wall 0WW8
  Cisterna Chyli 07WL
  Clavicle
    Left 0PWB
    Right 0PW9
  Coccyx 0QWS
  Diaphragm 0BWT
  Disc
    Cervical Vertebral 0RW3
    Cervicothoracic Vertebral 0RW5
    Lumbar Vertebral 0SW2
    Lumbosacral 0SW4

**Revision of device in** – *continued*
  Disc – *continued*
    Thoracic Vertebral 0RW9
    Thoracolumbar Vertebral 0RWB
  Duct
    Hepatobiliary 0FWB
    Pancreatic 0FWD
  Ear
    Inner
      Left 09WE
      Right 09WD
    Left 09WJ
    Right 09WH
  Epididymis and Spermatic Cord 0VWM
  Esophagus 0DW5
  Extremity
    Lower
      Left 0YWB
      Right 0YW9
    Upper
      Left 0XW7
      Right 0XW6
  Eye
    Left 08W1
    Right 08W0
  Face 0WW2
  Fallopian Tube 0UW8
  Femoral Shaft
    Left 0QW9
    Right 0QW8
  Femur
    Lower
      Left 0QWC
      Right 0QWB
    Upper
      Left 0QW7
      Right 0QW6
  Fibula
    Left 0QWK
    Right 0QWJ
  Finger Nail 0HWQX
  Gallbladder 0FW4
  Gastrointestinal Tract 0WWP
  Genitourinary Tract 0WWR
  Gland
    Adrenal 0GW5
    Endocrine 0GWS
    Pituitary 0GW0
    Salivary 0CWA
  Glenoid Cavity
    Left 0PW8
    Right 0PW7
  Great Vessel 02WY
  Hair 0HWSX
  Head 0WW0
  Heart 02WA
  Humeral Head
    Left 0PWD
    Right 0PWC
  Humeral Shaft
    Left 0PWG
    Right 0PWF
  Intestinal Tract
    Lower 0DWD
    Upper 0DW0
  Intestine
    Large 0DWE
    Small 0DW8
  Jaw
    Lower 0WW5
    Upper 0WW4
  Joint
    Acromioclavicular
      Left 0RWH
      Right 0RWG
    Ankle
      Left 0SWG
      Right 0SWF
    Carpal
      Left 0RWR
      Right 0RWQ
    Cervical Vertebral 0RW1
    Cervicothoracic Vertebral 0RW4
    Coccygeal 0SW6
    Elbow
      Left 0RWM
      Right 0RWL
    Finger Phalangeal
      Left 0RWX
      Right 0RWW
    Hip
      Left 0SWB
      Right 0SW9

**Revision of device in** – *continued*
  Joint – *continued*
    Knee
      Left 0SWD
      Right 0SWC
    Lumbar Vertebral 0SW0
    Lumbosacral 0SW3
    Metacarpocarpal
      Left 0RWT
      Right 0RWS
    Metacarpophalangeal
      Left 0RWV
      Right 0RWU
    Metatarsal–Phalangeal
      Left 0SWN
      Right 0SWM
    Metatarsal–Tarsal
      Left 0SWL
      Right 0SWK
    Occipital–cervical 0RW0
    Sacrococcygeal 0SW5
    Sacroiliac
      Left 0SW8
      Right 0SW7
    Shoulder
      Left 0RWK
      Right 0RWJ
    Sternoclavicular
      Left 0RWF
      Right 0RWE
    Tarsal
      Left 0SWJ
      Right 0SWH
    Temporomandibular
      Left 0RWD
      Right 0RWC
    Thoracic Vertebral 0RW6
    Thoracolumbar Vertebral 0RWA
    Toe Phalangeal
      Left 0SWQ
      Right 0SWP
    Wrist
      Left 0RWP
      Right 0RWN
  Kidney 0TW5
  Larynx 0CWS
  Lens
    Left 08WK
    Right 08WJ
  Liver 0FW0
  Lung
    Left 0BWL
    Right 0BWK
  Lymphatic 07WN
    Thoracic Duct 07WK
  Mediastinum 0WWC
  Mesentery 0DWV
  Metacarpal
    Left 0PWQ
    Right 0PWP
  Metatarsal
    Left 0QWP
    Right 0QWN
  Mouth and Throat 0CWY
  Muscle
    Extraocular
      Left 08WM
      Right 08WL
    Lower 0KWY
    Upper 0KWX
  Neck 0WW6
  Nerve
    Cranial 00WE
    Peripheral 01WY
  Nose 09WK
  Omentum 0DWU
  Ovary 0UW3
  Pancreas 0FWG
  Parathyroid Gland 0GWR
  Patella
    Left 0QWF
    Right 0QWD
  Pelvic Cavity 0WWJ
  Penis 0VWS
  Pericardial Cavity 0WWD
  Perineum
    Female 0WWN
    Male 0WWM
  Peritoneal Cavity 0WWG
  Peritoneum 0DWW
  Phalanx
    Finger
      Left 0PWV

**Revision of device in** – *continued*
  Phalanx – *continued*
    Finger – *continued*
      Right 0PWT
    Thumb
      Left 0PWS
      Right 0PWR
    Toe
      Left 0QWR
      Right 0QWQ
  Pineal Body 0GW1
  Pleura 0BWQ
  Pleural Cavity
    Left 0WWB
    Right 0WW9
  Prostate and Seminal Vesicles 0VW4
  Radius
    Left 0PWJ
    Right 0PWH
  Respiratory Tract 0WWQ
  Retroperitoneum 0WWH
  Rib
    Left 0PW2
    Right 0PW1
  Sacrum 0QW1
  Scapula
    Left 0PW6
    Right 0PW5
  Scrotum and Tunica Vaginalis 0VW8
  Septum
    Atrial 02W5
    Ventricular 02WM
  Sinus 09WY
  Skin 0HWPX
  Skull 0NW0
  Spinal Canal 00WU
  Spinal Cord 00WV
  Spleen 07WP
  Sternum 0PW0
  Stomach 0DW6
  Subcutaneous Tissue and Fascia
    Head and Neck 0JWS
    Lower Extremity 0JWW
    Trunk 0JWT
    Upper Extremity 0JWV
  Tarsal
    Left 0QWM
    Right 0QWL
  Tendon
    Lower 0LWY
    Upper 0LWX
  Testis 0VWD
  Thymus 07WM
  Thyroid Gland 0GWK
  Tibia
    Left 0QWH
    Right 0QWG
  Toe Nail 0HWRX
  Trachea 0BW1
  Tracheobronchial Tree 0BW0
  Tympanic Membrane
    Left 09W8
    Right 09W7
  Ulna
    Left 0PWL
    Right 0PWK
  Ureter 0TW9
  Urethra 0TWD
  Uterus and Cervix 0UWD
  Vagina and Cul-de-sac 0UWH
  Valve
    Aortic 02WF
    Mitral 02WG
    Pulmonary 02WH
    Tricuspid 02WJ
  Vas Deferens 0VWR
  Vein
    Lower 06WY
    Upper 05WY
  Vertebra
    Cervical 0PW3
    Lumbar 0QW0
    Thoracic 0PW4
  Vulva 0UWM
**Revo MRI™ SureScan® pacemaker** – *use* Pacemaker, Dual Chamber in 0JH
**rhBMP-2** – *use* Recombinant Bone Morphogenetic Protein
**Rheos® System device** – *use* Stimulator Generator in Subcutaneous Tissue and Fascia
**Rheos® System lead** – *use* Stimulator Lead in Upper Arteries
**Rhinopharynx** – *use* Nasopharynx

**Rhinoplasty**
  – *see* Alteration, Nose 090K
  – *see* Repair, Nose 09QK
  – *see* Replacement, Nose 09RK
  – *see* Supplement, Nose 09UK
**Rhinorrhaphy** – *see* Repair, Nose 09QK
**Rhinoscopy** 09JKXZZ
**Rhizotomy**
  – *see* Division, Central Nervous System 008
  – *see* Division, Peripheral Nervous System 018
**Rhomboid major muscle**
  – *use* Muscle, Trunk, Left
  – *use* Muscle, Trunk, Right
**Rhomboid minor muscle**
  – *use* Muscle, Trunk, Right
  – *use* Muscle, Trunk, Left
**Rhythm electrocardiogram** – *see* Measurement, Cardiac 4A02
**Rhytidectomy** – *see* Face lift
**Right ascending lumbar vein** – *use* Vein, Azygos
**Right atrioventricular valve** – *use* Valve, Tricuspid
**Right auricular appendix** – *use* Atrium, Right
**Right colic vein** – *use* Vein, Colic
**Right coronary sulcus** – *use* Heart, Right
**Right gastric artery** – *use* Artery, Gastric
**Right gastroepiploic vein** – *use* Vein, Superior Mesenteric
**Right inferior phrenic vein** – *use* Vena Cava, Inferior
**Right inferior pulmonary vein** – *use* Vein, Pulmonary, Right
**Right jugular trunk** – *use* Lymphatic, Neck, Right
**Right lateral ventricle** – *use* Cerebral Ventricle
**Right lymphatic duct** – *use* Lymphatic, Neck, Right
**Right ovarian vein** – *use* Vena Cava, Inferior
**Right second lumbar vein** – *use* Vena Cava, Inferior
**Right subclavian trunk** – *use* Lymphatic, Neck, Right
**Right subcostal vein** – *use* Vein, Azygos
**Right superior pulmonary vein** – *use* Vein, Pulmonary, Right
**Right suprarenal vein** – *use* Vena Cava, Inferior
**Right testicular vein** – *use* Vena Cava, Inferior
**Rima glottidis** – *use* Larynx
**Risorius muscle** – *use* Muscle, Facial
**RNS System lead** – *use* Neurostimulator Lead in Central Nervous System
**RNS system neurostimulator generator** – *use* Neurostimulator Generator in Head and Facial Bones
**Robotic Assisted Procedure**
  Extremity
    Lower 8E0Y
    Upper 8E0X
  Head and Neck Region 8E09
  Trunk Region 8E0W
**Rotation of fetal head**
  Forceps 10S07ZZ
  Manual 10S0XZZ
**Round ligament of uterus** – *use* Uterine Supporting Structure
**Round window**
  – *use* Ear, Inner, Right
  – *use* Ear, Inner, Left
**Roux-en-Y operation**
  – *see* Bypass, Gastrointestinal System 0D1
  – *see* Bypass, Hepatobiliary System and Pancreas 0F1
**Rupture**
  Adhesions – *see* Release
  Fluid collection – *see* Drainage

# S

**Sacral ganglion** – *use* Nerve, Sacral Sympathetic
**Sacral lymph node** – *use* Lymphatic, Pelvis
**Sacral nerve modulation (SNM) lead** – *use* Stimulator Lead in Urinary System
**Sacral neuromodulation lead** – *use* Stimulator Lead in Urinary System
**Sacral splanchnic nerve** – *use* Nerve, Sacral Sympathetic
**Sacrectomy** – *see* Excision, Lower Bones 0QB
**Sacrococcygeal ligament**
  – *use* Bursa and Ligament, Trunk, Right
  – *use* Bursa and Ligament, Trunk, Left
**Sacrococcygeal symphysis** – *use* Joint, Sacrococcygeal
**Sacroiliac ligament**
  – *use* Bursa and Ligament, Trunk, Left

**Sacroiliac ligament** – *continued*
– *use* Bursa and Ligament, Trunk, Right
**Sacrospinous ligament**
– *use* Bursa and Ligament, Trunk, Left
– *use* Bursa and Ligament, Trunk, Right
**Sacrotuberous ligament**
– *use* Bursa and Ligament, Trunk, Left
– *use* Bursa and Ligament, Trunk, Right
**Salpingectomy**
– *see* Excision, Female Reproductive System ØUB
– *see* Resection, Female Reproductive System ØUT
**Salpingolysis** – *see* Release, Female Reproductive System ØUN
**Salpingopexy**
– *see* Repair, Female Reproductive System ØUQ
– *see* Reposition, Female Reproductive System ØUS
**Salpingopharyngeus muscle** – *use* Muscle, Tongue, Palate, Pharynx
**Salpingoplasty**
– *see* Repair, Female Reproductive System ØUQ
– *see* Supplement, Female Reproductive System ØUU
**Salpingorrhaphy** – *see* Repair, Female Reproductive System ØUQ
**Salpingoscopy** ØUJ88ZZ
**Salpingostomy** – *see* Drainage, Female Reproductive System ØU9
**Salpingotomy** – *see* Drainage, Female Reproductive System ØU9
**Salpinx**
– *use* Fallopian Tube, Left
– *use* Fallopian Tube, Right
**Saphenous nerve** – *use* Nerve, Femoral
**SAPIEN transcatheter aortic valve** – *use* Zooplastic Tissue in Heart and Great Vessels
**Sartorius muscle**
– *use* Muscle, Upper Leg, Right
– *use* Muscle, Upper Leg, Left
**Scalene muscle**
– *use* Muscle, Neck, Right
– *use* Muscle, Neck, Left
**Scan**
Computerized Tomography (CT) – *see* Computerized Tomography (CT Scan)
Radioisotope – *see* Planar Nuclear Medicine Imaging
**Scaphoid bone**
– *use* Carpal, Left
– *use* Carpal, Right
**Scapholunate ligament**
– *use* Bursa and Ligament, Hand, Right
– *use* Bursa and Ligament, Hand, Left
**Scaphotrapezium ligament**
– *use* Bursa and Ligament, Hand, Right
– *use* Bursa and Ligament, Hand, Left
**Scapulectomy**
– *see* Excision, Upper Bones ØPB
– *see* Resection, Upper Bones ØPT
**Scapulopexy**
– *see* Repair, Upper Bones ØPQ
– *see* Reposition, Upper Bones ØPS
**Scarpa's** (vestibular) **ganglion** – *use* Nerve, Acoustic
**Sclerectomy** – *see* Excision, Eye Ø8B
**Sclerotherapy, mechanical** – *see* Destruction
**Sclerotomy** – *see* Drainage, Eye Ø89
**Scrotectomy**
– *see* Excision, Male Reproductive System ØVB
– *see* Resection, Male Reproductive System ØVT
**Scrotoplasty**
– *see* Repair, Male Reproductive System ØVQ
– *see* Supplement, Male Reproductive System ØVU
**Scrotorrhaphy** – *see* Repair, Male Reproductive System ØVQ
**Scrototomy** – *see* Drainage, Male Reproductive System ØV9
**Sebaceous gland** – *use* Skin
**Second cranial nerve** – *use* Nerve, Optic
**Section, cesarean** – *see* Extraction, Pregnancy 1ØD
**Secura** (DR) (VR) – *use* Defibrillator Generator in ØJH
**Sella Turcica**
– *use* Bone, Sphenoid, Right
– *use* Bone, Sphenoid, Left
**Semicircular canal**
– *use* Ear, Inner, Right
– *use* Ear, Inner, Left
**Semimembranosus muscle**
– *use* Muscle, Upper Leg, Left
– *use* Muscle, Upper Leg, Right

**Semitendinosus muscle**
– *use* Muscle, Upper Leg, Left
– *use* Muscle, Upper Leg, Right
**Seprafilm** – *use* Adhesion Barrier
**Septal cartilage** – *use* Septum, Nasal
**Septectomy**
– *see* Excision, Heart and Great Vessels Ø2B
– *see* Resection, Heart and Great Vessels Ø2T
– *see* Excision, Ear, Nose, Sinus Ø9B
– *see* Resection, Ear, Nose, Sinus Ø9T
**Septoplasty**
– *see* Repair, Ear, Nose, Sinus Ø9Q
– *see* Replacement, Ear, Nose, Sinus Ø9R
– *see* Supplement, Ear, Nose, Sinus Ø9U
– *see* Reposition, Ear, Nose, Sinus Ø9S
– *see* Repair, Heart and Great Vessels Ø2Q
– *see* Replacement, Heart and Great Vessels Ø2R
– *see* Supplement, Heart and Great Vessels Ø2U
**Septotomy** – *see* Drainage, Ear, Nose, Sinus Ø99
**Sequestrectomy, bone** – *see* Extirpation
**Serratus anterior muscle**
– *use* Muscle, Thorax, Left
– *use* Muscle, Thorax, Right
**Serratus posterior muscle**
– *use* Muscle, Trunk, Left
– *use* Muscle, Trunk, Right
**Seventh cranial nerve** – *use* Nerve, Facial
**Sheffield hybrid external fixator**
– *use* External Fixation Device, Hybrid in ØPH
– *use* External Fixation Device, Hybrid in ØPS
– *use* External Fixation Device, Hybrid in ØQH
– *use* External Fixation Device, Hybrid in ØQS
**Sheffield ring external fixator**
– *use* External Fixation Device, Ring in ØPH
– *use* External Fixation Device, Ring in ØPS
– *use* External Fixation Device, Ring in ØQH
– *use* External Fixation Device, Ring in ØQS
**Shirodkar cervical cerclage** ØUVC7ZZ
**Shock Wave Therapy, Musculoskeletal** 6A93
**Short gastric artery** – *use* Artery, Splenic
**Shortening**
– *see* Excision
– *see* Repair
– *see* Reposition
**Shunt creation** – *see* Bypass
**Sialoadenectomy**
Complete – *see* Resection, Mouth and Throat ØCT
Partial – *see* Excision, Mouth and Throat ØCB
**Sialodochoplasty**
– *see* Repair, Mouth and Throat ØCQ
– *see* Replacement, Mouth and Throat ØCR
– *see* Supplement, Mouth and Throat ØCU
**Sialoectomy**
– *see* Excision, Mouth and Throat ØCB
– *see* Resection, Mouth and Throat ØCT
**Sialography** – *see* Plain Radiography, Ear, Nose, Mouth and Throat B9Ø
**Sialolithotomy** – *see* Extirpation, Mouth and Throat ØCC
**Sigmoid artery** – *use* Artery, Inferior Mesenteric
**Sigmoid flexure** – *use* Colon, Sigmoid
**Sigmoid vein** – *use* Vein, Inferior Mesenteric
**Sigmoidectomy**
– *see* Excision, Gastrointestinal System ØDB
– *see* Resection, Gastrointestinal System ØDT
**Sigmoidorrhaphy** – *see* Repair, Gastrointestinal System ØDQ
**Sigmoidoscopy** ØDJD8ZZ
**Sigmoidotomy** – *see* Drainage, Gastrointestinal System ØD9
**Single lead pacemaker** (atrium)(ventricle) – *use* Pacemaker, Single Chamber in ØJH
**Single lead rate responsive pacemaker** (atrium) (ventricle) – *use* Pacemaker, Single Chamber Rate Responsive in ØJH
**Sinoatrial node** – *use* Conduction Mechanism
**Sinogram**
Abdominal Wall – *see* Fluoroscopy, Abdomen and Pelvis BW11
Chest Wall – *see* Plain Radiography, Chest BWØ3
Retroperitoneum – *see* Fluoroscopy, Abdomen and Pelvis BW11
**Sinus venosus** – *use* Atrium, Right
**Sinusectomy**
– *see* Excision, Ear, Nose, Sinus Ø9B
– *see* Resection, Ear, Nose, Sinus Ø9T
**Sinusoscopy** Ø9JY4ZZ
**Sinusotomy** – *see* Drainage, Ear, Nose, Sinus Ø99

**Sirolimus-eluting coronary stent** – *use* Intraluminal Device, Drug-eluting in Heart and Great Vessels
**Sixth cranial nerve** – *use* Nerve, Abducens
**Size reduction, breast** – *see* Excision, Skin and Breast ØHB
**SJM Biocor® Stented Valve System** – *use* Zooplastic Tissue in Heart and Great Vessels
**Skene's** (paraurethral) **gland** – *use* Gland, Vestibular
**Sling**
Fascial, orbicularis muscle (mouth) – *see* Supplement, Muscle, Facial ØKU1
Levator muscle, for urethral suspension – *see* Reposition, Bladder Neck ØTSC
Pubococcygeal, for urethral suspension – *see* Reposition, Bladder Neck ØTSC
Rectum – *see* Reposition, Rectum ØDSP
**Small bowel series** – *see* Fluoroscopy, Bowel, Small BD13
**Small saphenous vein**
– *use* Vein, Lesser Saphenous, Left
– *use* Vein, Lesser Saphenous, Right
**Snaring, polyp, colon** – *see* Excision, Gastrointestinal System ØDB
**Solar** (celiac) **plexus** – *use* Nerve, Abdominal Sympathetic
**Soleus muscle**
– *use* Muscle, Lower Leg, Left
– *use* Muscle, Lower Leg, Right
**Spacer**
Insertion of device in
Disc
Lumbar Vertebral ØSH2
Lumbosacral ØSH4
Joint
Acromioclavicular
Left ØRHH
Right ØRHG
Ankle
Left ØSHG
Right ØSHF
Carpal
Left ØRHR
Right ØRHQ
Cervical Vertebral ØRH1
Cervicothoracic Vertebral ØRH4
Coccygeal ØSH6
Elbow
Left ØRHM
Right ØRHL
Finger Phalangeal
Left ØRHX
Right ØRHW
Hip
Left ØSH3
Right ØSH9
Knee
Left ØSHD
Right ØSHC
Lumbar Vertebral ØSHØ
Lumbosacral ØSH3
Metacarpocarpal
Left ØRHT
Right ØRHS
Metacarpophalangeal
Left ØRHV
Right ØRHU
Metatarsal–Phalangeal
Left ØSHN
Right ØSHM
Metatarsal–Tarsal
Left ØSHL
Right ØSHK
Occipital–cervical ØRHØ
Sacrococcygeal ØSH5
Sacroiliac
Left ØSH8
Right ØSH7
Shoulder
Left ØRHK
Right ØRHJ
Sternoclavicular
Left ØRHF
Right ØRHE
Tarsal
Left ØSHJ
Right ØSHH
Temporomandibular
Left ØRHD
Right ØRHC
Thoracic Vertebral ØRH6
Thoracolumbar Vertebral ØRHA
Toe Phalangeal
Left ØSHQ
Right ØSHP

**Spacer** – continued
  Insertion of device in – continued
    Joint – continued
      Wrist
        Left ØRHP
        Right ØRHN
  Removal of device from
    Acromioclavicular
      Left ØRPH
      Right ØRPG
    Ankle
      Left ØSPG
      Right ØSPF
    Carpal
      Left ØRPR
      Right ØRPQ
    Cervical Vertebral ØRP1
    Cervicothoracic Vertebral ØRP4
    Coccygeal ØSP6
    Elbow
      Left ØRPM
      Right ØRPL
    Finger Phalangeal
      Left ØRPX
      Right ØRPW
    Hip
      Left ØSPB
      Right ØSP9
    Knee
      Left ØSPD
      Right ØSPC
    Lumbar Vertebral ØSPØ
    Lumbosacral ØSP3
    Metacarpocarpal
      Left ØRPT
      Right ØRPS
    Metacarpophalangeal
      Left ØRPV
      Right ØRPU
    Metatarsal–Phalangeal
      Left ØSPN
      Right ØSPM
    Metatarsal–Tarsal
      Left ØSPL
      Right ØSPK
    Occipital–cervical ØRPØ
    Sacrococcygeal ØSP5
    Sacroiliac
      Left ØSP8
      Right ØSP7
    Shoulder
      Left ØRPK
      Right ØRPJ
    Sternoclavicular
      Left ØRPF
      Right ØRPE
    Tarsal
      Left ØSPJ
      Right ØSPH
    Temporomandibular
      Left ØRPD
      Right ØRPC
    Thoracic Vertebral ØRP6
    Thoracolumbar Vertebral ØRPA
    Toe Phalangeal
      Left ØSPQ
      Right ØSPP
    Wrist
      Left ØRPP
      Right ØRPN
  Revision of device in
    Acromioclavicular
      Left ØRWH
      Right ØRWG
    Ankle
      Left ØSWG
      Right ØSWF
    Carpal
      Left ØRWR
      Right ØRWQ
    Cervical Vertebral ØRW1
    Cervicothoracic Vertebral ØRW4
    Coccygeal ØSW6
    Elbow
      Left ØRWM
      Right ØRWL
    Finger Phalangeal
      Left ØRWX
      Right ØRWW
    Hip
      Left ØSWB
      Right ØSW9

**Spacer** – continued
  Revision of device in – continued
    Knee
      Left ØSWD
      Right ØSWC
    Lumbar Vertebral ØSWØ
    Lumbosacral ØSW3
    Metacarpocarpal
      Left ØRWT
      Right ØRWS
    Metacarpophalangeal
      Left ØRWV
      Right ØRWU
    Metatarsal–Phalangeal
      Left ØSWN
      Right ØSWM
    Metatarsal–Tarsal
      Left ØSWL
      Right ØSWK
    Occipital–cervical ØRWØ
    Sacrococcygeal ØSW5
    Sacroiliac
      Left ØSW8
      Right ØSW7
    Shoulder
      Left ØRWK
      Right ØRWJ
    Sternoclavicular
      Left ØRWF
      Right ØRWE
    Tarsal
      Left ØSWJ
      Right ØSWH
    Temporomandibular
      Left ØRWD
      Right ØRWC
    Thoracic Vertebral ØRW6
    Thoracolumbar Vertebral ØRWA
    Toe Phalangeal
      Left ØSWQ
      Right ØSWP
    Wrist
      Left ØRWP
      Right ØRWN
**Spectroscopy**
  Intravascular 8E023DZ
  Near infrared 8E023DZ
**Speech Assessment** F00
**Speech therapy** – see Speech Treatment, Rehabilitation F06
**Speech Treatment** F06
**Sphenoidectomy**
  – see Excision, Ear, Nose, Sinus 09B
  – see Resection, Ear, Nose, Sinus 09T
  – see Excision, Head and Facial Bones 0NB
  – see Resection, Head and Facial Bones 0NT
**Sphenoidotomy** – see Drainage, Ear, Nose, Sinus 099
**Sphenomandibular ligament** – use Bursa and Ligament, Head and Neck
**Sphenopalatine** (pterygopalatine) **ganglion** – use Nerve, Head and Neck Sympathetic
**Sphincterorrhaphy, anal** – see Repair, Anal Sphincter 0DQR
**Sphincterotomy, anal**
  – see Drainage, Anal Sphincter 0D9R
  – see Division, Anal Sphincter 0D8R
**Spinal cord neurostimulator lead** – use Neurostimulator Lead in Central Nervous System
**Spinal dura mater** – use Dura Mater
**Spinal epidural space** – use Epidural Space
**Spinal nerve, cervical** – use Nerve, Cervical
**Spinal nerve, lumbar** – use Nerve, Lumbar
**Spinal nerve, sacral** – use Nerve, Sacral
**Spinal nerve, thoracic** – use Nerve, Thoracic
**Spinal Stabilization Device**
  Facet Replacement
    Cervical Vertebral ØRH1
    Cervicothoracic Vertebral ØRH4
    Lumbar Vertebral ØSHØ
    Lumbosacral ØSH3
    Occipital–cervical ØRHØ
    Thoracic Vertebral ØRH6
    Thoracolumbar Vertebral ØRHA
  Interspinous Process
    Cervical Vertebral ØRH1
    Cervicothoracic Vertebral ØRH4
    Lumbar Vertebral ØSHØ
    Lumbosacral ØSH3
    Occipital–cervical ØRHØ
    Thoracic Vertebral ØRH6
    Thoracolumbar Vertebral ØRHA

**Spinal Stabilization Device** – continued
  Pedicle–Based
    Cervical Vertebral ØRH1
    Cervicothoracic Vertebral ØRH4
    Lumbar Vertebral ØSHØ
    Lumbosacral ØSH3
    Occipital–cervical ØRHØ
    Thoracic Vertebral ØRH6
    Thoracolumbar Vertebral ØRHA
**Spinal subarachnoid space** – use Subarachnoid Space
**Spinal subdural space** – use Subdural Space
**Spinous process**
  – use Vertebra, Thoracic
  – use Vertebra, Lumbar
  – use Vertebra, Cervical
**Spiral ganglion** – use Nerve, Acoustic
**Spiration IBV™ Valve System** – use Intraluminal Device, Endobronchial Valve in Respiratory System
**Splenectomy**
  – see Excision, Lymphatic and Hemic Systems 07B
  – see Resection, Lymphatic and Hemic Systems 07T
**Splenic flexure** – use Colon, Transverse
**Splenic plexus** – use Nerve, Abdominal Sympathetic
**Splenius capitis muscle** – use Muscle, Head
**Splenius cervicis muscle**
  – use Muscle, Neck, Left
  – use Muscle, Neck, Right
**Splenolysis** – see Release, Lymphatic and Hemic Systems 07N
**Splenopexy**
  – see Repair, Lymphatic and Hemic Systems 07Q
  – see Reposition, Lymphatic and Hemic Systems 07S
**Splenoplasty** – see Repair, Lymphatic and Hemic Systems 07Q
**Splenorrhaphy** – see Repair, Lymphatic and Hemic Systems 07Q
**Splenotomy** – see Drainage, Lymphatic and Hemic Systems 079
**Splinting, musculoskeletal** – see Immobilization, Anatomical Regions 2W3
**Stapedectomy**
  – see Excision, Ear, Nose, Sinus 09B
  – see Resection, Ear, Nose, Sinus 09T
**Stapediolysis** – see Release, Ear, Nose, Sinus 09N
**Stapedioplasty**
  – see Repair, Ear, Nose, Sinus 09Q
  – see Replacement, Ear, Nose, Sinus 09R
  – see Supplement, Ear, Nose, Sinus 09U
**Stapedotomy** – see Drainage, Ear, Nose, Sinus 099
**Stapes**
  – use Auditory Ossicle, Right
  – use Auditory Ossicle, Left
**Stellate ganglion** – use Nerve, Head and Neck Sympathetic
**Stensen's duct**
  – use Duct, Parotid, Right
  – use Duct, Parotid, Left
**Stent, intraluminal (cardiovascular)(gastrointestinal) (hepatobiliary)(urinary)** – use Intraluminal Device
**Stented tissue valve** – use Zooplastic Tissue in Heart and Great Vessels
**Stereotactic Radiosurgery**
  Gamma Beam
    Abdomen DW23JZZ
    Adrenal Gland DG22JZZ
    Bile Ducts DF22JZZ
    Bladder DT22JZZ
    Bone Marrow D720JZZ
    Brain D020JZZ
    Brain Stem D021JZZ
    Breast
      Left DM20JZZ
      Right DM21JZZ
    Bronchus DB21JZZ
    Cervix DU21JZZ
    Chest DW22JZZ
    Chest Wall DB27JZZ
    Colon DD25JZZ
    Diaphragm DB28JZZ
    Duodenum DD22JZZ
    Ear D920JZZ
    Esophagus DD20JZZ
    Eye D820JZZ
    Gallbladder DF21JZZ
    Gland
      Adrenal DG22JZZ
      Parathyroid DG24JZZ
      Pituitary DG20JZZ
      Thyroid DG25JZZ

**Stereotactic Radiosurgery** – *continued*
  Gamma Beam – *continued*
    Glands, Salivary D926JZZ
    Head and Neck DW21JZZ
    Ileum DD24JZZ
    Jejunum DD23JZZ
    Kidney DT20JZZ
    Larynx D92BJZZ
    Liver DF20JZZ
    Lung DB22JZZ
    Lymphatics
      Abdomen D726JZZ
      Axillary D724JZZ
      Inguinal D728JZZ
      Neck D723JZZ
      Pelvis D727JZZ
      Thorax D725JZZ
    Mediastinum DB26JZZ
    Mouth D924JZZ
    Nasopharynx D92DJZZ
    Neck and Head DW21JZZ
    Nerve, Peripheral D027JZZ
    Nose D921JZZ
    Ovary DU20JZZ
    Palate
      Hard D928JZZ
      Soft D929JZZ
    Pancreas DF23JZZ
    Parathyroid Gland DG24JZZ
    Pelvic Region DW26JZZ
    Pharynx D92CJZZ
    Pineal Body DG21JZZ
    Pituitary Gland DG20JZZ
    Pleura DB25JZZ
    Prostate DV20JZZ
    Rectum DD27JZZ
    Sinuses D927JZZ
    Spinal Cord D026JZZ
    Spleen D722JZZ
    Stomach DD21JZZ
    Testis DV21JZZ
    Thymus D721JZZ
    Thyroid Gland DG25JZZ
    Tongue D925JZZ
    Trachea DB20JZZ
    Ureter DT21JZZ
    Urethra DT23JZZ
    Uterus DU22JZZ
  Other Photon
    Abdomen DW23DZZ
    Adrenal Gland DG22DZZ
    Bile Ducts DF22DZZ
    Bladder DT22DZZ
    Bone Marrow D720DZZ
    Brain D020DZZ
    Brain Stem D021DZZ
    Breast
      Left DM20DZZ
      Right DM21DZZ
    Bronchus DB21DZZ
    Cervix DU21DZZ
    Chest DW22DZZ
    Chest Wall DB27DZZ
    Colon DD25DZZ
    Diaphragm DB28DZZ
    Duodenum DD22DZZ
    Ear D920DZZ
    Esophagus DD20DZZ
    Eye D820DZZ
    Gallbladder DF21DZZ
    Gland
      Adrenal DG22DZZ
      Parathyroid DG24DZZ
      Pituitary DG20DZZ
      Thyroid DG25DZZ
    Glands, Salivary D926DZZ
    Head and Neck DW21DZZ
    Ileum DD24DZZ
    Jejunum DD23DZZ
    Kidney DT20DZZ
    Larynx D92BDZZ
    Liver DF20DZZ
    Lung DB22DZZ
    Lymphatics
      Abdomen D726DZZ
      Axillary D724DZZ
      Inguinal D728DZZ
      Neck D723DZZ
      Pelvis D727DZZ
      Thorax D725DZZ
    Mediastinum DB26DZZ
    Mouth D924DZZ
    Nasopharynx D92DDZZ
    Neck and Head DW21DZZ

**Stereotactic Radiosurgery** – *continued*
  Other Photon – *continued*
    Nerve, Peripheral D027DZZ
    Nose D921DZZ
    Ovary DU20DZZ
    Palate
      Hard D928DZZ
      Soft D929DZZ
    Pancreas DF23DZZ
    Parathyroid Gland DG24DZZ
    Pelvic Region DW26DZZ
    Pharynx D92CDZZ
    Pineal Body DG21DZZ
    Pituitary Gland DG20DZZ
    Pleura DB25DZZ
    Prostate DV20DZZ
    Rectum DD27DZZ
    Sinuses D927DZZ
    Spinal Cord D026DZZ
    Spleen D722DZZ
    Stomach DD21DZZ
    Testis DV21DZZ
    Thymus D721DZZ
    Thyroid Gland DG25DZZ
    Tongue D925DZZ
    Trachea DB20DZZ
    Ureter DT21DZZ
    Urethra DT23DZZ
    Uterus DU22DZZ
  Particulate
    Abdomen DW23HZZ
    Adrenal Gland DG22HZZ
    Bile Ducts DF22HZZ
    Bladder DT22HZZ
    Bone Marrow D720HZZ
    Brain D020HZZ
    Brain Stem D021HZZ
    Breast
      Left DM20HZZ
      Right DM21HZZ
    Bronchus DB21HZZ
    Cervix DU21HZZ
    Chest DW22HZZ
    Chest Wall DB27HZZ
    Colon DD25HZZ
    Diaphragm DB28HZZ
    Duodenum DD22HZZ
    Ear D920HZZ
    Esophagus DD20HZZ
    Eye D820HZZ
    Gallbladder DF21HZZ
    Gland
      Adrenal DG22HZZ
      Parathyroid DG24HZZ
      Pituitary DG20HZZ
      Thyroid DG25HZZ
    Glands, Salivary D926HZZ
    Head and Neck DW21HZZ
    Ileum DD24HZZ
    Jejunum DD23HZZ
    Kidney DT20HZZ
    Larynx D92BHZZ
    Liver DF20HZZ
    Lung DB22HZZ
    Lymphatics
      Abdomen D726HZZ
      Axillary D724HZZ
      Inguinal D728HZZ
      Neck D723HZZ
      Pelvis D727HZZ
      Thorax D725HZZ
    Mediastinum DB26HZZ
    Mouth D924HZZ
    Nasopharynx D92DHZZ
    Neck and Head DW21HZZ
    Nerve, Peripheral D027HZZ
    Nose D921HZZ
    Ovary DU20HZZ
    Palate
      Hard D928HZZ
      Soft D929HZZ
    Pancreas DF23HZZ
    Parathyroid Gland DG24HZZ
    Pelvic Region DW26HZZ
    Pharynx D92CHZZ
    Pineal Body DG21HZZ
    Pituitary Gland DG20HZZ
    Pleura DB25HZZ
    Prostate DV20HZZ
    Rectum DD27HZZ
    Sinuses D927HZZ
    Spinal Cord D026HZZ
    Spleen D722HZZ
    Stomach DD21HZZ

**Stereotactic Radiosurgery** – *continued*
  Particulate – *continued*
    Testis DV21HZZ
    Thymus D721HZZ
    Thyroid Gland DG25HZZ
    Tongue D925HZZ
    Trachea DB20HZZ
    Ureter DT21HZZ
    Urethra DT23HZZ
    Uterus DU22HZZ
**Sternoclavicular ligament**
  – *use* Bursa and Ligament, Shoulder, Left
  – *use* Bursa and Ligament, Shoulder, Right
**Sternocleidomastoid artery**
  – *use* Artery, Thyroid, Left
  – *use* Artery, Thyroid, Right
**Sternocleidomastoid muscle**
  – *use* Muscle, Neck, Left
  – *use* Muscle, Neck, Right
**Sternocostal ligament**
  – *use* Bursa and Ligament, Thorax, Right
  – *use* Bursa and Ligament, Thorax, Left
**Sternotomy**
  – *see* Division, Sternum 0P80
  – *see* Drainage, Sternum 0P90
**Stimulation, cardiac**
  Cardioversion 5A2204Z
  Electrophysiologic testing – *see* Measurement,
    Cardiac 4A02
**Stimulator Generator**
  Insertion of device in
    Abdomen 0JH8
    Back 0JH7
    Chest 0JH6
    Multiple Array
      Abdomen 0JH8
      Back 0JH7
      Chest 0JH6
    Multiple Array Rechargeable
      Abdomen 0JH8
      Back 0JH7
      Chest 0JH6
    Removal of device from, Subcutaneous Tissue and
      Fascia, Trunk 0JPT
    Revision of device in, Subcutaneous Tissue and
      Fascia, Trunk 0JWT
    Single Array
      Abdomen 0JH8
      Back 0JH7
      Chest 0JH6
    Single Array Rechargeable
      Abdomen 0JH8
      Back 0JH7
      Chest 0JH6
**Stimulator Lead**
  Insertion of device in
    Anal Sphincter 0DHR
    Artery
      Left 03HL
      Right 03HK
    Bladder 0THB
    Muscle
      Lower 0KHY
      Upper 0KHX
    Stomach 0DH6
    Ureter 0TH9
  Removal of device from
    Anal Sphincter 0DPR
    Artery, Upper 03PY
    Bladder 0TPB
    Muscle
      Lower 0KPY
      Upper 0KPX
    Stomach 0DP6
    Ureter 0TP9
  Revision of device in
    Anal Sphincter 0DWR
    Artery, Upper 03WY
    Bladder 0TWB
    Muscle
      Lower 0KWY
      Upper 0KWX
    Stomach 0DW6
    Ureter 0TW9
**Stoma**
  Excision
    Abdominal Wall 0WBFXZ2
    Neck 0WB6XZ2
  Repair
    Abdominal Wall 0WQFXZ2
    Neck 0WQ6XZ2

**Stomatoplasty**
- *see* Repair, Mouth and Throat ØCQ
- *see* Replacement, Mouth and Throat ØCR
- *see* Supplement, Mouth and Throat ØCU

**Stomatorrhaphy** – *see* Repair, Mouth and Throat ØCQ

**Stratos LV** – *use* Cardiac Resynchronization Pacemaker Pulse Generator in ØJH

**Stress test**
    4AØ2XM4
    4A12XM4

**Stripping** – *see* Extraction

**Study**
    Electrophysiologic stimulation, cardiac – *see* Measurement, Cardiac 4AØ2
    Ocular motility 4AØ7X7Z
    Pulmonary airway flow measurement – *see* Measurement, Respiratory 4AØ9
    Visual acuity 4AØ7XØZ

**Styloglossus muscle** – *use* Muscle, Tongue, Palate, Pharynx

**Stylomandibular ligament** – *use* Bursa and Ligament, Head and Neck

**Stylopharyngeus muscle** – *use* Muscle, Tongue, Palate, Pharynx

**Subacromial bursa**
- *use* Bursa and Ligament, Shoulder, Left
- *use* Bursa and Ligament, Shoulder, Right

**Subaortic** (common iliac) **lymph node** – *use* Lymphatic, Pelvis

**Subclavicular** (apical) **lymph node**
- *use* Lymphatic, Axillary, Left
- *use* Lymphatic, Axillary, Right

**Subclavius muscle**
- *use* Muscle, Thorax, Left
- *use* Muscle, Thorax, Right

**Subclavius nerve** – *use* Nerve, Brachial Plexus

**Subcostal artery** – *use* Aorta, Thoracic

**Subcostal muscle**
- *use* Muscle, Thorax, Left
- *use* Muscle, Thorax, Right

**Subcostal nerve** – *use* Nerve, Thoracic

**Subcutaneous injection reservoir, port** – *use* Vascular Access Device, Reservoir in Subcutaneous Tissue and Fascia

**Subcutaneous injection reservoir, pump** – *use* Infusion Device, Pump in Subcutaneous Tissue and Fascia

**Subdermal progesterone implant** – *use* Contraceptive Device in Subcutaneous Tissue and Fascia

**Submandibular ganglion**
- *use* Nerve, Head and Neck Sympathetic
- *use* Nerve, Facial

**Submandibular gland**
- *use* Gland, Submaxillary, Left
- *use* Gland, Submaxillary, Right

**Submandibular lymph node** – *use* Lymphatic, Head

**Submaxillary ganglion** – *use* Nerve, Head and Neck Sympathetic

**Submaxillary lymph node** – *use* Lymphatic, Head

**Submental artery** – *use* Artery, Face

**Submental lymph node** – *use* Lymphatic, Head

**Submucous** (Meissner's) **plexus** – *use* Nerve, Abdominal Sympathetic

**Suboccipital nerve** – *use* Nerve, Cervical

**Suboccipital venous plexus**
- *use* Vein, Vertebral, Left
- *use* Vein, Vertebral, Right

**Subparotid lymph node** – *use* Lymphatic, Head

**Subscapular** (posterior) **lymph node**
- *use* Lymphatic, Axillary, Left
- *use* Lymphatic, Axillary, Right

**Subscapular aponeurosis**
- *use* Subcutaneous Tissue and Fascia, Upper Arm, Right
- *use* Subcutaneous Tissue and Fascia, Upper Arm, Left

**Subscapular artery**
- *use* Artery, Axillary, Left
- *use* Artery, Axillary, Right

**Subscapularis muscle**
- *use* Muscle, Shoulder, Left
- *use* Muscle, Shoulder, Right

**Substance Abuse Treatment**
    Counseling
        Family, for substance abuse, Other Family Counseling HZ63ZZZ
        Group
            12–Step HZ43ZZZ
            Behavioral HZ41ZZZ

**Substance Abuse Treatment** – *continued*
    Counseling – *continued*
        Group – *continued*
            Cognitive HZ40ZZZ
            Cognitive–Behavioral HZ42ZZZ
            Confrontational HZ48ZZZ
            Continuing Care HZ49ZZZ
            Infectious Disease
                Post–Test HZ4CZZZ
                Pre–Test HZ4CZZZ
            Interpersonal HZ44ZZZ
            Motivational Enhancement HZ47ZZZ
            Psychoeducation HZ46ZZZ
            Spiritual HZ4BZZZ
            Vocational HZ45ZZZ
        Individual
            12–Step HZ33ZZZ
            Behavioral HZ31ZZZ
            Cognitive HZ30ZZZ
            Cognitive–Behavioral HZ32ZZZ
            Confrontational HZ38ZZZ
            Continuing Care HZ39ZZZ
            Infectious Disease
                Post–Test HZ3CZZZ
                Pre–Test HZ3CZZZ
            Interpersonal HZ34ZZZ
            Motivational Enhancement HZ37ZZZ
            Psychoeducation HZ36ZZZ
            Spiritual HZ3BZZZ
            Vocational HZ35ZZZ
    Detoxification Services, for substance abuse HZ2ZZZZ
    Medication Management
        Antabuse HZ83ZZZ
        Bupropion HZ87ZZZ
        Clonidine HZ86ZZZ
        Levo–alpha–acetyl–methadol (LAAM) HZ82ZZZ
        Methadone Maintenance HZ81ZZZ
        Naloxone HZ85ZZZ
        Naltrexone HZ84ZZZ
        Nicotine Replacement HZ80ZZZ
        Other Replacement Medication HZ89ZZZ
        Psychiatric Medication HZ88ZZZ
    Pharmacotherapy
        Antabuse HZ93ZZZ
        Bupropion HZ97ZZZ
        Clonidine HZ96ZZZ
        Levo–alpha–acetyl–methadol (LAAM) HZ92ZZZ
        Methadone Maintenance HZ91ZZZ
        Naloxone HZ95ZZZ
        Naltrexone HZ94ZZZ
        Nicotine Replacement HZ90ZZZ
        Psychiatric Medication HZ98ZZZ
        Replacement Medication, Other HZ99ZZZ
    Psychotherapy
        12–Step HZ53ZZZ
        Behavioral HZ51ZZZ
        Cognitive HZ50ZZZ
        Cognitive–Behavioral HZ52ZZZ
        Confrontational HZ58ZZZ
        Interactive HZ55ZZZ
        Interpersonal HZ54ZZZ
        Motivational Enhancement HZ57ZZZ
        Psychoanalysis HZ5BZZZ
        Psychodynamic HZ5CZZZ
        Psychoeducation HZ56ZZZ
        Psychophysiological HZ5DZZZ
        Supportive HZ59ZZZ

**Substantia nigra** – *use* Basal Ganglia

**Subtalar** (talocalcaneal) **joint**
- *use* Joint, Tarsal, Right
- *use* Joint, Tarsal, Left

**Subtalar ligament**
- *use* Bursa and Ligament, Foot, Left
- *use* Bursa and Ligament, Foot, Right

**Subthalamic nucleus** – *use* Basal Ganglia

**Suction** – *see* Drainage

**Suction curettage** (D&C), **nonobstetric** – *see* Extraction, Endometrium ØUDB

**Suction curettage, obstetric post-delivery** – *see* Extraction, Products of Conception, Retained 10D1

**Superficial circumflex iliac vein**
- *use* Vein, Greater Saphenous, Right
- *use* Vein, Greater Saphenous, Left

**Superficial epigastric artery**
- *use* Artery, Femoral, Left
- *use* Artery, Femoral, Right

**Superficial epigastric vein**
- *use* Vein, Greater Saphenous, Right
- *use* Vein, Greater Saphenous, Left

**Superficial Inferior Epigastric Artery Flap**
    Bilateral ØHRV078
    Left ØHRU078

**Superficial Inferior Epigastric Artery Flap** – *continued*
    Right ØHRT078

**Superficial palmar arch**
- *use* Artery, Hand, Left
- *use* Artery, Hand, Right

**Superficial palmar venous arch**
- *use* Vein, Hand, Left
- *use* Vein, Hand, Right

**Superficial temporal artery**
- *use* Artery, Temporal, Right
- *use* Artery, Temporal, Left

**Superficial transverse perineal muscle** – *use* Muscle, Perineum

**Superior cardiac nerve** – *use* Nerve, Thoracic Sympathetic

**Superior cerebellar vein** – *use* Vein, Intracranial

**Superior cerebral vein** – *use* Vein, Intracranial

**Superior clunic** (cluneal) **nerve** – *use* Nerve, Lumbar

**Superior epigastric artery**
- *use* Artery, Internal Mammary, Right
- *use* Artery, Internal Mammary, Left

**Superior genicular artery**
- *use* Artery, Popliteal, Left
- *use* Artery, Popliteal, Right

**Superior gluteal artery**
- *use* Artery, Internal Iliac, Left
- *use* Artery, Internal Iliac, Right

**Superior gluteal nerve** – *use* Nerve, Lumbar Plexus

**Superior hypogastric plexus** – *use* Nerve, Abdominal Sympathetic

**Superior labial artery** – *use* Artery, Face

**Superior laryngeal artery**
- *use* Artery, Thyroid, Left
- *use* Artery, Thyroid, Right

**Superior laryngeal nerve** – *use* Nerve, Vagus

**Superior longitudinal muscle** – *use* Muscle, Tongue, Palate, Pharynx

**Superior mesenteric ganglion** – *use* Nerve, Abdominal Sympathetic

**Superior mesenteric lymph node** – *use* Lymphatic, Mesenteric

**Superior mesenteric plexus** – *use* Nerve, Abdominal Sympathetic

**Superior oblique muscle**
- *use* Muscle, Extraocular, Left
- *use* Muscle, Extraocular, Right

**Superior olivary nucleus** – *use* Pons

**Superior rectal artery** – *use* Artery, Inferior Mesenteric

**Superior rectal vein** – *use* Vein, Inferior Mesenteric

**Superior rectus muscle**
- *use* Muscle, Extraocular, Left
- *use* Muscle, Extraocular, Right

**Superior tarsal plate**
- *use* Eyelid, Upper, Right
- *use* Eyelid, Upper, Left

**Superior thoracic artery**
- *use* Artery, Axillary, Left
- *use* Artery, Axillary, Right

**Superior thyroid artery**
- *use* Artery, Thyroid, Right
- *use* Artery, External Carotid, Right
- *use* Artery, Thyroid, Left
- *use* Artery, External Carotid, Left

**Superior turbinate** – *use* Turbinate, Nasal

**Superior ulnar collateral artery**
- *use* Artery, Brachial, Right
- *use* Artery, Brachial, Left

**Supplement**
    Abdominal Wall ØWUF
    Acetabulum
        Left ØQU5
        Right ØQU4
    Ampulla of Vater ØFUC
    Anal Sphincter ØDUR
    Ankle Region
        Left ØYUL
        Right ØYUK
    Anus ØDUQ
    Aorta
        Abdominal 04U0
        Thoracic 02UW
    Arm
        Lower
            Left ØXUF
            Right ØXUD
        Upper
            Left ØXU9
            Right ØXU8

**Supplement** – *continued*
- Artery
  - Anterior Tibial
    - Left Ø4UQ
    - Right Ø4UP
  - Axillary
    - Left Ø3U6
    - Right Ø3U5
  - Brachial
    - Left Ø3U8
    - Right Ø3U7
  - Celiac Ø4U1
  - Colic
    - Left Ø4U7
    - Middle Ø4U8
    - Right Ø4U6
  - Common Carotid
    - Left Ø3UJ
    - Right Ø3UH
  - Common Iliac
    - Left Ø4UD
    - Right Ø4UC
  - External Carotid
    - Left Ø3UN
    - Right Ø3UM
  - External Iliac
    - Left Ø4UJ
    - Right Ø4UH
  - Face Ø3UR
  - Femoral
    - Left Ø4UL
    - Right Ø4UK
  - Foot
    - Left Ø4UW
    - Right Ø4UV
  - Gastric Ø4U2
  - Hand
    - Left Ø3UF
    - Right Ø3UD
  - Hepatic Ø4U3
  - Inferior Mesenteric Ø4UB
  - Innominate Ø3U2
  - Internal Carotid
    - Left Ø3UL
    - Right Ø3UK
  - Internal Iliac
    - Left Ø4UF
    - Right Ø4UE
  - Internal Mammary
    - Left Ø3U1
    - Right Ø3UØ
  - Intracranial Ø3UG
  - Lower Ø4UY
  - Peroneal
    - Left Ø4UU
    - Right Ø4UT
  - Popliteal
    - Left Ø4UN
    - Right Ø4UM
  - Posterior Tibial
    - Left Ø4US
    - Right Ø4UR
  - Pulmonary
    - Left Ø2UR
    - Right Ø2UQ
  - Pulmonary Trunk Ø2UP
  - Radial
    - Left Ø3UC
    - Right Ø3UB
  - Renal
    - Left Ø4UA
    - Right Ø4U9
  - Splenic Ø4U4
  - Subclavian
    - Left Ø3U4
    - Right Ø3U3
  - Superior Mesenteric Ø4U5
  - Temporal
    - Left Ø3UT
    - Right Ø3US
  - Thyroid
    - Left Ø3UV
    - Right Ø3UU
  - Ulnar
    - Left Ø3UA
    - Right Ø3U9
  - Upper Ø3UY
  - Vertebral
    - Left Ø3UQ
    - Right Ø3UP
- Atrium
  - Left Ø2U7
  - Right Ø2U6

**Supplement** – *continued*
- Auditory Ossicle
  - Left Ø9UAØ
  - Right Ø9U9Ø
- Axilla
  - Left ØXU5
  - Right ØXU4
- Back
  - Lower ØWUL
  - Upper ØWUK
- Bladder ØTUB
- Bladder Neck ØTUC
- Bone
  - Ethmoid
    - Left ØNUG
    - Right ØNUF
  - Frontal
    - Left ØNU2
    - Right ØNU1
  - Hyoid ØNUX
  - Lacrimal
    - Left ØNUJ
    - Right ØNUH
  - Nasal ØNUB
  - Occipital
    - Left ØNU8
    - Right ØNU7
  - Palatine
    - Left ØNUL
    - Right ØNUK
  - Parietal
    - Left ØNU4
    - Right ØNU3
  - Pelvic
    - Left ØQU3
    - Right ØQU2
  - Sphenoid
    - Left ØNUD
    - Right ØNUC
  - Temporal
    - Left ØNU6
    - Right ØNU5
  - Zygomatic
    - Left ØNUN
    - Right ØNUM
- Breast
  - Bilateral ØHUV
  - Left ØHUU
  - Right ØHUT
- Bronchus
  - Lingula ØBU9
  - Lower Lobe
    - Left ØBUB
    - Right ØBU6
  - Main
    - Left ØBU7
    - Right ØBU3
  - Middle Lobe, Right ØBU5
  - Upper Lobe
    - Left ØBU8
    - Right ØBU4
- Buccal Mucosa ØCU4
- Bursa and Ligament
  - Abdomen
    - Left ØMUJ
    - Right ØMUH
  - Ankle
    - Left ØMUR
    - Right ØMUQ
  - Elbow
    - Left ØMU4
    - Right ØMU3
  - Foot
    - Left ØMUT
    - Right ØMUS
  - Hand
    - Left ØMU8
    - Right ØMU7
  - Head and Neck ØMUØ
  - Hip
    - Left ØMUM
    - Right ØMUL
  - Knee
    - Left ØMUP
    - Right ØMUN
  - Lower Extremity
    - Left ØMUW
    - Right ØMUV
  - Perineum ØMUK
  - Shoulder
    - Left ØMU2
    - Right ØMU1
  - Thorax
    - Left ØMUG

**Supplement** – *continued*
- Bursa and Ligament – *continued*
  - Thorax – *continued*
    - Right ØMUF
  - Trunk
    - Left ØMUD
    - Right ØMUC
  - Upper Extremity
    - Left ØMUB
    - Right ØMU9
  - Wrist
    - Left ØMU6
    - Right ØMU5
- Buttock
  - Left ØYU1
  - Right ØYUØ
- Carina ØBU2
- Carpal
  - Left ØPUN
  - Right ØPUM
- Cecum ØDUH
- Cerebral Meninges ØØU1
- Chest Wall ØWU8
- Chordae Tendineae Ø2U9
- Cisterna Chyli Ø7UL
- Clavicle
  - Left ØPUB
  - Right ØPU9
- Clitoris ØUUJ
- Coccyx ØQUS
- Colon
  - Ascending ØDUK
  - Descending ØDUM
  - Sigmoid ØDUN
  - Transverse ØDUL
- Cord
  - Bilateral ØVUH
  - Left ØVUG
  - Right ØVUF
- Cornea
  - Left Ø8U9
  - Right Ø8U8
- Cul-de-sac ØUUF
- Diaphragm
  - Left ØBUS
  - Right ØBUR
- Disc
  - Cervical Vertebral ØRU3
  - Cervicothoracic Vertebral ØRU5
  - Lumbar Vertebral ØSU2
  - Lumbosacral ØSU4
  - Thoracic Vertebral ØRU9
  - Thoracolumbar Vertebral ØRUB
- Duct
  - Common Bile ØFU9
  - Cystic ØFU8
  - Hepatic
    - Left ØFU6
    - Right ØFU5
  - Lacrimal
    - Left Ø8UY
    - Right Ø8UX
  - Pancreatic ØFUD
    - Accessory ØFUF
- Duodenum ØDU9
- Dura Mater ØØU2
- Ear
  - External
    - Bilateral Ø9U2
    - Left Ø9U1
    - Right Ø9UØ
  - Inner
    - Left Ø9UEØ
    - Right Ø9UDØ
  - Middle
    - Left Ø9U6Ø
    - Right Ø9U5Ø
- Elbow Region
  - Left ØXUC
  - Right ØXUB
- Epididymis
  - Bilateral ØVUL
  - Left ØVUK
  - Right ØVUJ
- Epiglottis ØCUR
- Esophagogastric Junction ØDU4
- Esophagus ØDU5
  - Lower ØDU3
  - Middle ØDU2
  - Upper ØDU1
- Extremity
  - Lower
    - Left ØYUB
    - Right ØYU9

**Supplement** – *continued*
Extremity – *continued*
Upper
Left 0XU7
Right 0XU6
Eye
Left 08U1
Right 08U0
Eyelid
Lower
Left 08UR
Right 08UQ
Upper
Left 08UP
Right 08UN
Face 0WU2
Fallopian Tube
Left 0UU6
Right 0UU5
Fallopian Tubes, Bilateral 0UU7
Femoral Region
Bilateral 0YUE
Left 0YU8
Right 0YU7
Femoral Shaft
Left 0QU9
Right 0QU8
Femur
Lower
Left 0QUC
Right 0QUB
Upper
Left 0QU7
Right 0QU6
Fibula
Left 0QUK
Right 0QUJ
Finger
Index
Left 0XUP
Right 0XUN
Little
Left 0XUW
Right 0XUV
Middle
Left 0XUR
Right 0XUQ
Ring
Left 0XUT
Right 0XUS
Foot
Left 0YUN
Right 0YUM
Gingiva
Lower 0CU6
Upper 0CU5
Glenoid Cavity
Left 0PU8
Right 0PU7
Hand
Left 0XUK
Right 0XUJ
Head 0WU0
Heart 02UA
Humeral Head
Left 0PUD
Right 0PUC
Humeral Shaft
Left 0PUG
Right 0PUF
Hymen 0UUK
Ileocecal Valve 0DUC
Ileum 0DUB
Inguinal Region
Bilateral 0YUA
Left 0YU6
Right 0YU5
Intestine
Large 0DUE
Left 0DUG
Right 0DUF
Small 0DU8
Iris
Left 08UD
Right 08UC
Jaw
Lower 0WU5
Upper 0WU4
Jejunum 0DUA
Joint
Acromioclavicular
Left 0RUH
Right 0RUG

**Supplement** – *continued*
Joint – *continued*
Ankle
Left 0SUG
Right 0SUF
Carpal
Left 0RUR
Right 0RUQ
Cervical Vertebral 0RU1
Cervicothoracic Vertebral 0RU4
Coccygeal 0SU6
Elbow
Left 0RUM
Right 0RUL
Finger Phalangeal
Left 0RUX
Right 0RUW
Hip
Left 0SUB
Acetabular Surface 0SUE
Femoral Surface 0SUS
Right 0SU9
Acetabular Surface 0SUA
Femoral Surface 0SUR
Knee
Left 0SUD
Femoral Surface 0SUU09Z
Tibial Surface 0SUW09Z
Right 0SUC
Femoral Surface 0SUT09Z
Tibial Surface 0SUV09Z
Lumbar Vertebral 0SU0
Lumbosacral 0SU3
Metacarpocarpal
Left 0RUT
Right 0RUS
Metacarpophalangeal
Left 0RUV
Right 0RUU
Metatarsal–Phalangeal
Left 0SUN
Right 0SUM
Metatarsal–Tarsal
Left 0SUL
Right 0SUK
Occipital–cervical 0RU0
Sacrococcygeal 0SU5
Sacroiliac
Left 0SU8
Right 0SU7
Shoulder
Left 0RUK
Right 0RUJ
Sternoclavicular
Left 0RUF
Right 0RUE
Tarsal
Left 0SUJ
Right 0SUH
Temporomandibular
Left 0RUD
Right 0RUC
Thoracic Vertebral 0RU6
Thoracolumbar Vertebral 0RUA
Toe Phalangeal
Left 0SUQ
Right 0SUP
Wrist
Left 0RUP
Right 0RUN
Kidney Pelvis
Left 0TU4
Right 0TU3
Knee Region
Left 0YUG
Right 0YUF
Larynx 0CUS
Leg
Lower
Left 0YUJ
Right 0YUH
Upper
Left 0YUD
Right 0YUC
Lip
Lower 0CU1
Upper 0CU0
Lymphatic
Aortic 07UD
Axillary
Left 07U6
Right 07U5
Head 07U0

**Supplement** – *continued*
Lymphatic – *continued*
Inguinal
Left 07UJ
Right 07UH
Internal Mammary
Left 07U9
Right 07U8
Lower Extremity
Left 07UG
Right 07UF
Mesenteric 07UB
Neck
Left 07U2
Right 07U1
Pelvis 07UC
Thoracic Duct 07UK
Thorax 07U7
Upper Extremity
Left 07U4
Right 07U3
Mandible
Left 0NUV
Right 0NUT
Maxilla
Left 0NUS
Right 0NUR
Mediastinum 0WUC
Mesentery 0DUV
Metacarpal
Left 0PUQ
Right 0PUP
Metatarsal
Left 0QUP
Right 0QUN
Muscle
Abdomen
Left 0KUL
Right 0KUK
Extraocular
Left 08UM
Right 08UL
Facial 0KU1
Foot
Left 0KUW
Right 0KUV
Hand
Left 0KUD
Right 0KUC
Head 0KU0
Hip
Left 0KUP
Right 0KUN
Lower Arm and Wrist
Left 0KUB
Right 0KU9
Lower Leg
Left 0KUT
Right 0KUS
Neck
Left 0KU3
Right 0KU2
Papillary 02UD
Perineum 0KUM
Shoulder
Left 0KU6
Right 0KU5
Thorax
Left 0KUJ
Right 0KUH
Tongue, Palate, Pharynx 0KU4
Trunk
Left 0KUG
Right 0KUF
Upper Arm
Left 0KU8
Right 0KU7
Upper Leg
Left 0KUR
Right 0KUQ
Nasopharynx 09UN
Neck 0WU6
Nerve
Abducens 00UL
Accessory 00UR
Acoustic 00UN
Cervical 01U1
Facial 00UM
Femoral 01UD
Glossopharyngeal 00UP
Hypoglossal 00US
Lumbar 01UB
Median 01U5

**Supplement** – *continued*
  Nerve – *continued*
    Oculomotor 00UH
    Olfactory 00UF
    Optic 00UG
    Peroneal 01UH
    Phrenic 01U2
    Pudendal 01UC
    Radial 01U6
    Sacral 01UR
    Sciatic 01UF
    Thoracic 01U8
    Tibial 01UG
    Trigeminal 00UK
    Trochlear 00UJ
    Ulnar 01U4
    Vagus 00UQ
  Nipple
    Left 0HUX
    Right 0HUW
  Nose 09UK
  Omentum
    Greater 0DUS
    Lesser 0DUT
  Orbit
    Left 0NUQ
    Right 0NUP
  Palate
    Hard 0CU2
    Soft 0CU3
  Patella
    Left 0QUF
    Right 0QUD
  Penis 0VUS
  Pericardium 02UN
  Perineum
    Female 0WUN
    Male 0WUM
  Peritoneum 0DUW
  Phalanx
    Finger
      Left 0PUV
      Right 0PUT
    Thumb
      Left 0PUS
      Right 0PUR
    Toe
      Left 0QUR
      Right 0QUQ
  Pharynx 0CUM
  Prepuce 0VUT
  Radius
    Left 0PUJ
    Right 0PUH
  Rectum 0DUP
  Retina
    Left 08UF
    Right 08UE
  Retinal Vessel
    Left 08UH
    Right 08UG
  Rib
    Left 0PU2
    Right 0PU1
  Sacrum 0QU1
  Scapula
    Left 0PU6
    Right 0PU5
  Scrotum 0VU5
  Septum
    Atrial 02U5
    Nasal 09UM
    Ventricular 02UM
  Shoulder Region
    Left 0XU3
    Right 0XU2
  Skull 0NU0
  Spinal Meninges 00UT
  Sternum 0PU0
  Stomach 0DU6
    Pylorus 0DU7
  Subcutaneous Tissue and Fascia
    Abdomen 0JU8
    Back 0JU7
    Buttock 0JU9
    Chest 0JU6
    Face 0JU1
    Foot
      Left 0JUR
      Right 0JUQ
    Hand
      Left 0JUK
      Right 0JUJ

**Supplement** – *continued*
  Subcutaneous Tissue and Fascia – *continued*
    Lower Arm
      Left 0JUH
      Right 0JUG
    Lower Leg
      Left 0JUP
      Right 0JUN
    Neck
      Anterior 0JU4
      Posterior 0JU5
    Pelvic Region 0JUC
    Perineum 0JUB
    Scalp 0JU0
    Upper Arm
      Left 0JUF
      Right 0JUD
    Upper Leg
      Left 0JUM
      Right 0JUL
  Tarsal
    Left 0QUM
    Right 0QUL
  Tendon
    Abdomen
      Left 0LUG
      Right 0LUF
    Ankle
      Left 0LUT
      Right 0LUS
    Foot
      Left 0LUW
      Right 0LUV
    Hand
      Left 0LU8
      Right 0LU7
    Head and Neck 0LU0
    Hip
      Left 0LUK
      Right 0LUJ
    Knee
      Left 0LUR
      Right 0LUQ
    Lower Arm and Wrist
      Left 0LU6
      Right 0LU5
    Lower Leg
      Left 0LUP
      Right 0LUN
    Perineum 0LUH
    Shoulder
      Left 0LU2
      Right 0LU1
    Thorax
      Left 0LUD
      Right 0LUC
    Trunk
      Left 0LUB
      Right 0LU9
    Upper Arm
      Left 0LU4
      Right 0LU3
    Upper Leg
      Left 0LUM
      Right 0LUL
  Testis
    Bilateral 0VUC0
    Left 0VUB0
    Right 0VU90
  Thumb
    Left 0XUM
    Right 0XUL
  Tibia
    Left 0QUH
    Right 0QUG
  Toe
    1st
      Left 0YUQ
      Right 0YUP
    2nd
      Left 0YUS
      Right 0YUR
    3rd
      Left 0YUU
      Right 0YUT
    4th
      Left 0YUW
      Right 0YUV
    5th
      Left 0YUY
      Right 0YUX
  Tongue 0CU7
  Trachea 0BU1

**Supplement** – *continued*
  Tunica Vaginalis
    Left 0VU7
    Right 0VU6
  Turbinate, Nasal 09UL
  Tympanic Membrane
    Left 09U8
    Right 09U7
  Ulna
    Left 0PUL
    Right 0PUK
  Ureter
    Left 0TU7
    Right 0TU6
  Urethra 0TUD
  Uterine Supporting Structure 0UU4
  Uvula 0CUN
  Vagina 0UUG
  Valve
    Aortic 02UF
    Mitral 02UG
    Pulmonary 02UH
    Tricuspid 02UJ
  Vas Deferens
    Bilateral 0VUQ
    Left 0VUP
    Right 0VUN
  Vein
    Axillary
      Left 05U8
      Right 05U7
    Azygos 05U0
    Basilic
      Left 05UC
      Right 05UB
    Brachial
      Left 05UA
      Right 05U9
    Cephalic
      Left 05UF
      Right 05UD
    Colic 06U7
    Common Iliac
      Left 06UD
      Right 06UC
    Esophageal 06U3
    External Iliac
      Left 06UG
      Right 06UF
    External Jugular
      Left 05UQ
      Right 05UP
    Face
      Left 05UV
      Right 05UT
    Femoral
      Left 06UN
      Right 06UM
    Foot
      Left 06UV
      Right 06UT
    Gastric 06U2
    Greater Saphenous
      Left 06UQ
      Right 06UP
    Hand
      Left 05UH
      Right 05UG
    Hemiazygos 05U1
    Hepatic 06U4
    Hypogastric
      Left 06UJ
      Right 06UH
    Inferior Mesenteric 06U6
    Innominate
      Left 05U4
      Right 05U3
    Internal Jugular
      Left 05UN
      Right 05UM
    Intracranial 05UL
    Lesser Saphenous
      Left 06US
      Right 06UR
    Lower 06UY
    Portal 06U8
    Pulmonary
      Left 02UT
      Right 02US
    Renal
      Left 06UB
      Right 06U9
    Splenic 06U1

**Supplement** – *continued*
  Vein – *continued*
    Subclavian
      Left 05U6
      Right 05U5
    Superior Mesenteric 06U5
    Upper 05UY
    Vertebral
      Left 05US
      Right 05UR
    Vena Cava
      Inferior 06U0
      Superior 02UV
    Ventricle
      Left 02UL
      Right 02UK
    Vertebra
      Cervical 0PU3
      Lumbar 0QU0
      Thoracic 0PU4
    Vesicle
      Bilateral 0VU3
      Left 0VU2
      Right 0VU1
    Vocal Cord
      Left 0CUV
      Right 0CUT
    Vulva 0UUM
    Wrist Region
      Left 0XUH
      Right 0XUG
**Supraclavicular** (Virchow's) **lymph node**
  – *use* Lymphatic, Neck, Left
  – *use* Lymphatic, Neck, Right
**Supraclavicular nerve** – *use* Nerve, Cervical Plexus
**Suprahyoid lymph node** – *use* Lymphatic, Head
**Suprahyoid muscle**
  – *use* Muscle, Neck, Right
  – *use* Muscle, Neck, Left
**Suprainguinal lymph node** – *use* Lymphatic, Pelvis
**Supraorbital vein**
  – *use* Vein, Face, Left
  – *use* Vein, Face, Right
**Suprarenal gland**
  – *use* Gland, Adrenal, Left
  – *use* Gland, Adrenal, Right
  – *use* Gland, Adrenal, Bilateral
  – *use* Gland, Adrenal
**Suprarenal plexus** – *use* Nerve, Abdominal Sympathetic
**Suprascapular nerve** – *use* Nerve, Brachial Plexus
**Supraspinatus fascia**
  – *use* Subcutaneous Tissue and Fascia, Upper Arm, Right
  – *use* Subcutaneous Tissue and Fascia, Upper Arm, Left
**Supraspinatus muscle**
  – *use* Muscle, Shoulder, Right
  – *use* Muscle, Shoulder, Left
**Supraspinous ligament**
  – *use* Bursa and Ligament, Trunk, Right
  – *use* Bursa and Ligament, Trunk, Left
**Suprasternal notch** – *use* Sternum
**Supratrochlear lymph node**
  – *use* Lymphatic, Upper Extremity, Right
  – *use* Lymphatic, Upper Extremity, Left
**Sural artery**
  – *use* Artery, Popliteal, Right
  – *use* Artery, Popliteal, Left
**Suspension**
  Bladder Neck – *see* Reposition, Bladder Neck 0TSC
  Kidney – *see* Reposition, Urinary System 0TS
  Urethra – *see* Reposition, Urinary System 0TS
  Urethrovesical – *see* Reposition, Bladder Neck 0TSC
  Uterus – *see* Reposition, Uterus 0US9
  Vagina – *see* Reposition, Vagina 0USG
**Suture**
  Laceration repair – *see* Repair
  Ligation – *see* Occlusion
**Suture Removal**
  Extremity
    Lower 8E0YXY8
    Upper 8E0XXY8
  Head and Neck Region 8E09XY8
  Trunk Region 8E0WXY8
**Sweat gland** – *use* Skin
**Sympathectomy** – *see* Excision, Peripheral Nervous System 01B
**SynCardia Total Artificial Heart** – *use* Synthetic Substitute

**Synchra CRT-P** – *use* Cardiac Resynchronization Pacemaker Pulse Generator in 0JH
**SynchroMed pump** – *use* Infusion Device, Pump in Subcutaneous Tissue and Fascia
**Synechiotomy, iris** – *see* Release, Eye 08N
**Synovectomy**
  Lower joint – *see* Excision, Lower Joints 0SB
  Upper joint – *see* Excision, Upper Joints 0RB
**Systemic Nuclear Medicine Therapy**
  Abdomen CW70
  Anatomical Regions, Multiple CW7YYZZ
  Chest CW73
  Thyroid CW7G
  Whole Body CW7N

# T

**Takedown**
  Arteriovenous shunt – *see* Removal of device from, Upper Arteries 03P
  Arteriovenous shunt, with creation of new shunt – *see* Bypass, Upper Arteries 031
  Stoma – *see* Repair
**Talent® Converter** – *use* Intraluminal Device
**Talent® Occluder** – *use* Intraluminal Device
**Talent® Stent Graft** (abdominal)(thoracic) – *use* Intraluminal Device
**Talocalcaneal** (subtalar) **joint**
  – *use* Joint, Tarsal, Left
  – *use* Joint, Tarsal, Right
**Talocalcaneal ligament**
  – *use* Bursa and Ligament, Foot, Left
  – *use* Bursa and Ligament, Foot, Right
**Talocalcaneonavicular joint**
  – *use* Joint, Tarsal, Right
  – *use* Joint, Tarsal, Left
**Talocalcaneonavicular ligament**
  – *use* Bursa and Ligament, Foot, Left
  – *use* Bursa and Ligament, Foot, Right
**Talocrural joint**
  – *use* Joint, Ankle, Right
  – *use* Joint, Ankle, Left
**Talofibular ligament**
  – *use* Bursa and Ligament, Ankle, Right
  – *use* Bursa and Ligament, Ankle, Left
**Talus bone**
  – *use* Tarsal, Right
  – *use* Tarsal, Left
**TandemHeart® System** – *use* External Heart Assist System in Heart and Great Vessels
**Tarsectomy**
  – *see* Excision, Lower Bones 0QB
  – *see* Resection, Lower Bones 0QT
**Tarsometatarsal joint**
  – *use* Joint, Metatarsal–Tarsal, Right
  – *use* Joint, Metatarsal–Tarsal, Left
**Tarsometatarsal ligament**
  – *use* Bursa and Ligament, Foot, Right
  – *use* Bursa and Ligament, Foot, Left
**Tarsorrhaphy** – *see* Repair, Eye 08Q
**Tattooing**
  Cornea 3E0CXMZ
  Skin – *use* Introduction of substance in or on, Skin 3E00
**TAXUS® Liberté® Paclitaxel-eluting Coronary Stent System** – *use* Intraluminal Device, Drug-eluting in Heart and Great Vessels
**TBNA (transbronchial needle aspiration)** – *see* Drainage, Respiratory System 0B9
**Telemetry** 4A12X4Z
  Ambulatory 4A12X45
**Temperature gradient study** 4A0ZXKZ
**Temporal lobe** – *use* Cerebral Hemisphere
**Temporalis muscle** – *use* Muscle, Head
**Temporoparietalis muscle** – *use* Muscle, Head
**Tendolysis** – *see* Release, Tendons 0LN
**Tendonectomy**
  – *see* Excision, Tendons 0LB
  – *see* Resection, Tendons 0LT
**Tendonoplasty, tenoplasty**
  – *see* Repair, Tendons 0LQ
  – *see* Replacement, Tendons 0LR
  – *see* Supplement, Tendons 0LU
**Tendorrhaphy** – *see* Repair, Tendons 0LQ
**Tendototomy**
  – *see* Division, Tendons 0L8
  – *see* Drainage, Tendons 0L9

**Tenectomy, tenonectomy**
  – *see* Excision, Tendons 0LB
  – *see* Resection, Tendons 0LT
**Tenolysis** – *see* Release, Tendons 0LN
**Tenontorrhaphy** – *see* Repair, Tendons 0LQ
**Tenontotomy**
  – *see* Division, Tendons 0L8
  – *see* Drainage, Tendons 0L9
**Tenorrhaphy** – *see* Repair, Tendons 0LQ
**Tenosynovectomy**
  – *see* Excision, Tendons 0LB
  – *see* Resection, Tendons 0LT
**Tenotomy**
  – *see* Division, Tendons 0L8
  – *see* Drainage, Tendons 0L9
**Tensor fasciae latae muscle**
  – *use* Muscle, Hip, Left
  – *use* Muscle, Hip, Right
**Tensor veli palatini muscle** – *use* Muscle, Tongue, Palate, Pharynx
**Tenth cranial nerve** – *use* Nerve, Vagus
**Tentorium cerebelli** – *use* Dura Mater
**Teres major muscle**
  – *use* Muscle, Shoulder, Left
  – *use* Muscle, Shoulder, Right
**Teres minor muscle**
  – *use* Muscle, Shoulder, Right
  – *use* Muscle, Shoulder, Left
**Termination of pregnancy**
  Aspiration curettage 10A07ZZ
  Dilation and curettage 10A07ZZ
  Hysterotomy 10A00ZZ
  Intra–amniotic injection 10A03ZZ
  Laminaria 10A07ZW
  Vacuum 10A07Z6
**Testectomy**
  – *see* Excision, Male Reproductive System 0VB
  – *see* Resection, Male Reproductive System 0VT
**Testicular artery** – *use* Aorta, Abdominal
**Testing**
  Glaucoma 4A07XBZ
  Hearing – *see* Hearing Assessment, Diagnostic Audiology F13
  Mental health – *see* Psychological Tests
  Muscle function, electromyography (EMG) – *see* Measurement, Musculoskeletal 4A0F
  Muscle function, manual – *see* Motor Function Assessment, Rehabilitation F01
  Neurophysiologic monitoring, intra–operative – *see* Monitoring, Physiological Systems 4A1
  Range of motion – *see* Motor Function Assessment, Rehabilitation F01
  Vestibular function – *see* Vestibular Assessment, Diagnostic Audiology F15
**Thalamectomy** – *see* Excision, Thalamus 00B9
**Thalamotomy** – *see* Drainage, Thalamus 0099
**Thenar muscle**
  – *use* Muscle, Hand, Right
  – *use* Muscle, Hand, Left
**Therapeutic Massage**
  Musculoskeletal System 8E0KX1Z
  Reproductive System
    Prostate 8E0VX1C
    Rectum 8E0VX1D
**Therapeutic occlusion coil(s)** – *use* Intraluminal Device
**Thermography** 4A0ZXKZ
**Thermotherapy, prostate** – *see* Destruction, Prostate 0V50
**Third cranial nerve** – *use* Nerve, Oculomotor
**Third occipital nerve** – *use* Nerve, Cervical
**Third ventricle** – *use* Cerebral Ventricle
**Thoracectomy** – *see* Excision, Anatomical Regions, General 0WB
**Thoracentesis** – *see* Drainage, Anatomical Regions, General 0W9
**Thoracic aortic plexus** – *use* Nerve, Thoracic Sympathetic
**Thoracic esophagus** – *use* Esophagus, Middle
**Thoracic facet joint** – *use* Joint, Thoracic Vertebral
**Thoracic ganglion** – *use* Nerve, Thoracic Sympathetic
**Thoracoacromial artery**
  – *use* Artery, Axillary, Right
  – *use* Artery, Axillary, Left
**Thoracocentesis** – *see* Drainage, Anatomical Regions, General 0W9
**Thoracolumbar facet joint** – *use* Joint, Thoracolumbar Vertebral

**Thoracoplasty**
– *see* Repair, Anatomical Regions, General 0WQ
– *see* Supplement, Anatomical Regions, General 0WU

**Thoracostomy tube** – *use* Drainage Device

**Thoracostomy, for lung collapse** – *see* Drainage, Respiratory System 0B9

**Thoracotomy** – *see* Drainage, Anatomical Regions, General 0W9

**Thoratec IVAD (Implantable Ventricular Assist Device)** – *use* Implantable Heart Assist System in Heart and Great Vessels

**Thoratec Paracorporeal Ventricular Assist Device** – *use* External Heart Assist System in Heart and Great Vessels

**Thrombectomy** – *see* Extirpation

**Thymectomy**
– *see* Excision, Lymphatic and Hemic Systems 07B
– *see* Resection, Lymphatic and Hemic Systems 07T

**Thymopexy**
– *see* Repair, Lymphatic and Hemic Systems 07Q
– *see* Reposition, Lymphatic and Hemic Systems 07S

**Thymus gland** – *use* Thymus

**Thyroarytenoid muscle**
– *use* Muscle, Neck, Right
– *use* Muscle, Neck, Left

**Thyrocervical trunk**
– *use* Artery, Thyroid, Right
– *use* Artery, Thyroid, Left

**Thyroid cartilage** – *use* Larynx

**Thyroidectomy**
– *see* Excision, Endocrine System 0GB
– *see* Resection, Endocrine System 0GT

**Thyroidorrhaphy** – *see* Repair, Endocrine System 0GQ

**Thyroidoscopy** 0GJK4ZZ

**Thyroidotomy** – *see* Drainage, Endocrine System 0G9

**Tibialis anterior muscle**
– *use* Muscle, Lower Leg, Right
– *use* Muscle, Lower Leg, Left

**Tibialis posterior muscle**
– *use* Muscle, Lower Leg, Right
– *use* Muscle, Lower Leg, Left

**Tibiofemoral joint**
– *use* Joint, Knee, Right, Tibial Surface
– *use* Joint, Knee, Left, Tibial Surface
– *use* Joint, Knee, Right
– *use* Joint, Knee, Left

**TigerPaw® system for closure of left atrial appendage** – *use* Extraluminal Device

**Tissue bank graft** – *use* Nonautologous Tissue Substitute

**Tissue Expander**
Insertion of device in
Breast
Bilateral 0HHV
Left 0HHU
Right 0HHT
Nipple
Left 0HHX
Right 0HHW
Subcutaneous Tissue and Fascia
Abdomen 0JH8
Back 0JH7
Buttock 0JH9
Chest 0JH6
Face 0JH1
Foot
Left 0JHR
Right 0JHQ
Hand
Left 0JHK
Right 0JHJ
Lower Arm
Left 0JHH
Right 0JHG
Lower Leg
Left 0JHP
Right 0JHN
Neck
Anterior 0JH4
Posterior 0JH5
Pelvic Region 0JHC
Perineum 0JHB
Scalp 0JH0
Upper Arm
Left 0JHF
Right 0JHD
Upper Leg
Left 0JHM
Right 0JHL

**Tissue Expander** – *continued*
Removal of device from
Breast
Left 0HPU
Right 0HPT
Subcutaneous Tissue and Fascia
Head and Neck 0JPS
Lower Extremity 0JPW
Trunk 0JPT
Upper Extremity 0JPV
Revision of device in
Breast
Left 0HWU
Right 0HWT
Subcutaneous Tissue and Fascia
Head and Neck 0JWS
Lower Extremity 0JWW
Trunk 0JWT
Upper Extremity 0JWV

**Tissue expander** (inflatable)(injectable)
– *use* Tissue Expander in Skin and Breast
– *use* Tissue Expander in Subcutaneous Tissue and Fascia

**Tissue Plasminogen Activator (tPA)(r-tPA)** – *use* Thrombolytic, Other

**Titanium Sternal Fixation System (TSFS)**
– *use* Internal Fixation Device, Rigid Plate in 0PS
– *use* Internal Fixation Device, Rigid Plate in 0PH

**Tomographic (Tomo) Nuclear Medicine Imaging** CP2YYZZ
Abdomen CW20
Abdomen and Chest CW24
Abdomen and Pelvis CW21
Anatomical Regions, Multiple CW2YYZZ
Bladder, Kidneys and Ureters CT23
Brain C020
Breast CH2YYZZ
Bilateral CH22
Left CH21
Right CH20
Bronchi and Lungs CB22
Central Nervous System C02YYZZ
Cerebrospinal Fluid C025
Chest CW23
Chest and Abdomen CW24
Chest and Neck CW26
Digestive System CD2YYZZ
Endocrine System CG2YYZZ
Extremity
Lower CW2D
Bilateral CP2F
Left CP2D
Right CP2C
Upper CW2M
Bilateral CP2B
Left CP29
Right CP28
Gallbladder CF24
Gastrointestinal Tract CD27
Gland, Parathyroid CG21
Head and Neck CW2B
Heart C22YYZZ
Right and Left C226
Hepatobiliary System and Pancreas CF2YYZZ
Kidneys, Ureters and Bladder CT23
Liver CF25
Liver and Spleen CF26
Lungs and Bronchi CB22
Lymphatics and Hematologic System C72YYZZ
Myocardium C22G
Neck and Chest CW26
Neck and Head CW2B
Pancreas and Hepatobiliary System CF2YYZZ
Pelvic Region CW2J
Pelvis CP26
Pelvis and Abdomen CW21
Pelvis and Spine CP27
Respiratory System CB2YYZZ
Skin CH2YYZZ
Skull CP21
Skull and Cervical Spine CP23
Spine
Cervical CP22
Cervical and Skull CP23
Lumbar CP2H
Thoracic CP2G
Thoracolumbar CP2J
Spine and Pelvis CP27
Spleen C722
Spleen and Liver CF26
Subcutaneous Tissue CH2YYZZ
Thorax CP24
Ureters, Kidneys and Bladder CT23
Urinary System CT2YYZZ

**Tomography, computerized** – *see* Computerized Tomography (CT Scan)

**Tonometry** 4A07XBZ

**Tonsillectomy**
– *see* Excision, Mouth and Throat 0CB
– *see* Resection, Mouth and Throat 0CT

**Tonsillotomy** – *see* Drainage, Mouth and Throat 0C9

**Total artificial** (replacement) **heart** – *use* Synthetic Substitute

**Total parenteral nutrition (TPN)** – *see* Introduction of Nutritional Substance

**Trachectomy**
– *see* Excision, Trachea 0BB1
– *see* Resection, Trachea 0BT1

**Trachelectomy**
– *see* Excision, Cervix 0UBC
– *see* Resection, Cervix 0UTC

**Trachelopexy**
– *see* Repair, Cervix 0UQC
– *see* Reposition, Cervix 0USC

**Tracheloplasty** – *see* Repair, Cervix 0UQC

**Trachelorrhaphy** – *see* Repair, Cervix 0UQC

**Trachelotomy** – *see* Drainage, Cervix 0U9C

**Tracheobronchial lymph node** – *use* Lymphatic, Thorax

**Tracheoesophageal fistulization** 0B110D6

**Tracheolysis** – *see* Release, Respiratory System 0BN

**Tracheoplasty**
– *see* Repair, Respiratory System 0BQ
– *see* Supplement, Respiratory System 0BU

**Tracheorrhaphy** – *see* Repair, Respiratory System 0BQ

**Tracheoscopy** 0BJ18ZZ

**Tracheostomy** – *see* Bypass, Respiratory System 0B1

**Tracheostomy Device**
Bypass, Trachea 0B11
Change device in, Trachea 0B21XFZ
Removal of device from, Trachea 0BP1
Revision of device in, Trachea 0BW1

**Tracheostomy tube** – *use* Tracheostomy Device in Respiratory System

**Tracheotomy** – *see* Drainage, Respiratory System 0B9

**Traction**
Abdominal Wall 2W63X
Arm
Lower
Left 2W6DX
Right 2W6CX
Upper
Left 2W6BX
Right 2W6AX
Back 2W65X
Chest Wall 2W64X
Extremity
Lower
Left 2W6MX
Right 2W6LX
Upper
Left 2W69X
Right 2W68X
Face 2W61X
Finger
Left 2W6KX
Right 2W6JX
Foot
Left 2W6TX
Right 2W6SX
Hand
Left 2W6FX
Right 2W6EX
Head 2W60X
Inguinal Region
Left 2W67X
Right 2W66X
Leg
Lower
Left 2W6RX
Right 2W6QX
Upper
Left 2W6PX
Right 2W6NX
Neck 2W62X
Thumb
Left 2W6HX
Right 2W6GX
Toe
Left 2W6VX
Right 2W6UX

**Tractotomy** – *see* Division, Central Nervous System 008

**Tragus**
– *use* Ear, External, Left
– *use* Ear, External, Right
– *use* Ear, External, Bilateral
**Training, caregiver** – *see* Caregiver Training
**TRAM (transverse rectus abdominis myocutaneous)**
**flap reconstruction**
Free – *see* Replacement, Skin and Breast ØHR
Pedicled – *see* Transfer, Muscles ØKX
**Transection** – *see* Division
**Transfer**
Buccal Mucosa ØCX4
Bursa and Ligament
Abdomen
Left ØMXJ
Right ØMXH
Ankle
Left ØMXR
Right ØMXQ
Elbow
Left ØMX4
Right ØMX3
Foot
Left ØMXT
Right ØMXS
Hand
Left ØMX8
Right ØMX7
Head and Neck ØMXØ
Hip
Left ØMXM
Right ØMXL
Knee
Left ØMXP
Right ØMXN
Lower Extremity
Left ØMXW
Right ØMXV
Perineum ØMXK
Shoulder
Left ØMX2
Right ØMX1
Thorax
Left ØMXG
Right ØMXF
Trunk
Left ØMXD
Right ØMXC
Upper Extremity
Left ØMXB
Right ØMX9
Wrist
Left ØMX6
Right ØMX5
Finger
Left ØXXPØZM
Right ØXXNØZL
Gingiva
Lower ØCX6
Upper ØCX5
Intestine
Large ØDXE
Small ØDX8
Lip
Lower ØCX1
Upper ØCXØ
Muscle
Abdomen
Left ØKXL
Right ØKXK
Extraocular
Left Ø8XM
Right Ø8XL
Facial ØKX1
Foot
Left ØKXW
Right ØKXV
Hand
Left ØKXD
Right ØKXC
Head ØKXØ
Hip
Left ØKXP
Right ØKXN
Lower Arm and Wrist
Left ØKXB
Right ØKX9
Lower Leg
Left ØKXT
Right ØKXS
Neck
Left ØKX3
Right ØKX2

**Transfer** – *continued*
Muscle – *continued*
Perineum ØKXM
Shoulder
Left ØKX6
Right ØKX5
Thorax
Left ØKXJ
Right ØKXH
Tongue, Palate, Pharynx ØKX4
Trunk
Left ØKXG
Right ØKXF
Upper Arm
Left ØKX8
Right ØKX7
Upper Leg
Left ØKXR
Right ØKXQ
Nerve
Abducens ØØXL
Accessory ØØXR
Acoustic ØØXN
Cervical Ø1X1
Facial ØØXM
Femoral Ø1XD
Glossopharyngeal ØØXP
Hypoglossal ØØXS
Lumbar Ø1XB
Median Ø1X5
Oculomotor ØØXH
Olfactory ØØXF
Optic ØØXG
Peroneal Ø1XH
Phrenic Ø1X2
Pudendal Ø1XC
Radial Ø1X6
Sciatic Ø1XF
Thoracic Ø1X8
Tibial Ø1XG
Trigeminal ØØXK
Trochlear ØØXJ
Ulnar Ø1X4
Vagus ØØXQ
Palate, Soft ØCX3
Skin
Abdomen ØHX7XZZ
Back ØHX6XZZ
Buttock ØHX8XZZ
Chest ØHX5XZZ
Ear
Left ØHX3XZZ
Right ØHX2XZZ
Face ØHX1XZZ
Foot
Left ØHXNXZZ
Right ØHXMXZZ
Genitalia ØHXAXZZ
Hand
Left ØHXGXZZ
Right ØHXFXZZ
Lower Arm
Left ØHXEXZZ
Right ØHXDXZZ
Lower Leg
Left ØHXLXZZ
Right ØHXKXZZ
Neck ØHX4XZZ
Perineum ØHX9XZZ
Scalp ØHXØXZZ
Upper Arm
Left ØHXCXZZ
Right ØHXBXZZ
Upper Leg
Left ØHXJXZZ
Right ØHXHXZZ
Stomach ØDX6
Subcutaneous Tissue and Fascia
Abdomen ØJX8
Back ØJX7
Buttock ØJX9
Chest ØJX6
Face ØJX1
Foot
Left ØJXR
Right ØJXQ
Hand
Left ØJXK
Right ØJXJ
Lower Arm
Left ØJXH
Right ØJXG

**Transfer** – *continued*
Subcutaneous Tissue and Fascia – *continued*
Lower Leg
Left ØJXP
Right ØJXN
Neck
Anterior ØJX4
Posterior ØJX5
Pelvic Region ØJXC
Perineum ØJXB
Scalp ØJXØ
Upper Arm
Left ØJXF
Right ØJXD
Upper Leg
Left ØJXM
Right ØJXL
Tendon
Abdomen
Left ØLXG
Right ØLXF
Ankle
Left ØLXT
Right ØLXS
Foot
Left ØLXW
Right ØLXV
Hand
Left ØLX8
Right ØLX7
Head and Neck ØLXØ
Hip
Left ØLXK
Right ØLXJ
Knee
Left ØLXR
Right ØLXQ
Lower Arm and Wrist
Left ØLX6
Right ØLX5
Lower Leg
Left ØLXP
Right ØLXN
Perineum ØLXH
Shoulder
Left ØLX2
Right ØLX1
Thorax
Left ØLXD
Right ØLXC
Trunk
Left ØLXB
Right ØLX9
Upper Arm
Left ØLX4
Right ØLX3
Upper Leg
Left ØLXM
Right ØLXL
Tongue ØCX7
**Transfusion**
Artery
Central
Antihemophilic Factors 3Ø26
Blood
Platelets 3Ø26
Red Cells 3Ø26
Frozen 3Ø26
White Cells 3Ø26
Whole 3Ø26
Bone Marrow 3Ø26
Factor IX 3Ø26
Fibrinogen 3Ø26
Globulin 3Ø26
Plasma
Fresh 3Ø26
Frozen 3Ø26
Plasma Cryoprecipitate 3Ø26
Serum Albumin 3Ø26
Stem Cells
Cord Blood 3Ø26
Hematopoietic 3Ø26
Peripheral
Antihemophilic Factors 3Ø25
Blood
Platelets 3Ø25
Red Cells 3Ø25
Frozen 3Ø25
White Cells 3Ø25
Whole 3Ø25
Bone Marrow 3Ø25
Factor IX 3Ø25
Fibrinogen 3Ø25

**Transfusion** – continued
  Artery – continued
    Peripheral – continued
      Globulin 3025
      Plasma
        Fresh 3025
        Frozen 3025
      Plasma Cryoprecipitate 3025
      Serum Albumin 3025
      Stem Cells
        Cord Blood 3025
        Hematopoietic 3025
  Products of Conception
    Antihemophilic Factors 3027
    Blood
      Platelets 3027
      Red Cells 3027
        Frozen 3027
      White Cells 3027
      Whole 3027
    Factor IX 3027
    Fibrinogen 3027
    Globulin 3027
    Plasma
      Fresh 3027
      Frozen 3027
    Plasma Cryoprecipitate 3027
    Serum Albumin 3027
  Vein
    4–Factor Prothrombin Complex Concentrate 3028
    Central
      Antihemophilic Factors 3024
      Blood
        Platelets 3024
        Red Cells 3024
          Frozen 3024
        White Cells 3024
        Whole 3024
      Bone Marrow 3024
      Factor IX 3024
      Fibrinogen 3024
      Globulin 3024
      Plasma
        Fresh 3024
        Frozen 3024
      Plasma Cryoprecipitate 3024
      Serum Albumin 3024
      Stem Cells
        Cord Blood 3024
        Embryonic 3024
        Hematopoietic 3024
    Peripheral
      Antihemophilic Factors 3023
      Blood
        Platelets 3023
        Red Cells 3023
          Frozen 3023
        White Cells 3023
        Whole 3023
      Bone Marrow 3023
      Factor IX 3023
      Fibrinogen 3023
      Globulin 3023
      Plasma
        Fresh 3023
        Frozen 3023
      Plasma Cryoprecipitate 3023
      Serum Albumin 3023
      Stem Cells
        Cord Blood 3023
        Embryonic 3023
        Hematopoietic 3023

**Transplantation**
  Esophagus 0DY50Z
  Heart 02YA0Z
  Intestine
    Large 0DYE0Z
    Small 0DY80Z
  Kidney
    Left 0TY10Z
    Right 0TY00Z
  Liver 0FY00Z
  Lung
    Bilateral 0BYM0Z
    Left 0BYL0Z
    Lower Lobe
      Left 0BYJ0Z
      Right 0BYF0Z
    Middle Lobe, Right 0BYD0Z
    Right 0BYK0Z
    Upper Lobe
      Left 0BYG0Z

**Transplantation** – continued
  Lung – continued
    Upper Lobe – continued
      Right 0BYC0Z
    Lung Lingula 0BYH0Z
  Ovary
    Left 0UY10Z
    Right 0UY00Z
  Pancreas 0FYG0Z
  Products of Conception 10Y0
  Spleen 07YP0Z
  Stomach 0DY60Z
  Thymus 07YM0Z
**Transposition**
  – see Reposition
  – see Transfer
**Transversalis fascia** – use Subcutaneous Tissue and Fascia, Trunk
**Transverse** (cutaneous) **cervical nerve** – use Nerve, Cervical Plexus
**Transverse acetabular ligament**
  – use Bursa and Ligament, Hip, Left
  – use Bursa and Ligament, Hip, Right
**Transverse facial artery**
  – use Artery, Temporal, Left
  – use Artery, Temporal, Right
**Transverse humeral ligament**
  – use Bursa and Ligament, Shoulder, Left
  – use Bursa and Ligament, Shoulder, Right
**Transverse ligament of atlas** – use Bursa and Ligament, Head and Neck
**Transverse Rectus Abdominis Myocutaneous Flap**
  Replacement
    Bilateral 0HRV076
    Left 0HRU076
    Right 0HRT076
  Transfer
    Left 0KXL
    Right 0KXK
**Transverse scapular ligament**
  – use Bursa and Ligament, Shoulder, Left
  – use Bursa and Ligament, Shoulder, Right
**Transverse thoracis muscle**
  – use Muscle, Thorax, Right
  – use Muscle, Thorax, Left
**Transversospinalis muscle**
  – use Muscle, Trunk, Right
  – use Muscle, Trunk, Left
**Transversus abdominis muscle**
  – use Muscle, Abdomen, Left
  – use Muscle, Abdomen, Right
**Trapezium bone**
  – use Carpal, Right
  – use Carpal, Left
**Trapezius muscle**
  – use Muscle, Trunk, Right
  – use Muscle, Trunk, Left
**Trapezoid bone**
  – use Carpal, Right
  – use Carpal, Left
**Triceps brachii muscle**
  – use Muscle, Upper Arm, Right
  – use Muscle, Upper Arm, Left
**Tricuspid annulus** – use Valve, Tricuspid
**Trifacial nerve** – use Nerve, Trigeminal
**Trifecta™ Valve** (aortic) – use Zooplastic Tissue in Heart and Great Vessels
**Trigone of bladder** – use Bladder
**Trimming, excisional** – see Excision
**Triquetral bone**
  – use Carpal, Right
  – use Carpal, Left
**Trochanteric bursa**
  – use Bursa and Ligament, Hip, Right
  – use Bursa and Ligament, Hip, Left
**TUMT (Transurethral microwave thermotherapy of prostate)** 0V507ZZ
**TUNA (transurethral needle ablation of prostate)** 0V507ZZ
**Tunneled central venous catheter** – use Vascular Access Device in Subcutaneous Tissue and Fascia
**Tunneled spinal** (intrathecal) **catheter** – use Infusion Device
**Turbinectomy**
  – see Excision, Ear, Nose, Sinus 09B
  – see Resection, Ear, Nose, Sinus 09T
**Turbinoplasty**
  – see Repair, Ear, Nose, Sinus 09Q
  – see Replacement, Ear, Nose, Sinus 09R

**Turbinoplasty** – continued
  – see Supplement, Ear, Nose, Sinus 09U
**Turbinotomy**
  – see Drainage, Ear, Nose, Sinus 099
  – see Division, Ear, Nose, Sinus 098
**TURP (transurethral resection of prostate)**
  – see Excision, Prostate 0VB0
  – see Resection, Prostate 0VT0
**Twelfth cranial nerve** – use Nerve, Hypoglossal
**Two lead pacemaker** – use Pacemaker, Dual Chamber in 0JH
**Tympanic cavity**
  – use Ear, Middle, Left
  – use Ear, Middle, Right
**Tympanic nerve** – use Nerve, Glossopharyngeal
**Tympanic part of temporal bone**
  – use Bone, Temporal, Right
  – use Bone, Temporal, Left
**Tympanogram** – see Hearing Assessment, Diagnostic Audiology F13
**Tympanoplasty**
  – see Repair, Ear, Nose, Sinus 09Q
  – see Replacement, Ear, Nose, Sinus 09R
  – see Supplement, Ear, Nose, Sinus 09U
**Tympanosympathectomy** – see Excision, Nerve, Head and Neck Sympathetic 01BK
**Tympanotomy** – see Drainage, Ear, Nose, Sinus 099

## U

**Ulnar collateral carpal ligament**
  – use Bursa and Ligament, Wrist, Left
  – use Bursa and Ligament, Wrist, Right
**Ulnar collateral ligament**
  – use Bursa and Ligament, Elbow, Right
  – use Bursa and Ligament, Elbow, Left
**Ulnar notch**
  – use Radius, Left
  – use Radius, Right
**Ulnar vein**
  – use Vein, Brachial, Left
  – use Vein, Brachial, Right
**Ultrafiltration**
  Hemodialysis – see Performance, Urinary 5A1D
  Therapeutic plasmapheresis – see Pheresis, Circulatory 6A55
**Ultraflex™ Precision Colonic Stent System** – use Intraluminal Device
**ULTRAPRO Hernia System (UHS)** – use Synthetic Substitute
**ULTRAPRO Partially Absorbable Lightweight Mesh** – use Synthetic Substitute
**ULTRAPRO Plug** – use Synthetic Substitute
**Ultrasonic osteogenic stimulator**
  – use Bone Growth Stimulator in Upper Bones
  – use Bone Growth Stimulator in Head and Facial Bones
  – use Bone Growth Stimulator in Lower Bones
**Ultrasonography**
  Abdomen BW40ZZZ
  Abdomen and Pelvis BW41ZZZ
  Abdominal Wall BH49ZZZ
  Aorta
    Abdominal, Intravascular B440ZZ3
    Thoracic, Intravascular B340ZZ3
  Appendix BD48ZZZ
  Artery
    Brachiocephalic–Subclavian, Right, Intravascular B341ZZ3
    Celiac and Mesenteric, Intravascular B44KZZ3
    Common Carotid
      Bilateral, Intravascular B345ZZ3
      Left, Intravascular B344ZZ3
      Right, Intravascular B343ZZ3
    Coronary
      Multiple B241YZZ
        Intravascular B241ZZ3
        Transesophageal B241ZZ4
      Single B240YZZ
        Intravascular B240ZZ3
        Transesophageal B240ZZ4
    Femoral, Intravascular B44LZZ3
    Inferior Mesenteric, Intravascular B445ZZ3
    Internal Carotid
      Bilateral, Intravascular B348ZZ3
      Left, Intravascular B347ZZ3
      Right, Intravascular B346ZZ3
    Intra–Abdominal, Other, Intravascular B44BZZ3
    Intracranial, Intravascular B34RZZ3

**Ultrasonography** – *continued*
  Artery – *continued*
    Lower Extremity
      Bilateral, Intravascular B44HZZ3
      Left, Intravascular B44GZZ3
      Right, Intravascular B44FZZ3
    Mesenteric and Celiac, Intravascular B44KZZ3
    Ophthalmic, Intravascular B34VZZ3
    Penile, Intravascular B44NZZ3
    Pulmonary
      Left, Intravascular B34TZZ3
      Right, Intravascular B34SZZ3
    Renal
      Bilateral, Intravascular B448ZZ3
      Left, Intravascular B447ZZ3
      Right, Intravascular B446ZZ3
    Subclavian, Left, Intravascular B342ZZ3
    Superior Mesenteric, Intravascular B444ZZ3
    Upper Extremity
      Bilateral, Intravascular B34KZZ3
      Left, Intravascular B34JZZ3
      Right, Intravascular B34HZZ3
  Bile Duct BF40ZZZ
  Bile Duct and Gallbladder BF43ZZZ
  Bladder BT40ZZZ
    and Kidney BT4JZZZ
  Brain B040ZZZ
  Breast
    Bilateral BH42ZZZ
    Left BH41ZZZ
    Right BH40ZZZ
  Chest Wall BH4BZZZ
  Coccyx BR4FZZZ
  Connective Tissue
    Lower Extremity BL41ZZZ
    Upper Extremity BL40ZZZ
  Duodenum BD49ZZZ
  Elbow
    Left, Densitometry BP4HZZ1
    Right, Densitometry BP4GZZ1
  Esophagus BD41ZZZ
  Extremity
    Lower BH48ZZZ
    Upper BH47ZZZ
  Eye
    Bilateral B847ZZZ
    Left B846ZZZ
    Right B845ZZZ
  Fallopian Tube
    Bilateral BU42
    Left BU41
    Right BU40
  Fetal Umbilical Cord BY47ZZZ
  Fetus
    First Trimester, Multiple Gestation BY4BZZZ
    Second Trimester, Multiple Gestation BY4DZZZ
    Single
      First Trimester BY49ZZZ
      Second Trimester BY4CZZZ
      Third Trimester BY4FZZZ
    Third Trimester, Multiple Gestation BY4GZZZ
  Gallbladder BF42ZZZ
  Gallbladder and Bile Duct BF43ZZZ
  Gastrointestinal Tract BD47ZZZ
  Gland
    Adrenal
      Bilateral BG42ZZZ
      Left BG41ZZZ
      Right BG40ZZZ
    Parathyroid BG43ZZZ
    Thyroid BG44ZZZ
  Hand
    Left, Densitometry BP4PZZ1
    Right, Densitometry BP4NZZ1
  Head and Neck BH4CZZZ
  Heart
    Left B245YZZ
      Intravascular B245ZZ3
      Transesophageal B245ZZ4
    Pediatric B24DYZZ
      Intravascular B24DZZ3
      Transesophageal B24DZZ4
    Right B244YZZ
      Intravascular B244ZZ3
      Transesophageal B244ZZ4
    Right and Left B246YZZ
      Intravascular B246ZZ3
      Transesophageal B246ZZ4
    Heart with Aorta B24BYZZ
      Intravascular B24BZZ3
      Transesophageal B24BZZ4
  Hepatobiliary System, All BF4CZZZ

**Ultrasonography** – *continued*
  Hip
    Bilateral BQ42ZZZ
    Left BQ41ZZZ
    Right BQ40ZZZ
  Kidney
    and Bladder BT4JZZZ
    Bilateral BT43ZZZ
    Left BT42ZZZ
    Right BT41ZZZ
    Transplant BT49ZZZ
  Knee
    Bilateral BQ49ZZZ
    Left BQ48ZZZ
    Right BQ47ZZZ
  Liver BF45ZZZ
  Liver and Spleen BF46ZZZ
  Mediastinum BB4CZZZ
  Neck BW4FZZZ
  Ovary
    Bilateral BU45
    Left BU44
    Right BU43
  Ovary and Uterus BU4C
  Pancreas BF47ZZZ
  Pelvic Region BW4GZZZ
  Pelvis and Abdomen BW41ZZZ
  Penis BV4BZZZ
  Pericardium B24CYZZ
    Intravascular B24CZZ3
    Transesophageal B24CZZ4
  Placenta BY48ZZZ
  Pleura BB4BZZZ
  Prostate and Seminal Vesicle BV49ZZZ
  Rectum BD4CZZZ
  Sacrum BR4FZZZ
  Scrotum BV44ZZZ
  Seminal Vesicle and Prostate BV49ZZZ
  Shoulder
    Left, Densitometry BP49ZZ1
    Right, Densitometry BP48ZZ1
  Spinal Cord B04BZZZ
  Spine
    Cervical BR40ZZZ
    Lumbar BR49ZZZ
    Thoracic BR47ZZZ
  Spleen and Liver BF46ZZZ
  Stomach BD42ZZZ
  Tendon
    Lower Extremity BL43ZZZ
    Upper Extremity BL42ZZZ
  Ureter
    Bilateral BT48ZZZ
    Left BT47ZZZ
    Right BT46ZZZ
  Urethra BT45ZZZ
  Uterus BU46
  Uterus and Ovary BU4C
  Vein
    Jugular
      Left, Intravascular B544ZZ3
      Right, Intravascular B543ZZ3
    Lower Extremity
      Bilateral, Intravascular B54DZZ3
      Left, Intravascular B54CZZ3
    Lower Extremity – *continued*
      Right, Intravascular B54BZZ3
    Portal, Intravascular B54TZZ3
    Renal
      Bilateral, Intravascular B54LZZ3
      Left, Intravascular B54KZZ3
      Right, Intravascular B54JZZ3
    Spanchnic, Intravascular B54TZZ3
    Subclavian
      Left, Intravascular B547ZZ3
      Right, Intravascular B546ZZ3
    Upper Extremity
      Bilateral, Intravascular B54PZZ3
      Left, Intravascular B54NZZ3
      Right, Intravascular B54MZZ3
    Vena Cava
      Inferior, Intravascular B549ZZ3
      Superior, Intravascular B548ZZ3
  Wrist
    Left, Densitometry BP4MZZ1
    Right, Densitometry BP4LZZ1
**Ultrasound bone healing system**
  – *use* Bone Growth Stimulator in Upper Bones
  – *use* Bone Growth Stimulator in Head and Facial Bones
  – *use* Bone Growth Stimulator in Lower Bones
**Ultrasound Therapy**
  Heart 6A75
  No Qualifier 6A75

**Ultrasound Therapy** – *continued*
  Vessels
    Head and Neck 6A75
    Other 6A75
    Peripheral 6A75
**Ultraviolet Light Therapy, Skin** 6A80
**Umbilical artery**
  – *use* Artery, Internal Iliac, Left
  – *use* Artery, Internal Iliac, Right
**Uniplanar external fixator**
  – *use* External Fixation Device, Monoplanar in 0PH
  – *use* External Fixation Device, Monoplanar in 0PS
  – *use* External Fixation Device, Monoplanar in 0QH
  – *use* External Fixation Device, Monoplanar in 0QS
**Upper GI series** – *see* Fluoroscopy, Gastrointestinal, Upper BD15
**Ureteral orifice**
  – *use* Ureter, Left
  – *use* Ureter
  – *use* Ureter, Right
  – *use* Ureters, Bilateral
**Ureterectomy**
  – *see* Excision, Urinary System 0TB
  – *see* Resection, Urinary System 0TT
**Ureterocolostomy** – *see* Bypass, Urinary System 0T1
**Ureterocystostomy** – *see* Bypass, Urinary System 0T1
**Ureteroenterostomy** – *see* Bypass, Urinary System 0T1
**Ureteroileostomy** – *see* Bypass, Urinary System 0T1
**Ureterolithotomy** – *see* Extirpation, Urinary System 0TC
**Ureterolysis** – *see* Release, Urinary System 0TN
**Ureteroneocystostomy**
  – *see* Bypass, Urinary System 0T1
  – *see* Reposition, Urinary System 0TS
**Ureteropelvic junction (UPJ)**
  – *use* Kidney Pelvis, Right
  – *use* Kidney Pelvis, Left
**Ureteropexy**
  – *see* Repair, Urinary System 0TQ
  – *see* Reposition, Urinary System 0TS
**Ureteroplasty**
  – *see* Repair, Urinary System 0TQ
  – *see* Replacement, Urinary System 0TR
  – *see* Supplement, Urinary System 0TU
**Ureteroplication** – *see* Restriction, Urinary System 0TV
**Ureteropyelography** – *see* Fluoroscopy, Urinary System BT1
**Ureterorrhaphy** – *see* Repair, Urinary System 0TQ
**Ureteroscopy** 0TJ98ZZ
**Ureterostomy**
  – *see* Bypass, Urinary System 0T1
  – *see* Drainage, Urinary System 0T9
**Ureterotomy** – *see* Drainage, Urinary System 0T9
**Ureteroureterostomy** – *see* Bypass, Urinary System 0T1
**Ureterovesical orifice**
  – *use* Ureter, Right
  – *use* Ureter, Left
  – *use* Ureters, Bilateral
  – *use* Ureter
**Urethral catheterization, indwelling** 0T9B70Z
**Urethrectomy**
  – *see* Excision, Urethra 0TBD
  – *see* Resection, Urethra 0TTD
**Urethrolithotomy** – *see* Extirpation, Urethra 0TCD
**Urethrolysis** – *see* Release, Urethra 0TND
**Urethropexy**
  – *see* Repair, Urethra 0TQD
  – *see* Reposition, Urethra 0TSD
**Urethroplasty**
  – *see* Repair, Urethra 0TQD
  – *see* Replacement, Urethra 0TRD
  – *see* Supplement, Urethra 0TUD
**Urethrorrhaphy** – *see* Repair, Urethra 0TQD
**Urethroscopy** 0TJD8ZZ
**Urethrotomy** – *see* Drainage, Urethra 0T9D
**Urinary incontinence stimulator lead** – *use* Stimulator Lead in Urinary System
**Urography** – *see* Fluoroscopy, Urinary System BT1
**Uterine Artery**
  – *use* Artery, Internal Iliac, Left
  – *use* Artery, Internal Iliac, Right
  Left, Occlusion, Artery, Internal Iliac, Left 04LF
  Right, Occlusion, Artery, Internal Iliac, Right 04LE
**Uterine artery embolization (UAE)** – *see* Occlusion, Lower Arteries 04L
**Uterine cornu** – *use* Uterus
**Uterine tube**
  – *use* Fallopian Tube, Left

**Zenith® Renu™ AAA Ancillary Graft** – *use* Intraluminal Device

**Zilver® PTX®** (paclitaxel) **Drug-Eluting Peripheral Stent**
  – *use* Intraluminal Device, Drug-eluting in Upper Arteries
  – *use* Intraluminal Device, Drug-eluting in Lower Arteries

**Zimmer® NexGen® LPS Mobile Bearing Knee** – *use* Synthetic Substitute

**Zimmer® NexGen® LPS-Flex Mobile Knee** – *use* Synthetic Substitute

**Zonule of Zinn**
  – *use* Lens, Left
  – *use* Lens, Right

**Zotarolimus-eluting coronary stent** – *use* Intraluminal Device, Drug-eluting in Heart and Great Vessels

**Zygomatic process of frontal bone**
  – *use* Bone, Frontal, Left
  – *use* Bone, Frontal, Right

**Zygomatic process of temporal bone**
  – *use* Bone, Temporal, Right
  – *use* Bone, Temporal, Left

**Zygomaticus muscle** – *use* Muscle, Facial

**Zyvox** – *use* Oxazolidinones

# Central Nervous System | 001-00X

| 0 Medical and Surgical | | | |
|---|---|---|---|
| 0 Central Nervous System | | | |
| 1 Bypass: Altering the route of passage of the contents of a tubular body part | | | |

| Character 4<br>Body Part | Character 5<br>Approach | Character 6<br>Device | Character 7<br>Qualifier |
|---|---|---|---|
| 6 Cerebral Ventricle | 0 Open<br>3 Percutaneous | 7 Autologous Tissue Substitute<br>J Synthetic Substitute<br>K Nonautologous Tissue Substitute | 0 Nasopharynx<br>1 Mastoid Sinus<br>2 Atrium<br>3 Blood Vessel<br>4 Pleural Cavity<br>5 Intestine<br>6 Peritoneal Cavity<br>7 Urinary Tract<br>8 Bone Marrow<br>B Cerebral Cisterns |
| U Spinal Canal | 0 Open<br>3 Percutaneous | 7 Autologous Tissue Substitute<br>J Synthetic Substitute<br>K Nonautologous Tissue Substitute | 4 Pleural Cavity<br>6 Peritoneal Cavity<br>7 Urinary Tract<br>9 Fallopian Tube |

**AHA:** 00163J6 - 2Q 2013, 37

| 0 Medical and Surgical | | | |
|---|---|---|---|
| 0 Central Nervous System | | | |
| 2 Change: Taking out or off a device from a body part and putting back an identical or similar device in or on the same body part without cutting or puncturing the skin or a mucous membrane | | | |

| Character 4<br>Body Part | Character 5<br>Approach | Character 6<br>Device | Character 7<br>Qualifier |
|---|---|---|---|
| 0 Brain<br>E Cranial Nerve<br>U Spinal Canal | X External | 0 Drainage Device<br>Y Other Device | Z No Qualifier |

| 0 Medical and Surgical | | | |
|---|---|---|---|
| 0 Central Nervous System | | | |
| 5 Destruction: Physical eradication of all or a portion of a body part by the direct use of energy, force, or a destructive agent | | | |

| Character 4<br>Body Part | Character 5<br>Approach | Character 6<br>Device | Character 7<br>Qualifier |
|---|---|---|---|
| 0 Brain<br>1 Cerebral Meninges<br>2 Dura Mater<br>6 Cerebral Ventricle<br>7 Cerebral Hemisphere<br>8 Basal Ganglia<br>9 Thalamus<br>A Hypothalamus<br>B Pons<br>C Cerebellum<br>D Medulla Oblongata<br>F Olfactory Nerve<br>G Optic Nerve<br>H Oculomotor Nerve<br>J Trochlear Nerve<br>K Trigeminal Nerve<br>L Abducens Nerve<br>M Facial Nerve<br>N Acoustic Nerve<br>P Glossopharyngeal Nerve<br>Q Vagus Nerve<br>R Accessory Nerve<br>S Hypoglossal Nerve<br>T Spinal Meninges<br>W Cervical Spinal Cord<br>X Thoracic Spinal Cord<br>Y Lumbar Spinal Cord | 0 Open<br>3 Percutaneous<br>4 Percutaneous Endoscopic | Z No Device | Z No Qualifier |

0  Medical and Surgical
0  Central Nervous System
8  Division: Cutting into a body part, without draining fluids and/or gases from the body part, in order to separate or transect a body part

| Character 4 Body Part | Character 5 Approach | Character 6 Device | Character 7 Qualifier |
|---|---|---|---|
| 0  Brain | 0  Open | Z  No Device | Z  No Qualifier |
| 7  Cerebral Hemisphere | 3  Percutaneous | | |
| 8  Basal Ganglia | 4  Percutaneous Endoscopic | | |
| F  Olfactory Nerve | | | |
| G  Optic Nerve | | | |
| H  Oculomotor Nerve | | | |
| J  Trochlear Nerve | | | |
| K  Trigeminal Nerve | | | |
| L  Abducens Nerve | | | |
| M  Facial Nerve | | | |
| N  Acoustic Nerve | | | |
| P  Glossopharyngeal Nerve | | | |
| Q  Vagus Nerve | | | |
| R  Accessory Nerve | | | |
| S  Hypoglossal Nerve | | | |
| W  Cervical Spinal Cord | | | |
| X  Thoracic Spinal Cord | | | |
| Y  Lumbar Spinal Cord | | | |

**0** Medical and Surgical
**0** Central Nervous System
**9** Drainage: Taking or letting out fluids and/or gases from a body part

| Character 4<br>Body Part | Character 5<br>Approach | Character 6<br>Device | Character 7<br>Qualifier |
|---|---|---|---|
| 0 Brain<br>1 Cerebral Meninges<br>2 Dura Mater<br>3 Epidural Space<br>4 Subdural Space<br>5 Subarachnoid Space<br>6 Cerebral Ventricle<br>7 Cerebral Hemisphere<br>8 Basal Ganglia<br>9 Thalamus<br>A Hypothalamus<br>B Pons<br>C Cerebellum<br>D Medulla Oblongata<br>F Olfactory Nerve<br>G Optic Nerve<br>H Oculomotor Nerve<br>J Trochlear Nerve<br>K Trigeminal Nerve<br>L Abducens Nerve<br>M Facial Nerve<br>N Acoustic Nerve<br>P Glossopharyngeal Nerve<br>Q Vagus Nerve<br>R Accessory Nerve<br>S Hypoglossal Nerve<br>T Spinal Meninges<br>U Spinal Canal<br>W Cervical Spinal Cord<br>X Thoracic Spinal Cord<br>Y Lumbar Spinal Cord | 0 Open<br>3 Percutaneous<br>4 Percutaneous Endoscopic | 0 Drainage Device | Z No Qualifier |
| 0 Brain<br>1 Cerebral Meninges<br>2 Dura Mater<br>3 Epidural Space<br>4 Subdural Space<br>5 Subarachnoid Space<br>6 Cerebral Ventricle<br>7 Cerebral Hemisphere<br>8 Basal Ganglia<br>9 Thalamus<br>A Hypothalamus<br>B Pons<br>C Cerebellum<br>D Medulla Oblongata<br>F Olfactory Nerve<br>G Optic Nerve<br>H Oculomotor Nerve<br>J Trochlear Nerve<br>K Trigeminal Nerve<br>L Abducens Nerve<br>M Facial Nerve<br>N Acoustic Nerve<br>P Glossopharyngeal Nerve<br>Q Vagus Nerve<br>R Accessory Nerve<br>S Hypoglossal Nerve<br>T Spinal Meninges<br>U Spinal Canal<br>W Cervical Spinal Cord<br>X Thoracic Spinal Cord<br>Y Lumbar Spinal Cord | 0 Open<br>3 Percutaneous<br>4 Percutaneous Endoscopic | Z No Device | X Diagnostic<br>Z No Qualifier |

**AHA:** 009U3ZX - 1Q 2014, 8

**0** Medical and Surgical
**0** Central Nervous System
**B** Excision: Cutting out or off, without replacement, a portion of a body part

| Character 4 Body Part | Character 5 Approach | Character 6 Device | Character 7 Qualifier |
|---|---|---|---|
| 0 Brain<br>1 Cerebral Meninges<br>2 Dura Mater<br>6 Cerebral Ventricle<br>7 Cerebral Hemisphere<br>8 Basal Ganglia<br>9 Thalamus<br>A Hypothalamus<br>B Pons<br>C Cerebellum<br>D Medulla Oblongata<br>F Olfactory Nerve<br>G Optic Nerve<br>H Oculomotor Nerve<br>J Trochlear Nerve<br>K Trigeminal Nerve<br>L Abducens Nerve<br>M Facial Nerve<br>N Acoustic Nerve<br>P Glossopharyngeal Nerve<br>Q Vagus Nerve<br>R Accessory Nerve<br>S Hypoglossal Nerve<br>T Spinal Meninges<br>W Cervical Spinal Cord<br>X Thoracic Spinal Cord<br>Y Lumbar Spinal Cord | 0 Open<br>3 Percutaneous<br>4 Percutaneous Endoscopic | Z No Device | X Diagnostic<br>Z No Qualifier |

**0** Medical and Surgical
**0** Central Nervous System
**C** Extirpation: Taking or cutting out solid matter from a body part

| Character 4 Body Part | Character 5 Approach | Character 6 Device | Character 7 Qualifier |
|---|---|---|---|
| 0 Brain<br>1 Cerebral Meninges<br>2 Dura Mater<br>3 Epidural Space<br>4 Subdural Space<br>5 Subarachnoid Space<br>6 Cerebral Ventricle<br>7 Cerebral Hemisphere<br>8 Basal Ganglia<br>9 Thalamus<br>A Hypothalamus<br>B Pons<br>C Cerebellum<br>D Medulla Oblongata<br>F Olfactory Nerve<br>G Optic Nerve<br>H Oculomotor Nerve<br>J Trochlear Nerve<br>K Trigeminal Nerve<br>L Abducens Nerve<br>M Facial Nerve<br>N Acoustic Nerve<br>P Glossopharyngeal Nerve<br>Q Vagus Nerve<br>R Accessory Nerve<br>S Hypoglossal Nerve<br>T Spinal Meninges<br>W Cervical Spinal Cord<br>X Thoracic Spinal Cord<br>Y Lumbar Spinal Cord | 0 Open<br>3 Percutaneous<br>4 Percutaneous Endoscopic | Z No Device | Z No Qualifier |

**0** Medical and Surgical
**0** Central Nervous System
**D** Extraction: Pulling or stripping out or off all or a portion of a body part by the use of force

| Character 4<br>Body Part | Character 5<br>Approach | Character 6<br>Device | Character 7<br>Qualifier |
|---|---|---|---|
| 1 Cerebral Meninges<br>2 Dura Mater<br>F Olfactory Nerve<br>G Optic Nerve<br>H Oculomotor Nerve<br>J Trochlear Nerve<br>K Trigeminal Nerve<br>L Abducens Nerve<br>M Facial Nerve<br>N Acoustic Nerve<br>P Glossopharyngeal Nerve<br>Q Vagus Nerve<br>R Accessory Nerve<br>S Hypoglossal Nerve<br>T Spinal Meninges | 0 Open<br>3 Percutaneous<br>4 Percutaneous Endoscopic | Z No Device | Z No Qualifier |

**0** Medical and Surgical
**0** Central Nervous System
**F** Fragmentation: Breaking solid matter in a body part into pieces

| Character 4<br>Body Part | Character 5<br>Approach | Character 6<br>Device | Character 7<br>Qualifier |
|---|---|---|---|
| 3 Epidural Space NC<br>4 Subdural Space NC<br>5 Subarachnoid Space NC<br>6 Cerebral Ventricle NC<br>U Spinal Canal | 0 Open<br>3 Percutaneous<br>4 Percutaneous Endoscopic<br>X External | Z No Device | Z No Qualifier |

NC 00F3XZZ, 00F4XZZ, 00F5XZZ, 00F6XZZ

**0** Medical and Surgical
**0** Central Nervous System
**H** Insertion: Putting in a nonbiological appliance that monitors, assists, performs, or prevents a physiological function but does not physically take the place of a body part

| Character 4<br>Body Part | Character 5<br>Approach | Character 6<br>Device | Character 7<br>Qualifier |
|---|---|---|---|
| 0 Brain<br>6 Cerebral Ventricle<br>E Cranial Nerve<br>U Spinal Canal<br>V Spinal Cord | 0 Open<br>3 Percutaneous<br>4 Percutaneous Endoscopic | 2 Monitoring Device<br>3 Infusion Device<br>M Neurostimulator Lead | Z No Qualifier |

**0** Medical and Surgical
**0** Central Nervous System
**J** Inspection: Visually and/or manually exploring a body part

| Character 4<br>Body Part | Character 5<br>Approach | Character 6<br>Device | Character 7<br>Qualifier |
|---|---|---|---|
| 0 Brain<br>E Cranial Nerve<br>U Spinal Canal<br>V Spinal Cord | 0 Open<br>3 Percutaneous<br>4 Percutaneous Endoscopic | Z No Device | Z No Qualifier |

**0** Medical and Surgical
**0** Central Nervous System
**K** Map: Locating the route of passage of electrical impulses and/or locating functional areas in a body part

| Character 4<br>Body Part | Character 5<br>Approach | Character 6<br>Device | Character 7<br>Qualifier |
|---|---|---|---|
| 0 Brain<br>7 Cerebral Hemisphere<br>8 Basal Ganglia<br>9 Thalamus<br>A Hypothalamus<br>B Pons<br>C Cerebellum<br>D Medulla Oblongata | 0 Open<br>3 Percutaneous<br>4 Percutaneous Endoscopic | Z No Device | Z No Qualifier |

**0** Medical and Surgical
**0** Central Nervous System
**N** Release: Freeing a body part from an abnormal physical constraint by cutting or by the use of force

| Character 4<br>Body Part | Character 5<br>Approach | Character 6<br>Device | Character 7<br>Qualifier |
|---|---|---|---|
| 0 Brain<br>1 Cerebral Meninges<br>2 Dura Mater<br>6 Cerebral Ventricle<br>7 Cerebral Hemisphere<br>8 Basal Ganglia<br>9 Thalamus<br>A Hypothalamus<br>B Pons<br>C Cerebellum<br>D Medulla Oblongata<br>F Olfactory Nerve<br>G Optic Nerve<br>H Oculomotor Nerve<br>J Trochlear Nerve<br>K Trigeminal Nerve<br>L Abducens Nerve<br>M Facial Nerve<br>N Acoustic Nerve<br>P Glossopharyngeal Nerve<br>Q Vagus Nerve<br>R Accessory Nerve<br>S Hypoglossal Nerve<br>T Spinal Meninges<br>W Cervical Spinal Cord<br>X Thoracic Spinal Cord<br>Y Lumbar Spinal Cord | 0 Open<br>3 Percutaneous<br>4 Percutaneous Endoscopic | Z No Device | Z No Qualifier |

**0** Medical and Surgical
**0** Central Nervous System
**P** Removal: Taking out or off a device from a body part

| Character 4<br>Body Part | Character 5<br>Approach | Character 6<br>Device | Character 7<br>Qualifier |
|---|---|---|---|
| 0 Brain<br>V Spinal Cord | 0 Open<br>3 Percutaneous<br>4 Percutaneous Endoscopic | 0 Drainage Device<br>2 Monitoring Device<br>3 Infusion Device<br>7 Autologous Tissue Substitute<br>J Synthetic Substitute<br>K Nonautologous Tissue Substitute<br>M Neurostimulator Lead | Z No Qualifier |
| 0 Brain<br>V Spinal Cord | X External | 0 Drainage Device<br>2 Monitoring Device<br>3 Infusion Device<br>M Neurostimulator Lead | Z No Qualifier |
| 6 Cerebral Ventricle<br>U Spinal Canal | 0 Open<br>3 Percutaneous<br>4 Percutaneous Endoscopic | 0 Drainage Device<br>2 Monitoring Device<br>3 Infusion Device<br>J Synthetic Substitute<br>M Neurostimulator Lead | Z No Qualifier |
| 6 Cerebral Ventricle<br>U Spinal Canal | X External | 0 Drainage Device<br>2 Monitoring Device<br>3 Infusion Device<br>M Neurostimulator Lead | Z No Qualifier |
| E Cranial Nerve | 0 Open<br>3 Percutaneous<br>4 Percutaneous Endoscopic | 0 Drainage Device<br>2 Monitoring Device<br>3 Infusion Device<br>7 Autologous Tissue Substitute<br>M Neurostimulator Lead | Z No Qualifier |
| E Cranial Nerve | X External | 0 Drainage Device<br>2 Monitoring Device<br>3 Infusion Device<br>M Neurostimulator Lead | Z No Qualifier |

**0** Medical and Surgical
**0** Central Nervous System
**Q** Repair: Restoring, to the extent possible, a body part to its normal anatomic structure and function

| Character 4<br>Body Part | Character 5<br>Approach | Character 6<br>Device | Character 7<br>Qualifier |
|---|---|---|---|
| 0 Brain<br>1 Cerebral Meninges<br>2 Dura Mater<br>6 Cerebral Ventricle<br>7 Cerebral Hemisphere<br>8 Basal Ganglia<br>9 Thalamus<br>A Hypothalamus<br>B Pons<br>C Cerebellum<br>D Medulla Oblongata<br>F Olfactory Nerve<br>G Optic Nerve<br>H Oculomotor Nerve<br>J Trochlear Nerve<br>K Trigeminal Nerve<br>L Abducens Nerve<br>M Facial Nerve<br>N Acoustic Nerve<br>P Glossopharyngeal Nerve<br>Q Vagus Nerve<br>R Accessory Nerve<br>S Hypoglossal Nerve<br>T Spinal Meninges<br>W Cervical Spinal Cord<br>X Thoracic Spinal Cord<br>Y Lumbar Spinal Cord | 0 Open<br>3 Percutaneous<br>4 Percutaneous Endoscopic | Z No Device | Z No Qualifier |

**AHA:** 00Q20ZZ - 3Q 2013, 25

**0** Medical and Surgical
**0** Central Nervous System
**S** Reposition: Moving to its normal location, or other suitable location, all or a portion of a body part

| Character 4<br>Body Part | Character 5<br>Approach | Character 6<br>Device | Character 7<br>Qualifier |
|---|---|---|---|
| F Olfactory Nerve<br>G Optic Nerve<br>H Oculomotor Nerve<br>J Trochlear Nerve<br>K Trigeminal Nerve<br>L Abducens Nerve<br>M Facial Nerve<br>N Acoustic Nerve<br>P Glossopharyngeal Nerve<br>Q Vagus Nerve<br>R Accessory Nerve<br>S Hypoglossal Nerve<br>W Cervical Spinal Cord<br>X Thoracic Spinal Cord<br>Y Lumbar Spinal Cord | 0 Open<br>3 Percutaneous<br>4 Percutaneous Endoscopic | Z No Device | Z No Qualifier |

**0** Medical and Surgical
**0** Central Nervous System
**T** Resection: Cutting out or off, without replacement, all of a body part

| Character 4<br>Body Part | Character 5<br>Approach | Character 6<br>Device | Character 7<br>Qualifier |
|---|---|---|---|
| 7 Cerebral Hemisphere | 0 Open<br>3 Percutaneous<br>4 Percutaneous Endoscopic | Z No Device | Z No Qualifier |

**0** Medical and Surgical
**0** Central Nervous System
**U** Supplement: Putting in or on biological or synthetic material that physically reinforces and/or augments the function of a portion of a body part

| Character 4<br>Body Part | Character 5<br>Approach | Character 6<br>Device | Character 7<br>Qualifier |
|---|---|---|---|
| 1  Cerebral Meninges<br>2  Dura Mater<br>T  Spinal Meninges | 0  Open<br>3  Percutaneous<br>4  Percutaneous Endoscopic | 7  Autologous Tissue Substitute<br>J  Synthetic Substitute<br>K  Nonautologous Tissue Substitute | Z  No Qualifier |
| F  Olfactory Nerve<br>G  Optic Nerve<br>H  Oculomotor Nerve<br>J  Trochlear Nerve<br>K  Trigeminal Nerve<br>L  Abducens Nerve<br>M  Facial Nerve<br>N  Acoustic Nerve<br>P  Glossopharyngeal Nerve<br>Q  Vagus Nerve<br>R  Accessory Nerve<br>S  Hypoglossal Nerve | 0  Open<br>3  Percutaneous<br>4  Percutaneous Endoscopic | 7  Autologous Tissue Substitute | Z  No Qualifier |

**0** Medical and Surgical
**0** Central Nervous System
**W** Revision: Correcting, to the extent possible, a portion of a malfunctioning device or the position of a displaced device

| Character 4<br>Body Part | Character 5<br>Approach | Character 6<br>Device | Character 7<br>Qualifier |
|---|---|---|---|
| 0  Brain<br>V  Spinal Cord | 0  Open<br>3  Percutaneous<br>4  Percutaneous Endoscopic<br>X  External | 0  Drainage Device<br>2  Monitoring Device<br>3  Infusion Device<br>7  Autologous Tissue Substitute<br>J  Synthetic Substitute<br>K  Nonautologous Tissue Substitute<br>M  Neurostimulator Lead | Z  No Qualifier |
| 6  Cerebral Ventricle<br>U  Spinal Canal | 0  Open<br>3  Percutaneous<br>4  Percutaneous Endoscopic<br>X  External | 0  Drainage Device<br>2  Monitoring Device<br>3  Infusion Device<br>J  Synthetic Substitute<br>M  Neurostimulator Lead | Z  No Qualifier |
| E  Cranial Nerve | 0  Open<br>3  Percutaneous<br>4  Percutaneous Endoscopic<br>X  External | 0  Drainage Device<br>2  Monitoring Device<br>3  Infusion Device<br>7  Autologous Tissue Substitute<br>M  Neurostimulator Lead | Z  No Qualifier |

**0** Medical and Surgical
**0** Central Nervous System
**X** Transfer: Moving, without taking out, all or a portion of a body part to another location to take over the function of all or a portion of a body part

| Character 4<br>Body Part | Character 5<br>Approach | Character 6<br>Device | Character 7<br>Qualifier |
|---|---|---|---|
| F  Olfactory Nerve<br>G  Optic Nerve<br>H  Oculomotor Nerve<br>J  Trochlear Nerve<br>K  Trigeminal Nerve<br>L  Abducens Nerve<br>M  Facial Nerve<br>N  Acoustic Nerve<br>P  Glossopharyngeal Nerve<br>Q  Vagus Nerve<br>R  Accessory Nerve<br>S  Hypoglossal Nerve | 0  Open<br>4  Percutaneous Endoscopic | Z  No Device | F  Olfactory Nerve<br>G  Optic Nerve<br>H  Oculomotor Nerve<br>J  Trochlear Nerve<br>K  Trigeminal Nerve<br>L  Abducens Nerve<br>M  Facial Nerve<br>N  Acoustic Nerve<br>P  Glossopharyngeal Nerve<br>Q  Vagus Nerve<br>R  Accessory Nerve<br>S  Hypoglossal Nerve |

# Peripheral Nervous System | 012-01X

| 0 Medical and Surgical |
|---|
| 1 Peripheral Nervous System |
| 2 Change: Taking out or off a device from a body part and putting back an identical or similar device in or on the same body part without cutting or puncturing the skin or a mucous membrane |

| Character 4<br>Body Part | Character 5<br>Approach | Character 6<br>Device | Character 7<br>Qualifier |
|---|---|---|---|
| Y Peripheral Nerve | X External | 0 Drainage Device<br>Y Other Device | Z No Qualifier |

| 0 Medical and Surgical |
|---|
| 1 Peripheral Nervous System |
| 5 Destruction: Physical eradication of all or a portion of a body part by the direct use of energy, force, or a destructive agent |

| Character 4<br>Body Part | Character 5<br>Approach | Character 6<br>Device | Character 7<br>Qualifier |
|---|---|---|---|
| 0 Cervical Plexus<br>1 Cervical Nerve<br>2 Phrenic Nerve<br>3 Brachial Plexus<br>4 Ulnar Nerve<br>5 Median Nerve<br>6 Radial Nerve<br>8 Thoracic Nerve<br>9 Lumbar Plexus<br>A Lumbosacral Plexus<br>B Lumbar Nerve<br>C Pudendal Nerve<br>D Femoral Nerve<br>F Sciatic Nerve<br>G Tibial Nerve<br>H Peroneal Nerve<br>K Head and Neck Sympathetic Nerve<br>L Thoracic Sympathetic Nerve<br>M Abdominal Sympathetic Nerve<br>N Lumbar Sympathetic Nerve<br>P Sacral Sympathetic Nerve<br>Q Sacral Plexus<br>R Sacral Nerve | 0 Open<br>3 Percutaneous<br>4 Percutaneous Endoscopic | Z No Device | Z No Qualifier |

| 0 Medical and Surgical |
|---|
| 1 Peripheral Nervous System |
| 8 Division: Cutting into a body part, without draining fluids and/or gases from the body part, in order to separate or transect a body part |

| Character 4<br>Body Part | Character 5<br>Approach | Character 6<br>Device | Character 7<br>Qualifier |
|---|---|---|---|
| 0 Cervical Plexus<br>1 Cervical Nerve<br>2 Phrenic Nerve<br>3 Brachial Plexus<br>4 Ulnar Nerve<br>5 Median Nerve<br>6 Radial Nerve<br>8 Thoracic Nerve<br>9 Lumbar Plexus<br>A Lumbosacral Plexus<br>B Lumbar Nerve<br>C Pudendal Nerve<br>D Femoral Nerve<br>F Sciatic Nerve<br>G Tibial Nerve<br>H Peroneal Nerve<br>K Head and Neck Sympathetic Nerve<br>L Thoracic Sympathetic Nerve<br>M Abdominal Sympathetic Nerve<br>N Lumbar Sympathetic Nerve<br>P Sacral Sympathetic Nerve<br>Q Sacral Plexus<br>R Sacral Nerve | 0 Open<br>3 Percutaneous<br>4 Percutaneous Endoscopic | Z No Device | Z No Qualifier |

**0** Medical and Surgical
**1** Peripheral Nervous System
**9** Drainage: Taking or letting out fluids and/or gases from a body part

| Character 4<br>Body Part | Character 5<br>Approach | Character 6<br>Device | Character 7<br>Qualifier |
|---|---|---|---|
| 0 Cervical Plexus<br>1 Cervical Nerve<br>2 Phrenic Nerve<br>3 Brachial Plexus<br>4 Ulnar Nerve<br>5 Median Nerve<br>6 Radial Nerve<br>8 Thoracic Nerve<br>9 Lumbar Plexus<br>A Lumbosacral Plexus<br>B Lumbar Nerve<br>C Pudendal Nerve<br>D Femoral Nerve<br>F Sciatic Nerve<br>G Tibial Nerve<br>H Peroneal Nerve<br>K Head and Neck Sympathetic Nerve<br>L Thoracic Sympathetic Nerve<br>M Abdominal Sympathetic Nerve<br>N Lumbar Sympathetic Nerve<br>P Sacral Sympathetic Nerve<br>Q Sacral Plexus<br>R Sacral Nerve | 0 Open<br>3 Percutaneous<br>4 Percutaneous Endoscopic | 0 Drainage Device | Z No Qualifier |
| 0 Cervical Plexus<br>1 Cervical Nerve<br>2 Phrenic Nerve<br>3 Brachial Plexus<br>4 Ulnar Nerve<br>5 Median Nerve<br>6 Radial Nerve<br>8 Thoracic Nerve<br>9 Lumbar Plexus<br>A Lumbosacral Plexus<br>B Lumbar Nerve<br>C Pudendal Nerve<br>D Femoral Nerve<br>F Sciatic Nerve<br>G Tibial Nerve<br>H Peroneal Nerve<br>K Head and Neck Sympathetic Nerve<br>L Thoracic Sympathetic Nerve<br>M Abdominal Sympathetic Nerve<br>N Lumbar Sympathetic Nerve<br>P Sacral Sympathetic Nerve<br>Q Sacral Plexus<br>R Sacral Nerve | 0 Open<br>3 Percutaneous<br>4 Percutaneous Endoscopic | Z No Device | X Diagnostic<br>Z No Qualifier |

**0** Medical and Surgical
**1** Peripheral Nervous System
**B** Excision: Cutting out or off, without replacement, a portion of a body part

| Character 4<br>Body Part | Character 5<br>Approach | Character 6<br>Device | Character 7<br>Qualifier |
|---|---|---|---|
| 0 Cervical Plexus<br>1 Cervical Nerve<br>2 Phrenic Nerve<br>3 Brachial Plexus<br>4 Ulnar Nerve<br>5 Median Nerve<br>6 Radial Nerve<br>8 Thoracic Nerve<br>9 Lumbar Plexus<br>A Lumbosacral Plexus<br>B Lumbar Nerve<br>C Pudendal Nerve<br>D Femoral Nerve<br>F Sciatic Nerve<br>G Tibial Nerve<br>H Peroneal Nerve<br>K Head and Neck Sympathetic Nerve<br>L Thoracic Sympathetic Nerve<br>M Abdominal Sympathetic Nerve<br>N Lumbar Sympathetic Nerve<br>P Sacral Sympathetic Nerve<br>Q Sacral Plexus<br>R Sacral Nerve | 0 Open<br>3 Percutaneous<br>4 Percutaneous Endoscopic | Z No Device | X Diagnostic<br>Z No Qualifier |

**0** Medical and Surgical
**1** Peripheral Nervous System
**C** Extirpation: Taking or cutting out solid matter from a body part

| Character 4<br>Body Part | Character 5<br>Approach | Character 6<br>Device | Character 7<br>Qualifier |
|---|---|---|---|
| 0 Cervical Plexus | 0 Open | Z No Device | Z No Qualifier |
| 1 Cervical Nerve | 3 Percutaneous | | |
| 2 Phrenic Nerve | 4 Percutaneous Endoscopic | | |
| 3 Brachial Plexus | | | |
| 4 Ulnar Nerve | | | |
| 5 Median Nerve | | | |
| 6 Radial Nerve | | | |
| 8 Thoracic Nerve | | | |
| 9 Lumbar Plexus | | | |
| A Lumbosacral Plexus | | | |
| B Lumbar Nerve | | | |
| C Pudendal Nerve | | | |
| D Femoral Nerve | | | |
| F Sciatic Nerve | | | |
| G Tibial Nerve | | | |
| H Peroneal Nerve | | | |
| K Head and Neck Sympathetic Nerve | | | |
| L Thoracic Sympathetic Nerve | | | |
| M Abdominal Sympathetic Nerve | | | |
| N Lumbar Sympathetic Nerve | | | |
| P Sacral Sympathetic Nerve | | | |
| Q Sacral Plexus | | | |
| R Sacral Nerve | | | |

**0** Medical and Surgical
**1** Peripheral Nervous System
**D** Extraction: Pulling or stripping out or off all or a portion of a body part by the use of force

| Character 4<br>Body Part | Character 5<br>Approach | Character 6<br>Device | Character 7<br>Qualifier |
|---|---|---|---|
| 0 Cervical Plexus | 0 Open | Z No Device | Z No Qualifier |
| 1 Cervical Nerve | 3 Percutaneous | | |
| 2 Phrenic Nerve | 4 Percutaneous Endoscopic | | |
| 3 Brachial Plexus | | | |
| 4 Ulnar Nerve | | | |
| 5 Median Nerve | | | |
| 6 Radial Nerve | | | |
| 8 Thoracic Nerve | | | |
| 9 Lumbar Plexus | | | |
| A Lumbosacral Plexus | | | |
| B Lumbar Nerve | | | |
| C Pudendal Nerve | | | |
| D Femoral Nerve | | | |
| F Sciatic Nerve | | | |
| G Tibial Nerve | | | |
| H Peroneal Nerve | | | |
| K Head and Neck Sympathetic Nerve | | | |
| L Thoracic Sympathetic Nerve | | | |
| M Abdominal Sympathetic Nerve | | | |
| N Lumbar Sympathetic Nerve | | | |
| P Sacral Sympathetic Nerve | | | |
| Q Sacral Plexus | | | |
| R Sacral Nerve | | | |

**0** Medical and Surgical
**1** Peripheral Nervous System
**H** Insertion: Putting in a nonbiological appliance that monitors, assists, performs, or prevents a physiological function but does not physically take the place of a body part

| Character 4<br>Body Part | Character 5<br>Approach | Character 6<br>Device | Character 7<br>Qualifier |
|---|---|---|---|
| Y Peripheral Nerve | 0 Open | 2 Monitoring Device | Z No Qualifier |
| | 3 Percutaneous | M Neurostimulator Lead | |
| | 4 Percutaneous Endoscopic | | |

**0** Medical and Surgical
**1** Peripheral Nervous System
**J** Inspection: Visually and/or manually exploring a body part

| Character 4<br>Body Part | Character 5<br>Approach | Character 6<br>Device | Character 7<br>Qualifier |
|---|---|---|---|
| Y Peripheral Nerve | 0 Open | Z No Device | Z No Qualifier |
| | 3 Percutaneous | | |
| | 4 Percutaneous Endoscopic | | |

**0** Medical and Surgical
**1** Peripheral Nervous System
**N** Release: Freeing a body part from an abnormal physical constraint by cutting or by the use of force

| Character 4<br>Body Part | Character 5<br>Approach | Character 6<br>Device | Character 7<br>Qualifier |
|---|---|---|---|
| 0 Cervical Plexus<br>1 Cervical Nerve<br>2 Phrenic Nerve<br>3 Brachial Plexus<br>4 Ulnar Nerve<br>5 Median Nerve<br>6 Radial Nerve<br>8 Thoracic Nerve<br>9 Lumbar Plexus<br>A Lumbosacral Plexus<br>B Lumbar Nerve<br>C Pudendal Nerve<br>D Femoral Nerve<br>F Sciatic Nerve<br>G Tibial Nerve<br>H Peroneal Nerve<br>K Head and Neck Sympathetic Nerve<br>L Thoracic Sympathetic Nerve<br>M Abdominal Sympathetic Nerve<br>N Lumbar Sympathetic Nerve<br>P Sacral Sympathetic Nerve<br>Q Sacral Plexus<br>R Sacral Nerve | 0 Open<br>3 Percutaneous<br>4 Percutaneous Endoscopic | Z No Device | Z No Qualifier |

**0** Medical and Surgical
**1** Peripheral Nervous System
**P** Removal: Taking out or off a device from a body part

| Character 4<br>Body Part | Character 5<br>Approach | Character 6<br>Device | Character 7<br>Qualifier |
|---|---|---|---|
| Y Peripheral Nerve | 0 Open<br>3 Percutaneous<br>4 Percutaneous Endoscopic | 0 Drainage Device<br>2 Monitoring Device<br>7 Autologous Tissue Substitute<br>M Neurostimulator Lead | Z No Qualifier |
| Y Peripheral Nerve | X External | 0 Drainage Device<br>2 Monitoring Device<br>M Neurostimulator Lead | Z No Qualifier |

**0** Medical and Surgical
**1** Peripheral Nervous System
**Q** Repair: Restoring, to the extent possible, a body part to its normal anatomic structure and function

| Character 4<br>Body Part | Character 5<br>Approach | Character 6<br>Device | Character 7<br>Qualifier |
|---|---|---|---|
| 0 Cervical Plexus<br>1 Cervical Nerve<br>2 Phrenic Nerve<br>3 Brachial Plexus<br>4 Ulnar Nerve<br>5 Median Nerve<br>6 Radial Nerve<br>8 Thoracic Nerve<br>9 Lumbar Plexus<br>A Lumbosacral Plexus<br>B Lumbar Nerve<br>C Pudendal Nerve<br>D Femoral Nerve<br>F Sciatic Nerve<br>G Tibial Nerve<br>H Peroneal Nerve<br>K Head and Neck Sympathetic Nerve<br>L Thoracic Sympathetic Nerve<br>M Abdominal Sympathetic Nerve<br>N Lumbar Sympathetic Nerve<br>P Sacral Sympathetic Nerve<br>Q Sacral Plexus<br>R Sacral Nerve | 0 Open<br>3 Percutaneous<br>4 Percutaneous Endoscopic | Z No Device | Z No Qualifier |

**0** Medical and Surgical
**1** Peripheral Nervous System
**S** Reposition: Moving to its normal location, or other suitable location, all or a portion of a body part

| Character 4<br>Body Part | Character 5<br>Approach | Character 6<br>Device | Character 7<br>Qualifier |
|---|---|---|---|
| 0 Cervical Plexus<br>1 Cervical Nerve<br>2 Phrenic Nerve<br>3 Brachial Plexus<br>4 Ulnar Nerve<br>5 Median Nerve<br>6 Radial Nerve<br>8 Thoracic Nerve<br>9 Lumbar Plexus<br>A Lumbosacral Plexus<br>B Lumbar Nerve<br>C Pudendal Nerve<br>D Femoral Nerve<br>F Sciatic Nerve<br>G Tibial Nerve<br>H Peroneal Nerve<br>Q Sacral Plexus<br>R Sacral Nerve | 0 Open<br>3 Percutaneous<br>4 Percutaneous Endoscopic | Z No Device | Z No Qualifier |

**0** Medical and Surgical
**1** Peripheral Nervous System
**U** Supplement: Putting in or on biological or synthetic material that physically reinforces and/or augments the function of a portion of a body part

| Character 4<br>Body Part | Character 5<br>Approach | Character 6<br>Device | Character 7<br>Qualifier |
|---|---|---|---|
| 1 Cervical Nerve<br>2 Phrenic Nerve<br>4 Ulnar Nerve<br>5 Median Nerve<br>6 Radial Nerve<br>8 Thoracic Nerve<br>B Lumbar Nerve<br>C Pudendal Nerve<br>D Femoral Nerve<br>F Sciatic Nerve<br>G Tibial Nerve<br>H Peroneal Nerve<br>R Sacral Nerve | 0 Open<br>3 Percutaneous<br>4 Percutaneous Endoscopic | 7 Autologous Tissue Substitute | Z No Qualifier |

**0** Medical and Surgical
**1** Peripheral Nervous System
**W** Revision: Correcting, to the extent possible, a portion of a malfunctioning device or the position of a displaced device

| Character 4<br>Body Part | Character 5<br>Approach | Character 6<br>Device | Character 7<br>Qualifier |
|---|---|---|---|
| Y Peripheral Nerve | 0 Open<br>3 Percutaneous<br>4 Percutaneous Endoscopic<br>X External | 0 Drainage Device<br>2 Monitoring Device<br>7 Autologous Tissue Substitute<br>M Neurostimulator Lead | Z No Qualifier |

**0** Medical and Surgical
**1** Peripheral Nervous System
**X** Transfer: Moving, without taking out, all or a portion of a body part to another location to take over the function of all or a portion of a body part

| Character 4<br>Body Part | Character 5<br>Approach | Character 6<br>Device | Character 7<br>Qualifier |
|---|---|---|---|
| 1 Cervical Nerve<br>2 Phrenic Nerve | 0 Open<br>4 Percutaneous Endoscopic | Z No Device | 1 Cervical Nerve<br>2 Phrenic Nerve |
| 4 Ulnar Nerve<br>5 Median Nerve<br>6 Radial Nerve | 0 Open<br>4 Percutaneous Endoscopic | Z No Device | 4 Ulnar Nerve<br>5 Median Nerve<br>6 Radial Nerve |
| 8 Thoracic Nerve | 0 Open<br>4 Percutaneous Endoscopic | Z No Device | 8 Thoracic Nerve |
| B Lumbar Nerve<br>C Pudendal Nerve | 0 Open<br>4 Percutaneous Endoscopic | Z No Device | B Lumbar Nerve<br>C Perineal Nerve |
| D Femoral Nerve<br>F Sciatic Nerve<br>G Tibial Nerve<br>H Peroneal Nerve | 0 Open<br>4 Percutaneous Endoscopic | Z No Device | D Femoral Nerve<br>F Sciatic Nerve<br>G Tibial Nerve<br>H Peroneal Nerve |

♂ Male          ♀ Female          N C Non-covered          L C Limited Coverage          **AHA** *AHA Coding Clinic*

# Heart and Great Vessels | 021-02Y

**0** Medical and Surgical
**2** Heart and Great Vessels
**1** Bypass: Altering the route of passage of the contents of a tubular body part

| Character 4<br>Body Part | Character 5<br>Approach | Character 6<br>Device | Character 7<br>Qualifier |
|---|---|---|---|
| 0 Coronary Artery, One Site<br>1 Coronary Artery, Two Sites<br>2 Coronary Artery, Three Sites<br>3 Coronary Artery, Four or More Sites | 0 Open | 9 Autologous Venous Tissue<br>A Autologous Arterial Tissue<br>J Synthetic Substitute<br>K Nonautologous Tissue Substitute | 3 Coronary Artery<br>8 Internal Mammary, Right<br>9 Internal Mammary, Left<br>C Thoracic Artery<br>F Abdominal Artery<br>W Aorta |
| 0 Coronary Artery, One Site<br>1 Coronary Artery, Two Sites<br>2 Coronary Artery, Three Sites<br>3 Coronary Artery, Four or More Sites | 0 Open | Z No Device | 3 Coronary Artery<br>8 Internal Mammary, Right<br>9 Internal Mammary, Left<br>C Thoracic Artery<br>F Abdominal Artery |
| 0 Coronary Artery, One Site<br>1 Coronary Artery, Two Sites<br>2 Coronary Artery, Three Sites<br>3 Coronary Artery, Four or More Sites | 3 Percutaneous | 4 Intraluminal Device, Drug-eluting<br>D Intraluminal Device | 4 Coronary Vein |
| 0 Coronary Artery, One Site<br>1 Coronary Artery, Two Sites<br>2 Coronary Artery, Three Sites<br>3 Coronary Artery, Four or More Sites | 4 Percutaneous Endoscopic | 4 Intraluminal Device, Drug-eluting<br>D Intraluminal Device | 4 Coronary Vein |
| 0 Coronary Artery, One Site<br>1 Coronary Artery, Two Sites<br>2 Coronary Artery, Three Sites<br>3 Coronary Artery, Four or More Sites | 4 Percutaneous Endoscopic | 9 Autologous Venous Tissue<br>A Autologous Arterial Tissue<br>J Synthetic Substitute<br>K Nonautologous Tissue Substitute | 3 Coronary Artery<br>8 Internal Mammary, Right<br>9 Internal Mammary, Left<br>C Thoracic Artery<br>F Abdominal Artery<br>W Aorta |
| 0 Coronary Artery, One Site<br>1 Coronary Artery, Two Sites<br>2 Coronary Artery, Three Sites<br>3 Coronary Artery, Four or More Sites | 4 Percutaneous Endoscopic | Z No Device | 3 Coronary Artery<br>8 Internal Mammary, Right<br>9 Internal Mammary, Left<br>C Thoracic Artery<br>F Abdominal Artery |
| 6 Atrium, Right | 0 Open<br>4 Percutaneous Endoscopic | 9 Autologous Venous Tissue<br>A Autologous Arterial Tissue<br>J Synthetic Substitute<br>K Nonautologous Tissue Substitute | P Pulmonary Trunk<br>Q Pulmonary Artery, Right<br>R Pulmonary Artery, Left |
| 6 Atrium, Right | 0 Open<br>4 Percutaneous Endoscopic | Z No Device | 7 Atrium, Left<br>P Pulmonary Trunk<br>Q Pulmonary Artery, Right<br>R Pulmonary Artery, Left |
| 7 Atrium, Left<br>V Superior Vena Cava | 0 Open<br>4 Percutaneous Endoscopic | 9 Autologous Venous Tissue<br>A Autologous Arterial Tissue<br>J Synthetic Substitute<br>K Nonautologous Tissue Substitute<br>Z No Device | P Pulmonary Trunk<br>Q Pulmonary Artery, Right<br>R Pulmonary Artery, Left |
| K Ventricle, Right<br>L Ventricle, Left | 0 Open<br>4 Percutaneous Endoscopic | 9 Autologous Venous Tissue<br>A Autologous Arterial Tissue<br>J Synthetic Substitute<br>K Nonautologous Tissue Substitute | P Pulmonary Trunk<br>Q Pulmonary Artery, Right<br>R Pulmonary Artery, Left |
| K Ventricle, Right<br>L Ventricle, Left | 0 Open<br>4 Percutaneous Endoscopic | Z No Device | 5 Coronary Circulation<br>8 Internal Mammary, Right<br>9 Internal Mammary, Left<br>C Thoracic Artery<br>F Abdominal Artery<br>P Pulmonary Trunk<br>Q Pulmonary Artery, Right<br>R Pulmonary Artery, Left<br>W Aorta |
| W Thoracic Aorta | 0 Open<br>4 Percutaneous Endoscopic | 9 Autologous Venous Tissue<br>A Autologous Arterial Tissue<br>J Synthetic Substitute<br>K Nonautologous Tissue Substitute<br>Z No Device | B Subclavian<br>D Carotid<br>P Pulmonary Trunk<br>Q Pulmonary Artery, Right<br>R Pulmonary Artery, Left |

**AHA:** 021009W - 1Q 2014, 11

**0** Medical and Surgical
**2** Heart and Great Vessels
**B** Excision: Cutting out or off, without replacement, a portion of a body part

| Character 4<br>Body Part | Character 5<br>Approach | Character 6<br>Device | Character 7<br>Qualifier |
|---|---|---|---|
| 4 Coronary Vein<br>5 Atrial Septum<br>6 Atrium, Right<br>8 Conduction Mechanism<br>9 Chordae Tendineae<br>D Papillary Muscle<br>F Aortic Valve<br>G Mitral Valve<br>H Pulmonary Valve<br>J Tricuspid Valve<br>K Ventricle, Right **NC**<br>L Ventricle, Left **NC**<br>M Ventricular Septum<br>N Pericardium<br>P Pulmonary Trunk<br>Q Pulmonary Artery, Right<br>R Pulmonary Artery, Left<br>S Pulmonary Vein, Right<br>T Pulmonary Vein, Left<br>V Superior Vena Cava<br>W Thoracic Aorta | 0 Open<br>3 Percutaneous<br>4 Percutaneous Endoscopic | Z No Device | X Diagnostic<br>Z No Qualifier |
| 7 Atrium, Left | 0 Open<br>3 Percutaneous<br>4 Percutaneous Endoscopic | Z No Device | K Left Atrial Appendage<br>X Diagnostic<br>Z No Qualifier |

**NC** 02BK(0,3,4)ZZ, 02BL(0,3,4)ZZ

**0** Medical and Surgical
**2** Heart and Great Vessels
**C** Extirpation: Taking or cutting out solid matter from a body part

| Character 4<br>Body Part | Character 5<br>Approach | Character 6<br>Device | Character 7<br>Qualifier |
|---|---|---|---|
| 0 Coronary Artery, One Site<br>1 Coronary Artery, Two Sites<br>2 Coronary Artery, Three Sites<br>3 Coronary Artery, Four or More Sites<br>4 Coronary Vein<br>5 Atrial Septum<br>6 Atrium, Right<br>7 Atrium, Left<br>8 Conduction Mechanism<br>9 Chordae Tendineae<br>D Papillary Muscle<br>F Aortic Valve<br>G Mitral Valve<br>H Pulmonary Valve<br>J Tricuspid Valve<br>K Ventricle, Right<br>L Ventricle, Left<br>M Ventricular Septum<br>N Pericardium<br>P Pulmonary Trunk<br>Q Pulmonary Artery, Right<br>R Pulmonary Artery, Left<br>S Pulmonary Vein, Right<br>T Pulmonary Vein, Left<br>V Superior Vena Cava<br>W Thoracic Aorta | 0 Open<br>3 Percutaneous<br>4 Percutaneous Endoscopic | Z No Device | Z No Qualifier |

**0** Medical and Surgical
**2** Heart and Great Vessels
**F** Fragmentation: Breaking solid matter in a body part into pieces

| Character 4<br>Body Part | Character 5<br>Approach | Character 6<br>Device | Character 7<br>Qualifier |
|---|---|---|---|
| N Pericardium **NC** | 0 Open<br>3 Percutaneous<br>4 Percutaneous Endoscopic<br>X External | Z No Device | Z No Qualifier |

**NC** 02FNXZZ

**0** Medical and Surgical
**2** Heart and Great Vessels
**H** Insertion: Putting in a nonbiological appliance that monitors, assists, performs, or prevents a physiological function but does not physically take the place of a body part

| Character 4<br>Body Part | Character 5<br>Approach | Character 6<br>Device | Character 7<br>Qualifier |
|---|---|---|---|
| 4 Coronary Vein<br>6 Atrium, Right<br>7 Atrium, Left<br>K Ventricle, Right<br>L Ventricle, Left | 0 Open<br>3 Percutaneous<br>4 Percutaneous Endoscopic | 0 Monitoring Device, Pressure Sensor<br>2 Monitoring Device<br>3 Infusion Device<br>D Intraluminal Device<br>J Cardiac Lead, Pacemaker<br>K Cardiac Lead, Defibrillator<br>M Cardiac Lead | Z No Qualifier |
| A Heart **L C** | 0 Open<br>3 Percutaneous<br>4 Percutaneous Endoscopic | Q Implantable Heart Assist System | Z No Qualifier |
| A Heart | 0 Open<br>3 Percutaneous<br>4 Percutaneous Endoscopic | R External Heart Assist System | S Biventricular<br>Z No Qualifier |
| N Pericardium | 0 Open<br>3 Percutaneous<br>4 Percutaneous Endoscopic | 0 Monitoring Device, Pressure Sensor<br>2 Monitoring Device<br>J Cardiac Lead, Pacemaker<br>K Cardiac Lead, Defibrillator<br>M Cardiac Lead | Z No Qualifier |
| P Pulmonary Trunk<br>Q Pulmonary Artery, Right<br>R Pulmonary Artery, Left<br>S Pulmonary Vein, Right<br>T Pulmonary Vein, Left<br>V Superior Vena Cava<br>W Thoracic Aorta | 0 Open<br>3 Percutaneous<br>4 Percutaneous Endoscopic | 0 Monitoring Device, Pressure Sensor<br>2 Monitoring Device<br>3 Infusion Device<br>D Intraluminal Device | Z No Qualifier |

**AHA:** 02HV33Z - 3Q 2013, 18

**L C** 02HA(0,3,4)QZ

**0** Medical and Surgical
**2** Heart and Great Vessels
**J** Inspection: Visually and/or manually exploring a body part

| Character 4<br>Body Part | Character 5<br>Approach | Character 6<br>Device | Character 7<br>Qualifier |
|---|---|---|---|
| A Heart<br>Y Great Vessel | 0 Open<br>3 Percutaneous<br>4 Percutaneous Endoscopic | Z No Device | Z No Qualifier |

**0** Medical and Surgical
**2** Heart and Great Vessels
**K** Map: Locating the route of passage of electrical impulses and/or locating functional areas in a body part

| Character 4<br>Body Part | Character 5<br>Approach | Character 6<br>Device | Character 7<br>Qualifier |
|---|---|---|---|
| 8 Conduction Mechanism | 0 Open<br>3 Percutaneous<br>4 Percutaneous Endoscopic | Z No Device | Z No Qualifier |

**0** Medical and Surgical
**2** Heart and Great Vessels
**L** Occlusion: Completely closing an orifice or the lumen of a tubular body part

| Character 4<br>Body Part | Character 5<br>Approach | Character 6<br>Device | Character 7<br>Qualifier |
|---|---|---|---|
| 7 Atrium, Left | 0 Open<br>3 Percutaneous<br>4 Percutaneous Endoscopic | C Extraluminal Device<br>D Intraluminal Device<br>Z No Device | K Left Atrial Appendage |
| R Pulmonary Artery, Left | 0 Open<br>3 Percutaneous<br>4 Percutaneous Endoscopic | C Extraluminal Device<br>D Intraluminal Device<br>Z No Device | T Ductus Arteriosus |
| S Pulmonary Vein, Right<br>T Pulmonary Vein, Left<br>V Superior Vena Cava | 0 Open<br>3 Percutaneous<br>4 Percutaneous Endoscopic | C Extraluminal Device<br>D Intraluminal Device<br>Z No Device | Z No Qualifier |

**0** Medical and Surgical
**2** Heart and Great Vessels
**N** Release: Freeing a body part from an abnormal physical constraint by cutting or by the use of force

| Character 4<br>Body Part | Character 5<br>Approach | Character 6<br>Device | Character 7<br>Qualifier |
|---|---|---|---|
| 4 Coronary Vein<br>5 Atrial Septum<br>6 Atrium, Right<br>7 Atrium, Left<br>8 Conduction Mechanism<br>9 Chordae Tendineae<br>D Papillary Muscle<br>F Aortic Valve<br>G Mitral Valve<br>H Pulmonary Valve<br>J Tricuspid Valve<br>K Ventricle, Right<br>L Ventricle, Left<br>M Ventricular Septum<br>N Pericardium<br>P Pulmonary Trunk<br>Q Pulmonary Artery, Right<br>R Pulmonary Artery, Left<br>S Pulmonary Vein, Right<br>T Pulmonary Vein, Left<br>V Superior Vena Cava<br>W Thoracic Aorta | 0 Open<br>3 Percutaneous<br>4 Percutaneous Endoscopic | Z No Device | Z No Qualifier |

**0** Medical and Surgical
**2** Heart and Great Vessels
**P** Removal: Taking out or off a device from a body part

| Character 4<br>Body Part | Character 5<br>Approach | Character 6<br>Device | Character 7<br>Qualifier |
|---|---|---|---|
| A Heart | 0 Open<br>3 Percutaneous Endoscopic<br>4 Percutaneous Endoscopic | 2 Monitoring Device<br>3 Infusion Device<br>7 Autologous Tissue Substitute<br>8 Zooplastic Tissue<br>C Extraluminal Device<br>D Intraluminal Device<br>J Synthetic Substitute<br>K Nonautologous Tissue Substitute<br>M Cardiac Lead<br>Q Implantable Heart Assist System<br>R External Heart Assist System | Z No Qualifier |
| A Heart | X External | 2 Monitoring Device<br>3 Infusion Device<br>D Intraluminal Device<br>M Cardiac Lead | Z No Qualifier |
| Y Great Vessel | 0 Open<br>3 Percutaneous<br>4 Percutaneous Endoscopic | 2 Monitoring Device<br>3 Infusion Device<br>7 Autologous Tissue Substitute<br>8 Zooplastic Tissue<br>C Extraluminal Device<br>D Intraluminal Device<br>J Synthetic Substitute<br>K Nonautologous Tissue Substitute | Z No Qualifier |
| Y Great Vessel | X External | 2 Monitoring Device<br>3 Infusion Device<br>D Intraluminal Device | Z No Qualifier |

**0** Medical and Surgical
**2** Heart and Great Vessels
**Q** Repair: Restoring, to the extent possible, a body part to its normal anatomic structure and function

| Character 4<br>Body Part | Character 5<br>Approach | Character 6<br>Device | Character 7<br>Qualifier |
|---|---|---|---|
| 0 Coronary Artery, One Site<br>1 Coronary Artery, Two Sites<br>2 Coronary Artery, Three Sites<br>3 Coronary Artery, Four or More Sites<br>4 Coronary Vein<br>5 Atrial Septum<br>6 Atrium, Right<br>7 Atrium, Left<br>8 Conduction Mechanism<br>9 Chordae Tendineae<br>A Heart<br>B Heart, Right<br>C Heart, Left<br>D Papillary Muscle<br>F Aortic Valve<br>G Mitral Valve<br>H Pulmonary Valve<br>J Tricuspid Valve<br>K Ventricle, Right<br>L Ventricle, Left<br>M Ventricular Septum<br>N Pericardium<br>P Pulmonary Trunk<br>Q Pulmonary Artery, Right<br>R Pulmonary Artery, Left<br>S Pulmonary Vein, Right<br>T Pulmonary Vein, Left<br>V Superior Vena Cava<br>W Thoracic Aorta | 0 Open<br>3 Percutaneous<br>4 Percutaneous Endoscopic | Z No Device | Z No Qualifier |

**0** Medical and Surgical
**2** Heart and Great Vessels
**R** Replacement: Putting in or on biological or synthetic material that physically takes the place and/or function of all or a portion of a body part

| Character 4<br>Body Part | Character 5<br>Approach | Character 6<br>Device | Character 7<br>Qualifier |
|---|---|---|---|
| 5 Atrial Septum<br>6 Atrium, Right<br>7 Atrium, Left<br>9 Chordae Tendineae<br>D Papillary Muscle<br>J Tricuspid Valve<br>K Ventricle, Right<br>L Ventricle, Left<br>M Ventricular Septum<br>N Pericardium<br>P Pulmonary Trunk<br>Q Pulmonary Artery, Right<br>R Pulmonary Artery, Left<br>S Pulmonary Vein, Right<br>T Pulmonary Vein, Left<br>V Superior Vena Cava<br>W Thoracic Aorta | 0 Open<br>4 Percutaneous Endoscopic | 7 Autologous Tissue Substitute<br>8 Zooplastic Tissue<br>J Synthetic Substitute<br>K Nonautologous Tissue Substitute | Z No Qualifier |
| F Aortic Valve<br>G Mitral Valve<br>H Pulmonary Valve | 0 Open<br>4 Percutaneous Endoscopic | 7 Autologous Tissue Substitute<br>8 Zooplastic Tissue<br>J Synthetic Substitute<br>K Nonautologous Tissue Substitute | Z No Qualifier |
| F Aortic Valve<br>G Mitral Valve<br>H Pulmonary Valve | 3 Percutaneous | 7 Autologous Tissue Substitute<br>8 Zooplastic Tissue<br>J Synthetic Substitute<br>K Nonautologous Tissue Substitute | H Transapical<br>Z No Qualifier |

**AHA:** 02RW0KZ - 1Q 2014, 11

**0** Medical and Surgical
**2** Heart and Great Vessels
**S** Reposition: Moving to its normal location, or other suitable location, all or a portion of a body part

| Character 4<br>Body Part | Character 5<br>Approach | Character 6<br>Device | Character 7<br>Qualifier |
|---|---|---|---|
| P Pulmonary Trunk<br>Q Pulmonary Artery, Right<br>R Pulmonary Artery, Left<br>S Pulmonary Vein, Right<br>T Pulmonary Vein, Left<br>V Superior Vena Cava<br>W Thoracic Aorta | 0 Open | Z No Device | Z No Qualifier |

---

♂ Male          ♀ Female          N C Non-covered          L C Limited Coverage          **AHA** AHA Coding Clinic

**0** Medical and Surgical
**2** Heart and Great Vessels
**T** Resection: Cutting out or off, without replacement, all of a body part

| Character 4<br>Body Part | Character 5<br>Approach | Character 6<br>Device | Character 7<br>Qualifier |
|---|---|---|---|
| 5 Atrial Septum<br>8 Conduction Mechanism<br>9 Chordae Tendineae<br>D Papillary Muscle<br>H Pulmonary Valve<br>M Ventricular Septum<br>N Pericardium | 0 Open<br>3 Percutaneous<br>4 Percutaneous Endoscopic | Z No Device | Z No Qualifier |

**0** Medical and Surgical
**2** Heart and Great Vessels
**U** Supplement: Putting in or on biological or synthetic material that physically reinforces and/or augments the function of a portion of a body part

| Character 4<br>Body Part | Character 5<br>Approach | Character 6<br>Device | Character 7<br>Qualifier |
|---|---|---|---|
| 5 Atrial Septum<br>6 Atrium, Right<br>7 Atrium, Left<br>9 Chordae Tendineae<br>A Heart<br>D Papillary Muscle<br>F Aortic Valve<br>G Mitral Valve<br>H Pulmonary Valve<br>J Tricuspid Valve<br>K Ventricle, Right<br>L Ventricle, Left<br>M Ventricular Septum<br>N Pericardium<br>P Pulmonary Trunk<br>Q Pulmonary Artery, Right<br>R Pulmonary Artery, Left<br>S Pulmonary Vein, Right<br>T Pulmonary Vein, Left<br>V Superior Vena Cava<br>W Thoracic Aorta | 0 Open<br>3 Percutaneous<br>4 Percutaneous Endoscopic | 7 Autologous Tissue Substitute<br>8 Zooplastic Tissue<br>J Synthetic Substitute<br>K Nonautologous Tissue Substitute | Z No Qualifier |

**0** Medical and Surgical
**2** Heart and Great Vessels
**V** Restriction: Partially closing an orifice or the lumen of a tubular body part

| Character 4<br>Body Part | Character 5<br>Approach | Character 6<br>Device | Character 7<br>Qualifier |
|---|---|---|---|
| A Heart | 0 Open<br>3 Percutaneous<br>4 Percutaneous Endoscopic | C Extraluminal Device<br>Z No Device | Z No Qualifier |
| P Pulmonary Trunk<br>Q Pulmonary Artery, Right<br>S Pulmonary Vein, Right<br>T Pulmonary Vein, Left<br>V Superior Vena Cava<br>W Thoracic Aorta | 0 Open<br>3 Percutaneous<br>4 Percutaneous Endoscopic | C Extraluminal Device<br>D Intraluminal Device<br>Z No Device | Z No Qualifier |
| R Pulmonary Artery, Left | 0 Open<br>3 Percutaneous<br>4 Percutaneous Endoscopic | C Extraluminal Device<br>D Intraluminal Device<br>Z No Device | T Ductus Arteriosus<br>Z No Qualifier |

**0** Medical and Surgical
**2** Heart and Great Vessels
**5** Destruction: Physical eradication of all or a portion of a body part by the direct use of energy, force, or a destructive agent

| Character 4<br>Body Part | Character 5<br>Approach | Character 6<br>Device | Character 7<br>Qualifier |
|---|---|---|---|
| 4 Coronary Vein<br>5 Atrial Septum<br>6 Atrium, Right<br>8 Conduction Mechanism<br>9 Chordae Tendineae<br>D Papillary Muscle<br>F Aortic Valve<br>G Mitral Valve<br>H Pulmonary Valve<br>J Tricuspid Valve<br>K Ventricle, Right<br>L Ventricle, Left<br>M Ventricular Septum<br>N Pericardium<br>P Pulmonary Trunk<br>Q Pulmonary Artery, Right<br>R Pulmonary Artery, Left<br>S Pulmonary Vein, Right<br>T Pulmonary Vein, Left<br>V Superior Vena Cava<br>W Thoracic Aorta | 0 Open<br>3 Percutaneous<br>4 Percutaneous Endoscopic | Z No Device | Z No Qualifier |
| 7 Atrium, Left | 0 Open<br>3 Percutaneous<br>4 Percutaneous Endoscopic | Z No Device | K Left Atrial Appendage<br>Z No Qualifier |

**AHA:** 025S3ZZ - 2Q 2013, 39; 025T3ZZ - 2Q 2013, 39

**0** Medical and Surgical
**2** Heart and Great Vessels
**7** Dilation: Expanding an orifice or the lumen of a tubular body part

| Character 4<br>Body Part | Character 5<br>Approach | Character 6<br>Device | Character 7<br>Qualifier |
|---|---|---|---|
| 0 Coronary Artery, One Site<br>1 Coronary Artery, Two Sites<br>2 Coronary Artery, Three Sites<br>3 Coronary Artery, Four or More Sites | 0 Open<br>3 Percutaneous<br>4 Percutaneous Endoscopic | 4 Intraluminal Device, Drug-eluting<br>D Intraluminal Device<br>T Intraluminal Device, Radioactive<br>Z No Device | 6 Bifurcation<br>Z No Qualifier |
| F Aortic Valve<br>G Mitral Valve<br>H Pulmonary Valve<br>J Tricuspid Valve<br>K Ventricle, Right<br>P Pulmonary Trunk<br>Q Pulmonary Artery, Right<br>S Pulmonary Vein, Right<br>T Pulmonary Vein, Left<br>V Superior Vena Cava<br>W Thoracic Aorta | 0 Open<br>3 Percutaneous<br>4 Percutaneous Endoscopic | 4 Intraluminal Device, Drug-eluting<br>D Intraluminal Device<br>Z No Device | Z No Qualifier |
| R Pulmonary Artery, Left | 0 Open<br>3 Percutaneous<br>4 Percutaneous Endoscopic | 4 Intraluminal Device, Drug-eluting<br>D Intraluminal Device<br>Z No Device | T Ductus Arteriosus<br>Z No Qualifier |

**AHA:** 027034Z - 2Q 2014, 4

**0** Medical and Surgical
**2** Heart and Great Vessels
**8** Division: Cutting into a body part, without draining fluids and/or gases from the body part, in order to separate or transect a body part

| Character 4<br>Body Part | Character 5<br>Approach | Character 6<br>Device | Character 7<br>Qualifier |
|---|---|---|---|
| 8 Conduction Mechanism<br>9 Chordae Tendineae<br>D Papillary Muscle | 0 Open<br>3 Percutaneous<br>4 Percutaneous Endoscopic | Z No Device | Z No Qualifier |

0  Medical and Surgical
2  Heart and Great Vessels
W  Revision: Correcting, to the extent possible, a portion of a malfunctioning device or the position of a displaced device

| Character 4<br>Body Part | Character 5<br>Approach | Character 6<br>Device | Character 7<br>Qualifier |
|---|---|---|---|
| 5  Atrial Septum<br>M  Ventricular Septum | 0  Open<br>4  Percutaneous Endoscopic | J  Synthetic Substitute | Z  No Qualifier |
| A  Heart  N C | 0  Open<br>3  Percutaneous<br>4  Percutaneous Endoscopic<br>X  External | 2  Monitoring Device<br>3  Infusion Device<br>7  Autologous Tissue Substitute<br>8  Zooplastic Tissue<br>C  Extraluminal Device<br>D  Intraluminal Device<br>J  Synthetic Substitute<br>K  Nonautologous Tissue Substitute<br>M  Cardiac Lead<br>Q  Implantable Heart Assist System<br>R  External Heart Assist System | Z  No Qualifier |
| F  Aortic Valve<br>G  Mitral Valve<br>H  Pulmonary Valve<br>J  Tricuspid Valve | 0  Open<br>4  Percutaneous Endoscopic | 7  Autologous Tissue Substitute<br>8  Zooplastic Tissue<br>J  Synthetic Substitute<br>K  Nonautologous Tissue Substitute | Z  No Qualifier |
| Y  Great Vessel | 0  Open<br>3  Percutaneous<br>4  Percutaneous Endoscopic<br>X  External | 2  Monitoring Device<br>3  Infusion Device<br>7  Autologous Tissue Substitute<br>8  Zooplastic Tissue<br>C  Extraluminal Device<br>D  Intraluminal Device<br>J  Synthetic Substitute<br>K  Nonautologous Tissue Substitute | Z  No Qualifier |

N C  02WA(0,3,4)QZ, 02WA0JZ

0  Medical and Surgical
2  Heart and Great Vessels
Y  Transplantation: Putting in or on all or a portion of a living body part taken from another individual or animal to physically take the place and/or function of all or a portion of a similar body part

| Character 4<br>Body Part | Character 5<br>Approach | Character 6<br>Device | Character 7<br>Qualifier |
|---|---|---|---|
| A  Heart  L C | 0  Open | Z  No Device | 0  Allogeneic<br>1  Syngeneic<br>2  Zooplastic |

AHA: 02YA0Z0 - 3Q 2013, 19
L C  02YA0Z(0,1,2)

# Upper Arteries | 031 – 03W

| 0 Medical and Surgical |
| 3 Upper Arteries |
| 1 Bypass: Altering the route of passage of the contents of a tubular body part |

| Character 4<br>Body Part | Character 5<br>Approach | Character 6<br>Device | Character 7<br>Qualifier |
|---|---|---|---|
| 2 Innominate Artery<br>5 Axillary Artery, Right<br>6 Axillary Artery, Left | 0 Open | 9 Autologous Venous Tissue<br>A Autologous Arterial Tissue<br>J Synthetic Substitute<br>K Nonautologous Tissue Substitute<br>Z No Device | 0 Upper Arm Artery, Right<br>1 Upper Arm Artery, Left<br>2 Upper Arm Artery, Bilateral<br>3 Lower Arm Artery, Right<br>4 Lower Arm Artery, Left<br>5 Lower Arm Artery, Bilateral<br>6 Upper Leg Artery, Right<br>7 Upper Leg Artery, Left<br>8 Upper Leg Artery, Bilateral<br>9 Lower Leg Artery, Right<br>B Lower Leg Artery, Left<br>C Lower Leg Artery, Bilateral<br>D Upper Arm Vein<br>F Lower Arm Vein<br>J Extracranial Artery, Right<br>K Extracranial Artery, Left |
| 3 Subclavian Artery, Right<br>4 Subclavian Artery, Left | 0 Open | 9 Autologous Venous Tissue<br>A Autologous Arterial Tissue<br>J Synthetic Substitute<br>K Nonautologous Tissue Substitute<br>Z No Device | 0 Upper Arm Artery, Right<br>1 Upper Arm Artery, Left<br>2 Upper Arm Artery, Bilateral<br>3 Lower Arm Artery, Right<br>4 Lower Arm Artery, Left<br>5 Lower Arm Artery, Bilateral<br>6 Upper Leg Artery, Right<br>7 Upper Leg Artery, Left<br>8 Upper Leg Artery, Bilateral<br>9 Lower Leg Artery, Right<br>B Lower Leg Artery, Left<br>C Lower Leg Artery, Bilateral<br>D Upper Arm Vein<br>F Lower Arm Vein<br>J Extracranial Artery, Right<br>K Extracranial Artery, Left<br>M Pulmonary Artery, Right<br>N Pulmonary Artery, Left |
| 7 Brachial Artery, Right | 0 Open | 9 Autologous Venous Tissue<br>A Autologous Arterial Tissue<br>J Synthetic Substitute<br>K Nonautologous Tissue Substitute<br>Z No Device | 0 Upper Arm Artery, Right<br>3 Lower Arm Artery, Right<br>D Upper Arm Vein<br>F Lower Arm Vein |
| 8 Brachial Artery, Left | 0 Open | 9 Autologous Venous Tissue<br>A Autologous Arterial Tissue<br>J Synthetic Substitute<br>K Nonautologous Tissue Substitute<br>Z No Device | 1 Upper Arm Artery, Left<br>4 Lower Arm Artery, Left<br>D Upper Arm Vein<br>F Lower Arm Vein |
| 9 Ulnar Artery, Right<br>B Radial Artery, Right | 0 Open | 9 Autologous Venous Tissue<br>A Autologous Arterial Tissue<br>J Synthetic Substitute<br>K Nonautologous Tissue Substitute<br>Z No Device | 3 Lower Arm Artery, Right<br>F Lower Arm Vein |
| A Ulnar Artery, Left<br>C Radial Artery, Left | 0 Open | 9 Autologous Venous Tissue<br>A Autologous Arterial Tissue<br>J Synthetic Substitute<br>K Nonautologous Tissue Substitute<br>Z No Device | 4 Lower Arm Artery, Left<br>F Lower Arm Vein |
| G Intracranial Artery<br>S Temporal Artery, Right NC<br>T Temporal Artery, Left NC | 0 Open | 9 Autologous Venous Tissue<br>A Autologous Arterial Tissue<br>J Synthetic Substitute<br>K Nonautologous Tissue Substitute<br>Z No Device | G Intracranial Artery |
| H Common Carotid Artery, Right NC | 0 Open | 9 Autologous Venous Tissue<br>A Autologous Arterial Tissue<br>J Synthetic Substitute<br>K Nonautologous Tissue Substitute<br>Z No Device | G Intracranial Artery<br>J Extracranial Artery, Right |
| J Common Carotid Artery, Left NC | 0 Open | 9 Autologous Venous Tissue<br>A Autologous Arterial Tissue<br>J Synthetic Substitute<br>K Nonautologous Tissue Substitute<br>Z No Device | G Intracranial Artery<br>K Extracranial Artery, Left |
| K Internal Carotid Artery, Right NC<br>M External Carotid Artery, Right NC | 0 Open | 9 Autologous Venous Tissue<br>A Autologous Arterial Tissue<br>J Synthetic Substitute<br>K Nonautologous Tissue Substitute<br>Z No Device | J Extracranial Artery, Right |

**031** continues on next page

| 0 Medical and Surgical – *continued*<br>3 Upper Arteries – *continued*<br>1 Bypass: Altering the route of passage of the contents of a tubular body part – *continued* | | | |
|---|---|---|---|
| Character 4<br>Body Part | Character 5<br>Approach | Character 6<br>Device | Character 7<br>Qualifier |
| L Internal Carotid Artery, Left N C<br>N External Carotid Artery, Left N C | 0 Open | 9 Autologous Venous Tissue<br>A Autologous Arterial Tissue<br>J Synthetic Substitute<br>K Nonautologous Tissue Substitute<br>Z No Device | K Extracranial Artery, Left |

**AHA:** 031C0ZF - 1Q 2013, 28; 03170ZD - 4Q 2013, 126

N C 031H0(9,A,J,K,Z)J, 031J0(9,A,J,K,Z)K, 031K0(9,A,J,K,Z)J, 031L0(9,A,J,K,Z)K, 031M0(9,A,J,K,Z)J, 031N0(9,A,J,K,Z)K, 031S0(9,A,J,K,Z)G, 031T0(9,A,J,K,Z)G

| 0 Medical and Surgical<br>3 Upper Arteries<br>5 Destruction: Physical eradication of all or a portion of a body part by the direct use of energy, force, or a destructive agent | | | |
|---|---|---|---|
| Character 4<br>Body Part | Character 5<br>Approach | Character 6<br>Device | Character 7<br>Qualifier |
| 0 Internal Mammary Artery, Right<br>1 Internal Mammary Artery, Left<br>2 Innominate Artery<br>3 Subclavian Artery, Right<br>4 Subclavian Artery, Left<br>5 Axillary Artery, Right<br>6 Axillary Artery, Left<br>7 Brachial Artery, Right<br>8 Brachial Artery, Left<br>9 Ulnar Artery, Right<br>A Ulnar Artery, Left<br>B Radial Artery, Right<br>C Radial Artery, Left<br>D Hand Artery, Right<br>F Hand Artery, Left<br>G Intracranial Artery<br>H Common Carotid Artery, Right<br>J Common Carotid Artery, Left<br>K Internal Carotid Artery, Right<br>L Internal Carotid Artery, Left<br>M External Carotid Artery, Right<br>N External Carotid Artery, Left<br>P Vertebral Artery, Right<br>Q Vertebral Artery, Left<br>R Face Artery<br>S Temporal Artery, Right<br>T Temporal Artery, Left<br>U Thyroid Artery, Right<br>V Thyroid Artery, Left<br>Y Upper Artery | 0 Open<br>3 Percutaneous<br>4 Percutaneous Endoscopic | Z No Device | Z No Qualifier |

**0** Medical and Surgical
**3** Upper Arteries
**7** Dilation: Expanding an orifice or the lumen of a tubular body part

| Character 4<br>Body Part | Character 5<br>Approach | Character 6<br>Device | Character 7<br>Qualifier |
|---|---|---|---|
| 0 Internal Mammary Artery, Right | 0 Open | 4 Intraluminal Device, Drug-eluting | Z No Qualifier |
| 1 Internal Mammary Artery, Left | 3 Percutaneous | D Intraluminal Device | |
| 2 Innominate Artery | 4 Percutaneous Endoscopic | Z No Device | |
| 3 Subclavian Artery, Right | | | |
| 4 Subclavian Artery, Left | | | |
| 5 Axillary Artery, Right | | | |
| 6 Axillary Artery, Left | | | |
| 7 Brachial Artery, Right | | | |
| 8 Brachial Artery, Left | | | |
| 9 Ulnar Artery, Right | | | |
| A Ulnar Artery, Left | | | |
| B Radial Artery, Right | | | |
| C Radial Artery, Left | | | |
| D Hand Artery, Right | | | |
| F Hand Artery, Left | | | |
| G Intracranial Artery  N C | | | |
| H Common Carotid Artery, Right | | | |
| J Common Carotid Artery, Left | | | |
| K Internal Carotid Artery, Right | | | |
| L Internal Carotid Artery, Left | | | |
| M External Carotid Artery, Right | | | |
| N External Carotid Artery, Left | | | |
| P Vertebral Artery, Right | | | |
| Q Vertebral Artery, Left | | | |
| R Face Artery | | | |
| S Temporal Artery, Right | | | |
| T Temporal Artery, Left | | | |
| U Thyroid Artery, Right | | | |
| V Thyroid Artery, Left | | | |
| Y Upper Artery | | | |

N C 037G(3,4)ZZ

**0** Medical and Surgical
**3** Upper Arteries
**9** Drainage: Taking or letting out fluids and/or gases from a body part

| Character 4 Body Part | Character 5 Approach | Character 6 Device | Character 7 Qualifier |
|---|---|---|---|
| 0 Internal Mammary Artery, Right | 0 Open | 0 Drainage Device | Z No Qualifier |
| 1 Internal Mammary Artery, Left | 3 Percutaneous | | |
| 2 Innominate Artery | 4 Percutaneous Endoscopic | | |
| 3 Subclavian Artery, Right | | | |
| 4 Subclavian Artery, Left | | | |
| 5 Axillary Artery, Right | | | |
| 6 Axillary Artery, Left | | | |
| 7 Brachial Artery, Right | | | |
| 8 Brachial Artery, Left | | | |
| 9 Ulnar Artery, Right | | | |
| A Ulnar Artery, Left | | | |
| B Radial Artery, Right | | | |
| C Radial Artery, Left | | | |
| D Hand Artery, Right | | | |
| F Hand Artery, Left | | | |
| G Intracranial Artery | | | |
| H Common Carotid Artery, Right | | | |
| J Common Carotid Artery, Left | | | |
| K Internal Carotid Artery, Right | | | |
| L Internal Carotid Artery, Left | | | |
| M External Carotid Artery, Right | | | |
| N External Carotid Artery, Left | | | |
| P Vertebral Artery, Right | | | |
| Q Vertebral Artery, Left | | | |
| R Face Artery | | | |
| S Temporal Artery, Right | | | |
| T Temporal Artery, Left | | | |
| U Thyroid Artery, Right | | | |
| V Thyroid Artery, Left | | | |
| Y Upper Artery | | | |

| Character 4 Body Part | Character 5 Approach | Character 6 Device | Character 7 Qualifier |
|---|---|---|---|
| 0 Internal Mammary Artery, Right | 0 Open | Z No Device | X Diagnostic |
| 1 Internal Mammary Artery, Left | 3 Percutaneous | | Z No Qualifier |
| 2 Innominate Artery | 4 Percutaneous Endoscopic | | |
| 3 Subclavian Artery, Right | | | |
| 4 Subclavian Artery, Left | | | |
| 5 Axillary Artery, Right | | | |
| 6 Axillary Artery, Left | | | |
| 7 Brachial Artery, Right | | | |
| 8 Brachial Artery, Left | | | |
| 9 Ulnar Artery, Right | | | |
| A Ulnar Artery, Left | | | |
| B Radial Artery, Right | | | |
| C Radial Artery, Left | | | |
| D Hand Artery, Right | | | |
| F Hand Artery, Left | | | |
| G Intracranial Artery | | | |
| H Common Carotid Artery, Right | | | |
| J Common Carotid Artery, Left | | | |
| K Internal Carotid Artery, Right | | | |
| L Internal Carotid Artery, Left | | | |
| M External Carotid Artery, Right | | | |
| N External Carotid Artery, Left | | | |
| P Vertebral Artery, Right | | | |
| Q Vertebral Artery, Left | | | |
| R Face Artery | | | |
| S Temporal Artery, Right | | | |
| T Temporal Artery, Left | | | |
| U Thyroid Artery, Right | | | |
| V Thyroid Artery, Left | | | |
| Y Upper Artery | | | |

**0** Medical and Surgical
**3** Upper Arteries
**B** Excision: Cutting out or off, without replacement, a portion of a body part

| Character 4<br>Body Part | Character 5<br>Approach | Character 6<br>Device | Character 7<br>Qualifier |
|---|---|---|---|
| 0 Internal Mammary Artery, Right | 0 Open | Z No Device | X Diagnostic |
| 1 Internal Mammary Artery, Left | 3 Percutaneous | | Z No Qualifier |
| 2 Innominate Artery | 4 Percutaneous Endoscopic | | |
| 3 Subclavian Artery, Right | | | |
| 4 Subclavian Artery, Left | | | |
| 5 Axillary Artery, Right | | | |
| 6 Axillary Artery, Left | | | |
| 7 Brachial Artery, Right | | | |
| 8 Brachial Artery, Left | | | |
| 9 Ulnar Artery, Right | | | |
| A Ulnar Artery, Left | | | |
| B Radial Artery, Right | | | |
| C Radial Artery, Left | | | |
| D Hand Artery, Right | | | |
| F Hand Artery, Left | | | |
| G Intracranial Artery | | | |
| H Common Carotid Artery, Right | | | |
| J Common Carotid Artery, Left | | | |
| K Internal Carotid Artery, Right | | | |
| L Internal Carotid Artery, Left | | | |
| M External Carotid Artery, Right | | | |
| N External Carotid Artery, Left | | | |
| P Vertebral Artery, Right | | | |
| Q Vertebral Artery, Left | | | |
| R Face Artery | | | |
| S Temporal Artery, Right | | | |
| T Temporal Artery, Left | | | |
| U Thyroid Artery, Right | | | |
| V Thyroid Artery, Left | | | |
| Y Upper Artery | | | |

**0** Medical and Surgical
**3** Upper Arteries
**C** Extirpation: Taking or cutting out solid matter from a body part

| Character 4<br>Body Part | Character 5<br>Approach | Character 6<br>Device | Character 7<br>Qualifier |
|---|---|---|---|
| 0 Internal Mammary Artery, Right | 0 Open | Z No Device | Z No Qualifier |
| 1 Internal Mammary Artery, Left | 3 Percutaneous | | |
| 2 Innominate Artery | 4 Percutaneous Endoscopic | | |
| 3 Subclavian Artery, Right | | | |
| 4 Subclavian Artery, Left | | | |
| 5 Axillary Artery, Right | | | |
| 6 Axillary Artery, Left | | | |
| 7 Brachial Artery, Right | | | |
| 8 Brachial Artery, Left | | | |
| 9 Ulnar Artery, Right | | | |
| A Ulnar Artery, Left | | | |
| B Radial Artery, Right | | | |
| C Radial Artery, Left | | | |
| D Hand Artery, Right | | | |
| F Hand Artery, Left | | | |
| G Intracranial Artery  N C | | | |
| H Common Carotid Artery, Right | | | |
| J Common Carotid Artery, Left | | | |
| K Internal Carotid Artery, Right | | | |
| L Internal Carotid Artery, Left | | | |
| M External Carotid Artery, Right | | | |
| N External Carotid Artery, Left | | | |
| P Vertebral Artery, Right | | | |
| Q Vertebral Artery, Left | | | |
| R Face Artery | | | |
| S Temporal Artery, Right | | | |
| T Temporal Artery, Left | | | |
| U Thyroid Artery, Right | | | |
| V Thyroid Artery, Left | | | |
| Y Upper Artery | | | |

N C 03CG(3,4)ZZ

**0** Medical and Surgical
**3** Upper Arteries
**H** Insertion: Putting in a nonbiological appliance that monitors, assists, performs, or prevents a physiological function but does not physically take the place of a body part

| Character 4<br>Body Part | Character 5<br>Approach | Character 6<br>Device | Character 7<br>Qualifier |
|---|---|---|---|
| 0 Internal Mammary Artery, Right<br>1 Internal Mammary Artery, Left<br>2 Innominate Artery<br>3 Subclavian Artery, Right<br>4 Subclavian Artery, Left<br>5 Axillary Artery, Right<br>6 Axillary Artery, Left<br>7 Brachial Artery, Right<br>8 Brachial Artery, Left<br>9 Ulnar Artery, Right<br>A Ulnar Artery, Left<br>B Radial Artery, Right<br>C Radial Artery, Left<br>D Hand Artery, Right<br>F Hand Artery, Left<br>G Intracranial Artery<br>H Common Carotid Artery, Right<br>J Common Carotid Artery, Left<br>M External Carotid Artery, Right<br>N External Carotid Artery, Left<br>P Vertebral Artery, Right<br>Q Vertebral Artery, Left<br>R Face Artery<br>S Temporal Artery, Right<br>T Temporal Artery, Left<br>U Thyroid Artery, Right<br>V Thyroid Artery, Left | 0 Open<br>3 Percutaneous<br>4 Percutaneous Endoscopic | 3 Infusion Device<br>D Intraluminal Device | Z No Qualifier |
| K Internal Carotid Artery, Right<br>L Internal Carotid Artery, Left | 0 Open<br>3 Percutaneous<br>4 Percutaneous Endoscopic | 3 Infusion Device<br>D Intraluminal Device<br>M Stimulator Lead | Z No Qualifier |
| Y Upper Artery | 0 Open<br>3 Percutaneous<br>4 Percutaneous Endoscopic | 2 Monitoring Device<br>3 Infusion Device<br>D Intraluminal Device | Z No Qualifier |

**0** Medical and Surgical
**3** Upper Arteries
**J** Inspection: Visually and/or manually exploring a body part

| Character 4<br>Body Part | Character 5<br>Approach | Character 6<br>Device | Character 7<br>Qualifier |
|---|---|---|---|
| Y Upper Artery | 0 Open<br>3 Percutaneous<br>4 Percutaneous Endoscopic<br>X External | Z No Device | Z No Qualifier |

**0** Medical and Surgical
**3** Upper Arteries
**L** Occlusion: Completely closing an orifice or the lumen of a tubular body part

| Character 4<br>Body Part | Character 5<br>Approach | Character 6<br>Device | Character 7<br>Qualifier |
|---|---|---|---|
| 0 Internal Mammary Artery, Right<br>1 Internal Mammary Artery, Left<br>2 Innominate Artery<br>3 Subclavian Artery, Right<br>4 Subclavian Artery, Left<br>5 Axillary Artery, Right<br>6 Axillary Artery, Left<br>7 Brachial Artery, Right<br>8 Brachial Artery, Left<br>9 Ulnar Artery, Right<br>A Ulnar Artery, Left<br>B Radial Artery, Right<br>C Radial Artery, Left<br>D Hand Artery, Right<br>F Hand Artery, Left<br>R Face Artery<br>S Temporal Artery, Right<br>T Temporal Artery, Left<br>U Thyroid Artery, Right<br>V Thyroid Artery, Left<br>Y Upper Artery | 0 Open<br>3 Percutaneous<br>4 Percutaneous Endoscopic | C Extraluminal Device<br>D Intraluminal Device<br>Z No Device | Z No Qualifier |
| G Intracranial Artery<br>H Common Carotid Artery, Right<br>J Common Carotid Artery, Left<br>K Internal Carotid Artery, Right<br>L Internal Carotid Artery, Left<br>M External Carotid Artery, Right<br>N External Carotid Artery, Left<br>P Vertebral Artery, Right<br>Q Vertebral Artery, Left | 0 Open<br>3 Percutaneous<br>4 Percutaneous Endoscopic | B Intraluminal Device, Bioactive<br>C Extraluminal Device<br>D Intraluminal Device<br>Z No Device | Z No Qualifier |

**0** Medical and Surgical
**3** Upper Arteries
**N** Release: Freeing a body part from an abnormal physical constraint by cutting or by the use of force

| Character 4<br>Body Part | Character 5<br>Approach | Character 6<br>Device | Character 7<br>Qualifier |
|---|---|---|---|
| 0 Internal Mammary Artery, Right<br>1 Internal Mammary Artery, Left<br>2 Innominate Artery<br>3 Subclavian Artery, Right<br>4 Subclavian Artery, Left<br>5 Axillary Artery, Right<br>6 Axillary Artery, Left<br>7 Brachial Artery, Right<br>8 Brachial Artery, Left<br>9 Ulnar Artery, Right<br>A Ulnar Artery, Left<br>B Radial Artery, Right<br>C Radial Artery, Left<br>D Hand Artery, Right<br>F Hand Artery, Left<br>G Intracranial Artery<br>H Common Carotid Artery, Right<br>J Common Carotid Artery, Left<br>K Internal Carotid Artery, Right<br>L Internal Carotid Artery, Left<br>M External Carotid Artery, Right<br>N External Carotid Artery, Left<br>P Vertebral Artery, Right<br>Q Vertebral Artery, Left<br>R Face Artery<br>S Temporal Artery, Right<br>T Temporal Artery, Left<br>U Thyroid Artery, Right<br>V Thyroid Artery, Left<br>Y Upper Artery | 0 Open<br>3 Percutaneous<br>4 Percutaneous Endoscopic | Z No Device | Z No Qualifier |

**0** Medical and Surgical
**3** Upper Arteries
**P** Removal: Taking out or off a device from a body part

| Character 4<br>Body Part | Character 5<br>Approach | Character 6<br>Device | Character 7<br>Qualifier |
|---|---|---|---|
| Y Upper Artery | 0 Open<br>3 Percutaneous<br>4 Percutaneous Endoscopic | 0 Drainage Device<br>2 Monitoring Device<br>3 Infusion Device<br>7 Autologous Tissue Substitute<br>C Extraluminal Device<br>D Intraluminal Device<br>J Synthetic Substitute<br>K Nonautologous Tissue Substitute<br>M Stimulator Lead | Z No Qualifier |
| Y Upper Artery | X External | 0 Drainage Device<br>2 Monitoring Device<br>3 Infusion Device<br>D Intraluminal Device<br>M Stimulator Lead | Z No Qualifier |

**0** Medical and Surgical
**3** Upper Arteries
**Q** Repair: Restoring, to the extent possible, a body part to its normal anatomic structure and function

| Character 4<br>Body Part | Character 5<br>Approach | Character 6<br>Device | Character 7<br>Qualifier |
|---|---|---|---|
| 0 Internal Mammary Artery, Right<br>1 Internal Mammary Artery, Left<br>2 Innominate Artery<br>3 Subclavian Artery, Right<br>4 Subclavian Artery, Left<br>5 Axillary Artery, Right<br>6 Axillary Artery, Left<br>7 Brachial Artery, Right<br>8 Brachial Artery, Left<br>9 Ulnar Artery, Right<br>A Ulnar Artery, Left<br>B Radial Artery, Right<br>C Radial Artery, Left<br>D Hand Artery, Right<br>F Hand Artery, Left<br>G Intracranial Artery<br>H Common Carotid Artery, Right<br>J Common Carotid Artery, Left<br>K Internal Carotid Artery, Right<br>L Internal Carotid Artery, Left<br>M External Carotid Artery, Right<br>N External Carotid Artery, Left<br>P Vertebral Artery, Right<br>Q Vertebral Artery, Left<br>R Face Artery<br>S Temporal Artery, Right<br>T Temporal Artery, Left<br>U Thyroid Artery, Right<br>V Thyroid Artery, Left<br>Y Upper Artery | 0 Open<br>3 Percutaneous<br>4 Percutaneous Endoscopic | Z No Device | Z No Qualifier |

**0** Medical and Surgical
**3** Upper Arteries
**R** Replacement: Putting in or on biological or synthetic material that physically takes the place and/or function of all or a portion of a body part

| Character 4<br>Body Part | Character 5<br>Approach | Character 6<br>Device | Character 7<br>Qualifier |
|---|---|---|---|
| 0 Internal Mammary Artery, Right<br>1 Internal Mammary Artery, Left<br>2 Innominate Artery<br>3 Subclavian Artery, Right<br>4 Subclavian Artery, Left<br>5 Axillary Artery, Right<br>6 Axillary Artery, Left<br>7 Brachial Artery, Right<br>8 Brachial Artery, Left<br>9 Ulnar Artery, Right<br>A Ulnar Artery, Left<br>B Radial Artery, Right<br>C Radial Artery, Left<br>D Hand Artery, Right<br>F Hand Artery, Left<br>G Intracranial Artery<br>H Common Carotid Artery, Right<br>J Common Carotid Artery, Left<br>K Internal Carotid Artery, Right<br>L Internal Carotid Artery, Left<br>M External Carotid Artery, Right<br>N External Carotid Artery, Left<br>P Vertebral Artery, Right<br>Q Vertebral Artery, Left<br>R Face Artery<br>S Temporal Artery, Right<br>T Temporal Artery, Left<br>U Thyroid Artery, Right<br>V Thyroid Artery, Left<br>Y Upper Artery | 0 Open<br>4 Percutaneous Endoscopic | 7 Autologous Tissue Substitute<br>J Synthetic Substitute<br>K Nonautologous Tissue Substitute | Z No Qualifier |

**0** Medical and Surgical
**3** Upper Arteries
**S** Reposition: Moving to its normal location, or other suitable location, all or a portion of a body part

| Character 4<br>Body Part | Character 5<br>Approach | Character 6<br>Device | Character 7<br>Qualifier |
|---|---|---|---|
| 0 Internal Mammary Artery, Right<br>1 Internal Mammary Artery, Left<br>2 Innominate Artery<br>3 Subclavian Artery, Right<br>4 Subclavian Artery, Left<br>5 Axillary Artery, Right<br>6 Axillary Artery, Left<br>7 Brachial Artery, Right<br>8 Brachial Artery, Left<br>9 Ulnar Artery, Right<br>A Ulnar Artery, Left<br>B Radial Artery, Right<br>C Radial Artery, Left<br>D Hand Artery, Right<br>F Hand Artery, Left<br>G Intracranial Artery<br>H Common Carotid Artery, Right<br>J Common Carotid Artery, Left<br>K Internal Carotid Artery, Right<br>L Internal Carotid Artery, Left<br>M External Carotid Artery, Right<br>N External Carotid Artery, Left<br>P Vertebral Artery, Right<br>Q Vertebral Artery, Left<br>R Face Artery<br>S Temporal Artery, Right<br>T Temporal Artery, Left<br>U Thyroid Artery, Right<br>V Thyroid Artery, Left<br>Y Upper Artery | 0 Open<br>3 Percutaneous<br>4 Percutaneous Endoscopic | Z No Device | Z No Qualifier |

**0** Medical and Surgical
**3** Upper Arteries
**U** Supplement: Putting in or on biological or synthetic material that physically reinforces and/or augments the function of a portion of a body part

| Character 4<br>Body Part | Character 5<br>Approach | Character 6<br>Device | Character 7<br>Qualifier |
|---|---|---|---|
| 0 Internal Mammary Artery, Right<br>1 Internal Mammary Artery, Left<br>2 Innominate Artery<br>3 Subclavian Artery, Right<br>4 Subclavian Artery, Left<br>5 Axillary Artery, Right<br>6 Axillary Artery, Left<br>7 Brachial Artery, Right<br>8 Brachial Artery, Left<br>9 Ulnar Artery, Right<br>A Ulnar Artery, Left<br>B Radial Artery, Right<br>C Radial Artery, Left<br>D Hand Artery, Right<br>F Hand Artery, Left<br>G Intracranial Artery<br>H Common Carotid Artery, Right<br>J Common Carotid Artery, Left<br>K Internal Carotid Artery, Right<br>L Internal Carotid Artery, Left<br>M External Carotid Artery, Right<br>N External Carotid Artery, Left<br>P Vertebral Artery, Right<br>Q Vertebral Artery, Left<br>R Face Artery<br>S Temporal Artery, Right<br>T Temporal Artery, Left<br>U Thyroid Artery, Right<br>V Thyroid Artery, Left<br>Y Upper Artery | 0 Open<br>3 Percutaneous<br>4 Percutaneous Endoscopic | 7 Autologous Tissue Substitute<br>J Synthetic Substitute<br>K Nonautologous Tissue Substitute | Z No Qualifier |

**0** Medical and Surgical
**3** Upper Arteries
**V** Restriction: Partially closing an orifice or the lumen of a tubular body part

| Character 4<br>Body Part | Character 5<br>Approach | Character 6<br>Device | Character 7<br>Qualifier |
|---|---|---|---|
| 0 Internal Mammary Artery, Right<br>1 Internal Mammary Artery, Left<br>2 Innominate Artery<br>3 Subclavian Artery, Right<br>4 Subclavian Artery, Left<br>5 Axillary Artery, Right<br>6 Axillary Artery, Left<br>7 Brachial Artery, Right<br>8 Brachial Artery, Left<br>9 Ulnar Artery, Right<br>A Ulnar Artery, Left<br>B Radial Artery, Right<br>C Radial Artery, Left<br>D Hand Artery, Right<br>F Hand Artery, Left<br>R Face Artery<br>S Temporal Artery, Right<br>T Temporal Artery, Left<br>U Thyroid Artery, Right<br>V Thyroid Artery, Left<br>Y Upper Artery | 0 Open<br>3 Percutaneous<br>4 Percutaneous Endoscopic | C Extraluminal Device<br>D Intraluminal Device<br>Z No Device | Z No Qualifier |
| G Intracranial Artery<br>H Common Carotid Artery, Right<br>J Common Carotid Artery, Left<br>K Internal Carotid Artery, Right<br>L Internal Carotid Artery, Left<br>M External Carotid Artery, Right<br>N External Carotid Artery, Left<br>P Vertebral Artery, Right<br>Q Vertebral Artery, Left | 0 Open<br>3 Percutaneous<br>4 Percutaneous Endoscopic | B Intraluminal Device, Bioactive<br>C Extraluminal Device<br>D Intraluminal Device<br>Z No Device | Z No Qualifier |

| | N C Non-covered | L C Limited Coverage | AHA AHA Coding Clinic |

**0** Medical and Surgical
**3** Upper Arteries
**W** Revision: Correcting, to the extent possible, a portion of a malfunctioning device or the position of a displaced device

| Character 4<br>Body Part | Character 5<br>Approach | Character 6<br>Device | Character 7<br>Qualifier |
|---|---|---|---|
| Y Upper Artery | 0 Open<br>3 Percutaneous<br>4 Percutaneous Endoscopic<br>X External | 0 Drainage Device<br>2 Monitoring Device<br>3 Infusion Device<br>7 Autologous Tissue Substitute<br>C Extraluminal Device<br>D Intraluminal Device<br>J Synthetic Substitute<br>K Nonautologous Tissue Substitute<br>M Stimulator Lead | Z No Qualifier |

# Lower Arteries | 041 – 04W

**0** Medical and Surgical
**4** Lower Arteries
**1** Bypass: Altering the route of passage of the contents of a tubular body part

| Character 4<br>Body Part | Character 5<br>Approach | Character 6<br>Device | Character 7<br>Qualifier |
|---|---|---|---|
| 0 Abdominal Aorta<br>C Common Iliac Artery, Right<br>D Common Iliac Artery, Left | 0 Open<br>4 Percutaneous Endoscopic | 9 Autologous Venous Tissue<br>A Autologous Arterial Tissue<br>J Synthetic Substitute<br>K Nonautologous Tissue Substitute<br>Z No Device | 0 Abdominal Aorta<br>1 Celiac Artery<br>2 Mesenteric Artery<br>3 Renal Artery, Right<br>4 Renal Artery, Left<br>5 Renal Artery, Bilateral<br>6 Common Iliac Artery, Right<br>7 Common Iliac Artery, Left<br>8 Common Iliac Arteries, Bilateral<br>9 Internal Iliac Artery, Right<br>B Internal Iliac Artery, Left<br>C Internal Iliac Arteries, Bilateral<br>D External Iliac Artery, Right<br>F External Iliac Artery, Left<br>G External Iliac Arteries, Bilateral<br>H Femoral Artery, Right<br>J Femoral Artery, Left<br>K Femoral Arteries, Bilateral<br>Q Lower Extremity Artery<br>R Lower Artery |
| 4 Splenic Artery | 0 Open<br>4 Percutaneous Endoscopic | 9 Autologous Venous Tissue<br>A Autologous Arterial Tissue<br>J Synthetic Substitute<br>K Nonautologous Tissue Substitute<br>Z No Device | 3 Renal Artery, Right<br>4 Renal Artery, Left<br>5 Renal Artery, Bilateral |
| E Internal Iliac Artery, Right<br>F Internal Iliac Artery, Left<br>H External Iliac Artery, Right<br>J External Iliac Artery, Left | 0 Open<br>4 Percutaneous Endoscopic | 9 Autologous Venous Tissue<br>A Autologous Arterial Tissue<br>J Synthetic Substitute<br>K Nonautologous Tissue Substitute<br>Z No Device | 9 Internal Iliac Artery, Right<br>B Internal Iliac Artery, Left<br>C Internal Iliac Arteries, Bilateral<br>D External Iliac Artery, Right<br>F External Iliac Artery, Left<br>G External Iliac Arteries, Bilateral<br>H Femoral Artery, Right<br>J Femoral Artery, Left<br>K Femoral Arteries, Bilateral<br>P Foot Artery<br>Q Lower Extremity Artery |
| K Femoral Artery, Right<br>L Femoral Artery, Left | 0 Open<br>4 Percutaneous Endoscopic | 9 Autologous Venous Tissue<br>A Autologous Arterial Tissue<br>J Synthetic Substitute<br>K Nonautologous Tissue Substitute<br>Z No Device | H Femoral Artery, Right<br>J Femoral Artery, Left<br>K Femoral Arteries, Bilateral<br>L Popliteal Artery<br>M Peroneal Artery<br>N Posterior Tibial Artery<br>P Foot Artery<br>Q Lower Extremity Artery<br>S Lower Extremity Vein |
| M Popliteal Artery, Right<br>N Popliteal Artery, Left | 0 Open<br>4 Percutaneous Endoscopic | 9 Autologous Venous Tissue<br>A Autologous Arterial Tissue<br>J Synthetic Substitute<br>K Nonautologous Tissue Substitute<br>Z No Device | L Popliteal Artery<br>M Peroneal Artery<br>P Foot Artery<br>Q Lower Extremity Artery<br>S Lower Extremity Vein |

**0** Medical and Surgical
**4** Lower Arteries
**5** Destruction: Physical eradication of all or a portion of a body part by the direct use of energy, force, or a destructive agent

| Character 4<br>Body Part | Character 5<br>Approach | Character 6<br>Device | Character 7<br>Qualifier |
|---|---|---|---|
| 0 Abdominal Aorta<br>1 Celiac Artery<br>2 Gastric Artery<br>3 Hepatic Artery<br>4 Splenic Artery<br>5 Superior Mesenteric Artery<br>6 Colic Artery, Right<br>7 Colic Artery, Left<br>8 Colic Artery, Middle<br>9 Renal Artery, Right<br>A Renal Artery, Left<br>B Inferior Mesenteric Artery<br>C Common Iliac Artery, Right<br>D Common Iliac Artery, Left<br>E Internal Iliac Artery, Right<br>F Internal Iliac Artery, Left<br>H External Iliac Artery, Right<br>J External Iliac Artery, Left<br>K Femoral Artery, Right<br>L Femoral Artery, Left<br>M Popliteal Artery, Right<br>N Popliteal Artery, Left<br>P Anterior Tibial Artery, Right<br>Q Anterior Tibial Artery, Left<br>R Posterior Tibial Artery, Right<br>S Posterior Tibial Artery, Left<br>T Peroneal Artery, Right<br>U Peroneal Artery, Left<br>V Foot Artery, Right<br>W Foot Artery, Left<br>Y Lower Artery | 0 Open<br>3 Percutaneous<br>4 Percutaneous Endoscopic | Z No Device | Z No Qualifier |

**0** Medical and Surgical
**4** Lower Arteries
**7** Dilation: Expanding an orifice or the lumen of a tubular body part

| Character 4<br>Body Part | Character 5<br>Approach | Character 6<br>Device | Character 7<br>Qualifier |
|---|---|---|---|
| 0 Abdominal Aorta<br>1 Celiac Artery<br>2 Gastric Artery<br>3 Hepatic Artery<br>4 Splenic Artery<br>5 Superior Mesenteric Artery<br>6 Colic Artery, Right<br>7 Colic Artery, Left<br>8 Colic Artery, Middle<br>9 Renal Artery, Right<br>A Renal Artery, Left<br>B Inferior Mesenteric Artery<br>C Common Iliac Artery, Right<br>D Common Iliac Artery, Left<br>E Internal Iliac Artery, Right<br>F Internal Iliac Artery, Left<br>H External Iliac Artery, Right<br>J External Iliac Artery, Left<br>K Femoral Artery, Right<br>L Femoral Artery, Left<br>M Popliteal Artery, Right<br>N Popliteal Artery, Left<br>P Anterior Tibial Artery, Right<br>Q Anterior Tibial Artery, Left<br>R Posterior Tibial Artery, Right<br>S Posterior Tibial Artery, Left<br>T Peroneal Artery, Right<br>U Peroneal Artery, Left<br>V Foot Artery, Right<br>W Foot Artery, Left<br>Y Lower Artery | 0 Open<br>3 Percutaneous<br>4 Percutaneous Endoscopic | 4 Intraluminal Device, Drug-eluting<br>D Intraluminal Device<br>Z No Device | Z No Qualifier |

**0** Medical and Surgical
**4** Lower Arteries
**9** Drainage: Taking or letting out fluids and/or gases from a body part

| Character 4<br>Body Part | Character 5<br>Approach | Character 6<br>Device | Character 7<br>Qualifier |
|---|---|---|---|
| 0 Abdominal Aorta<br>1 Celiac Artery<br>2 Gastric Artery<br>3 Hepatic Artery<br>4 Splenic Artery<br>5 Superior Mesenteric Artery<br>6 Colic Artery, Right<br>7 Colic Artery, Left<br>8 Colic Artery, Middle<br>9 Renal Artery, Right<br>A Renal Artery, Left<br>B Inferior Mesenteric Artery<br>C Common Iliac Artery, Right<br>D Common Iliac Artery, Left<br>E Internal Iliac Artery, Right<br>F Internal Iliac Artery, Left<br>H External Iliac Artery, Right<br>J External Iliac Artery, Left<br>K Femoral Artery, Right<br>L Femoral Artery, Left<br>M Popliteal Artery, Right<br>N Popliteal Artery, Left<br>P Anterior Tibial Artery, Right<br>Q Anterior Tibial Artery, Left<br>R Posterior Tibial Artery, Right<br>S Posterior Tibial Artery, Left<br>T Peroneal Artery, Right<br>U Peroneal Artery, Left<br>V Foot Artery, Right<br>W Foot Artery, Left<br>Y Lower Artery | 0 Open<br>3 Percutaneous<br>4 Percutaneous Endoscopic | 0 Drainage Device | Z No Qualifier |
| 0 Abdominal Aorta<br>1 Celiac Artery<br>2 Gastric Artery<br>3 Hepatic Artery<br>4 Splenic Artery<br>5 Superior Mesenteric Artery<br>6 Colic Artery, Right<br>7 Colic Artery, Left<br>8 Colic Artery, Middle<br>9 Renal Artery, Right<br>A Renal Artery, Left<br>B Inferior Mesenteric Artery<br>C Common Iliac Artery, Right<br>D Common Iliac Artery, Left<br>E Internal Iliac Artery, Right<br>F Internal Iliac Artery, Left<br>H External Iliac Artery, Right<br>J External Iliac Artery, Left<br>K Femoral Artery, Right<br>L Femoral Artery, Left<br>M Popliteal Artery, Right<br>N Popliteal Artery, Left<br>P Anterior Tibial Artery, Right<br>Q Anterior Tibial Artery, Left<br>R Posterior Tibial Artery, Right<br>S Posterior Tibial Artery, Left<br>T Peroneal Artery, Right<br>U Peroneal Artery, Left<br>V Foot Artery, Right<br>W Foot Artery, Left<br>Y Lower Artery | 0 Open<br>3 Percutaneous<br>4 Percutaneous Endoscopic | Z No Device | X Diagnostic<br>Z No Qualifier |

**0** Medical and Surgical
**4** Lower Arteries
**B** Excision: Cutting out or off, without replacement, a portion of a body part

| Character 4 Body Part | Character 5 Approach | Character 6 Device | Character 7 Qualifier |
|---|---|---|---|
| 0 Abdominal Aorta | 0 Open | Z No Device | X Diagnostic |
| 1 Celiac Artery | 3 Percutaneous | | Z No Qualifier |
| 2 Gastric Artery | 4 Percutaneous Endoscopic | | |
| 3 Hepatic Artery | | | |
| 4 Splenic Artery | | | |
| 5 Superior Mesenteric Artery | | | |
| 6 Colic Artery, Right | | | |
| 7 Colic Artery, Left | | | |
| 8 Colic Artery, Middle | | | |
| 9 Renal Artery, Right | | | |
| A Renal Artery, Left | | | |
| B Inferior Mesenteric Artery | | | |
| C Common Iliac Artery, Right | | | |
| D Common Iliac Artery, Left | | | |
| E Internal Iliac Artery, Right | | | |
| F Internal Iliac Artery, Left | | | |
| H External Iliac Artery, Right | | | |
| J External Iliac Artery, Left | | | |
| K Femoral Artery, Right | | | |
| L Femoral Artery, Left | | | |
| M Popliteal Artery, Right | | | |
| N Popliteal Artery, Left | | | |
| P Anterior Tibial Artery, Right | | | |
| Q Anterior Tibial Artery, Left | | | |
| R Posterior Tibial Artery, Right | | | |
| S Posterior Tibial Artery, Left | | | |
| T Peroneal Artery, Right | | | |
| U Peroneal Artery, Left | | | |
| V Foot Artery, Right | | | |
| W Foot Artery, Left | | | |
| Y Lower Artery | | | |

**0** Medical and Surgical
**4** Lower Arteries
**C** Extirpation: Taking or cutting out solid matter from a body part

| Character 4 Body Part | Character 5 Approach | Character 6 Device | Character 7 Qualifier |
|---|---|---|---|
| 0 Abdominal Aorta | 0 Open | Z No Device | Z No Qualifier |
| 1 Celiac Artery | 3 Percutaneous | | |
| 2 Gastric Artery | 4 Percutaneous Endoscopic | | |
| 3 Hepatic Artery | | | |
| 4 Splenic Artery | | | |
| 5 Superior Mesenteric Artery | | | |
| 6 Colic Artery, Right | | | |
| 7 Colic Artery, Left | | | |
| 8 Colic Artery, Middle | | | |
| 9 Renal Artery, Right | | | |
| A Renal Artery, Left | | | |
| B Inferior Mesenteric Artery | | | |
| C Common Iliac Artery, Right | | | |
| D Common Iliac Artery, Left | | | |
| E Internal Iliac Artery, Right | | | |
| F Internal Iliac Artery, Left | | | |
| H External Iliac Artery, Right | | | |
| J External Iliac Artery, Left | | | |
| K Femoral Artery, Right | | | |
| L Femoral Artery, Left | | | |
| M Popliteal Artery, Right | | | |
| N Popliteal Artery, Left | | | |
| P Anterior Tibial Artery, Right | | | |
| Q Anterior Tibial Artery, Left | | | |
| R Posterior Tibial Artery, Right | | | |
| S Posterior Tibial Artery, Left | | | |
| T Peroneal Artery, Right | | | |
| U Peroneal Artery, Left | | | |
| V Foot Artery, Right | | | |
| W Foot Artery, Left | | | |
| Y Lower Artery | | | |

**0** Medical and Surgical
**4** Lower Arteries
**H** Insertion: Putting in a nonbiological appliance that monitors, assists, performs, or prevents a physiological function but does not physically take the place of a body part

| Character 4<br>Body Part | Character 5<br>Approach | Character 6<br>Device | Character 7<br>Qualifier |
|---|---|---|---|
| 0  Abdominal Aorta<br>Y  Lower Artery | 0  Open<br>3  Percutaneous<br>4  Percutaneous Endoscopic | 2  Monitoring Device<br>3  Infusion Device<br>D  Intraluminal Device | Z  No Qualifier |
| 1  Celiac Artery<br>2  Gastric Artery<br>3  Hepatic Artery<br>4  Splenic Artery<br>5  Superior Mesenteric Artery<br>6  Colic Artery, Right<br>7  Colic Artery, Left<br>8  Colic Artery, Middle<br>9  Renal Artery, Right<br>A  Renal Artery, Left<br>B  Inferior Mesenteric Artery<br>C  Common Iliac Artery, Right<br>D  Common Iliac Artery, Left<br>E  Internal Iliac Artery, Right<br>F  Internal Iliac Artery, Left<br>H  External Iliac Artery, Right<br>J  External Iliac Artery, Left<br>K  Femoral Artery, Right<br>L  Femoral Artery, Left<br>M  Popliteal Artery, Right<br>N  Popliteal Artery, Left<br>P  Anterior Tibial Artery, Right<br>Q  Anterior Tibial Artery, Left<br>R  Posterior Tibial Artery, Right<br>S  Posterior Tibial Artery, Left<br>T  Peroneal Artery, Right<br>U  Peroneal Artery, Left<br>V  Foot Artery, Right<br>W  Foot Artery, Left | 0  Open<br>3  Percutaneous<br>4  Percutaneous Endoscopic | 3  Infusion Device<br>D  Intraluminal Device | Z  No Qualifier |

**0** Medical and Surgical
**4** Lower Arteries
**J** Inspection: Visually and/or manually exploring a body part

| Character 4<br>Body Part | Character 5<br>Approach | Character 6<br>Device | Character 7<br>Qualifier |
|---|---|---|---|
| Y  Lower Artery | 0  Open<br>3  Percutaneous<br>4  Percutaneous Endoscopic<br>X  External | Z  No Device | Z  No Qualifier |

**0** Medical and Surgical
**4** Lower Arteries
**L** Occlusion: Completely closing an orifice or the lumen of a tubular body part

| Character 4 Body Part | Character 5 Approach | Character 6 Device | Character 7 Qualifier |
|---|---|---|---|
| 0 Abdominal Aorta<br>1 Celiac Artery<br>2 Gastric Artery<br>3 Hepatic Artery<br>4 Splenic Artery<br>5 Superior Mesenteric Artery<br>6 Colic Artery, Right<br>7 Colic Artery, Left<br>8 Colic Artery, Middle<br>9 Renal Artery, Right<br>A Renal Artery, Left<br>B Inferior Mesenteric Artery<br>C Common Iliac Artery, Right<br>D Common Iliac Artery, Left<br>H External Iliac Artery, Right<br>J External Iliac Artery, Left<br>K Femoral Artery, Right<br>L Femoral Artery, Left<br>M Popliteal Artery, Right<br>N Popliteal Artery, Left<br>P Anterior Tibial Artery, Right<br>Q Anterior Tibial Artery, Left<br>R Posterior Tibial Artery, Right<br>S Posterior Tibial Artery, Left<br>T Peroneal Artery, Right<br>U Peroneal Artery, Left<br>V Foot Artery, Right<br>W Foot Artery, Left<br>Y Lower Artery | 0 Open<br>3 Percutaneous<br>4 Percutaneous Endoscopic | C Extraluminal Device<br>D Intraluminal Device<br>Z No Device | Z No Qualifier |
| E Internal Iliac Artery, Right | 0 Open<br>3 Percutaneous<br>4 Percutaneous Endoscopic | C Extraluminal Device<br>D Intraluminal Device<br>Z No Device | T Uterine Artery, Right ♀<br>Z No Qualifier |
| F Internal Iliac Artery, Left | 0 Open<br>3 Percutaneous<br>4 Percutaneous Endoscopic | C Extraluminal Device<br>D Intraluminal Device<br>Z No Device | U Uterine Artery, Left ♀<br>Z No Qualifier |

**AHA:** 04LB3DZ - 1Q 2014, 24; 04L73DZ - 1Q 2014, 24

**0** Medical and Surgical
**4** Lower Arteries
**N** Release: Freeing a body part from an abnormal physical constraint by cutting or by the use of force

| Character 4 Body Part | Character 5 Approach | Character 6 Device | Character 7 Qualifier |
|---|---|---|---|
| 0 Abdominal Aorta<br>1 Celiac Artery<br>2 Gastric Artery<br>3 Hepatic Artery<br>4 Splenic Artery<br>5 Superior Mesenteric Artery<br>6 Colic Artery, Right<br>7 Colic Artery, Left<br>8 Colic Artery, Middle<br>9 Renal Artery, Right<br>A Renal Artery, Left<br>B Inferior Mesenteric Artery<br>C Common Iliac Artery, Right<br>D Common Iliac Artery, Left<br>E Internal Iliac Artery, Right<br>F Internal Iliac Artery, Left<br>H External Iliac Artery, Right<br>J External Iliac Artery, Left<br>K Femoral Artery, Right<br>L Femoral Artery, Left<br>M Popliteal Artery, Right<br>N Popliteal Artery, Left<br>P Anterior Tibial Artery, Right<br>Q Anterior Tibial Artery, Left<br>R Posterior Tibial Artery, Right<br>S Posterior Tibial Artery, Left<br>T Peroneal Artery, Right<br>U Peroneal Artery, Left<br>V Foot Artery, Right<br>W Foot Artery, Left<br>Y Lower Artery | 0 Open<br>3 Percutaneous<br>4 Percutaneous Endoscopic | Z No Device | Z No Qualifier |

**0** Medical and Surgical
**4** Lower Arteries
**P** Removal: Taking out or off a device from a body part

| Character 4 Body Part | Character 5 Approach | Character 6 Device | Character 7 Qualifier |
|---|---|---|---|
| Y  Lower Artery | 0  Open<br>3  Percutaneous<br>4  Percutaneous Endoscopic | 0  Drainage Device<br>2  Monitoring Device<br>3  Infusion Device<br>7  Autologous Tissue Substitute<br>C  Extraluminal Device<br>D  Intraluminal Device<br>J  Synthetic Substitute<br>K  Nonautologous Tissue Substitute | Z  No Qualifier |
| Y  Lower Artery | X  External | 0  Drainage Device<br>1  Radioactive Element<br>2  Monitoring Device<br>3  Infusion Device<br>D  Intraluminal Device | Z  No Qualifier |

**0** Medical and Surgical
**4** Lower Arteries
**Q** Repair: Restoring, to the extent possible, a body part to its normal anatomic structure and function

| Character 4 Body Part | Character 5 Approach | Character 6 Device | Character 7 Qualifier |
|---|---|---|---|
| 0  Abdominal Aorta<br>1  Celiac Artery<br>2  Gastric Artery<br>3  Hepatic Artery<br>4  Splenic Artery<br>5  Superior Mesenteric Artery<br>6  Colic Artery, Right<br>7  Colic Artery, Left<br>8  Colic Artery, Middle<br>9  Renal Artery, Right<br>A  Renal Artery, Left<br>B  Inferior Mesenteric Artery<br>C  Common Iliac Artery, Right<br>D  Common Iliac Artery, Left<br>E  Internal Iliac Artery, Right<br>F  Internal Iliac Artery, Left<br>H  External Iliac Artery, Right<br>J  External Iliac Artery, Left<br>K  Femoral Artery, Right<br>L  Femoral Artery, Left<br>M  Popliteal Artery, Right<br>N  Popliteal Artery, Left<br>P  Anterior Tibial Artery, Right<br>Q  Anterior Tibial Artery, Left<br>R  Posterior Tibial Artery, Right<br>S  Posterior Tibial Artery, Left<br>T  Peroneal Artery, Right<br>U  Peroneal Artery, Left<br>V  Foot Artery, Right<br>W  Foot Artery, Left<br>Y  Lower Artery | 0  Open<br>3  Percutaneous<br>4  Percutaneous Endoscopic | Z  No Device | Z  No Qualifier |

**AHA:** 04QK0ZZ - 1Q 2014, 22

♂ Male          ♀ Female          Ⓝ Ⓒ Non-covered          Ⓛ Ⓒ Limited Coverage          **AHA** *AHA Coding Clinic*

**0** Medical and Surgical
**4** Lower Arteries
**R** Replacement: Putting in or on biological or synthetic material that physically takes the place and/or function of all or a portion of a body part

| Character 4<br>Body Part | Character 5<br>Approach | Character 6<br>Device | Character 7<br>Qualifier |
|---|---|---|---|
| 0 Abdominal Aorta<br>1 Celiac Artery<br>2 Gastric Artery<br>3 Hepatic Artery<br>4 Splenic Artery<br>5 Superior Mesenteric Artery<br>6 Colic Artery, Right<br>7 Colic Artery, Left<br>8 Colic Artery, Middle<br>9 Renal Artery, Right<br>A Renal Artery, Left<br>B Inferior Mesenteric Artery<br>C Common Iliac Artery, Right<br>D Common Iliac Artery, Left<br>E Internal Iliac Artery, Right<br>F Internal Iliac Artery, Left<br>H External Iliac Artery, Right<br>J External Iliac Artery, Left<br>K Femoral Artery, Right<br>L Femoral Artery, Left<br>M Popliteal Artery, Right<br>N Popliteal Artery, Left<br>P Anterior Tibial Artery, Right<br>Q Anterior Tibial Artery, Left<br>R Posterior Tibial Artery, Right<br>S Posterior Tibial Artery, Left<br>T Peroneal Artery, Right<br>U Peroneal Artery, Left<br>V Foot Artery, Right<br>W Foot Artery, Left<br>Y Lower Artery | 0 Open<br>4 Percutaneous Endoscopic | 7 Autologous Tissue Substitute<br>J Synthetic Substitute<br>K Nonautologous Tissue Substitute | Z No Qualifier |

**0** Medical and Surgical
**4** Lower Arteries
**S** Reposition: Moving to its normal location, or other suitable location, all or a portion of a body part

| Character 4<br>Body Part | Character 5<br>Approach | Character 6<br>Device | Character 7<br>Qualifier |
|---|---|---|---|
| 0 Abdominal Aorta<br>1 Celiac Artery<br>2 Gastric Artery<br>3 Hepatic Artery<br>4 Splenic Artery<br>5 Superior Mesenteric Artery<br>6 Colic Artery, Right<br>7 Colic Artery, Left<br>8 Colic Artery, Middle<br>9 Renal Artery, Right<br>A Renal Artery, Left<br>B Inferior Mesenteric Artery<br>C Common Iliac Artery, Right<br>D Common Iliac Artery, Left<br>E Internal Iliac Artery, Right<br>F Internal Iliac Artery, Left<br>H External Iliac Artery, Right<br>J External Iliac Artery, Left<br>K Femoral Artery, Right<br>L Femoral Artery, Left<br>M Popliteal Artery, Right<br>N Popliteal Artery, Left<br>P Anterior Tibial Artery, Right<br>Q Anterior Tibial Artery, Left<br>R Posterior Tibial Artery, Right<br>S Posterior Tibial Artery, Left<br>T Peroneal Artery, Right<br>U Peroneal Artery, Left<br>V Foot Artery, Right<br>W Foot Artery, Left<br>Y Lower Artery | 0 Open<br>3 Percutaneous<br>4 Percutaneous Endoscopic | Z No Device | Z No Qualifier |

**0 Medical and Surgical**
**4 Lower Arteries**
**U Supplement: Putting in or on biological or synthetic material that physically reinforces and/or augments the function of a portion of a body part**

| Character 4<br>Body Part | Character 5<br>Approach | Character 6<br>Device | Character 7<br>Qualifier |
|---|---|---|---|
| 0 Abdominal Aorta<br>1 Celiac Artery<br>2 Gastric Artery<br>3 Hepatic Artery<br>4 Splenic Artery<br>5 Superior Mesenteric Artery<br>6 Colic Artery, Right<br>7 Colic Artery, Left<br>8 Colic Artery, Middle<br>9 Renal Artery, Right<br>A Renal Artery, Left<br>B Inferior Mesenteric Artery<br>C Common Iliac Artery, Right<br>D Common Iliac Artery, Left<br>E Internal Iliac Artery, Right<br>F Internal Iliac Artery, Left<br>H External Iliac Artery, Right<br>J External Iliac Artery, Left<br>K Femoral Artery, Right<br>L Femoral Artery, Left<br>M Popliteal Artery, Right<br>N Popliteal Artery, Left<br>P Anterior Tibial Artery, Right<br>Q Anterior Tibial Artery, Left<br>R Posterior Tibial Artery, Right<br>S Posterior Tibial Artery, Left<br>T Peroneal Artery, Right<br>U Peroneal Artery, Left<br>V Foot Artery, Right<br>W Foot Artery, Left<br>Y Lower Artery | 0 Open<br>3 Percutaneous<br>4 Percutaneous Endoscopic | 7 Autologous Tissue Substitute<br>J Synthetic Substitute<br>K Nonautologous Tissue Substitute | Z No Qualifier |

**AHA:** 04UK3JZ - 1Q 2014, 23

**0 Medical and Surgical**
**4 Lower Arteries**
**V Restriction: Partially closing an orifice or the lumen of a tubular body part**

| Character 4<br>Body Part | Character 5<br>Approach | Character 6<br>Device | Character 7<br>Qualifier |
|---|---|---|---|
| 0 Abdominal Aorta | 0 Open<br>3 Percutaneous<br>4 Percutaneous Endoscopic | C Extraluminal Device<br>Z No Device | Z No Qualifier |
| 0 Abdominal Aorta | 0 Open<br>3 Percutaneous<br>4 Percutaneous Endoscopic | D Intraluminal Device | J Temporary<br>Z No Qualifier |
| 1 Celiac Artery<br>2 Gastric Artery<br>3 Hepatic Artery<br>4 Splenic Artery<br>5 Superior Mesenteric Artery<br>6 Colic Artery, Right<br>7 Colic Artery, Left<br>8 Colic Artery, Middle<br>9 Renal Artery, Right<br>A Renal Artery, Left<br>B Inferior Mesenteric Artery<br>C Common Iliac Artery, Right<br>D Common Iliac Artery, Left<br>E Internal Iliac Artery, Right<br>F Internal Iliac Artery, Left<br>H External Iliac Artery, Right<br>J External Iliac Artery, Left<br>K Femoral Artery, Right<br>L Femoral Artery, Left<br>M Popliteal Artery, Right<br>N Popliteal Artery, Left<br>P Anterior Tibial Artery, Right<br>Q Anterior Tibial Artery, Left<br>R Posterior Tibial Artery, Right<br>S Posterior Tibial Artery, Left<br>T Peroneal Artery, Right<br>U Peroneal Artery, Left<br>V Foot Artery, Right<br>W Foot Artery, Left<br>Y Lower Artery<br>3 Hepatic Artery | 0 Open<br>3 Percutaneous<br>4 Percutaneous Endoscopic | C Extraluminal Device<br>D Intraluminal Device<br>Z No Device | Z No Qualifier |

**AHA:** 04V03DZ - 1Q 2014, 9

**0** Medical and Surgical
**4** Lower Arteries
**W** Revision: Correcting, to the extent possible, a portion of a malfunctioning device or the position of a displaced device

| Character 4<br>Body Part | Character 5<br>Approach | Character 6<br>Device | Character 7<br>Qualifier |
|---|---|---|---|
| Y  Lower Artery | 0  Open<br>3  Percutaneous<br>4  Percutaneous Endoscopic<br>X  External | 0  Drainage Device<br>2  Monitoring Device<br>3  Infusion Device<br>7  Autologous Tissue Substitute<br>C  Extraluminal Device<br>D  Intraluminal Device<br>J  Synthetic Substitute<br>K  Nonautologous Tissue Substitute | Z  No Qualifier |

**AHA:** 04WY3DZ - 1Q 2014, 10; 04WY37Z - 1Q 2014, 23

# Upper Veins | 051-05W

**0** Medical and Surgical
**5** Upper Veins
**1** Bypass: Altering the route of passage of the contents of a tubular body part

| Character 4<br>Body Part | Character 5<br>Approach | Character 6<br>Device | Character 7<br>Qualifier |
|---|---|---|---|
| 0  Azygos Vein<br>1  Hemiazygos Vein<br>3  Innominate Vein, Right<br>4  Innominate Vein, Left<br>5  Subclavian Vein, Right<br>6  Subclavian Vein, Left<br>7  Axillary Vein, Right<br>8  Axillary Vein, Left<br>9  Brachial Vein, Right<br>A  Brachial Vein, Left<br>B  Basilic Vein, Right<br>C  Basilic Vein, Left<br>D  Cephalic Vein, Right<br>F  Cephalic Vein, Left<br>G  Hand Vein, Right<br>H  Hand Vein, Left<br>L  Intracranial Vein<br>M  Internal Jugular Vein, Right<br>N  Internal Jugular Vein, Left<br>P  External Jugular Vein, Right<br>Q  External Jugular Vein, Left<br>R  Vertebral Vein, Right<br>S  Vertebral Vein, Left<br>T  Face Vein, Right<br>V  Face Vein, Left | 0  Open<br>4  Percutaneous Endoscopic | 7  Autologous Tissue Substitute<br>9  Autologous Venous Tissue<br>A  Autologous Arterial Tissue<br>J  Synthetic Substitute<br>K  Nonautologous Tissue Substitute<br>Z  No Device | Y  Upper Vein |

**0** Medical and Surgical
**5** Upper Veins
**5** Destruction: Physical eradication of all or a portion of a body part by the direct use of energy, force, or a destructive agent

| Character 4<br>Body Part | Character 5<br>Approach | Character 6<br>Device | Character 7<br>Qualifier |
|---|---|---|---|
| 0  Azygos Vein<br>1  Hemiazygos Vein<br>3  Innominate Vein, Right<br>4  Innominate Vein, Left<br>5  Subclavian Vein, Right<br>6  Subclavian Vein, Left<br>7  Axillary Vein, Right<br>8  Axillary Vein, Left<br>9  Brachial Vein, Right<br>A  Brachial Vein, Left<br>B  Basilic Vein, Right<br>C  Basilic Vein, Left<br>D  Cephalic Vein, Right<br>F  Cephalic Vein, Left<br>G  Hand Vein, Right<br>H  Hand Vein, Left<br>L  Intracranial Vein<br>M  Internal Jugular Vein, Right<br>N  Internal Jugular Vein, Left<br>P  External Jugular Vein, Right<br>Q  External Jugular Vein, Left<br>R  Vertebral Vein, Right<br>S  Vertebral Vein, Left<br>T  Face Vein, Right<br>V  Face Vein, Left<br>Y  Upper Vein | 0  Open<br>3  Percutaneous<br>4  Percutaneous Endoscopic | Z  No Device | Z  No Qualifier |

**0** Medical and Surgical
**5** Upper Veins
**7** Dilation: Expanding an orifice or the lumen of a tubular body part

| Character 4 Body Part | Character 5 Approach | Character 6 Device | Character 7 Qualifier |
|---|---|---|---|
| 0 Azygos Vein | 0 Open | D Intraluminal Device | Z No Qualifier |
| 1 Hemiazygos Vein | 3 Percutaneous | Z No Device | |
| 3 Innominate Vein, Right | 4 Percutaneous Endoscopic | | |
| 4 Innominate Vein, Left | | | |
| 5 Subclavian Vein, Right | | | |
| 6 Subclavian Vein, Left | | | |
| 7 Axillary Vein, Right | | | |
| 8 Axillary Vein, Left | | | |
| 9 Brachial Vein, Right | | | |
| A Brachial Vein, Left | | | |
| B Basilic Vein, Right | | | |
| C Basilic Vein, Left | | | |
| D Cephalic Vein, Right | | | |
| F Cephalic Vein, Left | | | |
| G Hand Vein, Right | | | |
| H Hand Vein, Left | | | |
| L Intracranial Vein  NC | | | |
| M Internal Jugular Vein, Right | | | |
| N Internal Jugular Vein, Left | | | |
| P External Jugular Vein, Right | | | |
| Q External Jugular Vein, Left | | | |
| R Vertebral Vein, Right | | | |
| S Vertebral Vein, Left | | | |
| T Face Vein, Right | | | |
| V Face Vein, Left | | | |
| Y Upper Vein | | | |

NC 057L(3,4)ZZ

| | | | |
|---|---|---|---|
| **0** Medical and Surgical | | | |
| **5** Upper Veins | | | |
| **9** Drainage: Taking or letting out fluids and/or gases from a body part | | | |

| Character 4 Body Part | Character 5 Approach | Character 6 Device | Character 7 Qualifier |
|---|---|---|---|
| 0 Azygos Vein | 0 Open | 0 Drainage Device | Z No Qualifier |
| 1 Hemiazygos Vein | 3 Percutaneous | | |
| 3 Innominate Vein, Right | 4 Percutaneous Endoscopic | | |
| 4 Innominate Vein, Left | | | |
| 5 Subclavian Vein, Right | | | |
| 6 Subclavian Vein, Left | | | |
| 7 Axillary Vein, Right | | | |
| 8 Axillary Vein, Left | | | |
| 9 Brachial Vein, Right | | | |
| A Brachial Vein, Left | | | |
| B Basilic Vein, Right | | | |
| C Basilic Vein, Left | | | |
| D Cephalic Vein, Right | | | |
| F Cephalic Vein, Left | | | |
| G Hand Vein, Right | | | |
| H Hand Vein, Left | | | |
| L Intracranial Vein | | | |
| M Internal Jugular Vein, Right | | | |
| N Internal Jugular Vein, Left | | | |
| P External Jugular Vein, Right | | | |
| Q External Jugular Vein, Left | | | |
| R Vertebral Vein, Right | | | |
| S Vertebral Vein, Left | | | |
| T Face Vein, Right | | | |
| V Face Vein, Left | | | |
| Y Upper Vein | | | |

| Character 4 Body Part | Character 5 Approach | Character 6 Device | Character 7 Qualifier |
|---|---|---|---|
| 0 Azygos Vein | 0 Open | Z No Device | X Diagnostic |
| 1 Hemiazygos Vein | 3 Percutaneous | | Z No Qualifier |
| 3 Innominate Vein, Right | 4 Percutaneous Endoscopic | | |
| 4 Innominate Vein, Left | | | |
| 5 Subclavian Vein, Right | | | |
| 6 Subclavian Vein, Left | | | |
| 7 Axillary Vein, Right | | | |
| 8 Axillary Vein, Left | | | |
| 9 Brachial Vein, Right | | | |
| A Brachial Vein, Left | | | |
| B Basilic Vein, Right | | | |
| C Basilic Vein, Left | | | |
| D Cephalic Vein, Right | | | |
| F Cephalic Vein, Left | | | |
| G Hand Vein, Right | | | |
| H Hand Vein, Left | | | |
| L Intracranial Vein | | | |
| M Internal Jugular Vein, Right | | | |
| N Internal Jugular Vein, Left | | | |
| P External Jugular Vein, Right | | | |
| Q External Jugular Vein, Left | | | |
| R Vertebral Vein, Right | | | |
| S Vertebral Vein, Left | | | |
| T Face Vein, Right | | | |
| V Face Vein, Left | | | |
| Y Upper Vein | | | |

♂ Male     ♀ Female     N C Non-covered     L C Limited Coverage     **AHA** *AHA Coding Clinic*

**0** Medical and Surgical
**5** Upper Veins
**B** Excision: Cutting out or off, without replacement, a portion of a body part

| Character 4<br>Body Part | Character 5<br>Approach | Character 6<br>Device | Character 7<br>Qualifier |
|---|---|---|---|
| 0 Azygos Vein | 0 Open | Z No Device | X Diagnostic |
| 1 Hemiazygos Vein | 3 Percutaneous | | Z No Qualifier |
| 3 Innominate Vein, Right | 4 Percutaneous Endoscopic | | |
| 4 Innominate Vein, Left | | | |
| 5 Subclavian Vein, Right | | | |
| 6 Subclavian Vein, Left | | | |
| 7 Axillary Vein, Right | | | |
| 8 Axillary Vein, Left | | | |
| 9 Brachial Vein, Right | | | |
| A Brachial Vein, Left | | | |
| B Basilic Vein, Right | | | |
| C Basilic Vein, Left | | | |
| D Cephalic Vein, Right | | | |
| F Cephalic Vein, Left | | | |
| G Hand Vein, Right | | | |
| H Hand Vein, Left | | | |
| L Intracranial Vein | | | |
| M Internal Jugular Vein, Right | | | |
| N Internal Jugular Vein, Left | | | |
| P External Jugular Vein, Right | | | |
| Q External Jugular Vein, Left | | | |
| R Vertebral Vein, Right | | | |
| S Vertebral Vein, Left | | | |
| T Face Vein, Right | | | |
| V Face Vein, Left | | | |
| Y Upper Vein | | | |

**0** Medical and Surgical
**5** Upper Veins
**C** Extirpation: Taking or cutting out solid matter from a body part

| Character 4<br>Body Part | Character 5<br>Approach | Character 6<br>Device | Character 7<br>Qualifier |
|---|---|---|---|
| 0 Azygos Vein | 0 Open | Z No Device | Z No Qualifier |
| 1 Hemiazygos Vein | 3 Percutaneous | | |
| 3 Innominate Vein, Right | 4 Percutaneous Endoscopic | | |
| 4 Innominate Vein, Left | | | |
| 5 Subclavian Vein, Right | | | |
| 6 Subclavian Vein, Left | | | |
| 7 Axillary Vein, Right | | | |
| 8 Axillary Vein, Left | | | |
| 9 Brachial Vein, Right | | | |
| A Brachial Vein, Left | | | |
| B Basilic Vein, Right | | | |
| C Basilic Vein, Left | | | |
| D Cephalic Vein, Right | | | |
| F Cephalic Vein, Left | | | |
| G Hand Vein, Right | | | |
| H Hand Vein, Left | | | |
| L Intracranial Vein   N C | | | |
| M Internal Jugular Vein, Right | | | |
| N Internal Jugular Vein, Left | | | |
| P External Jugular Vein, Right | | | |
| Q External Jugular Vein, Left | | | |
| R Vertebral Vein, Right | | | |
| S Vertebral Vein, Left | | | |
| T Face Vein, Right | | | |
| V Face Vein, Left | | | |
| Y Upper Vein | | | |

N C 05CL(3,4)ZZ

**0** Medical and Surgical
**5** Upper Veins
**D** Extraction: Pulling or stripping out or off all or a portion of a body part by the use of force

| Character 4<br>Body Part | Character 5<br>Approach | Character 6<br>Device | Character 7<br>Qualifier |
|---|---|---|---|
| 9 Brachial Vein, Right | 0 Open | Z No Device | Z No Qualifier |
| A Brachial Vein, Left | 3 Percutaneous | | |
| B Basilic Vein, Right | | | |
| C Basilic Vein, Left | | | |
| D Cephalic Vein, Right | | | |
| F Cephalic Vein, Left | | | |
| G Hand Vein, Right | | | |
| H Hand Vein, Left | | | |
| Y Upper Vein | | | |

**0 Medical and Surgical**
**5 Upper Veins**
**H Insertion:** Putting in a nonbiological appliance that monitors, assists, performs, or prevents a physiological function but does not physically take the place of a body part

| Character 4<br>Body Part | Character 5<br>Approach | Character 6<br>Device | Character 7<br>Qualifier |
|---|---|---|---|
| 0 Azygos Vein<br>1 Hemiazygos Vein<br>3 Innominate Vein, Right<br>4 Innominate Vein, Left<br>5 Subclavian Vein, Right<br>6 Subclavian Vein, Left<br>7 Axillary Vein, Right<br>8 Axillary Vein, Left<br>9 Brachial Vein, Right<br>A Brachial Vein, Left<br>B Basilic Vein, Right<br>C Basilic Vein, Left<br>D Cephalic Vein, Right<br>F Cephalic Vein, Left<br>G Hand Vein, Right<br>H Hand Vein, Left<br>L Intracranial Vein<br>M Internal Jugular Vein, Right<br>N Internal Jugular Vein, Left<br>P External Jugular Vein, Right<br>Q External Jugular Vein, Left<br>R Vertebral Vein, Right<br>S Vertebral Vein, Left<br>T Face Vein, Right<br>V Face Vein, Left | 0 Open<br>3 Percutaneous<br>4 Percutaneous Endoscopic | 3 Infusion Device<br>D Intraluminal Device | Z No Qualifier |
| Y Upper Vein | 0 Open<br>3 Percutaneous<br>4 Percutaneous Endoscopic | 2 Monitoring Device<br>3 Infusion Device<br>D Intraluminal Device | Z No Qualifier |

**0 Medical and Surgical**
**5 Upper Veins**
**J Inspection:** Visually and/or manually exploring a body part

| Character 4<br>Body Part | Character 5<br>Approach | Character 6<br>Device | Character 7<br>Qualifier |
|---|---|---|---|
| Y Upper Vein | 0 Open<br>3 Percutaneous<br>4 Percutaneous Endoscopic<br>X External | Z No Device | Z No Qualifier |

**0 Medical and Surgical**
**5 Upper Veins**
**L Occlusion:** Completely closing an orifice or the lumen of a tubular body part

| Character 4<br>Body Part | Character 5<br>Approach | Character 6<br>Device | Character 7<br>Qualifier |
|---|---|---|---|
| 0 Azygos Vein<br>1 Hemiazygos Vein<br>3 Innominate Vein, Right<br>4 Innominate Vein, Left<br>5 Subclavian Vein, Right<br>6 Subclavian Vein, Left<br>7 Axillary Vein, Right<br>8 Axillary Vein, Left<br>9 Brachial Vein, Right<br>A Brachial Vein, Left<br>B Basilic Vein, Right<br>C Basilic Vein, Left<br>D Cephalic Vein, Right<br>F Cephalic Vein, Left<br>G Hand Vein, Right<br>H Hand Vein, Left<br>L Intracranial Vein<br>M Internal Jugular Vein, Right<br>N Internal Jugular Vein, Left<br>P External Jugular Vein, Right<br>Q External Jugular Vein, Left<br>R Vertebral Vein, Right<br>S Vertebral Vein, Left<br>T Face Vein, Right<br>V Face Vein, Left<br>Y Upper Vein | 0 Open<br>3 Percutaneous<br>4 Percutaneous Endoscopic | C Extraluminal Device<br>D Intraluminal Device<br>Z No Device | Z No Qualifier |

**0** Medical and Surgical
**5** Upper Veins
**N** Release: Freeing a body part from an abnormal physical constraint by cutting or by the use of force

| Character 4<br>Body Part | Character 5<br>Approach | Character 6<br>Device | Character 7<br>Qualifier |
|---|---|---|---|
| 0 Azygos Vein<br>1 Hemiazygos Vein<br>3 Innominate Vein, Right<br>4 Innominate Vein, Left<br>5 Subclavian Vein, Right<br>6 Subclavian Vein, Left<br>7 Axillary Vein, Right<br>8 Axillary Vein, Left<br>9 Brachial Vein, Right<br>A Brachial Vein, Left<br>B Basilic Vein, Right<br>C Basilic Vein, Left<br>D Cephalic Vein, Right<br>F Cephalic Vein, Left<br>G Hand Vein, Right<br>H Hand Vein, Left<br>L Intracranial Vein<br>M Internal Jugular Vein, Right<br>N Internal Jugular Vein, Left<br>P External Jugular Vein, Right<br>Q External Jugular Vein, Left<br>R Vertebral Vein, Right<br>S Vertebral Vein, Left<br>T Face Vein, Right<br>V Face Vein, Left<br>Y Upper Vein | 0 Open<br>3 Percutaneous<br>4 Percutaneous Endoscopic | Z No Device | Z No Qualifier |

**0** Medical and Surgical
**5** Upper Veins
**P** Removal: Taking out or off a device from a body part

| Character 4<br>Body Part | Character 5<br>Approach | Character 6<br>Device | Character 7<br>Qualifier |
|---|---|---|---|
| Y Upper Vein | 0 Open<br>3 Percutaneous<br>4 Percutaneous Endoscopic | 0 Drainage Device<br>2 Monitoring Device<br>3 Infusion Device<br>7 Autologous Tissue Substitute<br>C Extraluminal Device<br>D Intraluminal Device<br>J Synthetic Substitute<br>K Nonautologous Tissue Substitute | Z No Qualifier |
| Y Upper Vein | X External | 0 Drainage Device<br>2 Monitoring Device<br>3 Infusion Device<br>D Intraluminal Device | Z No Qualifier |

**0** Medical and Surgical
**5** Upper Veins
**Q** Repair: Restoring, to the extent possible, a body part to its normal anatomic structure and function

| Character 4 Body Part | Character 5 Approach | Character 6 Device | Character 7 Qualifier |
|---|---|---|---|
| 0 Azygos Vein | 0 Open | Z No Device | Z No Qualifier |
| 1 Hemiazygos Vein | 3 Percutaneous | | |
| 3 Innominate Vein, Right | 4 Percutaneous Endoscopic | | |
| 4 Innominate Vein, Left | | | |
| 5 Subclavian Vein, Right | | | |
| 6 Subclavian Vein, Left | | | |
| 7 Axillary Vein, Right | | | |
| 8 Axillary Vein, Left | | | |
| 9 Brachial Vein, Right | | | |
| A Brachial Vein, Left | | | |
| B Basilic Vein, Right | | | |
| C Basilic Vein, Left | | | |
| D Cephalic Vein, Right | | | |
| F Cephalic Vein, Left | | | |
| G Hand Vein, Right | | | |
| H Hand Vein, Left | | | |
| L Intracranial Vein | | | |
| M Internal Jugular Vein, Right | | | |
| N Internal Jugular Vein, Left | | | |
| P External Jugular Vein, Right | | | |
| Q External Jugular Vein, Left | | | |
| R Vertebral Vein, Right | | | |
| S Vertebral Vein, Left | | | |
| T Face Vein, Right | | | |
| V Face Vein, Left | | | |
| Y Upper Vein | | | |

**0** Medical and Surgical
**5** Upper Veins
**R** Replacement: Putting in or on biological or synthetic material that physically takes the place and/or function of all or a portion of a body part

| Character 4 Body Part | Character 5 Approach | Character 6 Device | Character 7 Qualifier |
|---|---|---|---|
| 0 Azygos Vein | 0 Open | 7 Autologous Tissue Substitute | Z No Qualifier |
| 1 Hemiazygos Vein | 4 Percutaneous Endoscopic | J Synthetic Substitute | |
| 3 Innominate Vein, Right | | K Nonautologous Tissue Substitute | |
| 4 Innominate Vein, Left | | | |
| 5 Subclavian Vein, Right | | | |
| 6 Subclavian Vein, Left | | | |
| 7 Axillary Vein, Right | | | |
| 8 Axillary Vein, Left | | | |
| 9 Brachial Vein, Right | | | |
| A Brachial Vein, Left | | | |
| B Basilic Vein, Right | | | |
| C Basilic Vein, Left | | | |
| D Cephalic Vein, Right | | | |
| F Cephalic Vein, Left | | | |
| G Hand Vein, Right | | | |
| H Hand Vein, Left | | | |
| L Intracranial Vein | | | |
| M Internal Jugular Vein, Right | | | |
| N Internal Jugular Vein, Left | | | |
| P External Jugular Vein, Right | | | |
| Q External Jugular Vein, Left | | | |
| R Vertebral Vein, Right | | | |
| S Vertebral Vein, Left | | | |
| T Face Vein, Right | | | |
| V Face Vein, Left | | | |
| Y Upper Vein | | | |

**0** Medical and Surgical
**5** Upper Veins
**S** Reposition: Moving to its normal location, or other suitable location, all or a portion of a body part

| Character 4<br>Body Part | Character 5<br>Approach | Character 6<br>Device | Character 7<br>Qualifier |
|---|---|---|---|
| 0 Azygos Vein<br>1 Hemiazygos Vein<br>3 Innominate Vein, Right<br>4 Innominate Vein, Left<br>5 Subclavian Vein, Right<br>6 Subclavian Vein, Left<br>7 Axillary Vein, Right<br>8 Axillary Vein, Left<br>9 Brachial Vein, Right<br>A Brachial Vein, Left<br>B Basilic Vein, Right<br>C Basilic Vein, Left<br>D Cephalic Vein, Right<br>F Cephalic Vein, Left<br>G Hand Vein, Right<br>H Hand Vein, Left<br>L Intracranial Vein<br>M Internal Jugular Vein, Right<br>N Internal Jugular Vein, Left<br>P External Jugular Vein, Right<br>Q External Jugular Vein, Left<br>R Vertebral Vein, Right<br>S Vertebral Vein, Left<br>T Face Vein, Right<br>V Face Vein, Left<br>Y Upper Vein | 0 Open<br>3 Percutaneous<br>4 Percutaneous Endoscopic | Z No Device | Z No Qualifier |

**AHA:** 05SD0ZZ - 4Q 2013, 126

**0** Medical and Surgical
**5** Upper Veins
**U** Supplement: Putting in or on biological or synthetic material that physically reinforces and/or augments the function of a portion of a body part

| Character 4<br>Body Part | Character 5<br>Approach | Character 6<br>Device | Character 7<br>Qualifier |
|---|---|---|---|
| 0 Azygos Vein<br>1 Hemiazygos Vein<br>3 Innominate Vein, Right<br>4 Innominate Vein, Left<br>5 Subclavian Vein, Right<br>6 Subclavian Vein, Left<br>7 Axillary Vein, Right<br>8 Axillary Vein, Left<br>9 Brachial Vein, Right<br>A Brachial Vein, Left<br>B Basilic Vein, Right<br>C Basilic Vein, Left<br>D Cephalic Vein, Right<br>F Cephalic Vein, Left<br>G Hand Vein, Right<br>H Hand Vein, Left<br>L Intracranial Vein<br>M Internal Jugular Vein, Right<br>N Internal Jugular Vein, Left<br>P External Jugular Vein, Right<br>Q External Jugular Vein, Left<br>R Vertebral Vein, Right<br>S Vertebral Vein, Left<br>T Face Vein, Right<br>V Face Vein, Left<br>Y Upper Vein | 0 Open<br>3 Percutaneous<br>4 Percutaneous Endoscopic | 7 Autologous Tissue Substitute<br>J Synthetic Substitute<br>K Nonautologous Tissue Substitute | Z No Qualifier |

**0** Medical and Surgical
**5** Upper Veins
**V** Restriction: Partially closing an orifice or the lumen of a tubular body part

| Character 4 Body Part | Character 5 Approach | Character 6 Device | Character 7 Qualifier |
|---|---|---|---|
| 0 Azygos Vein | 0 Open | C Extraluminal Device | Z No Qualifier |
| 1 Hemiazygos Vein | 3 Percutaneous | D Intraluminal Device | |
| 3 Innominate Vein, Right | 4 Percutaneous Endoscopic | Z No Device | |
| 4 Innominate Vein, Left | | | |
| 5 Subclavian Vein, Right | | | |
| 6 Subclavian Vein, Left | | | |
| 7 Axillary Vein, Right | | | |
| 8 Axillary Vein, Left | | | |
| 9 Brachial Vein, Right | | | |
| A Brachial Vein, Left | | | |
| B Basilic Vein, Right | | | |
| C Basilic Vein, Left | | | |
| D Cephalic Vein, Right | | | |
| F Cephalic Vein, Left | | | |
| G Hand Vein, Right | | | |
| H Hand Vein, Left | | | |
| L Intracranial Vein | | | |
| M Internal Jugular Vein, Right | | | |
| N Internal Jugular Vein, Left | | | |
| P External Jugular Vein, Right | | | |
| Q External Jugular Vein, Left | | | |
| R Vertebral Vein, Right | | | |
| S Vertebral Vein, Left | | | |
| T Face Vein, Right | | | |
| V Face Vein, Left | | | |
| Y Upper Vein | | | |

**0** Medical and Surgical
**5** Upper Veins
**W** Revision: Correcting, to the extent possible, a portion of a malfunctioning device or the position of a displaced device

| Character 4 Body Part | Character 5 Approach | Character 6 Device | Character 7 Qualifier |
|---|---|---|---|
| Y Upper Vein | 0 Open | 0 Drainage Device | Z No Qualifier |
| | 3 Percutaneous | 2 Monitoring Device | |
| | 4 Percutaneous Endoscopic | 3 Infusion Device | |
| | X External | 7 Autologous Tissue Substitute | |
| | | C Extraluminal Device | |
| | | D Intraluminal Device | |
| | | J Synthetic Substitute | |
| | | K Nonautologous Tissue Substitute | |

# Lower Veins | 061-06W

**0** Medical and Surgical
**6** Lower Veins
**1** Bypass: Altering the route of passage of the contents of a tubular body part

| Character 4<br>Body Part | Character 5<br>Approach | Character 6<br>Device | Character 7<br>Qualifier |
|---|---|---|---|
| 0 Inferior Vena Cava | 0 Open<br>4 Percutaneous Endoscopic | 7 Autologous Tissue Substitute<br>9 Autologous Venous Tissue<br>A Autologous Arterial Tissue<br>J Synthetic Substitute<br>K Nonautologous Tissue Substitute<br>Z No Device | 5 Superior Mesenteric Vein<br>6 Inferior Mesenteric Vein<br>Y Lower Vein |
| 1 Splenic Vein | 0 Open<br>4 Percutaneous Endoscopic | 7 Autologous Tissue Substitute<br>9 Autologous Venous Tissue<br>A Autologous Arterial Tissue<br>J Synthetic Substitute<br>K Nonautologous Tissue Substitute<br>Z No Device | 9 Renal Vein, Right<br>B Renal Vein, Left<br>Y Lower Vein |
| 2 Gastric Vein<br>3 Esophageal Vein<br>4 Hepatic Vein<br>5 Superior Mesenteric Vein<br>6 Inferior Mesenteric Vein<br>7 Colic Vein<br>9 Renal Vein, Right<br>B Renal Vein, Left<br>C Common Iliac Vein, Right<br>D Common Iliac Vein, Left<br>F External Iliac Vein, Right<br>G External Iliac Vein, Left<br>H Hypogastric Vein, Right<br>J Hypogastric Vein, Left<br>M Femoral Vein, Right<br>N Femoral Vein, Left<br>P Greater Saphenous Vein, Right<br>Q Greater Saphenous Vein, Left<br>R Lesser Saphenous Vein, Right<br>S Lesser Saphenous Vein, Left<br>T Foot Vein, Right<br>V Foot Vein, Left | 0 Open<br>4 Percutaneous Endoscopic | 7 Autologous Tissue Substitute<br>9 Autologous Venous Tissue<br>A Autologous Arterial Tissue<br>J Synthetic Substitute<br>K Nonautologous Tissue Substitute<br>Z No Device | Y Lower Vein |
| 8 Portal Vein | 0 Open | 7 Autologous Tissue Substitute<br>9 Autologous Venous Tissue<br>A Autologous Arterial Tissue<br>J Synthetic Substitute<br>K Nonautologous Tissue Substitute<br>Z No Device | 9 Renal Vein, Right<br>B Renal Vein, Left<br>Y Lower Vein |
| 8 Portal Vein | 3 Percutaneous | D Intraluminal Device | Y Lower Vein |
| 8 Portal Vein | 4 Percutaneous Endoscopic | 7 Autologous Tissue Substitute<br>9 Autologous Venous Tissue<br>A Autologous Arterial Tissue<br>J Synthetic Substitute<br>K Nonautologous Tissue Substitute<br>Z No Device | 9 Renal Vein, Right<br>3 Renal Vein, Left<br>Y Lower Vein |
| 8 Portal Vein | 4 Percutaneous Endoscopic | D Intraluminal Device | Y Lower Vein |

**0 Medical and Surgical**
**6 Lower Veins**
**5 Destruction:** Physical eradication of all or a portion of a body part by the direct use of energy, force, or a destructive agent

| Character 4 Body Part | Character 5 Approach | Character 6 Device | Character 7 Qualifier |
|---|---|---|---|
| 0 Inferior Vena Cava<br>1 Splenic Vein<br>2 Gastric Vein<br>3 Esophageal Vein<br>4 Hepatic Vein<br>5 Superior Mesenteric Vein<br>6 Inferior Mesenteric Vein<br>7 Colic Vein<br>8 Portal Vein<br>9 Renal Vein, Right<br>B Renal Vein, Left<br>C Common Iliac Vein, Right<br>D Common Iliac Vein, Left<br>F External Iliac Vein, Right<br>G External Iliac Vein, Left<br>H Hypogastric Vein, Right<br>J Hypogastric Vein, Left<br>M Femoral Vein, Right<br>N Femoral Vein, Left<br>P Greater Saphenous Vein, Right<br>Q Greater Saphenous Vein, Left<br>R Lesser Saphenous Vein, Right<br>S Lesser Saphenous Vein, Left<br>T Foot Vein, Right<br>V Foot Vein, Left | 0 Open<br>3 Percutaneous<br>4 Percutaneous Endoscopic | Z No Device | Z No Qualifier |
| Y Lower Vein | 0 Open<br>3 Percutaneous<br>4 Percutaneous Endoscopic | Z No Device | C Hemorrhoidal Plexus<br>Z No Qualifier |

**0 Medical and Surgical**
**6 Lower Veins**
**7 Dilation:** Expanding an orifice or the lumen of a tubular body part

| Character 4 Body Part | Character 5 Approach | Character 6 Device | Character 7 Qualifier |
|---|---|---|---|
| 0 Inferior Vena Cava<br>1 Splenic Vein<br>2 Gastric Vein<br>3 Esophageal Vein<br>4 Hepatic Vein<br>5 Superior Mesenteric Vein<br>6 Inferior Mesenteric Vein<br>7 Colic Vein<br>8 Portal Vein<br>9 Renal Vein, Right<br>B Renal Vein, Left<br>C Common Iliac Vein, Right<br>D Common Iliac Vein, Left<br>F External Iliac Vein, Right<br>G External Iliac Vein, Left<br>H Hypogastric Vein, Right<br>J Hypogastric Vein, Left<br>M Femoral Vein, Right<br>N Femoral Vein, Left<br>P Greater Saphenous Vein, Right<br>Q Greater Saphenous Vein, Left<br>R Lesser Saphenous Vein, Right<br>S Lesser Saphenous Vein, Left<br>T Foot Vein, Right<br>V Foot Vein, Left<br>Y Lower Vein | 0 Open<br>3 Percutaneous<br>4 Percutaneous Endoscopic | D Intraluminal Device<br>Z No Device | Z No Qualifier |

**0** Medical and Surgical
**6** Lower Veins
**9** Drainage: Taking or letting out fluids and/or gases from a body part

| Character 4 Body Part | Character 5 Approach | Character 6 Device | Character 7 Qualifier |
|---|---|---|---|
| 0 Inferior Vena Cava | 0 Open | 0 Drainage Device | Z No Qualifier |
| 1 Splenic Vein | 3 Percutaneous | | |
| 2 Gastric Vein | 4 Percutaneous Endoscopic | | |
| 3 Esophageal Vein | | | |
| 4 Hepatic Vein | | | |
| 5 Superior Mesenteric Vein | | | |
| 6 Inferior Mesenteric Vein | | | |
| 7 Colic Vein | | | |
| 8 Portal Vein | | | |
| 9 Renal Vein, Right | | | |
| B Renal Vein, Left | | | |
| C Common Iliac Vein, Right | | | |
| D Common Iliac Vein, Left | | | |
| F External Iliac Vein, Right | | | |
| G External Iliac Vein, Left | | | |
| H Hypogastric Vein, Right | | | |
| J Hypogastric Vein, Left | | | |
| M Femoral Vein, Right | | | |
| N Femoral Vein, Left | | | |
| P Greater Saphenous Vein, Right | | | |
| Q Greater Saphenous Vein, Left | | | |
| R Lesser Saphenous Vein, Right | | | |
| S Lesser Saphenous Vein, Left | | | |
| T Foot Vein, Right | | | |
| V Foot Vein, Left | | | |
| Y Lower Vein | | | |

| Character 4 Body Part | Character 5 Approach | Character 6 Device | Character 7 Qualifier |
|---|---|---|---|
| 0 Inferior Vena Cava | 0 Open | Z No Device | X Diagnostic |
| 1 Splenic Vein | 3 Percutaneous | | Z No Qualifier |
| 2 Gastric Vein | 4 Percutaneous Endoscopic | | |
| 3 Esophageal Vein | | | |
| 4 Hepatic Vein | | | |
| 5 Superior Mesenteric Vein | | | |
| 6 Inferior Mesenteric Vein | | | |
| 7 Colic Vein | | | |
| 8 Portal Vein | | | |
| 9 Renal Vein, Right | | | |
| B Renal Vein, Left | | | |
| C Common Iliac Vein, Right | | | |
| D Common Iliac Vein, Left | | | |
| F External Iliac Vein, Right | | | |
| G External Iliac Vein, Left | | | |
| H Hypogastric Vein, Right | | | |
| J Hypogastric Vein, Left | | | |
| M Femoral Vein, Right | | | |
| N Femoral Vein, Left | | | |
| P Greater Saphenous Vein, Right | | | |
| Q Greater Saphenous Vein, Left | | | |
| R Lesser Saphenous Vein, Right | | | |
| S Lesser Saphenous Vein, Left | | | |
| T Foot Vein, Right | | | |
| V Foot Vein, Left | | | |
| Y Lower Vein | | | |

**0** Medical and Surgical
**6** Lower Veins
**B** Excision: Cutting out or off, without replacement, a portion of a body part

| Character 4<br>Body Part | Character 5<br>Approach | Character 6<br>Device | Character 7<br>Qualifier |
|---|---|---|---|
| 0 Inferior Vena Cava<br>1 Splenic Vein<br>2 Gastric Vein<br>3 Esophageal Vein<br>4 Hepatic Vein<br>5 Superior Mesenteric Vein<br>6 Inferior Mesenteric Vein<br>7 Colic Vein<br>8 Portal Vein<br>9 Renal Vein, Right<br>B Renal Vein, Left<br>C Common Iliac Vein, Right<br>D Common Iliac Vein, Left<br>F External Iliac Vein, Right<br>G External Iliac Vein, Left<br>H Hypogastric Vein, Right<br>J Hypogastric Vein, Left<br>M Femoral Vein, Right<br>N Femoral Vein, Left<br>P Greater Saphenous Vein, Right<br>Q Greater Saphenous Vein, Left<br>R Lesser Saphenous Vein, Right<br>S Lesser Saphenous Vein, Left<br>T Foot Vein, Right<br>V Foot Vein, Left | 0 Open<br>3 Percutaneous<br>4 Percutaneous Endoscopic | Z No Device | X Diagnostic<br>Z No Qualifier |
| Y Lower Vein | 0 Open<br>3 Percutaneous<br>4 Percutaneous Endoscopic | Z No Device | C Hemorrhoidal Plexus<br>X Diagnostic<br>Z No Qualifier |

**AHA:** 06BP0ZZ - 1Q 2014, 11

**0** Medical and Surgical
**6** Lower Veins
**C** Extirpation: Taking or cutting out solid matter from a body part

| Character 4<br>Body Part | Character 5<br>Approach | Character 6<br>Device | Character 7<br>Qualifier |
|---|---|---|---|
| 0 Inferior Vena Cava<br>1 Splenic Vein<br>2 Gastric Vein<br>3 Esophageal Vein<br>4 Hepatic Vein<br>5 Superior Mesenteric Vein<br>6 Inferior Mesenteric Vein<br>7 Colic Vein<br>8 Portal Vein<br>9 Renal Vein, Right<br>B Renal Vein, Left<br>C Common Iliac Vein, Right<br>D Common Iliac Vein, Left<br>F External Iliac Vein, Right<br>G External Iliac Vein, Left<br>H Hypogastric Vein, Right<br>J Hypogastric Vein, Left<br>M Femoral Vein, Right<br>N Femoral Vein, Left<br>P Greater Saphenous Vein, Right<br>Q Greater Saphenous Vein, Left<br>R Lesser Saphenous Vein, Right<br>S Lesser Saphenous Vein, Left<br>T Foot Vein, Right<br>V Foot Vein, Left<br>Y Lower Vein | 0 Open<br>3 Percutaneous<br>4 Percutaneous Endoscopic | Z No Device | Z No Qualifier |

**0** Medical and Surgical
**6** Lower Veins
**D** Extraction: Pulling or stripping out or off all or a portion of a body part by the use of force

| Character 4 Body Part | Character 5 Approach | Character 6 Device | Character 7 Qualifier |
|---|---|---|---|
| M Femoral Vein, Right<br>N Femoral Vein, Left<br>P Greater Saphenous Vein, Right<br>Q Greater Saphenous Vein, Left<br>R Lesser Saphenous Vein, Right<br>S Lesser Saphenous Vein, Left<br>T Foot Vein, Right<br>V Foot Vein, Left<br>Y Lower Vein | 0 Open<br>3 Percutaneous<br>4 Percutaneous Endoscopic | Z No Device | Z No Qualifier |

**0** Medical and Surgical
**6** Lower Veins
**H** Insertion: Putting in a nonbiological appliance that monitors, assists, performs, or prevents a physiological function but does not physically take the place of a body part

| Character 4 Body Part | Character 5 Approach | Character 6 Device | Character 7 Qualifier |
|---|---|---|---|
| 0 Inferior Vena Cava | 0 Open<br>3 Percutaneous | 3 Infusion Device | T Via Umbilical Vein<br>Z No Qualifier |
| 0 Inferior Vena Cava | 0 Open<br>3 Percutaneous | D Intraluminal Device | Z No Qualifier |
| 0 Inferior Vena Cava | 4 Percutaneous Endoscopic | 3 Infusion Device<br>D Intraluminal Device | Z No Qualifier |
| 1 Splenic Vein<br>2 Gastric Vein<br>3 Esophageal Vein<br>4 Hepatic Vein<br>5 Superior Mesenteric Vein<br>6 Inferior Mesenteric Vein<br>7 Colic Vein<br>8 Portal Vein<br>9 Renal Vein, Right<br>B Renal Vein, Left<br>C Common Iliac Vein, Right<br>D Common Iliac Vein, Left<br>F External Iliac Vein, Right<br>G External Iliac Vein, Left<br>H Hypogastric Vein, Right<br>J Hypogastric Vein, Left<br>M Femoral Vein, Right<br>N Femoral Vein, Left<br>P Greater Saphenous Vein, Right<br>Q Greater Saphenous Vein, Left<br>R Lesser Saphenous Vein, Right<br>S Lesser Saphenous Vein, Left<br>T Foot Vein, Right<br>V Foot Vein, Left | 0 Open<br>3 Percutaneous<br>4 Percutaneous Endoscopic | 3 Infusion Device<br>D Intraluminal Device | Z No Qualifier |
| Y Lower Vein | 0 Open<br>3 Percutaneous<br>4 Percutaneous Endoscopic | 2 Monitoring Device<br>3 Infusion Device<br>D Intraluminal Device | Z No Qualifier |

**AHA:** 06H033Z - 3Q 2013, 19

**0** Medical and Surgical
**6** Lower Veins
**J** Inspection: Visually and/or manually exploring a body part

| Character 4 Body Part | Character 5 Approach | Character 6 Device | Character 7 Qualifier |
|---|---|---|---|
| Y Lower Vein | 0 Open<br>3 Percutaneous<br>4 Percutaneous Endoscopic<br>X External | Z No Device | Z No Qualifier |

**0 Medical and Surgical**
**6 Lower Veins**
**L Occlusion: Completely closing an orifice or the lumen of a tubular body part**

| Character 4<br>Body Part | Character 5<br>Approach | Character 6<br>Device | Character 7<br>Qualifier |
|---|---|---|---|
| 0 Inferior Vena Cava<br>1 Splenic Vein<br>2 Gastric Vein<br>3 Esophageal Vein<br>4 Hepatic Vein<br>5 Superior Mesenteric Vein<br>6 Inferior Mesenteric Vein<br>7 Colic Vein<br>8 Portal Vein<br>9 Renal Vein, Right<br>B Renal Vein, Left<br>C Common Iliac Vein, Right<br>D Common Iliac Vein, Left<br>F External Iliac Vein, Right<br>G External Iliac Vein, Left<br>H Hypogastric Vein, Right<br>J Hypogastric Vein, Left<br>M Femoral Vein, Right<br>N Femoral Vein, Left<br>P Greater Saphenous Vein, Right<br>Q Greater Saphenous Vein, Left<br>R Lesser Saphenous Vein, Right<br>S Lesser Saphenous Vein, Left<br>T Foot Vein, Right<br>V Foot Vein, Left | 0 Open<br>3 Percutaneous<br>4 Percutaneous Endoscopic | C Extraluminal Device<br>D Intraluminal Device<br>Z No Device | Z No Qualifier |
| Y Lower Vein | 0 Open<br>3 Percutaneous<br>4 Percutaneous Endoscopic | C Extraluminal Device<br>D Intraluminal Device<br>Z No Device | C Hemorrhoidal Plexus<br>Z No Qualifier |

**AHA:** 06L34CZ - 4Q 2013, 113

**0 Medical and Surgical**
**6 Lower Veins**
**N Release: Freeing a body part from an abnormal physical constraint by cutting or by the use of force**

| Character 4<br>Body Part | Character 5<br>Approach | Character 6<br>Device | Character 7<br>Qualifier |
|---|---|---|---|
| 0 Inferior Vena Cava<br>1 Splenic Vein<br>2 Gastric Vein<br>3 Esophageal Vein<br>4 Hepatic Vein<br>5 Superior Mesenteric Vein<br>6 Inferior Mesenteric Vein<br>7 Colic Vein<br>8 Portal Vein<br>9 Renal Vein, Right<br>B Renal Vein, Left<br>C Common Iliac Vein, Right<br>D Common Iliac Vein, Left<br>F External Iliac Vein, Right<br>G External Iliac Vein, Left<br>H Hypogastric Vein, Right<br>J Hypogastric Vein, Left<br>M Femoral Vein, Right<br>N Femoral Vein, Left<br>P Greater Saphenous Vein, Right<br>Q Greater Saphenous Vein, Left<br>R Lesser Saphenous Vein, Right<br>S Lesser Saphenous Vein, Left<br>T Foot Vein, Right<br>V Foot Vein, Left<br>Y Lower Vein | 0 Open<br>3 Percutaneous<br>4 Percutaneous Endoscopic | Z No Device | Z No Qualifier |

**0** Medical and Surgical
**6** Lower Veins
**P** Removal: Taking out or off a device from a body part

| Character 4<br>Body Part | Character 5<br>Approach | Character 6<br>Device | Character 7<br>Qualifier |
|---|---|---|---|
| Y Lower Vein | 0 Open<br>3 Percutaneous<br>4 Percutaneous Endoscopic | 0 Drainage Device<br>2 Monitoring Device<br>3 Infusion Device<br>7 Autologous Tissue Substitute<br>C Extraluminal Device<br>D Intraluminal Device<br>J Synthetic Substitute<br>K Nonautologous Tissue Substitute | Z No Qualifier |
| Y Lower Vein | X External | 0 Drainage Device<br>2 Monitoring Device<br>3 Infusion Device<br>D Intraluminal Device | Z No Qualifier |

**0** Medical and Surgical
**6** Lower Veins
**Q** Repair: Restoring, to the extent possible, a body part to its normal anatomic structure and function

| Character 4<br>Body Part | Character 5<br>Approach | Character 6<br>Device | Character 7<br>Qualifier |
|---|---|---|---|
| 0 Inferior Vena Cava<br>1 Splenic Vein<br>2 Gastric Vein<br>3 Esophageal Vein<br>4 Hepatic Vein<br>5 Superior Mesenteric Vein<br>6 Inferior Mesenteric Vein<br>7 Colic Vein<br>8 Portal Vein<br>9 Renal Vein, Right<br>B Renal Vein, Left<br>C Common Iliac Vein, Right<br>D Common Iliac Vein, Left<br>F External Iliac Vein, Right<br>G External Iliac Vein, Left<br>H Hypogastric Vein, Right<br>J Hypogastric Vein, Left<br>M Femoral Vein, Right<br>N Femoral Vein, Left<br>P Greater Saphenous Vein, Right<br>Q Greater Saphenous Vein, Left<br>R Lesser Saphenous Vein, Right<br>S Lesser Saphenous Vein, Left<br>T Foot Vein, Right<br>V Foot Vein, Left<br>Y Lower Vein | 0 Open<br>3 Percutaneous<br>4 Percutaneous Endoscopic | Z No Device | Z No Qualifier |

**0** Medical and Surgical
**6** Lower Veins
**R** Replacement: Putting in or on biological or synthetic material that physically takes the place and/or function of all or a portion of a body part

| Character 4<br>Body Part | Character 5<br>Approach | Character 6<br>Device | Character 7<br>Qualifier |
|---|---|---|---|
| 0 Inferior Vena Cava<br>1 Splenic Vein<br>2 Gastric Vein<br>3 Esophageal Vein<br>4 Hepatic Vein<br>5 Superior Mesenteric Vein<br>6 Inferior Mesenteric Vein<br>7 Colic Vein<br>8 Portal Vein<br>9 Renal Vein, Right<br>B Renal Vein, Left<br>C Common Iliac Vein, Right<br>D Common Iliac Vein, Left<br>F External Iliac Vein, Right<br>G External Iliac Vein, Left<br>H Hypogastric Vein, Right<br>J Hypogastric Vein, Left<br>M Femoral Vein, Right<br>N Femoral Vein, Left<br>P Greater Saphenous Vein, Right<br>Q Greater Saphenous Vein, Left<br>R Lesser Saphenous Vein, Right<br>S Lesser Saphenous Vein, Left<br>T Foot Vein, Right<br>V Foot Vein, Left<br>Y Lower Vein | 0 Open<br>4 Percutaneous Endoscopic | 7 Autologous Tissue Substitute<br>J Synthetic Substitute<br>K Nonautologous Tissue Substitute | Z No Qualifier |

**0** Medical and Surgical
**6** Lower Veins
**S** Reposition: Moving to its normal location, or other suitable location, all or a portion of a body part

| Character 4<br>Body Part | Character 5<br>Approach | Character 6<br>Device | Character 7<br>Qualifier |
|---|---|---|---|
| 0 Inferior Vena Cava<br>1 Splenic Vein<br>2 Gastric Vein<br>3 Esophageal Vein<br>4 Hepatic Vein<br>5 Superior Mesenteric Vein<br>6 Inferior Mesenteric Vein<br>7 Colic Vein<br>8 Portal Vein<br>9 Renal Vein, Right<br>B Renal Vein, Left<br>C Common Iliac Vein, Right<br>D Common Iliac Vein, Left<br>F External Iliac Vein, Right<br>G External Iliac Vein, Left<br>H Hypogastric Vein, Right<br>J Hypogastric Vein, Left<br>M Femoral Vein, Right<br>N Femoral Vein, Left<br>P Greater Saphenous Vein, Right<br>Q Greater Saphenous Vein, Left<br>R Lesser Saphenous Vein, Right<br>S Lesser Saphenous Vein, Left<br>T Foot Vein, Right<br>V Foot Vein, Left<br>Y Lower Vein | 0 Open<br>3 Percutaneous<br>4 Percutaneous Endoscopic | Z No Device | Z No Qualifier |

**0** Medical and Surgical
**6** Lower Veins
**U** Supplement: Putting in or on biological or synthetic material that physically reinforces and/or augments the function of a portion of a body part

| Character 4<br>Body Part | Character 5<br>Approach | Character 6<br>Device | Character 7<br>Qualifier |
|---|---|---|---|
| 0 Inferior Vena Cava | 0 Open | 7 Autologous Tissue Substitute | Z No Qualifier |
| 1 Splenic Vein | 3 Percutaneous | J Synthetic Substitute | |
| 2 Gastric Vein | 4 Percutaneous Endoscopic | K Nonautologous Tissue Substitute | |
| 3 Esophageal Vein | | | |
| 4 Hepatic Vein | | | |
| 5 Superior Mesenteric Vein | | | |
| 6 Inferior Mesenteric Vein | | | |
| 7 Colic Vein | | | |
| 8 Portal Vein | | | |
| 9 Renal Vein, Right | | | |
| B Renal Vein, Left | | | |
| C Common Iliac Vein, Right | | | |
| D Common Iliac Vein, Left | | | |
| F External Iliac Vein, Right | | | |
| G External Iliac Vein, Left | | | |
| H Hypogastric Vein, Right | | | |
| J Hypogastric Vein, Left | | | |
| M Femoral Vein, Right | | | |
| N Femoral Vein, Left | | | |
| P Greater Saphenous Vein, Right | | | |
| Q Greater Saphenous Vein, Left | | | |
| R Lesser Saphenous Vein, Right | | | |
| S Lesser Saphenous Vein, Left | | | |
| T Foot Vein, Right | | | |
| V Foot Vein, Left | | | |
| Y Lower Vein | | | |

**0** Medical and Surgical
**6** Lower Veins
**V** Restriction: Partially closing an orifice or the lumen of a tubular body part

| Character 4<br>Body Part | Character 5<br>Approach | Character 6<br>Device | Character 7<br>Qualifier |
|---|---|---|---|
| 0 Inferior Vena Cava | 0 Open | C Extraluminal Device | Z No Qualifier |
| 1 Splenic Vein | 3 Percutaneous | D Intraluminal Device | |
| 2 Gastric Vein | 4 Percutaneous Endoscopic | Z No Device | |
| 3 Esophageal Vein | | | |
| 4 Hepatic Vein | | | |
| 5 Superior Mesenteric Vein | | | |
| 6 Inferior Mesenteric Vein | | | |
| 7 Colic Vein | | | |
| 8 Portal Vein | | | |
| 9 Renal Vein, Right | | | |
| B Renal Vein, Left | | | |
| C Common Iliac Vein, Right | | | |
| D Common Iliac Vein, Left | | | |
| F External Iliac Vein, Right | | | |
| G External Iliac Vein, Left | | | |
| H Hypogastric Vein, Right | | | |
| J Hypogastric Vein, Left | | | |
| M Femoral Vein, Right | | | |
| N Femoral Vein, Left | | | |
| P Greater Saphenous Vein, Right | | | |
| Q Greater Saphenous Vein, Left | | | |
| R Lesser Saphenous Vein, Right | | | |
| S Lesser Saphenous Vein, Left | | | |
| T Foot Vein, Right | | | |
| V Foot Vein, Left | | | |
| Y Lower Vein | | | |

**0** Medical and Surgical
**6** Lower Veins
**W** Revision: Correcting, to the extent possible, a portion of a malfunctioning device or the position of a displaced device

| Character 4<br>Body Part | Character 5<br>Approach | Character 6<br>Device | Character 7<br>Qualifier |
|---|---|---|---|
| Y Lower Vein | 0 Open | 0 Drainage Device | Z No Qualifier |
| | 3 Percutaneous | 2 Monitoring Device | |
| | 4 Percutaneous Endoscopic | 3 Infusion Device | |
| | X External | 7 Autologous Tissue Substitute | |
| | | C Extraluminal Device | |
| | | D Intraluminal Device | |
| | | J Synthetic Substitute | |
| | | K Nonautologous Tissue Substitute | |

# Lymphatic and Hemic Systems | 072-07Y

**0** Medical and Surgical
**7** Lymphatic and Hemic Systems
**2** Change: Taking out or off a device from a body part and putting back an identical or similar device in or on the same body part without cutting or puncturing the skin or a mucous membrane

| Character 4<br>Body Part | Character 5<br>Approach | Character 6<br>Device | Character 7<br>Qualifier |
|---|---|---|---|
| K  Thoracic Duct<br>L  Cisterna Chyli<br>M  Thymus<br>N  Lymphatic<br>P  Spleen<br>T  Bone Marrow | X  External | 0  Drainage Device<br>Y  Other Device | Z  No Qualifier |

**0** Medical and Surgical
**7** Lymphatic and Hemic Systems
**5** Destruction: Physical eradication of all or a portion of a body part by the direct use of energy, force, or a destructive agent

| Character 4<br>Body Part | Character 5<br>Approach | Character 6<br>Device | Character 7<br>Qualifier |
|---|---|---|---|
| 0  Lymphatic, Head<br>1  Lymphatic, Right Neck<br>2  Lymphatic, Left Neck<br>3  Lymphatic, Right Upper Extremity<br>4  Lymphatic, Left Upper Extremity<br>5  Lymphatic, Right Axillary<br>6  Lymphatic, Left Axillary<br>7  Lymphatic, Thorax<br>8  Lymphatic, Internal Mammary, Right<br>9  Lymphatic, Internal Mammary, Left<br>B  Lymphatic, Mesenteric<br>C  Lymphatic, Pelvis<br>D  Lymphatic, Aortic<br>F  Lymphatic, Right Lower Extremity<br>G  Lymphatic, Left Lower Extremity<br>H  Lymphatic, Right Inguinal<br>J  Lymphatic, Left Inguinal<br>K  Thoracic Duct<br>L  Cisterna Chyli<br>M  Thymus<br>P  Spleen | 0  Open<br>3  Percutaneous<br>4  Percutaneous Endoscopic | Z  No Device | Z  No Qualifier |

**0** Medical and Surgical
**7** Lymphatic and Hemic Systems
**9** Drainage: Taking or letting out fluids and/or gases from a body part

| Character 4<br>Body Part | Character 5<br>Approach | Character 6<br>Device | Character 7<br>Qualifier |
|---|---|---|---|
| 0 Lymphatic, Head<br>1 Lymphatic, Right Neck<br>2 Lymphatic, Left Neck<br>3 Lymphatic, Right Upper Extremity<br>4 Lymphatic, Left Upper Extremity<br>5 Lymphatic, Right Axillary<br>6 Lymphatic, Left Axillary<br>7 Lymphatic, Thorax<br>8 Lymphatic, Internal Mammary, Right<br>9 Lymphatic, Internal Mammary, Left<br>B Lymphatic, Mesenteric<br>C Lymphatic, Pelvis<br>D Lymphatic, Aortic<br>F Lymphatic, Right Lower Extremity<br>G Lymphatic, Left Lower Extremity<br>H Lymphatic, Right Inguinal<br>J Lymphatic, Left Inguinal<br>K Thoracic Duct<br>L Cisterna Chyli<br>M Thymus<br>P Spleen<br>T Bone Marrow | 0 Open<br>3 Percutaneous<br>4 Percutaneous Endoscopic | 0 Drainage Device | Z No Qualifier |
| 0 Lymphatic, Head<br>1 Lymphatic, Right Neck<br>2 Lymphatic, Left Neck<br>3 Lymphatic, Right Upper Extremity<br>4 Lymphatic, Left Upper Extremity<br>5 Lymphatic, Right Axillary<br>6 Lymphatic, Left Axillary<br>7 Lymphatic, Thorax<br>8 Lymphatic, Internal Mammary, Right<br>9 Lymphatic, Internal Mammary, Left<br>B Lymphatic, Mesenteric<br>C Lymphatic, Pelvis<br>D Lymphatic, Aortic<br>F Lymphatic, Right Lower Extremity<br>G Lymphatic, Left Lower Extremity<br>H Lymphatic, Right Inguinal<br>J Lymphatic, Left Inguinal<br>K Thoracic Duct<br>L Cisterna Chyli<br>M Thymus<br>P Spleen<br>T Bone Marrow | 0 Open<br>3 Percutaneous<br>4 Percutaneous Endoscopic | Z No Device | X Diagnostic<br>Z No Qualifier |

**0** Medical and Surgical
**7** Lymphatic and Hemic Systems
**B** Excision: Cutting out or off, without replacement, a portion of a body part

| Character 4<br>Body Part | Character 5<br>Approach | Character 6<br>Device | Character 7<br>Qualifier |
|---|---|---|---|
| 0 Lymphatic, Head<br>1 Lymphatic, Right Neck<br>2 Lymphatic, Left Neck<br>3 Lymphatic, Right Upper Extremity<br>4 Lymphatic, Left Upper Extremity<br>5 Lymphatic, Right Axillary<br>6 Lymphatic, Left Axillary<br>7 Lymphatic, Thorax<br>8 Lymphatic, Internal Mammary, Right<br>9 Lymphatic, Internal Mammary, Left<br>B Lymphatic, Mesenteric<br>C Lymphatic, Pelvis<br>D Lymphatic, Aortic<br>F Lymphatic, Right Lower Extremity<br>G Lymphatic, Left Lower Extremity<br>H Lymphatic, Right Inguinal<br>J Lymphatic, Left Inguinal<br>K Thoracic Duct<br>L Cisterna Chyli<br>M Thymus<br>P Spleen | 0 Open<br>3 Percutaneous<br>4 Percutaneous Endoscopic | Z No Device | X Diagnostic<br>Z No Qualifier |

**AHA:** 07B74ZX - 1Q 2014, 21, 26

**0** Medical and Surgical
**7** Lymphatic and Hemic Systems
**C** Extirpation: Taking or cutting out solid matter from a body part

| Character 4<br>Body Part | Character 5<br>Approach | Character 6<br>Device | Character 7<br>Qualifier |
|---|---|---|---|
| 0 Lymphatic, Head<br>1 Lymphatic, Right Neck<br>2 Lymphatic, Left Neck<br>3 Lymphatic, Right Upper Extremity<br>4 Lymphatic, Left Upper Extremity<br>5 Lymphatic, Right Axillary<br>6 Lymphatic, Left Axillary<br>7 Lymphatic, Thorax<br>8 Lymphatic, Internal Mammary, Right<br>9 Lymphatic, Internal Mammary, Left<br>B Lymphatic, Mesenteric<br>C Lymphatic, Pelvis<br>D Lymphatic, Aortic<br>F Lymphatic, Right Lower Extremity<br>G Lymphatic, Left Lower Extremity<br>H Lymphatic, Right Inguinal<br>J Lymphatic, Left Inguinal<br>K Thoracic Duct<br>L Cisterna Chyli<br>M Thymus<br>P Spleen | 0 Open<br>3 Percutaneous<br>4 Percutaneous Endoscopic | Z No Device | Z No Qualifier |

**0** Medical and Surgical
**7** Lymphatic and Hemic Systems
**D** Extraction: Pulling or stripping out or off all or a portion of a body part by the use of force

| Character 4<br>Body Part | Character 5<br>Approach | Character 6<br>Device | Character 7<br>Qualifier |
|---|---|---|---|
| Q Bone Marrow, Sternum<br>R Bone Marrow, Iliac<br>S Bone Marrow, Vertebral | 0 Open<br>3 Percutaneous | Z No Device | X Diagnostic<br>Z No Qualifier |

**0** Medical and Surgical
**7** Lymphatic and Hemic Systems
**H** Insertion: Putting in a nonbiological appliance that monitors, assists, performs, or prevents a physiological function but does not physically take the place of a body part

| Character 4<br>Body Part | Character 5<br>Approach | Character 6<br>Device | Character 7<br>Qualifier |
|---|---|---|---|
| K Thoracic Duct<br>L Cisterna Chyli<br>M Thymus<br>N Lymphatic<br>P Spleen | 0 Open<br>3 Percutaneous<br>4 Percutaneous Endoscopic | 3 Infusion Device | Z No Qualifier |

**0** Medical and Surgical
**7** Lymphatic and Hemic Systems
**J** Inspection: Visually and/or manually exploring a body part

| Character 4<br>Body Part | Character 5<br>Approach | Character 6<br>Device | Character 7<br>Qualifier |
|---|---|---|---|
| K Thoracic Duct<br>L Cisterna Chyli<br>M Thymus<br>T Bone Marrow | 0 Open<br>3 Percutaneous<br>4 Percutaneous Endoscopic | Z No Device | Z No Qualifier |
| N Lymphatic<br>P Spleen | 0 Open<br>3 Percutaneous<br>4 Percutaneous Endoscopic<br>X External | Z No Device | Z No Qualifier |

**0** Medical and Surgical
**7** Lymphatic and Hemic Systems
**L** Occlusion: Completely closing an orifice or the lumen of a tubular body part

| Character 4 Body Part | Character 5 Approach | Character 6 Device | Character 7 Qualifier |
|---|---|---|---|
| 0 Lymphatic, Head | 0 Open | C Extraluminal Device | Z No Qualifier |
| 1 Lymphatic, Right Neck | 3 Percutaneous | D Intraluminal Device | |
| 2 Lymphatic, Left Neck | 4 Percutaneous Endoscopic | Z No Device | |
| 3 Lymphatic, Right Upper Extremity | | | |
| 4 Lymphatic, Left Upper Extremity | | | |
| 5 Lymphatic, Right Axillary | | | |
| 6 Lymphatic, Left Axillary | | | |
| 7 Lymphatic, Thorax | | | |
| 8 Lymphatic, Internal Mammary, Right | | | |
| 9 Lymphatic, Internal Mammary, Left | | | |
| B Lymphatic, Mesenteric | | | |
| C Lymphatic, Pelvis | | | |
| D Lymphatic, Aortic | | | |
| F Lymphatic, Right Lower Extremity | | | |
| G Lymphatic, Left Lower Extremity | | | |
| H Lymphatic, Right Inguinal | | | |
| J Lymphatic, Left Inguinal | | | |
| K Thoracic Duct | | | |
| L Cisterna Chyli | | | |

**0** Medical and Surgical
**7** Lymphatic and Hemic Systems
**N** Release: Freeing a body part from an abnormal physical constraint by cutting or by the use of force

| Character 4 Body Part | Character 5 Approach | Character 6 Device | Character 7 Qualifier |
|---|---|---|---|
| 0 Lymphatic, Head | 0 Open | Z No Device | Z No Qualifier |
| 1 Lymphatic, Right Neck | 3 Percutaneous | | |
| 2 Lymphatic, Left Neck | 4 Percutaneous Endoscopic | | |
| 3 Lymphatic, Right Upper Extremity | | | |
| 4 Lymphatic, Left Upper Extremity | | | |
| 5 Lymphatic, Right Axillary | | | |
| 6 Lymphatic, Left Axillary | | | |
| 7 Lymphatic, Thorax | | | |
| 8 Lymphatic, Internal Mammary, Right | | | |
| 9 Lymphatic, Internal Mammary, Left | | | |
| B Lymphatic, Mesenteric | | | |
| C Lymphatic, Pelvis | | | |
| D Lymphatic, Aortic | | | |
| F Lymphatic, Right Lower Extremity | | | |
| G Lymphatic, Left Lower Extremity | | | |
| H Lymphatic, Right Inguinal | | | |
| J Lymphatic, Left Inguinal | | | |
| K Thoracic Duct | | | |
| L Cisterna Chyli | | | |
| M Thymus | | | |
| P Spleen | | | |

**0** Medical and Surgical
**7** Lymphatic and Hemic Systems
**P** Removal: Taking out or off a device from a body part

| Character 4 Body Part | Character 5 Approach | Character 6 Device | Character 7 Qualifier |
|---|---|---|---|
| K Thoracic Duct | 0 Open | 0 Drainage Device | Z No Qualifier |
| L Cisterna Chyli | 3 Percutaneous | 3 Infusion Device | |
| N Lymphatic | 4 Percutaneous Endoscopic | 7 Autologous Tissue Substitute | |
| | | C Extraluminal Device | |
| | | D Intraluminal Device | |
| | | J Synthetic Substitute | |
| | | K Nonautologous Tissue Substitute | |
| K Thoracic Duct | X External | 0 Drainage Device | Z No Qualifier |
| L Cisterna Chyli | | 3 Infusion Device | |
| N Lymphatic | | D Intraluminal Device | |
| M Thymus | 0 Open | 0 Drainage Device | Z No Qualifier |
| P Spleen | 3 Percutaneous | 3 Infusion Device | |
| | 4 Percutaneous Endoscopic | | |
| | X External | | |
| T Bone Marrow | 0 Open | 0 Drainage Device | Z No Qualifier |
| | 3 Percutaneous | | |
| | 4 Percutaneous Endoscopic | | |
| | X External | | |

**0** Medical and Surgical
**7** Lymphatic and Hemic Systems
**Q** Repair: Restoring, to the extent possible, a body part to its normal anatomic structure and function

| Character 4<br>Body Part | Character 5<br>Approach | Character 6<br>Device | Character 7<br>Qualifier |
|---|---|---|---|
| 0 Lymphatic, Head<br>1 Lymphatic, Right Neck<br>2 Lymphatic, Left Neck<br>3 Lymphatic, Right Upper Extremity<br>4 Lymphatic, Left Upper Extremity<br>5 Lymphatic, Right Axillary<br>6 Lymphatic, Left Axillary<br>7 Lymphatic, Thorax<br>8 Lymphatic, Internal Mammary, Right<br>9 Lymphatic, Internal Mammary, Left<br>B Lymphatic, Mesenteric<br>C Lymphatic, Pelvis<br>D Lymphatic, Aortic<br>F Lymphatic, Right Lower Extremity<br>G Lymphatic, Left Lower Extremity<br>H Lymphatic, Right Inguinal<br>J Lymphatic, Left Inguinal<br>K Thoracic Duct<br>L Cisterna Chyli<br>M Thymus<br>P Spleen | 0 Open<br>3 Percutaneous<br>4 Percutaneous Endoscopic | Z No Device | Z No Qualifier |

**0** Medical and Surgical
**7** Lymphatic and Hemic Systems
**S** Reposition: Moving to its normal location, or other suitable location, all or a portion of a body part

| Character 4<br>Body Part | Character 5<br>Approach | Character 6<br>Device | Character 7<br>Qualifier |
|---|---|---|---|
| M Thymus<br>P Spleen | 0 Open | Z No Device | Z No Qualifier |

**0** Medical and Surgical
**7** Lymphatic and Hemic Systems
**T** Resection: Cutting out or off, without replacement, all of a body part

| Character 4<br>Body Part | Character 5<br>Approach | Character 6<br>Device | Character 7<br>Qualifier |
|---|---|---|---|
| 0 Lymphatic, Head<br>1 Lymphatic, Right Neck<br>2 Lymphatic, Left Neck<br>3 Lymphatic, Right Upper Extremity<br>4 Lymphatic, Left Upper Extremity<br>5 Lymphatic, Right Axillary<br>6 Lymphatic, Left Axillary<br>7 Lymphatic, Thorax<br>8 Lymphatic, Internal Mammary, Right<br>9 Lymphatic, Internal Mammary, Left<br>B Lymphatic, Mesenteric<br>C Lymphatic, Pelvis<br>D Lymphatic, Aortic<br>F Lymphatic, Right Lower Extremity<br>G Lymphatic, Left Lower Extremity<br>H Lymphatic, Right Inguinal<br>J Lymphatic, Left Inguinal<br>K Thoracic Duct<br>L Cisterna Chyli<br>M Thymus<br>P Spleen | 0 Open<br>4 Percutaneous Endoscopic | Z No Device | Z No Qualifier |

**0** Medical and Surgical
**7** Lymphatic and Hemic Systems
**U** Supplement: Putting in or on biological or synthetic material that physically reinforces and/or augments the function of a portion of a body part

| Character 4<br>Body Part | Character 5<br>Approach | Character 6<br>Device | Character 7<br>Qualifier |
|---|---|---|---|
| 0 Lymphatic, Head<br>1 Lymphatic, Right Neck<br>2 Lymphatic, Left Neck<br>3 Lymphatic, Right Upper Extremity<br>4 Lymphatic, Left Upper Extremity<br>5 Lymphatic, Right Axillary<br>6 Lymphatic, Left Axillary<br>7 Lymphatic, Thorax<br>8 Lymphatic, Internal Mammary, Right<br>9 Lymphatic, Internal Mammary, Left<br>B Lymphatic, Mesenteric<br>C Lymphatic, Pelvis<br>D Lymphatic, Aortic<br>F Lymphatic, Right Lower Extremity<br>G Lymphatic, Left Lower Extremity<br>H Lymphatic, Right Inguinal<br>J Lymphatic, Left Inguinal<br>K Thoracic Duct<br>L Cisterna Chyli | 0 Open<br>4 Percutaneous Endoscopic | 7 Autologous Tissue Substitute<br>J Synthetic Substitute<br>K Nonautologous Tissue Substitute | Z No Qualifier |

**0** Medical and Surgical
**7** Lymphatic and Hemic Systems
**V** Restriction: Partially closing an orifice or the lumen of a tubular body part

| Character 4<br>Body Part | Character 5<br>Approach | Character 6<br>Device | Character 7<br>Qualifier |
|---|---|---|---|
| 0 Lymphatic, Head<br>1 Lymphatic, Right Neck<br>2 Lymphatic, Left Neck<br>3 Lymphatic, Right Upper Extremity<br>4 Lymphatic, Left Upper Extremity<br>5 Lymphatic, Right Axillary<br>6 Lymphatic, Left Axillary<br>7 Lymphatic, Thorax<br>8 Lymphatic, Internal Mammary, Right<br>9 Lymphatic, Internal Mammary, Left<br>B Lymphatic, Mesenteric<br>C Lymphatic, Pelvis<br>D Lymphatic, Aortic<br>F Lymphatic, Right Lower Extremity<br>G Lymphatic, Left Lower Extremity<br>H Lymphatic, Right Inguinal<br>J Lymphatic, Left Inguinal<br>K Thoracic Duct<br>L Cisterna Chyli | 0 Open<br>3 Percutaneous<br>4 Percutaneous Endoscopic | C Extraluminal Device<br>D Intraluminal Device<br>Z No Device | Z No Qualifier |

**0** Medical and Surgical
**7** Lymphatic and Hemic Systems
**W** Revision: Correcting, to the extent possible, a portion of a malfunctioning device or the position of a displaced device

| Character 4<br>Body Part | Character 5<br>Approach | Character 6<br>Device | Character 7<br>Qualifier |
|---|---|---|---|
| K Thoracic Duct<br>L Cisterna Chyli<br>N Lymphatic | 0 Open<br>3 Percutaneous<br>4 Percutaneous Endoscopic<br>X External | 0 Drainage Device<br>3 Infusion Device<br>7 Autologous Tissue Substitute<br>C Extraluminal Device<br>D Intraluminal Device<br>J Synthetic Substitute<br>K Nonautologous Tissue Substitute | Z No Qualifier |
| M Thymus<br>P Spleen | 0 Open<br>3 Percutaneous<br>4 Percutaneous Endoscopic<br>X External | 0 Drainage Device<br>3 Infusion Device | Z No Qualifier |
| T Bone Marrow | 0 Open<br>3 Percutaneous<br>4 Percutaneous Endoscopic<br>X External | 0 Drainage Device | Z No Qualifier |

| 0 Medical and Surgical |
| 7 Lymphatic and Hemic Systems |
| Y Transplantation: Putting in or on all or a portion of a living body part taken from another individual or animal to physically take the place and/or function of all or a portion of a similar body part |

| Character 4<br>Body Part | Character 5<br>Approach | Character 6<br>Device | Character 7<br>Qualifier |
|---|---|---|---|
| M Thymus<br>P Spleen | 0 Open | Z No Device | 0 Allogeneic<br>1 Syngeneic<br>2 Zooplastic |

# EYE | 080-08X

| 0 Medical and Surgical |
| 8 Eye |
| 0 Alteration: Modifying the anatomic structure of a body part without affecting the function of the body part |

| Character 4<br>Body Part | Character 5<br>Approach | Character 6<br>Device | Character 7<br>Qualifier |
|---|---|---|---|
| N Upper Eyelid, Right<br>P Upper Eyelid, Left<br>Q Lower Eyelid, Right<br>R Lower Eyelid, Left | 0 Open<br>3 Percutaneous<br>X External | 7 Autologous Tissue Substitute<br>J Synthetic Substitute<br>K Nonautologous Tissue Substitute<br>Z No Device | Z No Qualifier |

| 0 Medical and Surgical |
| 8 Eye |
| 1 Bypass: Altering the route of passage of the contents of a tubular body part |

| Character 4<br>Body Part | Character 5<br>Approach | Character 6<br>Device | Character 7<br>Qualifier |
|---|---|---|---|
| 2 Anterior Chamber, Right<br>3 Anterior Chamber, Left | 3 Percutaneous | J Synthetic Substitute<br>K Nonautologous Tissue Substitute<br>Z No Device | 4 Sclera |
| X Lacrimal Duct, Right<br>Y Lacrimal Duct, Left | 0 Open<br>3 Percutaneous | J Synthetic Substitute<br>K Nonautologous Tissue Substitute<br>Z No Device | 3 Nasal Cavity |

| 0 Medical and Surgical |
| 8 Eye |
| 2 Change: Taking out or off a device from a body part and putting back an identical or similar device in or on the same body part without cutting or puncturing the skin or a mucous membrane |

| Character 4<br>Body Part | Character 5<br>Approach | Character 6<br>Device | Character 7<br>Qualifier |
|---|---|---|---|
| 0 Eye, Right<br>1 Eye, Left | X External | 0 Drainage Device<br>Y Other Device | Z No Qualifier |

**0** Medical and Surgical
**8** Eye
**5** Destruction: Physical eradication of all or a portion of a body part by the direct use of energy, force, or a destructive agent

| Character 4<br>Body Part | Character 5<br>Approach | Character 6<br>Device | Character 7<br>Qualifier |
|---|---|---|---|
| 0 Eye, Right<br>1 Eye, Left<br>6 Sclera, Right<br>7 Sclera, Left<br>8 Cornea, Right<br>9 Cornea, Left<br>S Conjunctiva, Right<br>T Conjunctiva, Left | X External | Z No Device | Z No Qualifier |
| 2 Anterior Chamber, Right<br>3 Anterior Chamber, Left<br>4 Vitreous, Right<br>5 Vitreous, Left<br>C Iris, Right<br>D Iris, Left<br>E Retina, Right<br>F Retina, Left<br>G Retinal Vessel, Right<br>H Retinal Vessel, Left<br>J Lens, Right<br>K Lens, Left | 3 Percutaneous | Z No Device | Z No Qualifier |
| A Choroid, Right<br>B Choroid, Left<br>L Extraocular Muscle, Right<br>M Extraocular Muscle, Left<br>V Lacrimal Gland, Right<br>W Lacrimal Gland, Left | 0 Open<br>3 Percutaneous | Z No Device | Z No Qualifier |
| N Upper Eyelid, Right<br>P Upper Eyelid, Left<br>Q Lower Eyelid, Right<br>R Lower Eyelid, Left | 0 Open<br>3 Percutaneous<br>X External | Z No Device | Z No Qualifier |
| X Lacrimal Duct, Right<br>Y Lacrimal Duct, Left | 0 Open<br>3 Percutaneous<br>7 Via Natural or Artificial Opening<br>8 Via Natural or Artificial Opening Endoscopic | Z No Device | Z No Qualifier |

**0** Medical and Surgical
**8** Eye
**7** Dilation: Expanding an orifice or the lumen of a tubular body part

| Character 4<br>Body Part | Character 5<br>Approach | Character 6<br>Device | Character 7<br>Qualifier |
|---|---|---|---|
| X Lacrimal Duct, Right<br>Y Lacrimal Duct, Left | 0 Open<br>3 Percutaneous<br>7 Via Natural or Artificial Opening<br>8 Via Natural or Artificial Opening Endoscopic | D Intraluminal Device<br>Z No Device | Z No Qualifier |

| 0 Medical and Surgical |
| --- |
| 8 Eye |
| 9 Drainage: Taking or letting out fluids and/or gases from a body part |

| Character 4<br>Body Part | Character 5<br>Approach | Character 6<br>Device | Character 7<br>Qualifier |
| --- | --- | --- | --- |
| 0 Eye, Right<br>1 Eye, Left<br>6 Sclera, Right<br>7 Sclera, Left<br>8 Cornea, Right<br>9 Cornea, Left<br>S Conjunctiva, Right<br>T Conjunctiva, Left | X External | 0 Drainage Device | Z No Qualifier |
| 0 Eye, Right<br>1 Eye, Left<br>6 Sclera, Right<br>7 Sclera, Left<br>8 Cornea, Right<br>9 Cornea, Left<br>S Conjunctiva, Right<br>T Conjunctiva, Left | X External | Z No Device | X Diagnostic<br>Z No Qualifier |
| 2 Anterior Chamber, Right<br>3 Anterior Chamber, Left<br>4 Vitreous, Right<br>5 Vitreous, Left<br>C Iris, Right<br>D Iris, Left<br>E Retina, Right<br>F Retina, Left<br>G Retinal Vessel, Right<br>H Retinal Vessel, Left<br>J Lens, Right<br>K Lens, Left | 3 Percutaneous | 0 Drainage Device | Z No Qualifier |
| 2 Anterior Chamber, Right<br>3 Anterior Chamber, Left<br>4 Vitreous, Right<br>5 Vitreous, Left<br>C Iris, Right<br>D Iris, Left<br>E Retina, Right<br>F Retina, Left<br>G Retinal Vessel, Right<br>H Retinal Vessel, Left<br>J Lens, Right<br>K Lens, Left | 3 Percutaneous | Z No Device | X Diagnostic<br>Z No Qualifier |
| A Choroid, Right<br>B Choroid, Left<br>L Extraocular Muscle, Right<br>M Extraocular Muscle, Left<br>V Lacrimal Gland, Right<br>W Lacrimal Gland, Left | 0 Open<br>3 Percutaneous | 0 Drainage Device | Z No Qualifier |
| A Choroid, Right<br>B Choroid, Left<br>L Extraocular Muscle, Right<br>M Extraocular Muscle, Left<br>V Lacrimal Gland, Right<br>W Lacrimal Gland, Left | 0 Open<br>3 Percutaneous | Z No Device | X Diagnostic<br>Z No Qualifier |
| N Upper Eyelid, Right<br>P Upper Eyelid, Left<br>Q Lower Eyelid, Right<br>R Lower Eyelid, Left | 0 Open<br>3 Percutaneous<br>X External | 0 Drainage Device | Z No Qualifier |
| N Upper Eyelid, Right<br>P Upper Eyelid, Left<br>Q Lower Eyelid, Right<br>R Lower Eyelid, Left | 0 Open<br>3 Percutaneous<br>X External | Z No Device | X Diagnostic<br>Z No Qualifier |
| X Lacrimal Duct, Right<br>Y Lacrimal Duct, Left | 0 Open<br>3 Percutaneous<br>7 Via Natural or Artificial Opening<br>8 Via Natural or Artificial Opening Endoscopic | 0 Drainage Device | Z No Qualifier |
| X Lacrimal Duct, Right<br>Y Lacrimal Duct, Left | 0 Open<br>3 Percutaneous<br>7 Via Natural or Artificial Opening<br>8 Via Natural or Artificial Opening Endoscopic | Z No Device | X Diagnostic<br>Z No Qualifier |

**0** Medical and Surgical
**8** Eye
**B** Excision: Cutting out or off, without replacement, a portion of a body part

| Character 4<br>Body Part | Character 5<br>Approach | Character 6<br>Device | Character 7<br>Qualifier |
|---|---|---|---|
| 0 Eye, Right<br>1 Eye, Left<br>N Upper Eyelid, Right<br>P Upper Eyelid, Left<br>Q Lower Eyelid, Right<br>R Lower Eyelid, Left | 0 Open<br>3 Percutaneous<br>X External | Z No Device | X Diagnostic<br>Z No Qualifier |
| 4 Vitreous, Right<br>5 Vitreous, Left<br>C Iris, Right<br>D Iris, Left<br>E Retina, Right<br>F Retina, Left<br>J Lens, Right<br>K Lens, Left | 3 Percutaneous | Z No Device | X Diagnostic<br>Z No Qualifier |
| 6 Sclera, Right<br>7 Sclera, Left<br>8 Cornea, Right<br>9 Cornea, Left<br>S Conjunctiva, Right<br>T Conjunctiva, Left | X External | Z No Device | X Diagnostic<br>Z No Qualifier |
| A Choroid, Right<br>B Choroid, Left<br>L Extraocular Muscle, Right<br>M Extraocular Muscle, Left<br>V Lacrimal Gland, Right<br>W Lacrimal Gland, Left | 0 Open<br>3 Percutaneous | Z No Device | X Diagnostic<br>Z No Qualifier |
| X Lacrimal Duct, Right<br>Y Lacrimal Duct, Left | 0 Open<br>3 Percutaneous<br>7 Via Natural or Artificial Opening<br>8 Via Natural or Artificial Opening<br>   Endoscopic | Z No Device | X Diagnostic<br>Z No Qualifier |

**0** Medical and Surgical
**8** Eye
**C** Extirpation: Taking or cutting out solid matter from a body part

| Character 4<br>Body Part | Character 5<br>Approach | Character 6<br>Device | Character 7<br>Qualifier |
|---|---|---|---|
| 0 Eye, Right<br>1 Eye, Left<br>6 Sclera, Right<br>7 Sclera, Left<br>8 Cornea, Right<br>9 Cornea, Left<br>S Conjunctiva, Right<br>T Conjunctiva, Left | X External | Z No Device | Z No Qualifier |
| 2 Anterior Chamber, Right<br>3 Anterior Chamber, Left<br>4 Vitreous, Right<br>5 Vitreous, Left<br>C Iris, Right<br>D Iris, Left<br>E Retina, Right<br>F Retina, Left<br>G Retinal Vessel, Right<br>H Retinal Vessel, Left<br>J Lens, Right<br>K Lens, Left | 3 Percutaneous<br>X External | Z No Device | Z No Qualifier |
| A Choroid, Right<br>B Choroid, Left<br>L Extraocular Muscle, Right<br>M Extraocular Muscle, Left<br>N Upper Eyelid, Right<br>P Upper Eyelid, Left<br>Q Lower Eyelid, Right<br>R Lower Eyelid, Left<br>V Lacrimal Gland, Right<br>W Lacrimal Gland, Left | 0 Open<br>3 Percutaneous<br>X External | Z No Device | Z No Qualifier |
| X Lacrimal Duct, Right<br>Y Lacrimal Duct, Left | 0 Open<br>3 Percutaneous<br>7 Via Natural or Artificial Opening<br>8 Via Natural or Artificial Opening<br>   Endoscopic | Z No Device | Z No Qualifier |

**0** Medical and Surgical
**8** Eye
**D** Extraction: Pulling or stripping out or off all or a portion of a body part by the use of force

| Character 4<br>Body Part | Character 5<br>Approach | Character 6<br>Device | Character 7<br>Qualifier |
|---|---|---|---|
| 8 Cornea, Right<br>9 Cornea, Left | X External | Z No Device | X Diagnostic<br>Z No Qualifier |
| J Lens, Right<br>K Lens, Left | 3 Percutaneous | Z No Device | Z No Qualifier |

**0** Medical and Surgical
**8** Eye
**F** Fragmentation: Breaking solid matter in a body part into pieces

| Character 4<br>Body Part | Character 5<br>Approach | Character 6<br>Device | Character 7<br>Qualifier |
|---|---|---|---|
| 4 Vitreous, Right  N C<br>5 Vitreous, Left  N C | 3 Percutaneous<br>X External | Z No Device | Z No Qualifier |

N C 08F(4,5)XZZ

**0** Medical and Surgical
**8** Eye
**H** Insertion: Putting in a nonbiological appliance that monitors, assists, performs, or prevents a physiological function but does not physically take the place of a body part

| Character 4 Body Part | Character 5 Approach | Character 6 Device | Character 7 Qualifier |
|---|---|---|---|
| 0  Eye, Right<br>1  Eye, Left | 0  Open | 5  Epiretinal Visual Prosthesis | Z  No Qualifier |
| 0  Eye, Right<br>1  Eye, Left | 3  Percutaneous<br>X  External | 1  Radioactive Element<br>3  Infusion Device | Z  No Qualifier |

**0** Medical and Surgical
**8** Eye
**J** Inspection: Visually and/or manually exploring a body part

| Character 4 Body Part | Character 5 Approach | Character 6 Device | Character 7 Qualifier |
|---|---|---|---|
| 0  Eye, Right<br>1  Eye, Left<br>J  Lens, Right<br>K  Lens, Left | X  External | Z  No Device | Z  No Qualifier |
| L  Extraocular Muscle, Right<br>M  Extraocular Muscle, Left | 0  Open<br>X  External | Z  No Device | Z  No Qualifier |

**0** Medical and Surgical
**8** Eye
**L** Occlusion: Completely closing an orifice or the lumen of a tubular body part

| Character 4 Body Part | Character 5 Approach | Character 6 Device | Character 7 Qualifier |
|---|---|---|---|
| X  Lacrimal Duct, Right<br>Y  Lacrimal Duct, Left | 0  Open<br>3  Percutaneous | C  Extraluminal Device<br>D  Intraluminal Device<br>Z  No Device | Z  No Qualifier |
| X  Lacrimal Duct, Right<br>Y  Lacrimal Duct, Left | 7  Via Natural or Artificial Opening<br>8  Via Natural or Artificial Opening Endoscopic | D  Intraluminal Device<br>Z  No Device | Z  No Qualifier |

**0** Medical and Surgical
**8** Eye
**M** Reattachment: Putting back in or on all or a portion of a separated body part to its normal location or other suitable location

| Character 4 Body Part | Character 5 Approach | Character 6 Device | Character 7 Qualifier |
|---|---|---|---|
| N  Upper Eyelid, Right<br>P  Upper Eyelid, Left<br>Q  Lower Eyelid, Right<br>R  Lower Eyelid, Left | X  External | Z  No Device | Z  No Qualifier |

**0** Medical and Surgical
**8** Eye
**N** Release: Freeing a body part from an abnormal physical constraint by cutting or by the use of force

| Character 4<br>Body Part | Character 5<br>Approach | Character 6<br>Device | Character 7<br>Qualifier |
|---|---|---|---|
| 0 Eye, Right<br>1 Eye, Left<br>6 Sclera, Right<br>7 Sclera, Left<br>8 Cornea, Right<br>9 Cornea, Left<br>S Conjunctiva, Right<br>T Conjunctiva, Left | X External | Z No Device | Z No Qualifier |
| 2 Anterior Chamber, Right<br>3 Anterior Chamber, Left<br>4 Vitreous, Right<br>5 Vitreous, Left<br>C Iris, Right<br>D Iris, Left<br>E Retina, Right<br>F Retina, Left<br>G Retinal Vessel, Right<br>H Retinal Vessel, Left<br>J Lens, Right<br>K Lens, Left | 3 Percutaneous | Z No Device | Z No Qualifier |
| A Choroid, Right<br>B Choroid, Left<br>L Extraocular Muscle, Right<br>M Extraocular Muscle, Left<br>V Lacrimal Gland, Right<br>W Lacrimal Gland, Left | 0 Open<br>3 Percutaneous | Z No Device | Z No Qualifier |
| N Upper Eyelid, Right<br>P Upper Eyelid, Left<br>Q Lower Eyelid, Right<br>R Lower Eyelid, Left | 0 Open<br>3 Percutaneous<br>X External | Z No Device | Z No Qualifier |
| X Lacrimal Duct, Right<br>Y Lacrimal Duct, Left | 0 Open<br>3 Percutaneous<br>7 Via Natural or Artificial Opening<br>8 Via Natural or Artificial Opening<br>Endoscopic | Z No Device | Z No Qualifier |

**0** Medical and Surgical
**8** Eye
**P** Removal: Taking out or off a device from a body part

| Character 4<br>Body Part | Character 5<br>Approach | Character 6<br>Device | Character 7<br>Qualifier |
|---|---|---|---|
| 0 Eye, Right<br>1 Eye, Left | 0 Open<br>3 Percutaneous<br>7 Via Natural or Artificial Opening<br>8 Via Natural or Artificial Opening<br>Endoscopic<br>X External | 0 Drainage Device<br>1 Radioactive Element<br>3 Infusion Device<br>7 Autologous Tissue Substitute<br>C Extraluminal Device<br>D Intraluminal Device<br>J Synthetic Substitute<br>K Nonautologous Tissue Substitute | Z No Qualifier |
| J Lens, Right<br>K Lens, Left | 3 Percutaneous | J Synthetic Substitute | Z No Qualifier |
| L Extraocular Muscle, Right<br>M Extraocular Muscle, Left | 0 Open<br>3 Percutaneous | 0 Drainage Device<br>7 Autologous Tissue Substitute<br>J Synthetic Substitute<br>K Nonautologous Tissue Substitute | Z No Qualifier |

**0** Medical and Surgical
**8** Eye
**Q** Repair: Restoring, to the extent possible, a body part to its normal anatomic structure and function

| Character 4<br>Body Part | Character 5<br>Approach | Character 6<br>Device | Character 7<br>Qualifier |
|---|---|---|---|
| 0 Eye, Right<br>1 Eye, Left<br>6 Sclera, Right<br>7 Sclera, Left<br>8 Cornea, Right N C<br>9 Cornea, Left N C<br>S Conjunctiva, Right<br>T Conjunctiva, Left | X External | Z No Device | Z No Qualifier |
| 2 Anterior Chamber, Right<br>3 Anterior Chamber, Left<br>4 Vitreous, Right<br>5 Vitreous, Left<br>C Iris, Right<br>D Iris, Left<br>E Retina, Right<br>F Retina, Left<br>G Retinal Vessel, Right<br>H Retinal Vessel, Left<br>J Lens, Right<br>K Lens, Left | 3 Percutaneous | Z No Device | Z No Qualifier |
| A Choroid, Right<br>B Choroid, Left<br>L Extraocular Muscle, Right<br>M Extraocular Muscle, Left<br>V Lacrimal Gland, Right<br>W Lacrimal Gland, Left | 0 Open<br>3 Percutaneous | Z No Device | Z No Qualifier |
| N Upper Eyelid, Right<br>P Upper Eyelid, Left<br>Q Lower Eyelid, Right<br>R Lower Eyelid, Left | 0 Open<br>3 Percutaneous<br>X External | Z No Device | Z No Qualifier |
| X Lacrimal Duct, Right<br>Y Lacrimal Duct, Left | 0 Open<br>3 Percutaneous<br>7 Via Natural or Artificial Opening<br>8 Via Natural or Artificial Opening<br>Endoscopic | Z No Device | Z No Qualifier |

N C 08Q(8,9)XZZ

**0** Medical and Surgical
**8** Eye
**R** Replacement: Putting in or on biological or synthetic material that physically takes the place and/or function of all or a portion of a body part

| Character 4<br>Body Part | Character 5<br>Approach | Character 6<br>Device | Character 7<br>Qualifier |
|---|---|---|---|
| 0 Eye, Right<br>1 Eye, Left<br>A Choroid, Right<br>B Choroid, Left | 0 Open<br>3 Percutaneous | 7 Autologous Tissue Substitute<br>J Synthetic Substitute<br>K Nonautologous Tissue Substitute | Z No Qualifier |
| 4 Vitreous, Right<br>5 Vitreous, Left<br>C Iris, Right<br>D Iris, Left<br>G Retinal Vessel, Right<br>H Retinal Vessel, Left | 3 Percutaneous | 7 Autologous Tissue Substitute<br>J Synthetic Substitute<br>K Nonautologous Tissue Substitute | Z No Qualifier |
| 6 Sclera, Right<br>7 Sclera, Left<br>S Conjunctiva, Right<br>T Conjunctiva, Left | X External | 7 Autologous Tissue Substitute<br>J Synthetic Substitute<br>K Nonautologous Tissue Substitute | Z No Qualifier |
| 8 Cornea, Right<br>9 Cornea, Left | 3 Percutaneous<br>X External | 7 Autologous Tissue Substitute<br>J Synthetic Substitute<br>K Nonautologous Tissue Substitute | Z No Qualifier |
| J Lens, Right<br>K Lens, Left | 3 Percutaneous | 0 Synthetic Substitute, Intraocular Telescope<br>7 Autologous Tissue Substitute<br>J Synthetic Substitute<br>K Nonautologous Tissue Substitute | Z No Qualifier |
| N Upper Eyelid, Right<br>P Upper Eyelid, Left<br>Q Lower Eyelid, Right<br>R Lower Eyelid, Left | 0 Open<br>3 Percutaneous<br>X External | 7 Autologous Tissue Substitute<br>J Synthetic Substitute<br>K Nonautologous Tissue Substitute | Z No Qualifier |
| X Lacrimal Duct, Right<br>Y Lacrimal Duct, Left | 0 Open<br>3 Percutaneous<br>7 Via Natural or Artificial Opening<br>8 Via Natural or Artificial Opening Endoscopic | 7 Autologous Tissue Substitute<br>J Synthetic Substitute<br>K Nonautologous Tissue Substitute | Z No Qualifier |

**0** Medical and Surgical
**8** Eye
**S** Reposition: Moving to its normal location, or other suitable location, all or a portion of a body part

| Character 4<br>Body Part | Character 5<br>Approach | Character 6<br>Device | Character 7<br>Qualifier |
|---|---|---|---|
| C Iris, Right<br>D Iris, Left<br>G Retinal Vessel, Right<br>H Retinal Vessel, Left<br>J Lens, Right<br>K Lens, Left | 3 Percutaneous | Z No Device | Z No Qualifier |
| L Extraocular Muscle, Right<br>M Extraocular Muscle, Left<br>V Lacrimal Gland, Right<br>W Lacrimal Gland, Left | 0 Open<br>3 Percutaneous | Z No Device | Z No Qualifier |
| N Upper Eyelid, Right<br>P Upper Eyelid, Left<br>Q Lower Eyelid, Right<br>R Lower Eyelid, Left | 0 Open<br>3 Percutaneous<br>X External | Z No Device | Z No Qualifier |
| X Lacrimal Duct, Right<br>Y Lacrimal Duct, Left | 0 Open<br>3 Percutaneous<br>7 Via Natural or Artificial Opening<br>8 Via Natural or Artificial Opening Endoscopic | Z No Device | Z No Qualifier |

**0** Medical and Surgical
**8** Eye
**T** Resection: Cutting out or off, without replacement, all of a body part

| Character 4<br>Body Part | Character 5<br>Approach | Character 6<br>Device | Character 7<br>Qualifier |
|---|---|---|---|
| 0 Eye, Right<br>1 Eye, Left<br>8 Cornea, Right<br>9 Cornea, Left | X External | Z No Device | Z No Qualifier |
| 4 Vitreous, Right<br>5 Vitreous, Left<br>C Iris, Right<br>D Iris, Left<br>J Lens, Right<br>K Lens, Left | 3 Percutaneous | Z No Device | Z No Qualifier |
| L Extraocular Muscle, Right<br>M Extraocular Muscle, Left<br>V Lacrimal Gland, Right<br>W Lacrimal Gland, Left | 0 Open<br>3 Percutaneous | Z No Device | Z No Qualifier |
| N Upper Eyelid, Right<br>P Upper Eyelid, Left<br>Q Lower Eyelid, Right<br>R Lower Eyelid, Left | 0 Open<br>X External | Z No Device | Z No Qualifier |
| X Lacrimal Duct, Right<br>Y Lacrimal Duct, Left | 0 Open<br>3 Percutaneous<br>7 Via Natural or Artificial Opening<br>8 Via Natural or Artificial Opening Endoscopic | Z No Device | Z No Qualifier |

**0** Medical and Surgical
**8** Eye
**U** Supplement: Putting in or on biological or synthetic material that physically reinforces and/or augments the function of a portion of a body part

| Character 4<br>Body Part | Character 5<br>Approach | Character 6<br>Device | Character 7<br>Qualifier |
|---|---|---|---|
| 0 Eye, Right<br>1 Eye, Left<br>C Iris, Right<br>D Iris, Left<br>E Retina, Right<br>F Retina, Left<br>G Retinal Vessel, Right<br>H Retinal Vessel, Left<br>L Extraocular Muscle, Right<br>M Extraocular Muscle, Left | 0 Open<br>3 Percutaneous | 7 Autologous Tissue Substitute<br>J Synthetic Substitute<br>K Nonautologous Tissue Substitute | Z No Qualifier |
| 8 Cornea, Right **N C**<br>9 Cornea, Left **N C**<br>N Upper Eyelid, Right<br>P Upper Eyelid, Left<br>Q Lower Eyelid, Right<br>R Lower Eyelid, Left | 0 Open<br>3 Percutaneous<br>X External | 7 Autologous Tissue Substitute<br>J Synthetic Substitute<br>K Nonautologous Tissue Substitute | Z No Qualifier |
| X Lacrimal Duct, Right<br>Y Lacrimal Duct, Left | 0 Open<br>3 Percutaneous<br>7 Via Natural or Artificial Opening<br>8 Via Natural or Artificial Opening Endoscopic | 7 Autologous Tissue Substitute<br>J Synthetic Substitute<br>K Nonautologous Tissue Substitute | Z No Qualifier |

**N C** 08U8(0,3,X)KZ , 08U9(0,3,X)KZ

**0** Medical and Surgical
**8** Eye
**V** Restriction: Partially closing an orifice or the lumen of a tubular body part

| Character 4<br>Body Part | Character 5<br>Approach | Character 6<br>Device | Character 7<br>Qualifier |
|---|---|---|---|
| X Lacrimal Duct, Right<br>Y Lacrimal Duct, Left | 0 Open<br>3 Percutaneous | C Extraluminal Device<br>D Intraluminal Device<br>Z No Device | Z No Qualifier |
| X Lacrimal Duct, Right<br>Y Lacrimal Duct, Left | 7 Via Natural or Artificial Opening<br>8 Via Natural or Artificial Opening Endoscopic | D Intraluminal Device<br>Z No Device | Z No Qualifier |

**0** Medical and Surgical
**8** Eye
**W** Revision: Correcting, to the extent possible, a portion of a malfunctioning device or the position of a displaced device

| Character 4<br>Body Part | Character 5<br>Approach | Character 6<br>Device | Character 7<br>Qualifier |
|---|---|---|---|
| 0  Eye, Right<br>1  Eye, Left | 0  Open<br>3  Percutaneous<br>7  Via Natural or Artificial Opening<br>8  Via Natural or Artificial Opening<br>   Endoscopic<br>X  External | 0  Drainage Device<br>3  Infusion Device<br>7  Autologous Tissue Substitute<br>C  Extraluminal Device<br>D  Intraluminal Device<br>J  Synthetic Substitute<br>K  Nonautologous Tissue Substitute | Z  No Qualifier |
| J  Lens, Right<br>K  Lens, Left | 3  Percutaneous<br>X  External | J  Synthetic Substitute | Z  No Qualifier |
| L  Extraocular Muscle, Right<br>M  Extraocular Muscle, Left | 0  Open<br>3  Percutaneous | 0  Drainage Device<br>7  Autologous Tissue Substitute<br>J  Synthetic Substitute<br>K  Nonautologous Tissue Substitute | Z  No Qualifier |

**0** Medical and Surgical
**8** Eye
**X** Transfer: Moving, without taking out, all or a portion of a body part to another location to take over the function of all or a portion of a body part

| Character 4<br>Body Part | Character 5<br>Approach | Character 6<br>Device | Character 7<br>Qualifier |
|---|---|---|---|
| L  Extraocular Muscle, Right<br>M  Extraocular Muscle, Left | 0  Open<br>3  Percutaneous | Z  No Device | Z  No Qualifier |

# Ear, Nose, Sinus | 090-09W

**0** Medical and Surgical
**9** Ear, Nose, Sinus
**0** Alteration: Modifying the anatomic structure of a body part without affecting the function of the body part

| Character 4<br>Body Part | Character 5<br>Approach | Character 6<br>Device | Character 7<br>Qualifier |
|---|---|---|---|
| 0 External Ear, Right<br>1 External Ear, Left<br>2 External Ear, Bilateral<br>K Nose | 0 Open<br>3 Percutaneous<br>4 Percutaneous Endoscopic<br>X External | 7 Autologous Tissue Substitute<br>J Synthetic Substitute<br>K Nonautologous Tissue Substitute<br>Z No Device | Z No Qualifier |

**0** Medical and Surgical
**9** Ear, Nose, Sinus
**1** Bypass: Altering the route of passage of the contents of a tubular body part

| Character 4<br>Body Part | Character 5<br>Approach | Character 6<br>Device | Character 7<br>Qualifier |
|---|---|---|---|
| D Inner Ear, Right<br>E Inner Ear, Left | 0 Open | 7 Autologous Tissue Substitute<br>J Synthetic Substitute<br>K Nonautologous Tissue Substitute<br>Z No Device | 0 Endolymphatic |

**0** Medical and Surgical
**9** Ear, Nose, Sinus
**2** Change: Taking out or off a device from a body part and putting back an identical or similar device in or on the same body part without cutting or puncturing the skin or a mucous membrane

| Character 4<br>Body Part | Character 5<br>Approach | Character 6<br>Device | Character 7<br>Qualifier |
|---|---|---|---|
| H Ear, Right<br>J Ear, Left<br>K Nose<br>Y Sinus | X External | 0 Drainage Device<br>Y Other Device | Z No Qualifier |

**0 Medical and Surgical**
**9 Ear, Nose, Sinus**
**5 Destruction:** Physical eradication of all or a portion of a body part by the direct use of energy, force, or a destructive agent

| Character 4<br>Body Part | Character 5<br>Approach | Character 6<br>Device | Character 7<br>Qualifier |
|---|---|---|---|
| 0 External Ear, Right<br>1 External Ear, Left<br>K Nose | 0 Open<br>3 Percutaneous<br>4 Percutaneous Endoscopic<br>X External | Z No Device | Z No Qualifier |
| 3 External Auditory Canal, Right<br>4 External Auditory Canal, Left | 0 Open<br>3 Percutaneous<br>4 Percutaneous Endoscopic<br>7 Via Natural or Artificial Opening<br>8 Via Natural or Artificial Opening<br>  Endoscopic<br>X External | Z No Device | Z No Qualifier |
| 5 Middle Ear, Right<br>6 Middle Ear, Left<br>9 Auditory Ossicle, Right<br>A Auditory Ossicle, Left<br>D Inner Ear, Right<br>E Inner Ear, Left | 0 Open | Z No Device | Z No Qualifier |
| 7 Tympanic Membrane, Right<br>8 Tympanic Membrane, Left<br>F Eustachian Tube, Right<br>G Eustachian Tube, Left<br>L Nasal Turbinate<br>N Nasopharynx | 0 Open<br>3 Percutaneous<br>4 Percutaneous Endoscopic<br>7 Via Natural or Artificial Opening<br>8 Via Natural or Artificial Opening<br>  Endoscopic | Z No Device | Z No Qualifier |
| B Mastoid Sinus, Right<br>C Mastoid Sinus, Left<br>M Nasal Septum<br>P Accessory Sinus<br>Q Maxillary Sinus, Right<br>R Maxillary Sinus, Left<br>S Frontal Sinus, Right<br>T Frontal Sinus, Left<br>U Ethmoid Sinus, Right<br>V Ethmoid Sinus, Left<br>W Sphenoid Sinus, Right<br>X Sphenoid Sinus, Left | 0 Open<br>3 Percutaneous<br>4 Percutaneous Endoscopic | Z No Device | Z No Qualifier |

**0 Medical and Surgical**
**9 Ear, Nose, Sinus**
**7 Dilation:** Expanding an orifice or the lumen of a tubular body part

| Character 4<br>Body Part | Character 5<br>Approach | Character 6<br>Device | Character 7<br>Qualifier |
|---|---|---|---|
| F Eustachian Tube, Right<br>G Eustachian Tube, Left | 0 Open<br>7 Via Natural or Artificial Opening<br>8 Via Natural or Artificial Opening<br>  Endoscopic | D Intraluminal Device<br>Z No Device | Z No Qualifier |
| F Eustachian Tube, Right<br>G Eustachian Tube, Left | 3 Percutaneous<br>4 Percutaneous Endoscopic | Z No Device | Z No Qualifier |

**0 Medical and Surgical**
**9 Ear, Nose, Sinus**
**8 Division:** Cutting into a body part, without draining fluids and/or gases from the body part, in order to separate or transect a body part

| Character 4<br>Body Part | Character 5<br>Approach | Character 6<br>Device | Character 7<br>Qualifier |
|---|---|---|---|
| L Nasal Turbinate | 0 Open<br>3 Percutaneous<br>4 Percutaneous Endoscopic<br>7 Via Natural or Artificial Opening<br>8 Via Natural or Artificial Opening<br>  Endoscopic | Z No Device | Z No Qualifier |

**0** Medical and Surgical
**9** Ear, Nose, Sinus
**9** Drainage: Taking or letting out fluids and/or gases from a body part

| Character 4<br>Body Part | Character 5<br>Approach | Character 6<br>Device | Character 7<br>Qualifier |
|---|---|---|---|
| 0 External Ear, Right<br>1 External Ear, Left<br>K Nose | 0 Open<br>3 Percutaneous<br>4 Percutaneous Endoscopic<br>X External | 0 Drainage Device | Z No Qualifier |
| 0 External Ear, Right<br>1 External Ear, Left<br>K Nose | 0 Open<br>3 Percutaneous<br>4 Percutaneous Endoscopic<br>X External | Z No Device | X Diagnostic<br>Z No Qualifier |
| 3 External Auditory Canal, Right<br>4 External Auditory Canal, Left | 0 Open<br>3 Percutaneous<br>4 Percutaneous Endoscopic<br>7 Via Natural or Artificial Opening<br>8 Via Natural or Artificial Opening<br>  Endoscopic<br>X External | 0 Drainage Device | Z No Qualifier |
| 3 External Auditory Canal, Right<br>4 External Auditory Canal, Left | 0 Open<br>3 Percutaneous<br>4 Percutaneous Endoscopic<br>7 Via Natural or Artificial Opening<br>8 Via Natural or Artificial Opening<br>  Endoscopic<br>X External | Z No Device | X Diagnostic<br>Z No Qualifier |
| 5 Middle Ear, Right<br>6 Middle Ear, Left<br>9 Auditory Ossicle, Right<br>A Auditory Ossicle, Left<br>D Inner Ear, Right<br>E Inner Ear, Left | 0 Open | 0 Drainage Device | Z No Qualifier |
| 5 Middle Ear, Right<br>6 Middle Ear, Left<br>9 Auditory Ossicle, Right<br>A Auditory Ossicle, Left<br>D Inner Ear, Right<br>E Inner Ear, Left | 0 Open | Z No Device | X Diagnostic<br>Z No Qualifier |
| 7 Tympanic Membrane, Right<br>8 Tympanic Membrane, Left<br>F Eustachian Tube, Right<br>G Eustachian Tube, Left<br>L Nasal Turbinate<br>N Nasopharynx | 0 Open<br>3 Percutaneous<br>4 Percutaneous Endoscopic<br>7 Via Natural or Artificial Opening<br>8 Via Natural or Artificial Opening<br>  Endoscopic | 0 Drainage Device | Z No Qualifier |
| 7 Tympanic Membrane, Right<br>8 Tympanic Membrane, Left<br>F Eustachian Tube, Right<br>G Eustachian Tube, Left<br>L Nasal Turbinate<br>N Nasopharynx | 0 Open<br>3 Percutaneous<br>4 Percutaneous Endoscopic<br>7 Via Natural or Artificial Opening<br>8 Via Natural or Artificial Opening<br>  Endoscopic | Z No Device | X Diagnostic<br>Z No Qualifier |
| B Mastoid Sinus, Right<br>C Mastoid Sinus, Left<br>M Nasal Septum<br>P Accessory Sinus<br>Q Maxillary Sinus, Right<br>R Maxillary Sinus, Left<br>S Frontal Sinus, Right<br>T Frontal Sinus, Left<br>U Ethmoid Sinus, Right<br>V Ethmoid Sinus, Left<br>W Sphenoid Sinus, Right<br>X Sphenoid Sinus, Left | 0 Open<br>3 Percutaneous<br>4 Percutaneous Endoscopic | 0 Drainage Device | Z No Qualifier |
| B Mastoid Sinus, Right<br>C Mastoid Sinus, Left<br>M Nasal Septum<br>P Accessory Sinus<br>Q Maxillary Sinus, Right<br>R Maxillary Sinus, Left<br>S Frontal Sinus, Right<br>T Frontal Sinus, Left<br>U Ethmoid Sinus, Right<br>V Ethmoid Sinus, Left<br>W Sphenoid Sinus, Right<br>X Sphenoid Sinus, Left | 0 Open<br>3 Percutaneous<br>4 Percutaneous Endoscopic | Z No Device | X Diagnostic<br>Z No Qualifier |

**0** Medical and Surgical
**9** Ear, Nose, Sinus
**B** Excision: Cutting out or off, without replacement, a portion of a body part

| Character 4<br>Body Part | Character 5<br>Approach | Character 6<br>Device | Character 7<br>Qualifier |
|---|---|---|---|
| 0 External Ear, Right<br>1 External Ear, Left<br>K Nose | 0 Open<br>3 Percutaneous<br>4 Percutaneous Endoscopic<br>X External | Z No Device | X Diagnostic<br>Z No Qualifier |
| 3 External Auditory Canal, Right<br>4 External Auditory Canal, Left | 0 Open<br>3 Percutaneous<br>4 Percutaneous Endoscopic<br>7 Via Natural or Artificial Opening<br>8 Via Natural or Artificial Opening<br>  Endoscopic<br>X External | Z No Device | X Diagnostic<br>Z No Qualifier |
| 5 Middle Ear, Right<br>6 Middle Ear, Left<br>9 Auditory Ossicle, Right<br>A Auditory Ossicle, Left<br>D Inner Ear, Right<br>E Inner Ear, Left | 0 Open | Z No Device | X Diagnostic<br>Z No Qualifier |
| 7 Tympanic Membrane, Right<br>8 Tympanic Membrane, Left<br>F Eustachian Tube, Right<br>G Eustachian Tube, Left<br>L Nasal Turbinate<br>N Nasopharynx | 0 Open<br>3 Percutaneous<br>4 Percutaneous Endoscopic<br>7 Via Natural or Artificial Opening<br>8 Via Natural or Artificial Opening<br>  Endoscopic | Z No Device | X Diagnostic<br>Z No Qualifier |
| B Mastoid Sinus, Right<br>C Mastoid Sinus, Left<br>M Nasal Septum<br>P Accessory Sinus<br>Q Maxillary Sinus, Right<br>R Maxillary Sinus, Left<br>S Frontal Sinus, Right<br>T Frontal Sinus, Left<br>U Ethmoid Sinus, Right<br>V Ethmoid Sinus, Left<br>W Sphenoid Sinus, Right<br>X Sphenoid Sinus, Left | 0 Open<br>3 Percutaneous<br>4 Percutaneous Endoscopic | Z No Device | X Diagnostic<br>Z No Qualifier |

**0** Medical and Surgical
**9** Ear, Nose, Sinus
**C** Extirpation: Taking or cutting out solid matter from a body part

| Character 4<br>Body Part | Character 5<br>Approach | Character 6<br>Device | Character 7<br>Qualifier |
|---|---|---|---|
| 0 External Ear, Right<br>1 External Ear, Left<br>K Nose | 0 Open<br>3 Percutaneous<br>4 Percutaneous Endoscopic<br>X External | Z No Device | Z No Qualifier |
| 3 External Auditory Canal, Right<br>4 External Auditory Canal, Left | 0 Open<br>3 Percutaneous<br>4 Percutaneous Endoscopic<br>7 Via Natural or Artificial Opening<br>8 Via Natural or Artificial Opening<br>   Endoscopic<br>X External | Z No Device | Z No Qualifier |
| 5 Middle Ear, Right<br>6 Middle Ear, Left<br>9 Auditory Ossicle, Right<br>A Auditory Ossicle, Left<br>D Inner Ear, Right<br>E Inner Ear, Left | 0 Open | Z No Device | Z No Qualifier |
| 7 Tympanic Membrane, Right<br>8 Tympanic Membrane, Left<br>F Eustachian Tube, Right<br>G Eustachian Tube, Left<br>L Nasal Turbinate<br>N Nasopharynx | 0 Open<br>3 Percutaneous<br>4 Percutaneous Endoscopic<br>7 Via Natural or Artificial Opening<br>8 Via Natural or Artificial Opening<br>   Endoscopic | Z No Device | Z No Qualifier |
| B Mastoid Sinus, Right<br>C Mastoid Sinus, Left<br>M Nasal Septum<br>P Accessory Sinus<br>Q Maxillary Sinus, Right<br>R Maxillary Sinus, Left<br>S Frontal Sinus, Right<br>T Frontal Sinus, Left<br>U Ethmoid Sinus, Right<br>V Ethmoid Sinus, Left<br>W Sphenoid Sinus, Right<br>X Sphenoid Sinus, Left | 0 Open<br>3 Percutaneous<br>4 Percutaneous Endoscopic | Z No Device | Z No Qualifier |

**0** Medical and Surgical
**9** Ear, Nose, Sinus
**D** Extraction: Pulling or stripping out or off all or a portion of a body part by the use of force

| Character 4<br>Body Part | Character 5<br>Approach | Character 6<br>Device | Character 7<br>Qualifier |
|---|---|---|---|
| 7 Tympanic Membrane, Right<br>8 Tympanic Membrane, Left<br>L Nasal Turbinate | 0 Open<br>3 Percutaneous<br>4 Percutaneous Endoscopic<br>7 Via Natural or Artificial Opening<br>8 Via Natural or Artificial Opening<br>   Endoscopic | Z No Device | Z No Qualifier |
| 9 Auditory Ossicle, Right<br>A Auditory Ossicle, Left | 0 Open | Z No Device | Z No Qualifier |
| B Mastoid Sinus, Right<br>C Mastoid Sinus, Left<br>M Nasal Septum<br>P Accessory Sinus<br>Q Maxillary Sinus, Right<br>R Maxillary Sinus, Left<br>S Frontal Sinus, Right<br>T Frontal Sinus, Left<br>U Ethmoid Sinus, Right<br>V Ethmoid Sinus, Left<br>W Sphenoid Sinus, Right<br>X Sphenoid Sinus, Left | 0 Open<br>3 Percutaneous<br>4 Percutaneous Endoscopic | Z No Device | Z No Qualifier |

**0** Medical and Surgical
**9** Ear, Nose, Sinus
**H** Insertion: Putting in a nonbiological appliance that monitors, assists, performs, or prevents a physiological function but does not physically take the place of a body part

| Character 4<br>Body Part | Character 5<br>Approach | Character 6<br>Device | Character 7<br>Qualifier |
|---|---|---|---|
| D Inner Ear, Right<br>E Inner Ear, Left | 0 Open<br>3 Percutaneous<br>4 Percutaneous Endoscopic | 4 Hearing Device, Bone Conduction<br>5 Hearing Device, Single Channel<br>  Cochlear Prosthesis<br>6 Hearing Device, Multiple Channel<br>  Cochlear Prosthesis<br>S Hearing Device | Z No Qualifier |
| N Nasopharynx | 7 Via Natural or Artificial Opening<br>8 Via Natural or Artificial Opening<br>  Endoscopic | B Intraluminal Device, Airway | Z No Qualifier |

**0** Medical and Surgical
**9** Ear, Nose, Sinus
**J** Inspection: Visually and/or manually exploring a body part

| Character 4<br>Body Part | Character 5<br>Approach | Character 6<br>Device | Character 7<br>Qualifier |
|---|---|---|---|
| 7 Tympanic Membrane, Right<br>8 Tympanic Membrane, Left<br>H Ear, Right<br>J Ear, Left | 0 Open<br>3 Percutaneous<br>4 Percutaneous Endoscopic<br>7 Via Natural or Artificial Opening<br>8 Via Natural or Artificial Opening<br>  Endoscopic<br>X External | Z No Device | Z No Qualifier |
| D Inner Ear, Right<br>E Inner Ear, Left<br>K Nose<br>Y Sinus | 0 Open<br>3 Percutaneous<br>4 Percutaneous Endoscopic<br>X External | Z No Device | Z No Qualifier |

**0** Medical and Surgical
**9** Ear, Nose, Sinus
**M** Reattachment: Putting back in or on all or a portion of a separated body part to its normal location or other suitable location

| Character 4<br>Body Part | Character 5<br>Approach | Character 6<br>Device | Character 7<br>Qualifier |
|---|---|---|---|
| 0 External Ear, Right<br>1 External Ear, Left<br>K Nose | X External | Z No Device | Z No Qualifier |

**0** Medical and Surgical
**9** Ear, Nose, Sinus
**N** Release: Freeing a body part from an abnormal physical constraint by cutting or by the use of force

| Character 4<br>Body Part | Character 5<br>Approach | Character 6<br>Device | Character 7<br>Qualifier |
|---|---|---|---|
| 0 External Ear, Right<br>1 External Ear, Left<br>K Nose | 0 Open<br>3 Percutaneous<br>4 Percutaneous Endoscopic<br>X External | Z No Device | Z No Qualifier |
| 3 External Auditory Canal, Right<br>4 External Auditory Canal, Left | 0 Open<br>3 Percutaneous<br>4 Percutaneous Endoscopic<br>7 Via Natural or Artificial Opening<br>8 Via Natural or Artificial Opening Endoscopic<br>X External | Z No Device | Z No Qualifier |
| 5 Middle Ear, Right<br>6 Middle Ear, Left<br>9 Auditory Ossicle, Right<br>A Auditory Ossicle, Left<br>D Inner Ear, Right<br>E Inner Ear, Left | 0 Open | Z No Device | Z No Qualifier |
| 7 Tympanic Membrane, Right<br>8 Tympanic Membrane, Left<br>F Eustachian Tube, Right<br>G Eustachian Tube, Left<br>L Nasal Turbinate<br>N Nasopharynx | 0 Open<br>3 Percutaneous<br>4 Percutaneous Endoscopic<br>7 Via Natural or Artificial Opening<br>8 Via Natural or Artificial Opening Endoscopic | Z No Device | Z No Qualifier |
| B Mastoid Sinus, Right<br>C Mastoid Sinus, Left<br>M Nasal Septum<br>P Accessory Sinus<br>Q Maxillary Sinus, Right<br>R Maxillary Sinus, Left<br>S Frontal Sinus, Right<br>T Frontal Sinus, Left<br>U Ethmoid Sinus, Right<br>V Ethmoid Sinus, Left<br>W Sphenoid Sinus, Right<br>X Sphenoid Sinus, Left | 0 Open<br>3 Percutaneous<br>4 Percutaneous Endoscopic | Z No Device | Z No Qualifier |

**0** Medical and Surgical
**9** Ear, Nose, Sinus
**P** Removal: Taking out or off a device from a body part

| Character 4<br>Body Part | Character 5<br>Approach | Character 6<br>Device | Character 7<br>Qualifier |
|---|---|---|---|
| 7 Tympanic Membrane, Right<br>8 Tympanic Membrane, Left | 0 Open<br>7 Via Natural or Artificial Opening<br>8 Via Natural or Artificial Opening Endoscopic<br>X External | 0 Drainage Device | Z No Qualifier |
| D Inner Ear, Right<br>E Inner Ear, Left | 0 Open<br>7 Via Natural or Artificial Opening<br>8 Via Natural or Artificial Opening Endoscopic | S Hearing Device | Z No Qualifier |
| H Ear, Right<br>J Ear, Left<br>K Nose | 0 Open<br>3 Percutaneous<br>4 Percutaneous Endoscopic<br>7 Via Natural or Artificial Opening<br>8 Via Natural or Artificial Opening Endoscopic<br>X External | 0 Drainage Device<br>7 Autologous Tissue Substitute<br>D Intraluminal Device<br>J Synthetic Substitute<br>K Nonautologous Tissue Substitute | Z No Qualifier |
| Y Sinus | 0 Open<br>3 Percutaneous<br>4 Percutaneous Endoscopic<br>X External | 0 Drainage Device | Z No Qualifier |

**0** Medical and Surgical
**9** Ear, Nose, Sinus
**Q** Repair: Restoring, to the extent possible, a body part to its normal anatomic structure and function

| Character 4<br>Body Part | Character 5<br>Approach | Character 6<br>Device | Character 7<br>Qualifier |
|---|---|---|---|
| 0  External Ear, Right<br>1  External Ear, Left<br>2  External Ear, Bilateral<br>K  Nose | 0  Open<br>3  Percutaneous<br>4  Percutaneous Endoscopic<br>X  External | Z  No Device | Z  No Qualifier |
| 3  External Auditory Canal, Right<br>4  External Auditory Canal, Left<br>F  Eustachian Tube, Right<br>G  Eustachian Tube, Left | 0  Open<br>3  Percutaneous<br>4  Percutaneous Endoscopic<br>7  Via Natural or Artificial Opening<br>8  Via Natural or Artificial Opening<br>   Endoscopic<br>X  External | Z  No Device | Z  No Qualifier |
| 5  Middle Ear, Right<br>6  Middle Ear, Left<br>9  Auditory Ossicle, Right<br>A  Auditory Ossicle, Left<br>D  Inner Ear, Right<br>E  Inner Ear, Left | 0  Open | Z  No Device | Z  No Qualifier |
| 7  Tympanic Membrane, Right<br>8  Tympanic Membrane, Left<br>L  Nasal Turbinate<br>N  Nasopharynx | 0  Open<br>3  Percutaneous<br>4  Percutaneous Endoscopic<br>7  Via Natural or Artificial Opening<br>8  Via Natural or Artificial Opening<br>   Endoscopic | Z  No Device | Z  No Qualifier |
| B  Mastoid Sinus, Right<br>C  Mastoid Sinus, Left<br>M  Nasal Septum<br>P  Accessory Sinus<br>Q  Maxillary Sinus, Right<br>R  Maxillary Sinus, Left<br>S  Frontal Sinus, Right<br>T  Frontal Sinus, Left<br>U  Ethmoid Sinus, Right<br>V  Ethmoid Sinus, Left<br>W  Sphenoid Sinus, Right<br>X  Sphenoid Sinus, Left | 0  Open<br>3  Percutaneous<br>4  Percutaneous Endoscopic | Z  No Device | Z  No Qualifier |

**AHA:** 09QT4ZZ - 4Q 2013, 114

**0** Medical and Surgical
**9** Ear, Nose, Sinus
**R** Replacement: Putting in or on biological or synthetic material that physically takes the place and/or function of all or a portion of a body part

| Character 4<br>Body Part | Character 5<br>Approach | Character 6<br>Device | Character 7<br>Qualifier |
|---|---|---|---|
| 0  External Ear, Right<br>1  External Ear, Left<br>2  External Ear, Bilateral<br>K  Nose | 0  Open<br>X  External | 7  Autologous Tissue Substitute<br>J  Synthetic Substitute<br>K  Nonautologous Tissue Substitute | Z  No Qualifier |
| 5  Middle Ear, Right<br>6  Middle Ear, Left<br>9  Auditory Ossicle, Right<br>A  Auditory Ossicle, Left<br>D  Inner Ear, Right<br>E  Inner Ear, Left | 0  Open | 7  Autologous Tissue Substitute<br>J  Synthetic Substitute<br>K  Nonautologous Tissue Substitute | Z  No Qualifier |
| 7  Tympanic Membrane, Right<br>8  Tympanic Membrane, Left<br>N  Nasopharynx | 0  Open<br>7  Via Natural or Artificial Opening<br>8  Via Natural or Artificial Opening<br>   Endoscopic | 7  Autologous Tissue Substitute<br>J  Synthetic Substitute<br>K  Nonautologous Tissue Substitute | Z  No Qualifier |
| L  Nasal Turbinate | 0  Open<br>3  Percutaneous<br>4  Percutaneous Endoscopic<br>7  Via Natural or Artificial Opening<br>8  Via Natural or Artificial Opening<br>   Endoscopic | 7  Autologous Tissue Substitute<br>J  Synthetic Substitute<br>K  Nonautologous Tissue Substitute | Z  No Qualifier |
| M  Nasal Septum | 0  Open<br>3  Percutaneous<br>4  Percutaneous Endoscopic | 7  Autologous Tissue Substitute<br>J  Synthetic Substitute<br>K  Nonautologous Tissue Substitute | Z  No Qualifier |

**0 Medical and Surgical**
**9 Ear, Nose, Sinus**
**S Reposition: Moving to its normal location, or other suitable location, all or a portion of a body part**

| Character 4<br>Body Part | Character 5<br>Approach | Character 6<br>Device | Character 7<br>Qualifier |
|---|---|---|---|
| 0 External Ear, Right<br>1 External Ear, Left<br>2 External Ear, Bilateral<br>K Nose | 0 Open<br>4 Percutaneous Endoscopic<br>X External | Z No Device | Z No Qualifier |
| 7 Tympanic Membrane, Right<br>8 Tympanic Membrane, Left<br>F Eustachian Tube, Right<br>G Eustachian Tube, Left<br>L Nasal Turbinate | 0 Open<br>4 Percutaneous Endoscopic<br>7 Via Natural or Artificial Opening<br>8 Via Natural or Artificial Opening<br>   Endoscopic | Z No Device | Z No Qualifier |
| 9 Auditory Ossicle, Right<br>A Auditory Ossicle, Left<br>M Nasal Septum | 0 Open<br>4 Percutaneous Endoscopic | Z No Device | Z No Qualifier |

**0 Medical and Surgical**
**9 Ear, Nose, Sinus**
**T Resection: Cutting out or off, without replacement, all of a body part**

| Character 4<br>Body Part | Character 5<br>Approach | Character 6<br>Device | Character 7<br>Qualifier |
|---|---|---|---|
| 0 External Ear, Right<br>1 External Ear, Left<br>K Nose | 0 Open<br>4 Percutaneous Endoscopic<br>X External | Z No Device | Z No Qualifier |
| 5 Middle Ear, Right<br>6 Middle Ear, Left<br>9 Auditory Ossicle, Right<br>A Auditory Ossicle, Left<br>D Inner Ear, Right<br>E Inner Ear, Left | 0 Open | Z No Device | Z No Qualifier |
| 7 Tympanic Membrane, Right<br>8 Tympanic Membrane, Left<br>F Eustachian Tube, Right<br>G Eustachian Tube, Left<br>L Nasal Turbinate<br>N Nasopharynx | 0 Open<br>4 Percutaneous Endoscopic<br>7 Via Natural or Artificial Opening<br>8 Via Natural or Artificial Opening<br>   Endoscopic | Z No Device | Z No Qualifier |
| B Mastoid Sinus, Right<br>C Mastoid Sinus, Left<br>M Nasal Septum<br>P Accessory Sinus<br>Q Maxillary Sinus, Right<br>R Maxillary Sinus, Left<br>S Frontal Sinus, Right<br>T Frontal Sinus, Left<br>U Ethmoid Sinus, Right<br>V Ethmoid Sinus, Left<br>W Sphenoid Sinus, Right<br>X Sphenoid Sinus, Left | 0 Open<br>4 Percutaneous Endoscopic | Z No Device | Z No Qualifier |

**0** Medical and Surgical
**9** Ear, Nose, Sinus
**U** Supplement: Putting in or on biological or synthetic material that physically reinforces and/or augments the function of a portion of a body part

| Character 4 Body Part | Character 5 Approach | Character 6 Device | Character 7 Qualifier |
|---|---|---|---|
| 0 External Ear, Right<br>1 External Ear, Left<br>2 External Ear, Bilateral<br>K Nose | 0 Open<br>X External | 7 Autologous Tissue Substitute<br>J Synthetic Substitute<br>K Nonautologous Tissue Substitute | Z No Qualifier |
| 5 Middle Ear, Right<br>6 Middle Ear, Left<br>9 Auditory Ossicle, Right<br>A Auditory Ossicle, Left<br>D Inner Ear, Right<br>E Inner Ear, Left | 0 Open | 7 Autologous Tissue Substitute<br>J Synthetic Substitute<br>K Nonautologous Tissue Substitute | Z No Qualifier |
| 7 Tympanic Membrane, Right<br>8 Tympanic Membrane, Left<br>N Nasopharynx | 0 Open<br>7 Via Natural or Artificial Opening<br>8 Via Natural or Artificial Opening Endoscopic | 7 Autologous Tissue Substitute<br>J Synthetic Substitute<br>K Nonautologous Tissue Substitute | Z No Qualifier |
| L Nasal Turbinate | 0 Open<br>3 Percutaneous<br>4 Percutaneous Endoscopic<br>7 Via Natural or Artificial Opening<br>8 Via Natural or Artificial Opening Endoscopic | 7 Autologous Tissue Substitute<br>J Synthetic Substitute<br>K Nonautologous Tissue Substitute | Z No Qualifier |
| M Nasal Septum | 0 Open<br>3 Percutaneous<br>4 Percutaneous Endoscopic | 7 Autologous Tissue Substitute<br>J Synthetic Substitute<br>K Nonautologous Tissue Substitute | Z No Qualifier |

**0** Medical and Surgical
**9** Ear, Nose, Sinus
**W** Revision: Correcting, to the extent possible, a portion of a malfunctioning device or the position of a displaced device

| Character 4 Body Part | Character 5 Approach | Character 6 Device | Character 7 Qualifier |
|---|---|---|---|
| 7 Tympanic Membrane, Right<br>8 Tympanic Membrane, Left<br>9 Auditory Ossicle, Right<br>A Auditory Ossicle, Left | 0 Open<br>7 Via Natural or Artificial Opening<br>8 Via Natural or Artificial Opening Endoscopic | 7 Autologous Tissue Substitute<br>J Synthetic Substitute<br>K Nonautologous Tissue Substitute | Z No Qualifier |
| D Inner Ear, Right<br>E Inner Ear, Left | 0 Open<br>7 Via Natural or Artificial Opening<br>8 Via Natural or Artificial Opening Endoscopic | S Hearing Device | Z No Qualifier |
| H Ear, Right<br>J Ear, Left<br>K Nose | 0 Open<br>3 Percutaneous<br>4 Percutaneous Endoscopic<br>7 Via Natural or Artificial Opening<br>8 Via Natural or Artificial Opening Endoscopic<br>X External | 0 Drainage Device<br>7 Autologous Tissue Substitute<br>D Intraluminal Device<br>J Synthetic Substitute<br>K Nonautologous Tissue Substitute | Z No Qualifier |
| Y Sinus | 0 Open<br>3 Percutaneous<br>4 Percutaneous Endoscopic<br>X External | 0 Drainage Device | Z No Qualifier |

# Respiratory System | 0B1-0BY

**0** Medical and Surgical
**B** Respiratory System
**1** Bypass: Altering the route of passage of the contents of a tubular body part

| Character 4<br>Body Part | Character 5<br>Approach | Character 6<br>Device | Character 7<br>Qualifier |
|---|---|---|---|
| 1 Trachea | 0 Open | D Intraluminal Device | 6 Esophagus |
| 1 Trachea | 0 Open | F Tracheostomy Device<br>Z No Device | 4 Cutaneous |
| 1 Trachea | 3 Percutaneous<br>4 Percutaneous Endoscopic | F Tracheostomy Device<br>Z No Device | 4 Cutaneous |

**0** Medical and Surgical
**B** Respiratory System
**2** Change: Taking out or off a device from a body part and putting back an identical or similar device in or on the same body part without cutting or puncturing the skin or a mucous membrane

| Character 4<br>Body Part | Character 5<br>Approach | Character 6<br>Device | Character 7<br>Qualifier |
|---|---|---|---|
| 0 Tracheobronchial Tree<br>K Lung, Right<br>L Lung, Left<br>Q Pleura<br>T Diaphragm | X External | 0 Drainage Device<br>Y Other Device | Z No Qualifier |
| 1 Trachea | X External | 0 Drainage Device<br>E Intraluminal Device, Endotracheal Airway<br>F Tracheostomy Device<br>Y Other Device | Z No Qualifier |

**0** Medical and Surgical
**B** Respiratory System
**5** Destruction: Physical eradication of all or a portion of a body part by the direct use of energy, force, or a destructive agent

| Character 4<br>Body Part | Character 5<br>Approach | Character 6<br>Device | Character 7<br>Qualifier |
|---|---|---|---|
| 1 Trachea<br>2 Carina<br>3 Main Bronchus, Right<br>4 Upper Lobe Bronchus, Right<br>5 Middle Lobe Bronchus, Right<br>6 Lower Lobe Bronchus, Right<br>7 Main Bronchus, Left<br>8 Upper Lobe Bronchus, Left<br>9 Lingula Bronchus<br>B Lower Lobe Bronchus, Left<br>C Upper Lung Lobe, Right<br>D Middle Lung Lobe, Right<br>F Lower Lung Lobe, Right<br>G Upper Lung Lobe, Left<br>H Lung Lingula<br>J Lower Lung Lobe, Left<br>K Lung, Right<br>L Lung, Left<br>M Lungs, Bilateral | 0 Open<br>3 Percutaneous<br>4 Percutaneous Endoscopic<br>7 Via Natural or Artificial Opening<br>8 Via Natural or Artificial Opening Endoscopic | Z No Device | Z No Qualifier |
| N Pleura, Right<br>P Pleura, Left<br>R Diaphragm, Right<br>S Diaphragm, Left | 0 Open<br>3 Percutaneous<br>4 Percutaneous Endoscopic | Z No Device | Z No Qualifier |

**0** Medical and Surgical
**B** Respiratory System
**7** Dilation: Expanding an orifice or the lumen of a tubular body part

| Character 4<br>Body Part | Character 5<br>Approach | Character 6<br>Device | Character 7<br>Qualifier |
|---|---|---|---|
| 1 Trachea<br>2 Carina<br>3 Main Bronchus, Right<br>4 Upper Lobe Bronchus, Right<br>5 Middle Lobe Bronchus, Right<br>6 Lower Lobe Bronchus, Right<br>7 Main Bronchus, Left<br>8 Upper Lobe Bronchus, Left<br>9 Lingula Bronchus<br>B Lower Lobe Bronchus, Left | 0 Open<br>3 Percutaneous<br>4 Percutaneous Endoscopic<br>7 Via Natural or Artificial Opening<br>8 Via Natural or Artificial Opening<br>   Endoscopic | D Intraluminal Device<br>Z No Device | Z No Qualifier |

**0** Medical and Surgical
**B** Respiratory System
**9** Drainage: Taking or letting out fluids and/or gases from a body part

| Character 4<br>Body Part | Character 5<br>Approach | Character 6<br>Device | Character 7<br>Qualifier |
|---|---|---|---|
| 1 Trachea<br>2 Carina<br>3 Main Bronchus, Right<br>4 Upper Lobe Bronchus, Right<br>5 Middle Lobe Bronchus, Right<br>6 Lower Lobe Bronchus, Right<br>7 Main Bronchus, Left<br>8 Upper Lobe Bronchus, Left<br>9 Lingula Bronchus<br>B Lower Lobe Bronchus, Left<br>C Upper Lung Lobe, Right<br>D Middle Lung Lobe, Right<br>F Lower Lung Lobe, Right<br>G Upper Lung Lobe, Left<br>H Lung Lingula<br>J Lower Lung Lobe, Left<br>K Lung, Right<br>L Lung, Left<br>M Lungs, Bilateral | 0 Open<br>3 Percutaneous<br>4 Percutaneous Endoscopic<br>7 Via Natural or Artificial Opening<br>8 Via Natural or Artificial Opening<br>   Endoscopic | 0 Drainage Device | Z No Qualifier |
| 1 Trachea<br>2 Carina<br>3 Main Bronchus, Right<br>4 Upper Lobe Bronchus, Right<br>5 Middle Lobe Bronchus, Right<br>6 Lower Lobe Bronchus, Right<br>7 Main Bronchus, Left<br>8 Upper Lobe Bronchus, Left<br>9 Lingula Bronchus<br>B Lower Lobe Bronchus, Left<br>C Upper Lung Lobe, Right<br>D Middle Lung Lobe, Right<br>F Lower Lung Lobe, Right<br>G Upper Lung Lobe, Left<br>H Lung Lingula<br>J Lower Lung Lobe, Left<br>K Lung, Right<br>L Lung, Left<br>M Lungs, Bilateral | 0 Open<br>3 Percutaneous<br>4 Percutaneous Endoscopic<br>7 Via Natural or Artificial Opening<br>8 Via Natural or Artificial Opening<br>   Endoscopic | Z No Device | X Diagnostic<br>Z No Qualifier |
| N Pleura, Right<br>P Pleura, Left<br>R Diaphragm, Right<br>S Diaphragm, Left | 0 Open<br>3 Percutaneous<br>4 Percutaneous Endoscopic | 0 Drainage Device | Z No Qualifier |
| N Pleura, Right<br>P Pleura, Left<br>R Diaphragm, Right<br>S Diaphragm, Left | 0 Open<br>3 Percutaneous<br>4 Percutaneous Endoscopic | Z No Device | X Diagnostic<br>Z No Qualifier |

**0BB–0BD**

**Respiratory System | 0BB–0BD**

**0** Medical and Surgical
**B** Respiratory System
**B** Excision: Cutting out or off, without replacement, a portion of a body part

| Character 4 Body Part | Character 5 Approach | Character 6 Device | Character 7 Qualifier |
|---|---|---|---|
| 1 Trachea<br>2 Carina<br>3 Main Bronchus, Right<br>4 Upper Lobe Bronchus, Right<br>5 Middle Lobe Bronchus, Right<br>6 Lower Lobe Bronchus, Right<br>7 Main Bronchus, Left<br>8 Upper Lobe Bronchus, Left<br>9 Lingula Bronchus<br>B Lower Lobe Bronchus, Left<br>C Upper Lung Lobe, Right<br>D Middle Lung Lobe, Right<br>F Lower Lung Lobe, Right<br>G Upper Lung Lobe, Left<br>H Lung Lingula<br>J Lower Lung Lobe, Left<br>K Lung, Right<br>L Lung, Left<br>M Lungs, Bilateral | 0 Open<br>3 Percutaneous<br>4 Percutaneous Endoscopic<br>7 Via Natural or Artificial Opening<br>8 Via Natural or Artificial Opening Endoscopic | Z No Device | X Diagnostic<br>Z No Qualifier |
| N Pleura, Right<br>P Pleura, Left<br>R Diaphragm, Right<br>S Diaphragm, Left | 0 Open<br>3 Percutaneous<br>4 Percutaneous Endoscopic | Z No Device | X Diagnostic<br>Z No Qualifier |

**AHA:** 0BBK8ZX - 1Q 2014, 21

**0** Medical and Surgical
**B** Respiratory System
**C** Extirpation: Taking or cutting out solid matter from a body part

| Character 4 Body Part | Character 5 Approach | Character 6 Device | Character 7 Qualifier |
|---|---|---|---|
| 1 Trachea<br>2 Carina<br>3 Main Bronchus, Right<br>4 Upper Lobe Bronchus, Right<br>5 Middle Lobe Bronchus, Right<br>6 Lower Lobe Bronchus, Right<br>7 Main Bronchus, Left<br>8 Upper Lobe Bronchus, Left<br>9 Lingula Bronchus<br>B Lower Lobe Bronchus, Left<br>C Upper Lung Lobe, Right<br>D Middle Lung Lobe, Right<br>F Lower Lung Lobe, Right<br>G Upper Lung Lobe, Left<br>H Lung Lingula<br>J Lower Lung Lobe, Left<br>K Lung, Right<br>L Lung, Left<br>M Lungs, Bilateral | 0 Open<br>3 Percutaneous<br>4 Percutaneous Endoscopic<br>7 Via Natural or Artificial Opening<br>8 Via Natural or Artificial Opening Endoscopic | Z No Device | Z No Qualifier |
| N Pleura, Right<br>P Pleura, Left<br>R Diaphragm, Right<br>S Diaphragm, Left | 0 Open<br>3 Percutaneous<br>4 Percutaneous Endoscopic | Z No Device | Z No Qualifier |

**0** Medical and Surgical
**B** Respiratory System
**D** Extraction: Pulling or stripping out or off all or a portion of a body part by the use of force

| Character 4 Body Part | Character 5 Approach | Character 6 Device | Character 7 Qualifier |
|---|---|---|---|
| N Pleura, Right<br>P Pleura, Left | 0 Open<br>3 Percutaneous<br>4 Percutaneous Endoscopic | Z No Device | X Diagnostic<br>Z No Qualifier |

**0** Medical and Surgical
**B** Respiratory System
**F** Fragmentation: Breaking solid matter in a body part into pieces

| Character 4<br>Body Part | Character 5<br>Approach | Character 6<br>Device | Character 7<br>Qualifier |
|---|---|---|---|
| 1  Trachea  N C<br>2  Carina  N C<br>3  Main Bronchus, Right  N C<br>4  Upper Lobe Bronchus, Right  N C<br>5  Middle Lobe Bronchus, Right  N C<br>6  Lower Lobe Bronchus, Right  N C<br>7  Main Bronchus, Left  N C<br>8  Upper Lobe Bronchus, Left  N C<br>9  Lingula Bronchus  N C<br>B  Lower Lobe Bronchus, Left  N C | 0  Open<br>3  Percutaneous<br>4  Percutaneous Endoscopic<br>7  Via Natural or Artificial Opening<br>8  Via Natural or Artificial Opening<br>   Endoscopic<br>X  External | Z  No Device | Z  No Qualifier |

N C  0BF(1-9,B)XZZ

---

**0** Medical and Surgical
**B** Respiratory System
**H** Insertion: Putting in a nonbiological appliance that monitors, assists, performs, or prevents a physiological function but does not physically take the place of a body part

| Character 4<br>Body Part | Character 5<br>Approach | Character 6<br>Device | Character 7<br>Qualifier |
|---|---|---|---|
| 0  Tracheobronchial Tree | 0  Open<br>3  Percutaneous<br>4  Percutaneous Endoscopic<br>7  Via Natural or Artificial Opening<br>8  Via Natural or Artificial Opening<br>   Endoscopic | 1  Radioactive Element<br>2  Monitoring Device<br>3  Infusion Device<br>D  Intraluminal Device | Z  No Qualifier |
| 1  Trachea | 0  Open | 2  Monitoring Device<br>D  Intraluminal Device | Z  No Qualifier |
| 1  Trachea | 3  Percutaneous | D  Intraluminal Device<br>E  Intraluminal Device, Endotracheal<br>   Airway | Z  No Qualifier |
| 1  Trachea | 4  Percutaneous Endoscopic | D  Intraluminal Device | Z  No Qualifier |
| 1  Trachea | 7  Via Natural or Artificial Opening<br>8  Via Natural or Artificial Opening<br>   Endoscopic | 2  Monitoring Device<br>D  Intraluminal Device<br>E  Intraluminal Device, Endotracheal<br>   Airway | Z  No Qualifier |
| 3  Main Bronchus, Right<br>4  Upper Lobe Bronchus, Right<br>5  Middle Lobe Bronchus, Right<br>6  Lower Lobe Bronchus, Right<br>7  Main Bronchus, Left<br>8  Upper Lobe Bronchus, Left<br>9  Lingula Bronchus<br>B  Lower Lobe Bronchus, Left | 0  Open<br>3  Percutaneous<br>4  Percutaneous Endoscopic<br>7  Via Natural or Artificial Opening<br>8  Via Natural or Artificial Opening<br>   Endoscopic | G  Intraluminal Device, Endobronchial<br>   Valve | Z  No Qualifier |
| K  Lung, Right<br>L  Lung, Left | 0  Open<br>3  Percutaneous<br>4  Percutaneous Endoscopic<br>7  Via Natural or Artificial Opening<br>8  Via Natural or Artificial Opening<br>   Endoscopic | 1  Radioactive Element<br>2  Monitoring Device<br>3  Infusion Device | Z  No Qualifier |
| R  Diaphragm, Right<br>S  Diaphragm, Left | 0  Open<br>3  Percutaneous<br>4  Percutaneous Endoscopic | 2  Monitoring Device<br>M  Diaphragmatic Pacemaker Lead | Z  No Qualifier |

---

**0** Medical and Surgical
**B** Respiratory System
**J** Inspection: Visually and/or manually exploring a body part

| Character 4<br>Body Part | Character 5<br>Approach | Character 6<br>Device | Character 7<br>Qualifier |
|---|---|---|---|
| 0  Tracheobronchial Tree<br>1  Trachea<br>K  Lung, Right<br>L  Lung, Left<br>Q  Pleura<br>T  Diaphragm | 0  Open<br>3  Percutaneous<br>4  Percutaneous Endoscopic<br>7  Via Natural or Artificial Opening<br>8  Via Natural or Artificial Opening<br>   Endoscopic<br>X  External | Z  No Device | Z  No Qualifier |

**AHA:** 0BJL8ZZ - 1Q 2014, 20

---

**0** Medical and Surgical
**B** Respiratory System
**L** Occlusion: Completely closing an orifice or the lumen of a tubular body part

| Character 4<br>Body Part | Character 5<br>Approach | Character 6<br>Device | Character 7<br>Qualifier |
|---|---|---|---|
| 1 Trachea<br>2 Carina<br>3 Main Bronchus, Right<br>4 Upper Lobe Bronchus, Right<br>5 Middle Lobe Bronchus, Right<br>6 Lower Lobe Bronchus, Right<br>7 Main Bronchus, Left<br>8 Upper Lobe Bronchus, Left<br>9 Lingula Bronchus<br>B Lower Lobe Bronchus, Left | 0 Open<br>3 Percutaneous<br>4 Percutaneous Endoscopic | C Extraluminal Device<br>D Intraluminal Device<br>Z No Device | Z No Qualifier |
| 1 Trachea<br>2 Carina<br>3 Main Bronchus, Right<br>4 Upper Lobe Bronchus, Right<br>5 Middle Lobe Bronchus, Right<br>6 Lower Lobe Bronchus, Right<br>7 Main Bronchus, Left<br>8 Upper Lobe Bronchus, Left<br>9 Lingula Bronchus<br>B Lower Lobe Bronchus, Left | 7 Via Natural or Artificial Opening<br>8 Via Natural or Artificial Opening<br>  Endoscopic | D Intraluminal Device<br>Z No Device | Z No Qualifier |

**0** Medical and Surgical
**B** Respiratory System
**M** Reattachment: Putting back in or on all or a portion of a separated body part to its normal location or other suitable location

| Character 4<br>Body Part | Character 5<br>Approach | Character 6<br>Device | Character 7<br>Qualifier |
|---|---|---|---|
| 1 Trachea<br>2 Carina<br>3 Main Bronchus, Right<br>4 Upper Lobe Bronchus, Right<br>5 Middle Lobe Bronchus, Right<br>6 Lower Lobe Bronchus, Right<br>7 Main Bronchus, Left<br>8 Upper Lobe Bronchus, Left<br>9 Lingula Bronchus<br>B Lower Lobe Bronchus, Left<br>C Upper Lung Lobe, Right<br>D Middle Lung Lobe, Right<br>F Lower Lung Lobe, Right<br>G Upper Lung Lobe, Left<br>H Lung Lingula<br>J Lower Lung Lobe, Left<br>K Lung, Right<br>L Lung, Left<br>R Diaphragm, Right<br>S Diaphragm, Left | 0 Open | Z No Device | Z No Qualifier |

| 0 | Medical and Surgical |
|---|---|
| B | Respiratory System |
| N | Release: Freeing a body part from an abnormal physical constraint by cutting or by the use of force |

| Character 4<br>Body Part | Character 5<br>Approach | Character 6<br>Device | Character 7<br>Qualifier |
|---|---|---|---|
| 1 Trachea<br>2 Carina<br>3 Main Bronchus, Right<br>4 Upper Lobe Bronchus, Right<br>5 Middle Lobe Bronchus, Right<br>6 Lower Lobe Bronchus, Right<br>7 Main Bronchus, Left<br>8 Upper Lobe Bronchus, Left<br>9 Lingula Bronchus<br>B Lower Lobe Bronchus, Left<br>C Upper Lung Lobe, Right<br>D Middle Lung Lobe, Right<br>F Lower Lung Lobe, Right<br>G Upper Lung Lobe, Left<br>H Lung Lingula<br>J Lower Lung Lobe, Left<br>K Lung, Right<br>L Lung, Left<br>M Lungs, Bilateral | 0 Open<br>3 Percutaneous<br>4 Percutaneous Endoscopic<br>7 Via Natural or Artificial Opening<br>8 Via Natural or Artificial Opening Endoscopic | Z No Device | Z No Qualifier |
| N Pleura, Right<br>P Pleura, Left<br>R Diaphragm, Right<br>S Diaphragm, Left | 0 Open<br>3 Percutaneous<br>4 Percutaneous Endoscopic | Z No Device | Z No Qualifier |

**Respiratory System | 0BP–0BP**

0 Medical and Surgical
B Respiratory System
P Removal: Taking out or off a device from a body part

| Character 4 Body Part | Character 5 Approach | Character 6 Device | Character 7 Qualifier |
|---|---|---|---|
| 0 Tracheobronchial Tree | 0 Open<br>3 Percutaneous<br>4 Percutaneous Endoscopic<br>7 Via Natural or Artificial Opening<br>8 Via Natural or Artificial Opening Endoscopic | 0 Drainage Device<br>1 Radioactive Element<br>2 Monitoring Device<br>3 Infusion Device<br>7 Autologous Tissue Substitute<br>C Extraluminal Device<br>D Intraluminal Device<br>J Synthetic Substitute<br>K Nonautologous Tissue Substitute | Z No Qualifier |
| 0 Tracheobronchial Tree | X External | 0 Drainage Device<br>1 Radioactive Element<br>2 Monitoring Device<br>3 Infusion Device<br>D Intraluminal Device | Z No Qualifier |
| 1 Trachea | 0 Open<br>3 Percutaneous<br>4 Percutaneous Endoscopic<br>7 Via Natural or Artificial Opening<br>8 Via Natural or Artificial Opening Endoscopic | 0 Drainage Device<br>2 Monitoring Device<br>7 Autologous Tissue Substitute<br>C Extraluminal Device<br>D Intraluminal Device<br>F Tracheostomy Device<br>J Synthetic Substitute<br>K Nonautologous Tissue Substitute | Z No Qualifier |
| 1 Trachea | X External | 0 Drainage Device<br>2 Monitoring Device<br>D Intraluminal Device<br>F Tracheostomy Device | Z No Qualifier |
| K Lung, Right<br>L Lung, Left | 0 Open<br>3 Percutaneous<br>4 Percutaneous Endoscopic<br>7 Via Natural or Artificial Opening<br>8 Via Natural or Artificial Opening Endoscopic<br>X External | 0 Drainage Device<br>1 Radioactive Element<br>2 Monitoring Device<br>3 Infusion Device | Z No Qualifier |
| Q Pleura | 0 Open<br>3 Percutaneous<br>4 Percutaneous Endoscopic<br>7 Via Natural or Artificial Opening<br>8 Via Natural or Artificial Opening Endoscopic<br>X External | 0 Drainage Device<br>1 Radioactive Element<br>2 Monitoring Device | Z No Qualifier |
| T Diaphragm | 0 Open<br>3 Percutaneous<br>4 Percutaneous Endoscopic<br>7 Via Natural or Artificial Opening<br>8 Via Natural or Artificial Opening Endoscopic | 0 Drainage Device<br>2 Monitoring Device<br>7 Autologous Tissue Substitute<br>J Synthetic Substitute<br>K Nonautologous Tissue Substitute<br>M Diaphragmatic Pacemaker Lead | Z No Qualifier |
| T Diaphragm | X External | 0 Drainage Device<br>2 Monitoring Device<br>M Diaphragmatic Pacemaker Lead | Z No Qualifier |

**0** Medical and Surgical
**B** Respiratory System
**Q** Repair: Restoring, to the extent possible, a body part to its normal anatomic structure and function

| Character 4<br>Body Part | Character 5<br>Approach | Character 6<br>Device | Character 7<br>Qualifier |
|---|---|---|---|
| 1 Trachea<br>2 Carina<br>3 Main Bronchus, Right<br>4 Upper Lobe Bronchus, Right<br>5 Middle Lobe Bronchus, Right<br>6 Lower Lobe Bronchus, Right<br>7 Main Bronchus, Left<br>8 Upper Lobe Bronchus, Left<br>9 Lingula Bronchus<br>B Lower Lobe Bronchus, Left<br>C Upper Lung Lobe, Right<br>D Middle Lung Lobe, Right<br>F Lower Lung Lobe, Right<br>G Upper Lung Lobe, Left<br>H Lung Lingula<br>J Lower Lung Lobe, Left<br>K Lung, Right<br>L Lung, Left<br>M Lungs, Bilateral | 0 Open<br>3 Percutaneous<br>4 Percutaneous Endoscopic<br>7 Via Natural or Artificial Opening<br>8 Via Natural or Artificial Opening Endoscopic | Z No Device | Z No Qualifier |
| N Pleura, Right<br>P Pleura, Left<br>R Diaphragm, Right<br>S Diaphragm, Left | 0 Open<br>3 Percutaneous<br>4 Percutaneous Endoscopic | Z No Device | Z No Qualifier |

**0** Medical and Surgical
**B** Respiratory System
**S** Reposition: Moving to its normal location, or other suitable location, all or a portion of a body part

| Character 4<br>Body Part | Character 5<br>Approach | Character 6<br>Device | Character 7<br>Qualifier |
|---|---|---|---|
| 1 Trachea<br>2 Carina<br>3 Main Bronchus, Right<br>4 Upper Lobe Bronchus, Right<br>5 Middle Lobe Bronchus, Right<br>6 Lower Lobe Bronchus, Right<br>7 Main Bronchus, Left<br>8 Upper Lobe Bronchus, Left<br>9 Lingula Bronchus<br>B Lower Lobe Bronchus, Left<br>C Upper Lung Lobe, Right<br>D Middle Lung Lobe, Right<br>F Lower Lung Lobe, Right<br>G Upper Lung Lobe, Left<br>H Lung Lingula<br>J Lower Lung Lobe, Left<br>K Lung, Right<br>L Lung, Left<br>R Diaphragm, Right<br>S Diaphragm, Left | 0 Open | Z No Device | Z No Qualifier |

**0** Medical and Surgical
**B** Respiratory System
**T** Resection: Cutting out or off, without replacement, all of a body part

| Character 4<br>Body Part | Character 5<br>Approach | Character 6<br>Device | Character 7<br>Qualifier |
|---|---|---|---|
| 1 Trachea<br>2 Carina<br>3 Main Bronchus, Right<br>4 Upper Lobe Bronchus, Right<br>5 Middle Lobe Bronchus, Right<br>6 Lower Lobe Bronchus, Right<br>7 Main Bronchus, Left<br>8 Upper Lobe Bronchus, Left<br>9 Lingula Bronchus<br>B Lower Lobe Bronchus, Left<br>C Upper Lung Lobe, Right<br>D Middle Lung Lobe, Right<br>F Lower Lung Lobe, Right<br>G Upper Lung Lobe, Left<br>H Lung Lingula<br>J Lower Lung Lobe, Left<br>K Lung, Right<br>L Lung, Left<br>M Lungs, Bilateral<br>R Diaphragm, Right<br>S Diaphragm, Left | 0 Open<br>4 Percutaneous Endoscopic | Z No Device | Z No Qualifier |

**0** Medical and Surgical
**B** Respiratory System
**U** Supplement: Putting in or on biological or synthetic material that physically reinforces and/or augments the function of a portion of a body part

| Character 4<br>Body Part | Character 5<br>Approach | Character 6<br>Device | Character 7<br>Qualifier |
|---|---|---|---|
| 1 Trachea<br>2 Carina<br>3 Main Bronchus, Right<br>4 Upper Lobe Bronchus, Right<br>5 Middle Lobe Bronchus, Right<br>6 Lower Lobe Bronchus, Right<br>7 Main Bronchus, Left<br>8 Upper Lobe Bronchus, Left<br>9 Lingula Bronchus<br>B Lower Lobe Bronchus, Left<br>R Diaphragm, Right<br>S Diaphragm, Left | 0 Open<br>4 Percutaneous Endoscopic | 7 Autologous Tissue Substitute<br>J Synthetic Substitute<br>K Nonautologous Tissue Substitute | Z No Qualifier |

**0** Medical and Surgical
**B** Respiratory System
**V** Restriction: Partially closing an orifice or the lumen of a tubular body part

| Character 4<br>Body Part | Character 5<br>Approach | Character 6<br>Device | Character 7<br>Qualifier |
|---|---|---|---|
| 1 Trachea<br>2 Carina<br>3 Main Bronchus, Right<br>4 Upper Lobe Bronchus, Right<br>5 Middle Lobe Bronchus, Right<br>6 Lower Lobe Bronchus, Right<br>7 Main Bronchus, Left<br>8 Upper Lobe Bronchus, Left<br>9 Lingula Bronchus<br>B Lower Lobe Bronchus, Left | 0 Open<br>3 Percutaneous<br>4 Percutaneous Endoscopic | C Extraluminal Device<br>D Intraluminal Device<br>Z No Device | Z No Qualifier |
| 1 Trachea<br>2 Carina<br>3 Main Bronchus, Right<br>4 Upper Lobe Bronchus, Right<br>5 Middle Lobe Bronchus, Right<br>6 Lower Lobe Bronchus, Right<br>7 Main Bronchus, Left<br>8 Upper Lobe Bronchus, Left<br>9 Lingula Bronchus<br>B Lower Lobe Bronchus, Left | 7 Via Natural or Artificial Opening<br>8 Via Natural or Artificial Opening Endoscopic | D Intraluminal Device<br>Z No Device | Z No Qualifier |

**0** Medical and Surgical
**B** Respiratory System
**W** Revision: Correcting, to the extent possible, a portion of a malfunctioning device or the position of a displaced device

| Character 4<br>Body Part | Character 5<br>Approach | Character 6<br>Device | Character 7<br>Qualifier |
|---|---|---|---|
| 0 Tracheobronchial Tree | 0 Open<br>3 Percutaneous<br>4 Percutaneous Endoscopic<br>7 Via Natural or Artificial Opening<br>8 Via Natural or Artificial Opening Endoscopic<br>X External | 0 Drainage Device<br>2 Monitoring Device<br>3 Infusion Device<br>7 Autologous Tissue Substitute<br>C Extraluminal Device<br>D Intraluminal Device<br>J Synthetic Substitute<br>K Nonautologous Tissue Substitute | Z No Qualifier |
| 1 Trachea | 0 Open<br>3 Percutaneous<br>4 Percutaneous Endoscopic<br>7 Via Natural or Artificial Opening<br>8 Via Natural or Artificial Opening Endoscopic<br>X External | 0 Drainage Device<br>2 Monitoring Device<br>7 Autologous Tissue Substitute<br>C Extraluminal Device<br>D Intraluminal Device<br>F Tracheostomy Device<br>J Synthetic Substitute<br>K Nonautologous Tissue Substitute | Z No Qualifier |
| K Lung, Right<br>L Lung, Left | 0 Open<br>3 Percutaneous<br>4 Percutaneous Endoscopic<br>7 Via Natural or Artificial Opening<br>8 Via Natural or Artificial Opening Endoscopic<br>X External | 0 Drainage Device<br>2 Monitoring Device<br>3 Infusion Device | Z No Qualifier |
| Q Pleura | 0 Open<br>3 Percutaneous<br>4 Percutaneous Endoscopic<br>7 Via Natural or Artificial Opening<br>8 Via Natural or Artificial Opening Endoscopic<br>X External | 0 Drainage Device<br>2 Monitoring Device | Z No Qualifier |
| T Diaphragm | 0 Open<br>3 Percutaneous<br>4 Percutaneous Endoscopic<br>7 Via Natural or Artificial Opening<br>8 Via Natural or Artificial Opening Endoscopic<br>X External | 0 Drainage Device<br>2 Monitoring Device<br>7 Autologous Tissue Substitute<br>J Synthetic Substitute<br>K Nonautologous Tissue Substitute<br>M Diaphragmatic Pacemaker Lead | Z No Qualifier |

**0** Medical and Surgical
**B** Respiratory System
**Y** Transplantation: Putting in or on all or a portion of a living body part taken from another individual or animal to physically take the place and/or function of all or a portion of a similar body part

| Character 4<br>Body Part | Character 5<br>Approach | Character 6<br>Device | Character 7<br>Qualifier |
|---|---|---|---|
| C Upper Lung Lobe, Right **LC**<br>D Middle Lung Lobe, Right **LC**<br>F Lower Lung Lobe, Right **LC**<br>G Upper Lung Lobe, Left **LC**<br>H Lung Lingula **LC**<br>J Lower Lung Lobe, Left **LC**<br>K Lung, Right **LC**<br>L Lung, Left **LC**<br>M Lungs, Bilateral **LC** | 0 Open | Z No Device | 0 Allogeneic<br>1 Syngeneic<br>2 Zooplastic |

**LC** 0BYC0Z(0,1,2), 0BYD0Z(0,1,2), 0BYF0Z(0,1,2), 0BYG0Z(0,1,2), 0BYH0Z(0,1,2), 0BYJ0Z(0,1,2), 0BYK0Z(0,1,2), 0BYL0Z(0,1,2), 0BYM0Z(0,1,2)

# Mouth and Throat | 0C0-0CX

**0** Medical and Surgical
**C** Mouth and Throat
**0** Alteration: Modifying the anatomic structure of a body part without affecting the function of the body part

| Character 4 Body Part | Character 5 Approach | Character 6 Device | Character 7 Qualifier |
|---|---|---|---|
| 0  Upper Lip<br>1  Lower Lip | X  External | 7  Autologous Tissue Substitute<br>J  Synthetic Substitute<br>K  Nonautologous Tissue Substitute<br>Z  No Device | Z  No Qualifier |

**0** Medical and Surgical
**C** Mouth and Throat
**2** Change: Taking out or off a device from a body part and putting back an identical or similar device in or on the same body part without cutting or puncturing the skin or a mucous membrane

| Character 4 Body Part | Character 5 Approach | Character 6 Device | Character 7 Qualifier |
|---|---|---|---|
| A  Salivary Gland<br>S  Larynx<br>Y  Mouth and Throat | X  External | 0  Drainage Device<br>Y  Other Device | Z  No Qualifier |

**0** Medical and Surgical
**C** Mouth and Throat
**5** Destruction: Physical eradication of all or a portion of a body part by the direct use of energy, force, or a destructive agent

| Character 4 Body Part | Character 5 Approach | Character 6 Device | Character 7 Qualifier |
|---|---|---|---|
| 0  Upper Lip<br>1  Lower Lip<br>2  Hard Palate<br>3  Soft Palate<br>4  Buccal Mucosa<br>5  Upper Gingiva<br>6  Lower Gingiva<br>7  Tongue<br>N  Uvula<br>P  Tonsils<br>Q  Adenoids | 0  Open<br>3  Percutaneous<br>X  External | Z  No Device | Z  No Qualifier |
| 8  Parotid Gland, Right<br>9  Parotid Gland, Left<br>B  Parotid Duct, Right<br>C  Parotid Duct, Left<br>D  Sublingual Gland, Right<br>F  Sublingual Gland, Left<br>G  Submaxillary Gland, Right<br>H  Submaxillary Gland, Left<br>J  Minor Salivary Gland | 0  Open<br>3  Percutaneous | Z  No Device | Z  No Qualifier |
| M  Pharynx<br>R  Epiglottis<br>S  Larynx<br>T  Vocal Cord, Right<br>V  Vocal Cord, Left | 0  Open<br>3  Percutaneous<br>4  Percutaneous Endoscopic<br>7  Via Natural or Artificial Opening<br>8  Via Natural or Artificial Opening Endoscopic | Z  No Device | Z  No Qualifier |
| W  Upper Tooth<br>X  Lower Tooth | 0  Open<br>X  External | Z  No Device | 0  Single<br>1  Multiple<br>2  All |

| 0 Medical and Surgical |
| C Mouth and Throat |
| 7 Dilation: Expanding an orifice or the lumen of a tubular body part |

| Character 4<br>Body Part | Character 5<br>Approach | Character 6<br>Device | Character 7<br>Qualifier |
|---|---|---|---|
| B Parotid Duct, Right<br>C Parotid Duct, Left | 0 Open<br>3 Percutaneous<br>7 Via Natural or Artificial Opening | D Intraluminal Device<br>Z No Device | Z No Qualifier |
| M Pharynx | 7 Via Natural or Artificial Opening<br>8 Via Natural or Artificial Opening<br>   Endoscopic | D Intraluminal Device<br>Z No Device | Z No Qualifier |
| S Larynx | 0 Open<br>3 Percutaneous<br>4 Percutaneous Endoscopic<br>7 Via Natural or Artificial Opening<br>8 Via Natural or Artificial Opening<br>   Endoscopic | D Intraluminal Device<br>Z No Device | Z No Qualifier |

**0** Medical and Surgical
**C** Mouth and Throat
**9** Drainage: Taking or letting out fluids and/or gases from a body part

| Character 4 Body Part | Character 5 Approach | Character 6 Device | Character 7 Qualifier |
|---|---|---|---|
| 0 Upper Lip<br>1 Lower Lip<br>2 Hard Palate<br>3 Soft Palate<br>4 Buccal Mucosa<br>5 Upper Gingiva<br>6 Lower Gingiva<br>7 Tongue<br>N Uvula<br>P Tonsils<br>Q Adenoids | 0 Open<br>3 Percutaneous<br>X External | 0 Drainage Device | Z No Qualifier |
| 0 Upper Lip<br>1 Lower Lip<br>2 Hard Palate<br>3 Soft Palate<br>4 Buccal Mucosa<br>5 Upper Gingiva<br>6 Lower Gingiva<br>7 Tongue<br>N Uvula<br>P Tonsils<br>Q Adenoids | 0 Open<br>3 Percutaneous<br>X External | Z No Device | X Diagnostic<br>Z No Qualifier |
| 8 Parotid Gland, Right<br>9 Parotid Gland, Left<br>B Parotid Duct, Right<br>C Parotid Duct, Left<br>D Sublingual Gland, Right<br>F Sublingual Gland, Left<br>G Submaxillary Gland, Right<br>H Submaxillary Gland, Left<br>J Minor Salivary Gland | 0 Open<br>3 Percutaneous | 0 Drainage Device | Z No Qualifier |
| 8 Parotid Gland, Right<br>9 Parotid Gland, Left<br>B Parotid Duct, Right<br>C Parotid Duct, Left<br>D Sublingual Gland, Right<br>F Sublingual Gland, Left<br>G Submaxillary Gland, Right<br>H Submaxillary Gland, Left<br>J Minor Salivary Gland | 0 Open<br>3 Percutaneous | Z No Device | X Diagnostic<br>Z No Qualifier |
| M Pharynx<br>R Epiglottis<br>S Larynx<br>T Vocal Cord, Right<br>V Vocal Cord, Left | 0 Open<br>3 Percutaneous<br>4 Percutaneous Endoscopic<br>7 Via Natural or Artificial Opening<br>8 Via Natural or Artificial Opening Endoscopic | 0 Drainage Device | Z No Qualifier |
| M Pharynx<br>R Epiglottis<br>S Larynx<br>T Vocal Cord, Right<br>V Vocal Cord, Left | 0 Open<br>3 Percutaneous<br>4 Percutaneous Endoscopic<br>7 Via Natural or Artificial Opening<br>8 Via Natural or Artificial Opening Endoscopic | Z No Device | X Diagnostic<br>Z No Qualifier |
| W Upper Tooth<br>X Lower Tooth | 0 Open<br>X External | 0 Drainage Device<br>Z No Device | 0 Single<br>1 Multiple<br>2 All |

**0** Medical and Surgical
**C** Mouth and Throat
**B** Excision: Cutting out or off, without replacement, a portion of a body part

| Character 4<br>Body Part | Character 5<br>Approach | Character 6<br>Device | Character 7<br>Qualifier |
|---|---|---|---|
| 0 Upper Lip<br>1 Lower Lip<br>2 Hard Palate<br>3 Soft Palate<br>4 Buccal Mucosa<br>5 Upper Gingiva<br>6 Lower Gingiva<br>7 Tongue<br>N Uvula<br>P Tonsils<br>Q Adenoids | 0 Open<br>3 Percutaneous<br>X External | Z No Device | X Diagnostic<br>Z No Qualifier |
| 8 Parotid Gland, Right<br>9 Parotid Gland, Left<br>B Parotid Duct, Right<br>C Parotid Duct, Left<br>D Sublingual Gland, Right<br>F Sublingual Gland, Left<br>G Submaxillary Gland, Right<br>H Submaxillary Gland, Left<br>J Minor Salivary Gland | 0 Open<br>3 Percutaneous | Z No Device | X Diagnostic<br>Z No Qualifier |
| M Pharynx<br>R Epiglottis<br>S Larynx<br>T Vocal Cord, Right<br>V Vocal Cord, Left | 0 Open<br>3 Percutaneous<br>4 Percutaneous Endoscopic<br>7 Via Natural or Artificial Opening<br>8 Via Natural or Artificial Opening<br>Endoscopic | Z No Device | X Diagnostic<br>Z No Qualifier |
| W Upper Tooth<br>X Lower Tooth | 0 Open<br>X External | Z No Device | 0 Single<br>1 Multiple<br>2 All |

**0** Medical and Surgical
**C** Mouth and Throat
**C** Extirpation: Taking or cutting out solid matter from a body part

| Character 4<br>Body Part | Character 5<br>Approach | Character 6<br>Device | Character 7<br>Qualifier |
|---|---|---|---|
| 0 Upper Lip<br>1 Lower Lip<br>2 Hard Palate<br>3 Soft Palate<br>4 Buccal Mucosa<br>5 Upper Gingiva<br>6 Lower Gingiva<br>7 Tongue<br>N Uvula<br>P Tonsils<br>Q Adenoids | 0 Open<br>3 Percutaneous<br>X External | Z No Device | Z No Qualifier |
| 8 Parotid Gland, Right<br>9 Parotid Gland, Left<br>B Parotid Duct, Right<br>C Parotid Duct, Left<br>D Sublingual Gland, Right<br>F Sublingual Gland, Left<br>G Submaxillary Gland, Right<br>H Submaxillary Gland, Left<br>J Minor Salivary Gland | 0 Open<br>3 Percutaneous | Z No Device | Z No Qualifier |
| M Pharynx<br>R Epiglottis<br>S Larynx<br>T Vocal Cord, Right<br>V Vocal Cord, Left | 0 Open<br>3 Percutaneous<br>4 Percutaneous Endoscopic<br>7 Via Natural or Artificial Opening<br>8 Via Natural or Artificial Opening<br>Endoscopic | Z No Device | Z No Qualifier |
| W Upper Tooth<br>X Lower Tooth | 0 Open<br>X External | Z No Device | 0 Single<br>1 Multiple<br>2 All |

**0 Medical and Surgical**
**C Mouth and Throat**
**D Extraction:** Pulling or stripping out or off all or a portion of a body part by the use of force

| Character 4<br>Body Part | Character 5<br>Approach | Character 6<br>Device | Character 7<br>Qualifier |
|---|---|---|---|
| T Vocal Cord, Right<br>V Vocal Cord, Left | 0 Open<br>3 Percutaneous<br>4 Percutaneous Endoscopic<br>7 Via Natural or Artificial Opening<br>8 Via Natural or Artificial Opening<br>  Endoscopic | Z No Device | Z No Qualifier |
| W Upper Tooth<br>X Lower Tooth | X External | Z No Device | 0 Single<br>1 Multiple<br>2 All |

**0 Medical and Surgical**
**C Mouth and Throat**
**F Fragmentation:** Breaking solid matter in a body part into pieces

| Character 4<br>Body Part | Character 5<br>Approach | Character 6<br>Device | Character 7<br>Qualifier |
|---|---|---|---|
| B Parotid Duct, Right   N C<br>C Parotid Duct, Left   N C | 0 Open<br>3 Percutaneous<br>7 Via Natural or Artificial Opening<br>X External | Z No Device | Z No Qualifier |

N C  0CF(B,C)XZZ

**0 Medical and Surgical**
**C Mouth and Throat**
**H Insertion:** Putting in a nonbiological appliance that monitors, assists, performs, or prevents a physiological function but does not physically take the place of a body part

| Character 4<br>Body Part | Character 5<br>Approach | Character 6<br>Device | Character 7<br>Qualifier |
|---|---|---|---|
| 7 Tongue | 0 Open<br>3 Percutaneous<br>X External | 1 Radioactive Element | Z No Qualifier |
| Y Mouth and Throat | 7 Via Natural or Artificial Opening<br>8 Via Natural or Artificial Opening<br>  Endoscopic | B Intraluminal Device, Airway | Z No Qualifier |

**0 Medical and Surgical**
**C Mouth and Throat**
**J Inspection:** Visually and/or manually exploring a body part

| Character 4<br>Body Part | Character 5<br>Approach | Character 6<br>Device | Character 7<br>Qualifier |
|---|---|---|---|
| A Salivary Gland | 0 Open<br>3 Percutaneous<br>X External | Z No Device | Z No Qualifier |
| S Larynx<br>Y Mouth and Throat | 0 Open<br>3 Percutaneous<br>4 Percutaneous Endoscopic<br>7 Via Natural or Artificial Opening<br>8 Via Natural or Artificial Opening<br>  Endoscopic<br>X External | Z No Device | Z No Qualifier |

**0** Medical and Surgical
**C** Mouth and Throat
**L** Occlusion: Completely closing an orifice or the lumen of a tubular body part

| Character 4 Body Part | Character 5 Approach | Character 6 Device | Character 7 Qualifier |
|---|---|---|---|
| B Parotid Duct, Right<br>C Parotid Duct, Left | 0 Open<br>3 Percutaneous<br>4 Percutaneous Endoscopic | C Extraluminal Device<br>D Intraluminal Device<br>Z No Device | Z No Qualifier |
| B Parotid Duct, Right<br>C Parotid Duct, Left | 7 Via Natural or Artificial Opening<br>8 Via Natural or Artificial Opening Endoscopic | D Intraluminal Device<br>Z No Device | Z No Qualifier |

**0** Medical and Surgical
**C** Mouth and Throat
**M** Reattachment: Putting back in or on all or a portion of a separated body part to its normal location or other suitable location

| Character 4 Body Part | Character 5 Approach | Character 6 Device | Character 7 Qualifier |
|---|---|---|---|
| 0 Upper Lip<br>1 Lower Lip<br>3 Soft Palate<br>7 Tongue<br>N Uvula | 0 Open | Z No Device | Z No Qualifier |
| W Upper Tooth<br>X Lower Tooth | 0 Open<br>X External | Z No Device | 0 Single<br>1 Multiple<br>2 All |

**0** Medical and Surgical
**C** Mouth and Throat
**N** Release: Freeing a body part from an abnormal physical constraint by cutting or by the use of force

| Character 4 Body Part | Character 5 Approach | Character 6 Device | Character 7 Qualifier |
|---|---|---|---|
| 0 Upper Lip<br>1 Lower Lip<br>2 Hard Palate<br>3 Soft Palate<br>4 Buccal Mucosa<br>5 Upper Gingiva<br>6 Lower Gingiva<br>7 Tongue<br>N Uvula<br>P Tonsils<br>Q Adenoids | 0 Open<br>3 Percutaneous<br>X External | Z No Device | Z No Qualifier |
| 8 Parotid Gland, Right<br>9 Parotid Gland, Left<br>B Parotid Duct, Right<br>C Parotid Duct, Left<br>D Sublingual Gland, Right<br>F Sublingual Gland, Left<br>G Submaxillary Gland, Right<br>H Submaxillary Gland, Left<br>J Minor Salivary Gland | 0 Open<br>3 Percutaneous | Z No Device | Z No Qualifier |
| M Pharynx<br>R Epiglottis<br>S Larynx<br>T Vocal Cord, Right<br>V Vocal Cord, Left | 0 Open<br>3 Percutaneous<br>4 Percutaneous Endoscopic<br>7 Via Natural or Artificial Opening<br>8 Via Natural or Artificial Opening Endoscopic | Z No Device | Z No Qualifier |
| W Upper Tooth<br>X Lower Tooth | 0 Open<br>X External | Z No Device | 0 Single<br>1 Multiple<br>2 All |

**0** Medical and Surgical
**C** Mouth and Throat
**P** Removal: Taking out or off a device from a body part

| Character 4<br>Body Part | Character 5<br>Approach | Character 6<br>Device | Character 7<br>Qualifier |
|---|---|---|---|
| A Salivary Gland | 0 Open<br>3 Percutaneous | 0 Drainage Device<br>C Extraluminal Device | Z No Qualifier |
| S Larynx | 0 Open<br>3 Percutaneous<br>7 Via Natural or Artificial Opening<br>8 Via Natural or Artificial Opening<br>   Endoscopic<br>X External | 0 Drainage Device<br>7 Autologous Tissue Substitute<br>D Intraluminal Device<br>J Synthetic Substitute<br>K Nonautologous Tissue Substitute | Z No Qualifier |
| Y Mouth and Throat | 0 Open<br>3 Percutaneous<br>7 Via Natural or Artificial Opening<br>8 Via Natural or Artificial Opening<br>   Endoscopic<br>X External | 0 Drainage Device<br>1 Radioactive Element<br>7 Autologous Tissue Substitute<br>D Intraluminal Device<br>J Synthetic Substitute<br>K Nonautologous Tissue Substitute | Z No Qualifier |

**0** Medical and Surgical
**C** Mouth and Throat
**Q** Repair: Restoring, to the extent possible, a body part to its normal anatomic structure and function

| Character 4<br>Body Part | Character 5<br>Approach | Character 6<br>Device | Character 7<br>Qualifier |
|---|---|---|---|
| 0 Upper Lip<br>1 Lower Lip<br>2 Hard Palate<br>3 Soft Palate<br>4 Buccal Mucosa<br>5 Upper Gingiva<br>6 Lower Gingiva<br>7 Tongue<br>N Uvula<br>P Tonsils<br>Q Adenoids | 0 Open<br>3 Percutaneous<br>X External | Z No Device | Z No Qualifier |
| 8 Parotid Gland, Right<br>9 Parotid Gland, Left<br>B Parotid Duct, Right<br>C Parotid Duct, Left<br>D Sublingual Gland, Right<br>F Sublingual Gland, Left<br>G Submaxillary Gland, Right<br>H Submaxillary Gland, Left<br>J Minor Salivary Gland | 0 Open<br>3 Percutaneous | Z No Device | Z No Qualifier |
| M Pharynx<br>R Epiglottis<br>S Larynx<br>T Vocal Cord, Right<br>V Vocal Cord, Left | 0 Open<br>3 Percutaneous<br>4 Percutaneous Endoscopic<br>7 Via Natural or Artificial Opening<br>8 Via Natural or Artificial Opening<br>   Endoscopic | Z No Device | Z No Qualifier |
| W Upper Tooth<br>X Lower Tooth | 0 Open<br>X External | Z No Device | 0 Single<br>1 Multiple<br>2 All |

**0** Medical and Surgical
**C** Mouth and Throat
**R** Replacement: Putting in or on biological or synthetic material that physically takes the place and/or function of all or a portion of a body part

| Character 4<br>Body Part | Character 5<br>Approach | Character 6<br>Device | Character 7<br>Qualifier |
|---|---|---|---|
| 0 Upper Lip<br>1 Lower Lip<br>2 Hard Palate<br>3 Soft Palate<br>4 Buccal Mucosa<br>5 Upper Gingiva<br>6 Lower Gingiva<br>7 Tongue<br>N Uvula | 0 Open<br>3 Percutaneous<br>X External | 7 Autologous Tissue Substitute<br>J Synthetic Substitute<br>K Nonautologous Tissue Substitute | Z No Qualifier |
| B Parotid Duct, Right<br>C Parotid Duct, Left | 0 Open<br>3 Percutaneous | 7 Autologous Tissue Substitute<br>J Synthetic Substitute<br>K Nonautologous Tissue Substitute | Z No Qualifier |
| M Pharynx<br>R Epiglottis<br>S Larynx<br>T Vocal Cord, Right<br>V Vocal Cord, Left | 0 Open<br>7 Via Natural or Artificial Opening<br>8 Via Natural or Artificial Opening<br>   Endoscopic | 7 Autologous Tissue Substitute<br>J Synthetic Substitute<br>K Nonautologous Tissue Substitute | Z No Qualifier |
| W Upper Tooth<br>X Lower Tooth | 0 Open<br>X External | 7 Autologous Tissue Substitute<br>J Synthetic Substitute<br>K Nonautologous Tissue Substitute | 0 Single<br>1 Multiple<br>2 All |

**AHA:** 0CR4XKZ - 2Q 2014, 6

**0** Medical and Surgical
**C** Mouth and Throat
**S** Reposition: Moving to its normal location, or other suitable location, all or a portion of a body part

| Character 4<br>Body Part | Character 5<br>Approach | Character 6<br>Device | Character 7<br>Qualifier |
|---|---|---|---|
| 0 Upper Lip<br>1 Lower Lip<br>2 Hard Palate<br>3 Soft Palate<br>7 Tongue<br>N Uvula | 0 Open<br>X External | Z No Device | Z No Qualifier |
| B Parotid Duct, Right<br>C Parotid Duct, Left | 0 Open<br>3 Percutaneous | Z No Device | Z No Qualifier |
| R Epiglottis<br>T Vocal Cord, Right<br>V Vocal Cord, Left | 0 Open<br>7 Via Natural or Artificial Opening<br>8 Via Natural or Artificial Opening<br>   Endoscopic | Z No Device | Z No Qualifier |
| W Upper Tooth<br>X Lower Tooth | 0 Open<br>X External | 5 External Fixation Device<br>Z No Device | 0 Single<br>1 Multiple<br>2 All |

**0** Medical and Surgical
**C** Mouth and Throat
**T** Resection: Cutting out or off, without replacement, all of a body part

| Character 4<br>Body Part | Character 5<br>Approach | Character 6<br>Device | Character 7<br>Qualifier |
|---|---|---|---|
| 0 Upper Lip<br>1 Lower Lip<br>2 Hard Palate<br>3 Soft Palate<br>7 Tongue<br>N Uvula<br>P Tonsils<br>Q Adenoids | 0 Open<br>X External | Z No Device | Z No Qualifier |
| 8 Parotid Gland, Right<br>9 Parotid Gland, Left<br>B Parotid Duct, Right<br>C Parotid Duct, Left<br>D Sublingual Gland, Right<br>F Sublingual Gland, Left<br>G Submaxillary Gland, Right<br>H Submaxillary Gland, Left<br>J Minor Salivary Gland | 0 Open | Z No Device | Z No Qualifier |
| M Pharynx<br>R Epiglottis<br>S Larynx<br>T Vocal Cord, Right<br>V Vocal Cord, Left | 0 Open<br>4 Percutaneous Endoscopic<br>7 Via Natural or Artificial Opening<br>8 Via Natural or Artificial Opening<br>Endoscopic | Z No Device | Z No Qualifier |
| W Upper Tooth<br>X Lower Tooth | 0 Open | Z No Device | 0 Single<br>1 Multiple<br>2 All |

**0** Medical and Surgical
**C** Mouth and Throat
**U** Supplement: Putting in or on biological or synthetic material that physically reinforces and/or augments the function of a portion of a body part

| Character 4<br>Body Part | Character 5<br>Approach | Character 6<br>Device | Character 7<br>Qualifier |
|---|---|---|---|
| 0 Upper Lip<br>1 Lower Lip<br>2 Hard Palate<br>3 Soft Palate<br>4 Buccal Mucosa<br>5 Upper Gingiva<br>6 Lower Gingiva<br>7 Tongue<br>N Uvula | 0 Open<br>3 Percutaneous<br>X External | 7 Autologous Tissue Substitute<br>J Synthetic Substitute<br>K Nonautologous Tissue Substitute | Z No Qualifier |
| M Pharynx<br>R Epiglottis<br>S Larynx<br>T Vocal Cord, Right<br>V Vocal Cord, Left | 0 Open<br>7 Via Natural or Artificial Opening<br>8 Via Natural or Artificial Opening<br>Endoscopic | 7 Autologous Tissue Substitute<br>J Synthetic Substitute<br>K Nonautologous Tissue Substitute | Z No Qualifier |

**0** Medical and Surgical
**C** Mouth and Throat
**V** Restriction: Partially closing an orifice or the lumen of a tubular body part

| Character 4<br>Body Part | Character 5<br>Approach | Character 6<br>Device | Character 7<br>Qualifier |
|---|---|---|---|
| B Parotid Duct, Right<br>C Parotid Duct, Left | 0 Open<br>3 Percutaneous | C Extraluminal Device<br>D Intraluminal Device<br>Z No Device | Z No Qualifier |
| B Parotid Duct, Right<br>C Parotid Duct, Left | 7 Via Natural or Artificial Opening<br>8 Via Natural or Artificial Opening<br>Endoscopic | D Intraluminal Device<br>Z No Device | Z No Qualifier |

**0** Medical and Surgical
**C** Mouth and Throat
**W** Revision: Correcting, to the extent possible, a portion of a malfunctioning device or the position of a displaced device

| Character 4<br>Body Part | Character 5<br>Approach | Character 6<br>Device | Character 7<br>Qualifier |
|---|---|---|---|
| A Salivary Gland | 0 Open<br>3 Percutaneous<br>X External | 0 Drainage Device<br>C Extraluminal Device | Z No Qualifier |
| S Larynx | 0 Open<br>3 Percutaneous<br>7 Via Natural or Artificial Opening<br>8 Via Natural or Artificial Opening Endoscopic<br>X External | 0 Drainage Device<br>7 Autologous Tissue Substitute<br>D Intraluminal Device<br>J Synthetic Substitute<br>K Nonautologous Tissue Substitute | Z No Qualifier |
| Y Mouth and Throat | 0 Open<br>3 Percutaneous<br>7 Via Natural or Artificial Opening<br>8 Via Natural or Artificial Opening Endoscopic<br>X External | 0 Drainage Device<br>1 Radioactive Element<br>7 Autologous Tissue Substitute<br>D Intraluminal Device<br>J Synthetic Substitute<br>K Nonautologous Tissue Substitute | Z No Qualifier |

**0** Medical and Surgical
**C** Mouth and Throat
**X** Transfer: Moving, without taking out, all or a portion of a body part to another location to take over the function of all or a portion of a body part

| Character 4<br>Body Part | Character 5<br>Approach | Character 6<br>Device | Character 7<br>Qualifier |
|---|---|---|---|
| 0 Upper Lip<br>1 Lower Lip<br>3 Soft Palate<br>4 Buccal Mucosa<br>5 Upper Gingiva<br>6 Lower Gingiva<br>7 Tongue | 0 Open<br>X External | Z No Device | Z No Qualifier |

# Gastronintestinal System | 0D1-0DY

**0** Medical and Surgical
**D** Gastrointestinal System
**1** Bypass: Altering the route of passage of the contents of a tubular body part

| Character 4 Body Part | Character 5 Approach | Character 6 Device | Character 7 Qualifier |
|---|---|---|---|
| 1 Esophagus, Upper<br>2 Esophagus, Middle<br>3 Esophagus, Lower<br>5 Esophagus | 0 Open<br>4 Percutaneous Endoscopic<br>8 Via Natural or Artificial Opening Endoscopic | 7 Autologous Tissue Substitute<br>J Synthetic Substitute<br>K Nonautologous Tissue Substitute<br>Z No Device | 4 Cutaneous<br>6 Stomach<br>9 Duodenum<br>A Jejunum<br>B Ileum |
| 1 Esophagus, Upper<br>2 Esophagus, Middle<br>3 Esophagus, Lower<br>5 Esophagus | 3 Percutaneous | J Synthetic Substitute | 4 Cutaneous |
| 6 Stomach<br>9 Duodenum | 0 Open<br>4 Percutaneous Endoscopic<br>8 Via Natural or Artificial Opening Endoscopic | 7 Autologous Tissue Substitute<br>J Synthetic Substitute<br>K Nonautologous Tissue Substitute<br>Z No Device | 4 Cutaneous<br>9 Duodenum<br>A Jejunum<br>B Ileum<br>L Transverse Colon |
| 6 Stomach<br>9 Duodenum | 3 Percutaneous | J Synthetic Substitute | 4 Cutaneous |
| A Jejunum | 0 Open<br>4 Percutaneous Endoscopic<br>8 Via Natural or Artificial Opening Endoscopic | 7 Autologous Tissue Substitute<br>J Synthetic Substitute<br>K Nonautologous Tissue Substitute<br>Z No Device | 4 Cutaneous<br>A Jejunum<br>B Ileum<br>H Cecum<br>K Ascending Colon<br>L Transverse Colon<br>M Descending Colon<br>N Sigmoid Colon<br>P Rectum<br>Q Anus |
| A Jejunum | 3 Percutaneous | J Synthetic Substitute | 4 Cutaneous |
| B Ileum | 0 Open<br>4 Percutaneous Endoscopic<br>8 Via Natural or Artificial Opening Endoscopic | 7 Autologous Tissue Substitute<br>J Synthetic Substitute<br>K Nonautologous Tissue Substitute<br>Z No Device | 4 Cutaneous<br>B Ileum<br>H Cecum<br>K Ascending Colon<br>L Transverse Colon<br>M Descending Colon<br>N Sigmoid Colon<br>P Rectum<br>Q Anus |
| B Ileum | 3 Percutaneous | J Synthetic Substitute | 4 Cutaneous |
| H Cecum | 0 Open<br>4 Percutaneous Endoscopic<br>8 Via Natural or Artificial Opening Endoscopic | 7 Autologous Tissue Substitute<br>J Synthetic Substitute<br>K Nonautologous Tissue Substitute<br>Z No Device | 4 Cutaneous<br>H Cecum<br>K Ascending Colon<br>L Transverse Colon<br>M Descending Colon<br>N Sigmoid Colon<br>P Rectum |
| H Cecum | 3 Percutaneous | J Synthetic Substitute | 4 Cutaneous |
| K Ascending Colon | 0 Open<br>4 Percutaneous Endoscopic<br>8 Via Natural or Artificial Opening Endoscopic | 7 Autologous Tissue Substitute<br>J Synthetic Substitute<br>K Nonautologous Tissue Substitute<br>Z No Device | 4 Cutaneous<br>K Ascending Colon<br>L Transverse Colon<br>M Descending Colon<br>N Sigmoid Colon<br>P Rectum |
| K Ascending Colon | 3 Percutaneous | J Synthetic Substitute | 4 Cutaneous |
| L Transverse Colon | 0 Open<br>4 Percutaneous Endoscopic<br>8 Via Natural or Artificial Opening Endoscopic | 7 Autologous Tissue Substitute<br>J Synthetic Substitute<br>K Nonautologous Tissue Substitute<br>Z No Device | 4 Cutaneous<br>L Transverse Colon<br>M Descending Colon<br>N Sigmoid Colon<br>P Rectum |
| L Transverse Colon | 3 Percutaneous | J Synthetic Substitute | 4 Cutaneous |
| M Descending Colon | 0 Open<br>4 Percutaneous Endoscopic<br>8 Via Natural or Artificial Opening Endoscopic | 7 Autologous Tissue Substitute<br>J Synthetic Substitute<br>K Nonautologous Tissue Substitute<br>Z No Device | 4 Cutaneous<br>M Descending Colon<br>N Sigmoid Colon<br>P Rectum |
| M Descending Colon | 3 Percutaneous | J Synthetic Substitute | 4 Cutaneous |
| N Sigmoid Colon | 0 Open<br>4 Percutaneous Endoscopic<br>8 Via Natural or Artificial Opening Endoscopic | 7 Autologous Tissue Substitute<br>J Synthetic Substitute<br>K Nonautologous Tissue Substitute<br>Z No Device | 4 Cutaneous<br>N Sigmoid Colon<br>P Rectum |

**0D1** continues on next page

**0** Medical and Surgical – *continued*
**D** Gastrointestinal System – *continued*
**1** Bypass: Altering the route of passage of the contents of a tubular body part – *continued*

| Character 4 Body Part | Character 5 Approach | Character 6 Device | Character 7 Qualifier |
|---|---|---|---|
| N Sigmoid Colon | 3 Percutaneous | J Synthetic Substitute | 4 Cutaneous |

**0** Medical and Surgical
**D** Gastrointestinal System
**2** Change: Taking out or off a device from a body part and putting back an identical or similar device in or on the same body part without cutting or puncturing the skin or a mucous membrane

| Character 4 Body Part | Character 5 Approach | Character 6 Device | Character 7 Qualifier |
|---|---|---|---|
| 0 Upper Intestinal Tract<br>D Lower Intestinal Tract | X External | 0 Drainage Device<br>U Feeding Device<br>Y Other Device | Z No Qualifier |
| U Omentum<br>V Mesentery<br>W Peritoneum | X External | 0 Drainage Device<br>Y Other Device | Z No Qualifier |

**0** Medical and Surgical
**D** Gastrointestinal System
**5** Destruction: Physical eradication of all or a portion of a body part by the direct use of energy, force, or a destructive agent

| Character 4 Body Part | Character 5 Approach | Character 6 Device | Character 7 Qualifier |
|---|---|---|---|
| 1 Esophagus, Upper<br>2 Esophagus, Middle<br>3 Esophagus, Lower<br>4 Esophagogastric Junction<br>5 Esophagus<br>6 Stomach<br>7 Stomach, Pylorus<br>8 Small Intestine<br>9 Duodenum<br>A Jejunum<br>B Ileum<br>C Ileocecal Valve<br>E Large Intestine<br>F Large Intestine, Right<br>G Large Intestine, Left<br>H Cecum<br>J Appendix<br>K Ascending Colon<br>L Transverse Colon<br>M Descending Colon<br>N Sigmoid Colon<br>P Rectum | 0 Open<br>3 Percutaneous<br>4 Percutaneous Endoscopic<br>7 Via Natural or Artificial Opening<br>8 Via Natural or Artificial Opening Endoscopic | Z No Device | Z No Qualifier |
| Q Anus | 0 Open<br>3 Percutaneous<br>4 Percutaneous Endoscopic<br>7 Via Natural or Artificial Opening<br>8 Via Natural or Artificial Opening Endoscopic<br>X External | Z No Device | Z No Qualifier |
| R Anal Sphincter<br>S Greater Omentum<br>T Lesser Omentum<br>V Mesentery<br>W Peritoneum | 0 Open<br>3 Percutaneous<br>4 Percutaneous Endoscopic | Z No Device | Z No Qualifier |

**0** Medical and Surgical
**D** Gastrointestinal System
**7** Dilation: Expanding an orifice or the lumen of a tubular body part

| Character 4 Body Part | Character 5 Approach | Character 6 Device | Character 7 Qualifier |
|---|---|---|---|
| 1 Esophagus, Upper<br>2 Esophagus, Middle<br>3 Esophagus, Lower<br>4 Esophagogastric Junction<br>5 Esophagus<br>6 Stomach<br>7 Stomach, Pylorus<br>8 Small Intestine<br>9 Duodenum<br>A Jejunum<br>B Ileum<br>C Ileocecal Valve<br>E Large Intestine<br>F Large Intestine, Right<br>G Large Intestine, Left<br>H Cecum<br>K Ascending Colon<br>L Transverse Colon<br>M Descending Colon<br>N Sigmoid Colon<br>P Rectum<br>Q Anus | 0 Open<br>3 Percutaneous<br>4 Percutaneous Endoscopic<br>7 Via Natural or Artificial Opening<br>8 Via Natural or Artificial Opening Endoscopic | D Intraluminal Device<br>Z No Device | Z No Qualifier |

**0** Medical and Surgical
**D** Gastrointestinal System
**8** Division: Cutting into a body part, without draining fluids and/or gases from the body part, in order to separate or transect a body part

| Character 4 Body Part | Character 5 Approach | Character 6 Device | Character 7 Qualifier |
|---|---|---|---|
| 4 Esophagogastric Junction<br>7 Stomach, Pylorus | 0 Open<br>3 Percutaneous<br>4 Percutaneous Endoscopic<br>7 Via Natural or Artificial Opening<br>8 Via Natural or Artificial Opening Endoscopic | Z No Device | Z No Qualifier |
| R Anal Sphincter | 0 Open<br>3 Percutaneous | Z No Device | Z No Qualifier |

**0** Medical and Surgical
**D** Gastrointestinal System
**9** Drainage: Taking or letting out fluids and/or gases from a body part

| Character 4 Body Part | Character 5 Approach | Character 6 Device | Character 7 Qualifier |
|---|---|---|---|
| 1 Esophagus, Upper<br>2 Esophagus, Middle<br>3 Esophagus, Lower<br>4 Esophagogastric Junction<br>5 Esophagus<br>6 Stomach<br>7 Stomach, Pylorus<br>8 Small Intestine<br>9 Duodenum<br>A Jejunum<br>B Ileum<br>C Ileocecal Valve<br>E Large Intestine<br>F Large Intestine, Right<br>G Large Intestine, Left<br>H Cecum<br>J Appendix<br>K Ascending Colon<br>L Transverse Colon<br>M Descending Colon<br>N Sigmoid Colon<br>P Rectum | 0 Open<br>3 Percutaneous<br>4 Percutaneous Endoscopic<br>7 Via Natural or Artificial Opening<br>8 Via Natural or Artificial Opening Endoscopic | 0 Drainage Device | Z No Qualifier |
| 1 Esophagus, Upper<br>2 Esophagus, Middle<br>3 Esophagus, Lower<br>4 Esophagogastric Junction<br>5 Esophagus<br>6 Stomach<br>7 Stomach, Pylorus<br>8 Small Intestine<br>9 Duodenum<br>A Jejunum<br>B Ileum<br>C Ileocecal Valve<br>E Large Intestine<br>F Large Intestine, Right<br>G Large Intestine, Left<br>H Cecum<br>J Appendix<br>K Ascending Colon<br>L Transverse Colon<br>M Descending Colon<br>N Sigmoid Colon<br>P Rectum | 0 Open<br>3 Percutaneous<br>4 Percutaneous Endoscopic<br>7 Via Natural or Artificial Opening<br>8 Via Natural or Artificial Opening Endoscopic | Z No Device | X Diagnostic<br>Z No Qualifier |
| Q Anus | 0 Open<br>3 Percutaneous<br>4 Percutaneous Endoscopic<br>7 Via Natural or Artificial Opening<br>8 Via Natural or Artificial Opening Endoscopic<br>X External | 0 Drainage Device | Z No Qualifier |
| Q Anus | 0 Open<br>3 Percutaneous<br>4 Percutaneous Endoscopic<br>7 Via Natural or Artificial Opening<br>8 Via Natural or Artificial Opening Endoscopic<br>X External | Z No Device | X Diagnostic<br>Z No Qualifier |
| R Anal Sphincter<br>S Greater Omentum<br>T Lesser Omentum<br>V Mesentery<br>W Peritoneum | 0 Open<br>3 Percutaneous<br>4 Percutaneous Endoscopic | 0 Drainage Device | Z No Qualifier |
| R Anal Sphincter<br>S Greater Omentum<br>T Lesser Omentum<br>V Mesentery<br>W Peritoneum | 0 Open<br>3 Percutaneous<br>4 Percutaneous Endoscopic | Z No Device | X Diagnostic<br>Z No Qualifier |

**0** Medical and Surgical
**D** Gastrointestinal System
**B** Excision: Cutting out or off, without replacement, a portion of a body part

| Character 4<br>Body Part | Character 5<br>Approach | Character 6<br>Device | Character 7<br>Qualifier |
|---|---|---|---|
| 1 Esophagus, Upper<br>2 Esophagus, Middle<br>3 Esophagus, Lower<br>4 Esophagogastric Junction<br>5 Esophagus<br>7 Stomach, Pylorus<br>8 Small Intestine<br>9 Duodenum<br>A Jejunum<br>B Ileum<br>C Ileocecal Valve<br>E Large Intestine<br>F Large Intestine, Right<br>G Large Intestine, Left<br>H Cecum<br>J Appendix<br>K Ascending Colon<br>L Transverse Colon<br>M Descending Colon<br>N Sigmoid Colon<br>P Rectum | 0 Open<br>3 Percutaneous<br>4 Percutaneous Endoscopic<br>7 Via Natural or Artificial Opening<br>8 Via Natural or Artificial Opening<br>  Endoscopic | Z No Device | X Diagnostic<br>Z No Qualifier |
| 6 Stomach | 0 Open<br>3 Percutaneous<br>4 Percutaneous Endoscopic<br>7 Via Natural or Artificial Opening<br>8 Via Natural or Artificial Opening<br>  Endoscopic | Z No Device | 3 Vertical<br>X Diagnostic<br>Z No Qualifier |
| Q Anus | 0 Open<br>3 Percutaneous<br>4 Percutaneous Endoscopic<br>7 Via Natural or Artificial Opening<br>8 Via Natural or Artificial Opening<br>  Endoscopic<br>X External | Z No Device | X Diagnostic<br>Z No Qualifier |
| R Anal Sphincter<br>S Greater Omentum<br>T Lesser Omentum<br>V Mesentery<br>W Peritoneum | 0 Open<br>3 Percutaneous<br>4 Percutaneous Endoscopic | Z No Device | X Diagnostic<br>Z No Qualifier |

**0** Medical and Surgical
**D** Gastrointestinal System
**C** Extirpation: Taking or cutting out solid matter from a body part

| Character 4<br>Body Part | Character 5<br>Approach | Character 6<br>Device | Character 7<br>Qualifier |
|---|---|---|---|
| 1 Esophagus, Upper<br>2 Esophagus, Middle<br>3 Esophagus, Lower<br>4 Esophagogastric Junction<br>5 Esophagus<br>6 Stomach<br>7 Stomach, Pylorus<br>8 Small Intestine<br>9 Duodenum<br>A Jejunum<br>B Ileum<br>C Ileocecal Valve<br>E Large Intestine<br>F Large Intestine, Right<br>G Large Intestine, Left<br>H Cecum<br>J Appendix<br>K Ascending Colon<br>L Transverse Colon<br>M Descending Colon<br>N Sigmoid Colon<br>P Rectum | 0 Open<br>3 Percutaneous<br>4 Percutaneous Endoscopic<br>7 Via Natural or Artificial Opening<br>8 Via Natural or Artificial Opening<br>  Endoscopic | Z No Device | Z No Qualifier |
| Q Anus | 0 Open<br>3 Percutaneous<br>4 Percutaneous Endoscopic<br>7 Via Natural or Artificial Opening<br>8 Via Natural or Artificial Opening<br>  Endoscopic<br>X External | Z No Device | Z No Qualifier |
| R Anal Sphincter<br>S Greater Omentum<br>T Lesser Omentum<br>V Mesentery<br>W Peritoneum | 0 Open<br>3 Percutaneous<br>4 Percutaneous Endoscopic | Z No Device | Z No Qualifier |

**0** Medical and Surgical
**D** Gastrointestinal System
**F** Fragmentation: Breaking solid matter in a body part into pieces

| Character 4<br>Body Part | Character 5<br>Approach | Character 6<br>Device | Character 7<br>Qualifier |
|---|---|---|---|
| 5 Esophagus NC<br>6 Stomach NC<br>8 Small Intestine NC<br>9 Duodenum NC<br>A Jejunum NC<br>B Ileum NC<br>E Large Intestine NC<br>F Large Intestine, Right NC<br>G Large Intestine, Left NC<br>H Cecum NC<br>J Appendix NC<br>K Ascending Colon NC<br>L Transverse Colon NC<br>M Descending Colon NC<br>N Sigmoid Colon NC<br>P Rectum NC<br>Q Anus NC | 0 Open<br>3 Percutaneous<br>4 Percutaneous Endoscopic<br>7 Via Natural or Artificial Opening<br>8 Via Natural or Artificial Opening<br>  Endoscopic<br>X External | Z No Device | Z No Qualifier |

NC 0DF(5,6,8,9,A,B,E,F,G,H,J,K,L,M,N,P,Q)XZZ

**Gastrointestinal System | 0DH–0DJ**

0 Medical and Surgical
D Gastrointestinal System
H Insertion: Putting in a nonbiological appliance that monitors, assists, performs, or prevents a physiological function but does not physically take the place of a body part

| Character 4<br>Body Part | Character 5<br>Approach | Character 6<br>Device | Character 7<br>Qualifier |
|---|---|---|---|
| 5 Esophagus | 0 Open<br>3 Percutaneous<br>4 Percutaneous Endoscopic | 1 Radioactive Element<br>2 Monitoring Device<br>3 Infusion Device<br>D Intraluminal Device<br>U Feeding Device | Z No Qualifier |
| 5 Esophagus | 7 Via Natural or Artificial Opening<br>8 Via Natural or Artificial Opening<br>   Endoscopic | 1 Radioactive Element<br>2 Monitoring Device<br>3 Infusion Device<br>B Intraluminal Device, Airway<br>D Intraluminal Device<br>U Feeding Device | Z No Qualifier |
| 6 Stomach | 0 Open<br>3 Percutaneous<br>4 Percutaneous Endoscopic | 2 Monitoring Device<br>3 Infusion Device<br>D Intraluminal Device<br>M Stimulator Lead<br>U Feeding Device | Z No Qualifier |
| 6 Stomach | 7 Via Natural or Artificial Opening<br>8 Via Natural or Artificial Opening<br>   Endoscopic | 2 Monitoring Device<br>3 Infusion Device<br>D Intraluminal Device<br>U Feeding Device | Z No Qualifier |
| 8 Small Intestine<br>9 Duodenum<br>A Jejunum<br>B Ileum | 0 Open<br>3 Percutaneous<br>4 Percutaneous Endoscopic<br>7 Via Natural or Artificial Opening<br>8 Via Natural or Artificial Opening<br>   Endoscopic | 2 Monitoring Device<br>3 Infusion Device<br>D Intraluminal Device<br>U Feeding Device | Z No Qualifier |
| E Large Intestine | 0 Open<br>3 Percutaneous<br>4 Percutaneous Endoscopic<br>7 Via Natural or Artificial Opening<br>8 Via Natural or Artificial Opening<br>   Endoscopic | D Intraluminal Device | Z No Qualifier |
| P Rectum | 0 Open<br>3 Percutaneous<br>4 Percutaneous Endoscopic<br>7 Via Natural or Artificial Opening<br>8 Via Natural or Artificial Opening<br>   Endoscopic | 1 Radioactive Element<br>D Intraluminal Device | Z No Qualifier |
| Q Anus | 0 Open<br>3 Percutaneous<br>4 Percutaneous Endoscopic | D Intraluminal Device<br>L Artificial Sphincter | Z No Qualifier |
| Q Anus | 7 Via Natural or Artificial Opening<br>8 Via Natural or Artificial Opening<br>   Endoscopic | D Intraluminal Device | Z No Qualifier |
| R Anal Sphincter | 0 Open<br>3 Percutaneous<br>4 Percutaneous Endoscopic | M Stimulator Lead | Z No Qualifier |

**AHA:** 0DH63UZ - 4Q 2013, 117

0 Medical and Surgical
D Gastrointestinal System
J Inspection: Visually and/or manually exploring a body part

| Character 4<br>Body Part | Character 5<br>Approach | Character 6<br>Device | Character 7<br>Qualifier |
|---|---|---|---|
| 0 Upper Intestinal Tract<br>6 Stomach<br>D Lower Intestinal Tract | 0 Open<br>3 Percutaneous<br>4 Percutaneous Endoscopic<br>7 Via Natural or Artificial Opening<br>8 Via Natural or Artificial Opening<br>   Endoscopic<br>X External | Z No Device | Z No Qualifier |
| U Omentum<br>V Mesentery<br>W Peritoneum | 0 Open<br>3 Percutaneous<br>4 Percutaneous Endoscopic<br>X External | Z No Device | Z No Qualifier |

**0** Medical and Surgical
**D** Gastrointestinal System
**L** Occlusion: Completely closing an orifice or the lumen of a tubular body part

| Character 4<br>Body Part | Character 5<br>Approach | Character 6<br>Device | Character 7<br>Qualifier |
|---|---|---|---|
| 1 Esophagus, Upper<br>2 Esophagus, Middle<br>3 Esophagus, Lower<br>4 Esophagogastric Junction<br>5 Esophagus<br>6 Stomach<br>7 Stomach, Pylorus<br>8 Small Intestine<br>9 Duodenum<br>A Jejunum<br>B Ileum<br>C Ileocecal Valve<br>E Large Intestine<br>F Large Intestine, Right<br>G Large Intestine, Left<br>H Cecum<br>K Ascending Colon<br>L Transverse Colon<br>M Descending Colon<br>N Sigmoid Colon<br>P Rectum | 0 Open<br>3 Percutaneous<br>4 Percutaneous Endoscopic | C Extraluminal Device<br>D Intraluminal Device<br>Z No Device | Z No Qualifier |
| 1 Esophagus, Upper<br>2 Esophagus, Middle<br>3 Esophagus, Lower<br>4 Esophagogastric Junction<br>5 Esophagus<br>6 Stomach<br>7 Stomach, Pylorus<br>8 Small Intestine<br>9 Duodenum<br>A Jejunum<br>B Ileum<br>C Ileocecal Valve<br>E Large Intestine<br>F Large Intestine, Right<br>G Large Intestine, Left<br>H Cecum<br>K Ascending Colon<br>L Transverse Colon<br>M Descending Colon<br>N Sigmoid Colon<br>P Rectum | 7 Via Natural or Artificial Opening<br>8 Via Natural or Artificial Opening<br>  Endoscopic | D Intraluminal Device<br>Z No Device | Z No Qualifier |
| Q Anus | 0 Open<br>3 Percutaneous<br>4 Percutaneous Endoscopic<br>X External | C Extraluminal Device<br>D Intraluminal Device<br>Z No Device | Z No Qualifier |
| Q Anus | 7 Via Natural or Artificial Opening<br>8 Via Natural or Artificial Opening<br>  Endoscopic | D Intraluminal Device<br>Z No Device | Z No Qualifier |

**0** Medical and Surgical
**D** Gastrointestinal System
**M** Reattachment: Putting back in or on all or a portion of a separated body part to its normal location or other suitable location

| Character 4<br>Body Part | Character 5<br>Approach | Character 6<br>Device | Character 7<br>Qualifier |
|---|---|---|---|
| 5 Esophagus<br>6 Stomach<br>8 Small Intestine<br>9 Duodenum<br>A Jejunum<br>B Ileum<br>E Large Intestine<br>F Large Intestine, Right<br>G Large Intestine, Left<br>H Cecum<br>K Ascending Colon<br>L Transverse Colon<br>M Descending Colon<br>N Sigmoid Colon<br>P Rectum | 0 Open<br>4 Percutaneous Endoscopic | Z No Device | Z No Qualifier |

**0** Medical and Surgical
**D** Gastrointestinal System
**N** Release: Freeing a body part from an abnormal physical constraint by cutting or by the use of force

| Character 4<br>Body Part | Character 5<br>Approach | Character 6<br>Device | Character 7<br>Qualifier |
|---|---|---|---|
| 1 Esophagus, Upper<br>2 Esophagus, Middle<br>3 Esophagus, Lower<br>4 Esophagogastric Junction<br>5 Esophagus<br>6 Stomach<br>7 Stomach, Pylorus<br>8 Small Intestine<br>9 Duodenum<br>A Jejunum<br>B Ileum<br>C Ileocecal Valve<br>E Large Intestine<br>F Large Intestine, Right<br>G Large Intestine, Left<br>H Cecum<br>J Appendix<br>K Ascending Colon<br>L Transverse Colon<br>M Descending Colon<br>N Sigmoid Colon<br>P Rectum | 0 Open<br>3 Percutaneous<br>4 Percutaneous Endoscopic<br>7 Via Natural or Artificial Opening<br>8 Via Natural or Artificial Opening<br>  Endoscopic | Z No Device | Z No Qualifier |
| Q Anus | 0 Open<br>3 Percutaneous<br>4 Percutaneous Endoscopic<br>7 Via Natural or Artificial Opening<br>8 Via Natural or Artificial Opening<br>  Endoscopic<br>X External | Z No Device | Z No Qualifier |
| R Anal Sphincter<br>S Greater Omentum<br>T Lesser Omentum<br>V Mesentery<br>W Peritoneum | 0 Open<br>3 Percutaneous<br>4 Percutaneous Endoscopic | Z No Device | Z No Qualifier |

**0** Medical and Surgical
**D** Gastrointestinal System
**P** Removal: Taking out or off a device from a body part

| Character 4<br>Body Part | Character 5<br>Approach | Character 6<br>Device | Character 7<br>Qualifier |
|---|---|---|---|
| 0 Upper Intestinal Tract<br>D Lower Intestinal Tract | 0 Open<br>3 Percutaneous<br>4 Percutaneous Endoscopic<br>7 Via Natural or Artificial Opening<br>8 Via Natural or Artificial Opening<br>  Endoscopic | 0 Drainage Device<br>2 Monitoring Device<br>3 Infusion Device<br>7 Autologous Tissue Substitute<br>C Extraluminal Device<br>D Intraluminal Device<br>J Synthetic Substitute<br>K Nonautologous Tissue Substitute<br>U Feeding Device | Z No Qualifier |
| 0 Upper Intestinal Tract<br>D Lower Intestinal Tract | X External | 0 Drainage Device<br>2 Monitoring Device<br>3 Infusion Device<br>D Intraluminal Device<br>U Feeding Device | Z No Qualifier |
| 5 Esophagus | 0 Open<br>3 Percutaneous<br>4 Percutaneous Endoscopic | 1 Radioactive Element<br>2 Monitoring Device<br>3 Infusion Device<br>U Feeding Device | Z No Qualifier |
| 5 Esophagus | 7 Via Natural or Artificial Opening<br>8 Via Natural or Artificial Opening<br>  Endoscopic | 1 Radioactive Element<br>D Intraluminal Device | Z No Qualifier |
| 5 Esophagus | X External | 1 Radioactive Element<br>2 Monitoring Device<br>3 Infusion Device<br>D Intraluminal Device<br>U Feeding Device | Z No Qualifier |
| 6 Stomach | 0 Open<br>3 Percutaneous<br>4 Percutaneous Endoscopic | 0 Drainage Device<br>2 Monitoring Device<br>3 Infusion Device<br>7 Autologous Tissue Substitute<br>C Extraluminal Device<br>D Intraluminal Device<br>J Synthetic Substitute<br>K Nonautologous Tissue Substitute<br>M Stimulator Lead<br>U Feeding Device | Z No Qualifier |
| 6 Stomach | 7 Via Natural or Artificial Opening<br>8 Via Natural or Artificial Opening<br>  Endoscopic | 0 Drainage Device<br>2 Monitoring Device<br>3 Infusion Device<br>7 Autologous Tissue Substitute<br>C Extraluminal Device<br>D Intraluminal Device<br>J Synthetic Substitute<br>K Nonautologous Tissue Substitute<br>U Feeding Device | Z No Qualifier |
| 6 Stomach | X External | 0 Drainage Device<br>2 Monitoring Device<br>3 Infusion Device<br>D Intraluminal Device<br>U Feeding Device | Z No Qualifier |
| P Rectum | 0 Open<br>3 Percutaneous<br>4 Percutaneous Endoscopic<br>7 Via Natural or Artificial Opening<br>8 Via Natural or Artificial Opening<br>  Endoscopic<br>X External | 1 Radioactive Element | Z No Qualifier |
| Q Anus | 0 Open<br>3 Percutaneous<br>4 Percutaneous Endoscopic<br>7 Via Natural or Artificial Opening<br>8 Via Natural or Artificial Opening<br>  Endoscopic | L Artificial Sphincter | Z No Qualifier |
| R Anal Sphincter | 0 Open<br>3 Percutaneous<br>4 Percutaneous Endoscopic | M Stimulator Lead | Z No Qualifier |
| U Omentum<br>V Mesentery<br>W Peritoneum | 0 Open<br>3 Percutaneous<br>4 Percutaneous Endoscopic | 0 Drainage Device<br>1 Radioactive Element<br>7 Autologous Tissue Substitute<br>J Synthetic Substitute<br>K Nonautologous Tissue Substitute | Z No Qualifier |

**0** Medical and Surgical
**D** Gastrointestinal System
**Q** Repair: Restoring, to the extent possible, a body part to its normal anatomic structure and function

| Character 4 Body Part | Character 5 Approach | Character 6 Device | Character 7 Qualifier |
|---|---|---|---|
| 1 Esophagus, Upper<br>2 Esophagus, Middle<br>3 Esophagus, Lower<br>4 Esophagogastric Junction<br>5 Esophagus<br>6 Stomach<br>7 Stomach, Pylorus<br>8 Small Intestine<br>9 Duodenum<br>A Jejunum<br>B Ileum<br>C Ileocecal Valve<br>E Large Intestine<br>F Large Intestine, Right<br>G Large Intestine, Left<br>H Cecum<br>J Appendix<br>K Ascending Colon<br>L Transverse Colon<br>M Descending Colon<br>N Sigmoid Colon<br>P Rectum | 0 Open<br>3 Percutaneous<br>4 Percutaneous Endoscopic<br>7 Via Natural or Artificial Opening<br>8 Via Natural or Artificial Opening<br>  Endoscopic | Z No Device | Z No Qualifier |
| Q Anus | 0 Open<br>3 Percutaneous<br>4 Percutaneous Endoscopic<br>7 Via Natural or Artificial Opening<br>8 Via Natural or Artificial Opening<br>  Endoscopic<br>X External | Z No Device | Z No Qualifier |
| R Anal Sphincter<br>S Greater Omentum<br>T Lesser Omentum<br>V Mesentery<br>W Peritoneum | 0 Open<br>3 Percutaneous<br>4 Percutaneous Endoscopic | Z No Device | Z No Qualifier |

**0** Medical and Surgical
**D** Gastrointestinal System
**R** Replacement: Putting in or on biological or synthetic material that physically takes the place and/or function of all or a portion of a body part

| Character 4 Body Part | Character 5 Approach | Character 6 Device | Character 7 Qualifier |
|---|---|---|---|
| 5 Esophagus | 0 Open<br>4 Percutaneous Endoscopic<br>7 Via Natural or Artificial Opening<br>8 Via Natural or Artificial Opening<br>  Endoscopic | 7 Autologous Tissue Substitute<br>J Synthetic Substitute<br>K Nonautologous Tissue Substitute | Z No Qualifier |
| R Anal Sphincter<br>S Greater Omentum<br>T Lesser Omentum<br>V Mesentery<br>W Peritoneum | 0 Open<br>4 Percutaneous Endoscopic | 7 Autologous Tissue Substitute<br>J Synthetic Substitute<br>K Nonautologous Tissue Substitute | Z No Qualifier |

**0** Medical and Surgical
**D** Gastrointestinal System
**S** Reposition: Moving to its normal location, or other suitable location, all or a portion of a body part

| Character 4 Body Part | Character 5 Approach | Character 6 Device | Character 7 Qualifier |
|---|---|---|---|
| 5 Esophagus<br>6 Stomach<br>9 Duodenum<br>A Jejunum<br>B Ileum<br>H Cecum<br>K Ascending Colon<br>L Transverse Colon<br>M Descending Colon<br>N Sigmoid Colon<br>P Rectum<br>Q Anus | 0 Open<br>4 Percutaneous Endoscopic<br>7 Via Natural or Artificial Opening<br>8 Via Natural or Artificial Opening<br>  Endoscopic<br>X External | Z No Device | Z No Qualifier |

**0** Medical and Surgical
**D** Gastrointestinal System
**T** Resection: Cutting out or off, without replacement, all of a body part

| Character 4<br>Body Part | Character 5<br>Approach | Character 6<br>Device | Character 7<br>Qualifier |
|---|---|---|---|
| 1 Esophagus, Upper<br>2 Esophagus, Middle<br>3 Esophagus, Lower<br>4 Esophagogastric Junction<br>5 Esophagus<br>6 Stomach<br>7 Stomach, Pylorus<br>8 Small Intestine<br>9 Duodenum<br>A Jejunum<br>B Ileum<br>C Ileocecal Valve<br>E Large Intestine<br>F Large Intestine, Right<br>G Large Intestine, Left<br>H Cecum<br>J Appendix<br>K Ascending Colon<br>L Transverse Colon<br>M Descending Colon<br>N Sigmoid Colon<br>P Rectum<br>Q Anus | 0 Open<br>4 Percutaneous Endoscopic<br>7 Via Natural or Artificial Opening<br>8 Via Natural or Artificial Opening Endoscopic | Z No Device | Z No Qualifier |
| R Anal Sphincter<br>S Greater Omentum<br>T Lesser Omentum | 0 Open<br>4 Percutaneous Endoscopic | Z No Device | Z No Qualifier |

**0** Medical and Surgical
**D** Gastrointestinal System
**U** Supplement: Putting in or on biological or synthetic material that physically reinforces and/or augments the function of a portion of a body part

| Character 4<br>Body Part | Character 5<br>Approach | Character 6<br>Device | Character 7<br>Qualifier |
|---|---|---|---|
| 1 Esophagus, Upper<br>2 Esophagus, Middle<br>3 Esophagus, Lower<br>4 Esophagogastric Junction<br>5 Esophagus<br>6 Stomach<br>7 Stomach, Pylorus<br>8 Small Intestine<br>9 Duodenum<br>A Jejunum<br>B Ileum<br>C Ileocecal Valve<br>E Large Intestine<br>F Large Intestine, Right<br>G Large Intestine, Left<br>H Cecum<br>K Ascending Colon<br>L Transverse Colon<br>M Descending Colon<br>N Sigmoid Colon<br>P Rectum | 0 Open<br>4 Percutaneous Endoscopic<br>7 Via Natural or Artificial Opening<br>8 Via Natural or Artificial Opening Endoscopic | 7 Autologous Tissue Substitute<br>J Synthetic Substitute<br>K Nonautologous Tissue Substitute | Z No Qualifier |
| Q Anus | 0 Open<br>4 Percutaneous Endoscopic<br>7 Via Natural or Artificial Opening<br>8 Via Natural or Artificial Opening Endoscopic<br>X External | 7 Autologous Tissue Substitute<br>J Synthetic Substitute<br>K Nonautologous Tissue Substitute | Z No Qualifier |
| R Anal Sphincter<br>S Greater Omentum<br>T Lesser Omentum<br>V Mesentery<br>W Peritoneum | 0 Open<br>4 Percutaneous Endoscopic | 7 Autologous Tissue Substitute<br>J Synthetic Substitute<br>K Nonautologous Tissue Substitute | Z No Qualifier |

**0** Medical and Surgical
**D** Gastrointestinal System
**V** Restriction: Partially closing an orifice or the lumen of a tubular body part

| Character 4<br>Body Part | Character 5<br>Approach | Character 6<br>Device | Character 7<br>Qualifier |
|---|---|---|---|
| 1 Esophagus, Upper<br>2 Esophagus, Middle<br>3 Esophagus, Lower<br>4 Esophagogastric Junction<br>5 Esophagus<br>6 Stomach<br>7 Stomach, Pylorus<br>8 Small Intestine<br>9 Duodenum<br>A Jejunum<br>B Ileum<br>C Ileocecal Valve<br>E Large Intestine<br>F Large Intestine, Right<br>G Large Intestine, Left<br>H Cecum<br>K Ascending Colon<br>L Transverse Colon<br>M Descending Colon<br>N Sigmoid Colon<br>P Rectum | 0 Open<br>3 Percutaneous<br>4 Percutaneous Endoscopic | C Extraluminal Device<br>D Intraluminal Device<br>Z No Device | Z No Qualifier |
| 1 Esophagus, Upper<br>2 Esophagus, Middle<br>3 Esophagus, Lower<br>4 Esophagogastric Junction<br>5 Esophagus<br>6 Stomach  Ⓝ Ⓒ<br>7 Stomach, Pylorus<br>8 Small Intestine<br>9 Duodenum<br>A Jejunum<br>B Ileum<br>C Ileocecal Valve<br>E Large Intestine<br>F Large Intestine, Right<br>G Large Intestine, Left<br>H Cecum<br>K Ascending Colon<br>L Transverse Colon<br>M Descending Colon<br>N Sigmoid Colon<br>P Rectum | 7 Via Natural or Artificial Opening<br>8 Via Natural or Artificial Opening Endoscopic | D Intraluminal Device<br>Z No Device | Z No Qualifier |
| Q Anus | 0 Open<br>3 Percutaneous<br>4 Percutaneous Endoscopic<br>X External | C Extraluminal Device<br>D Intraluminal Device<br>Z No Device | Z No Qualifier |
| Q Anus | 7 Via Natural or Artificial Opening<br>8 Via Natural or Artificial Opening Endoscopic | D Intraluminal Device<br>Z No Device | Z No Qualifier |

Ⓝ Ⓒ 0DV6(7,8)DZ

**0** Medical and Surgical
**D** Gastrointestinal System
**W** Revision: Correcting, to the extent possible, a portion of a malfunctioning device or the position of a displaced device

| Character 4<br>Body Part | Character 5<br>Approach | Character 6<br>Device | Character 7<br>Qualifier |
|---|---|---|---|
| 0 Upper Intestinal Tract<br>D Lower Intestinal Tract | 0 Open<br>3 Percutaneous<br>4 Percutaneous Endoscopic<br>7 Via Natural or Artificial Opening<br>8 Via Natural or Artificial Opening Endoscopic<br>X External | 0 Drainage Device<br>2 Monitoring Device<br>3 Infusion Device<br>7 Autologous Tissue Substitute<br>C Extraluminal Device<br>D Intraluminal Device<br>J Synthetic Substitute<br>K Nonautologous Tissue Substitute<br>U Feeding Device | Z No Qualifier |
| 5 Esophagus | 7 Via Natural or Artificial Opening<br>8 Via Natural or Artificial Opening Endoscopic<br>X External | D Intraluminal Device | Z No Qualifier |
| 6 Stomach | 0 Open<br>3 Percutaneous<br>4 Percutaneous Endoscopic | 0 Drainage Device<br>2 Monitoring Device<br>3 Infusion Device<br>7 Autologous Tissue Substitute<br>C Extraluminal Device<br>D Intraluminal Device<br>J Synthetic Substitute<br>K Nonautologous Tissue Substitute<br>M Stimulator Lead<br>U Feeding Device | Z No Qualifier |
| 6 Stomach | 7 Via Natural or Artificial Opening<br>8 Via Natural or Artificial Opening Endoscopic<br>X External | 0 Drainage Device<br>2 Monitoring Device<br>3 Infusion Device<br>7 Autologous Tissue Substitute<br>C Extraluminal Device<br>D Intraluminal Device<br>J Synthetic Substitute<br>K Nonautologous Tissue Substitute<br>U Feeding Device | Z No Qualifier |
| 8 Small Intestine<br>E Large Intestine | 0 Open<br>4 Percutaneous Endoscopic<br>7 Via Natural or Artificial Opening<br>8 Via Natural or Artificial Opening Endoscopic | 7 Autologous Tissue Substitute<br>J Synthetic Substitute<br>K Nonautologous Tissue Substitute | Z No Qualifier |
| Q Anus | 0 Open<br>3 Percutaneous<br>4 Percutaneous Endoscopic<br>7 Via Natural or Artificial Opening<br>8 Via Natural or Artificial Opening Endoscopic | L Artificial Sphincter | Z No Qualifier |
| R Anal Sphincter | 0 Open<br>3 Percutaneous<br>4 Percutaneous Endoscopic | M Stimulator Lead | Z No Qualifier |
| U Omentum<br>V Mesentery<br>W Peritoneum | 0 Open<br>3 Percutaneous<br>4 Percutaneous Endoscopic | 0 Drainage Device<br>7 Autologous Tissue Substitute<br>J Synthetic Substitute<br>K Nonautologous Tissue Substitute | Z No Qualifier |

**0** Medical and Surgical
**D** Gastrointestinal System
**X** Transfer: Moving, without taking out, all or a portion of a body part to another location to take over the function of all or a portion of a body part

| Character 4<br>Body Part | Character 5<br>Approach | Character 6<br>Device | Character 7<br>Qualifier |
|---|---|---|---|
| 6 Stomach<br>8 Small Intestine<br>E Large Intestine | 0 Open<br>4 Percutaneous Endoscopic | Z No Device | 5 Esophagus |

**0** Medical and Surgical
**D** Gastrointestinal System
**Y** Transplantation: Putting in or on all or a portion of a living body part taken from another individual or animal to physically take the place and/or function of all or a portion of a similar body part

| Character 4<br>Body Part | Character 5<br>Approach | Character 6<br>Device | Character 7<br>Qualifier |
|---|---|---|---|
| 5 Esophagus<br>6 Stomach<br>8 Small Intestine **L C**<br>E Large Intestine **L C** | 0 Open | Z No Device | 0 Allogeneic<br>1 Syngeneic<br>2 Zooplastic |

**L C** 0DY80Z(0,1,2), 0DYE0Z(0,1,2)

# Hepatobiliary System and Pancreas | 0F1-0FY

**0** Medical and Surgical
**F** Hepatobiliary System and Pancreas
**1** Bypass: Altering the route of passage of the contents of a tubular body part

| Character 4<br>Body Part | Character 5<br>Approach | Character 6<br>Device | Character 7<br>Qualifier |
|---|---|---|---|
| 4 Gallbladder<br>5 Hepatic Duct, Right<br>6 Hepatic Duct, Left<br>8 Cystic Duct<br>9 Common Bile Duct | 0 Open<br>4 Percutaneous Endoscopic | D Intraluminal Device<br>Z No Device | 3 Duodenum<br>4 Stomach<br>5 Hepatic Duct, Right<br>6 Hepatic Duct, Left<br>7 Hepatic Duct, Caudate<br>8 Cystic Duct<br>9 Common Bile Duct<br>B Small Intestine |
| D Pancreatic Duct<br>F Pancreatic Duct, Accessory<br>G Pancreas | 0 Open<br>4 Percutaneous Endoscopic | D Intraluminal Device<br>Z No Device | 3 Duodenum<br>B Small Intestine<br>C Large Intestine |

**0** Medical and Surgical
**F** Hepatobiliary System and Pancreas
**2** Change: Taking out or off a device from a body part and putting back an identical or similar device in or on the same body part without cutting or puncturing the skin or a mucous membrane

| Character 4<br>Body Part | Character 5<br>Approach | Character 6<br>Device | Character 7<br>Qualifier |
|---|---|---|---|
| 0 Liver<br>4 Gallbladder<br>B Hepatobiliary Duct<br>D Pancreatic Duct<br>G Pancreas | X External | 0 Drainage Device<br>Y Other Device | Z No Qualifier |

**0** Medical and Surgical
**F** Hepatobiliary System and Pancreas
**5** Destruction: Physical eradication of all or a portion of a body part by the direct use of energy, force, or a destructive agent

| Character 4<br>Body Part | Character 5<br>Approach | Character 6<br>Device | Character 7<br>Qualifier |
|---|---|---|---|
| 0 Liver<br>1 Liver, Right Lobe<br>2 Liver, Left Lobe<br>4 Gallbladder<br>G Pancreas | 0 Open<br>3 Percutaneous<br>4 Percutaneous Endoscopic | Z No Device | Z No Qualifier |
| 5 Hepatic Duct, Right<br>6 Hepatic Duct, Left<br>8 Cystic Duct<br>9 Common Bile Duct<br>C Ampulla of Vater<br>D Pancreatic Duct<br>F Pancreatic Duct, Accessory | 0 Open<br>3 Percutaneous<br>4 Percutaneous Endoscopic<br>7 Via Natural or Artificial Opening<br>8 Via Natural or Artificial Opening Endoscopic | Z No Device | Z No Qualifier |

**0** Medical and Surgical
**F** Hepatobiliary System and Pancreas
**7** Dilation: Expanding an orifice or the lumen of a tubular body part

| Character 4<br>Body Part | Character 5<br>Approach | Character 6<br>Device | Character 7<br>Qualifier |
|---|---|---|---|
| 5  Hepatic Duct, Right<br>6  Hepatic Duct, Left<br>8  Cystic Duct<br>9  Common Bile Duct<br>C  Ampulla of Vater<br>D  Pancreatic Duct<br>F  Pancreatic Duct, Accessory | 0  Open<br>3  Percutaneous<br>4  Percutaneous Endoscopic<br>7  Via Natural or Artificial Opening<br>8  Via Natural or Artificial Opening<br>   Endoscopic | D  Intraluminal Device<br>Z  No Device | Z  No Qualifier |

**0** Medical and Surgical
**F** Hepatobiliary System and Pancreas
**8** Division: Cutting into a body part, without draining fluids and/or gases from the body part, in order to separate or transect a body part

| Character 4<br>Body Part | Character 5<br>Approach | Character 6<br>Device | Character 7<br>Qualifier |
|---|---|---|---|
| G  Pancreas | 0  Open<br>3  Percutaneous<br>4  Percutaneous Endoscopic | Z  No Device | Z  No Qualifier |

**0** Medical and Surgical
**F** Hepatobiliary System and Pancreas
**9** Drainage: Taking or letting out fluids and/or gases from a body part

| Character 4<br>Body Part | Character 5<br>Approach | Character 6<br>Device | Character 7<br>Qualifier |
|---|---|---|---|
| 0  Liver<br>1  Liver, Right Lobe<br>2  Liver, Left Lobe<br>4  Gallbladder<br>G  Pancreas | 0  Open<br>3  Percutaneous<br>4  Percutaneous Endoscopic | 0  Drainage Device | Z  No Qualifier |
| 0  Liver<br>1  Liver, Right Lobe<br>2  Liver, Left Lobe<br>4  Gallbladder<br>G  Pancreas | 0  Open<br>3  Percutaneous<br>4  Percutaneous Endoscopic | Z  No Device | X  Diagnostic<br>Z  No Qualifier |
| 5  Hepatic Duct, Right<br>6  Hepatic Duct, Left<br>8  Cystic Duct<br>9  Common Bile Duct<br>C  Ampulla of Vater<br>D  Pancreatic Duct<br>F  Pancreatic Duct, Accessory | 0  Open<br>3  Percutaneous<br>4  Percutaneous Endoscopic<br>7  Via Natural or Artificial Opening<br>8  Via Natural or Artificial Opening<br>   Endoscopic | 0  Drainage Device | Z  No Qualifier |
| 5  Hepatic Duct, Right<br>6  Hepatic Duct, Left<br>8  Cystic Duct<br>9  Common Bile Duct<br>C  Ampulla of Vater<br>D  Pancreatic Duct<br>F  Pancreatic Duct, Accessory | 0  Open<br>3  Percutaneous<br>4  Percutaneous Endoscopic<br>7  Via Natural or Artificial Opening<br>8  Via Natural or Artificial Opening<br>   Endoscopic | Z  No Device | X  Diagnostic<br>Z  No Qualifier |

**0** Medical and Surgical
**F** Hepatobiliary System and Pancreas
**B** Excision: Cutting out or off, without replacement, a portion of a body part

| Character 4<br>Body Part | Character 5<br>Approach | Character 6<br>Device | Character 7<br>Qualifier |
|---|---|---|---|
| 0 Liver<br>1 Liver, Right Lobe<br>2 Liver, Left Lobe<br>4 Gallbladder<br>G Pancreas | 0 Open<br>3 Percutaneous<br>4 Percutaneous Endoscopic | Z No Device | X Diagnostic<br>Z No Qualifier |
| 5 Hepatic Duct, Right<br>6 Hepatic Duct, Left<br>8 Cystic Duct<br>9 Common Bile Duct<br>C Ampulla of Vater<br>D Pancreatic Duct<br>F Pancreatic Duct, Accessory | 0 Open<br>3 Percutaneous<br>4 Percutaneous Endoscopic<br>7 Via Natural or Artificial Opening<br>8 Via Natural or Artificial Opening<br>   Endoscopic | Z No Device | X Diagnostic<br>Z No Qualifier |

**0** Medical and Surgical
**F** Hepatobiliary System and Pancreas
**C** Extirpation: Taking or cutting out solid matter from a body part

| Character 4<br>Body Part | Character 5<br>Approach | Character 6<br>Device | Character 7<br>Qualifier |
|---|---|---|---|
| 0 Liver<br>1 Liver, Right Lobe<br>2 Liver, Left Lobe<br>4 Gallbladder<br>G Pancreas | 0 Open<br>3 Percutaneous<br>4 Percutaneous Endoscopic | Z No Device | Z No Qualifier |
| 5 Hepatic Duct, Right<br>6 Hepatic Duct, Left<br>8 Cystic Duct<br>9 Common Bile Duct<br>C Ampulla of Vater<br>D Pancreatic Duct<br>F Pancreatic Duct, Accessory | 0 Open<br>3 Percutaneous<br>4 Percutaneous Endoscopic<br>7 Via Natural or Artificial Opening<br>8 Via Natural or Artificial Opening<br>   Endoscopic | Z No Device | Z No Qualifier |

**0** Medical and Surgical
**F** Hepatobiliary System and Pancreas
**F** Fragmentation: Breaking solid matter in a body part into pieces

| Character 4<br>Body Part | Character 5<br>Approach | Character 6<br>Device | Character 7<br>Qualifier |
|---|---|---|---|
| 4 Gallbladder NC<br>5 Hepatic Duct, Right NC<br>6 Hepatic Duct, Left NC<br>8 Cystic Duct NC<br>9 Common Bile Duct NC<br>C Ampulla of Vater NC<br>D Pancreatic Duct NC<br>F Pancreatic Duct, Accessory NC | 0 Open<br>3 Percutaneous<br>4 Percutaneous Endoscopic<br>7 Via Natural or Artificial Opening<br>8 Via Natural or Artificial Opening<br>   Endoscopic<br>X External | Z No Device | Z No Qualifier |

NC 0FF(4-6,8-9,C,D,F)XZZ

**0** Medical and Surgical
**F** Hepatobiliary System and Pancreas
**H** Insertion: Putting in a nonbiological appliance that monitors, assists, performs, or prevents a physiological function but does not physically take the place of a body part

| Character 4<br>Body Part | Character 5<br>Approach | Character 6<br>Device | Character 7<br>Qualifier |
|---|---|---|---|
| 0 Liver<br>1 Liver, Right Lobe<br>2 Liver, Left Lobe<br>4 Gallbladder<br>G Pancreas | 0 Open<br>3 Percutaneous<br>4 Percutaneous Endoscopic | 2 Monitoring Device<br>3 Infusion Device | Z No Qualifier |
| B Hepatobiliary Duct<br>D Pancreatic Duct | 0 Open<br>3 Percutaneous<br>4 Percutaneous Endoscopic<br>7 Via Natural or Artificial Opening<br>8 Via Natural or Artificial Opening<br>   Endoscopic | 1 Radioactive Element<br>2 Monitoring Device<br>3 Infusion Device<br>D Intraluminal Device | Z No Qualifier |

0  Medical and Surgical
F  Hepatobiliary System and Pancreas
J  Inspection: Visually and/or manually exploring a body part

| Character 4<br>Body Part | Character 5<br>Approach | Character 6<br>Device | Character 7<br>Qualifier |
|---|---|---|---|
| 0  Liver<br>4  Gallbladder<br>G  Pancreas | 0  Open<br>3  Percutaneous<br>4  Percutaneous Endoscopic<br>X  External | Z  No Device | Z  No Qualifier |
| B  Hepatobiliary Duct<br>D  Pancreatic Duct | 0  Open<br>3  Percutaneous<br>4  Percutaneous Endoscopic<br>7  Via Natural or Artificial Opening<br>8  Via Natural or Artificial Opening<br>   Endoscopic | Z  No Device | Z  No Qualifier |

0  Medical and Surgical
F  Hepatobiliary System and Pancreas
L  Occlusion: Completely closing an orifice or the lumen of a tubular body part

| Character 4<br>Body Part | Character 5<br>Approach | Character 6<br>Device | Character 7<br>Qualifier |
|---|---|---|---|
| 5  Hepatic Duct, Right<br>6  Hepatic Duct, Left<br>8  Cystic Duct<br>9  Common Bile Duct<br>C  Ampulla of Vater<br>D  Pancreatic Duct<br>F  Pancreatic Duct, Accessory | 0  Open<br>3  Percutaneous<br>4  Percutaneous Endoscopic | C  Extraluminal Device<br>D  Intraluminal Device<br>Z  No Device | Z  No Qualifier |
| 5  Hepatic Duct, Right<br>6  Hepatic Duct, Left<br>8  Cystic Duct<br>9  Common Bile Duct<br>C  Ampulla of Vater<br>D  Pancreatic Duct<br>F  Pancreatic Duct, Accessory | 7  Via Natural or Artificial Opening<br>8  Via Natural or Artificial Opening<br>   Endoscopic | D  Intraluminal Device<br>Z  No Device | Z  No Qualifier |

0  Medical and Surgical
F  Hepatobiliary System and Pancreas
M  Reattachment: Putting back in or on all or a portion of a separated body part to its normal location or other suitable location

| Character 4<br>Body Part | Character 5<br>Approach | Character 6<br>Device | Character 7<br>Qualifier |
|---|---|---|---|
| 0  Liver<br>1  Liver, Right Lobe<br>2  Liver, Left Lobe<br>4  Gallbladder<br>5  Hepatic Duct, Right<br>6  Hepatic Duct, Left<br>8  Cystic Duct<br>9  Common Bile Duct<br>C  Ampulla of Vater<br>D  Pancreatic Duct<br>F  Pancreatic Duct, Accessory<br>G  Pancreas | 0  Open<br>4  Percutaneous Endoscopic | Z  No Device | Z  No Qualifier |

0  Medical and Surgical
F  Hepatobiliary System and Pancreas
N  Release: Freeing a body part from an abnormal physical constraint by cutting or by the use of force

| Character 4<br>Body Part | Character 5<br>Approach | Character 6<br>Device | Character 7<br>Qualifier |
|---|---|---|---|
| 0  Liver<br>1  Liver, Right Lobe<br>2  Liver, Left Lobe<br>4  Gallbladder<br>G  Pancreas | 0  Open<br>3  Percutaneous<br>4  Percutaneous Endoscopic | Z  No Device | Z  No Qualifier |
| 5  Hepatic Duct, Right<br>6  Hepatic Duct, Left<br>8  Cystic Duct<br>9  Common Bile Duct<br>C  Ampulla of Vater<br>D  Pancreatic Duct<br>F  Pancreatic Duct, Accessory | 0  Open<br>3  Percutaneous<br>4  Percutaneous Endoscopic<br>7  Via Natural or Artificial Opening<br>8  Via Natural or Artificial Opening<br>   Endoscopic | Z  No Device | Z  No Qualifier |

**0** Medical and Surgical
**F** Hepatobiliary System and Pancreas
**P** Removal: Taking out or off a device from a body part

| Character 4 Body Part | Character 5 Approach | Character 6 Device | Character 7 Qualifier |
|---|---|---|---|
| 0 Liver | 0 Open<br>3 Percutaneous<br>4 Percutaneous Endoscopic<br>X External | 0 Drainage Device<br>2 Monitoring Device<br>3 Infusion Device | Z No Qualifier |
| 4 Gallbladder<br>G Pancreas | 0 Open<br>3 Percutaneous<br>4 Percutaneous Endoscopic<br>X External | 0 Drainage Device<br>2 Monitoring Device<br>3 Infusion Device<br>D Intraluminal Device | Z No Qualifier |
| B Hepatobiliary Duct<br>D Pancreatic Duct | 0 Open<br>3 Percutaneous<br>4 Percutaneous Endoscopic<br>7 Via Natural or Artificial Opening<br>8 Via Natural or Artificial Opening Endoscopic | 0 Drainage Device<br>1 Radioactive Element<br>2 Monitoring Device<br>3 Infusion Device<br>7 Autologous Tissue Substitute<br>C Extraluminal Device<br>D Intraluminal Device<br>J Synthetic Substitute<br>K Nonautologous Tissue Substitute | Z No Qualifier |
| B Hepatobiliary Duct<br>D Pancreatic Duct | X External | 0 Drainage Device<br>1 Radioactive Element<br>2 Monitoring Device<br>3 Infusion Device<br>D Intraluminal Device | Z No Qualifier |

**0** Medical and Surgical
**F** Hepatobiliary System and Pancreas
**Q** Repair: Restoring, to the extent possible, a body part to its normal anatomic structure and function

| Character 4 Body Part | Character 5 Approach | Character 6 Device | Character 7 Qualifier |
|---|---|---|---|
| 0 Liver<br>1 Liver, Right Lobe<br>2 Liver, Left Lobe<br>4 Gallbladder<br>G Pancreas | 0 Open<br>3 Percutaneous<br>4 Percutaneous Endoscopic | Z No Device | Z No Qualifier |
| 5 Hepatic Duct, Right<br>6 Hepatic Duct, Left<br>8 Cystic Duct<br>9 Common Bile Duct<br>C Ampulla of Vater<br>D Pancreatic Duct<br>F Pancreatic Duct, Accessory | 0 Open<br>3 Percutaneous<br>4 Percutaneous Endoscopic<br>7 Via Natural or Artificial Opening<br>8 Via Natural or Artificial Opening Endoscopic | Z No Device | Z No Qualifier |

**AHA:** 0FQ00ZZ - 4Q 2013, 110

**0** Medical and Surgical
**F** Hepatobiliary System and Pancreas
**R** Replacement: Putting in or on biological or synthetic material that physically takes the place and/or function of all or a portion of a body part

| Character 4 Body Part | Character 5 Approach | Character 6 Device | Character 7 Qualifier |
|---|---|---|---|
| 5 Hepatic Duct, Right<br>6 Hepatic Duct, Left<br>8 Cystic Duct<br>9 Common Bile Duct<br>C Ampulla of Vater<br>D Pancreatic Duct<br>F Pancreatic Duct, Accessory | 0 Open<br>4 Percutaneous Endoscopic | 7 Autologous Tissue Substitute<br>J Synthetic Substitute<br>K Nonautologous Tissue Substitute | Z No Qualifier |

**0** Medical and Surgical
**F** Hepatobiliary System and Pancreas
**S** Reposition: Moving to its normal location, or other suitable location, all or a portion of a body part

| Character 4 Body Part | Character 5 Approach | Character 6 Device | Character 7 Qualifier |
|---|---|---|---|
| 0 Liver<br>4 Gallbladder<br>5 Hepatic Duct, Right<br>6 Hepatic Duct, Left<br>8 Cystic Duct<br>9 Common Bile Duct<br>C Ampulla of Vater<br>D Pancreatic Duct<br>F Pancreatic Duct, Accessory<br>G Pancreas | 0 Open<br>4 Percutaneous Endoscopic | Z No Device | Z No Qualifier |

**0** Medical and Surgical
**F** Hepatobiliary System and Pancreas
**T** Resection: Cutting out or off, without replacement, all of a body part

| Character 4 Body Part | Character 5 Approach | Character 6 Device | Character 7 Qualifier |
|---|---|---|---|
| 0 Liver<br>1 Liver, Right Lobe<br>2 Liver, Left Lobe<br>4 Gallbladder<br>G Pancreas | 0 Open<br>4 Percutaneous Endoscopic | Z No Device | Z No Qualifier |
| 5 Hepatic Duct, Right<br>6 Hepatic Duct, Left<br>8 Cystic Duct<br>9 Common Bile Duct<br>C Ampulla of Vater<br>D Pancreatic Duct<br>F Pancreatic Duct, Accessory | 0 Open<br>4 Percutaneous Endoscopic<br>7 Via Natural or Artificial Opening<br>8 Via Natural or Artificial Opening Endoscopic | Z No Device | Z No Qualifier |

**0** Medical and Surgical
**F** Hepatobiliary System and Pancreas
**U** Supplement: Putting in or on biological or synthetic material that physically reinforces and/or augments the function of a portion of a body part

| Character 4 Body Part | Character 5 Approach | Character 6 Device | Character 7 Qualifier |
|---|---|---|---|
| 5 Hepatic Duct, Right<br>6 Hepatic Duct, Left<br>8 Cystic Duct<br>9 Common Bile Duct<br>C Ampulla of Vater<br>D Pancreatic Duct<br>F Pancreatic Duct, Accessory | 0 Open<br>3 Percutaneous<br>4 Percutaneous Endoscopic | 7 Autologous Tissue Substitute<br>J Synthetic Substitute<br>K Nonautologous Tissue Substitute | Z No Qualifier |

**0** Medical and Surgical
**F** Hepatobiliary System and Pancreas
**V** Restriction: Partially closing an orifice or the lumen of a tubular body part

| Character 4 Body Part | Character 5 Approach | Character 6 Device | Character 7 Qualifier |
|---|---|---|---|
| 5 Hepatic Duct, Right<br>6 Hepatic Duct, Left<br>8 Cystic Duct<br>9 Common Bile Duct<br>C Ampulla of Vater<br>D Pancreatic Duct<br>F Pancreatic Duct, Accessory | 0 Open<br>3 Percutaneous<br>4 Percutaneous Endoscopic | C Extraluminal Device<br>D Intraluminal Device<br>Z No Device | Z No Qualifier |
| 5 Hepatic Duct, Right<br>6 Hepatic Duct, Left<br>8 Cystic Duct<br>9 Common Bile Duct<br>C Ampulla of Vater<br>D Pancreatic Duct<br>F Pancreatic Duct, Accessory | 7 Via Natural or Artificial Opening<br>8 Via Natural or Artificial Opening Endoscopic | D Intraluminal Device<br>Z No Device | Z No Qualifier |

**0** Medical and Surgical
**F** Hepatobiliary System and Pancreas
**W** Revision: Correcting, to the extent possible, a portion of a malfunctioning device or the position of a displaced device

| Character 4 Body Part | Character 5 Approach | Character 6 Device | Character 7 Qualifier |
|---|---|---|---|
| 0 Liver | 0 Open<br>3 Percutaneous<br>4 Percutaneous Endoscopic<br>X External | 0 Drainage Device<br>2 Monitoring Device<br>3 Infusion Device | Z No Qualifier |
| 4 Gallbladder<br>G Pancreas | 0 Open<br>3 Percutaneous<br>4 Percutaneous Endoscopic<br>X External | 0 Drainage Device<br>2 Monitoring Device<br>3 Infusion Device<br>D Intraluminal Device | Z No Qualifier |
| B Hepatobiliary Duct<br>D Pancreatic Duct | 0 Open<br>3 Percutaneous<br>4 Percutaneous Endoscopic<br>7 Via Natural or Artificial Opening<br>8 Via Natural or Artificial Opening Endoscopic<br>X External | 0 Drainage Device<br>2 Monitoring Device<br>3 Infusion Device<br>7 Autologous Tissue Substitute<br>C Extraluminal Device<br>D Intraluminal Device<br>J Synthetic Substitute<br>K Nonautologous Tissue Substitute | Z No Qualifier |

**0** Medical and Surgical
**F** Hepatobiliary System and Pancreas
**Y** Transplantation: Putting in or on all or a portion of a living body part taken from another individual or animal to physically take the place and/or function of all or a portion of a similar body part

| Character 4 Body Part | Character 5 Approach | Character 6 Device | Character 7 Qualifier |
|---|---|---|---|
| 0 Liver **L C**<br>G Pancreas **L C**  **N C** | 0 Open | Z No Device | 0 Allogeneic<br>1 Syngeneic<br>2 Zooplastic |

**L C** 0FY00Z(0,1,2), 0FYG0Z(0,1)
**N C** 0FYG0Z 2

# Endocrine System | 062-06W

**0** Medical and Surgical
**G** Endocrine System
**2** Change: Taking out or off a device from a body part and putting back an identical or similar device in or on the same body part without cutting or puncturing the skin or a mucous membrane

| Character 4 Body Part | Character 5 Approach | Character 6 Device | Character 7 Qualifier |
|---|---|---|---|
| 0 Pituitary Gland | X External | 0 Drainage Device | Z No Qualifier |
| 1 Pineal Body | | Y Other Device | |
| 5 Adrenal Gland | | | |
| K Thyroid Gland | | | |
| R Parathyroid Gland | | | |
| S Endocrine Gland | | | |

**0** Medical and Surgical
**G** Endocrine System
**5** Destruction: Physical eradication of all or a portion of a body part by the direct use of energy, force, or a destructive agent

| Character 4 Body Part | Character 5 Approach | Character 6 Device | Character 7 Qualifier |
|---|---|---|---|
| 0 Pituitary Gland | 0 Open | Z No Device | Z No Qualifier |
| 1 Pineal Body | 3 Percutaneous | | |
| 2 Adrenal Gland, Left | 4 Percutaneous Endoscopic | | |
| 3 Adrenal Gland, Right | | | |
| 4 Adrenal Glands, Bilateral | | | |
| 6 Carotid Body, Left | | | |
| 7 Carotid Body, Right | | | |
| 8 Carotid Bodies, Bilateral | | | |
| 9 Para-aortic Body | | | |
| B Coccygeal Glomus | | | |
| C Glomus Jugulare | | | |
| D Aortic Body | | | |
| F Paraganglion Extremity | | | |
| G Thyroid Gland Lobe, Left | | | |
| H Thyroid Gland Lobe, Right | | | |
| K Thyroid Gland | | | |
| L Superior Parathyroid Gland, Right | | | |
| M Superior Parathyroid Gland, Left | | | |
| N Inferior Parathyroid Gland, Right | | | |
| P Inferior Parathyroid Gland, Left | | | |
| Q Parathyroid Glands, Multiple | | | |
| R Parathyroid Gland | | | |

**0** Medical and Surgical
**G** Endocrine System
**8** Division: Cutting into a body part, without draining fluids and/or gases from the body part, in order to separate or transect a body part

| Character 4 Body Part | Character 5 Approach | Character 6 Device | Character 7 Qualifier |
|---|---|---|---|
| 0 Pituitary Gland | 0 Open | Z No Device | Z No Qualifier |
| J Thyroid Gland Isthmus | 3 Percutaneous | | |
| | 4 Percutaneous Endoscopic | | |

**0** Medical and Surgical
**G** Endocrine System
**9** Drainage: Taking or letting out fluids and/or gases from a body part

| Character 4 Body Part | Character 5 Approach | Character 6 Device | Character 7 Qualifier |
|---|---|---|---|
| 0 Pituitary Gland | 0 Open | 0 Drainage Device | Z No Qualifier |
| 1 Pineal Body | 3 Percutaneous | | |
| 2 Adrenal Gland, Left | 4 Percutaneous Endoscopic | | |
| 3 Adrenal Gland, Right | | | |
| 4 Adrenal Glands, Bilateral | | | |
| 6 Carotid Body, Left | | | |
| 7 Carotid Body, Right | | | |
| 8 Carotid Bodies, Bilateral | | | |
| 9 Para-aortic Body | | | |
| B Coccygeal Glomus | | | |
| C Glomus Jugulare | | | |
| D Aortic Body | | | |
| F Paraganglion Extremity | | | |
| G Thyroid Gland Lobe, Left | | | |
| H Thyroid Gland Lobe, Right | | | |
| K Thyroid Gland | | | |
| L Superior Parathyroid Gland, Right | | | |
| M Superior Parathyroid Gland, Left | | | |
| N Inferior Parathyroid Gland, Right | | | |
| P Inferior Parathyroid Gland, Left | | | |
| Q Parathyroid Glands, Multiple | | | |
| R Parathyroid Gland | | | |
| 0 Pituitary Gland | 0 Open | Z No Device | X Diagnostic |
| 1 Pineal Body | 3 Percutaneous | | Z No Qualifier |
| 2 Adrenal Gland, Left | 4 Percutaneous Endoscopic | | |
| 3 Adrenal Gland, Right | | | |
| 4 Adrenal Glands, Bilateral | | | |
| 6 Carotid Body, Left | | | |
| 7 Carotid Body, Right | | | |
| 8 Carotid Bodies, Bilateral | | | |
| 9 Para-aortic Body | | | |
| B Coccygeal Glomus | | | |
| C Glomus Jugulare | | | |
| D Aortic Body | | | |
| F Paraganglion Extremity | | | |
| G Thyroid Gland Lobe, Left | | | |
| H Thyroid Gland Lobe, Right | | | |
| K Thyroid Gland | | | |
| L Superior Parathyroid Gland, Right | | | |
| M Superior Parathyroid Gland, Left | | | |
| N Inferior Parathyroid Gland, Right | | | |
| P Inferior Parathyroid Gland, Left | | | |
| Q Parathyroid Glands, Multiple | | | |
| R Parathyroid Gland | | | |

**0** Medical and Surgical
**G** Endocrine System
**B** Excision: Cutting out or off, without replacement, a portion of a body part

| Character 4 Body Part | Character 5 Approach | Character 6 Device | Character 7 Qualifier |
|---|---|---|---|
| 0 Pituitary Gland | 0 Open | Z No Device | X Diagnostic |
| 1 Pineal Body | 3 Percutaneous | | Z No Qualifier |
| 2 Adrenal Gland, Left | 4 Percutaneous Endoscopic | | |
| 3 Adrenal Gland, Right | | | |
| 4 Adrenal Glands, Bilateral | | | |
| 6 Carotid Body, Left | | | |
| 7 Carotid Body, Right | | | |
| 8 Carotid Bodies, Bilateral | | | |
| 9 Para-aortic Body | | | |
| B Coccygeal Glomus | | | |
| C Glomus Jugulare | | | |
| D Aortic Body | | | |
| F Paraganglion Extremity | | | |
| G Thyroid Gland Lobe, Left | | | |
| H Thyroid Gland Lobe, Right | | | |
| L Superior Parathyroid Gland, Right | | | |
| M Superior Parathyroid Gland, Left | | | |
| N Inferior Parathyroid Gland, Right | | | |
| P Inferior Parathyroid Gland, Left | | | |
| Q Parathyroid Glands, Multiple | | | |
| R Parathyroid Gland | | | |

**0** Medical and Surgical
**G** Endocrine System
**C** Extirpation: Taking or cutting out solid matter from a body part

| Character 4<br>Body Part | Character 5<br>Approach | Character 6<br>Device | Character 7<br>Qualifier |
| --- | --- | --- | --- |
| 0 Pituitary Gland<br>1 Pineal Body<br>2 Adrenal Gland, Left<br>3 Adrenal Gland, Right<br>4 Adrenal Glands, Bilateral<br>6 Carotid Body, Left<br>7 Carotid Body, Right<br>8 Carotid Bodies, Bilateral<br>9 Para-aortic Body<br>B Coccygeal Glomus<br>C Glomus Jugulare<br>D Aortic Body<br>F Paraganglion Extremity<br>G Thyroid Gland Lobe, Left<br>H Thyroid Gland Lobe, Right<br>K Thyroid Gland<br>L Superior Parathyroid Gland, Right<br>M Superior Parathyroid Gland, Left<br>N Inferior Parathyroid Gland, Right<br>P Inferior Parathyroid Gland, Left<br>Q Parathyroid Glands, Multiple<br>R Parathyroid Gland | 0 Open<br>3 Percutaneous<br>4 Percutaneous Endoscopic | Z No Device | Z No Qualifier |

**0** Medical and Surgical
**G** Endocrine System
**H** Insertion: Putting in a nonbiological appliance that monitors, assists, performs, or prevents a physiological function but does not physically take the place of a body part

| Character 4<br>Body Part | Character 5<br>Approach | Character 6<br>Device | Character 7<br>Qualifier |
| --- | --- | --- | --- |
| S Endocrine Gland | 0 Open<br>3 Percutaneous<br>4 Percutaneous Endoscopic | 2 Monitoring Device<br>3 Infusion Device | Z No Qualifier |

**0** Medical and Surgical
**G** Endocrine System
**J** Inspection: Visually and/or manually exploring a body part

| Character 4<br>Body Part | Character 5<br>Approach | Character 6<br>Device | Character 7<br>Qualifier |
| --- | --- | --- | --- |
| 0 Pituitary Gland<br>1 Pineal Body<br>5 Adrenal Gland<br>K Thyroid Gland<br>R Parathyroid Gland<br>S Endocrine Gland | 0 Open<br>3 Percutaneous<br>4 Percutaneous Endoscopic | Z No Device | Z No Qualifier |

**0** Medical and Surgical
**G** Endocrine System
**M** Reattachment: Putting back in or on all or a portion of a separated body part to its normal location or other suitable location

| Character 4<br>Body Part | Character 5<br>Approach | Character 6<br>Device | Character 7<br>Qualifier |
| --- | --- | --- | --- |
| 2 Adrenal Gland, Left<br>3 Adrenal Gland, Right<br>G Thyroid Gland Lobe, Left<br>H Thyroid Gland Lobe, Right<br>L Superior Parathyroid Gland, Right<br>M Superior Parathyroid Gland, Left<br>N Inferior Parathyroid Gland, Right<br>P Inferior Parathyroid Gland, Left<br>Q Parathyroid Glands, Multiple<br>R Parathyroid Gland | 0 Open<br>4 Percutaneous Endoscopic | Z No Device | Z No Qualifier |

**0** Medical and Surgical
**G** Endocrine System
**N** Release: Freeing a body part from an abnormal physical constraint by cutting or by the use of force

| Character 4<br>Body Part | Character 5<br>Approach | Character 6<br>Device | Character 7<br>Qualifier |
|---|---|---|---|
| 0 Pituitary Gland<br>1 Pineal Body<br>2 Adrenal Gland, Left<br>3 Adrenal Gland, Right<br>4 Adrenal Glands, Bilateral<br>6 Carotid Body, Left<br>7 Carotid Body, Right<br>8 Carotid Bodies, Bilateral<br>9 Para-aortic Body<br>B Coccygeal Glomus<br>C Glomus Jugulare<br>D Aortic Body<br>F Paraganglion Extremity<br>G Thyroid Gland Lobe, Left<br>H Thyroid Gland Lobe, Right<br>K Thyroid Gland<br>L Superior Parathyroid Gland, Right<br>M Superior Parathyroid Gland, Left<br>N Inferior Parathyroid Gland, Right<br>P Inferior Parathyroid Gland, Left<br>Q Parathyroid Glands, Multiple<br>R Parathyroid Gland | 0 Open<br>3 Percutaneous<br>4 Percutaneous Endoscopic | Z No Device | Z No Qualifier |

**0** Medical and Surgical
**G** Endocrine System
**P** Removal: Taking out or off a device from a body part

| Character 4<br>Body Part | Character 5<br>Approach | Character 6<br>Device | Character 7<br>Qualifier |
|---|---|---|---|
| 0 Pituitary Gland<br>1 Pineal Body<br>5 Adrenal Gland<br>K Thyroid Gland<br>R Parathyroid Gland | 0 Open<br>3 Percutaneous<br>4 Percutaneous Endoscopic<br>X External | 0 Drainage Device | Z No Qualifier |
| S Endocrine Gland | 0 Open<br>3 Percutaneous<br>4 Percutaneous Endoscopic<br>X External | 0 Drainage Device<br>2 Monitoring Device<br>3 Infusion Device | Z No Qualifier |

**0** Medical and Surgical
**G** Endocrine System
**Q** Repair: Restoring, to the extent possible, a body part to its normal anatomic structure and function

| Character 4<br>Body Part | Character 5<br>Approach | Character 6<br>Device | Character 7<br>Qualifier |
|---|---|---|---|
| 0 Pituitary Gland<br>1 Pineal Body<br>2 Adrenal Gland, Left<br>3 Adrenal Gland, Right<br>4 Adrenal Glands, Bilateral<br>6 Carotid Body, Left<br>7 Carotid Body, Right<br>8 Carotid Bodies, Bilateral<br>9 Para-aortic Body<br>B Coccygeal Glomus<br>C Glomus Jugulare<br>D Aortic Body<br>F Paraganglion Extremity<br>G Thyroid Gland Lobe, Left<br>H Thyroid Gland Lobe, Right<br>J Thyroid Gland Isthmus<br>K Thyroid Gland<br>L Superior Parathyroid Gland, Right<br>M Superior Parathyroid Gland, Left<br>N Inferior Parathyroid Gland, Right<br>P Inferior Parathyroid Gland, Left<br>Q Parathyroid Glands, Multiple<br>R Parathyroid Gland | 0 Open<br>3 Percutaneous<br>4 Percutaneous Endoscopic | Z No Device | Z No Qualifier |

**0** Medical and Surgical
**G** Endocrine System
**S** Reposition: Moving to its normal location, or other suitable location, all or a portion of a body part

| Character 4<br>Body Part | Character 5<br>Approach | Character 6<br>Device | Character 7<br>Qualifier |
|---|---|---|---|
| 2 Adrenal Gland, Left<br>3 Adrenal Gland, Right<br>G Thyroid Gland Lobe, Left<br>H Thyroid Gland Lobe, Right<br>L Superior Parathyroid Gland, Right<br>M Superior Parathyroid Gland, Left<br>N Inferior Parathyroid Gland, Right<br>P Inferior Parathyroid Gland, Left<br>Q Parathyroid Glands, Multiple<br>R Parathyroid Gland | 0 Open<br>4 Percutaneous Endoscopic | Z No Device | Z No Qualifier |

**0** Medical and Surgical
**G** Endocrine System
**T** Resection: Cutting out or off, without replacement, all of a body part

| Character 4<br>Body Part | Character 5<br>Approach | Character 6<br>Device | Character 7<br>Qualifier |
|---|---|---|---|
| 0 Pituitary Gland<br>1 Pineal Body<br>2 Adrenal Gland, Left<br>3 Adrenal Gland, Right<br>4 Adrenal Glands, Bilateral<br>6 Carotid Body, Left<br>7 Carotid Body, Right<br>8 Carotid Bodies, Bilateral<br>9 Para-aortic Body<br>B Coccygeal Glomus<br>C Glomus Jugulare<br>D Aortic Body<br>F Paraganglion Extremity<br>G Thyroid Gland Lobe, Left<br>H Thyroid Gland Lobe, Right<br>K Thyroid Gland<br>L Superior Parathyroid Gland, Right<br>M Superior Parathyroid Gland, Left<br>N Inferior Parathyroid Gland, Right<br>P Inferior Parathyroid Gland, Left<br>Q Parathyroid Glands, Multiple<br>R Parathyroid Gland | 0 Open<br>4 Percutaneous Endoscopic | Z No Device | Z No Qualifier |

**0** Medical and Surgical
**G** Endocrine System
**W** Revision: Correcting, to the extent possible, a portion of a malfunctioning device or the position of a displaced device

| Character 4<br>Body Part | Character 5<br>Approach | Character 6<br>Device | Character 7<br>Qualifier |
|---|---|---|---|
| 0 Pituitary Gland<br>1 Pineal Body<br>5 Adrenal Gland<br>K Thyroid Gland<br>R Parathyroid Gland | 0 Open<br>3 Percutaneous<br>4 Percutaneous Endoscopic<br>X External | 0 Drainage Device | Z No Qualifier |
| S Endocrine Gland | 0 Open<br>3 Percutaneous<br>4 Percutaneous Endoscopic<br>X External | 0 Drainage Device<br>2 Monitoring Device<br>3 Infusion Device | Z No Qualifier |

# Skin and Breast | 0H0-0HX

**0** Medical and Surgical
**H** Skin and Breast
**0** Alteration: Modifying the anatomic structure of a body part without affecting the function of the body part

| Character 4<br>Body Part | Character 5<br>Approach | Character 6<br>Device | Character 7<br>Qualifier |
|---|---|---|---|
| T  Breast, Right<br>U  Breast, Left<br>V  Breast, Bilateral | 0  Open<br>3  Percutaneous<br>X  External | 7  Autologous Tissue Substitute<br>J  Synthetic Substitute<br>K  Nonautologous Tissue Substitute<br>Z  No Device | Z  No Qualifier |

**0** Medical and Surgical
**H** Skin and Breast
**2** Change: Taking out or off a device from a body part and putting back an identical or similar device in or on the same body part without cutting or puncturing the skin or a mucous membrane

| Character 4<br>Body Part | Character 5<br>Approach | Character 6<br>Device | Character 7<br>Qualifier |
|---|---|---|---|
| P  Skin<br>T  Breast, Right<br>U  Breast, Left | X  External | 0  Drainage Device<br>Y  Other Device | Z  No Qualifier |

**0** Medical and Surgical
**H** Skin and Breast
**5** Destruction: Physical eradication of all or a portion of a body part by the direct use of energy, force, or a destructive agent

| Character 4<br>Body Part | Character 5<br>Approach | Character 6<br>Device | Character 7<br>Qualifier |
|---|---|---|---|
| 0  Skin, Scalp<br>1  Skin, Face<br>2  Skin, Right Ear<br>3  Skin, Left Ear<br>4  Skin, Neck<br>5  Skin, Chest<br>6  Skin, Back<br>7  Skin, Abdomen<br>8  Skin, Buttock<br>9  Skin, Perineum<br>A  Skin, Genitalia<br>B  Skin, Right Upper Arm<br>C  Skin, Left Upper Arm<br>D  Skin, Right Lower Arm<br>E  Skin, Left Lower Arm<br>F  Skin, Right Hand<br>G  Skin, Left Hand<br>H  Skin, Right Upper Leg<br>J  Skin, Left Upper Leg<br>K  Skin, Right Lower Leg<br>L  Skin, Left Lower Leg<br>M  Skin, Right Foot<br>N  Skin, Left Foot | X  External | Z  No Device | D  Multiple<br>Z  No Qualifier |
| Q  Finger Nail<br>R  Toe Nail | X  External | Z  No Device | Z  No Qualifier |
| T  Breast, Right<br>U  Breast, Left<br>V  Breast, Bilateral<br>W  Nipple, Right<br>X  Nipple, Left | 0  Open<br>3  Percutaneous<br>7  Via Natural or Artificial Opening<br>8  Via Natural or Artificial Opening Endoscopic<br>X  External | Z  No Device | Z  No Qualifier |

| 0 | Medical and Surgical |
|---|---|
| H | Skin and Breast |
| 8 | Division: Cutting into a body part, without draining fluids and/or gases from the body part, in order to separate or transect a body part |

| Character 4<br>Body Part | Character 5<br>Approach | Character 6<br>Device | Character 7<br>Qualifier |
|---|---|---|---|
| 0 Skin, Scalp | X External | Z No Device | Z No Qualifier |
| 1 Skin, Face | | | |
| 2 Skin, Right Ear | | | |
| 3 Skin, Left Ear | | | |
| 4 Skin, Neck | | | |
| 5 Skin, Chest | | | |
| 6 Skin, Back | | | |
| 7 Skin, Abdomen | | | |
| 8 Skin, Buttock | | | |
| 9 Skin, Perineum | | | |
| A Skin, Genitalia | | | |
| B Skin, Right Upper Arm | | | |
| C Skin, Left Upper Arm | | | |
| D Skin, Right Lower Arm | | | |
| E Skin, Left Lower Arm | | | |
| F Skin, Right Hand | | | |
| G Skin, Left Hand | | | |
| H Skin, Right Upper Leg | | | |
| J Skin, Left Upper Leg | | | |
| K Skin, Right Lower Leg | | | |
| L Skin, Left Lower Leg | | | |
| M Skin, Right Foot | | | |
| N Skin, Left Foot | | | |

**0** Medical and Surgical
**H** Skin and Breast
**9** Drainage: Taking or letting out fluids and/or gases from a body part

| Character 4<br>Body Part | Character 5<br>Approach | Character 6<br>Device | Character 7<br>Qualifier |
|---|---|---|---|
| 0 Skin, Scalp<br>1 Skin, Face<br>2 Skin, Right Ear<br>3 Skin, Left Ear<br>4 Skin, Neck<br>5 Skin, Chest<br>6 Skin, Back<br>7 Skin, Abdomen<br>8 Skin, Buttock<br>9 Skin, Perineum<br>A Skin, Genitalia<br>B Skin, Right Upper Arm<br>C Skin, Left Upper Arm<br>D Skin, Right Lower Arm<br>E Skin, Left Lower Arm<br>F Skin, Right Hand<br>G Skin, Left Hand<br>H Skin, Right Upper Leg<br>J Skin, Left Upper Leg<br>K Skin, Right Lower Leg<br>L Skin, Left Lower Leg<br>M Skin, Right Foot<br>N Skin, Left Foot<br>Q Finger Nail<br>R Toe Nail | X External | 0 Drainage Device | Z No Qualifier |
| 0 Skin, Scalp<br>1 Skin, Face<br>2 Skin, Right Ear<br>3 Skin, Left Ear<br>4 Skin, Neck<br>5 Skin, Chest<br>6 Skin, Back<br>7 Skin, Abdomen<br>8 Skin, Buttock<br>9 Skin, Perineum<br>A Skin, Genitalia<br>B Skin, Right Upper Arm<br>C Skin, Left Upper Arm<br>D Skin, Right Lower Arm<br>E Skin, Left Lower Arm<br>F Skin, Right Hand<br>G Skin, Left Hand<br>H Skin, Right Upper Leg<br>J Skin, Left Upper Leg<br>K Skin, Right Lower Leg<br>L Skin, Left Lower Leg<br>M Skin, Right Foot<br>N Skin, Left Foot<br>Q Finger Nail<br>R Toe Nail | X External | Z No Device | X Diagnostic<br>Z No Qualifier |
| T Breast, Right<br>U Breast, Left<br>V Breast, Bilateral<br>W Nipple, Right<br>X Nipple, Left | 0 Open<br>3 Percutaneous<br>7 Via Natural or Artificial Opening<br>8 Via Natural or Artificial Opening Endoscopic<br>X External | 0 Drainage Device | Z No Qualifier |
| T Breast, Right<br>U Breast, Left<br>V Breast, Bilateral<br>W Nipple, Right<br>X Nipple, Left | 0 Open<br>3 Percutaneous<br>7 Via Natural or Artificial Opening<br>8 Via Natural or Artificial Opening Endoscopic<br>X External | Z No Device | X Diagnostic<br>Z No Qualifier |

**0 Medical and Surgical**
**H Skin and Breast**
**B Excision: Cutting out or off, without replacement, a portion of a body part**

| Character 4<br>Body Part | Character 5<br>Approach | Character 6<br>Device | Character 7<br>Qualifier |
|---|---|---|---|
| 0 Skin, Scalp<br>1 Skin, Face<br>2 Skin, Right Ear<br>3 Skin, Left Ear<br>4 Skin, Neck<br>5 Skin, Chest<br>6 Skin, Back<br>7 Skin, Abdomen<br>8 Skin, Buttock<br>9 Skin, Perineum<br>A Skin, Genitalia<br>B Skin, Right Upper Arm<br>C Skin, Left Upper Arm<br>D Skin, Right Lower Arm<br>E Skin, Left Lower Arm<br>F Skin, Right Hand<br>G Skin, Left Hand<br>H Skin, Right Upper Leg<br>J Skin, Left Upper Leg<br>K Skin, Right Lower Leg<br>L Skin, Left Lower Leg<br>M Skin, Right Foot<br>N Skin, Left Foot<br>Q Finger Nail<br>R Toe Nail | X External | Z No Device | X Diagnostic<br>Z No Qualifier |
| T Breast, Right<br>U Breast, Left<br>V Breast, Bilateral<br>W Nipple, Right<br>X Nipple, Left<br>Y Supernumerary Breast | 0 Open<br>3 Percutaneous<br>7 Via Natural or Artificial Opening<br>8 Via Natural or Artificial Opening<br>   Endoscopic<br>X External | Z No Device | X Diagnostic<br>Z No Qualifier |

**0 Medical and Surgical**
**H Skin and Breast**
**C Extirpation: Taking or cutting out solid matter from a body part**

| Character 4<br>Body Part | Character 5<br>Approach | Character 6<br>Device | Character 7<br>Qualifier |
|---|---|---|---|
| 0 Skin, Scalp<br>1 Skin, Face<br>2 Skin, Right Ear<br>3 Skin, Left Ear<br>4 Skin, Neck<br>5 Skin, Chest<br>6 Skin, Back<br>7 Skin, Abdomen<br>8 Skin, Buttock<br>9 Skin, Perineum<br>A Skin, Genitalia<br>B Skin, Right Upper Arm<br>C Skin, Left Upper Arm<br>D Skin, Right Lower Arm<br>E Skin, Left Lower Arm<br>F Skin, Right Hand<br>G Skin, Left Hand<br>H Skin, Right Upper Leg<br>J Skin, Left Upper Leg<br>K Skin, Right Lower Leg<br>L Skin, Left Lower Leg<br>M Skin, Right Foot<br>N Skin, Left Foot<br>Q Finger Nail<br>R Toe Nail | X External | Z No Device | Z No Qualifier |
| T Breast, Right<br>U Breast, Left<br>V Breast, Bilateral<br>W Nipple, Right<br>X Nipple, Left | 0 Open<br>3 Percutaneous<br>7 Via Natural or Artificial Opening<br>8 Via Natural or Artificial Opening<br>   Endoscopic<br>X External | Z No Device | Z No Qualifier |

**0 Medical and Surgical**
**H Skin and Breast**
**D Extraction: Pulling or stripping out or off all or a portion of a body part by the use of force**

| Character 4<br>Body Part | Character 5<br>Approach | Character 6<br>Device | Character 7<br>Qualifier |
|---|---|---|---|
| 0 Skin, Scalp<br>1 Skin, Face<br>2 Skin, Right Ear<br>3 Skin, Left Ear<br>4 Skin, Neck<br>5 Skin, Chest<br>6 Skin, Back<br>7 Skin, Abdomen<br>8 Skin, Buttock<br>9 Skin, Perineum<br>A Skin, Genitalia<br>B Skin, Right Upper Arm<br>C Skin, Left Upper Arm<br>D Skin, Right Lower Arm<br>E Skin, Left Lower Arm<br>F Skin, Right Hand<br>G Skin, Left Hand<br>H Skin, Right Upper Leg<br>J Skin, Left Upper Leg<br>K Skin, Right Lower Leg<br>L Skin, Left Lower Leg<br>M Skin, Right Foot<br>N Skin, Left Foot<br>Q Finger Nail<br>R Toe Nail<br>S Hair | X External | Z No Device | Z No Qualifier |

**0 Medical and Surgical**
**H Skin and Breast**
**H Insertion: Putting in a nonbiological appliance that monitors, assists, performs, or prevents a physiological function but does not physically take the place of a body part**

| Character 4<br>Body Part | Character 5<br>Approach | Character 6<br>Device | Character 7<br>Qualifier |
|---|---|---|---|
| T Breast, Right<br>U Breast, Left<br>V Breast, Bilateral<br>W Nipple, Right<br>X Nipple, Left | 0 Open<br>3 Percutaneous<br>7 Via Natural or Artificial Opening<br>8 Via Natural or Artificial Opening<br>   Endoscopic | 1 Radioactive Element<br>N Tissue Expander | Z No Qualifier |
| T Breast, Right<br>U Breast, Left<br>V Breast, Bilateral<br>W Nipple, Right<br>X Nipple, Left | X External | 1 Radioactive Element | Z No Qualifier |

**AHA:** 0HHU0NZ - 4Q 2013, 107; 0HHV0NZ - 2Q 2014, 12

**0 Medical and Surgical**
**H Skin and Breast**
**J Inspection: Visually and/or manually exploring a body part**

| Character 4<br>Body Part | Character 5<br>Approach | Character 6<br>Device | Character 7<br>Qualifier |
|---|---|---|---|
| P Skin<br>Q Finger Nail<br>R Toe Nail | X External | Z No Device | Z No Qualifier |
| T Breast, Right<br>U Breast, Left | 0 Open<br>3 Percutaneous<br>7 Via Natural or Artificial Opening<br>8 Via Natural or Artificial Opening<br>   Endoscopic<br>X External | Z No Device | Z No Qualifier |

**0** Medical and Surgical
**H** Skin and Breast
**M** Reattachment: Putting back in or on all or a portion of a separated body part to its normal location or other suitable location

| Character 4 Body Part | Character 5 Approach | Character 6 Device | Character 7 Qualifier |
|---|---|---|---|
| 0 Skin, Scalp | X External | Z No Device | Z No Qualifier |
| 1 Skin, Face | | | |
| 2 Skin, Right Ear | | | |
| 3 Skin, Left Ear | | | |
| 4 Skin, Neck | | | |
| 5 Skin, Chest | | | |
| 6 Skin, Back | | | |
| 7 Skin, Abdomen | | | |
| 8 Skin, Buttock | | | |
| 9 Skin, Perineum | | | |
| A Skin, Genitalia | | | |
| B Skin, Right Upper Arm | | | |
| C Skin, Left Upper Arm | | | |
| D Skin, Right Lower Arm | | | |
| E Skin, Left Lower Arm | | | |
| F Skin, Right Hand | | | |
| G Skin, Left Hand | | | |
| H Skin, Right Upper Leg | | | |
| J Skin, Left Upper Leg | | | |
| K Skin, Right Lower Leg | | | |
| L Skin, Left Lower Leg | | | |
| M Skin, Right Foot | | | |
| N Skin, Left Foot | | | |
| T Breast, Right | | | |
| U Breast, Left | | | |
| V Breast, Bilateral | | | |
| W Nipple, Right | | | |
| X Nipple, Left | | | |

**0** Medical and Surgical
**H** Skin and Breast
**N** Release: Freeing a body part from an abnormal physical constraint by cutting or by the use of force

| Character 4 Body Part | Character 5 Approach | Character 6 Device | Character 7 Qualifier |
|---|---|---|---|
| 0 Skin, Scalp | X External | Z No Device | Z No Qualifier |
| 1 Skin, Face | | | |
| 2 Skin, Right Ear | | | |
| 3 Skin, Left Ear | | | |
| 4 Skin, Neck | | | |
| 5 Skin, Chest | | | |
| 6 Skin, Back | | | |
| 7 Skin, Abdomen | | | |
| 8 Skin, Buttock | | | |
| 9 Skin, Perineum | | | |
| A Skin, Genitalia | | | |
| B Skin, Right Upper Arm | | | |
| C Skin, Left Upper Arm | | | |
| D Skin, Right Lower Arm | | | |
| E Skin, Left Lower Arm | | | |
| F Skin, Right Hand | | | |
| G Skin, Left Hand | | | |
| H Skin, Right Upper Leg | | | |
| J Skin, Left Upper Leg | | | |
| K Skin, Right Lower Leg | | | |
| L Skin, Left Lower Leg | | | |
| M Skin, Right Foot | | | |
| N Skin, Left Foot | | | |
| Q Finger Nail | | | |
| R Toe Nail | | | |
| T Breast, Right | 0 Open | Z No Device | Z No Qualifier |
| U Breast, Left | 3 Percutaneous | | |
| V Breast, Bilateral | 7 Via Natural or Artificial Opening | | |
| W Nipple, Right | 8 Via Natural or Artificial Opening Endoscopic | | |
| X Nipple, Left | X External | | |

**0** Medical and Surgical
**H** Skin and Breast
**P** Removal: Taking out or off a device from a body part

| Character 4<br>Body Part | Character 5<br>Approach | Character 6<br>Device | Character 7<br>Qualifier |
|---|---|---|---|
| P  Skin<br>Q  Finger Nail<br>R  Toe Nail | X  External | 0  Drainage Device<br>7  Autologous Tissue Substitute<br>J  Synthetic Substitute<br>K  Nonautologous Tissue Substitute | Z  No Qualifier |
| S  Hair | X  External | 7  Autologous Tissue Substitute<br>J  Synthetic Substitute<br>K  Nonautologous Tissue Substitute | Z  No Qualifier |
| T  Breast, Right<br>U  Breast, Left | 0  Open<br>3  Percutaneous<br>7  Via Natural or Artificial Opening<br>8  Via Natural or Artificial Opening<br>    Endoscopic | 0  Drainage Device<br>1  Radioactive Element<br>7  Autologous Tissue Substitute<br>J  Synthetic Substitute<br>K  Nonautologous Tissue Substitute<br>N  Tissue Expander | Z  No Qualifier |
| T  Breast, Right<br>U  Breast, Left | X  External | 0  Drainage Device<br>1  Radioactive Element<br>7  Autologous Tissue Substitute<br>J  Synthetic Substitute<br>K  Nonautologous Tissue Substitute | Z  No Qualifier |

**0** Medical and Surgical
**H** Skin and Breast
**Q** Repair: Restoring, to the extent possible, a body part to its normal anatomic structure and function

| Character 4<br>Body Part | Character 5<br>Approach | Character 6<br>Device | Character 7<br>Qualifier |
|---|---|---|---|
| 0  Skin, Scalp<br>1  Skin, Face<br>2  Skin, Right Ear<br>3  Skin, Left Ear<br>4  Skin, Neck<br>5  Skin, Chest<br>6  Skin, Back<br>7  Skin, Abdomen<br>8  Skin, Buttock<br>9  Skin, Perineum<br>A  Skin, Genitalia<br>B  Skin, Right Upper Arm<br>C  Skin, Left Upper Arm<br>D  Skin, Right Lower Arm<br>E  Skin, Left Lower Arm<br>F  Skin, Right Hand<br>G  Skin, Left Hand<br>H  Skin, Right Upper Leg<br>J  Skin, Left Upper Leg<br>K  Skin, Right Lower Leg<br>L  Skin, Left Lower Leg<br>M  Skin, Right Foot<br>N  Skin, Left Foot<br>Q  Finger Nail<br>R  Toe Nail | X  External | Z  No Device | Z  No Qualifier |
| T  Breast, Right<br>U  Breast, Left<br>V  Breast, Bilateral<br>W  Nipple, Right<br>X  Nipple, Left<br>Y  Supernumerary Breast | 0  Open<br>3  Percutaneous<br>7  Via Natural or Artificial Opening<br>8  Via Natural or Artificial Opening<br>    Endoscopic<br>X  External | Z  No Device | Z  No Qualifier |

| | Character 4 Body Part | | Character 5 Approach | | Character 6 Device | | Character 7 Qualifier |
|---|---|---|---|---|---|---|---|

**0** Medical and Surgical
**H** Skin and Breast
**R** Replacement: Putting in or on biological or synthetic material that physically takes the place and/or function of all or a portion of a body part

| Character 4 — Body Part | Character 5 — Approach | Character 6 — Device | Character 7 — Qualifier |
|---|---|---|---|
| 0 Skin, Scalp<br>1 Skin, Face<br>2 Skin, Right Ear<br>3 Skin, Left Ear<br>4 Skin, Neck<br>5 Skin, Chest<br>6 Skin, Back<br>7 Skin, Abdomen<br>8 Skin, Buttock<br>9 Skin, Perineum<br>A Skin, Genitalia<br>B Skin, Right Upper Arm<br>C Skin, Left Upper Arm<br>D Skin, Right Lower Arm<br>E Skin, Left Lower Arm<br>F Skin, Right Hand<br>G Skin, Left Hand<br>H Skin, Right Upper Leg<br>J Skin, Left Upper Leg<br>K Skin, Right Lower Leg<br>L Skin, Left Lower Leg<br>M Skin, Right Foot<br>N Skin, Left Foot | X External | 7 Autologous Tissue Substitute<br>K Nonautologous Tissue Substitute | 3 Full Thickness<br>4 Partial Thickness |
| 0 Skin, Scalp<br>1 Skin, Face<br>2 Skin, Right Ear<br>3 Skin, Left Ear<br>4 Skin, Neck<br>5 Skin, Chest<br>6 Skin, Back<br>7 Skin, Abdomen<br>8 Skin, Buttock<br>9 Skin, Perineum<br>A Skin, Genitalia<br>B Skin, Right Upper Arm<br>C Skin, Left Upper Arm<br>D Skin, Right Lower Arm<br>E Skin, Left Lower Arm<br>F Skin, Right Hand<br>G Skin, Left Hand<br>H Skin, Right Upper Leg<br>J Skin, Left Upper Leg<br>K Skin, Right Lower Leg<br>L Skin, Left Lower Leg<br>M Skin, Right Foot<br>N Skin, Left Foot | X External | J Synthetic Substitute | 3 Full Thickness<br>4 Partial Thickness<br>Z No Qualifier |
| Q Finger Nail<br>R Toe Nail<br>S Hair | X External | 7 Autologous Tissue Substitute<br>J Synthetic Substitute<br>K Nonautologous Tissue Substitute | Z No Qualifier |
| T Breast, Right<br>U Breast, Left<br>V Breast, Bilateral | 0 Open | 7 Autologous Tissue Substitute | 5 Latissimus Dorsi Myocutaneous Flap<br>6 Transverse Rectus Abdominis Myocutaneous Flap<br>7 Deep Inferior Epigastric Artery Perforator Flap<br>8 Superficial Inferior Epigastric Artery Flap<br>9 Gluteal Artery Perforator Flap<br>Z No Qualifier |
| T Breast, Right<br>U Breast, Left<br>V Breast, Bilateral | 0 Open | J Synthetic Substitute<br>K Nonautologous Tissue Substitute | Z No Qualifier |
| T Breast, Right<br>U Breast, Left<br>V Breast, Bilateral | 3 Percutaneous<br>X External | 7 Autologous Tissue Substitute<br>J Synthetic Substitute<br>K Nonautologous Tissue Substitute | Z No Qualifier |
| W Nipple, Right<br>X Nipple, Left | 0 Open<br>3 Percutaneous<br>X External | 7 Autologous Tissue Substitute<br>J Synthetic Substitute<br>K Nonautologous Tissue Substitute | Z No Qualifier |

**0** Medical and Surgical
**H** Skin and Breast
**S** Reposition: Moving to its normal location, or other suitable location, all or a portion of a body part

| Character 4<br>Body Part | Character 5<br>Approach | Character 6<br>Device | Character 7<br>Qualifier |
|---|---|---|---|
| S Hair<br>W Nipple, Right<br>X Nipple, Left | X External | Z No Device | Z No Qualifier |
| T Breast, Right<br>U Breast, Left<br>V Breast, Bilateral | 0 Open | Z No Device | Z No Qualifier |

**0** Medical and Surgical
**H** Skin and Breast
**T** Resection: Cutting out or off, without replacement, all of a body part

| Character 4<br>Body Part | Character 5<br>Approach | Character 6<br>Device | Character 7<br>Qualifier |
|---|---|---|---|
| Q Finger Nail<br>R Toe Nail<br>W Nipple, Right<br>X Nipple, Left | X External | Z No Device | Z No Qualifier |
| T Breast, Right<br>U Breast, Left<br>V Breast, Bilateral<br>Y Supernumerary Breast | 0 Open | Z No Device | Z No Qualifier |

**0** Medical and Surgical
**H** Skin and Breast
**U** Supplement: Putting in or on biological or synthetic material that physically reinforces and/or augments the function of a portion of a body part

| Character 4<br>Body Part | Character 5<br>Approach | Character 6<br>Device | Character 7<br>Qualifier |
|---|---|---|---|
| T Breast, Right<br>U Breast, Left<br>V Breast, Bilateral<br>W Nipple, Right<br>X Nipple, Left | 0 Open<br>3 Percutaneous<br>7 Via Natural or Artificial Opening<br>8 Via Natural or Artificial Opening<br>   Endoscopic<br>X External | 7 Autologous Tissue Substitute<br>J Synthetic Substitute<br>K Nonautologous Tissue Substitute | Z No Qualifier |

**0** Medical and Surgical
**H** Skin and Breast
**W** Revision: Correcting, to the extent possible, a portion of a malfunctioning device or the position of a displaced device

| Character 4<br>Body Part | Character 5<br>Approach | Character 6<br>Device | Character 7<br>Qualifier |
|---|---|---|---|
| P Skin<br>Q Finger Nail<br>R Toe Nail | X External | 0 Drainage Device<br>7 Autologous Tissue Substitute<br>J Synthetic Substitute<br>K Nonautologous Tissue Substitute | Z No Qualifier |
| S Hair | X External | 7 Autologous Tissue Substitute<br>J Synthetic Substitute<br>K Nonautologous Tissue Substitute | Z No Qualifier |
| T Breast, Right<br>U Breast, Left | 0 Open<br>3 Percutaneous<br>7 Via Natural or Artificial Opening<br>8 Via Natural or Artificial Opening<br>   Endoscopic | 0 Drainage Device<br>7 Autologous Tissue Substitute<br>J Synthetic Substitute<br>K Nonautologous Tissue Substitute<br>N Tissue Expander | Z No Qualifier |
| T Breast, Right<br>U Breast, Left | X External | 0 Drainage Device<br>7 Autologous Tissue Substitute<br>J Synthetic Substitute<br>K Nonautologous Tissue Substitute | Z No Qualifier |

**0** Medical and Surgical
**H** Skin and Breast
**X** Transfer: Moving, without taking out, all or a portion of a body part to another location to take over the function of all or a portion of a body part

| Character 4<br>Body Part | Character 5<br>Approach | Character 6<br>Device | Character 7<br>Qualifier |
|---|---|---|---|
| 0 Skin, Scalp | X External | Z No Device | Z No Qualifier |
| 1 Skin, Face | | | |
| 2 Skin, Right Ear | | | |
| 3 Skin, Left Ear | | | |
| 4 Skin, Neck | | | |
| 5 Skin, Chest | | | |
| 6 Skin, Back | | | |
| 7 Skin, Abdomen | | | |
| 8 Skin, Buttock | | | |
| 9 Skin, Perineum | | | |
| A Skin, Genitalia | | | |
| B Skin, Right Upper Arm | | | |
| C Skin, Left Upper Arm | | | |
| D Skin, Right Lower Arm | | | |
| E Skin, Left Lower Arm | | | |
| F Skin, Right Hand | | | |
| G Skin, Left Hand | | | |
| H Skin, Right Upper Leg | | | |
| J Skin, Left Upper Leg | | | |
| K Skin, Right Lower Leg | | | |
| L Skin, Left Lower Leg | | | |
| M Skin, Right Foot | | | |
| N Skin, Left Foot | | | |

# Subcutaneous Tissue and Fascia | 0J0 – 0JX

**0** Medical and Surgical
**J** Subcutaneous Tissue and Fascia
**0** Alteration: Modifying the anatomic structure of a body part without affecting the function of the body part

| Character 4<br>Body Part | Character 5<br>Approach | Character 6<br>Device | Character 7<br>Qualifier |
|---|---|---|---|
| 1 Subcutaneous Tissue and Fascia, Face | 0 Open | Z No Device | Z No Qualifier |
| 4 Subcutaneous Tissue and Fascia, Anterior Neck | 3 Percutaneous | | |
| 5 Subcutaneous Tissue and Fascia, Posterior Neck | | | |
| 6 Subcutaneous Tissue and Fascia, Chest | | | |
| 7 Subcutaneous Tissue and Fascia, Back | | | |
| 8 Subcutaneous Tissue and Fascia, Abdomen | | | |
| 9 Subcutaneous Tissue and Fascia, Buttock | | | |
| D Subcutaneous Tissue and Fascia, Right Upper Arm | | | |
| F Subcutaneous Tissue and Fascia, Left Upper Arm | | | |
| G Subcutaneous Tissue and Fascia, Right Lower Arm | | | |
| H Subcutaneous Tissue and Fascia, Left Lower Arm | | | |
| L Subcutaneous Tissue and Fascia, Right Upper Leg | | | |
| M Subcutaneous Tissue and Fascia, Left Upper Leg | | | |
| N Subcutaneous Tissue and Fascia, Right Lower Leg | | | |
| P Subcutaneous Tissue and Fascia, Left Lower Leg | | | |

**0** Medical and Surgical
**J** Subcutaneous Tissue and Fascia
**2** Change: Taking out or off a device from a body part and putting back an identical or similar device in or on the same body part without cutting or puncturing the skin or a mucous membrane

| Character 4 Body Part | Character 5 Approach | Character 6 Device | Character 7 Qualifier |
|---|---|---|---|
| S  Subcutaneous Tissue and Fascia, Head and Neck<br>T  Subcutaneous Tissue and Fascia, Trunk<br>V  Subcutaneous Tissue and Fascia, Upper Extremity<br>W Subcutaneous Tissue and Fascia, Lower Extremity | X  External | 0  Drainage Device<br>Y  Other Device | Z  No Qualifier |

**0** Medical and Surgical
**J** Subcutaneous Tissue and Fascia
**5** Destruction: Physical eradication of all or a portion of a body part by the direct use of energy, force, or a destructive agent

| Character 4 Body Part | Character 5 Approach | Character 6 Device | Character 7 Qualifier |
|---|---|---|---|
| 0  Subcutaneous Tissue and Fascia, Scalp<br>1  Subcutaneous Tissue and Fascia, Face<br>4  Subcutaneous Tissue and Fascia, Anterior Neck<br>5  Subcutaneous Tissue and Fascia, Posterior Neck<br>6  Subcutaneous Tissue and Fascia, Chest<br>7  Subcutaneous Tissue and Fascia, Back<br>8  Subcutaneous Tissue and Fascia, Abdomen<br>9  Subcutaneous Tissue and Fascia, Buttock<br>B  Subcutaneous Tissue and Fascia, Perineum<br>C  Subcutaneous Tissue and Fascia, Pelvic Region<br>D  Subcutaneous Tissue and Fascia, Right Upper Arm<br>F  Subcutaneous Tissue and Fascia, Left Upper Arm<br>G  Subcutaneous Tissue and Fascia, Right Lower Arm<br>H  Subcutaneous Tissue and Fascia, Left Lower Arm<br>J  Subcutaneous Tissue and Fascia, Right Hand<br>K  Subcutaneous Tissue and Fascia, Left Hand<br>L  Subcutaneous Tissue and Fascia, Right Upper Leg<br>M Subcutaneous Tissue and Fascia, Left Upper Leg<br>N  Subcutaneous Tissue and Fascia, Right Lower Leg<br>P  Subcutaneous Tissue and Fascia, Left Lower Leg<br>Q  Subcutaneous Tissue and Fascia, Right Foot<br>R  Subcutaneous Tissue and Fascia, Left Foot | 0  Open<br>3  Percutaneous | Z  No Device | Z  No Qualifier |

**0** Medical and Surgical
**J** Subcutaneous Tissue and Fascia
**8** Division: Cutting into a body part, without draining fluids and/or gases from the body part, in order to separate or transect a body part

| Character 4<br>Body Part | Character 5<br>Approach | Character 6<br>Device | Character 7<br>Qualifier |
|---|---|---|---|
| 0 Subcutaneous Tissue and Fascia, Scalp | 0 Open<br>3 Percutaneous | Z No Device | Z No Qualifier |
| 1 Subcutaneous Tissue and Fascia, Face | | | |
| 4 Subcutaneous Tissue and Fascia, Anterior Neck | | | |
| 5 Subcutaneous Tissue and Fascia, Posterior Neck | | | |
| 6 Subcutaneous Tissue and Fascia, Chest | | | |
| 7 Subcutaneous Tissue and Fascia, Back | | | |
| 8 Subcutaneous Tissue and Fascia, Abdomen | | | |
| 9 Subcutaneous Tissue and Fascia, Buttock | | | |
| B Subcutaneous Tissue and Fascia, Perineum | | | |
| C Subcutaneous Tissue and Fascia, Pelvic Region | | | |
| D Subcutaneous Tissue and Fascia, Right Upper Arm | | | |
| F Subcutaneous Tissue and Fascia, Left Upper Arm | | | |
| G Subcutaneous Tissue and Fascia, Right Lower Arm | | | |
| H Subcutaneous Tissue and Fascia, Left Lower Arm | | | |
| J Subcutaneous Tissue and Fascia, Right Hand | | | |
| K Subcutaneous Tissue and Fascia, Left Hand | | | |
| L Subcutaneous Tissue and Fascia, Right Upper Leg | | | |
| M Subcutaneous Tissue and Fascia, Left Upper Leg | | | |
| N Subcutaneous Tissue and Fascia, Right Lower Leg | | | |
| P Subcutaneous Tissue and Fascia, Left Lower Leg | | | |
| Q Subcutaneous Tissue and Fascia, Right Foot | | | |
| R Subcutaneous Tissue and Fascia, Left Foot | | | |
| S Subcutaneous Tissue and Fascia, Head and Neck | | | |
| T Subcutaneous Tissue and Fascia, Trunk | | | |
| V Subcutaneous Tissue and Fascia, Upper Extremity | | | |
| W Subcutaneous Tissue and Fascia, Lower Extremity | | | |

**0** Medical and Surgical
**J** Subcutaneous Tissue and Fascia
**9** Drainage: Taking or letting out fluids and/or gases from a body part

| Character 4<br>Body Part | Character 5<br>Approach | Character 6<br>Device | Character 7<br>Qualifier |
|---|---|---|---|
| 0 Subcutaneous Tissue and Fascia, Scalp<br>1 Subcutaneous Tissue and Fascia, Face<br>4 Subcutaneous Tissue and Fascia, Anterior Neck<br>5 Subcutaneous Tissue and Fascia, Posterior Neck<br>6 Subcutaneous Tissue and Fascia, Chest<br>7 Subcutaneous Tissue and Fascia, Back<br>8 Subcutaneous Tissue and Fascia, Abdomen<br>9 Subcutaneous Tissue and Fascia, Buttock<br>B Subcutaneous Tissue and Fascia, Perineum<br>C Subcutaneous Tissue and Fascia, Pelvic Region<br>D Subcutaneous Tissue and Fascia, Right Upper Arm<br>F Subcutaneous Tissue and Fascia, Left Upper Arm<br>G Subcutaneous Tissue and Fascia, Right Lower Arm<br>H Subcutaneous Tissue and Fascia, Left Lower Arm<br>J Subcutaneous Tissue and Fascia, Right Hand<br>K Subcutaneous Tissue and Fascia, Left Hand<br>L Subcutaneous Tissue and Fascia, Right Upper Leg<br>M Subcutaneous Tissue and Fascia, Left Upper Leg<br>N Subcutaneous Tissue and Fascia, Right Lower Leg<br>P Subcutaneous Tissue and Fascia, Left Lower Leg<br>Q Subcutaneous Tissue and Fascia, Right Foot<br>R Subcutaneous Tissue and Fascia, Left Foot | 0 Open<br>3 Percutaneous | 0 Drainage Device | Z No Qualifier |
| 0 Subcutaneous Tissue and Fascia, Scalp<br>1 Subcutaneous Tissue and Fascia, Face<br>4 Subcutaneous Tissue and Fascia, Anterior Neck<br>5 Subcutaneous Tissue and Fascia, Posterior Neck<br>6 Subcutaneous Tissue and Fascia, Chest<br>7 Subcutaneous Tissue and Fascia, Back<br>8 Subcutaneous Tissue and Fascia, Abdomen<br>9 Subcutaneous Tissue and Fascia, Buttock<br>B Subcutaneous Tissue and Fascia, Perineum<br>C Subcutaneous Tissue and Fascia, Pelvic Region<br>D Subcutaneous Tissue and Fascia, Right Upper Arm<br>F Subcutaneous Tissue and Fascia, Left Upper Arm<br>G Subcutaneous Tissue and Fascia, Right Lower Arm<br>H Subcutaneous Tissue and Fascia, Left Lower Arm<br>J Subcutaneous Tissue and Fascia, Right Hand<br>K Subcutaneous Tissue and Fascia, Left Hand<br>L Subcutaneous Tissue and Fascia, Right Upper Leg<br>M Subcutaneous Tissue and Fascia, Left Upper Leg<br>N Subcutaneous Tissue and Fascia, Right Lower Leg<br>P Subcutaneous Tissue and Fascia, Left Lower Leg<br>Q Subcutaneous Tissue and Fascia, Right Foot<br>R Subcutaneous Tissue and Fascia, Left Foot | 0 Open<br>3 Percutaneous | Z No Device | X Diagnostic<br>Z No Qualifier |

**0** Medical and Surgical
**J** Subcutaneous Tissue and Fascia
**B** Excision: Cutting out or off, without replacement, a portion of a body part

| Character 4<br>Body Part | Character 5<br>Approach | Character 6<br>Device | Character 7<br>Qualifier |
|---|---|---|---|
| 0 Subcutaneous Tissue and Fascia, Scalp | 0 Open | Z No Device | X Diagnostic |
| 1 Subcutaneous Tissue and Fascia, Face | 3 Percutaneous | | Z No Qualifier |
| 4 Subcutaneous Tissue and Fascia, Anterior Neck | | | |
| 5 Subcutaneous Tissue and Fascia, Posterior Neck | | | |
| 6 Subcutaneous Tissue and Fascia, Chest | | | |
| 7 Subcutaneous Tissue and Fascia, Back | | | |
| 8 Subcutaneous Tissue and Fascia, Abdomen | | | |
| 9 Subcutaneous Tissue and Fascia, Buttock | | | |
| B Subcutaneous Tissue and Fascia, Perineum | | | |
| C Subcutaneous Tissue and Fascia, Pelvic Region | | | |
| D Subcutaneous Tissue and Fascia, Right Upper Arm | | | |
| F Subcutaneous Tissue and Fascia, Left Upper Arm | | | |
| G Subcutaneous Tissue and Fascia, Right Lower Arm | | | |
| H Subcutaneous Tissue and Fascia, Left Lower Arm | | | |
| J Subcutaneous Tissue and Fascia, Right Hand | | | |
| K Subcutaneous Tissue and Fascia, Left Hand | | | |
| L Subcutaneous Tissue and Fascia, Right Upper Leg | | | |
| M Subcutaneous Tissue and Fascia, Left Upper Leg | | | |
| N Subcutaneous Tissue and Fascia, Right Lower Leg | | | |
| P Subcutaneous Tissue and Fascia, Left Lower Leg | | | |
| Q Subcutaneous Tissue and Fascia, Right Foot | | | |
| R Subcutaneous Tissue and Fascia, Left Foot | | | |

| **0** Medical and Surgical **J** Subcutaneous Tissue and Fascia **C** Extirpation: Taking or cutting out solid matter from a body part | | | |
|---|---|---|---|
| **N C** Non-covered | | **L C** Limited Coverage | **AHA** AHA Coding Clinic |

| Character 4<br>Body Part | Character 5<br>Approach | Character 6<br>Device | Character 7<br>Qualifier |
|---|---|---|---|
| 0 Subcutaneous Tissue and Fascia, Scalp<br>1 Subcutaneous Tissue and Fascia, Face<br>4 Subcutaneous Tissue and Fascia, Anterior Neck<br>5 Subcutaneous Tissue and Fascia, Posterior Neck<br>6 Subcutaneous Tissue and Fascia, Chest<br>7 Subcutaneous Tissue and Fascia, Back<br>8 Subcutaneous Tissue and Fascia, Abdomen<br>9 Subcutaneous Tissue and Fascia, Buttock<br>B Subcutaneous Tissue and Fascia, Perineum<br>C Subcutaneous Tissue and Fascia, Pelvic Region<br>D Subcutaneous Tissue and Fascia, Right Upper Arm<br>F Subcutaneous Tissue and Fascia, Left Upper Arm<br>G Subcutaneous Tissue and Fascia, Right Lower Arm<br>H Subcutaneous Tissue and Fascia, Left Lower Arm<br>J Subcutaneous Tissue and Fascia, Right Hand<br>K Subcutaneous Tissue and Fascia, Left Hand<br>L Subcutaneous Tissue and Fascia, Right Upper Leg<br>M Subcutaneous Tissue and Fascia, Left Upper Leg<br>N Subcutaneous Tissue and Fascia, Right Lower Leg<br>P Subcutaneous Tissue and Fascia, Left Lower Leg<br>Q Subcutaneous Tissue and Fascia, Right Foot<br>R Subcutaneous Tissue and Fascia, Left Foot | 0 Open<br>3 Percutaneous | Z No Device | Z No Qualifier |

**0** Medical and Surgical
**J** Subcutaneous Tissue and Fascia
**D** Extraction: Pulling or stripping out or off all or a portion of a body part by the use of force

| Character 4 Body Part | Character 5 Approach | Character 6 Device | Character 7 Qualifier |
|---|---|---|---|
| 0 Subcutaneous Tissue and Fascia, Scalp | 0 Open | Z No Device | Z No Qualifier |
| 1 Subcutaneous Tissue and Fascia, Face | 3 Percutaneous | | |
| 4 Subcutaneous Tissue and Fascia, Anterior Neck | | | |
| 5 Subcutaneous Tissue and Fascia, Posterior Neck | | | |
| 6 Subcutaneous Tissue and Fascia, Chest | | | |
| 7 Subcutaneous Tissue and Fascia, Back | | | |
| 8 Subcutaneous Tissue and Fascia, Abdomen | | | |
| 9 Subcutaneous Tissue and Fascia, Buttock | | | |
| B Subcutaneous Tissue and Fascia, Perineum | | | |
| C Subcutaneous Tissue and Fascia, Pelvic Region | | | |
| D Subcutaneous Tissue and Fascia, Right Upper Arm | | | |
| F Subcutaneous Tissue and Fascia, Left Upper Arm | | | |
| G Subcutaneous Tissue and Fascia, Right Lower Arm | | | |
| H Subcutaneous Tissue and Fascia, Left Lower Arm | | | |
| J Subcutaneous Tissue and Fascia, Right Hand | | | |
| K Subcutaneous Tissue and Fascia, Left Hand | | | |
| L Subcutaneous Tissue and Fascia, Right Upper Leg | | | |
| M Subcutaneous Tissue and Fascia, Left Upper Leg | | | |
| N Subcutaneous Tissue and Fascia, Right Lower Leg | | | |
| P Subcutaneous Tissue and Fascia, Left Lower Leg | | | |
| Q Subcutaneous Tissue and Fascia, Right Foot | | | |
| R Subcutaneous Tissue and Fascia, Left Foot | | | |

**0** Medical and Surgical
**J** Subcutaneous Tissue and Fascia
**H** Insertion: Putting in a nonbiological appliance that monitors, assists, performs, or prevents a physiological function but does not physically take the place of a body part

| Character 4<br>Body Part | Character 5<br>Approach | Character 6<br>Device | Character 7<br>Qualifier |
|---|---|---|---|
| 0 Subcutaneous Tissue and Fascia, Scalp<br>1 Subcutaneous Tissue and Fascia, Face<br>4 Subcutaneous Tissue and Fascia, Anterior Neck<br>5 Subcutaneous Tissue and Fascia, Posterior Neck<br>9 Subcutaneous Tissue and Fascia, Buttock<br>B Subcutaneous Tissue and Fascia, Perineum<br>C Subcutaneous Tissue and Fascia, Pelvic Region<br>J Subcutaneous Tissue and Fascia, Right Hand<br>K Subcutaneous Tissue and Fascia, Left Hand<br>Q Subcutaneous Tissue and Fascia, Right Foot<br>R Subcutaneous Tissue and Fascia, Left Foot | 0 Open<br>3 Percutaneous | N Tissue Expander | Z No Qualifier |
| 6 Subcutaneous Tissue and Fascia, Chest<br>8 Subcutaneous Tissue and Fascia, Abdomen **N C** | 0 Open<br>3 Percutaneous | 0 Monitoring Device, Hemodynamic<br>2 Monitoring Device<br>4 Pacemaker, Single Chamber<br>5 Pacemaker, Single Chamber Rate Responsive<br>6 Pacemaker, Dual Chamber<br>7 Cardiac Resynchronization Pacemaker Pulse Generator<br>8 Defibrillator Generator<br>9 Cardiac Resynchronization Defibrillator Pulse Generator<br>A Contractility Modulation Device<br>B Stimulator Generator, Single Array<br>C Stimulator Generator, Single Array Rechargeable<br>D Stimulator Generator, Multiple Array<br>E Stimulator Generator, Multiple Array Rechargeable<br>H Contraceptive Device<br>M Stimulator Generator<br>N Tissue Expander<br>P Cardiac Rhythm Related Device<br>V Infusion Device, Pump<br>W Vascular Access Device, Reservoir<br>X Vascular Access Device | Z No Qualifier |
| 7 Subcutaneous Tissue and Fascia, Back **N C** | 0 Open<br>3 Percutaneous | B Stimulator Generator, Single Array<br>C Stimulator Generator, Single Array Rechargeable<br>D Stimulator Generator, Multiple Array<br>E Stimulator Generator, Multiple Array Rechargeable<br>M Stimulator Generator<br>N Tissue Expander<br>V Infusion Device, Pump | Z No Qualifier |
| D Subcutaneous Tissue and Fascia, Right Upper Arm<br>F Subcutaneous Tissue and Fascia, Left Upper Arm<br>G Subcutaneous Tissue and Fascia, Right Lower Arm<br>H Subcutaneous Tissue and Fascia, Left Lower Arm<br>L Subcutaneous Tissue and Fascia, Right Upper Leg<br>M Subcutaneous Tissue and Fascia, Left Upper Leg<br>N Subcutaneous Tissue and Fascia, Right Lower Leg<br>P Subcutaneous Tissue and Fascia, Left Lower Leg | 0 Open<br>3 Percutaneous | H Contraceptive Device<br>N Tissue Expander<br>V Infusion Device, Pump<br>W Vascular Access Device, Reservoir<br>X Vascular Access Device | Z No Qualifier |
| S Subcutaneous Tissue and Fascia, Head and Neck<br>V Subcutaneous Tissue and Fascia, Upper Extremity<br>W Subcutaneous Tissue and Fascia, Lower Extremity | 0 Open<br>3 Percutaneous | 1 Radioactive Element<br>3 Infusion Device | Z No Qualifier |
| T Subcutaneous Tissue and Fascia, Trunk | 0 Open<br>3 Percutaneous | 1 Radioactive Element<br>3 Infusion Device<br>V Infusion Device, Pump | Z No Qualifier |

**0JH** *continues on next page*

**0** Medical and Surgical – *continued*
**J** Subcutaneous Tissue and Fascia – *continued*
**H** Insertion: Putting in a nonbiological appliance that monitors, assists, performs, or prevents a physiological function but does not physically take the place of a body part
  – *continued*

| Character 4<br>Body Part | Character 5<br>Approach | Character 6<br>Device | Character 7<br>Qualifier |
|---|---|---|---|

**AHA:** 0JH63XZ - 4Q 2013, 117
N C 0JH7(0,3)MZ, 0JH8(0,3)MZ

---

**0** Medical and Surgical
**J** Subcutaneous Tissue and Fascia
**J** Inspection: Visually and/or manually exploring a body part

| Character 4<br>Body Part | Character 5<br>Approach | Character 6<br>Device | Character 7<br>Qualifier |
|---|---|---|---|
| S Subcutaneous Tissue and Fascia, Head and Neck<br>T Subcutaneous Tissue and Fascia, Trunk<br>V Subcutaneous Tissue and Fascia, Upper Extremity<br>W Subcutaneous Tissue and Fascia, Lower Extremity | 0 Open<br>3 Percutaneous<br>X External | Z No Device | Z No Qualifier |

---

**0** Medical and Surgical
**J** Subcutaneous Tissue and Fascia
**N** Release: Freeing a body part from an abnormal physical constraint by cutting or by the use of force

| Character 4<br>Body Part | Character 5<br>Approach | Character 6<br>Device | Character 7<br>Qualifier |
|---|---|---|---|
| 0 Subcutaneous Tissue and Fascia, Scalp<br>1 Subcutaneous Tissue and Fascia, Face<br>4 Subcutaneous Tissue and Fascia, Anterior Neck<br>5 Subcutaneous Tissue and Fascia, Posterior Neck<br>6 Subcutaneous Tissue and Fascia, Chest<br>7 Subcutaneous Tissue and Fascia, Back<br>8 Subcutaneous Tissue and Fascia, Abdomen<br>9 Subcutaneous Tissue and Fascia, Buttock<br>B Subcutaneous Tissue and Fascia, Perineum<br>C Subcutaneous Tissue and Fascia, Pelvic Region<br>D Subcutaneous Tissue and Fascia, Right Upper Arm<br>F Subcutaneous Tissue and Fascia, Left Upper Arm<br>G Subcutaneous Tissue and Fascia, Right Lower Arm<br>H Subcutaneous Tissue and Fascia, Left Lower Arm<br>J Subcutaneous Tissue and Fascia, Right Hand<br>K Subcutaneous Tissue and Fascia, Left Hand<br>L Subcutaneous Tissue and Fascia, Right Upper Leg<br>M Subcutaneous Tissue and Fascia, Left Upper Leg<br>N Subcutaneous Tissue and Fascia, Right Lower Leg<br>P Subcutaneous Tissue and Fascia, Left Lower Leg<br>Q Subcutaneous Tissue and Fascia, Right Foot<br>R Subcutaneous Tissue and Fascia, Left Foot | 0 Open<br>3 Percutaneous<br>X External | Z No Device | Z No Qualifier |

**0** Medical and Surgical
**J** Subcutaneous Tissue and Fascia
**P** Removal: Taking out or off a device from a body part

| Character 4<br>Body Part | Character 5<br>Approach | Character 6<br>Device | Character 7<br>Qualifier |
|---|---|---|---|
| S Subcutaneous Tissue and Fascia, Head and Neck | 0 Open<br>3 Percutaneous | 0 Drainage Device<br>1 Radioactive Element<br>3 Infusion Device<br>7 Autologous Tissue Substitute<br>J Synthetic Substitute<br>K Nonautologous Tissue Substitute<br>N Tissue Expander | Z No Qualifier |
| S Subcutaneous Tissue and Fascia, Head and Neck | X External | 0 Drainage Device<br>1 Radioactive Element<br>3 Infusion Device | Z No Qualifier |
| T Subcutaneous Tissue and Fascia, Trunk | 0 Open<br>3 Percutaneous | 0 Drainage Device<br>1 Radioactive Element<br>2 Monitoring Device<br>3 Infusion Device<br>7 Autologous Tissue Substitute<br>H Contraceptive Device<br>J Synthetic Substitute<br>K Nonautologous Tissue Substitute<br>M Stimulator Generator<br>N Tissue Expander<br>P Cardiac Rhythm Related Device<br>V Infusion Device, Pump<br>W Vascular Access Device, Reservoir<br>X Vascular Access Device | Z No Qualifier |
| T Subcutaneous Tissue and Fascia, Trunk | X External | 0 Drainage Device<br>1 Radioactive Element<br>2 Monitoring Device<br>3 Infusion Device<br>H Contraceptive Device<br>V Infusion Device, Pump<br>X Vascular Access Device | Z No Qualifier |
| V Subcutaneous Tissue and Fascia, Upper Extremity<br>W Subcutaneous Tissue and Fascia, Lower Extremity | 0 Open<br>3 Percutaneous | 0 Drainage Device<br>1 Radioactive Element<br>3 Infusion Device<br>7 Autologous Tissue Substitute<br>H Contraceptive Device<br>J Synthetic Substitute<br>K Nonautologous Tissue Substitute<br>N Tissue Expander<br>V Infusion Device, Pump<br>W Vascular Access Device, Reservoir<br>X Vascular Access Device | Z No Qualifier |
| V Subcutaneous Tissue and Fascia, Upper Extremity<br>W Subcutaneous Tissue and Fascia, Lower Extremity | X External | 0 Drainage Device<br>1 Radioactive Element<br>3 Infusion Device<br>H Contraceptive Device<br>V Infusion Device, Pump<br>X Vascular Access Device | Z No Qualifier |

**AHA:** 0JPT0NZ - 4Q 2013, 111

**0** Medical and Surgical
**J** Subcutaneous Tissue and Fascia
**Q** Repair: Restoring, to the extent possible, a body part to its normal anatomic structure and function

| Character 4<br>Body Part | Character 5<br>Approach | Character 6<br>Device | Character 7<br>Qualifier |
|---|---|---|---|
| 0 Subcutaneous Tissue and Fascia, Scalp<br>1 Subcutaneous Tissue and Fascia, Face<br>4 Subcutaneous Tissue and Fascia, Anterior Neck<br>5 Subcutaneous Tissue and Fascia, Posterior Neck<br>6 Subcutaneous Tissue and Fascia, Chest<br>7 Subcutaneous Tissue and Fascia, Back<br>8 Subcutaneous Tissue and Fascia, Abdomen<br>9 Subcutaneous Tissue and Fascia, Buttock<br>B Subcutaneous Tissue and Fascia, Perineum<br>C Subcutaneous Tissue and Fascia, Pelvic Region<br>D Subcutaneous Tissue and Fascia, Right Upper Arm<br>F Subcutaneous Tissue and Fascia, Left Upper Arm<br>G Subcutaneous Tissue and Fascia, Right Lower Arm<br>H Subcutaneous Tissue and Fascia, Left Lower Arm<br>J Subcutaneous Tissue and Fascia, Right Hand<br>K Subcutaneous Tissue and Fascia, Left Hand<br>L Subcutaneous Tissue and Fascia, Right Upper Leg<br>M Subcutaneous Tissue and Fascia, Left Upper Leg<br>N Subcutaneous Tissue and Fascia, Right Lower Leg<br>P Subcutaneous Tissue and Fascia, Left Lower Leg<br>Q Subcutaneous Tissue and Fascia, Right Foot<br>R Subcutaneous Tissue and Fascia, Left Foot | 0 Open<br>3 Percutaneous | Z No Device | Z No Qualifier |

**0** Medical and Surgical
**J** Subcutaneous Tissue and Fascia
**R** Replacement: Putting in or on biological or synthetic material that physically takes the place and/or function of all or a portion of a body part

| Character 4 Body Part | Character 5 Approach | Character 6 Device | Character 7 Qualifier |
|---|---|---|---|
| 0 Subcutaneous Tissue and Fascia, Scalp | 0 Open | 7 Autologous Tissue Substitute | Z No Qualifier |
| 1 Subcutaneous Tissue and Fascia, Face | 3 Percutaneous | J Synthetic Substitute | |
| 4 Subcutaneous Tissue and Fascia, Anterior Neck | | K Nonautologous Tissue Substitute | |
| 5 Subcutaneous Tissue and Fascia, Posterior Neck | | | |
| 6 Subcutaneous Tissue and Fascia, Chest | | | |
| 7 Subcutaneous Tissue and Fascia, Back | | | |
| 8 Subcutaneous Tissue and Fascia, Abdomen | | | |
| 9 Subcutaneous Tissue and Fascia, Buttock | | | |
| B Subcutaneous Tissue and Fascia, Perineum | | | |
| C Subcutaneous Tissue and Fascia, Pelvic Region | | | |
| D Subcutaneous Tissue and Fascia, Right Upper Arm | | | |
| F Subcutaneous Tissue and Fascia, Left Upper Arm | | | |
| G Subcutaneous Tissue and Fascia, Right Lower Arm | | | |
| H Subcutaneous Tissue and Fascia, Left Lower Arm | | | |
| J Subcutaneous Tissue and Fascia, Right Hand | | | |
| K Subcutaneous Tissue and Fascia, Left Hand | | | |
| L Subcutaneous Tissue and Fascia, Right Upper Leg | | | |
| M Subcutaneous Tissue and Fascia, Left Upper Leg | | | |
| N Subcutaneous Tissue and Fascia, Right Lower Leg | | | |
| P Subcutaneous Tissue and Fascia, Left Lower Leg | | | |
| Q Subcutaneous Tissue and Fascia, Right Foot | | | |
| R Subcutaneous Tissue and Fascia, Left Foot | | | |

**0** Medical and Surgical
**J** Subcutaneous Tissue and Fascia
**U** Supplement: Putting in or on biological or synthetic material that physically reinforces and/or augments the function of a portion of a body part

| Character 4<br>Body Part | Character 5<br>Approach | Character 6<br>Device | Character 7<br>Qualifier |
|---|---|---|---|
| 0 Subcutaneous Tissue and Fascia,<br>  Scalp<br>1 Subcutaneous Tissue and Fascia, Face<br>4 Subcutaneous Tissue and Fascia,<br>  Anterior Neck<br>5 Subcutaneous Tissue and Fascia,<br>  Posterior Neck<br>6 Subcutaneous Tissue and Fascia,<br>  Chest<br>7 Subcutaneous Tissue and Fascia,<br>  Back<br>8 Subcutaneous Tissue and Fascia,<br>  Abdomen<br>9 Subcutaneous Tissue and Fascia,<br>  Buttock<br>B Subcutaneous Tissue and Fascia,<br>  Perineum<br>C Subcutaneous Tissue and Fascia,<br>  Pelvic Region<br>D Subcutaneous Tissue and Fascia,<br>  Right Upper Arm<br>F Subcutaneous Tissue and Fascia, Left<br>  Upper Arm<br>G Subcutaneous Tissue and Fascia,<br>  Right Lower Arm<br>H Subcutaneous Tissue and Fascia, Left<br>  Lower Arm<br>J Subcutaneous Tissue and Fascia,<br>  Right Hand<br>K Subcutaneous Tissue and Fascia, Left<br>  Hand<br>L Subcutaneous Tissue and Fascia,<br>  Right Upper Leg<br>M Subcutaneous Tissue and Fascia, Left<br>  Upper Leg<br>N Subcutaneous Tissue and Fascia,<br>  Right Lower Leg<br>P Subcutaneous Tissue and Fascia, Left<br>  Lower Leg<br>Q Subcutaneous Tissue and Fascia,<br>  Right Foot<br>R Subcutaneous Tissue and Fascia, Left<br>  Foot | 0 Open<br>3 Percutaneous | 7 Autologous Tissue Substitute<br>J Synthetic Substitute<br>K Nonautologous Tissue Substitute | Z No Qualifier |

**0** Medical and Surgical
**J** Subcutaneous Tissue and Fascia
**W** Revision: Correcting, to the extent possible, a portion of a malfunctioning device or the position of a displaced device

| Character 4<br>Body Part | Character 5<br>Approach | Character 6<br>Device | Character 7<br>Qualifier |
|---|---|---|---|
| S Subcutaneous Tissue and Fascia,<br>  Head and Neck | 0 Open<br>3 Percutaneous<br>X External | 0 Drainage Device<br>3 Infusion Device<br>7 Autologous Tissue Substitute<br>J Synthetic Substitute<br>K Nonautologous Tissue Substitute<br>N Tissue Expander | Z No Qualifier |
| T Subcutaneous Tissue and Fascia,<br>  Trunk | 0 Open<br>3 Percutaneous<br>X External | 0 Drainage Device<br>2 Monitoring Device<br>3 Infusion Device<br>7 Autologous Tissue Substitute<br>H Contraceptive Device<br>J Synthetic Substitute<br>K Nonautologous Tissue Substitute<br>M Stimulator Generator<br>N Tissue Expander<br>P Cardiac Rhythm Related Device<br>V Infusion Device, Pump<br>W Vascular Access Device, Reservoir<br>X Vascular Access Device | Z No Qualifier |
| V Subcutaneous Tissue and Fascia,<br>  Upper Extremity<br>W Subcutaneous Tissue and Fascia,<br>  Lower Extremity | 0 Open<br>3 Percutaneous<br>X External | 0 Drainage Device<br>3 Infusion Device<br>7 Autologous Tissue Substitute<br>H Contraceptive Device<br>J Synthetic Substitute<br>K Nonautologous Tissue Substitute<br>N Tissue Expander<br>V Infusion Device, Pump<br>W Vascular Access Device, Reservoir<br>X Vascular Access Device | Z No Qualifier |

♂ Male          ♀ Female          N C Non-covered          L C Limited Coverage          **AHA** AHA Coding Clinic

**0**  Medical and Surgical
**J**  Subcutaneous Tissue and Fascia
**X**  Transfer: Moving, without taking out, all or a portion of a body part to another location to take over the function of all or a portion of a body part

| Character 4<br>Body Part | Character 5<br>Approach | Character 6<br>Device | Character 7<br>Qualifier |
|---|---|---|---|
| 0 Subcutaneous Tissue and Fascia, Scalp<br>1 Subcutaneous Tissue and Fascia, Face<br>4 Subcutaneous Tissue and Fascia, Anterior Neck<br>5 Subcutaneous Tissue and Fascia, Posterior Neck<br>6 Subcutaneous Tissue and Fascia, Chest<br>7 Subcutaneous Tissue and Fascia, Back<br>8 Subcutaneous Tissue and Fascia, Abdomen<br>9 Subcutaneous Tissue and Fascia, Buttock<br>B Subcutaneous Tissue and Fascia, Perineum<br>C Subcutaneous Tissue and Fascia, Pelvic Region<br>D Subcutaneous Tissue and Fascia, Right Upper Arm<br>F Subcutaneous Tissue and Fascia, Left Upper Arm<br>G Subcutaneous Tissue and Fascia, Right Lower Arm<br>H Subcutaneous Tissue and Fascia, Left Lower Arm<br>J Subcutaneous Tissue and Fascia, Right Hand<br>K Subcutaneous Tissue and Fascia, Left Hand<br>L Subcutaneous Tissue and Fascia, Right Upper Leg<br>M Subcutaneous Tissue and Fascia, Left Upper Leg<br>N Subcutaneous Tissue and Fascia, Right Lower Leg<br>P Subcutaneous Tissue and Fascia, Left Lower Leg<br>Q Subcutaneous Tissue and Fascia, Right Foot<br>R Subcutaneous Tissue and Fascia, Left Foot | 0 Open<br>3 Percutaneous | Z No Device | B Skin and Subcutaneous Tissue<br>C Skin, Subcutaneous Tissue and Fascia<br>Z No Qualifier |

**AHA:** 0JX60ZB - 4Q 2013, 11; 0JX80ZB - 4Q 2013, 111; 1

# Muscles | 0K2-0KX

**0** Medical and Surgical
**K** Muscles
**2** Change: Taking out or off a device from a body part and putting back an identical or similar device in or on the same body part without cutting or puncturing the skin or a mucous membrane

| Character 4 Body Part | Character 5 Approach | Character 6 Device | Character 7 Qualifier |
|---|---|---|---|
| X Upper Muscle<br>Y Lower Muscle | X External | 0 Drainage Device<br>Y Other Device | Z No Qualifier |

**0** Medical and Surgical
**K** Muscles
**5** Destruction: Physical eradication of all or a portion of a body part by the direct use of energy, force, or a destructive agent

| Character 4 Body Part | Character 5 Approach | Character 6 Device | Character 7 Qualifier |
|---|---|---|---|
| 0 Head Muscle<br>1 Facial Muscle<br>2 Neck Muscle, Right<br>3 Neck Muscle, Left<br>4 Tongue, Palate, Pharynx Muscle<br>5 Shoulder Muscle, Right<br>6 Shoulder Muscle, Left<br>7 Upper Arm Muscle, Right<br>8 Upper Arm Muscle, Left<br>9 Lower Arm and Wrist Muscle, Right<br>B Lower Arm and Wrist Muscle, Left<br>C Hand Muscle, Right<br>D Hand Muscle, Left<br>F Trunk Muscle, Right<br>G Trunk Muscle, Left<br>H Thorax Muscle, Right<br>J Thorax Muscle, Left<br>K Abdomen Muscle, Right<br>L Abdomen Muscle, Left<br>M Perineum Muscle<br>N Hip Muscle, Right<br>P Hip Muscle, Left<br>Q Upper Leg Muscle, Right<br>R Upper Leg Muscle, Left<br>S Lower Leg Muscle, Right<br>T Lower Leg Muscle, Left<br>V Foot Muscle, Right<br>W Foot Muscle, Left | 0 Open<br>3 Percutaneous<br>4 Percutaneous Endoscopic | Z No Device | Z No Qualifier |

**0** Medical and Surgical
**K** Muscles
**8** Division: Cutting into a body part, without draining fluids and/or gases from the body part, in order to separate or transect a body part

| Character 4 Body Part | Character 5 Approach | Character 6 Device | Character 7 Qualifier |
|---|---|---|---|
| 0 Head Muscle<br>1 Facial Muscle<br>2 Neck Muscle, Right<br>3 Neck Muscle, Left<br>4 Tongue, Palate, Pharynx Muscle<br>5 Shoulder Muscle, Right<br>6 Shoulder Muscle, Left<br>7 Upper Arm Muscle, Right<br>8 Upper Arm Muscle, Left<br>9 Lower Arm and Wrist Muscle, Right<br>B Lower Arm and Wrist Muscle, Left<br>C Hand Muscle, Right<br>D Hand Muscle, Left<br>F Trunk Muscle, Right<br>G Trunk Muscle, Left<br>H Thorax Muscle, Right<br>J Thorax Muscle, Left<br>K Abdomen Muscle, Right<br>L Abdomen Muscle, Left<br>M Perineum Muscle<br>N Hip Muscle, Right<br>P Hip Muscle, Left<br>Q Upper Leg Muscle, Right<br>R Upper Leg Muscle, Left<br>S Lower Leg Muscle, Right<br>T Lower Leg Muscle, Left<br>V Foot Muscle, Right<br>W Foot Muscle, Left | 0 Open<br>3 Percutaneous<br>4 Percutaneous Endoscopic | Z No Device | Z No Qualifier |

♂ Male　　♀ Female　　Ⓝ Ⓒ Non-covered　　Ⓛ Ⓒ Limited Coverage　　**AHA** *AHA Coding Clinic*

**0** Medical and Surgical
**K** Muscles
**9** Drainage: Taking or letting out fluids and/or gases from a body part

| Character 4<br>Body Part | Character 5<br>Approach | Character 6<br>Device | Character 7<br>Qualifier |
|---|---|---|---|
| 0 Head Muscle<br>1 Facial Muscle<br>2 Neck Muscle, Right<br>3 Neck Muscle, Left<br>4 Tongue, Palate, Pharynx Muscle<br>5 Shoulder Muscle, Right<br>6 Shoulder Muscle, Left<br>7 Upper Arm Muscle, Right<br>8 Upper Arm Muscle, Left<br>9 Lower Arm and Wrist Muscle, Right<br>B Lower Arm and Wrist Muscle, Left<br>C Hand Muscle, Right<br>D Hand Muscle, Left<br>F Trunk Muscle, Right<br>G Trunk Muscle, Left<br>H Thorax Muscle, Right<br>J Thorax Muscle, Left<br>K Abdomen Muscle, Right<br>L Abdomen Muscle, Left<br>M Perineum Muscle<br>N Hip Muscle, Right<br>P Hip Muscle, Left<br>Q Upper Leg Muscle, Right<br>R Upper Leg Muscle, Left<br>S Lower Leg Muscle, Right<br>T Lower Leg Muscle, Left<br>V Foot Muscle, Right<br>W Foot Muscle, Left | 0 Open<br>3 Percutaneous<br>4 Percutaneous Endoscopic | 0 Drainage Device | Z No Qualifier |
| 0 Head Muscle<br>1 Facial Muscle<br>2 Neck Muscle, Right<br>3 Neck Muscle, Left<br>4 Tongue, Palate, Pharynx Muscle<br>5 Shoulder Muscle, Right<br>6 Shoulder Muscle, Left<br>7 Upper Arm Muscle, Right<br>8 Upper Arm Muscle, Left<br>9 Lower Arm and Wrist Muscle, Right<br>B Lower Arm and Wrist Muscle, Left<br>C Hand Muscle, Right<br>D Hand Muscle, Left<br>F Trunk Muscle, Right<br>G Trunk Muscle, Left<br>H Thorax Muscle, Right<br>J Thorax Muscle, Left<br>K Abdomen Muscle, Right<br>L Abdomen Muscle, Left<br>M Perineum Muscle<br>N Hip Muscle, Right<br>P Hip Muscle, Left<br>Q Upper Leg Muscle, Right<br>R Upper Leg Muscle, Left<br>S Lower Leg Muscle, Right<br>T Lower Leg Muscle, Left<br>V Foot Muscle, Right<br>W Foot Muscle, Left | 0 Open<br>3 Percutaneous<br>4 Percutaneous Endoscopic | Z No Device | X Diagnostic<br>Z No Qualifier |

**0** Medical and Surgical
**K** Muscles
**B** Excision: Cutting out or off, without replacement, a portion of a body part

| Character 4<br>Body Part | Character 5<br>Approach | Character 6<br>Device | Character 7<br>Qualifier |
|---|---|---|---|
| 0 Head Muscle<br>1 Facial Muscle<br>2 Neck Muscle, Right<br>3 Neck Muscle, Left<br>4 Tongue, Palate, Pharynx Muscle<br>5 Shoulder Muscle, Right<br>6 Shoulder Muscle, Left<br>7 Upper Arm Muscle, Right<br>8 Upper Arm Muscle, Left<br>9 Lower Arm and Wrist Muscle, Right<br>B Lower Arm and Wrist Muscle, Left<br>C Hand Muscle, Right<br>D Hand Muscle, Left<br>F Trunk Muscle, Right<br>G Trunk Muscle, Left<br>H Thorax Muscle, Right<br>J Thorax Muscle, Left<br>K Abdomen Muscle, Right<br>L Abdomen Muscle, Left<br>M Perineum Muscle<br>N Hip Muscle, Right<br>P Hip Muscle, Left<br>Q Upper Leg Muscle, Right<br>R Upper Leg Muscle, Left<br>S Lower Leg Muscle, Right<br>T Lower Leg Muscle, Left<br>V Foot Muscle, Right<br>W Foot Muscle, Left | 0 Open<br>3 Percutaneous<br>4 Percutaneous Endoscopic | Z No Device | X Diagnostic<br>Z No Qualifier |

**0** Medical and Surgical
**K** Muscles
**C** Extirpation: Taking or cutting out solid matter from a body part

| Character 4<br>Body Part | Character 5<br>Approach | Character 6<br>Device | Character 7<br>Qualifier |
|---|---|---|---|
| 0 Head Muscle<br>1 Facial Muscle<br>2 Neck Muscle, Right<br>3 Neck Muscle, Left<br>4 Tongue, Palate, Pharynx Muscle<br>5 Shoulder Muscle, Right<br>6 Shoulder Muscle, Left<br>7 Upper Arm Muscle, Right<br>8 Upper Arm Muscle, Left<br>9 Lower Arm and Wrist Muscle, Right<br>B Lower Arm and Wrist Muscle, Left<br>C Hand Muscle, Right<br>D Hand Muscle, Left<br>F Trunk Muscle, Right<br>G Trunk Muscle, Left<br>H Thorax Muscle, Right<br>J Thorax Muscle, Left<br>K Abdomen Muscle, Right<br>L Abdomen Muscle, Left<br>M Perineum Muscle<br>N Hip Muscle, Right<br>P Hip Muscle, Left<br>Q Upper Leg Muscle, Right<br>R Upper Leg Muscle, Left<br>S Lower Leg Muscle, Right<br>T Lower Leg Muscle, Left<br>V Foot Muscle, Right<br>W Foot Muscle, Left | 0 Open<br>3 Percutaneous<br>4 Percutaneous Endoscopic | Z No Device | Z No Qualifier |

**0** Medical and Surgical
**K** Muscles
**H** Insertion: Putting in a nonbiological appliance that monitors, assists, performs, or prevents a physiological function but does not physically take the place of a body part

| Character 4<br>Body Part | Character 5<br>Approach | Character 6<br>Device | Character 7<br>Qualifier |
|---|---|---|---|
| X Upper Muscle<br>Y Lower Muscle | 0 Open<br>3 Percutaneous<br>4 Percutaneous Endoscopic | M Stimulator Lead | Z No Qualifier |

**0** Medical and Surgical
**K** Muscles
**J** Inspection: Visually and/or manually exploring a body part

| Character 4<br>Body Part | Character 5<br>Approach | Character 6<br>Device | Character 7<br>Qualifier |
|---|---|---|---|
| X Upper Muscle<br>Y Lower Muscle | 0 Open<br>3 Percutaneous<br>4 Percutaneous Endoscopic<br>X External | Z No Device | Z No Qualifier |

**0** Medical and Surgical
**K** Muscles
**M** Reattachment: Putting back in or on all or a portion of a separated body part to its normal location or other suitable location

| Character 4<br>Body Part | Character 5<br>Approach | Character 6<br>Device | Character 7<br>Qualifier |
|---|---|---|---|
| 0 Head Muscle<br>1 Facial Muscle<br>2 Neck Muscle, Right<br>3 Neck Muscle, Left<br>4 Tongue, Palate, Pharynx Muscle<br>5 Shoulder Muscle, Right<br>6 Shoulder Muscle, Left<br>7 Upper Arm Muscle, Right<br>8 Upper Arm Muscle, Left<br>9 Lower Arm and Wrist Muscle, Right<br>B Lower Arm and Wrist Muscle, Left<br>C Hand Muscle, Right<br>D Hand Muscle, Left<br>F Trunk Muscle, Right<br>G Trunk Muscle, Left<br>H Thorax Muscle, Right<br>J Thorax Muscle, Left<br>K Abdomen Muscle, Right<br>L Abdomen Muscle, Left<br>M Perineum Muscle<br>N Hip Muscle, Right<br>P Hip Muscle, Left<br>Q Upper Leg Muscle, Right<br>R Upper Leg Muscle, Left<br>S Lower Leg Muscle, Right<br>T Lower Leg Muscle, Left<br>V Foot Muscle, Right<br>W Foot Muscle, Left | 0 Open<br>4 Percutaneous Endoscopic | Z No Device | Z No Qualifier |

**0** Medical and Surgical
**K** Muscles
**N** Release: Freeing a body part from an abnormal physical constraint by cutting or by the use of force

| Character 4<br>Body Part | Character 5<br>Approach | Character 6<br>Device | Character 7<br>Qualifier |
|---|---|---|---|
| 0 Head Muscle<br>1 Facial Muscle<br>2 Neck Muscle, Right<br>3 Neck Muscle, Left<br>4 Tongue, Palate, Pharynx Muscle<br>5 Shoulder Muscle, Right<br>6 Shoulder Muscle, Left<br>7 Upper Arm Muscle, Right<br>8 Upper Arm Muscle, Left<br>9 Lower Arm and Wrist Muscle, Right<br>B Lower Arm and Wrist Muscle, Left<br>C Hand Muscle, Right<br>D Hand Muscle, Left<br>F Trunk Muscle, Right<br>G Trunk Muscle, Left<br>H Thorax Muscle, Right<br>J Thorax Muscle, Left<br>K Abdomen Muscle, Right<br>L Abdomen Muscle, Left<br>M Perineum Muscle<br>N Hip Muscle, Right<br>P Hip Muscle, Left<br>Q Upper Leg Muscle, Right<br>R Upper Leg Muscle, Left<br>S Lower Leg Muscle, Right<br>T Lower Leg Muscle, Left<br>V Foot Muscle, Right<br>W Foot Muscle, Left | 0 Open<br>3 Percutaneous<br>4 Percutaneous Endoscopic<br>X External | Z No Device | Z No Qualifier |

---

**0** Medical and Surgical
**K** Muscles
**P** Removal: Taking out or off a device from a body part

| Character 4 Body Part | Character 5 Approach | Character 6 Device | Character 7 Qualifier |
|---|---|---|---|
| X Upper Muscle<br>Y Lower Muscle | 0 Open<br>3 Percutaneous<br>4 Percutaneous Endoscopic | 0 Drainage Device<br>7 Autologous Tissue Substitute<br>J Synthetic Substitute<br>K Nonautologous Tissue Substitute<br>M Stimulator Lead | Z No Qualifier |
| X Upper Muscle<br>Y Lower Muscle | X External | 0 Drainage Device<br>M Stimulator Lead | Z No Qualifier |

---

**0** Medical and Surgical
**K** Muscles
**Q** Repair: Restoring, to the extent possible, a body part to its normal anatomic structure and function

| Character 4 Body Part | Character 5 Approach | Character 6 Device | Character 7 Qualifier |
|---|---|---|---|
| 0 Head Muscle<br>1 Facial Muscle<br>2 Neck Muscle, Right<br>3 Neck Muscle, Left<br>4 Tongue, Palate, Pharynx Muscle<br>5 Shoulder Muscle, Right<br>6 Shoulder Muscle, Left<br>7 Upper Arm Muscle, Right<br>8 Upper Arm Muscle, Left<br>9 Lower Arm and Wrist Muscle, Right<br>B Lower Arm and Wrist Muscle, Left<br>C Hand Muscle, Right<br>D Hand Muscle, Left<br>F Trunk Muscle, Right<br>G Trunk Muscle, Left<br>H Thorax Muscle, Right<br>J Thorax Muscle, Left<br>K Abdomen Muscle, Right<br>L Abdomen Muscle, Left<br>M Perineum Muscle<br>N Hip Muscle, Right<br>P Hip Muscle, Left<br>Q Upper Leg Muscle, Right<br>R Upper Leg Muscle, Left<br>S Lower Leg Muscle, Right<br>T Lower Leg Muscle, Left<br>V Foot Muscle, Right<br>W Foot Muscle, Left | 0 Open<br>3 Percutaneous<br>4 Percutaneous Endoscopic | Z No Device | Z No Qualifier |

**AHA:** 0KQM0ZZ - 4Q 2013, 120

---

**0 Medical and Surgical**
**K Muscles**
**S Reposition:** Moving to its normal location, or other suitable location, all or a portion of a body part

| Character 4<br>Body Part | Character 5<br>Approach | Character 6<br>Device | Character 7<br>Qualifier |
|---|---|---|---|
| 0 Head Muscle<br>1 Facial Muscle<br>2 Neck Muscle, Right<br>3 Neck Muscle, Left<br>4 Tongue, Palate, Pharynx Muscle<br>5 Shoulder Muscle, Right<br>6 Shoulder Muscle, Left<br>7 Upper Arm Muscle, Right<br>8 Upper Arm Muscle, Left<br>9 Lower Arm and Wrist Muscle, Right<br>B Lower Arm and Wrist Muscle, Left<br>C Hand Muscle, Right<br>D Hand Muscle, Left<br>F Trunk Muscle, Right<br>G Trunk Muscle, Left<br>H Thorax Muscle, Right<br>J Thorax Muscle, Left<br>K Abdomen Muscle, Right<br>L Abdomen Muscle, Left<br>M Perineum Muscle<br>N Hip Muscle, Right<br>P Hip Muscle, Left<br>Q Upper Leg Muscle, Right<br>R Upper Leg Muscle, Left<br>S Lower Leg Muscle, Right<br>T Lower Leg Muscle, Left<br>V Foot Muscle, Right<br>W Foot Muscle, Left | 0 Open<br>4 Percutaneous Endoscopic | Z No Device | Z No Qualifier |

**0 Medical and Surgical**
**K Muscles**
**T Resection:** Cutting out or off, without replacement, all of a body part

| Character 4<br>Body Part | Character 5<br>Approach | Character 6<br>Device | Character 7<br>Qualifier |
|---|---|---|---|
| 0 Head Muscle<br>1 Facial Muscle<br>2 Neck Muscle, Right<br>3 Neck Muscle, Left<br>4 Tongue, Palate, Pharynx Muscle<br>5 Shoulder Muscle, Right<br>6 Shoulder Muscle, Left<br>7 Upper Arm Muscle, Right<br>8 Upper Arm Muscle, Left<br>9 Lower Arm and Wrist Muscle, Right<br>B Lower Arm and Wrist Muscle, Left<br>C Hand Muscle, Right<br>D Hand Muscle, Left<br>F Trunk Muscle, Right<br>G Trunk Muscle, Left<br>H Thorax Muscle, Right<br>J Thorax Muscle, Left<br>K Abdomen Muscle, Right<br>L Abdomen Muscle, Left<br>M Perineum Muscle<br>N Hip Muscle, Right<br>P Hip Muscle, Left<br>Q Upper Leg Muscle, Right<br>R Upper Leg Muscle, Left<br>S Lower Leg Muscle, Right<br>T Lower Leg Muscle, Left<br>V Foot Muscle, Right<br>W Foot Muscle, Left | 0 Open<br>4 Percutaneous Endoscopic | Z No Device | Z No Qualifier |

| 0 Medical and Surgical | | | |
| K Muscles | | | |
| U Supplement: Putting in or on biological or synthetic material that physically reinforces and/or augments the function of a portion of a body part | | | |

| Character 4<br>Body Part | Character 5<br>Approach | Character 6<br>Device | Character 7<br>Qualifier |
|---|---|---|---|
| 0 Head Muscle<br>1 Facial Muscle<br>2 Neck Muscle, Right<br>3 Neck Muscle, Left<br>4 Tongue, Palate, Pharynx Muscle<br>5 Shoulder Muscle, Right<br>6 Shoulder Muscle, Left<br>7 Upper Arm Muscle, Right<br>8 Upper Arm Muscle, Left<br>9 Lower Arm and Wrist Muscle, Right<br>B Lower Arm and Wrist Muscle, Left<br>C Hand Muscle, Right<br>D Hand Muscle, Left<br>F Trunk Muscle, Right<br>G Trunk Muscle, Left<br>H Thorax Muscle, Right<br>J Thorax Muscle, Left<br>K Abdomen Muscle, Right<br>L Abdomen Muscle, Left<br>M Perineum Muscle<br>N Hip Muscle, Right<br>P Hip Muscle, Left<br>Q Upper Leg Muscle, Right<br>R Upper Leg Muscle, Left<br>S Lower Leg Muscle, Right<br>T Lower Leg Muscle, Left<br>V Foot Muscle, Right<br>W Foot Muscle, Left | 0 Open<br>4 Percutaneous Endoscopic | 7 Autologous Tissue Substitute<br>J Synthetic Substitute<br>K Nonautologous Tissue Substitute | Z No Qualifier |

| 0 Medical and Surgical | | | |
| K Muscles | | | |
| W Revision: Correcting, to the extent possible, a portion of a malfunctioning device or the position of a displaced device | | | |

| Character 4<br>Body Part | Character 5<br>Approach | Character 6<br>Device | Character 7<br>Qualifier |
|---|---|---|---|
| X Upper Muscle<br>Y Lower Muscle | 0 Open<br>3 Percutaneous<br>4 Percutaneous Endoscopic<br>X External | 0 Drainage Device<br>7 Autologous Tissue Substitute<br>J Synthetic Substitute<br>K Nonautologous Tissue Substitute<br>M Stimulator Lead | Z No Qualifier |

**0** Medical and Surgical
**K** Muscles
**X** Transfer: Moving, without taking out, all or a portion of a body part to another location to take over the function of all or a portion of a body part

| Character 4<br>Body Part | Character 5<br>Approach | Character 6<br>Device | Character 7<br>Qualifier |
|---|---|---|---|
| 0 Head Muscle<br>1 Facial Muscle<br>2 Neck Muscle, Right<br>3 Neck Muscle, Left<br>4 Tongue, Palate, Pharynx Muscle<br>5 Shoulder Muscle, Right<br>6 Shoulder Muscle, Left<br>7 Upper Arm Muscle, Right<br>8 Upper Arm Muscle, Left<br>9 Lower Arm and Wrist Muscle, Right<br>B Lower Arm and Wrist Muscle, Left<br>C Hand Muscle, Right<br>D Hand Muscle, Left<br>F Trunk Muscle, Right<br>G Trunk Muscle, Left<br>H Thorax Muscle, Right<br>J Thorax Muscle, Left<br>M Perineum Muscle<br>N Hip Muscle, Right<br>P Hip Muscle, Left<br>Q Upper Leg Muscle, Right<br>R Upper Leg Muscle, Left<br>S Lower Leg Muscle, Right<br>T Lower Leg Muscle, Left<br>V Foot Muscle, Right<br>W Foot Muscle, Left | 0 Open<br>4 Percutaneous Endoscopic | Z No Device | 0 Skin<br>1 Subcutaneous Tissue<br>2 Skin and Subcutaneous Tissue<br>Z No Qualifier |
| K Abdomen Muscle, Right<br>L Abdomen Muscle, Left | 0 Open<br>4 Percutaneous Endoscopic | Z No Device | 0 Skin<br>1 Subcutaneous Tissue<br>2 Skin and Subcutaneous Tissue<br>6 Transverse Rectus Abdominis Myocutaneous Flap<br>Z No Qualifier |

**AHA:** 0KXL0Z6 - 2Q 2014, 11; 0KXF0Z2 - 2Q 2014, 12

# Tendons | 0L2-0LX

**0** Medical and Surgical
**L** Tendons
**2** Change: Taking out or off a device from a body part and putting back an identical or similar device in or on the same body part without cutting or puncturing the skin or a mucous membrane

| Character 4<br>Body Part | Character 5<br>Approach | Character 6<br>Device | Character 7<br>Qualifier |
|---|---|---|---|
| X Upper Tendon<br>Y Lower Tendon | X External | 0 Drainage Device<br>Y Other Device | Z No Qualifier |

**0** Medical and Surgical
**L** Tendons
**5** Destruction: Physical eradication of all or a portion of a body part by the direct use of energy, force, or a destructive agent

| Character 4<br>Body Part | Character 5<br>Approach | Character 6<br>Device | Character 7<br>Qualifier |
|---|---|---|---|
| 0 Head and Neck Tendon<br>1 Shoulder Tendon, Right<br>2 Shoulder Tendon, Left<br>3 Upper Arm Tendon, Right<br>4 Upper Arm Tendon, Left<br>5 Lower Arm and Wrist Tendon, Right<br>6 Lower Arm and Wrist Tendon, Left<br>7 Hand Tendon, Right<br>8 Hand Tendon, Left<br>9 Trunk Tendon, Right<br>B Trunk Tendon, Left<br>C Thorax Tendon, Right<br>D Thorax Tendon, Left<br>F Abdomen Tendon, Right<br>G Abdomen Tendon, Left<br>H Perineum Tendon<br>J Hip Tendon, Right<br>K Hip Tendon, Left<br>L Upper Leg Tendon, Right<br>M Upper Leg Tendon, Left<br>N Lower Leg Tendon, Right<br>P Lower Leg Tendon, Left<br>Q Knee Tendon, Right<br>R Knee Tendon, Left<br>S Ankle Tendon, Right<br>T Ankle Tendon, Left<br>V Foot Tendon, Right<br>W Foot Tendon, Left | 0 Open<br>3 Percutaneous<br>4 Percutaneous Endoscopic | Z No Device | Z No Qualifier |

**0** Medical and Surgical
**L** Tendons
**8** Division: Cutting into a body part, without draining fluids and/or gases from the body part, in order to separate or transect a body part

| Character 4<br>Body Part | Character 5<br>Approach | Character 6<br>Device | Character 7<br>Qualifier |
|---|---|---|---|
| 0 Head and Neck Tendon<br>1 Shoulder Tendon, Right<br>2 Shoulder Tendon, Left<br>3 Upper Arm Tendon, Right<br>4 Upper Arm Tendon, Left<br>5 Lower Arm and Wrist Tendon, Right<br>6 Lower Arm and Wrist Tendon, Left<br>7 Hand Tendon, Right<br>8 Hand Tendon, Left<br>9 Trunk Tendon, Right<br>B Trunk Tendon, Left<br>C Thorax Tendon, Right<br>D Thorax Tendon, Left<br>F Abdomen Tendon, Right<br>G Abdomen Tendon, Left<br>H Perineum Tendon<br>J Hip Tendon, Right<br>K Hip Tendon, Left<br>L Upper Leg Tendon, Right<br>M Upper Leg Tendon, Left<br>N Lower Leg Tendon, Right<br>P Lower Leg Tendon, Left<br>Q Knee Tendon, Right<br>R Knee Tendon, Left<br>S Ankle Tendon, Right<br>T Ankle Tendon, Left<br>V Foot Tendon, Right<br>W Foot Tendon, Left | 0 Open<br>3 Percutaneous<br>4 Percutaneous Endoscopic | Z No Device | Z No Qualifier |

♂ Male     ♀ Female     N C Non-covered     L C Limited Coverage     **AHA** *AHA Coding Clinic*

**0** Medical and Surgical
**L** Tendons
**9** Drainage: Taking or letting out fluids and/or gases from a body part

| Character 4<br>Body Part | Character 5<br>Approach | Character 6<br>Device | Character 7<br>Qualifier |
|---|---|---|---|
| 0 Head and Neck Tendon<br>1 Shoulder Tendon, Right<br>2 Shoulder Tendon, Left<br>3 Upper Arm Tendon, Right<br>4 Upper Arm Tendon, Left<br>5 Lower Arm and Wrist Tendon, Right<br>6 Lower Arm and Wrist Tendon, Left<br>7 Hand Tendon, Right<br>8 Hand Tendon, Left<br>9 Trunk Tendon, Right<br>B Trunk Tendon, Left<br>C Thorax Tendon, Right<br>D Thorax Tendon, Left<br>F Abdomen Tendon, Right<br>G Abdomen Tendon, Left<br>H Perineum Tendon<br>J Hip Tendon, Right<br>K Hip Tendon, Left<br>L Upper Leg Tendon, Right<br>M Upper Leg Tendon, Left<br>N Lower Leg Tendon, Right<br>P Lower Leg Tendon, Left<br>Q Knee Tendon, Right<br>R Knee Tendon, Left<br>S Ankle Tendon, Right<br>T Ankle Tendon, Left<br>V Foot Tendon, Right<br>W Foot Tendon, Left | 0 Open<br>3 Percutaneous<br>4 Percutaneous Endoscopic | 0 Drainage Device | Z No Qualifier |
| 0 Head and Neck Tendon<br>1 Shoulder Tendon, Right<br>2 Shoulder Tendon, Left<br>3 Upper Arm Tendon, Right<br>4 Upper Arm Tendon, Left<br>5 Lower Arm and Wrist Tendon, Right<br>6 Lower Arm and Wrist Tendon, Left<br>7 Hand Tendon, Right<br>8 Hand Tendon, Left<br>9 Trunk Tendon, Right<br>B Trunk Tendon, Left<br>C Thorax Tendon, Right<br>D Thorax Tendon, Left<br>F Abdomen Tendon, Right<br>G Abdomen Tendon, Left<br>H Perineum Tendon<br>J Hip Tendon, Right<br>K Hip Tendon, Left<br>L Upper Leg Tendon, Right<br>M Upper Leg Tendon, Left<br>N Lower Leg Tendon, Right<br>P Lower Leg Tendon, Left<br>Q Knee Tendon, Right<br>R Knee Tendon, Left<br>S Ankle Tendon, Right<br>T Ankle Tendon, Left<br>V Foot Tendon, Right<br>W Foot Tendon, Left | 0 Open<br>3 Percutaneous<br>4 Percutaneous Endoscopic | Z No Device | X Diagnostic<br>Z No Qualifier |

0 Medical and Surgical
L Tendons
B Excision: Cutting out or off, without replacement, a portion of a body part

| Character 4<br>Body Part | Character 5<br>Approach | Character 6<br>Device | Character 7<br>Qualifier |
|---|---|---|---|
| 0 Head and Neck Tendon<br>1 Shoulder Tendon, Right<br>2 Shoulder Tendon, Left<br>3 Upper Arm Tendon, Right<br>4 Upper Arm Tendon, Left<br>5 Lower Arm and Wrist Tendon, Right<br>6 Lower Arm and Wrist Tendon, Left<br>7 Hand Tendon, Right<br>8 Hand Tendon, Left<br>9 Trunk Tendon, Right<br>B Trunk Tendon, Left<br>C Thorax Tendon, Right<br>D Thorax Tendon, Left<br>F Abdomen Tendon, Right<br>G Abdomen Tendon, Left<br>H Perineum Tendon<br>J Hip Tendon, Right<br>K Hip Tendon, Left<br>L Upper Leg Tendon, Right<br>M Upper Leg Tendon, Left<br>N Lower Leg Tendon, Right<br>P Lower Leg Tendon, Left<br>Q Knee Tendon, Right<br>R Knee Tendon, Left<br>S Ankle Tendon, Right<br>T Ankle Tendon, Left<br>V Foot Tendon, Right<br>W Foot Tendon, Left | 0 Open<br>3 Percutaneous<br>4 Percutaneous Endoscopic | Z No Device | X Diagnostic<br>Z No Qualifier |

0 Medical and Surgical
L Tendons
C Extirpation: Taking or cutting out solid matter from a body part

| Character 4<br>Body Part | Character 5<br>Approach | Character 6<br>Device | Character 7<br>Qualifier |
|---|---|---|---|
| 0 Head and Neck Tendon<br>1 Shoulder Tendon, Right<br>2 Shoulder Tendon, Left<br>3 Upper Arm Tendon, Right<br>4 Upper Arm Tendon, Left<br>5 Lower Arm and Wrist Tendon, Right<br>6 Lower Arm and Wrist Tendon, Left<br>7 Hand Tendon, Right<br>8 Hand Tendon, Left<br>9 Trunk Tendon, Right<br>B Trunk Tendon, Left<br>C Thorax Tendon, Right<br>D Thorax Tendon, Left<br>F Abdomen Tendon, Right<br>G Abdomen Tendon, Left<br>H Perineum Tendon<br>J Hip Tendon, Right<br>K Hip Tendon, Left<br>L Upper Leg Tendon, Right<br>M Upper Leg Tendon, Left<br>N Lower Leg Tendon, Right<br>P Lower Leg Tendon, Left<br>Q Knee Tendon, Right<br>R Knee Tendon, Left<br>S Ankle Tendon, Right<br>T Ankle Tendon, Left<br>V Foot Tendon, Right<br>W Foot Tendon, Left | 0 Open<br>3 Percutaneous<br>4 Percutaneous Endoscopic | Z No Device | Z No Qualifier |

0 Medical and Surgical
L Tendons
J Inspection: Visually and/or manually exploring a body part

| Character 4<br>Body Part | Character 5<br>Approach | Character 6<br>Device | Character 7<br>Qualifier |
|---|---|---|---|
| X Upper Tendon<br>Y Lower Tendon | 0 Open<br>3 Percutaneous<br>4 Percutaneous Endoscopic<br>X External | Z No Device | Z No Qualifier |

**0** Medical and Surgical
**L** Tendons
**M** Reattachment: Putting back in or on all or a portion of a separated body part to its normal location or other suitable location

| Character 4 Body Part | Character 5 Approach | Character 6 Device | Character 7 Qualifier |
|---|---|---|---|
| 0 Head and Neck Tendon | 0 Open | Z No Device | Z No Qualifier |
| 1 Shoulder Tendon, Right | 4 Percutaneous Endoscopic | | |
| 2 Shoulder Tendon, Left | | | |
| 3 Upper Arm Tendon, Right | | | |
| 4 Upper Arm Tendon, Left | | | |
| 5 Lower Arm and Wrist Tendon, Right | | | |
| 6 Lower Arm and Wrist Tendon, Left | | | |
| 7 Hand Tendon, Right | | | |
| 8 Hand Tendon, Left | | | |
| 9 Trunk Tendon, Right | | | |
| B Trunk Tendon, Left | | | |
| C Thorax Tendon, Right | | | |
| D Thorax Tendon, Left | | | |
| F Abdomen Tendon, Right | | | |
| G Abdomen Tendon, Left | | | |
| H Perineum Tendon | | | |
| J Hip Tendon, Right | | | |
| K Hip Tendon, Left | | | |
| L Upper Leg Tendon, Right | | | |
| M Upper Leg Tendon, Left | | | |
| N Lower Leg Tendon, Right | | | |
| P Lower Leg Tendon, Left | | | |
| Q Knee Tendon, Right | | | |
| R Knee Tendon, Left | | | |
| S Ankle Tendon, Right | | | |
| T Ankle Tendon, Left | | | |
| V Foot Tendon, Right | | | |
| W Foot Tendon, Left | | | |

**0** Medical and Surgical
**L** Tendons
**N** Release: Freeing a body part from an abnormal physical constraint by cutting or by the use of force

| Character 4 Body Part | Character 5 Approach | Character 6 Device | Character 7 Qualifier |
|---|---|---|---|
| 0 Head and Neck Tendon | 0 Open | Z No Device | Z No Qualifier |
| 1 Shoulder Tendon, Right | 3 Percutaneous | | |
| 2 Shoulder Tendon, Left | 4 Percutaneous Endoscopic | | |
| 3 Upper Arm Tendon, Right | X External | | |
| 4 Upper Arm Tendon, Left | | | |
| 5 Lower Arm and Wrist Tendon, Right | | | |
| 6 Lower Arm and Wrist Tendon, Left | | | |
| 7 Hand Tendon, Right | | | |
| 8 Hand Tendon, Left | | | |
| 9 Trunk Tendon, Right | | | |
| B Trunk Tendon, Left | | | |
| C Thorax Tendon, Right | | | |
| D Thorax Tendon, Left | | | |
| F Abdomen Tendon, Right | | | |
| G Abdomen Tendon, Left | | | |
| H Perineum Tendon | | | |
| J Hip Tendon, Right | | | |
| K Hip Tendon, Left | | | |
| L Upper Leg Tendon, Right | | | |
| M Upper Leg Tendon, Left | | | |
| N Lower Leg Tendon, Right | | | |
| P Lower Leg Tendon, Left | | | |
| Q Knee Tendon, Right | | | |
| R Knee Tendon, Left | | | |
| S Ankle Tendon, Right | | | |
| T Ankle Tendon, Left | | | |
| V Foot Tendon, Right | | | |
| W Foot Tendon, Left | | | |

**0** Medical and Surgical
**L** Tendons
**P** Removal: Taking out or off a device from a body part

| Character 4 Body Part | Character 5 Approach | Character 6 Device | Character 7 Qualifier |
|---|---|---|---|
| X Upper Tendon<br>Y Lower Tendon | 0 Open<br>3 Percutaneous<br>4 Percutaneous Endoscopic | 0 Drainage Device<br>7 Autologous Tissue Substitute<br>J Synthetic Substitute<br>K Nonautologous Tissue Substitute | Z No Qualifier |
| X Upper Tendon<br>Y Lower Tendon | X External | 0 Drainage Device | Z No Qualifier |

**0** Medical and Surgical
**L** Tendons
**Q** Repair: Restoring, to the extent possible, a body part to its normal anatomic structure and function

| Character 4 Body Part | Character 5 Approach | Character 6 Device | Character 7 Qualifier |
|---|---|---|---|
| 0 Head and Neck Tendon<br>1 Shoulder Tendon, Right<br>2 Shoulder Tendon, Left<br>3 Upper Arm Tendon, Right<br>4 Upper Arm Tendon, Left<br>5 Lower Arm and Wrist Tendon, Right<br>6 Lower Arm and Wrist Tendon, Left<br>7 Hand Tendon, Right<br>8 Hand Tendon, Left<br>9 Trunk Tendon, Right<br>B Trunk Tendon, Left<br>C Thorax Tendon, Right<br>D Thorax Tendon, Left<br>F Abdomen Tendon, Right<br>G Abdomen Tendon, Left<br>H Perineum Tendon<br>J Hip Tendon, Right<br>K Hip Tendon, Left<br>L Upper Leg Tendon, Right<br>M Upper Leg Tendon, Left<br>N Lower Leg Tendon, Right<br>P Lower Leg Tendon, Left<br>Q Knee Tendon, Right<br>R Knee Tendon, Left<br>S Ankle Tendon, Right<br>T Ankle Tendon, Left<br>V Foot Tendon, Right<br>W Foot Tendon, Left | 0 Open<br>3 Percutaneous<br>4 Percutaneous Endoscopic | Z No Device | Z No Qualifier |

**AHA:** 0LQ14ZZ - 3Q 2013, 21

**0** Medical and Surgical
**L** Tendons
**R** Replacement: Putting in or on biological or synthetic material that physically takes the place and/or function of all or a portion of a body part

| Character 4 Body Part | Character 5 Approach | Character 6 Device | Character 7 Qualifier |
|---|---|---|---|
| 0 Head and Neck Tendon<br>1 Shoulder Tendon, Right<br>2 Shoulder Tendon, Left<br>3 Upper Arm Tendon, Right<br>4 Upper Arm Tendon, Left<br>5 Lower Arm and Wrist Tendon, Right<br>6 Lower Arm and Wrist Tendon, Left<br>7 Hand Tendon, Right<br>8 Hand Tendon, Left<br>9 Trunk Tendon, Right<br>B Trunk Tendon, Left<br>C Thorax Tendon, Right<br>D Thorax Tendon, Left<br>F Abdomen Tendon, Right<br>G Abdomen Tendon, Left<br>H Perineum Tendon<br>J Hip Tendon, Right<br>K Hip Tendon, Left<br>L Upper Leg Tendon, Right<br>M Upper Leg Tendon, Left<br>N Lower Leg Tendon, Right<br>P Lower Leg Tendon, Left<br>Q Knee Tendon, Right<br>R Knee Tendon, Left<br>S Ankle Tendon, Right<br>T Ankle Tendon, Left<br>V Foot Tendon, Right<br>W Foot Tendon, Left | 0 Open<br>4 Percutaneous Endoscopic | 7 Autologous Tissue Substitute<br>J Synthetic Substitute<br>K Nonautologous Tissue Substitute | Z No Qualifier |

**0** Medical and Surgical
**L** Tendons
**S** Reposition: Moving to its normal location, or other suitable location, all or a portion of a body part

| Character 4<br>Body Part | Character 5<br>Approach | Character 6<br>Device | Character 7<br>Qualifier |
|---|---|---|---|
| 0 Head and Neck Tendon | 0 Open | Z No Device | Z No Qualifier |
| 1 Shoulder Tendon, Right | 4 Percutaneous Endoscopic | | |
| 2 Shoulder Tendon, Left | | | |
| 3 Upper Arm Tendon, Right | | | |
| 4 Upper Arm Tendon, Left | | | |
| 5 Lower Arm and Wrist Tendon, Right | | | |
| 6 Lower Arm and Wrist Tendon, Left | | | |
| 7 Hand Tendon, Right | | | |
| 8 Hand Tendon, Left | | | |
| 9 Trunk Tendon, Right | | | |
| B Trunk Tendon, Left | | | |
| C Thorax Tendon, Right | | | |
| D Thorax Tendon, Left | | | |
| F Abdomen Tendon, Right | | | |
| G Abdomen Tendon, Left | | | |
| H Perineum Tendon | | | |
| J Hip Tendon, Right | | | |
| K Hip Tendon, Left | | | |
| L Upper Leg Tendon, Right | | | |
| M Upper Leg Tendon, Left | | | |
| N Lower Leg Tendon, Right | | | |
| P Lower Leg Tendon, Left | | | |
| Q Knee Tendon, Right | | | |
| R Knee Tendon, Left | | | |
| S Ankle Tendon, Right | | | |
| T Ankle Tendon, Left | | | |
| V Foot Tendon, Right | | | |
| W Foot Tendon, Left | | | |

**0** Medical and Surgical
**L** Tendons
**T** Resection: Cutting out or off, without replacement, all of a body part

| Character 4<br>Body Part | Character 5<br>Approach | Character 6<br>Device | Character 7<br>Qualifier |
|---|---|---|---|
| 0 Head and Neck Tendon | 0 Open | Z No Device | Z No Qualifier |
| 1 Shoulder Tendon, Right | 4 Percutaneous Endoscopic | | |
| 2 Shoulder Tendon, Left | | | |
| 3 Upper Arm Tendon, Right | | | |
| 4 Upper Arm Tendon, Left | | | |
| 5 Lower Arm and Wrist Tendon, Right | | | |
| 6 Lower Arm and Wrist Tendon, Left | | | |
| 7 Hand Tendon, Right | | | |
| 8 Hand Tendon, Left | | | |
| 9 Trunk Tendon, Right | | | |
| B Trunk Tendon, Left | | | |
| C Thorax Tendon, Right | | | |
| D Thorax Tendon, Left | | | |
| F Abdomen Tendon, Right | | | |
| G Abdomen Tendon, Left | | | |
| H Perineum Tendon | | | |
| J Hip Tendon, Right | | | |
| K Hip Tendon, Left | | | |
| L Upper Leg Tendon, Right | | | |
| M Upper Leg Tendon, Left | | | |
| N Lower Leg Tendon, Right | | | |
| P Lower Leg Tendon, Left | | | |
| Q Knee Tendon, Right | | | |
| R Knee Tendon, Left | | | |
| S Ankle Tendon, Right | | | |
| T Ankle Tendon, Left | | | |
| V Foot Tendon, Right | | | |
| W Foot Tendon, Left | | | |

**0** Medical and Surgical
**L** Tendons
**U** Supplement: Putting in or on biological or synthetic material that physically reinforces and/or augments the function of a portion of a body part

| Character 4 Body Part | | Character 5 Approach | | Character 6 Device | | Character 7 Qualifier | |
|---|---|---|---|---|---|---|---|
| 0 | Head and Neck Tendon | 0 | Open | 7 | Autologous Tissue Substitute | Z | No Qualifier |
| 1 | Shoulder Tendon, Right | 4 | Percutaneous Endoscopic | J | Synthetic Substitute | | |
| 2 | Shoulder Tendon, Left | | | K | Nonautologous Tissue Substitute | | |
| 3 | Upper Arm Tendon, Right | | | | | | |
| 4 | Upper Arm Tendon, Left | | | | | | |
| 5 | Lower Arm and Wrist Tendon, Right | | | | | | |
| 6 | Lower Arm and Wrist Tendon, Left | | | | | | |
| 7 | Hand Tendon, Right | | | | | | |
| 8 | Hand Tendon, Left | | | | | | |
| 9 | Trunk Tendon, Right | | | | | | |
| B | Trunk Tendon, Left | | | | | | |
| C | Thorax Tendon, Right | | | | | | |
| D | Thorax Tendon, Left | | | | | | |
| F | Abdomen Tendon, Right | | | | | | |
| G | Abdomen Tendon, Left | | | | | | |
| H | Perineum Tendon | | | | | | |
| J | Hip Tendon, Right | | | | | | |
| K | Hip Tendon, Left | | | | | | |
| L | Upper Leg Tendon, Right | | | | | | |
| M | Upper Leg Tendon, Left | | | | | | |
| N | Lower Leg Tendon, Right | | | | | | |
| P | Lower Leg Tendon, Left | | | | | | |
| Q | Knee Tendon, Right | | | | | | |
| R | Knee Tendon, Left | | | | | | |
| S | Ankle Tendon, Right | | | | | | |
| T | Ankle Tendon, Left | | | | | | |
| V | Foot Tendon, Right | | | | | | |
| W | Foot Tendon, Left | | | | | | |

**0** Medical and Surgical
**L** Tendons
**W** Revision: Correcting, to the extent possible, a portion of a malfunctioning device or the position of a displaced device

| Character 4 Body Part | | Character 5 Approach | | Character 6 Device | | Character 7 Qualifier | |
|---|---|---|---|---|---|---|---|
| X | Upper Tendon | 0 | Open | 0 | Drainage Device | Z | No Qualifier |
| Y | Lower Tendon | 3 | Percutaneous | 7 | Autologous Tissue Substitute | | |
| | | 4 | Percutaneous Endoscopic | J | Synthetic Substitute | | |
| | | X | External | K | Nonautologous Tissue Substitute | | |

**0** Medical and Surgical
**L** Tendons
**X** Transfer: Moving, without taking out, all or a portion of a body part to another location to take over the function of all or a portion of a body part

| Character 4 Body Part | | Character 5 Approach | | Character 6 Device | | Character 7 Qualifier | |
|---|---|---|---|---|---|---|---|
| 0 | Head and Neck Tendon | 0 | Open | Z | No Device | Z | No Qualifier |
| 1 | Shoulder Tendon, Right | 4 | Percutaneous Endoscopic | | | | |
| 2 | Shoulder Tendon, Left | | | | | | |
| 3 | Upper Arm Tendon, Right | | | | | | |
| 4 | Upper Arm Tendon, Left | | | | | | |
| 5 | Lower Arm and Wrist Tendon, Right | | | | | | |
| 6 | Lower Arm and Wrist Tendon, Left | | | | | | |
| 7 | Hand Tendon, Right | | | | | | |
| 8 | Hand Tendon, Left | | | | | | |
| 9 | Trunk Tendon, Right | | | | | | |
| B | Trunk Tendon, Left | | | | | | |
| C | Thorax Tendon, Right | | | | | | |
| D | Thorax Tendon, Left | | | | | | |
| F | Abdomen Tendon, Right | | | | | | |
| G | Abdomen Tendon, Left | | | | | | |
| H | Perineum Tendon | | | | | | |
| J | Hip Tendon, Right | | | | | | |
| K | Hip Tendon, Left | | | | | | |
| L | Upper Leg Tendon, Right | | | | | | |
| M | Upper Leg Tendon, Left | | | | | | |
| N | Lower Leg Tendon, Right | | | | | | |
| P | Lower Leg Tendon, Left | | | | | | |
| Q | Knee Tendon, Right | | | | | | |
| R | Knee Tendon, Left | | | | | | |
| S | Ankle Tendon, Right | | | | | | |
| T | Ankle Tendon, Left | | | | | | |
| V | Foot Tendon, Right | | | | | | |
| W | Foot Tendon, Left | | | | | | |

# Bursae and Ligaments | 0M2-0MX

**0** Medical and Surgical
**M** Bursae and Ligaments
**2** Change: Taking out or off a device from a body part and putting back an identical or similar device in or on the same body part without cutting or puncturing the skin or a mucous membrane

| Character 4<br>Body Part | Character 5<br>Approach | Character 6<br>Device | Character 7<br>Qualifier |
|---|---|---|---|
| X   Upper Bursa and Ligament<br>Y   Lower Bursa and Ligament | X   External | 0   Drainage Device<br>Y   Other Device | Z   No Qualifier |

**0** Medical and Surgical
**M** Bursae and Ligaments
**5** Destruction: Physical eradication of all or a portion of a body part by the direct use of energy, force, or a destructive agent

| Character 4<br>Body Part | Character 5<br>Approach | Character 6<br>Device | Character 7<br>Qualifier |
|---|---|---|---|
| 0   Head and Neck Bursa and Ligament<br>1   Shoulder Bursa and Ligament, Right<br>2   Shoulder Bursa and Ligament, Left<br>3   Elbow Bursa and Ligament, Right<br>4   Elbow Bursa and Ligament, Left<br>5   Wrist Bursa and Ligament, Right<br>6   Wrist Bursa and Ligament, Left<br>7   Hand Bursa and Ligament, Right<br>8   Hand Bursa and Ligament, Left<br>9   Upper Extremity Bursa and Ligament, Right<br>B   Upper Extremity Bursa and Ligament, Left<br>C   Trunk Bursa and Ligament, Right<br>D   Trunk Bursa and Ligament, Left<br>F   Thorax Bursa and Ligament, Right<br>G   Thorax Bursa and Ligament, Left<br>H   Abdomen Bursa and Ligament, Right<br>J   Abdomen Bursa and Ligament, Left<br>K   Perineum Bursa and Ligament<br>L   Hip Bursa and Ligament, Right<br>M   Hip Bursa and Ligament, Left<br>N   Knee Bursa and Ligament, Right<br>P   Knee Bursa and Ligament, Left<br>Q   Ankle Bursa and Ligament, Right<br>R   Ankle Bursa and Ligament, Left<br>S   Foot Bursa and Ligament, Right<br>T   Foot Bursa and Ligament, Left<br>V   Lower Extremity Bursa and Ligament, Right<br>W   Lower Extremity Bursa and Ligament, Left | 0   Open<br>3   Percutaneous<br>4   Percutaneous Endoscopic | Z   No Device | Z   No Qualifier |

**0 Medical and Surgical**
**M Bursae and Ligaments**
**8 Division: Cutting into a body part, without draining fluids and/or gases from the body part, in order to separate or transect a body part**

| Character 4<br>Body Part | Character 5<br>Approach | Character 6<br>Device | Character 7<br>Qualifier |
|---|---|---|---|
| 0 Head and Neck Bursa and Ligament | 0 Open | Z No Device | Z No Qualifier |
| 1 Shoulder Bursa and Ligament, Right | 3 Percutaneous | | |
| 2 Shoulder Bursa and Ligament, Left | 4 Percutaneous Endoscopic | | |
| 3 Elbow Bursa and Ligament, Right | | | |
| 4 Elbow Bursa and Ligament, Left | | | |
| 5 Wrist Bursa and Ligament, Right | | | |
| 6 Wrist Bursa and Ligament, Left | | | |
| 7 Hand Bursa and Ligament, Right | | | |
| 8 Hand Bursa and Ligament, Left | | | |
| 9 Upper Extremity Bursa and Ligament, Right | | | |
| B Upper Extremity Bursa and Ligament, Left | | | |
| C Trunk Bursa and Ligament, Right | | | |
| D Trunk Bursa and Ligament, Left | | | |
| F Thorax Bursa and Ligament, Right | | | |
| G Thorax Bursa and Ligament, Left | | | |
| H Abdomen Bursa and Ligament, Right | | | |
| J Abdomen Bursa and Ligament, Left | | | |
| K Perineum Bursa and Ligament | | | |
| L Hip Bursa and Ligament, Right | | | |
| M Hip Bursa and Ligament, Left | | | |
| N Knee Bursa and Ligament, Right | | | |
| P Knee Bursa and Ligament, Left | | | |
| Q Ankle Bursa and Ligament, Right | | | |
| R Ankle Bursa and Ligament, Left | | | |
| S Foot Bursa and Ligament, Right | | | |
| T Foot Bursa and Ligament, Left | | | |
| V Lower Extremity Bursa and Ligament, Right | | | |
| W Lower Extremity Bursa and Ligament, Left | | | |

**0** Medical and Surgical
**M** Bursae and Ligaments
**9** Drainage: Taking or letting out fluids and/or gases from a body part

| Character 4 Body Part | Character 5 Approach | Character 6 Device | Character 7 Qualifier |
|---|---|---|---|
| 0 Head and Neck Bursa and Ligament | 0 Open | 0 Drainage Device | Z No Qualifier |
| 1 Shoulder Bursa and Ligament, Right | 3 Percutaneous | | |
| 2 Shoulder Bursa and Ligament, Left | 4 Percutaneous Endoscopic | | |
| 3 Elbow Bursa and Ligament, Right | | | |
| 4 Elbow Bursa and Ligament, Left | | | |
| 5 Wrist Bursa and Ligament, Right | | | |
| 6 Wrist Bursa and Ligament, Left | | | |
| 7 Hand Bursa and Ligament, Right | | | |
| 8 Hand Bursa and Ligament, Left | | | |
| 9 Upper Extremity Bursa and Ligament, Right | | | |
| B Upper Extremity Bursa and Ligament, Left | | | |
| C Trunk Bursa and Ligament, Right | | | |
| D Trunk Bursa and Ligament, Left | | | |
| F Thorax Bursa and Ligament, Right | | | |
| G Thorax Bursa and Ligament, Left | | | |
| H Abdomen Bursa and Ligament, Right | | | |
| J Abdomen Bursa and Ligament, Left | | | |
| K Perineum Bursa and Ligament | | | |
| L Hip Bursa and Ligament, Right | | | |
| M Hip Bursa and Ligament, Left | | | |
| N Knee Bursa and Ligament, Right | | | |
| P Knee Bursa and Ligament, Left | | | |
| Q Ankle Bursa and Ligament, Right | | | |
| R Ankle Bursa and Ligament, Left | | | |
| S Foot Bursa and Ligament, Right | | | |
| T Foot Bursa and Ligament, Left | | | |
| V Lower Extremity Bursa and Ligament, Right | | | |
| W Lower Extremity Bursa and Ligament, Left | | | |

| Character 4 Body Part | Character 5 Approach | Character 6 Device | Character 7 Qualifier |
|---|---|---|---|
| 0 Head and Neck Bursa and Ligament | 0 Open | Z No Device | X Diagnostic |
| 1 Shoulder Bursa and Ligament, Right | 3 Percutaneous | | Z No Qualifier |
| 2 Shoulder Bursa and Ligament, Left | 4 Percutaneous Endoscopic | | |
| 3 Elbow Bursa and Ligament, Right | | | |
| 4 Elbow Bursa and Ligament, Left | | | |
| 5 Wrist Bursa and Ligament, Right | | | |
| 6 Wrist Bursa and Ligament, Left | | | |
| 7 Hand Bursa and Ligament, Right | | | |
| 8 Hand Bursa and Ligament, Left | | | |
| 9 Upper Extremity Bursa and Ligament, Right | | | |
| B Upper Extremity Bursa and Ligament, Left | | | |
| C Trunk Bursa and Ligament, Right | | | |
| D Trunk Bursa and Ligament, Left | | | |
| F Thorax Bursa and Ligament, Right | | | |
| G Thorax Bursa and Ligament, Left | | | |
| H Abdomen Bursa and Ligament, Right | | | |
| J Abdomen Bursa and Ligament, Left | | | |
| K Perineum Bursa and Ligament | | | |
| L Hip Bursa and Ligament, Right | | | |
| M Hip Bursa and Ligament, Left | | | |
| N Knee Bursa and Ligament, Right | | | |
| P Knee Bursa and Ligament, Left | | | |
| Q Ankle Bursa and Ligament, Right | | | |
| R Ankle Bursa and Ligament, Left | | | |
| S Foot Bursa and Ligament, Right | | | |
| T Foot Bursa and Ligament, Left | | | |
| V Lower Extremity Bursa and Ligament, Right | | | |
| W Lower Extremity Bursa and Ligament, Left | | | |

**0** Medical and Surgical
**M** Bursae and Ligaments
**B** Excision: Cutting out or off, without replacement, a portion of a body part

| Character 4<br>Body Part | Character 5<br>Approach | Character 6<br>Device | Character 7<br>Qualifier |
|---|---|---|---|
| 0 Head and Neck Bursa and Ligament | 0 Open | Z No Device | X Diagnostic |
| 1 Shoulder Bursa and Ligament, Right | 3 Percutaneous | | Z No Qualifier |
| 2 Shoulder Bursa and Ligament, Left | 4 Percutaneous Endoscopic | | |
| 3 Elbow Bursa and Ligament, Right | | | |
| 4 Elbow Bursa and Ligament, Left | | | |
| 5 Wrist Bursa and Ligament, Right | | | |
| 6 Wrist Bursa and Ligament, Left | | | |
| 7 Hand Bursa and Ligament, Right | | | |
| 8 Hand Bursa and Ligament, Left | | | |
| 9 Upper Extremity Bursa and Ligament, Right | | | |
| B Upper Extremity Bursa and Ligament, Left | | | |
| C Trunk Bursa and Ligament, Right | | | |
| D Trunk Bursa and Ligament, Left | | | |
| F Thorax Bursa and Ligament, Right | | | |
| G Thorax Bursa and Ligament, Left | | | |
| H Abdomen Bursa and Ligament, Right | | | |
| J Abdomen Bursa and Ligament, Left | | | |
| K Perineum Bursa and Ligament | | | |
| L Hip Bursa and Ligament, Right | | | |
| M Hip Bursa and Ligament, Left | | | |
| N Knee Bursa and Ligament, Right | | | |
| P Knee Bursa and Ligament, Left | | | |
| Q Ankle Bursa and Ligament, Right | | | |
| R Ankle Bursa and Ligament, Left | | | |
| S Foot Bursa and Ligament, Right | | | |
| T Foot Bursa and Ligament, Left | | | |
| V Lower Extremity Bursa and Ligament, Right | | | |
| W Lower Extremity Bursa and Ligament, Left | | | |

**0** Medical and Surgical
**M** Bursae and Ligaments
**C** Extirpation: Taking or cutting out solid matter from a body part

| Character 4<br>Body Part | Character 5<br>Approach | Character 6<br>Device | Character 7<br>Qualifier |
|---|---|---|---|
| 0 Head and Neck Bursa and Ligament | 0 Open | Z No Device | Z No Qualifier |
| 1 Shoulder Bursa and Ligament, Right | 3 Percutaneous | | |
| 2 Shoulder Bursa and Ligament, Left | 4 Percutaneous Endoscopic | | |
| 3 Elbow Bursa and Ligament, Right | | | |
| 4 Elbow Bursa and Ligament, Left | | | |
| 5 Wrist Bursa and Ligament, Right | | | |
| 6 Wrist Bursa and Ligament, Left | | | |
| 7 Hand Bursa and Ligament, Right | | | |
| 8 Hand Bursa and Ligament, Left | | | |
| 9 Upper Extremity Bursa and Ligament, Right | | | |
| B Upper Extremity Bursa and Ligament, Left | | | |
| C Trunk Bursa and Ligament, Right | | | |
| D Trunk Bursa and Ligament, Left | | | |
| F Thorax Bursa and Ligament, Right | | | |
| G Thorax Bursa and Ligament, Left | | | |
| H Abdomen Bursa and Ligament, Right | | | |
| J Abdomen Bursa and Ligament, Left | | | |
| K Perineum Bursa and Ligament | | | |
| L Hip Bursa and Ligament, Right | | | |
| M Hip Bursa and Ligament, Left | | | |
| N Knee Bursa and Ligament, Right | | | |
| P Knee Bursa and Ligament, Left | | | |
| Q Ankle Bursa and Ligament, Right | | | |
| R Ankle Bursa and Ligament, Left | | | |
| S Foot Bursa and Ligament, Right | | | |
| T Foot Bursa and Ligament, Left | | | |
| V Lower Extremity Bursa and Ligament, Right | | | |
| W Lower Extremity Bursa and Ligament, Left | | | |

0   Medical and Surgical
M   Bursae and Ligaments
D   Extraction: Pulling or stripping out or off all or a portion of a body part by the use of force

| Character 4<br>Body Part | Character 5<br>Approach | Character 6<br>Device | Character 7<br>Qualifier |
|---|---|---|---|
| 0   Head and Neck Bursa and Ligament<br>1   Shoulder Bursa and Ligament, Right<br>2   Shoulder Bursa and Ligament, Left<br>3   Elbow Bursa and Ligament, Right<br>4   Elbow Bursa and Ligament, Left<br>5   Wrist Bursa and Ligament, Right<br>6   Wrist Bursa and Ligament, Left<br>7   Hand Bursa and Ligament, Right<br>8   Hand Bursa and Ligament, Left<br>9   Upper Extremity Bursa and Ligament,<br>      Right<br>B   Upper Extremity Bursa and Ligament,<br>      Left<br>C   Trunk Bursa and Ligament, Right<br>D   Trunk Bursa and Ligament, Left<br>F   Thorax Bursa and Ligament, Right<br>G   Thorax Bursa and Ligament, Left<br>H   Abdomen Bursa and Ligament, Right<br>J   Abdomen Bursa and Ligament, Left<br>K   Perineum Bursa and Ligament<br>L   Hip Bursa and Ligament, Right<br>M   Hip Bursa and Ligament, Left<br>N   Knee Bursa and Ligament, Right<br>P   Knee Bursa and Ligament, Left<br>Q   Ankle Bursa and Ligament, Right<br>R   Ankle Bursa and Ligament, Left<br>S   Foot Bursa and Ligament, Right<br>T   Foot Bursa and Ligament, Left<br>V   Lower Extremity Bursa and Ligament,<br>      Right<br>W   Lower Extremity Bursa and Ligament,<br>      Left | 0   Open<br>3   Percutaneous<br>4   Percutaneous Endoscopic | Z   No Device | Z   No Qualifier |

0   Medical and Surgical
M   Bursae and Ligaments
J   Inspection: Visually and/or manually exploring a body part

| Character 4<br>Body Part | Character 5<br>Approach | Character 6<br>Device | Character 7<br>Qualifier |
|---|---|---|---|
| X   Upper Bursa and Ligament<br>Y   Lower Bursa and Ligament | 0   Open<br>3   Percutaneous<br>4   Percutaneous Endoscopic<br>X   External | Z   No Device | Z   No Qualifier |

**0 Medical and Surgical**
**M Bursae and Ligaments**
**M Reattachment:** Putting back in or on all or a portion of a separated body part to its normal location or other suitable location

| Character 4<br>Body Part | Character 5<br>Approach | Character 6<br>Device | Character 7<br>Qualifier |
|---|---|---|---|
| 0 Head and Neck Bursa and Ligament<br>1 Shoulder Bursa and Ligament, Right<br>2 Shoulder Bursa and Ligament, Left<br>3 Elbow Bursa and Ligament, Right<br>4 Elbow Bursa and Ligament, Left<br>5 Wrist Bursa and Ligament, Right<br>6 Wrist Bursa and Ligament, Left<br>7 Hand Bursa and Ligament, Right<br>8 Hand Bursa and Ligament, Left<br>9 Upper Extremity Bursa and Ligament,<br>   Right<br>B Upper Extremity Bursa and Ligament,<br>   Left<br>C Trunk Bursa and Ligament, Right<br>D Trunk Bursa and Ligament, Left<br>F Thorax Bursa and Ligament, Right<br>G Thorax Bursa and Ligament, Left<br>H Abdomen Bursa and Ligament, Right<br>J Abdomen Bursa and Ligament, Left<br>K Perineum Bursa and Ligament<br>L Hip Bursa and Ligament, Right<br>M Hip Bursa and Ligament, Left<br>N Knee Bursa and Ligament, Right<br>P Knee Bursa and Ligament, Left<br>Q Ankle Bursa and Ligament, Right<br>R Ankle Bursa and Ligament, Left<br>S Foot Bursa and Ligament, Right<br>T Foot Bursa and Ligament, Left<br>V Lower Extremity Bursa and Ligament,<br>   Right<br>W Lower Extremity Bursa and Ligament,<br>   Left | 0 Open<br>4 Percutaneous Endoscopic | Z No Device | Z No Qualifier |

**AHA:** 0MM14ZZ - 3Q 2013, 22

**0 Medical and Surgical**
**M Bursae and Ligaments**
**N Release:** Freeing a body part from an abnormal physical constraint by cutting or by the use of force

| Character 4<br>Body Part | Character 5<br>Approach | Character 6<br>Device | Character 7<br>Qualifier |
|---|---|---|---|
| 0 Head and Neck Bursa and Ligament<br>1 Shoulder Bursa and Ligament, Right<br>2 Shoulder Bursa and Ligament, Left<br>3 Elbow Bursa and Ligament, Right<br>4 Elbow Bursa and Ligament, Left<br>5 Wrist Bursa and Ligament, Right<br>6 Wrist Bursa and Ligament, Left<br>7 Hand Bursa and Ligament, Right<br>8 Hand Bursa and Ligament, Left<br>9 Upper Extremity Bursa and Ligament,<br>   Right<br>B Upper Extremity Bursa and Ligament,<br>   Left<br>C Trunk Bursa and Ligament, Right<br>D Trunk Bursa and Ligament, Left<br>F Thorax Bursa and Ligament, Right<br>G Thorax Bursa and Ligament, Left<br>H Abdomen Bursa and Ligament, Right<br>J Abdomen Bursa and Ligament, Left<br>K Perineum Bursa and Ligament<br>L Hip Bursa and Ligament, Right<br>M Hip Bursa and Ligament, Left<br>N Knee Bursa and Ligament, Right<br>P Knee Bursa and Ligament, Left<br>Q Ankle Bursa and Ligament, Right<br>R Ankle Bursa and Ligament, Left<br>S Foot Bursa and Ligament, Right<br>T Foot Bursa and Ligament, Left<br>V Lower Extremity Bursa and Ligament,<br>   Right<br>W Lower Extremity Bursa and Ligament,<br>   Left | 0 Open<br>3 Percutaneous<br>4 Percutaneous Endoscopic<br>X External | Z No Device | Z No Qualifier |

**0** Medical and Surgical
**M** Bursae and Ligaments
**P** Removal: Taking out or off a device from a body part

| Character 4<br>Body Part | Character 5<br>Approach | Character 6<br>Device | Character 7<br>Qualifier |
|---|---|---|---|
| X Upper Bursa and Ligament<br>Y Lower Bursa and Ligament | 0 Open<br>3 Percutaneous<br>4 Percutaneous Endoscopic | 0 Drainage Device<br>7 Autologous Tissue Substitute<br>J Synthetic Substitute<br>K Nonautologous Tissue Substitute | Z No Qualifier |
| X Upper Bursa and Ligament<br>Y Lower Bursa and Ligament | X External | 0 Drainage Device | Z No Qualifier |

**0** Medical and Surgical
**M** Bursae and Ligaments
**Q** Repair: Restoring, to the extent possible, a body part to its normal anatomic structure and function

| Character 4<br>Body Part | Character 5<br>Approach | Character 6<br>Device | Character 7<br>Qualifier |
|---|---|---|---|
| 0 Head and Neck Bursa and Ligament<br>1 Shoulder Bursa and Ligament, Right<br>2 Shoulder Bursa and Ligament, Left<br>3 Elbow Bursa and Ligament, Right<br>4 Elbow Bursa and Ligament, Left<br>5 Wrist Bursa and Ligament, Right<br>6 Wrist Bursa and Ligament, Left<br>7 Hand Bursa and Ligament, Right<br>8 Hand Bursa and Ligament, Left<br>9 Upper Extremity Bursa and Ligament, Right<br>B Upper Extremity Bursa and Ligament, Left<br>C Trunk Bursa and Ligament, Right<br>D Trunk Bursa and Ligament, Left<br>F Thorax Bursa and Ligament, Right<br>G Thorax Bursa and Ligament, Left<br>H Abdomen Bursa and Ligament, Right<br>J Abdomen Bursa and Ligament, Left<br>K Perineum Bursa and Ligament<br>L Hip Bursa and Ligament, Right<br>M Hip Bursa and Ligament, Left<br>N Knee Bursa and Ligament, Right<br>P Knee Bursa and Ligament, Left<br>Q Ankle Bursa and Ligament, Right<br>R Ankle Bursa and Ligament, Left<br>S Foot Bursa and Ligament, Right<br>T Foot Bursa and Ligament, Left<br>V Lower Extremity Bursa and Ligament, Right<br>W Lower Extremity Bursa and Ligament, Left | 0 Open<br>3 Percutaneous<br>4 Percutaneous Endoscopic | Z No Device | Z No Qualifier |

**0** Medical and Surgical
**M** Bursae and Ligaments
**S** Reposition: Moving to its normal location, or other suitable location, all or a portion of a body part

| Character 4 Body Part | Character 5 Approach | Character 6 Device | Character 7 Qualifier |
|---|---|---|---|
| 0 Head and Neck Bursa and Ligament | 0 Open | Z No Device | Z No Qualifier |
| 1 Shoulder Bursa and Ligament, Right | 4 Percutaneous Endoscopic | | |
| 2 Shoulder Bursa and Ligament, Left | | | |
| 3 Elbow Bursa and Ligament, Right | | | |
| 4 Elbow Bursa and Ligament, Left | | | |
| 5 Wrist Bursa and Ligament, Right | | | |
| 6 Wrist Bursa and Ligament, Left | | | |
| 7 Hand Bursa and Ligament, Right | | | |
| 8 Hand Bursa and Ligament, Left | | | |
| 9 Upper Extremity Bursa and Ligament, Right | | | |
| B Upper Extremity Bursa and Ligament, Left | | | |
| C Trunk Bursa and Ligament, Right | | | |
| D Trunk Bursa and Ligament, Left | | | |
| F Thorax Bursa and Ligament, Right | | | |
| G Thorax Bursa and Ligament, Left | | | |
| H Abdomen Bursa and Ligament, Right | | | |
| J Abdomen Bursa and Ligament, Left | | | |
| K Perineum Bursa and Ligament | | | |
| L Hip Bursa and Ligament, Right | | | |
| M Hip Bursa and Ligament, Left | | | |
| N Knee Bursa and Ligament, Right | | | |
| P Knee Bursa and Ligament, Left | | | |
| Q Ankle Bursa and Ligament, Right | | | |
| R Ankle Bursa and Ligament, Left | | | |
| S Foot Bursa and Ligament, Right | | | |
| T Foot Bursa and Ligament, Left | | | |
| V Lower Extremity Bursa and Ligament, Right | | | |
| W Lower Extremity Bursa and Ligament, Left | | | |

**0** Medical and Surgical
**M** Bursae and Ligaments
**T** Resection: Cutting out or off, without replacement, all of a body part

| Character 4 Body Part | Character 5 Approach | Character 6 Device | Character 7 Qualifier |
|---|---|---|---|
| 0 Head and Neck Bursa and Ligament | 0 Open | Z No Device | Z No Qualifier |
| 1 Shoulder Bursa and Ligament, Right | 4 Percutaneous Endoscopic | | |
| 2 Shoulder Bursa and Ligament, Left | | | |
| 3 Elbow Bursa and Ligament, Right | | | |
| 4 Elbow Bursa and Ligament, Left | | | |
| 5 Wrist Bursa and Ligament, Right | | | |
| 6 Wrist Bursa and Ligament, Left | | | |
| 7 Hand Bursa and Ligament, Right | | | |
| 8 Hand Bursa and Ligament, Left | | | |
| 9 Upper Extremity Bursa and Ligament, Right | | | |
| B Upper Extremity Bursa and Ligament, Left | | | |
| C Trunk Bursa and Ligament, Right | | | |
| D Trunk Bursa and Ligament, Left | | | |
| F Thorax Bursa and Ligament, Right | | | |
| G Thorax Bursa and Ligament, Left | | | |
| H Abdomen Bursa and Ligament, Right | | | |
| J Abdomen Bursa and Ligament, Left | | | |
| K Perineum Bursa and Ligament | | | |
| L Hip Bursa and Ligament, Right | | | |
| M Hip Bursa and Ligament, Left | | | |
| N Knee Bursa and Ligament, Right | | | |
| P Knee Bursa and Ligament, Left | | | |
| Q Ankle Bursa and Ligament, Right | | | |
| R Ankle Bursa and Ligament, Left | | | |
| S Foot Bursa and Ligament, Right | | | |
| T Foot Bursa and Ligament, Left | | | |
| V Lower Extremity Bursa and Ligament, Right | | | |
| W Lower Extremity Bursa and Ligament, Left | | | |

**0** Medical and Surgical
**M** Bursae and Ligaments
**U** Supplement: Putting in or on biological or synthetic material that physically reinforces and/or augments the function of a portion of a body part

| Character 4<br>Body Part | Character 5<br>Approach | Character 6<br>Device | Character 7<br>Qualifier |
|---|---|---|---|
| 0 Head and Neck Bursa and Ligament<br>1 Shoulder Bursa and Ligament, Right<br>2 Shoulder Bursa and Ligament, Left<br>3 Elbow Bursa and Ligament, Right<br>4 Elbow Bursa and Ligament, Left<br>5 Wrist Bursa and Ligament, Right<br>6 Wrist Bursa and Ligament, Left<br>7 Hand Bursa and Ligament, Right<br>8 Hand Bursa and Ligament, Left<br>9 Upper Extremity Bursa and Ligament, Right<br>B Upper Extremity Bursa and Ligament, Left<br>C Trunk Bursa and Ligament, Right<br>D Trunk Bursa and Ligament, Left<br>F Thorax Bursa and Ligament, Right<br>G Thorax Bursa and Ligament, Left<br>H Abdomen Bursa and Ligament, Right<br>J Abdomen Bursa and Ligament, Left<br>K Perineum Bursa and Ligament<br>L Hip Bursa and Ligament, Right<br>M Hip Bursa and Ligament, Left<br>N Knee Bursa and Ligament, Right<br>P Knee Bursa and Ligament, Left<br>Q Ankle Bursa and Ligament, Right<br>R Ankle Bursa and Ligament, Left<br>S Foot Bursa and Ligament, Right<br>T Foot Bursa and Ligament, Left<br>V Lower Extremity Bursa and Ligament, Right<br>W Lower Extremity Bursa and Ligament, Left | 0 Open<br>4 Percutaneous Endoscopic | 7 Autologous Tissue Substitute<br>J Synthetic Substitute<br>K Nonautologous Tissue Substitute | Z No Qualifier |

**0** Medical and Surgical
**M** Bursae and Ligaments
**W** Revision: Correcting, to the extent possible, a portion of a malfunctioning device or the position of a displaced device

| Character 4<br>Body Part | Character 5<br>Approach | Character 6<br>Device | Character 7<br>Qualifier |
|---|---|---|---|
| X Upper Bursa and Ligament<br>Y Lower Bursa and Ligament | 0 Open<br>3 Percutaneous<br>4 Percutaneous Endoscopic<br>X External | 0 Drainage Device<br>7 Autologous Tissue Substitute<br>J Synthetic Substitute<br>K Nonautologous Tissue Substitute | Z No Qualifier |

**0** Medical and Surgical
**M** Bursae and Ligaments
**X** Transfer: Moving, without taking out, all or a portion of a body part to another location to take over the function of all or a portion of a body part

| Character 4<br>Body Part | Character 5<br>Approach | Character 6<br>Device | Character 7<br>Qualifier |
|---|---|---|---|
| 0 Head and Neck Bursa and Ligament | 0 Open | Z No Device | Z No Qualifier |
| 1 Shoulder Bursa and Ligament, Right | 4 Percutaneous Endoscopic | | |
| 2 Shoulder Bursa and Ligament, Left | | | |
| 3 Elbow Bursa and Ligament, Right | | | |
| 4 Elbow Bursa and Ligament, Left | | | |
| 5 Wrist Bursa and Ligament, Right | | | |
| 6 Wrist Bursa and Ligament, Left | | | |
| 7 Hand Bursa and Ligament, Right | | | |
| 8 Hand Bursa and Ligament, Left | | | |
| 9 Upper Extremity Bursa and Ligament, Right | | | |
| B Upper Extremity Bursa and Ligament, Left | | | |
| C Trunk Bursa and Ligament, Right | | | |
| D Trunk Bursa and Ligament, Left | | | |
| F Thorax Bursa and Ligament, Right | | | |
| G Thorax Bursa and Ligament, Left | | | |
| H Abdomen Bursa and Ligament, Right | | | |
| J Abdomen Bursa and Ligament, Left | | | |
| K Perineum Bursa and Ligament | | | |
| L Hip Bursa and Ligament, Right | | | |
| M Hip Bursa and Ligament, Left | | | |
| N Knee Bursa and Ligament, Right | | | |
| P Knee Bursa and Ligament, Left | | | |
| Q Ankle Bursa and Ligament, Right | | | |
| R Ankle Bursa and Ligament, Left | | | |
| S Foot Bursa and Ligament, Right | | | |
| T Foot Bursa and Ligament, Left | | | |
| V Lower Extremity Bursa and Ligament, Right | | | |
| W Lower Extremity Bursa and Ligament, Left | | | |

# Head and Facial Bones | 0N2-0NW

**0** Medical and Surgical
**N** Head and Facial Bones
**2** Change: Taking out or off a device from a body part and putting back an identical or similar device in or on the same body part without cutting or puncturing the skin or a mucous membrane

| Character 4 Body Part | Character 5 Approach | Character 6 Device | Character 7 Qualifier |
|---|---|---|---|
| 0 Skull<br>B Nasal Bone<br>W Facial Bone | X External | 0 Drainage Device<br>Y Other Device | Z No Qualifier |

**0** Medical and Surgical
**N** Head and Facial Bones
**5** Destruction: Physical eradication of all or a portion of a body part by the direct use of energy, force, or a destructive agent

| Character 4 Body Part | Character 5 Approach | Character 6 Device | Character 7 Qualifier |
|---|---|---|---|
| 0 Skull<br>1 Frontal Bone, Right<br>2 Frontal Bone, Left<br>3 Parietal Bone, Right<br>4 Parietal Bone, Left<br>5 Temporal Bone, Right<br>6 Temporal Bone, Left<br>7 Occipital Bone, Right<br>8 Occipital Bone, Left<br>B Nasal Bone<br>C Sphenoid Bone, Right<br>D Sphenoid Bone, Left<br>F Ethmoid Bone, Right<br>G Ethmoid Bone, Left<br>H Lacrimal Bone, Right<br>J Lacrimal Bone, Left<br>K Palatine Bone, Right<br>L Palatine Bone, Left<br>M Zygomatic Bone, Right<br>N Zygomatic Bone, Left<br>P Orbit, Right<br>Q Orbit, Left<br>R Maxilla, Right<br>S Maxilla, Left<br>T Mandible, Right<br>V Mandible, Left<br>X Hyoid Bone | 0 Open<br>3 Percutaneous<br>4 Percutaneous Endoscopic | Z No Device | Z No Qualifier |

**0** Medical and Surgical
**N** Head and Facial Bones
**8** Division: Cutting into a body part, without draining fluids and/or gases from the body part, in order to separate or transect a body part

| Character 4 Body Part | Character 5 Approach | Character 6 Device | Character 7 Qualifier |
|---|---|---|---|
| 0 Skull<br>1 Frontal Bone, Right<br>2 Frontal Bone, Left<br>3 Parietal Bone, Right<br>4 Parietal Bone, Left<br>5 Temporal Bone, Right<br>6 Temporal Bone, Left<br>7 Occipital Bone, Right<br>8 Occipital Bone, Left<br>B Nasal Bone<br>C Sphenoid Bone, Right<br>D Sphenoid Bone, Left<br>F Ethmoid Bone, Right<br>G Ethmoid Bone, Left<br>H Lacrimal Bone, Right<br>J Lacrimal Bone, Left<br>K Palatine Bone, Right<br>L Palatine Bone, Left<br>M Zygomatic Bone, Right<br>N Zygomatic Bone, Left<br>P Orbit, Right<br>Q Orbit, Left<br>R Maxilla, Right<br>S Maxilla, Left<br>T Mandible, Right<br>V Mandible, Left<br>X Hyoid Bone | 0 Open<br>3 Percutaneous<br>4 Percutaneous Endoscopic | Z No Device | Z No Qualifier |

| 0 Medical and Surgical |
| N Head and Facial Bones |
| 9 Drainage: Taking or letting out fluids and/or gases from a body part |

| Character 4<br>Body Part | Character 5<br>Approach | Character 6<br>Device | Character 7<br>Qualifier |
|---|---|---|---|
| 0 Skull<br>1 Frontal Bone, Right<br>2 Frontal Bone, Left<br>3 Parietal Bone, Right<br>4 Parietal Bone, Left<br>5 Temporal Bone, Right<br>6 Temporal Bone, Left<br>7 Occipital Bone, Right<br>8 Occipital Bone, Left<br>B Nasal Bone<br>C Sphenoid Bone, Right<br>D Sphenoid Bone, Left<br>F Ethmoid Bone, Right<br>G Ethmoid Bone, Left<br>H Lacrimal Bone, Right<br>J Lacrimal Bone, Left<br>K Palatine Bone, Right<br>L Palatine Bone, Left<br>M Zygomatic Bone, Right<br>N Zygomatic Bone, Left<br>P Orbit, Right<br>Q Orbit, Left<br>R Maxilla, Right<br>S Maxilla, Left<br>T Mandible, Right<br>V Mandible, Left<br>X Hyoid Bone | 0 Open<br>3 Percutaneous<br>4 Percutaneous Endoscopic | 0 Drainage Device | Z No Qualifier |
| 0 Skull<br>1 Frontal Bone, Right<br>2 Frontal Bone, Left<br>3 Parietal Bone, Right<br>4 Parietal Bone, Left<br>5 Temporal Bone, Right<br>6 Temporal Bone, Left<br>7 Occipital Bone, Right<br>8 Occipital Bone, Left<br>B Nasal Bone<br>C Sphenoid Bone, Right<br>D Sphenoid Bone, Left<br>F Ethmoid Bone, Right<br>G Ethmoid Bone, Left<br>H Lacrimal Bone, Right<br>J Lacrimal Bone, Left<br>K Palatine Bone, Right<br>L Palatine Bone, Left<br>M Zygomatic Bone, Right<br>N Zygomatic Bone, Left<br>P Orbit, Right<br>Q Orbit, Left<br>R Maxilla, Right<br>S Maxilla, Left<br>T Mandible, Right<br>V Mandible, Left<br>X Hyoid Bone | 0 Open<br>3 Percutaneous<br>4 Percutaneous Endoscopic | Z No Device | X Diagnostic<br>Z No Qualifier |

**0** Medical and Surgical
**N** Head and Facial Bones
**B** Excision: Cutting out or off, without replacement, a portion of a body part

| Character 4<br>Body Part | Character 5<br>Approach | Character 6<br>Device | Character 7<br>Qualifier |
|---|---|---|---|
| 0 Skull<br>1 Frontal Bone, Right<br>2 Frontal Bone, Left<br>3 Parietal Bone, Right<br>4 Parietal Bone, Left<br>5 Temporal Bone, Right<br>6 Temporal Bone, Left<br>7 Occipital Bone, Right<br>8 Occipital Bone, Left<br>B Nasal Bone<br>C Sphenoid Bone, Right<br>D Sphenoid Bone, Left<br>F Ethmoid Bone, Right<br>G Ethmoid Bone, Left<br>H Lacrimal Bone, Right<br>J Lacrimal Bone, Left<br>K Palatine Bone, Right<br>L Palatine Bone, Left<br>M Zygomatic Bone, Right<br>N Zygomatic Bone, Left<br>P Orbit, Right<br>Q Orbit, Left<br>R Maxilla, Right<br>S Maxilla, Left<br>T Mandible, Right<br>V Mandible, Left<br>X Hyoid Bone | 0 Open<br>3 Percutaneous<br>4 Percutaneous Endoscopic | Z No Device | X Diagnostic<br>Z No Qualifier |

**0** Medical and Surgical
**N** Head and Facial Bones
**C** Extirpation: Taking or cutting out solid matter from a body part

| Character 4<br>Body Part | Character 5<br>Approach | Character 6<br>Device | Character 7<br>Qualifier |
|---|---|---|---|
| 1 Frontal Bone, Right<br>2 Frontal Bone, Left<br>3 Parietal Bone, Right<br>4 Parietal Bone, Left<br>5 Temporal Bone, Right<br>6 Temporal Bone, Left<br>7 Occipital Bone, Right<br>8 Occipital Bone, Left<br>B Nasal Bone<br>C Sphenoid Bone, Right<br>D Sphenoid Bone, Left<br>F Ethmoid Bone, Right<br>G Ethmoid Bone, Left<br>H Lacrimal Bone, Right<br>J Lacrimal Bone, Left<br>K Palatine Bone, Right<br>L Palatine Bone, Left<br>M Zygomatic Bone, Right<br>N Zygomatic Bone, Left<br>P Orbit, Right<br>Q Orbit, Left<br>R Maxilla, Right<br>S Maxilla, Left<br>T Mandible, Right<br>V Mandible, Left<br>X Hyoid Bone | 0 Open<br>3 Percutaneous<br>4 Percutaneous Endoscopic | Z No Device | Z No Qualifier |

**0** Medical and Surgical
**N** Head and Facial Bones
**H** Insertion: Putting in a nonbiological appliance that monitors, assists, performs, or prevents a physiological function but does not physically take the place of a body part

| Character 4<br>Body Part | Character 5<br>Approach | Character 6<br>Device | Character 7<br>Qualifier |
|---|---|---|---|
| 0 Skull | 0 Open | 4 Internal Fixation Device<br>5 External Fixation Device<br>M Bone Growth Stimulator<br>N Neurostimulator Generator | Z No Qualifier |
| 0 Skull | 3 Percutaneous<br>4 Percutaneous Endoscopic | 4 Internal Fixation Device<br>5 External Fixation Device<br>M Bone Growth Stimulator | Z No Qualifier |
| 1 Frontal Bone, Right<br>2 Frontal Bone, Left<br>3 Parietal Bone, Right<br>4 Parietal Bone, Left<br>7 Occipital Bone, Right<br>8 Occipital Bone, Left<br>C Sphenoid Bone, Right<br>D Sphenoid Bone, Left<br>F Ethmoid Bone, Right<br>G Ethmoid Bone, Left<br>H Lacrimal Bone, Right<br>J Lacrimal Bone, Left<br>K Palatine Bone, Right<br>L Palatine Bone, Left<br>M Zygomatic Bone, Right<br>N Zygomatic Bone, Left<br>P Orbit, Right<br>Q Orbit, Left<br>X Hyoid Bone | 0 Open<br>3 Percutaneous<br>4 Percutaneous Endoscopic | 4 Internal Fixation Device | Z No Qualifier |
| 5 Temporal Bone, Right<br>6 Temporal Bone, Left | 0 Open<br>3 Percutaneous<br>4 Percutaneous Endoscopic | 4 Internal Fixation Device<br>S Hearing Device | Z No Qualifier |
| B Nasal Bone | 0 Open<br>3 Percutaneous<br>4 Percutaneous Endoscopic | 4 Internal Fixation Device<br>M Bone Growth Stimulator | Z No Qualifier |
| R Maxilla, Right<br>S Maxilla, Left<br>T Mandible, Right<br>V Mandible, Left | 0 Open<br>3 Percutaneous<br>4 Percutaneous Endoscopic | 4 Internal Fixation Device<br>5 External Fixation Device | Z No Qualifier |
| W Facial Bone | 0 Open<br>3 Percutaneous<br>4 Percutaneous Endoscopic | M Bone Growth Stimulator | Z No Qualifier |

**0** Medical and Surgical
**N** Head and Facial Bones
**J** Inspection: Visually and/or manually exploring a body part

| Character 4<br>Body Part | Character 5<br>Approach | Character 6<br>Device | Character 7<br>Qualifier |
|---|---|---|---|
| 0 Skull<br>B Nasal Bone<br>W Facial Bone | 0 Open<br>3 Percutaneous<br>4 Percutaneous Endoscopic<br>X External | Z No Device | Z No Qualifier |

**0** Medical and Surgical
**N** Head and Facial Bones
**N** Release: Freeing a body part from an abnormal physical constraint by cutting or by the use of force

| Character 4<br>Body Part | Character 5<br>Approach | Character 6<br>Device | Character 7<br>Qualifier |
|---|---|---|---|
| 1 Frontal Bone, Right<br>2 Frontal Bone, Left<br>3 Parietal Bone, Right<br>4 Parietal Bone, Left<br>5 Temporal Bone, Right<br>6 Temporal Bone, Left<br>7 Occipital Bone, Right<br>8 Occipital Bone, Left<br>B Nasal Bone<br>C Sphenoid Bone, Right<br>D Sphenoid Bone, Left<br>F Ethmoid Bone, Right<br>G Ethmoid Bone, Left<br>H Lacrimal Bone, Right<br>J Lacrimal Bone, Left<br>K Palatine Bone, Right<br>L Palatine Bone, Left<br>M Zygomatic Bone, Right<br>N Zygomatic Bone, Left<br>P Orbit, Right<br>Q Orbit, Left<br>R Maxilla, Right<br>S Maxilla, Left<br>T Mandible, Right<br>V Mandible, Left<br>X Hyoid Bone | 0 Open<br>3 Percutaneous<br>4 Percutaneous Endoscopic | Z No Device | Z No Qualifier |

**0** Medical and Surgical
**N** Head and Facial Bones
**P** Removal: Taking out or off a device from a body part

| Character 4<br>Body Part | Character 5<br>Approach | Character 6<br>Device | Character 7<br>Qualifier |
|---|---|---|---|
| 0 Skull | 0 Open | 0 Drainage Device<br>4 Internal Fixation Device<br>5 External Fixation Device<br>7 Autologous Tissue Substitute<br>J Synthetic Substitute<br>K Nonautologous Tissue Substitute<br>M Bone Growth Stimulator<br>N Neurostimulator Generator<br>S Hearing Device | Z No Qualifier |
| 0 Skull | 3 Percutaneous<br>4 Percutaneous Endoscopic | 0 Drainage Device<br>4 Internal Fixation Device<br>5 External Fixation Device<br>7 Autologous Tissue Substitute<br>J Synthetic Substitute<br>K Nonautologous Tissue Substitute<br>M Bone Growth Stimulator<br>S Hearing Device | Z No Qualifier |
| 0 Skull | X External | 0 Drainage Device<br>4 Internal Fixation Device<br>5 External Fixation Device<br>M Bone Growth Stimulator<br>S Hearing Device | Z No Qualifier |
| B Nasal Bone<br>W Facial Bone | 0 Open<br>3 Percutaneous<br>4 Percutaneous Endoscopic | 0 Drainage Device<br>4 Internal Fixation Device<br>7 Autologous Tissue Substitute<br>J Synthetic Substitute<br>K Nonautologous Tissue Substitute<br>M Bone Growth Stimulator | Z No Qualifier |
| B Nasal Bone<br>W Facial Bone | X External | 0 Drainage Device<br>4 Internal Fixation Device<br>M Bone Growth Stimulator | Z No Qualifier |

**0** Medical and Surgical
**N** Head and Facial Bones
**Q** Repair: Restoring, to the extent possible, a body part to its normal anatomic structure and function

| Character 4 Body Part | Character 5 Approach | Character 6 Device | Character 7 Qualifier |
|---|---|---|---|
| 0 Skull | 0 Open | Z No Device | Z No Qualifier |
| 1 Frontal Bone, Right | 3 Percutaneous | | |
| 2 Frontal Bone, Left | 4 Percutaneous Endoscopic | | |
| 3 Parietal Bone, Right | X External | | |
| 4 Parietal Bone, Left | | | |
| 5 Temporal Bone, Right | | | |
| 6 Temporal Bone, Left | | | |
| 7 Occipital Bone, Right | | | |
| 8 Occipital Bone, Left | | | |
| B Nasal Bone | | | |
| C Sphenoid Bone, Right | | | |
| D Sphenoid Bone, Left | | | |
| F Ethmoid Bone, Right | | | |
| G Ethmoid Bone, Left | | | |
| H Lacrimal Bone, Right | | | |
| J Lacrimal Bone, Left | | | |
| K Palatine Bone, Right | | | |
| L Palatine Bone, Left | | | |
| M Zygomatic Bone, Right | | | |
| N Zygomatic Bone, Left | | | |
| P Orbit, Right | | | |
| Q Orbit, Left | | | |
| R Maxilla, Right | | | |
| S Maxilla, Left | | | |
| T Mandible, Right | | | |
| V Mandible, Left | | | |
| X Hyoid Bone | | | |

**0** Medical and Surgical
**N** Head and Facial Bones
**R** Replacement: Putting in or on biological or synthetic material that physically takes the place and/or function of all or a portion of a body part

| Character 4 Body Part | Character 5 Approach | Character 6 Device | Character 7 Qualifier |
|---|---|---|---|
| 0 Skull | 0 Open | 7 Autologous Tissue Substitute | Z No Qualifier |
| 1 Frontal Bone, Right | 3 Percutaneous | J Synthetic Substitute | |
| 2 Frontal Bone, Left | 4 Percutaneous Endoscopic | K Nonautologous Tissue Substitute | |
| 3 Parietal Bone, Right | | | |
| 4 Parietal Bone, Left | | | |
| 5 Temporal Bone, Right | | | |
| 6 Temporal Bone, Left | | | |
| 7 Occipital Bone, Right | | | |
| 8 Occipital Bone, Left | | | |
| B Nasal Bone | | | |
| C Sphenoid Bone, Right | | | |
| D Sphenoid Bone, Left | | | |
| F Ethmoid Bone, Right | | | |
| G Ethmoid Bone, Left | | | |
| H Lacrimal Bone, Right | | | |
| J Lacrimal Bone, Left | | | |
| K Palatine Bone, Right | | | |
| L Palatine Bone, Left | | | |
| M Zygomatic Bone, Right | | | |
| N Zygomatic Bone, Left | | | |
| P Orbit, Right | | | |
| Q Orbit, Left | | | |
| R Maxilla, Right | | | |
| S Maxilla, Left | | | |
| T Mandible, Right | | | |
| V Mandible, Left | | | |
| X Hyoid Bone | | | |

**0** Medical and Surgical
**N** Head and Facial Bones
**S** Reposition: Moving to its normal location, or other suitable location, all or a portion of a body part

| Character 4 Body Part | Character 5 Approach | Character 6 Device | Character 7 Qualifier |
|---|---|---|---|
| 0 Skull<br>R Maxilla, Right<br>S Maxilla, Left<br>T Mandible, Right<br>V Mandible, Left | 0 Open<br>3 Percutaneous<br>4 Percutaneous Endoscopic | 4 Internal Fixation Device<br>5 External Fixation Device<br>Z No Device | Z No Qualifier |
| 0 Skull<br>R Maxilla, Right<br>S Maxilla, Left<br>T Mandible, Right<br>V Mandible, Left | X External | Z No Device | Z No Qualifier |
| 1 Frontal Bone, Right<br>2 Frontal Bone, Left<br>3 Parietal Bone, Right<br>4 Parietal Bone, Left<br>5 Temporal Bone, Right<br>6 Temporal Bone, Left<br>7 Occipital Bone, Right<br>8 Occipital Bone, Left<br>B Nasal Bone<br>C Sphenoid Bone, Right<br>D Sphenoid Bone, Left<br>F Ethmoid Bone, Right<br>G Ethmoid Bone, Left<br>H Lacrimal Bone, Right<br>J Lacrimal Bone, Left<br>K Palatine Bone, Right<br>L Palatine Bone, Left<br>M Zygomatic Bone, Right<br>N Zygomatic Bone, Left<br>P Orbit, Right<br>Q Orbit, Left<br>X Hyoid Bone | 0 Open<br>3 Percutaneous<br>4 Percutaneous Endoscopic | 4 Internal Fixation Device<br>Z No Device | Z No Qualifier |
| 1 Frontal Bone, Right<br>2 Frontal Bone, Left<br>3 Parietal Bone, Right<br>4 Parietal Bone, Left<br>5 Temporal Bone, Right<br>6 Temporal Bone, Left<br>7 Occipital Bone, Right<br>8 Occipital Bone, Left<br>B Nasal Bone<br>C Sphenoid Bone, Right<br>D Sphenoid Bone, Left<br>F Ethmoid Bone, Right<br>G Ethmoid Bone, Left<br>H Lacrimal Bone, Right<br>J Lacrimal Bone, Left<br>K Palatine Bone, Right<br>L Palatine Bone, Left<br>M Zygomatic Bone, Right<br>N Zygomatic Bone, Left<br>P Orbit, Right<br>Q Orbit, Left<br>X Hyoid Bone | X External | Z No Device | Z No Qualifier |

**AHA:** 0NS005Z - 3Q 2013, 25; 0NS104Z - 3Q 2013, 25

0 Medical and Surgical
N Head and Facial Bones
T Resection: Cutting out or off, without replacement, all of a body part

| Character 4<br>Body Part | Character 5<br>Approach | Character 6<br>Device | Character 7<br>Qualifier |
|---|---|---|---|
| 1 Frontal Bone, Right | 0 Open | Z No Device | Z No Qualifier |
| 2 Frontal Bone, Left | | | |
| 3 Parietal Bone, Right | | | |
| 4 Parietal Bone, Left | | | |
| 5 Temporal Bone, Right | | | |
| 6 Temporal Bone, Left | | | |
| 7 Occipital Bone, Right | | | |
| 8 Occipital Bone, Left | | | |
| B Nasal Bone | | | |
| C Sphenoid Bone, Right | | | |
| D Sphenoid Bone, Left | | | |
| F Ethmoid Bone, Right | | | |
| G Ethmoid Bone, Left | | | |
| H Lacrimal Bone, Right | | | |
| J Lacrimal Bone, Left | | | |
| K Palatine Bone, Right | | | |
| L Palatine Bone, Left | | | |
| M Zygomatic Bone, Right | | | |
| N Zygomatic Bone, Left | | | |
| P Orbit, Right | | | |
| Q Orbit, Left | | | |
| R Maxilla, Right | | | |
| S Maxilla, Left | | | |
| T Mandible, Right | | | |
| V Mandible, Left | | | |
| X Hyoid Bone | | | |

0 Medical and Surgical
N Head and Facial Bones
U Supplement: Putting in or on biological or synthetic material that physically reinforces and/or augments the function of a portion of a body part

| Character 4<br>Body Part | Character 5<br>Approach | Character 6<br>Device | Character 7<br>Qualifier |
|---|---|---|---|
| 0 Skull | 0 Open | 7 Autologous Tissue Substitute | Z No Qualifier |
| 1 Frontal Bone, Right | 3 Percutaneous | J Synthetic Substitute | |
| 2 Frontal Bone, Left | 4 Percutaneous Endoscopic | K Nonautologous Tissue Substitute | |
| 3 Parietal Bone, Right | | | |
| 4 Parietal Bone, Left | | | |
| 5 Temporal Bone, Right | | | |
| 6 Temporal Bone, Left | | | |
| 7 Occipital Bone, Right | | | |
| 8 Occipital Bone, Left | | | |
| B Nasal Bone | | | |
| C Sphenoid Bone, Right | | | |
| D Sphenoid Bone, Left | | | |
| F Ethmoid Bone, Right | | | |
| G Ethmoid Bone, Left | | | |
| H Lacrimal Bone, Right | | | |
| J Lacrimal Bone, Left | | | |
| K Palatine Bone, Right | | | |
| L Palatine Bone, Left | | | |
| M Zygomatic Bone, Right | | | |
| N Zygomatic Bone, Left | | | |
| P Orbit, Right | | | |
| Q Orbit, Left | | | |
| R Maxilla, Right | | | |
| S Maxilla, Left | | | |
| T Mandible, Right | | | |
| V Mandible, Left | | | |
| X Hyoid Bone | | | |

**AHA:** 0NU00JZ - 3Q 2013, 25

**0** Medical and Surgical
**N** Head and Facial Bones
**W** Revision: Correcting, to the extent possible, a portion of a malfunctioning device or the position of a displaced device

| Character 4<br>Body Part | Character 5<br>Approach | Character 6<br>Device | Character 7<br>Qualifier |
|---|---|---|---|
| 0 Skull | 0 Open | 0 Drainage Device<br>4 Internal Fixation Device<br>5 External Fixation Device<br>7 Autologous Tissue Substitute<br>J Synthetic Substitute<br>K Nonautologous Tissue Substitute<br>M Bone Growth Stimulator<br>N Neurostimulator Generator<br>S Hearing Device | Z No Qualifier |
| 0 Skull | 3 Percutaneous<br>4 Percutaneous Endoscopic<br>X External | 0 Drainage Device<br>4 Internal Fixation Device<br>5 External Fixation Device<br>7 Autologous Tissue Substitute<br>J Synthetic Substitute<br>K Nonautologous Tissue Substitute<br>M Bone Growth Stimulator<br>S Hearing Device | Z No Qualifier |
| B Nasal Bone<br>W Facial Bone | 0 Open<br>3 Percutaneous<br>4 Percutaneous Endoscopic<br>X External | 0 Drainage Device<br>4 Internal Fixation Device<br>7 Autologous Tissue Substitute<br>J Synthetic Substitute<br>K Nonautologous Tissue Substitute<br>M Bone Growth Stimulator | Z No Qualifier |

# Upper Bones | 0P2-0PW

**0** Medical and Surgical
**P** Upper Bones
**2** Change: Taking out or off a device from a body part and putting back an identical or similar device in or on the same body part without cutting or puncturing the skin or a mucous membrane

| Character 4<br>Body Part | Character 5<br>Approach | Character 6<br>Device | Character 7<br>Qualifier |
|---|---|---|---|
| Y Upper Bone | X External | 0 Drainage Device<br>Y Other Device | Z No Qualifier |

**0** Medical and Surgical
**P** Upper Bones
**5** Destruction: Physical eradication of all or a portion of a body part by the direct use of energy, force, or a destructive agent

| Character 4<br>Body Part | Character 5<br>Approach | Character 6<br>Device | Character 7<br>Qualifier |
|---|---|---|---|
| 0 Sternum<br>1 Rib, Right<br>2 Rib, Left<br>3 Cervical Vertebra<br>4 Thoracic Vertebra<br>5 Scapula, Right<br>6 Scapula, Left<br>7 Glenoid Cavity, Right<br>8 Glenoid Cavity, Left<br>9 Clavicle, Right<br>B Clavicle, Left<br>C Humeral Head, Right<br>D Humeral Head, Left<br>F Humeral Shaft, Right<br>G Humeral Shaft, Left<br>H Radius, Right<br>J Radius, Left<br>K Ulna, Right<br>L Ulna, Left<br>M Carpal, Right<br>N Carpal, Left<br>P Metacarpal, Right<br>Q Metacarpal, Left<br>R Thumb Phalanx, Right<br>S Thumb Phalanx, Left<br>T Finger Phalanx, Right<br>V Finger Phalanx, Left | 0 Open<br>3 Percutaneous<br>4 Percutaneous Endoscopic | Z No Device | Z No Qualifier |

**0 Medical and Surgical**
**P Upper Bones**
**8 Division:** Cutting into a body part, without draining fluids and/or gases from the body part, in order to separate or transect a body part

| Character 4<br>Body Part | Character 5<br>Approach | Character 6<br>Device | Character 7<br>Qualifier |
|---|---|---|---|
| 0 Sternum | 0 Open | Z No Device | Z No Qualifier |
| 1 Rib, Right | 3 Percutaneous | | |
| 2 Rib, Left | 4 Percutaneous Endoscopic | | |
| 3 Cervical Vertebra | | | |
| 4 Thoracic Vertebra | | | |
| 5 Scapula, Right | | | |
| 6 Scapula, Left | | | |
| 7 Glenoid Cavity, Right | | | |
| 8 Glenoid Cavity, Left | | | |
| 9 Clavicle, Right | | | |
| B Clavicle, Left | | | |
| C Humeral Head, Right | | | |
| D Humeral Head, Left | | | |
| F Humeral Shaft, Right | | | |
| G Humeral Shaft, Left | | | |
| H Radius, Right | | | |
| J Radius, Left | | | |
| K Ulna, Right | | | |
| L Ulna, Left | | | |
| M Carpal, Right | | | |
| N Carpal, Left | | | |
| P Metacarpal, Right | | | |
| Q Metacarpal, Left | | | |
| R Thumb Phalanx, Right | | | |
| S Thumb Phalanx, Left | | | |
| T Finger Phalanx, Right | | | |
| V Finger Phalanx, Left | | | |

**0** Medical and Surgical
**P** Upper Bones
**9** Drainage: Taking or letting out fluids and/or gases from a body part

| Character 4<br>Body Part | Character 5<br>Approach | Character 6<br>Device | Character 7<br>Qualifier |
|---|---|---|---|
| 0 Sternum<br>1 Rib, Right<br>2 Rib, Left<br>3 Cervical Vertebra<br>4 Thoracic Vertebra<br>5 Scapula, Right<br>6 Scapula, Left<br>7 Glenoid Cavity, Right<br>8 Glenoid Cavity, Left<br>9 Clavicle, Right<br>B Clavicle, Left<br>C Humeral Head, Right<br>D Humeral Head, Left<br>F Humeral Shaft, Right<br>G Humeral Shaft, Left<br>H Radius, Right<br>J Radius, Left<br>K Ulna, Right<br>L Ulna, Left<br>M Carpal, Right<br>N Carpal, Left<br>P Metacarpal, Right<br>Q Metacarpal, Left<br>R Thumb Phalanx, Right<br>S Thumb Phalanx, Left<br>T Finger Phalanx, Right<br>V Finger Phalanx, Left | 0 Open<br>3 Percutaneous<br>4 Percutaneous Endoscopic | 0 Drainage Device | Z No Qualifier |
| 0 Sternum<br>1 Rib, Right<br>2 Rib, Left<br>3 Cervical Vertebra<br>4 Thoracic Vertebra<br>5 Scapula, Right<br>6 Scapula, Left<br>7 Glenoid Cavity, Right<br>8 Glenoid Cavity, Left<br>9 Clavicle, Right<br>B Clavicle, Left<br>C Humeral Head, Right<br>D Humeral Head, Left<br>F Humeral Shaft, Right<br>G Humeral Shaft, Left<br>H Radius, Right<br>J Radius, Left<br>K Ulna, Right<br>L Ulna, Left<br>M Carpal, Right<br>N Carpal, Left<br>P Metacarpal, Right<br>Q Metacarpal, Left<br>R Thumb Phalanx, Right<br>S Thumb Phalanx, Left<br>T Finger Phalanx, Right<br>V Finger Phalanx, Left | 0 Open<br>3 Percutaneous<br>4 Percutaneous Endoscopic | Z No Device | X Diagnostic<br>Z No Qualifier |

**0** Medical and Surgical
**P** Upper Bones
**B** Excision: Cutting out or off, without replacement, a portion of a body part

| Character 4<br>Body Part | Character 5<br>Approach | Character 6<br>Device | Character 7<br>Qualifier |
|---|---|---|---|
| 0 Sternum | 0 Open | Z No Device | X Diagnostic |
| 1 Rib, Right | 3 Percutaneous | | Z No Qualifier |
| 2 Rib, Left | 4 Percutaneous Endoscopic | | |
| 3 Cervical Vertebra | | | |
| 4 Thoracic Vertebra | | | |
| 5 Scapula, Right | | | |
| 6 Scapula, Left | | | |
| 7 Glenoid Cavity, Right | | | |
| 8 Glenoid Cavity, Left | | | |
| 9 Clavicle, Right | | | |
| B Clavicle, Left | | | |
| C Humeral Head, Right | | | |
| D Humeral Head, Left | | | |
| F Humeral Shaft, Right | | | |
| G Humeral Shaft, Left | | | |
| H Radius, Right | | | |
| J Radius, Left | | | |
| K Ulna, Right | | | |
| L Ulna, Left | | | |
| M Carpal, Right | | | |
| N Carpal, Left | | | |
| P Metacarpal, Right | | | |
| Q Metacarpal, Left | | | |
| R Thumb Phalanx, Right | | | |
| S Thumb Phalanx, Left | | | |
| T Finger Phalanx, Right | | | |
| V Finger Phalanx, Left | | | |

**AHA:** 0PB54ZZ - 3Q 2013, 22; 0PB10ZZ - 4Q 2013, 110; 0PB20ZZ - 4Q 2013, 110; 0PB - 4Q 2013, 116

**0** Medical and Surgical
**P** Upper Bones
**C** Extirpation: Taking or cutting out solid matter from a body part

| Character 4<br>Body Part | Character 5<br>Approach | Character 6<br>Device | Character 7<br>Qualifier |
|---|---|---|---|
| 0 Sternum | 0 Open | Z No Device | Z No Qualifier |
| 1 Rib, Right | 3 Percutaneous | | |
| 2 Rib, Left | 4 Percutaneous Endoscopic | | |
| 3 Cervical Vertebra | | | |
| 4 Thoracic Vertebra | | | |
| 5 Scapula, Right | | | |
| 6 Scapula, Left | | | |
| 7 Glenoid Cavity, Right | | | |
| 8 Glenoid Cavity, Left | | | |
| 9 Clavicle, Right | | | |
| B Clavicle, Left | | | |
| C Humeral Head, Right | | | |
| D Humeral Head, Left | | | |
| F Humeral Shaft, Right | | | |
| G Humeral Shaft, Left | | | |
| H Radius, Right | | | |
| J Radius, Left | | | |
| K Ulna, Right | | | |
| L Ulna, Left | | | |
| M Carpal, Right | | | |
| N Carpal, Left | | | |
| P Metacarpal, Right | | | |
| Q Metacarpal, Left | | | |
| R Thumb Phalanx, Right | | | |
| S Thumb Phalanx, Left | | | |
| T Finger Phalanx, Right | | | |
| V Finger Phalanx, Left | | | |

**0** Medical and Surgical
**P** Upper Bones
**H** Insertion: Putting in a nonbiological appliance that monitors, assists, performs, or prevents a physiological function but does not physically take the place of a body part

| Character 4<br>Body Part | Character 5<br>Approach | Character 6<br>Device | Character 7<br>Qualifier |
|---|---|---|---|
| 0 Sternum | 0 Open<br>3 Percutaneous<br>4 Percutaneous Endoscopic | 0 Internal Fixation Device, Rigid Plate<br>4 Internal Fixation Device | Z No Qualifier |
| 1 Rib, Right<br>2 Rib, Left<br>3 Cervical Vertebra<br>4 Thoracic Vertebra<br>5 Scapula, Right<br>6 Scapula, Left<br>7 Glenoid Cavity, Right<br>8 Glenoid Cavity, Left<br>9 Clavicle, Right<br>B Clavicle, Left | 0 Open<br>3 Percutaneous<br>4 Percutaneous Endoscopic | 4 Internal Fixation Device | Z No Qualifier |
| C Humeral Head, Right<br>D Humeral Head, Left<br>F Humeral Shaft, Right<br>G Humeral Shaft, Left<br>H Radius, Right<br>J Radius, Left<br>K Ulna, Right<br>L Ulna, Left | 0 Open<br>3 Percutaneous<br>4 Percutaneous Endoscopic | 4 Internal Fixation Device<br>5 External Fixation Device<br>6 Internal Fixation Device,<br>　Intramedullary<br>8 External Fixation Device, Limb<br>　Lengthening<br>B External Fixation Device, Monoplanar<br>C External Fixation Device, Ring<br>D External Fixation Device, Hybrid | Z No Qualifier |
| M Carpal, Right<br>N Carpal, Left<br>P Metacarpal, Right<br>Q Metacarpal, Left<br>R Thumb Phalanx, Right<br>S Thumb Phalanx, Left<br>T Finger Phalanx, Right<br>V Finger Phalanx, Left | 0 Open<br>3 Percutaneous<br>4 Percutaneous Endoscopic | 4 Internal Fixation Device<br>5 External Fixation Device | Z No Qualifier |
| Y Upper Bone | 0 Open<br>3 Percutaneous<br>4 Percutaneous Endoscopic | M Bone Growth Stimulator | Z No Qualifier |

**0** Medical and Surgical
**P** Upper Bones
**J** Inspection: Visually and/or manually exploring a body part

| Character 4<br>Body Part | Character 5<br>Approach | Character 6<br>Device | Character 7<br>Qualifier |
|---|---|---|---|
| Y Upper Bone | 0 Open<br>3 Percutaneous<br>4 Percutaneous Endoscopic<br>X External | Z No Device | Z No Qualifier |

| | | | |
|---|---|---|---|
| **0** Medical and Surgical | | **N C** Non-covered | **L C** Limited Coverage |
| **P** Upper Bones | | | |
| **N** Release: Freeing a body part from an abnormal physical constraint by cutting or by the use of force | | | |

| Character 4<br>Body Part | Character 5<br>Approach | Character 6<br>Device | Character 7<br>Qualifier |
|---|---|---|---|
| 0 Sternum<br>1 Rib, Right<br>2 Rib, Left<br>3 Cervical Vertebra<br>4 Thoracic Vertebra<br>5 Scapula, Right<br>6 Scapula, Left<br>7 Glenoid Cavity, Right<br>8 Glenoid Cavity, Left<br>9 Clavicle, Right<br>B Clavicle, Left<br>C Humeral Head, Right<br>D Humeral Head, Left<br>F Humeral Shaft, Right<br>G Humeral Shaft, Left<br>H Radius, Right<br>J Radius, Left<br>K Ulna, Right<br>L Ulna, Left<br>M Carpal, Right<br>N Carpal, Left<br>P Metacarpal, Right<br>Q Metacarpal, Left<br>R Thumb Phalanx, Right<br>S Thumb Phalanx, Left<br>T Finger Phalanx, Right<br>V Finger Phalanx, Left | 0 Open<br>3 Percutaneous<br>4 Percutaneous Endoscopic | Z No Device | Z No Qualifier |

**0** Medical and Surgical
**P** Upper Bones
**P** Removal: Taking out or off a device from a body part

| Character 4 Body Part | Character 5 Approach | Character 6 Device | Character 7 Qualifier |
|---|---|---|---|
| 0 Sternum<br>1 Rib, Right<br>2 Rib, Left<br>3 Cervical Vertebra<br>4 Thoracic Vertebra<br>5 Scapula, Right<br>6 Scapula, Left<br>7 Glenoid Cavity, Right<br>8 Glenoid Cavity, Left<br>9 Clavicle, Right<br>B Clavicle, Left | 0 Open<br>3 Percutaneous<br>4 Percutaneous Endoscopic | 4 Internal Fixation Device<br>7 Autologous Tissue Substitute<br>J Synthetic Substitute<br>K Nonautologous Tissue Substitute | Z No Qualifier |
| 0 Sternum<br>1 Rib, Right<br>2 Rib, Left<br>3 Cervical Vertebra<br>4 Thoracic Vertebra<br>5 Scapula, Right<br>6 Scapula, Left<br>7 Glenoid Cavity, Right<br>8 Glenoid Cavity, Left<br>9 Clavicle, Right<br>B Clavicle, Left | X External | 4 Internal Fixation Device | Z No Qualifier |
| C Humeral Head, Right<br>D Humeral Head, Left<br>F Humeral Shaft, Right<br>G Humeral Shaft, Left<br>H Radius, Right<br>J Radius, Left<br>K Ulna, Right<br>L Ulna, Left<br>M Carpal, Right<br>N Carpal, Left<br>P Metacarpal, Right<br>Q Metacarpal, Left<br>R Thumb Phalanx, Right<br>S Thumb Phalanx, Left<br>T Finger Phalanx, Right<br>V Finger Phalanx, Left | 0 Open<br>3 Percutaneous<br>4 Percutaneous Endoscopic | 4 Internal Fixation Device<br>5 External Fixation Device<br>7 Autologous Tissue Substitute<br>J Synthetic Substitute<br>K Nonautologous Tissue Substitute | Z No Qualifier |
| C Humeral Head, Right<br>D Humeral Head, Left<br>F Humeral Shaft, Right<br>G Humeral Shaft, Left<br>H Radius, Right<br>J Radius, Left<br>K Ulna, Right<br>L Ulna, Left<br>M Carpal, Right<br>N Carpal, Left<br>P Metacarpal, Right<br>Q Metacarpal, Left<br>R Thumb Phalanx, Right<br>S Thumb Phalanx, Left<br>T Finger Phalanx, Right<br>V Finger Phalanx, Left | X External | 4 Internal Fixation Device<br>5 External Fixation Device | Z No Qualifier |
| Y Upper Bone | 0 Open<br>3 Percutaneous<br>4 Percutaneous Endoscopic<br>X External | 0 Drainage Device<br>M Bone Growth Stimulator | Z No Qualifier |

**0** Medical and Surgical
**P** Upper Bones
**Q** Repair: Restoring, to the extent possible, a body part to its normal anatomic structure and function

| Character 4 Body Part | Character 5 Approach | Character 6 Device | Character 7 Qualifier |
|---|---|---|---|
| 0 Sternum | 0 Open | Z No Device | Z No Qualifier |
| 1 Rib, Right | 3 Percutaneous | | |
| 2 Rib, Left | 4 Percutaneous Endoscopic | | |
| 3 Cervical Vertebra | X External | | |
| 4 Thoracic Vertebra | | | |
| 5 Scapula, Right | | | |
| 6 Scapula, Left | | | |
| 7 Glenoid Cavity, Right | | | |
| 8 Glenoid Cavity, Left | | | |
| 9 Clavicle, Right | | | |
| B Clavicle, Left | | | |
| C Humeral Head, Right | | | |
| D Humeral Head, Left | | | |
| F Humeral Shaft, Right | | | |
| G Humeral Shaft, Left | | | |
| H Radius, Right | | | |
| J Radius, Left | | | |
| K Ulna, Right | | | |
| L Ulna, Left | | | |
| M Carpal, Right | | | |
| N Carpal, Left | | | |
| P Metacarpal, Right | | | |
| Q Metacarpal, Left | | | |
| R Thumb Phalanx, Right | | | |
| S Thumb Phalanx, Left | | | |
| T Finger Phalanx, Right | | | |
| V Finger Phalanx, Left | | | |

**0** Medical and Surgical
**P** Upper Bones
**R** Replacement: Putting in or on biological or synthetic material that physically takes the place and/or function of all or a portion of a body part

| Character 4 Body Part | Character 5 Approach | Character 6 Device | Character 7 Qualifier |
|---|---|---|---|
| 0 Sternum | 0 Open | 7 Autologous Tissue Substitute | Z No Qualifier |
| 1 Rib, Right | 3 Percutaneous | J Synthetic Substitute | |
| 2 Rib, Left | 4 Percutaneous Endoscopic | K Nonautologous Tissue Substitute | |
| 3 Cervical Vertebra | | | |
| 4 Thoracic Vertebra | | | |
| 5 Scapula, Right | | | |
| 6 Scapula, Left | | | |
| 7 Glenoid Cavity, Right | | | |
| 8 Glenoid Cavity, Left | | | |
| 9 Clavicle, Right | | | |
| B Clavicle, Left | | | |
| C Humeral Head, Right | | | |
| D Humeral Head, Left | | | |
| F Humeral Shaft, Right | | | |
| G Humeral Shaft, Left | | | |
| H Radius, Right | | | |
| J Radius, Left | | | |
| K Ulna, Right | | | |
| L Ulna, Left | | | |
| M Carpal, Right | | | |
| N Carpal, Left | | | |
| P Metacarpal, Right | | | |
| Q Metacarpal, Left | | | |
| R Thumb Phalanx, Right | | | |
| S Thumb Phalanx, Left | | | |
| T Finger Phalanx, Right | | | |
| V Finger Phalanx, Left | | | |

**0** Medical and Surgical
**P** Upper Bones
**S** Reposition: Moving to its normal location, or other suitable location, all or a portion of a body part

| Character 4<br>Body Part | Character 5<br>Approach | Character 6<br>Device | Character 7<br>Qualifier |
|---|---|---|---|
| 0 Sternum | 0 Open<br>3 Percutaneous<br>4 Percutaneous Endoscopic | 0 Internal Fixation Device, Rigid Plate<br>4 Internal Fixation Device<br>Z No Device | Z No Qualifier |
| 0 Sternum | X External | Z No Device | Z No Qualifier |
| 1 Rib, Right<br>2 Rib, Left<br>3 Cervical Vertebra<br>4 Thoracic Vertebra<br>5 Scapula, Right<br>6 Scapula, Left<br>7 Glenoid Cavity, Right<br>8 Glenoid Cavity, Left<br>9 Clavicle, Right<br>B Clavicle, Left | 0 Open<br>3 Percutaneous<br>4 Percutaneous Endoscopic | 4 Internal Fixation Device<br>Z No Device | Z No Qualifier |
| 1 Rib, Right<br>2 Rib, Left<br>3 Cervical Vertebra<br>4 Thoracic Vertebra<br>5 Scapula, Right<br>6 Scapula, Left<br>7 Glenoid Cavity, Right<br>8 Glenoid Cavity, Left<br>9 Clavicle, Right<br>B Clavicle, Left | X External | Z No Device | Z No Qualifier |
| C Humeral Head, Right<br>D Humeral Head, Left<br>F Humeral Shaft, Right<br>G Humeral Shaft, Left<br>H Radius, Right<br>J Radius, Left<br>K Ulna, Right<br>L Ulna, Left | 0 Open<br>3 Percutaneous<br>4 Percutaneous Endoscopic | 4 Internal Fixation Device<br>5 External Fixation Device<br>6 Internal Fixation Device, Intramedullary<br>B External Fixation Device, Monoplanar<br>C External Fixation Device, Ring<br>D External Fixation Device, Hybrid<br>Z No Device | Z No Qualifier |
| C Humeral Head, Right<br>D Humeral Head, Left<br>F Humeral Shaft, Right<br>G Humeral Shaft, Left<br>H Radius, Right<br>J Radius, Left<br>K Ulna, Right<br>L Ulna, Left | X External | Z No Device | Z No Qualifier |
| M Carpal, Right<br>N Carpal, Left<br>P Metacarpal, Right<br>Q Metacarpal, Left<br>R Thumb Phalanx, Right<br>S Thumb Phalanx, Left<br>T Finger Phalanx, Right<br>V Finger Phalanx, Left | 0 Open<br>3 Percutaneous<br>4 Percutaneous Endoscopic | 4 Internal Fixation Device<br>5 External Fixation Device<br>Z No Device | Z No Qualifier |
| M Carpal, Right<br>N Carpal, Left<br>P Metacarpal, Right<br>Q Metacarpal, Left<br>R Thumb Phalanx, Right<br>S Thumb Phalanx, Left<br>T Finger Phalanx, Right<br>V Finger Phalanx, Left | X External | Z No Device | Z No Qualifier |

| 0 Medical and Surgical |
| P Upper Bones |
| T Resection: Cutting out or off, without replacement, all of a body part |

| Character 4<br>Body Part | Character 5<br>Approach | Character 6<br>Device | Character 7<br>Qualifier |
|---|---|---|---|
| 0 Sternum | 0 Open | Z No Device | Z No Qualifier |
| 1 Rib, Right | | | |
| 2 Rib, Left | | | |
| 5 Scapula, Right | | | |
| 6 Scapula, Left | | | |
| 7 Glenoid Cavity, Right | | | |
| 8 Glenoid Cavity, Left | | | |
| 9 Clavicle, Right | | | |
| B Clavicle, Left | | | |
| C Humeral Head, Right | | | |
| D Humeral Head, Left | | | |
| F Humeral Shaft, Right | | | |
| G Humeral Shaft, Left | | | |
| H Radius, Right | | | |
| J Radius, Left | | | |
| K Ulna, Right | | | |
| L Ulna, Left | | | |
| M Carpal, Right | | | |
| N Carpal, Left | | | |
| P Metacarpal, Right | | | |
| Q Metacarpal, Left | | | |
| R Thumb Phalanx, Right | | | |
| S Thumb Phalanx, Left | | | |
| T Finger Phalanx, Right | | | |
| V Finger Phalanx, Left | | | |

| 0 Medical and Surgical |
| P Upper Bones |
| U Supplement: Putting in or on biological or synthetic material that physically reinforces and/or augments the function of a portion of a body part |

| Character 4<br>Body Part | Character 5<br>Approach | Character 6<br>Device | Character 7<br>Qualifier |
|---|---|---|---|
| 0 Sternum | 0 Open | 7 Autologous Tissue Substitute | Z No Qualifier |
| 1 Rib, Right | 3 Percutaneous | J Synthetic Substitute | |
| 2 Rib, Left | 4 Percutaneous Endoscopic | K Nonautologous Tissue Substitute | |
| 3 Cervical Vertebra | | | |
| 4 Thoracic Vertebra | | | |
| 5 Scapula, Right | | | |
| 6 Scapula, Left | | | |
| 7 Glenoid Cavity, Right | | | |
| 8 Glenoid Cavity, Left | | | |
| 9 Clavicle, Right | | | |
| B Clavicle, Left | | | |
| C Humeral Head, Right | | | |
| D Humeral Head, Left | | | |
| F Humeral Shaft, Right | | | |
| G Humeral Shaft, Left | | | |
| H Radius, Right | | | |
| J Radius, Left | | | |
| K Ulna, Right | | | |
| L Ulna, Left | | | |
| M Carpal, Right | | | |
| N Carpal, Left | | | |
| P Metacarpal, Right | | | |
| Q Metacarpal, Left | | | |
| R Thumb Phalanx, Right | | | |
| S Thumb Phalanx, Left | | | |
| T Finger Phalanx, Right | | | |
| V Finger Phalanx, Left | | | |

**AHA:** 0PU00JZ - 4Q 2013, 111

**0** Medical and Surgical
**P** Upper Bones
**W** Revision: Correcting, to the extent possible, a portion of a malfunctioning device or the position of a displaced device

| Character 4 Body Part | Character 5 Approach | Character 6 Device | Character 7 Qualifier |
|---|---|---|---|
| 0 Sternum<br>1 Rib, Right<br>2 Rib, Left<br>3 Cervical Vertebra<br>4 Thoracic Vertebra<br>5 Scapula, Right<br>6 Scapula, Left<br>7 Glenoid Cavity, Right<br>8 Glenoid Cavity, Left<br>9 Clavicle, Right<br>B Clavicle, Left | 0 Open<br>3 Percutaneous<br>4 Percutaneous Endoscopic<br>X External | 4 Internal Fixation Device<br>7 Autologous Tissue Substitute<br>J Synthetic Substitute<br>K Nonautologous Tissue Substitute | Z No Qualifier |
| C Humeral Head, Right<br>D Humeral Head, Left<br>F Humeral Shaft, Right<br>G Humeral Shaft, Left<br>H Radius, Right<br>J Radius, Left<br>K Ulna, Right<br>L Ulna, Left<br>M Carpal, Right<br>N Carpal, Left<br>P Metacarpal, Right<br>Q Metacarpal, Left<br>R Thumb Phalanx, Right<br>S Thumb Phalanx, Left<br>T Finger Phalanx, Right<br>V Finger Phalanx, Left | 0 Open<br>3 Percutaneous<br>4 Percutaneous Endoscopic<br>X External | 4 Internal Fixation Device<br>5 External Fixation Device<br>7 Autologous Tissue Substitute<br>J Synthetic Substitute<br>K Nonautologous Tissue Substitute | Z No Qualifier |
| Y Upper Bone | 0 Open<br>3 Percutaneous<br>4 Percutaneous Endoscopic<br>X External | 0 Drainage Device<br>M Bone Growth Stimulator | Z No Qualifier |

# Lower Bones | 0Q2-0QW

**0** Medical and Surgical
**Q** Lower Bones
**2** Change: Taking out or off a device from a body part and putting back an identical or similar device in or on the same body part without cutting or puncturing the skin or a mucous membrane

| Character 4<br>Body Part | Character 5<br>Approach | Character 6<br>Device | Character 7<br>Qualifier |
| --- | --- | --- | --- |
| Y Lower Bone | X External | 0 Drainage Device<br>Y Other Device | Z No Qualifier |

**0** Medical and Surgical
**Q** Lower Bones
**5** Destruction: Physical eradication of all or a portion of a body part by the direct use of energy, force, or a destructive agent

| Character 4<br>Body Part | Character 5<br>Approach | Character 6<br>Device | Character 7<br>Qualifier |
| --- | --- | --- | --- |
| 0 Lumbar Vertebra<br>1 Sacrum<br>2 Pelvic Bone, Right<br>3 Pelvic Bone, Left<br>4 Acetabulum, Right<br>5 Acetabulum, Left<br>6 Upper Femur, Right<br>7 Upper Femur, Left<br>8 Femoral Shaft, Right<br>9 Femoral Shaft, Left<br>B Lower Femur, Right<br>C Lower Femur, Left<br>D Patella, Right<br>F Patella, Left<br>G Tibia, Right<br>H Tibia, Left<br>J Fibula, Right<br>K Fibula, Left<br>L Tarsal, Right<br>M Tarsal, Left<br>N Metatarsal, Right<br>P Metatarsal, Left<br>Q Toe Phalanx, Right<br>R Toe Phalanx, Left<br>S Coccyx | 0 Open<br>3 Percutaneous<br>4 Percutaneous Endoscopic | Z No Device | Z No Qualifier |

**0** Medical and Surgical
**Q** Lower Bones
**8** Division: Cutting into a body part, without draining fluids and/or gases from the body part, in order to separate or transect a body part

| Character 4<br>Body Part | Character 5<br>Approach | Character 6<br>Device | Character 7<br>Qualifier |
| --- | --- | --- | --- |
| 0 Lumbar Vertebra<br>1 Sacrum<br>2 Pelvic Bone, Right<br>3 Pelvic Bone, Left<br>4 Acetabulum, Right<br>5 Acetabulum, Left<br>6 Upper Femur, Right<br>7 Upper Femur, Left<br>8 Femoral Shaft, Right<br>9 Femoral Shaft, Left<br>B Lower Femur, Right<br>C Lower Femur, Left<br>D Patella, Right<br>F Patella, Left<br>G Tibia, Right<br>H Tibia, Left<br>J Fibula, Right<br>K Fibula, Left<br>L Tarsal, Right<br>M Tarsal, Left<br>N Metatarsal, Right<br>P Metatarsal, Left<br>Q Toe Phalanx, Right<br>R Toe Phalanx, Left<br>S Coccyx | 0 Open<br>3 Percutaneous<br>4 Percutaneous Endoscopic | Z No Device | Z No Qualifier |

♂ Male          ♀ Female          N C Non-covered          L C Limited Coverage          **AHA** AHA Coding Clinic

**0Q9–0Q9** *(side tab)*

**0** Medical and Surgical
**Q** Lower Bones
**9** Drainage: Taking or letting out fluids and/or gases from a body part

| Character 4<br>Body Part | Character 5<br>Approach | Character 6<br>Device | Character 7<br>Qualifier |
|---|---|---|---|
| 0 Lumbar Vertebra<br>1 Sacrum<br>2 Pelvic Bone, Right<br>3 Pelvic Bone, Left<br>4 Acetabulum, Right<br>5 Acetabulum, Left<br>6 Upper Femur, Right<br>7 Upper Femur, Left<br>8 Femoral Shaft, Right<br>9 Femoral Shaft, Left<br>B Lower Femur, Right<br>C Lower Femur, Left<br>D Patella, Right<br>F Patella, Left<br>G Tibia, Right<br>H Tibia, Left<br>J Fibula, Right<br>K Fibula, Left<br>L Tarsal, Right<br>M Tarsal, Left<br>N Metatarsal, Right<br>P Metatarsal, Left<br>Q Toe Phalanx, Right<br>R Toe Phalanx, Left<br>S Coccyx | 0 Open<br>3 Percutaneous<br>4 Percutaneous Endoscopic | 0 Drainage Device | Z No Qualifier |
| 0 Lumbar Vertebra<br>1 Sacrum<br>2 Pelvic Bone, Right<br>3 Pelvic Bone, Left<br>4 Acetabulum, Right<br>5 Acetabulum, Left<br>6 Upper Femur, Right<br>7 Upper Femur, Left<br>8 Femoral Shaft, Right<br>9 Femoral Shaft, Left<br>B Lower Femur, Right<br>C Lower Femur, Left<br>D Patella, Right<br>F Patella, Left<br>G Tibia, Right<br>H Tibia, Left<br>J Fibula, Right<br>K Fibula, Left<br>L Tarsal, Right<br>M Tarsal, Left<br>N Metatarsal, Right<br>P Metatarsal, Left<br>Q Toe Phalanx, Right<br>R Toe Phalanx, Left<br>S Coccyx | 0 Open<br>3 Percutaneous<br>4 Percutaneous Endoscopic | Z No Device | X Diagnostic<br>Z No Qualifier |

**0** Medical and Surgical
**Q** Lower Bones
**B** Excision: Cutting out or off, without replacement, a portion of a body part

| Character 4<br>Body Part | Character 5<br>Approach | Character 6<br>Device | Character 7<br>Qualifier |
|---|---|---|---|
| 0 Lumbar Vertebra | 0 Open | Z No Device | X Diagnostic |
| 1 Sacrum | 3 Percutaneous | | Z No Qualifier |
| 2 Pelvic Bone, Right | 4 Percutaneous Endoscopic | | |
| 3 Pelvic Bone, Left | | | |
| 4 Acetabulum, Right | | | |
| 5 Acetabulum, Left | | | |
| 6 Upper Femur, Right | | | |
| 7 Upper Femur, Left | | | |
| 8 Femoral Shaft, Right | | | |
| 9 Femoral Shaft, Left | | | |
| B Lower Femur, Right | | | |
| C Lower Femur, Left | | | |
| D Patella, Right | | | |
| F Patella, Left | | | |
| G Tibia, Right | | | |
| H Tibia, Left | | | |
| J Fibula, Right | | | |
| K Fibula, Left | | | |
| L Tarsal, Right | | | |
| M Tarsal, Left | | | |
| N Metatarsal, Right | | | |
| P Metatarsal, Left | | | |
| Q Toe Phalanx, Right | | | |
| R Toe Phalanx, Left | | | |
| S Coccyx | | | |

**AHA:** 0QBK0ZZ - 2Q 2013, 40; 0QB - 4Q 2013, 116; 0QB20ZZ - 2Q 2014, 7

**0** Medical and Surgical
**Q** Lower Bones
**C** Extirpation: Taking or cutting out solid matter from a body part

| Character 4<br>Body Part | Character 5<br>Approach | Character 6<br>Device | Character 7<br>Qualifier |
|---|---|---|---|
| 0 Lumbar Vertebra | 0 Open | Z No Device | Z No Qualifier |
| 1 Sacrum | 3 Percutaneous | | |
| 2 Pelvic Bone, Right | 4 Percutaneous Endoscopic | | |
| 3 Pelvic Bone, Left | | | |
| 4 Acetabulum, Right | | | |
| 5 Acetabulum, Left | | | |
| 6 Upper Femur, Right | | | |
| 7 Upper Femur, Left | | | |
| 8 Femoral Shaft, Right | | | |
| 9 Femoral Shaft, Left | | | |
| B Lower Femur, Right | | | |
| C Lower Femur, Left | | | |
| D Patella, Right | | | |
| F Patella, Left | | | |
| G Tibia, Right | | | |
| H Tibia, Left | | | |
| J Fibula, Right | | | |
| K Fibula, Left | | | |
| L Tarsal, Right | | | |
| M Tarsal, Left | | | |
| N Metatarsal, Right | | | |
| P Metatarsal, Left | | | |
| Q Toe Phalanx, Right | | | |
| R Toe Phalanx, Left | | | |
| S Coccyx | | | |

**0** Medical and Surgical
**Q** Lower Bones
**H** Insertion: Putting in a nonbiological appliance that monitors, assists, performs, or prevents a physiological function but does not physically take the place of a body part

| Character 4<br>Body Part | Character 5<br>Approach | Character 6<br>Device | Character 7<br>Qualifier |
|---|---|---|---|
| 0 Lumbar Vertebra<br>1 Sacrum<br>2 Pelvic Bone, Right<br>3 Pelvic Bone, Left<br>4 Acetabulum, Right<br>5 Acetabulum, Left<br>D Patella, Right<br>F Patella, Left<br>L Tarsal, Right<br>M Tarsal, Left<br>N Metatarsal, Right<br>P Metatarsal, Left<br>Q Toe Phalanx, Right<br>R Toe Phalanx, Left<br>S Coccyx | 0 Open<br>3 Percutaneous<br>4 Percutaneous Endoscopic | 4 Internal Fixation Device<br>5 External Fixation Device | Z No Qualifier |
| 6 Upper Femur, Right<br>7 Upper Femur, Left<br>8 Femoral Shaft, Right<br>9 Femoral Shaft, Left<br>B Lower Femur, Right<br>C Lower Femur, Left<br>G Tibia, Right<br>H Tibia, Left<br>J Fibula, Right<br>K Fibula, Left | 0 Open<br>3 Percutaneous<br>4 Percutaneous Endoscopic | 4 Internal Fixation Device<br>5 External Fixation Device<br>6 Internal Fixation Device, Intramedullary<br>8 External Fixation Device, Limb Lengthening<br>B External Fixation Device, Monoplanar<br>C External Fixation Device, Ring<br>D External Fixation Device, Hybrid | Z No Qualifier |
| Y Lower Bone | 0 Open<br>3 Percutaneous<br>4 Percutaneous Endoscopic | M Bone Growth Stimulator | Z No Qualifier |

**0** Medical and Surgical
**Q** Lower Bones
**J** Inspection: Visually and/or manually exploring a body part

| Character 4<br>Body Part | Character 5<br>Approach | Character 6<br>Device | Character 7<br>Qualifier |
|---|---|---|---|
| Y Lower Bone | 0 Open<br>3 Percutaneous<br>4 Percutaneous Endoscopic<br>X External | Z No Device | Z No Qualifier |

**0** Medical and Surgical
**Q** Lower Bones
**N** Release: Freeing a body part from an abnormal physical constraint by cutting or by the use of force

| Character 4<br>Body Part | Character 5<br>Approach | Character 6<br>Device | Character 7<br>Qualifier |
|---|---|---|---|
| 0 Lumbar Vertebra<br>1 Sacrum<br>2 Pelvic Bone, Right<br>3 Pelvic Bone, Left<br>4 Acetabulum, Right<br>5 Acetabulum, Left<br>6 Upper Femur, Right<br>7 Upper Femur, Left<br>8 Femoral Shaft, Right<br>9 Femoral Shaft, Left<br>B Lower Femur, Right<br>C Lower Femur, Left<br>D Patella, Right<br>F Patella, Left<br>G Tibia, Right<br>H Tibia, Left<br>J Fibula, Right<br>K Fibula, Left<br>L Tarsal, Right<br>M Tarsal, Left<br>N Metatarsal, Right<br>P Metatarsal, Left<br>Q Toe Phalanx, Right<br>R Toe Phalanx, Left<br>S Coccyx | 0 Open<br>3 Percutaneous<br>4 Percutaneous Endoscopic | Z No Device | Z No Qualifier |

**0 Medical and Surgical**
**Q Lower Bones**
**P Removal: Taking out or off a device from a body part**

| Character 4<br>Body Part | Character 5<br>Approach | Character 6<br>Device | Character 7<br>Qualifier |
|---|---|---|---|
| 0 Lumbar Vertebra<br>1 Sacrum<br>4 Acetabulum, Right<br>5 Acetabulum, Left<br>S Coccyx | 0 Open<br>3 Percutaneous<br>4 Percutaneous Endoscopic | 4 Internal Fixation Device<br>7 Autologous Tissue Substitute<br>J Synthetic Substitute<br>K Nonautologous Tissue Substitute | Z No Qualifier |
| 0 Lumbar Vertebra<br>1 Sacrum<br>4 Acetabulum, Right<br>5 Acetabulum, Left<br>S Coccyx | X External | 4 Internal Fixation Device | Z No Qualifier |
| 2 Pelvic Bone, Right<br>3 Pelvic Bone, Left<br>6 Upper Femur, Right<br>7 Upper Femur, Left<br>8 Femoral Shaft, Right<br>9 Femoral Shaft, Left<br>B Lower Femur, Right<br>C Lower Femur, Left<br>D Patella, Right<br>F Patella, Left<br>G Tibia, Right<br>H Tibia, Left<br>J Fibula, Right<br>K Fibula, Left<br>L Tarsal, Right<br>M Tarsal, Left<br>N Metatarsal, Right<br>P Metatarsal, Left<br>Q Toe Phalanx, Right<br>R Toe Phalanx, Left | 0 Open<br>3 Percutaneous<br>4 Percutaneous Endoscopic | 4 Internal Fixation Device<br>5 External Fixation Device<br>7 Autologous Tissue Substitute<br>J Synthetic Substitute<br>K Nonautologous Tissue Substitute | Z No Qualifier |
| 2 Pelvic Bone, Right<br>3 Pelvic Bone, Left<br>6 Upper Femur, Right<br>7 Upper Femur, Left<br>8 Femoral Shaft, Right<br>9 Femoral Shaft, Left<br>B Lower Femur, Right<br>C Lower Femur, Left<br>D Patella, Right<br>F Patella, Left<br>G Tibia, Right<br>H Tibia, Left<br>J Fibula, Right<br>K Fibula, Left<br>L Tarsal, Right<br>M Tarsal, Left<br>N Metatarsal, Right<br>P Metatarsal, Left<br>Q Toe Phalanx, Right<br>R Toe Phalanx, Left | X External | 4 Internal Fixation Device<br>5 External Fixation Device | Z No Qualifier |
| Y Lower Bone | 0 Open<br>3 Percutaneous<br>4 Percutaneous Endoscopic<br>X External | 0 Drainage Device<br>M Bone Growth Stimulator | Z No Qualifier |

**0** Medical and Surgical
**Q** Lower Bones
**Q** Repair: Restoring, to the extent possible, a body part to its normal anatomic structure and function

| Character 4<br>Body Part | Character 5<br>Approach | Character 6<br>Device | Character 7<br>Qualifier |
|---|---|---|---|
| 0 Lumbar Vertebra<br>1 Sacrum<br>2 Pelvic Bone, Right<br>3 Pelvic Bone, Left<br>4 Acetabulum, Right<br>5 Acetabulum, Left<br>6 Upper Femur, Right<br>7 Upper Femur, Left<br>8 Femoral Shaft, Right<br>9 Femoral Shaft, Left<br>B Lower Femur, Right<br>C Lower Femur, Left<br>D Patella, Right<br>F Patella, Left<br>G Tibia, Right<br>H Tibia, Left<br>J Fibula, Right<br>K Fibula, Left<br>L Tarsal, Right<br>M Tarsal, Left<br>N Metatarsal, Right<br>P Metatarsal, Left<br>Q Toe Phalanx, Right<br>R Toe Phalanx, Left<br>S Coccyx | 0 Open<br>3 Percutaneous<br>4 Percutaneous Endoscopic<br>X External | Z No Device | Z No Qualifier |

**0** Medical and Surgical
**Q** Lower Bones
**R** Replacement: Putting in or on biological or synthetic material that physically takes the place and/or function of all or a portion of a body part

| Character 4<br>Body Part | Character 5<br>Approach | Character 6<br>Device | Character 7<br>Qualifier |
|---|---|---|---|
| 0 Lumbar Vertebra<br>1 Sacrum<br>2 Pelvic Bone, Right<br>3 Pelvic Bone, Left<br>4 Acetabulum, Right<br>5 Acetabulum, Left<br>6 Upper Femur, Right<br>7 Upper Femur, Left<br>8 Femoral Shaft, Right<br>9 Femoral Shaft, Left<br>B Lower Femur, Right<br>C Lower Femur, Left<br>D Patella, Right<br>F Patella, Left<br>G Tibia, Right<br>H Tibia, Left<br>J Fibula, Right<br>K Fibula, Left<br>L Tarsal, Right<br>M Tarsal, Left<br>N Metatarsal, Right<br>P Metatarsal, Left<br>Q Toe Phalanx, Right<br>R Toe Phalanx, Left<br>S Coccyx | 0 Open<br>3 Percutaneous<br>4 Percutaneous Endoscopic | 7 Autologous Tissue Substitute<br>J Synthetic Substitute<br>K Nonautologous Tissue Substitute | Z No Qualifier |

**0** Medical and Surgical
**Q** Lower Bones
**S** Reposition: Moving to its normal location, or other suitable location, all or a portion of a body part

| Character 4 Body Part | Character 5 Approach | Character 6 Device | Character 7 Qualifier |
|---|---|---|---|
| 0 Lumbar Vertebra<br>1 Sacrum<br>4 Acetabulum, Right<br>5 Acetabulum, Left<br>S Coccyx | 0 Open<br>3 Percutaneous<br>4 Percutaneous Endoscopic | 4 Internal Fixation Device<br>Z No Device | Z No Qualifier |
| 0 Lumbar Vertebra<br>1 Sacrum<br>4 Acetabulum, Right<br>5 Acetabulum, Left<br>S Coccyx | X External | Z No Device | Z No Qualifier |
| 2 Pelvic Bone, Right<br>3 Pelvic Bone, Left<br>D Patella, Right<br>F Patella, Left<br>L Tarsal, Right<br>M Tarsal, Left<br>N Metatarsal, Right<br>P Metatarsal, Left<br>Q Toe Phalanx, Right<br>R Toe Phalanx, Left | 0 Open<br>3 Percutaneous<br>4 Percutaneous Endoscopic | 4 Internal Fixation Device<br>5 External Fixation Device<br>Z No Device | Z No Qualifier |
| 2 Pelvic Bone, Right<br>3 Pelvic Bone, Left<br>D Patella, Right<br>F Patella, Left<br>L Tarsal, Right<br>M Tarsal, Left<br>N Metatarsal, Right<br>P Metatarsal, Left<br>Q Toe Phalanx, Right<br>R Toe Phalanx, Left | X External | Z No Device | Z No Qualifier |
| 6 Upper Femur, Right<br>7 Upper Femur, Left<br>8 Femoral Shaft, Right<br>9 Femoral Shaft, Left<br>B Lower Femur, Right<br>C Lower Femur, Left<br>G Tibia, Right<br>H Tibia, Left<br>J Fibula, Right<br>K Fibula, Left | 0 Open<br>3 Percutaneous<br>4 Percutaneous Endoscopic | 4 Internal Fixation Device<br>5 External Fixation Device<br>6 Internal Fixation Device, Intramedullary<br>B External Fixation Device, Monoplanar<br>C External Fixation Device, Ring<br>D External Fixation Device, Hybrid<br>Z No Device | Z No Qualifier |
| 6 Upper Femur, Right<br>7 Upper Femur, Left<br>8 Femoral Shaft, Right<br>9 Femoral Shaft, Left<br>B Lower Femur, Right<br>C Lower Femur, Left<br>G Tibia, Right<br>H Tibia, Left<br>J Fibula, Right<br>K Fibula, Left | X External | Z No Device | Z No Qualifier |

**0** Medical and Surgical
**Q** Lower Bones
**T** Resection: Cutting out or off, without replacement, all of a body part

| Character 4 Body Part | Character 5 Approach | Character 6 Device | Character 7 Qualifier |
|---|---|---|---|
| 2 Pelvic Bone, Right | 0 Open | Z No Device | Z No Qualifier |
| 3 Pelvic Bone, Left | | | |
| 4 Acetabulum, Right | | | |
| 5 Acetabulum, Left | | | |
| 6 Upper Femur, Right | | | |
| 7 Upper Femur, Left | | | |
| 8 Femoral Shaft, Right | | | |
| 9 Femoral Shaft, Left | | | |
| B Lower Femur, Right | | | |
| C Lower Femur, Left | | | |
| D Patella, Right | | | |
| F Patella, Left | | | |
| G Tibia, Right | | | |
| H Tibia, Left | | | |
| J Fibula, Right | | | |
| K Fibula, Left | | | |
| L Tarsal, Right | | | |
| M Tarsal, Left | | | |
| N Metatarsal, Right | | | |
| P Metatarsal, Left | | | |
| Q Toe Phalanx, Right | | | |
| R Toe Phalanx, Left | | | |
| S Coccyx | | | |

**0** Medical and Surgical
**Q** Lower Bones
**U** Supplement: Putting in or on biological or synthetic material that physically reinforces and/or augments the function of a portion of a body part

| Character 4 Body Part | Character 5 Approach | Character 6 Device | Character 7 Qualifier |
|---|---|---|---|
| 0 Lumbar Vertebra | 0 Open | 7 Autologous Tissue Substitute | Z No Qualifier |
| 1 Sacrum | 3 Percutaneous | J Synthetic Substitute | |
| 2 Pelvic Bone, Right | 4 Percutaneous Endoscopic | K Nonautologous Tissue Substitute | |
| 3 Pelvic Bone, Left | | | |
| 4 Acetabulum, Right | | | |
| 5 Acetabulum, Left | | | |
| 6 Upper Femur, Right | | | |
| 7 Upper Femur, Left | | | |
| 8 Femoral Shaft, Right | | | |
| 9 Femoral Shaft, Left | | | |
| B Lower Femur, Right | | | |
| C Lower Femur, Left | | | |
| D Patella, Right | | | |
| F Patella, Left | | | |
| G Tibia, Right | | | |
| H Tibia, Left | | | |
| J Fibula, Right | | | |
| K Fibula, Left | | | |
| L Tarsal, Right | | | |
| M Tarsal, Left | | | |
| N Metatarsal, Right | | | |
| P Metatarsal, Left | | | |
| Q Toe Phalanx, Right | | | |
| R Toe Phalanx, Left | | | |
| S Coccyx | | | |

**AHA:** 0QU20JZ - 2Q 2013, 36;0QU03JZ - 2Q 2014, 13

**0** Medical and Surgical
**Q** Lower Bones
**W** Revision: Correcting, to the extent possible, a portion of a malfunctioning device or the position of a displaced device

| Character 4<br>Body Part | Character 5<br>Approach | Character 6<br>Device | Character 7<br>Qualifier |
|---|---|---|---|
| 0 Lumbar Vertebra<br>1 Sacrum<br>4 Acetabulum, Right<br>5 Acetabulum, Left<br>S Coccyx | 0 Open<br>3 Percutaneous<br>4 Percutaneous Endoscopic<br>X External | 4 Internal Fixation Device<br>7 Autologous Tissue Substitute<br>J Synthetic Substitute<br>K Nonautologous Tissue Substitute | Z No Qualifier |
| 2 Pelvic Bone, Right<br>3 Pelvic Bone, Left<br>6 Upper Femur, Right<br>7 Upper Femur, Left<br>8 Femoral Shaft, Right<br>9 Femoral Shaft, Left<br>B Lower Femur, Right<br>C Lower Femur, Left<br>D Patella, Right<br>F Patella, Left<br>G Tibia, Right<br>H Tibia, Left<br>J Fibula, Right<br>K Fibula, Left<br>L Tarsal, Right<br>M Tarsal, Left<br>N Metatarsal, Right<br>P Metatarsal, Left<br>Q Toe Phalanx, Right<br>R Toe Phalanx, Left | 0 Open<br>3 Percutaneous<br>4 Percutaneous Endoscopic<br>X External | 4 Internal Fixation Device<br>5 External Fixation Device<br>7 Autologous Tissue Substitute<br>J Synthetic Substitute<br>K Nonautologous Tissue Substitute | Z No Qualifier |
| Y Lower Bone | 0 Open<br>3 Percutaneous<br>4 Percutaneous Endoscopic<br>X External | 0 Drainage Device<br>M Bone Growth Stimulator | Z No Qualifier |

# Upper Joints | 0R2-0RX

**0** Medical and Surgical
**R** Upper Joints
**2** Change: Taking out or off a device from a body part and putting back an identical or similar device in or on the same body part without cutting or puncturing the skin or a mucous membrane

| Character 4<br>Body Part | Character 5<br>Approach | Character 6<br>Device | Character 7<br>Qualifier |
|---|---|---|---|
| Y  Upper Joint | X  External | 0  Drainage Device<br>Y  Other Device | Z  No Qualifier |

**0** Medical and Surgical
**R** Upper Joints
**5** Destruction: Physical eradication of all or a portion of a body part by the direct use of energy, force, or a destructive agent

| Character 4<br>Body Part | Character 5<br>Approach | Character 6<br>Device | Character 7<br>Qualifier |
|---|---|---|---|
| 0  Occipital-cervical Joint<br>1  Cervical Vertebral Joint<br>3  Cervical Vertebral Disc<br>4  Cervicothoracic Vertebral Joint<br>5  Cervicothoracic Vertebral Disc<br>6  Thoracic Vertebral Joint<br>9  Thoracic Vertebral Disc<br>A  Thoracolumbar Vertebral Joint<br>B  Thoracolumbar Vertebral Disc<br>C  Temporomandibular Joint, Right<br>D  Temporomandibular Joint, Left<br>E  Sternoclavicular Joint, Right<br>F  Sternoclavicular Joint, Left<br>G  Acromioclavicular Joint, Right<br>H  Acromioclavicular Joint, Left<br>J  Shoulder Joint, Right<br>K  Shoulder Joint, Left<br>L  Elbow Joint, Right<br>M  Elbow Joint, Left<br>N  Wrist Joint, Right<br>P  Wrist Joint, Left<br>Q  Carpal Joint, Right<br>R  Carpal Joint, Left<br>S  Metacarpocarpal Joint, Right<br>T  Metacarpocarpal Joint, Left<br>U  Metacarpophalangeal Joint, Right<br>V  Metacarpophalangeal Joint, Left<br>W  Finger Phalangeal Joint, Right<br>X  Finger Phalangeal Joint, Left | 0  Open<br>3  Percutaneous<br>4  Percutaneous Endoscopic | Z  No Device | Z  No Qualifier |

**0** Medical and Surgical
**R** Upper Joints
**9** Drainage: Taking or letting out fluids and/or gases from a body part

| Character 4<br>Body Part | Character 5<br>Approach | Character 6<br>Device | Character 7<br>Qualifier |
|---|---|---|---|
| 0 Occipital-cervical Joint<br>1 Cervical Vertebral Joint<br>3 Cervical Vertebral Disc<br>4 Cervicothoracic Vertebral Joint<br>5 Cervicothoracic Vertebral Disc<br>6 Thoracic Vertebral Joint<br>9 Thoracic Vertebral Disc<br>A Thoracolumbar Vertebral Joint<br>B Thoracolumbar Vertebral Disc<br>C Temporomandibular Joint, Right<br>D Temporomandibular Joint, Left<br>E Sternoclavicular Joint, Right<br>F Sternoclavicular Joint, Left<br>G Acromioclavicular Joint, Right<br>H Acromioclavicular Joint, Left<br>J Shoulder Joint, Right<br>K Shoulder Joint, Left<br>L Elbow Joint, Right<br>M Elbow Joint, Left<br>N Wrist Joint, Right<br>P Wrist Joint, Left<br>Q Carpal Joint, Right<br>R Carpal Joint, Left<br>S Metacarpocarpal Joint, Right<br>T Metacarpocarpal Joint, Left<br>U Metacarpophalangeal Joint, Right<br>V Metacarpophalangeal Joint, Left<br>W Finger Phalangeal Joint, Right<br>X Finger Phalangeal Joint, Left | 0 Open<br>3 Percutaneous<br>4 Percutaneous Endoscopic | 0 Drainage Device | Z No Qualifier |
| 0 Occipital-cervical Joint<br>1 Cervical Vertebral Joint<br>3 Cervical Vertebral Disc<br>4 Cervicothoracic Vertebral Joint<br>5 Cervicothoracic Vertebral Disc<br>6 Thoracic Vertebral Joint<br>9 Thoracic Vertebral Disc<br>A Thoracolumbar Vertebral Joint<br>B Thoracolumbar Vertebral Disc<br>C Temporomandibular Joint, Right<br>D Temporomandibular Joint, Left<br>E Sternoclavicular Joint, Right<br>F Sternoclavicular Joint, Left<br>G Acromioclavicular Joint, Right<br>H Acromioclavicular Joint, Left<br>J Shoulder Joint, Right<br>K Shoulder Joint, Left<br>L Elbow Joint, Right<br>M Elbow Joint, Left<br>N Wrist Joint, Right<br>P Wrist Joint, Left<br>Q Carpal Joint, Right<br>R Carpal Joint, Left<br>S Metacarpocarpal Joint, Right<br>T Metacarpocarpal Joint, Left<br>U Metacarpophalangeal Joint, Right<br>V Metacarpophalangeal Joint, Left<br>W Finger Phalangeal Joint, Right<br>X Finger Phalangeal Joint, Left | 0 Open<br>3 Percutaneous<br>4 Percutaneous Endoscopic | Z No Device | X Diagnostic<br>Z No Qualifier |

**0** Medical and Surgical
**R** Upper Joints
**B** Excision: Cutting out or off, without replacement, a portion of a body part

| Character 4<br>Body Part | Character 5<br>Approach | Character 6<br>Device | Character 7<br>Qualifier |
|---|---|---|---|
| 0 Occipital-cervical Joint | 0 Open | Z No Device | X Diagnostic |
| 1 Cervical Vertebral Joint | 3 Percutaneous | | Z No Qualifier |
| 3 Cervical Vertebral Disc | 4 Percutaneous Endoscopic | | |
| 4 Cervicothoracic Vertebral Joint | | | |
| 5 Cervicothoracic Vertebral Disc | | | |
| 6 Thoracic Vertebral Joint | | | |
| 9 Thoracic Vertebral Disc | | | |
| A Thoracolumbar Vertebral Joint | | | |
| B Thoracolumbar Vertebral Disc | | | |
| C Temporomandibular Joint, Right | | | |
| D Temporomandibular Joint, Left | | | |
| E Sternoclavicular Joint, Right | | | |
| F Sternoclavicular Joint, Left | | | |
| G Acromioclavicular Joint, Right | | | |
| H Acromioclavicular Joint, Left | | | |
| J Shoulder Joint, Right | | | |
| K Shoulder Joint, Left | | | |
| L Elbow Joint, Right | | | |
| M Elbow Joint, Left | | | |
| N Wrist Joint, Right | | | |
| P Wrist Joint, Left | | | |
| Q Carpal Joint, Right | | | |
| R Carpal Joint, Left | | | |
| S Metacarpocarpal Joint, Right | | | |
| T Metacarpocarpal Joint, Left | | | |
| U Metacarpophalangeal Joint, Right | | | |
| V Metacarpophalangeal Joint, Left | | | |
| W Finger Phalangeal Joint, Right | | | |
| X Finger Phalangeal Joint, Left | | | |

**0** Medical and Surgical
**R** Upper Joints
**C** Extirpation: Taking or cutting out solid matter from a body part

| Character 4<br>Body Part | Character 5<br>Approach | Character 6<br>Device | Character 7<br>Qualifier |
|---|---|---|---|
| 0 Occipital-cervical Joint | 0 Open | Z No Device | Z No Qualifier |
| 1 Cervical Vertebral Joint | 3 Percutaneous | | |
| 3 Cervical Vertebral Disc | 4 Percutaneous Endoscopic | | |
| 4 Cervicothoracic Vertebral Joint | | | |
| 5 Cervicothoracic Vertebral Disc | | | |
| 6 Thoracic Vertebral Joint | | | |
| 9 Thoracic Vertebral Disc | | | |
| A Thoracolumbar Vertebral Joint | | | |
| B Thoracolumbar Vertebral Disc | | | |
| C Temporomandibular Joint, Right | | | |
| D Temporomandibular Joint, Left | | | |
| E Sternoclavicular Joint, Right | | | |
| F Sternoclavicular Joint, Left | | | |
| G Acromioclavicular Joint, Right | | | |
| H Acromioclavicular Joint, Left | | | |
| J Shoulder Joint, Right | | | |
| K Shoulder Joint, Left | | | |
| L Elbow Joint, Right | | | |
| M Elbow Joint, Left | | | |
| N Wrist Joint, Right | | | |
| P Wrist Joint, Left | | | |
| Q Carpal Joint, Right | | | |
| R Carpal Joint, Left | | | |
| S Metacarpocarpal Joint, Right | | | |
| T Metacarpocarpal Joint, Left | | | |
| U Metacarpophalangeal Joint, Right | | | |
| V Metacarpophalangeal Joint, Left | | | |
| W Finger Phalangeal Joint, Right | | | |
| X Finger Phalangeal Joint, Left | | | |

**0 Medical and Surgical**
**R Upper Joints**
**G Fusion:** Joining together portions of an articular body part rendering the articular body part immobile

| Character 4<br>Body Part | Character 5<br>Approach | Character 6<br>Device | Character 7<br>Qualifier |
|---|---|---|---|
| 0 Occipital-cervical Joint<br>1 Cervical Vertebral Joint<br>2 Cervical Vertebral Joints, 2 or more<br>4 Cervicothoracic Vertebral Joint<br>6 Thoracic Vertebral Joint<br>7 Thoracic Vertebral Joints, 2 to 7<br>8 Thoracic Vertebral Joints, 8 or more<br>A Thoracolumbar Vertebral Joint | 0 Open<br>3 Percutaneous<br>4 Percutaneous Endoscopic | 7 Autologous Tissue Substitute<br>A Interbody Fusion Device<br>J Synthetic Substitute<br>K Nonautologous Tissue Substitute<br>Z No Device | 0 Anterior Approach, Anterior Column<br>1 Posterior Approach, Posterior Column<br>J Posterior Approach, Anterior Column |
| C Temporomandibular Joint, Right<br>D Temporomandibular Joint, Left<br>E Sternoclavicular Joint, Right<br>F Sternoclavicular Joint, Left<br>G Acromioclavicular Joint, Right<br>H Acromioclavicular Joint, Left<br>J Shoulder Joint, Right<br>K Shoulder Joint, Left | 0 Open<br>3 Percutaneous<br>4 Percutaneous Endoscopic | 4 Internal Fixation Device<br>7 Autologous Tissue Substitute<br>J Synthetic Substitute<br>K Nonautologous Tissue Substitute<br>Z No Device | Z No Qualifier |
| L Elbow Joint, Right<br>M Elbow Joint, Left<br>N Wrist Joint, Right<br>P Wrist Joint, Left<br>Q Carpal Joint, Right<br>R Carpal Joint, Left<br>S Metacarpocarpal Joint, Right<br>T Metacarpocarpal Joint, Left<br>U Metacarpophalangeal Joint, Right<br>V Metacarpophalangeal Joint, Left<br>W Finger Phalangeal Joint, Right<br>X Finger Phalangeal Joint, Left | 0 Open<br>3 Percutaneous<br>4 Percutaneous Endoscopic | 4 Internal Fixation Device<br>5 External Fixation Device<br>7 Autologous Tissue Substitute<br>J Synthetic Substitute<br>K Nonautologous Tissue Substitute<br>Z No Device | Z No Qualifier |

**AHA:** 0RG7071 - 1Q 2013, 22; 0RGA071 - 1Q 2013, 22; 0RG40A0 - 1Q 2013, 29; 0RG40A0 - 2Q 2014, 7

**0 Medical and Surgical**
**R Upper Joints**
**H Insertion:** Putting in a nonbiological appliance that monitors, assists, performs, or prevents a physiological function but does not physically take the place of a body part

| Character 4<br>Body Part | Character 5<br>Approach | Character 6<br>Device | Character 7<br>Qualifier |
|---|---|---|---|
| 0 Occipital-cervical Joint<br>1 Cervical Vertebral Joint<br>4 Cervicothoracic Vertebral Joint<br>6 Thoracic Vertebral Joint<br>A Thoracolumbar Vertebral Joint | 0 Open<br>3 Percutaneous<br>4 Percutaneous Endoscopic | 3 Infusion Device<br>4 Internal Fixation Device<br>8 Spacer<br>B Spinal Stabilization Device, Interspinous Process<br>C Spinal Stabilization Device, Pedicle-Based<br>D Spinal Stabilization Device, Facet Replacement | Z No Qualifier |
| 3 Cervical Vertebral Disc<br>5 Cervicothoracic Vertebral Disc<br>9 Thoracic Vertebral Disc<br>B Thoracolumbar Vertebral Disc | 0 Open<br>3 Percutaneous<br>4 Percutaneous Endoscopic | 3 Infusion Device | Z No Qualifier |
| C Temporomandibular Joint, Right<br>D Temporomandibular Joint, Left<br>E Sternoclavicular Joint, Right<br>F Sternoclavicular Joint, Left<br>G Acromioclavicular Joint, Right<br>H Acromioclavicular Joint, Left<br>J Shoulder Joint, Right<br>K Shoulder Joint, Left | 0 Open<br>3 Percutaneous<br>4 Percutaneous Endoscopic | 3 Infusion Device<br>4 Internal Fixation Device<br>8 Spacer | Z No Qualifier |
| L Elbow Joint, Right<br>M Elbow Joint, Left<br>N Wrist Joint, Right<br>P Wrist Joint, Left<br>Q Carpal Joint, Right<br>R Carpal Joint, Left<br>S Metacarpocarpal Joint, Right<br>T Metacarpocarpal Joint, Left<br>U Metacarpophalangeal Joint, Right<br>V Metacarpophalangeal Joint, Left<br>W Finger Phalangeal Joint, Right<br>X Finger Phalangeal Joint, Left | 0 Open<br>3 Percutaneous<br>4 Percutaneous Endoscopic | 3 Infusion Device<br>4 Internal Fixation Device<br>5 External Fixation Device<br>8 Spacer | Z No Qualifier |

♂ Male          ♀ Female          N C Non-covered          L C Limited Coverage          **AHA** *AHA Coding Clinic*

**0** Medical and Surgical
**R** Upper Joints
**J** Inspection: Visually and/or manually exploring a body part

| Character 4<br>Body Part | Character 5<br>Approach | Character 6<br>Device | Character 7<br>Qualifier |
|---|---|---|---|
| 0 Occipital-cervical Joint<br>1 Cervical Vertebral Joint<br>3 Cervical Vertebral Disc<br>4 Cervicothoracic Vertebral Joint<br>5 Cervicothoracic Vertebral Disc<br>6 Thoracic Vertebral Joint<br>9 Thoracic Vertebral Disc<br>A Thoracolumbar Vertebral Joint<br>B Thoracolumbar Vertebral Disc<br>C Temporomandibular Joint, Right<br>D Temporomandibular Joint, Left<br>E Sternoclavicular Joint, Right<br>F Sternoclavicular Joint, Left<br>G Acromioclavicular Joint, Right<br>H Acromioclavicular Joint, Left<br>J Shoulder Joint, Right<br>K Shoulder Joint, Left<br>L Elbow Joint, Right<br>M Elbow Joint, Left<br>N Wrist Joint, Right<br>P Wrist Joint, Left<br>Q Carpal Joint, Right<br>R Carpal Joint, Left<br>S Metacarpocarpal Joint, Right<br>T Metacarpocarpal Joint, Left<br>U Metacarpophalangeal Joint, Right<br>V Metacarpophalangeal Joint, Left<br>W Finger Phalangeal Joint, Right<br>X Finger Phalangeal Joint, Left | 0 Open<br>3 Percutaneous<br>4 Percutaneous Endoscopic<br>X External | Z No Device | Z No Qualifier |

**0** Medical and Surgical
**R** Upper Joints
**N** Release: Freeing a body part from an abnormal physical constraint by cutting or by the use of force

| Character 4<br>Body Part | Character 5<br>Approach | Character 6<br>Device | Character 7<br>Qualifier |
|---|---|---|---|
| 0 Occipital-cervical Joint<br>1 Cervical Vertebral Joint<br>3 Cervical Vertebral Disc<br>4 Cervicothoracic Vertebral Joint<br>5 Cervicothoracic Vertebral Disc<br>6 Thoracic Vertebral Joint<br>9 Thoracic Vertebral Disc<br>A Thoracolumbar Vertebral Joint<br>B Thoracolumbar Vertebral Disc<br>C Temporomandibular Joint, Right<br>D Temporomandibular Joint, Left<br>E Sternoclavicular Joint, Right<br>F Sternoclavicular Joint, Left<br>G Acromioclavicular Joint, Right<br>H Acromioclavicular Joint, Left<br>J Shoulder Joint, Right<br>K Shoulder Joint, Left<br>L Elbow Joint, Right<br>M Elbow Joint, Left<br>N Wrist Joint, Right<br>P Wrist Joint, Left<br>Q Carpal Joint, Right<br>R Carpal Joint, Left<br>S Metacarpocarpal Joint, Right<br>T Metacarpocarpal Joint, Left<br>U Metacarpophalangeal Joint, Right<br>V Metacarpophalangeal Joint, Left<br>W Finger Phalangeal Joint, Right<br>X Finger Phalangeal Joint, Left | 0 Open<br>3 Percutaneous<br>4 Percutaneous Endoscopic<br>X External | Z No Device | Z No Qualifier |

**0** Medical and Surgical
**R** Upper Joints
**P** Removal: Taking out or off a device from a body part

| Character 4<br>Body Part | Character 5<br>Approach | Character 6<br>Device | Character 7<br>Qualifier |
|---|---|---|---|
| 0 Occipital-cervical Joint<br>1 Cervical Vertebral Joint<br>4 Cervicothoracic Vertebral Joint<br>6 Thoracic Vertebral Joint<br>A Thoracolumbar Vertebral Joint | 0 Open<br>3 Percutaneous<br>4 Percutaneous Endoscopic | 0 Drainage Device<br>3 Infusion Device<br>4 Internal Fixation Device<br>7 Autologous Tissue Substitute<br>8 Spacer<br>A Interbody Fusion Device<br>J Synthetic Substitute<br>K Nonautologous Tissue Substitute | Z No Qualifier |
| 0 Occipital-cervical Joint<br>1 Cervical Vertebral Joint<br>4 Cervicothoracic Vertebral Joint<br>6 Thoracic Vertebral Joint<br>A Thoracolumbar Vertebral Joint | X External | 0 Drainage Device<br>3 Infusion Device<br>4 Internal Fixation Device | Z No Qualifier |
| 3 Cervical Vertebral Disc<br>5 Cervicothoracic Vertebral Disc<br>9 Thoracic Vertebral Disc<br>B Thoracolumbar Vertebral Disc | 0 Open<br>3 Percutaneous<br>4 Percutaneous Endoscopic | 0 Drainage Device<br>3 Infusion Device<br>7 Autologous Tissue Substitute<br>J Synthetic Substitute<br>K Nonautologous Tissue Substitute | Z No Qualifier |
| 3 Cervical Vertebral Disc<br>5 Cervicothoracic Vertebral Disc<br>9 Thoracic Vertebral Disc<br>B Thoracolumbar Vertebral Disc | X External | 0 Drainage Device<br>3 Infusion Device | Z No Qualifier |
| C Temporomandibular Joint, Right<br>D Temporomandibular Joint, Left<br>E Sternoclavicular Joint, Right<br>F Sternoclavicular Joint, Left<br>G Acromioclavicular Joint, Right<br>H Acromioclavicular Joint, Left<br>J Shoulder Joint, Right<br>K Shoulder Joint, Left | 0 Open<br>3 Percutaneous<br>4 Percutaneous Endoscopic | 0 Drainage Device<br>3 Infusion Device<br>4 Internal Fixation Device<br>7 Autologous Tissue Substitute<br>8 Spacer<br>J Synthetic Substitute<br>K Nonautologous Tissue Substitute | Z No Qualifier |
| C Temporomandibular Joint, Right<br>D Temporomandibular Joint, Left<br>E Sternoclavicular Joint, Right<br>F Sternoclavicular Joint, Left<br>G Acromioclavicular Joint, Right<br>H Acromioclavicular Joint, Left<br>J Shoulder Joint, Right<br>K Shoulder Joint, Left | X External | 0 Drainage Device<br>3 Infusion Device<br>4 Internal Fixation Device | Z No Qualifier |
| L Elbow Joint, Right<br>M Elbow Joint, Left<br>N Wrist Joint, Right<br>P Wrist Joint, Left<br>Q Carpal Joint, Right<br>R Carpal Joint, Left<br>S Metacarpocarpal Joint, Right<br>T Metacarpocarpal Joint, Left<br>U Metacarpophalangeal Joint, Right<br>V Metacarpophalangeal Joint, Left<br>W Finger Phalangeal Joint, Right<br>X Finger Phalangeal Joint, Left | 0 Open<br>3 Percutaneous<br>4 Percutaneous Endoscopic | 0 Drainage Device<br>3 Infusion Device<br>4 Internal Fixation Device<br>5 External Fixation Device<br>7 Autologous Tissue Substitute<br>8 Spacer<br>J Synthetic Substitute<br>K Nonautologous Tissue Substitute | Z No Qualifier |
| L Elbow Joint, Right<br>M Elbow Joint, Left<br>N Wrist Joint, Right<br>P Wrist Joint, Left<br>Q Carpal Joint, Right<br>R Carpal Joint, Left<br>S Metacarpocarpal Joint, Right<br>T Metacarpocarpal Joint, Left<br>U Metacarpophalangeal Joint, Right<br>V Metacarpophalangeal Joint, Left<br>W Finger Phalangeal Joint, Right<br>X Finger Phalangeal Joint, Left | X External | 0 Drainage Device<br>3 Infusion Device<br>4 Internal Fixation Device<br>5 External Fixation Device | Z No Qualifier |

**0** Medical and Surgical
**R** Upper Joints
**Q** Repair: Restoring, to the extent possible, a body part to its normal anatomic structure and function

| Character 4<br>Body Part | Character 5<br>Approach | Character 6<br>Device | Character 7<br>Qualifier |
|---|---|---|---|
| 0 Occipital-cervical Joint<br>1 Cervical Vertebral Joint<br>3 Cervical Vertebral Disc<br>4 Cervicothoracic Vertebral Joint<br>5 Cervicothoracic Vertebral Disc<br>6 Thoracic Vertebral Joint<br>9 Thoracic Vertebral Disc<br>A Thoracolumbar Vertebral Joint<br>B Thoracolumbar Vertebral Disc<br>C Temporomandibular Joint, Right<br>D Temporomandibular Joint, Left<br>E Sternoclavicular Joint, Right<br>F Sternoclavicular Joint, Left<br>G Acromioclavicular Joint, Right<br>H Acromioclavicular Joint, Left<br>J Shoulder Joint, Right<br>K Shoulder Joint, Left<br>L Elbow Joint, Right<br>M Elbow Joint, Left<br>N Wrist Joint, Right<br>P Wrist Joint, Left<br>Q Carpal Joint, Right<br>R Carpal Joint, Left<br>S Metacarpocarpal Joint, Right<br>T Metacarpocarpal Joint, Left<br>U Metacarpophalangeal Joint, Right<br>V Metacarpophalangeal Joint, Left<br>W Finger Phalangeal Joint, Right<br>X Finger Phalangeal Joint, Left | 0 Open<br>3 Percutaneous<br>4 Percutaneous Endoscopic<br>X External | Z No Device | Z No Qualifier |

**0** Medical and Surgical
**R** Upper Joints
**R** Replacement: Putting in or on biological or synthetic material that physically takes the place and/or function of all or a portion of a body part

| Character 4<br>Body Part | Character 5<br>Approach | Character 6<br>Device | Character 7<br>Qualifier |
|---|---|---|---|
| 0 Occipital-cervical Joint<br>1 Cervical Vertebral Joint<br>3 Cervical Vertebral Disc<br>4 Cervicothoracic Vertebral Joint<br>5 Cervicothoracic Vertebral Disc<br>6 Thoracic Vertebral Joint<br>9 Thoracic Vertebral Disc<br>A Thoracolumbar Vertebral Joint<br>B Thoracolumbar Vertebral Disc<br>C Temporomandibular Joint, Right<br>D Temporomandibular Joint, Left<br>E Sternoclavicular Joint, Right<br>F Sternoclavicular Joint, Left<br>G Acromioclavicular Joint, Right<br>H Acromioclavicular Joint, Left<br>L Elbow Joint, Right<br>M Elbow Joint, Left<br>N Wrist Joint, Right<br>P Wrist Joint, Left<br>Q Carpal Joint, Right<br>R Carpal Joint, Left<br>S Metacarpocarpal Joint, Right<br>T Metacarpocarpal Joint, Left<br>U Metacarpophalangeal Joint, Right<br>V Metacarpophalangeal Joint, Left<br>W Finger Phalangeal Joint, Right<br>X Finger Phalangeal Joint, Left | 0 Open | 7 Autologous Tissue Substitute<br>J Synthetic Substitute<br>K Nonautologous Tissue Substitute | Z No Qualifier |
| J Shoulder Joint, Right<br>K Shoulder Joint, Left | 0 Open | 0 Synthetic Substitute, Reverse Ball<br>   and Socket<br>7 Autologous Tissue Substitute<br>K Nonautologous Tissue Substitute | Z No Qualifier |
| J Shoulder Joint, Right<br>K Shoulder Joint, Left | 0 Open | J Synthetic Substitute | 6 Humeral Surface<br>7 Glenoid Surface<br>Z No Qualifier |

**0** Medical and Surgical
**R** Upper Joints
**S** Reposition: Moving to its normal location, or other suitable location, all or a portion of a body part

| Character 4<br>Body Part | Character 5<br>Approach | Character 6<br>Device | Character 7<br>Qualifier |
|---|---|---|---|
| 0 Occipital-cervical Joint<br>1 Cervical Vertebral Joint<br>4 Cervicothoracic Vertebral Joint<br>6 Thoracic Vertebral Joint<br>A Thoracolumbar Vertebral Joint<br>C Temporomandibular Joint, Right<br>D Temporomandibular Joint, Left<br>E Sternoclavicular Joint, Right<br>F Sternoclavicular Joint, Left<br>G Acromioclavicular Joint, Right<br>H Acromioclavicular Joint, Left<br>J Shoulder Joint, Right<br>K Shoulder Joint, Left | 0 Open<br>3 Percutaneous<br>4 Percutaneous Endoscopic<br>X External | 4 Internal Fixation Device<br>Z No Device | Z No Qualifier |
| L Elbow Joint, Right<br>M Elbow Joint, Left<br>N Wrist Joint, Right<br>P Wrist Joint, Left<br>Q Carpal Joint, Right<br>R Carpal Joint, Left<br>S Metacarpocarpal Joint, Right<br>T Metacarpocarpal Joint, Left<br>U Metacarpophalangeal Joint, Right<br>V Metacarpophalangeal Joint, Left<br>W Finger Phalangeal Joint, Right<br>X Finger Phalangeal Joint, Left | 0 Open<br>3 Percutaneous<br>4 Percutaneous Endoscopic<br>X External | 4 Internal Fixation Device<br>5 External Fixation Device<br>Z No Device | Z No Qualifier |

**AHA:** 0RS1XZZ - 2Q 2013, 39

**0** Medical and Surgical
**R** Upper Joints
**T** Resection: Cutting out or off, without replacement, all of a body part

| Character 4<br>Body Part | Character 5<br>Approach | Character 6<br>Device | Character 7<br>Qualifier |
|---|---|---|---|
| 3 Cervical Vertebral Disc<br>4 Cervicothoracic Vertebral Joint<br>5 Cervicothoracic Vertebral Disc<br>9 Thoracic Vertebral Disc<br>B Thoracolumbar Vertebral Disc<br>C Temporomandibular Joint, Right<br>D Temporomandibular Joint, Left<br>E Sternoclavicular Joint, Right<br>F Sternoclavicular Joint, Left<br>G Acromioclavicular Joint, Right<br>H Acromioclavicular Joint, Left<br>J Shoulder Joint, Right<br>K Shoulder Joint, Left<br>L Elbow Joint, Right<br>M Elbow Joint, Left<br>N Wrist Joint, Right<br>P Wrist Joint, Left<br>Q Carpal Joint, Right<br>R Carpal Joint, Left<br>S Metacarpocarpal Joint, Right<br>T Metacarpocarpal Joint, Left<br>U Metacarpophalangeal Joint, Right<br>V Metacarpophalangeal Joint, Left<br>W Finger Phalangeal Joint, Right<br>X Finger Phalangeal Joint, Left | 0 Open | Z No Device | Z No Qualifier |

**AHA:** 0RT50ZZ - 2Q 2014, 8

♂ Male    ♀ Female    N C Non-covered    L C Limited Coverage    **AHA** *AHA Coding Clinic*

**0** Medical and Surgical
**R** Upper Joints
**U** Supplement: Putting in or on biological or synthetic material that physically reinforces and/or augments the function of a portion of a body part

| Character 4<br>Body Part | Character 5<br>Approach | Character 6<br>Device | Character 7<br>Qualifier |
|---|---|---|---|
| 0 Occipital-cervical Joint<br>1 Cervical Vertebral Joint<br>3 Cervical Vertebral Disc<br>4 Cervicothoracic Vertebral Joint<br>5 Cervicothoracic Vertebral Disc<br>6 Thoracic Vertebral Joint<br>9 Thoracic Vertebral Disc<br>A Thoracolumbar Vertebral Joint<br>B Thoracolumbar Vertebral Disc<br>C Temporomandibular Joint, Right<br>D Temporomandibular Joint, Left<br>E Sternoclavicular Joint, Right<br>F Sternoclavicular Joint, Left<br>G Acromioclavicular Joint, Right<br>H Acromioclavicular Joint, Left<br>J Shoulder Joint, Right<br>K Shoulder Joint, Left<br>L Elbow Joint, Right<br>M Elbow Joint, Left<br>N Wrist Joint, Right<br>P Wrist Joint, Left<br>Q Carpal Joint, Right<br>R Carpal Joint, Left<br>S Metacarpocarpal Joint, Right<br>T Metacarpocarpal Joint, Left<br>U Metacarpophalangeal Joint, Right<br>V Metacarpophalangeal Joint, Left<br>W Finger Phalangeal Joint, Right<br>X Finger Phalangeal Joint, Left | 0 Open<br>3 Percutaneous<br>4 Percutaneous Endoscopic | 7 Autologous Tissue Substitute<br>J Synthetic Substitute<br>K Nonautologous Tissue Substitute | Z No Qualifier |

**0** Medical and Surgical
**R** Upper Joints
**W** Revision: Correcting, to the extent possible, a portion of a malfunctioning device or the position of a displaced device

| Character 4<br>Body Part | Character 5<br>Approach | Character 6<br>Device | Character 7<br>Qualifier |
|---|---|---|---|
| 0 Occipital-cervical Joint<br>1 Cervical Vertebral Joint<br>4 Cervicothoracic Vertebral Joint<br>6 Thoracic Vertebral Joint<br>A Thoracolumbar Vertebral Joint | 0 Open<br>3 Percutaneous<br>4 Percutaneous Endoscopic<br>X External | 0 Drainage Device<br>3 Infusion Device<br>4 Internal Fixation Device<br>7 Autologous Tissue Substitute<br>8 Spacer<br>A Interbody Fusion Device<br>J Synthetic Substitute<br>K Nonautologous Tissue Substitute | Z No Qualifier |
| 3 Cervical Vertebral Disc<br>5 Cervicothoracic Vertebral Disc<br>9 Thoracic Vertebral Disc<br>B Thoracolumbar Vertebral Disc | 0 Open<br>3 Percutaneous<br>4 Percutaneous Endoscopic<br>X External | 0 Drainage Device<br>3 Infusion Device<br>7 Autologous Tissue Substitute<br>J Synthetic Substitute<br>K Nonautologous Tissue Substitute | Z No Qualifier |
| C Temporomandibular Joint, Right<br>D Temporomandibular Joint, Left<br>E Sternoclavicular Joint, Right<br>F Sternoclavicular Joint, Left<br>G Acromioclavicular Joint, Right<br>H Acromioclavicular Joint, Left<br>J Shoulder Joint, Right<br>K Shoulder Joint, Left | 0 Open<br>3 Percutaneous<br>4 Percutaneous Endoscopic<br>X External | 0 Drainage Device<br>3 Infusion Device<br>4 Internal Fixation Device<br>7 Autologous Tissue Substitute<br>8 Spacer<br>J Synthetic Substitute<br>K Nonautologous Tissue Substitute | Z No Qualifier |
| L Elbow Joint, Right<br>M Elbow Joint, Left<br>N Wrist Joint, Right<br>P Wrist Joint, Left<br>Q Carpal Joint, Right<br>R Carpal Joint, Left<br>S Metacarpocarpal Joint, Right<br>T Metacarpocarpal Joint, Left<br>U Metacarpophalangeal Joint, Right<br>V Metacarpophalangeal Joint, Left<br>W Finger Phalangeal Joint, Right<br>X Finger Phalangeal Joint, Left | 0 Open<br>3 Percutaneous<br>4 Percutaneous Endoscopic<br>X External | 0 Drainage Device<br>3 Infusion Device<br>4 Internal Fixation Device<br>5 External Fixation Device<br>7 Autologous Tissue Substitute<br>8 Spacer<br>J Synthetic Substitute<br>K Nonautologous Tissue Substitute | Z No Qualifier |

# Lower Joints | 0S2-0SW

| 0 | Medical and Surgical |
|---|---|
| S | Lower Joints |
| 2 | Change: Taking out or off a device from a body part and putting back an identical or similar device in or on the same body part without cutting or puncturing the skin or a mucous membrane |

| Character 4<br>Body Part | Character 5<br>Approach | Character 6<br>Device | Character 7<br>Qualifier |
|---|---|---|---|
| Y   Lower Joint | X   External | 0   Drainage Device<br>Y   Other Device | Z   No Qualifier |

| 0 | Medical and Surgical |
|---|---|
| S | Lower Joints |
| 5 | Destruction: Physical eradication of all or a portion of a body part by the direct use of energy, force, or a destructive agent |

| Character 4<br>Body Part | Character 5<br>Approach | Character 6<br>Device | Character 7<br>Qualifier |
|---|---|---|---|
| 0   Lumbar Vertebral Joint<br>2   Lumbar Vertebral Disc<br>3   Lumbosacral Joint<br>4   Lumbosacral Disc<br>5   Sacrococcygeal Joint<br>6   Coccygeal Joint<br>7   Sacroiliac Joint, Right<br>8   Sacroiliac Joint, Left<br>9   Hip Joint, Right<br>B   Hip Joint, Left<br>C   Knee Joint, Right<br>D   Knee Joint, Left<br>F   Ankle Joint, Right<br>G   Ankle Joint, Left<br>H   Tarsal Joint, Right<br>J   Tarsal Joint, Left<br>K   Metatarsal-Tarsal Joint, Right<br>L   Metatarsal-Tarsal Joint, Left<br>M   Metatarsal-Phalangeal Joint, Right<br>N   Metatarsal-Phalangeal Joint, Left<br>P   Toe Phalangeal Joint, Right<br>Q   Toe Phalangeal Joint, Left | 0   Open<br>3   Percutaneous<br>4   Percutaneous Endoscopic | Z   No Device | Z   No Qualifier |

**0** Medical and Surgical
**S** Lower Joints
**9** Drainage: Taking or letting out fluids and/or gases from a body part

| Character 4<br>Body Part | Character 5<br>Approach | Character 6<br>Device | Character 7<br>Qualifier |
|---|---|---|---|
| 0 Lumbar Vertebral Joint<br>2 Lumbar Vertebral Disc<br>3 Lumbosacral Joint<br>4 Lumbosacral Disc<br>5 Sacrococcygeal Joint<br>6 Coccygeal Joint<br>7 Sacroiliac Joint, Right<br>8 Sacroiliac Joint, Left<br>9 Hip Joint, Right<br>B Hip Joint, Left<br>C Knee Joint, Right<br>D Knee Joint, Left<br>F Ankle Joint, Right<br>G Ankle Joint, Left<br>H Tarsal Joint, Right<br>J Tarsal Joint, Left<br>K Metatarsal-Tarsal Joint, Right<br>L Metatarsal-Tarsal Joint, Left<br>M Metatarsal-Phalangeal Joint, Right<br>N Metatarsal-Phalangeal Joint, Left<br>P Toe Phalangeal Joint, Right<br>Q Toe Phalangeal Joint, Left | 0 Open<br>3 Percutaneous<br>4 Percutaneous Endoscopic | 0 Drainage Device | Z No Qualifier |
| 0 Lumbar Vertebral Joint<br>2 Lumbar Vertebral Disc<br>3 Lumbosacral Joint<br>4 Lumbosacral Disc<br>5 Sacrococcygeal Joint<br>6 Coccygeal Joint<br>7 Sacroiliac Joint, Right<br>8 Sacroiliac Joint, Left<br>9 Hip Joint, Right<br>B Hip Joint, Left<br>C Knee Joint, Right<br>D Knee Joint, Left<br>F Ankle Joint, Right<br>G Ankle Joint, Left<br>H Tarsal Joint, Right<br>J Tarsal Joint, Left<br>K Metatarsal-Tarsal Joint, Right<br>L Metatarsal-Tarsal Joint, Left<br>M Metatarsal-Phalangeal Joint, Right<br>N Metatarsal-Phalangeal Joint, Left<br>P Toe Phalangeal Joint, Right<br>Q Toe Phalangeal Joint, Left | 0 Open<br>3 Percutaneous<br>4 Percutaneous Endoscopic | Z No Device | X Diagnostic<br>Z No Qualifier |

**0** Medical and Surgical
**S** Lower Joints
**B** Excision: Cutting out or off, without replacement, a portion of a body part

| Character 4<br>Body Part | Character 5<br>Approach | Character 6<br>Device | Character 7<br>Qualifier |
|---|---|---|---|
| 0 Lumbar Vertebral Joint<br>2 Lumbar Vertebral Disc<br>3 Lumbosacral Joint<br>4 Lumbosacral Disc<br>5 Sacrococcygeal Joint<br>6 Coccygeal Joint<br>7 Sacroiliac Joint, Right<br>8 Sacroiliac Joint, Left<br>9 Hip Joint, Right<br>B Hip Joint, Left<br>C Knee Joint, Right<br>D Knee Joint, Left<br>F Ankle Joint, Right<br>G Ankle Joint, Left<br>H Tarsal Joint, Right<br>J Tarsal Joint, Left<br>K Metatarsal-Tarsal Joint, Right<br>L Metatarsal-Tarsal Joint, Left<br>M Metatarsal-Phalangeal Joint, Right<br>N Metatarsal-Phalangeal Joint, Left<br>P Toe Phalangeal Joint, Right<br>Q Toe Phalangeal Joint, Left | 0 Open<br>3 Percutaneous<br>4 Percutaneous Endoscopic | Z No Device | X Diagnostic<br>Z No Qualifier |

**AHA:** 0SB20ZZ - 2Q 2014, 7

**0** Medical and Surgical
**S** Lower Joints
**C** Extirpation: Taking or cutting out solid matter from a body part

| Character 4<br>Body Part | Character 5<br>Approach | Character 6<br>Device | Character 7<br>Qualifier |
|---|---|---|---|
| 0 Lumbar Vertebral Joint<br>2 Lumbar Vertebral Disc<br>3 Lumbosacral Joint<br>4 Lumbosacral Disc<br>5 Sacrococcygeal Joint<br>6 Coccygeal Joint<br>7 Sacroiliac Joint, Right<br>8 Sacroiliac Joint, Left<br>9 Hip Joint, Right<br>B Hip Joint, Left<br>C Knee Joint, Right<br>D Knee Joint, Left<br>F Ankle Joint, Right<br>G Ankle Joint, Left<br>H Tarsal Joint, Right<br>J Tarsal Joint, Left<br>K Metatarsal-Tarsal Joint, Right<br>L Metatarsal-Tarsal Joint, Left<br>M Metatarsal-Phalangeal Joint, Right<br>N Metatarsal-Phalangeal Joint, Left<br>P Toe Phalangeal Joint, Right<br>Q Toe Phalangeal Joint, Left | 0 Open<br>3 Percutaneous<br>4 Percutaneous Endoscopic | Z No Device | Z No Qualifier |

**0** Medical and Surgical
**S** Lower Joints
**G** Fusion: Joining together portions of an articular body part rendering the articular body part immobile

| Character 4<br>Body Part | Character 5<br>Approach | Character 6<br>Device | Character 7<br>Qualifier |
|---|---|---|---|
| 0 Lumbar Vertebral Joint<br>1 Lumbar Vertebral Joints, 2 or more<br>3 Lumbosacral Joint | 0 Open<br>3 Percutaneous<br>4 Percutaneous Endoscopic | 7 Autologous Tissue Substitute<br>A Interbody Fusion Device<br>J Synthetic Substitute<br>K Nonautologous Tissue Substitute<br>Z No Device | 0 Anterior Approach, Anterior Column<br>1 Posterior Approach, Posterior Column<br>J Posterior Approach, Anterior Column |
| 5 Sacrococcygeal Joint<br>6 Coccygeal Joint<br>7 Sacroiliac Joint, Right<br>8 Sacroiliac Joint, Left | 0 Open<br>3 Percutaneous<br>4 Percutaneous Endoscopic | 4 Internal Fixation Device<br>7 Autologous Tissue Substitute<br>J Synthetic Substitute<br>K Nonautologous Tissue Substitute<br>Z No Device | Z No Qualifier |
| 9 Hip Joint, Right<br>B Hip Joint, Left<br>C Knee Joint, Right<br>D Knee Joint, Left<br>F Ankle Joint, Right<br>G Ankle Joint, Left<br>H Tarsal Joint, Right<br>J Tarsal Joint, Left<br>K Metatarsal-Tarsal Joint, Right<br>L Metatarsal-Tarsal Joint, Left<br>M Metatarsal-Phalangeal Joint, Right<br>N Metatarsal-Phalangeal Joint, Left<br>P Toe Phalangeal Joint, Right<br>Q Toe Phalangeal Joint, Left | 0 Open<br>3 Percutaneous<br>4 Percutaneous Endoscopic | 4 Internal Fixation Device<br>5 External Fixation Device<br>7 Autologous Tissue Substitute<br>J Synthetic Substitute<br>K Nonautologous Tissue Substitute<br>Z No Device | Z No Qualifier |

**AHA:** 0SG0071 - 1Q 2013, 23, 3Q 2013, 26; 0SGG04Z - 2Q 2013, 40; 0SGG07Z - 2Q 2013, 40; 0SG00AJ - 3Q 2013, 26; 0SG007J - 2Q 2014, 7

**0** Medical and Surgical
**S** Lower Joints
**H** Insertion: Putting in a nonbiological appliance that monitors, assists, performs, or prevents a physiological function but does not physically take the place of a body part

| Character 4<br>Body Part | Character 5<br>Approach | Character 6<br>Device | Character 7<br>Qualifier |
|---|---|---|---|
| 0 Lumbar Vertebral Joint<br>3 Lumbosacral Joint | 0 Open<br>3 Percutaneous<br>4 Percutaneous Endoscopic | 3 Infusion Device<br>4 Internal Fixation Device<br>8 Spacer<br>B Spinal Stabilization Device,<br>　Interspinous Process<br>C Spinal Stabilization Device, Pedicle-<br>　Based<br>D Spinal Stabilization Device, Facet<br>　Replacement | Z No Qualifier |
| 2 Lumbar Vertebral Disc<br>4 Lumbosacral Disc | 0 Open<br>3 Percutaneous<br>4 Percutaneous Endoscopic | 3 Infusion Device<br>8 Spacer | Z No Qualifier |
| 5 Sacrococcygeal Joint<br>6 Coccygeal Joint<br>7 Sacroiliac Joint, Right<br>8 Sacroiliac Joint, Left | 0 Open<br>3 Percutaneous<br>4 Percutaneous Endoscopic | 3 Infusion Device<br>4 Internal Fixation Device<br>8 Spacer | Z No Qualifier |
| 9 Hip Joint, Right<br>B Hip Joint, Left<br>C Knee Joint, Right<br>D Knee Joint, Left<br>F Ankle Joint, Right<br>G Ankle Joint, Left<br>H Tarsal Joint, Right<br>J Tarsal Joint, Left<br>K Metatarsal-Tarsal Joint, Right<br>L Metatarsal-Tarsal Joint, Left<br>M Metatarsal-Phalangeal Joint, Right<br>N Metatarsal-Phalangeal Joint, Left<br>P Toe Phalangeal Joint, Right<br>Q Toe Phalangeal Joint, Left | 0 Open<br>3 Percutaneous<br>4 Percutaneous Endoscopic | 3 Infusion Device<br>4 Internal Fixation Device<br>5 External Fixation Device<br>8 Spacer | Z No Qualifier |

**0** Medical and Surgical
**S** Lower Joints
**J** Inspection: Visually and/or manually exploring a body part

| Character 4<br>Body Part | Character 5<br>Approach | Character 6<br>Device | Character 7<br>Qualifier |
|---|---|---|---|
| 0 Lumbar Vertebral Joint<br>2 Lumbar Vertebral Disc<br>3 Lumbosacral Joint<br>4 Lumbosacral Disc<br>5 Sacrococcygeal Joint<br>6 Coccygeal Joint<br>7 Sacroiliac Joint, Right<br>8 Sacroiliac Joint, Left<br>9 Hip Joint, Right<br>B Hip Joint, Left<br>C Knee Joint, Right<br>D Knee Joint, Left<br>F Ankle Joint, Right<br>G Ankle Joint, Left<br>H Tarsal Joint, Right<br>J Tarsal Joint, Left<br>K Metatarsal-Tarsal Joint, Right<br>L Metatarsal-Tarsal Joint, Left<br>M Metatarsal-Phalangeal Joint, Right<br>N Metatarsal-Phalangeal Joint, Left<br>P Toe Phalangeal Joint, Right<br>Q Toe Phalangeal Joint, Left | 0 Open<br>3 Percutaneous<br>4 Percutaneous Endoscopic<br>X External | Z No Device | Z No Qualifier |

| 0 | Medical and Surgical |
| S | Lower Joints |
| N | Release: Freeing a body part from an abnormal physical constraint by cutting or by the use of force |

| Character 4<br>Body Part | Character 5<br>Approach | Character 6<br>Device | Character 7<br>Qualifier |
|---|---|---|---|
| 0 Lumbar Vertebral Joint | 0 Open | Z No Device | Z No Qualifier |
| 2 Lumbar Vertebral Disc | 3 Percutaneous | | |
| 3 Lumbosacral Joint | 4 Percutaneous Endoscopic | | |
| 4 Lumbosacral Disc | X External | | |
| 5 Sacrococcygeal Joint | | | |
| 6 Coccygeal Joint | | | |
| 7 Sacroiliac Joint, Right | | | |
| 8 Sacroiliac Joint, Left | | | |
| 9 Hip Joint, Right | | | |
| B Hip Joint, Left | | | |
| C Knee Joint, Right | | | |
| D Knee Joint, Left | | | |
| F Ankle Joint, Right | | | |
| G Ankle Joint, Left | | | |
| H Tarsal Joint, Right | | | |
| J Tarsal Joint, Left | | | |
| K Metatarsal-Tarsal Joint, Right | | | |
| L Metatarsal-Tarsal Joint, Left | | | |
| M Metatarsal-Phalangeal Joint, Right | | | |
| N Metatarsal-Phalangeal Joint, Left | | | |
| P Toe Phalangeal Joint, Right | | | |
| Q Toe Phalangeal Joint, Left | | | |

**0** Medical and Surgical
**S** Lower Joints
**P** Removal: Taking out or off a device from a body part

| Character 4<br>Body Part | Character 5<br>Approach | Character 6<br>Device | Character 7<br>Qualifier |
|---|---|---|---|
| 0 Lumbar Vertebral Joint<br>3 Lumbosacral Joint | 0 Open<br>3 Percutaneous<br>4 Percutaneous Endoscopic | 0 Drainage Device<br>3 Infusion Device<br>4 Internal Fixation Device<br>7 Autologous Tissue Substitute<br>8 Spacer<br>A Interbody Fusion Device<br>J Synthetic Substitute<br>K Nonautologous Tissue Substitute | Z No Qualifier |
| 0 Lumbar Vertebral Joint<br>3 Lumbosacral Joint | X External | 0 Drainage Device<br>3 Infusion Device<br>4 Internal Fixation Device | Z No Qualifier |
| 2 Lumbar Vertebral Disc<br>4 Lumbosacral Disc | 0 Open<br>3 Percutaneous<br>4 Percutaneous Endoscopic | 0 Drainage Device<br>3 Infusion Device<br>7 Autologous Tissue Substitute<br>J Synthetic Substitute<br>K Nonautologous Tissue Substitute | Z No Qualifier |
| 2 Lumbar Vertebral Disc<br>4 Lumbosacral Disc | X External | 0 Drainage Device<br>3 Infusion Device | Z No Qualifier |
| 5 Sacrococcygeal Joint<br>6 Coccygeal Joint<br>7 Sacroiliac Joint, Right<br>8 Sacroiliac Joint, Left | 0 Open<br>3 Percutaneous<br>4 Percutaneous Endoscopic | 0 Drainage Device<br>3 Infusion Device<br>4 Internal Fixation Device<br>7 Autologous Tissue Substitute<br>8 Spacer<br>J Synthetic Substitute<br>K Nonautologous Tissue Substitute | Z No Qualifier |
| 5 Sacrococcygeal Joint<br>6 Coccygeal Joint<br>7 Sacroiliac Joint, Right<br>8 Sacroiliac Joint, Left | X External | 0 Drainage Device<br>3 Infusion Device<br>4 Internal Fixation Device | Z No Qualifier |
| 9 Hip Joint, Right<br>B Hip Joint, Left | 0 Open | 0 Drainage Device<br>3 Infusion Device<br>4 Internal Fixation Device<br>5 External Fixation Device<br>7 Autologous Tissue Substitute<br>8 Spacer<br>9 Liner<br>B Resurfacing Device<br>J Synthetic Substitute<br>K Nonautologous Tissue Substitute | Z No Qualifier |
| 9 Hip Joint, Right<br>B Hip Joint, Left | 3 Percutaneous<br>4 Percutaneous Endoscopic | 0 Drainage Device<br>3 Infusion Device<br>4 Internal Fixation Device<br>5 External Fixation Device<br>7 Autologous Tissue Substitute<br>8 Spacer<br>J Synthetic Substitute<br>K Nonautologous Tissue Substitute | Z No Qualifier |
| 9 Hip Joint, Right<br>B Hip Joint, Left | X External | 0 Drainage Device<br>3 Infusion Device<br>4 Internal Fixation Device<br>5 External Fixation Device | Z No Qualifier |
| C Knee Joint, Right<br>D Knee Joint, Left | 0 Open | 0 Drainage Device<br>3 Infusion Device<br>4 Internal Fixation Device<br>5 External Fixation Device<br>7 Autologous Tissue Substitute<br>8 Spacer<br>9 Liner<br>J Synthetic Substitute<br>K Nonautologous Tissue Substitute | Z No Qualifier |
| C Knee Joint, Right<br>D Knee Joint, Left | 3 Percutaneous<br>4 Percutaneous Endoscopic | 0 Drainage Device<br>3 Infusion Device<br>4 Internal Fixation Device<br>5 External Fixation Device<br>7 Autologous Tissue Substitute<br>8 Spacer<br>J Synthetic Substitute<br>K Nonautologous Tissue Substitute | Z No Qualifier |
| C Knee Joint, Right<br>D Knee Joint, Left | X External | 0 Drainage Device<br>3 Infusion Device<br>4 Internal Fixation Device<br>5 External Fixation Device | Z No Qualifier |

**0SP** *continues on next page*

**0** Medical and Surgical – *continued*
**S** Lower Joints – *continued*
**P** Removal: Taking out or off a device from a body part – *continued*

| Character 4 Body Part | Character 5 Approach | Character 6 Device | Character 7 Qualifier |
|---|---|---|---|
| F Ankle Joint, Right<br>G Ankle Joint, Left<br>H Tarsal Joint, Right<br>J Tarsal Joint, Left<br>K Metatarsal-Tarsal Joint, Right<br>L Metatarsal-Tarsal Joint, Left<br>M Metatarsal-Phalangeal Joint, Right<br>N Metatarsal-Phalangeal Joint, Left<br>P Toe Phalangeal Joint, Right<br>Q Toe Phalangeal Joint, Left | 0 Open<br>3 Percutaneous<br>4 Percutaneous Endoscopic | 0 Drainage Device<br>3 Infusion Device<br>4 Internal Fixation Device<br>5 External Fixation Device<br>7 Autologous Tissue Substitute<br>8 Spacer<br>J Synthetic Substitute<br>K Nonautologous Tissue Substitute | Z No Qualifier |
| F Ankle Joint, Right<br>G Ankle Joint, Left<br>H Tarsal Joint, Right<br>J Tarsal Joint, Left<br>K Metatarsal-Tarsal Joint, Right<br>L Metatarsal-Tarsal Joint, Left<br>M Metatarsal-Phalangeal Joint, Right<br>N Metatarsal-Phalangeal Joint, Left<br>P Toe Phalangeal Joint, Right<br>Q Toe Phalangeal Joint, Left | X External | 0 Drainage Device<br>3 Infusion Device<br>4 Internal Fixation Device<br>5 External Fixation Device | Z No Qualifier |

**AHA:** 0SPG042 - 2Q 2013, 40

**0** Medical and Surgical
**S** Lower Joints
**Q** Repair: Restoring, to the extent possible, a body part to its normal anatomic structure and function

| Character 4 Body Part | Character 5 Approach | Character 6 Device | Character 7 Qualifier |
|---|---|---|---|
| 0 Lumbar Vertebral Joint<br>2 Lumbar Vertebral Disc<br>3 Lumbosacral Joint<br>4 Lumbosacral Disc<br>5 Sacrococcygeal Joint<br>6 Coccygeal Joint<br>7 Sacroiliac Joint, Right<br>8 Sacroiliac Joint, Left<br>9 Hip Joint, Right<br>B Hip Joint, Left<br>C Knee Joint, Right<br>D Knee Joint, Left<br>F Ankle Joint, Right<br>G Ankle Joint, Left<br>H Tarsal Joint, Right<br>J Tarsal Joint, Left<br>K Metatarsal-Tarsal Joint, Right<br>L Metatarsal-Tarsal Joint, Left<br>M Metatarsal-Phalangeal Joint, Right<br>N Metatarsal-Phalangeal Joint, Left<br>P Toe Phalangeal Joint, Right<br>Q Toe Phalangeal Joint, Left | 0 Open<br>3 Percutaneous<br>4 Percutaneous Endoscopic<br>X External | Z No Device | Z No Qualifier |

**0** Medical and Surgical
**S** Lower Joints
**R** Replacement: Putting in or on biological or synthetic material that physically takes the place and/or function of all or a portion of a body part

| Character 4<br>Body Part | Character 5<br>Approach | Character 6<br>Device | Character 7<br>Qualifier |
|---|---|---|---|
| 0 Lumbar Vertebral Joint<br>2 Lumbar Vertebral Disc<br>3 Lumbosacral Joint<br>4 Lumbosacral Disc<br>5 Sacrococcygeal Joint<br>6 Coccygeal Joint<br>7 Sacroiliac Joint, Right<br>8 Sacroiliac Joint, Left<br>H Tarsal Joint, Right<br>J Tarsal Joint, Left<br>K Metatarsal-Tarsal Joint, Right<br>L Metatarsal-Tarsal Joint, Left<br>M Metatarsal-Phalangeal Joint, Right<br>N Metatarsal-Phalangeal Joint, Left<br>P Toe Phalangeal Joint, Right<br>Q Toe Phalangeal Joint, Left | 0 Open | 7 Autologous Tissue Substitute<br>J Synthetic Substitute<br>K Nonautologous Tissue Substitute | Z No Qualifier |
| 9 Hip Joint, Right<br>B Hip Joint, Left | 0 Open | 1 Synthetic Substitute, Metal<br>2 Synthetic Substitute, Metal on Polyethylene<br>3 Synthetic Substitute, Ceramic<br>4 Synthetic Substitute, Ceramic on Polyethylene<br>J Synthetic Substitute | 9 Cemented<br>A Uncemented<br>Z No Qualifier |
| 9 Hip Joint, Right<br>B Hip Joint, Left | 0 Open | 7 Autologous Tissue Substitute<br>K Nonautologous Tissue Substitute | Z No Qualifier |
| A Hip Joint, Acetabular Surface, Right<br>E Hip Joint, Acetabular Surface, Left | 0 Open | 0 Synthetic Substitute, Polyethylene<br>1 Synthetic Substitute, Metal<br>3 Synthetic Substitute, Ceramic<br>J Synthetic Substitute | 9 Cemented<br>A Uncemented<br>Z No Qualifier |
| A Hip Joint, Acetabular Surface, Right<br>E Hip Joint, Acetabular Surface, Left | 0 Open | 7 Autologous Tissue Substitute<br>K Nonautologous Tissue Substitute | Z No Qualifier |
| C Knee Joint, Right<br>D Knee Joint, Left<br>F Ankle Joint, Right<br>G Ankle Joint, Left<br>T Knee Joint, Femoral Surface, Right<br>U Knee Joint, Femoral Surface, Left<br>V Knee Joint, Tibial Surface, Right<br>W Knee Joint, Tibial Surface, Left | 0 Open | 7 Autologous Tissue Substitute<br>K Nonautologous Tissue Substitute | Z No Qualifier |
| C Knee Joint, Right<br>D Knee Joint, Left<br>F Ankle Joint, Right<br>G Ankle Joint, Left<br>T Knee Joint, Femoral Surface, Right<br>U Knee Joint, Femoral Surface, Left<br>V Knee Joint, Tibial Surface, Right<br>W Knee Joint, Tibial Surface, Left | 0 Open | J Synthetic Substitute | 9 Cemented<br>A Uncemented<br>Z No Qualifier |
| R Hip Joint, Femoral Surface, Right<br>S Hip Joint, Femoral Surface, Left | 0 Open | 1 Synthetic Substitute, Metal<br>3 Synthetic Substitute, Ceramic<br>J Synthetic Substitute | 9 Cemented<br>A Uncemented<br>Z No Qualifier |
| R Hip Joint, Femoral Surface, Right<br>S Hip Joint, Femoral Surface, Left | 0 Open | 7 Autologous Tissue Substitute<br>K Nonautologous Tissue Substitute | Z No Qualifier |

**0** Medical and Surgical
**S** Lower Joints
**S** Reposition: Moving to its normal location, or other suitable location, all or a portion of a body part

| Character 4<br>Body Part | Character 5<br>Approach | Character 6<br>Device | Character 7<br>Qualifier |
|---|---|---|---|
| 0 Lumbar Vertebral Joint<br>3 Lumbosacral Joint<br>5 Sacrococcygeal Joint<br>6 Coccygeal Joint<br>7 Sacroiliac Joint, Right<br>8 Sacroiliac Joint, Left | 0 Open<br>3 Percutaneous<br>4 Percutaneous Endoscopic<br>X External | 4 Internal Fixation Device<br>Z No Device | Z No Qualifier |
| 9 Hip Joint, Right<br>B Hip Joint, Left<br>C Knee Joint, Right<br>D Knee Joint, Left<br>F Ankle Joint, Right<br>G Ankle Joint, Left<br>H Tarsal Joint, Right<br>J Tarsal Joint, Left<br>K Metatarsal-Tarsal Joint, Right<br>L Metatarsal-Tarsal Joint, Left<br>M Metatarsal-Phalangeal Joint, Right<br>N Metatarsal-Phalangeal Joint, Left<br>P Toe Phalangeal Joint, Right<br>Q Toe Phalangeal Joint, Left | 0 Open<br>3 Percutaneous<br>4 Percutaneous Endoscopic<br>X External | 4 Internal Fixation Device<br>5 External Fixation Device<br>Z No Device | Z No Qualifier |

**0** Medical and Surgical
**S** Lower Joints
**T** Resection: Cutting out or off, without replacement, all of a body part

| Character 4<br>Body Part | Character 5<br>Approach | Character 6<br>Device | Character 7<br>Qualifier |
|---|---|---|---|
| 2 Lumbar Vertebral Disc<br>4 Lumbosacral Disc<br>5 Sacrococcygeal Joint<br>6 Coccygeal Joint<br>7 Sacroiliac Joint, Right<br>8 Sacroiliac Joint, Left<br>9 Hip Joint, Right<br>B Hip Joint, Left<br>C Knee Joint, Right<br>D Knee Joint, Left<br>F Ankle Joint, Right<br>G Ankle Joint, Left<br>H Tarsal Joint, Right<br>J Tarsal Joint, Left<br>K Metatarsal-Tarsal Joint, Right<br>L Metatarsal-Tarsal Joint, Left<br>M Metatarsal-Phalangeal Joint, Right<br>N Metatarsal-Phalangeal Joint, Left<br>P Toe Phalangeal Joint, Right<br>Q Toe Phalangeal Joint, Left | 0 Open | Z No Device | Z No Qualifier |

**0** Medical and Surgical
**S** Lower Joints
**U** Supplement: Putting in or on biological or synthetic material that physically reinforces and/or augments the function of a portion of a body part

| Character 4 Body Part | Character 5 Approach | Character 6 Device | Character 7 Qualifier |
|---|---|---|---|
| 0 Lumbar Vertebral Joint<br>2 Lumbar Vertebral Disc<br>3 Lumbosacral Joint<br>4 Lumbosacral Disc<br>5 Sacrococcygeal Joint<br>6 Coccygeal Joint<br>7 Sacroiliac Joint, Right<br>8 Sacroiliac Joint, Left<br>F Ankle Joint, Right<br>G Ankle Joint, Left<br>H Tarsal Joint, Right<br>J Tarsal Joint, Left<br>K Metatarsal-Tarsal Joint, Right<br>L Metatarsal-Tarsal Joint, Left<br>M Metatarsal-Phalangeal Joint, Right<br>N Metatarsal-Phalangeal Joint, Left<br>P Toe Phalangeal Joint, Right<br>Q Toe Phalangeal Joint, Left | 0 Open<br>3 Percutaneous<br>4 Percutaneous Endoscopic | 7 Autologous Tissue Substitute<br>J Synthetic Substitute<br>K Nonautologous Tissue Substitute | Z No Qualifier |
| 9 Hip Joint, Right<br>B Hip Joint, Left | 0 Open | 7 Autologous Tissue Substitute<br>9 Liner<br>B Resurfacing Device<br>J Synthetic Substitute<br>K Nonautologous Tissue Substitute | Z No Qualifier |
| 9 Hip Joint, Right<br>B Hip Joint, Left | 3 Percutaneous<br>4 Percutaneous Endoscopic | 7 Autologous Tissue Substitute<br>J Synthetic Substitute<br>K Nonautologous Tissue Substitute | Z No Qualifier |
| A Hip Joint, Acetabular Surface, Right<br>E Hip Joint, Acetabular Surface, Left<br>R Hip Joint, Femoral Surface, Right<br>S Hip Joint, Femoral Surface, Left | 0 Open | 9 Liner<br>B Resurfacing Device | Z No Qualifier |
| C Knee Joint, Right<br>D Knee Joint, Left | 0 Open | 7 Autologous Tissue Substitute<br>J Synthetic Substitute<br>K Nonautologous Tissue Substitute | Z No Qualifier |
| C Knee Joint, Right<br>D Knee Joint, Left | 0 Open | 9 Liner | C Patellar Surface<br>Z No Qualifier |
| C Knee Joint, Right<br>D Knee Joint, Left | 3 Percutaneous<br>4 Percutaneous Endoscopic | 7 Autologous Tissue Substitute<br>J Synthetic Substitute<br>K Nonautologous Tissue Substitute | Z No Qualifier |
| T Knee Joint, Femoral Surface, Right<br>U Knee Joint, Femoral Surface, Left<br>V Knee Joint, Tibial Surface, Right<br>W Knee Joint, Tibial Surface, Left | 0 Open | 9 Liner | Z No Qualifier |

**0** Medical and Surgical
**S** Lower Joints
**W** Revision: Correcting, to the extent possible, a portion of a malfunctioning device or the position of a displaced device

| Character 4<br>Body Part | Character 5<br>Approach | Character 6<br>Device | Character 7<br>Qualifier |
|---|---|---|---|
| 0 Lumbar Vertebral Joint<br>3 Lumbosacral Joint | 0 Open<br>3 Percutaneous<br>4 Percutaneous Endoscopic<br>X External | 0 Drainage Device<br>3 Infusion Device<br>4 Internal Fixation Device<br>7 Autologous Tissue Substitute<br>8 Spacer<br>A Interbody Fusion Device<br>J Synthetic Substitute<br>K Nonautologous Tissue Substitute | Z No Qualifier |
| 2 Lumbar Vertebral Disc<br>4 Lumbosacral Disc | 0 Open<br>3 Percutaneous<br>4 Percutaneous Endoscopic<br>X External | 0 Drainage Device<br>3 Infusion Device<br>7 Autologous Tissue Substitute<br>J Synthetic Substitute<br>K Nonautologous Tissue Substitute | Z No Qualifier |
| 5 Sacrococcygeal Joint<br>6 Coccygeal Joint<br>7 Sacroiliac Joint, Right<br>8 Sacroiliac Joint, Left | 0 Open<br>3 Percutaneous<br>4 Percutaneous Endoscopic<br>X External | 0 Drainage Device<br>3 Infusion Device<br>4 Internal Fixation Device<br>7 Autologous Tissue Substitute<br>8 Spacer<br>J Synthetic Substitute<br>K Nonautologous Tissue Substitute | Z No Qualifier |
| 9 Hip Joint, Right<br>B Hip Joint, Left | 0 Open | 0 Drainage Device<br>3 Infusion Device<br>4 Internal Fixation Device<br>5 External Fixation Device<br>7 Autologous Tissue Substitute<br>8 Spacer<br>9 Liner<br>B Resurfacing Device<br>J Synthetic Substitute<br>K Nonautologous Tissue Substitute | Z No Qualifier |
| 9 Hip Joint, Right<br>B Hip Joint, Left | 3 Percutaneous<br>4 Percutaneous Endoscopic<br>X External | 0 Drainage Device<br>3 Infusion Device<br>4 Internal Fixation Device<br>5 External Fixation Device<br>7 Autologous Tissue Substitute<br>8 Spacer<br>J Synthetic Substitute<br>K Nonautologous Tissue Substitute | Z No Qualifier |
| C Knee Joint, Right<br>D Knee Joint, Left | 0 Open | 0 Drainage Device<br>3 Infusion Device<br>4 Internal Fixation Device<br>5 External Fixation Device<br>7 Autologous Tissue Substitute<br>8 Spacer<br>9 Liner<br>J Synthetic Substitute<br>K Nonautologous Tissue Substitute | Z No Qualifier |
| C Knee Joint, Right<br>D Knee Joint, Left | 3 Percutaneous<br>4 Percutaneous Endoscopic<br>X External | 0 Drainage Device<br>3 Infusion Device<br>4 Internal Fixation Device<br>5 External Fixation Device<br>7 Autologous Tissue Substitute<br>8 Spacer<br>J Synthetic Substitute<br>K Nonautologous Tissue Substitute | Z No Qualifier |
| F Ankle Joint, Right<br>G Ankle Joint, Left<br>H Tarsal Joint, Right<br>J Tarsal Joint, Left<br>K Metatarsal-Tarsal Joint, Right<br>L Metatarsal-Tarsal Joint, Left<br>M Metatarsal-Phalangeal Joint, Right<br>N Metatarsal-Phalangeal Joint, Left<br>P Toe Phalangeal Joint, Right<br>Q Toe Phalangeal Joint, Left | 0 Open<br>3 Percutaneous<br>4 Percutaneous Endoscopic<br>X External | 0 Drainage Device<br>3 Infusion Device<br>4 Internal Fixation Device<br>5 External Fixation Device<br>7 Autologous Tissue Substitute<br>8 Spacer<br>J Synthetic Substitute<br>K Nonautologous Tissue Substitute | Z No Qualifier |

# Urinary System | 0T1-0TY

**0** Medical and Surgical
**T** Urinary System
**1** Bypass: Altering the route of passage of the contents of a tubular body part

| Character 4<br>Body Part | Character 5<br>Approach | Character 6<br>Device | Character 7<br>Qualifier |
|---|---|---|---|
| 3 Kidney Pelvis, Right<br>4 Kidney Pelvis, Left | 0 Open<br>4 Percutaneous Endoscopic | 7 Autologous Tissue Substitute<br>J Synthetic Substitute<br>K Nonautologous Tissue Substitute<br>Z No Device | 3 Kidney Pelvis, Right<br>4 Kidney Pelvis, Left<br>6 Ureter, Right<br>7 Ureter, Left<br>8 Colon<br>9 Colocutaneous<br>A Ileum<br>B Bladder<br>C Ileocutaneous<br>D Cutaneous |
| 3 Kidney Pelvis, Right<br>4 Kidney Pelvis, Left | 3 Percutaneous | J Synthetic Substitute | D Cutaneous |
| 6 Ureter, Right<br>7 Ureter, Left<br>8 Ureters, Bilateral | 0 Open<br>4 Percutaneous Endoscopic | 7 Autologous Tissue Substitute<br>J Synthetic Substitute<br>K Nonautologous Tissue Substitute<br>Z No Device | 6 Ureter, Right<br>7 Ureter, Left<br>8 Colon<br>9 Colocutaneous<br>A Ileum<br>B Bladder<br>C Ileocutaneous<br>D Cutaneous |
| 6 Ureter, Right<br>7 Ureter, Left<br>8 Ureters, Bilateral | 3 Percutaneous | J Synthetic Substitute | D Cutaneous |
| B Bladder | 0 Open<br>4 Percutaneous Endoscopic | 7 Autologous Tissue Substitute<br>J Synthetic Substitute<br>K Nonautologous Tissue Substitute<br>Z No Device | 9 Colocutaneous<br>C Ileocutaneous<br>D Cutaneous |
| B Bladder | 3 Percutaneous | J Synthetic Substitute | D Cutaneous |

**0** Medical and Surgical
**T** Urinary System
**2** Change: Taking out or off a device from a body part and putting back an identical or similar device in or on the same body part without cutting or puncturing the skin or a mucous membrane

| Character 4<br>Body Part | Character 5<br>Approach | Character 6<br>Device | Character 7<br>Qualifier |
|---|---|---|---|
| 5 Kidney<br>9 Ureter<br>B Bladder<br>D Urethra | X External | 0 Drainage Device<br>Y Other Device | Z No Qualifier |

**0** Medical and Surgical
**T** Urinary System
**5** Destruction: Physical eradication of all or a portion of a body part by the direct use of energy, force, or a destructive agent

| Character 4<br>Body Part | Character 5<br>Approach | Character 6<br>Device | Character 7<br>Qualifier |
|---|---|---|---|
| 0 Kidney, Right<br>1 Kidney, Left<br>3 Kidney Pelvis, Right<br>4 Kidney Pelvis, Left<br>6 Ureter, Right<br>7 Ureter, Left<br>B Bladder<br>C Bladder Neck | 0 Open<br>3 Percutaneous<br>4 Percutaneous Endoscopic<br>7 Via Natural or Artificial Opening<br>8 Via Natural or Artificial Opening Endoscopic | Z No Device | Z No Qualifier |
| D Urethra | 0 Open<br>3 Percutaneous<br>4 Percutaneous Endoscopic<br>7 Via Natural or Artificial Opening<br>8 Via Natural or Artificial Opening Endoscopic<br>X External | Z No Device | Z No Qualifier |

| 0 | Medical and Surgical |
|---|---|
| T | Urinary System |
| 7 | Dilation: Expanding an orifice or the lumen of a tubular body part |

| Character 4<br>Body Part | Character 5<br>Approach | Character 6<br>Device | Character 7<br>Qualifier |
|---|---|---|---|
| 3 Kidney Pelvis, Right<br>4 Kidney Pelvis, Left<br>6 Ureter, Right<br>7 Ureter, Left<br>8 Ureters, Bilateral<br>B Bladder<br>C Bladder Neck<br>D Urethra | 0 Open<br>3 Percutaneous<br>4 Percutaneous Endoscopic<br>7 Via Natural or Artificial Opening<br>8 Via Natural or Artificial Opening<br>　Endoscopic | D Intraluminal Device<br>Z No Device | Z No Qualifier |

**AHA:** 0T7D8DZ - 4Q 2013, 123

| 0 | Medical and Surgical |
|---|---|
| T | Urinary System |
| 8 | Division: Cutting into a body part, without draining fluids and/or gases from the body part, in order to separate or transect a body part |

| Character 4<br>Body Part | Character 5<br>Approach | Character 6<br>Device | Character 7<br>Qualifier |
|---|---|---|---|
| 2 Kidneys, Bilateral<br>C Bladder Neck | 0 Open<br>3 Percutaneous<br>4 Percutaneous Endoscopic | Z No Device | Z No Qualifier |

| 0 | Medical and Surgical |
|---|---|
| T | Urinary System |
| 9 | Drainage: Taking or letting out fluids and/or gases from a body part |

| Character 4<br>Body Part | Character 5<br>Approach | Character 6<br>Device | Character 7<br>Qualifier |
|---|---|---|---|
| 0 Kidney, Right<br>1 Kidney, Left<br>3 Kidney Pelvis, Right<br>4 Kidney Pelvis, Left<br>6 Ureter, Right<br>7 Ureter, Left<br>8 Ureters, Bilateral<br>B Bladder<br>C Bladder Neck | 0 Open<br>3 Percutaneous<br>4 Percutaneous Endoscopic<br>7 Via Natural or Artificial Opening<br>8 Via Natural or Artificial Opening<br>　Endoscopic | 0 Drainage Device | Z No Qualifier |
| 0 Kidney, Right<br>1 Kidney, Left<br>3 Kidney Pelvis, Right<br>4 Kidney Pelvis, Left<br>6 Ureter, Right<br>7 Ureter, Left<br>8 Ureters, Bilateral<br>B Bladder<br>C Bladder Neck | 0 Open<br>3 Percutaneous<br>4 Percutaneous Endoscopic<br>7 Via Natural or Artificial Opening<br>8 Via Natural or Artificial Opening<br>　Endoscopic | Z No Device | X Diagnostic<br>Z No Qualifier |
| D Urethra | 0 Open<br>3 Percutaneous<br>4 Percutaneous Endoscopic<br>7 Via Natural or Artificial Opening<br>8 Via Natural or Artificial Opening<br>　Endoscopic<br>X External | 0 Drainage Device | Z No Qualifier |
| D Urethra | 0 Open<br>3 Percutaneous<br>4 Percutaneous Endoscopic<br>7 Via Natural or Artificial Opening<br>8 Via Natural or Artificial Opening<br>　Endoscopic<br>X External | Z No Device | X Diagnostic<br>Z No Qualifier |

**0** Medical and Surgical
**T** Urinary System
**B** Excision: Cutting out or off, without replacement, a portion of a body part

| Character 4<br>Body Part | Character 5<br>Approach | Character 6<br>Device | Character 7<br>Qualifier |
|---|---|---|---|
| 0 Kidney, Right<br>1 Kidney, Left<br>3 Kidney Pelvis, Right<br>4 Kidney Pelvis, Left<br>6 Ureter, Right<br>7 Ureter, Left<br>B Bladder<br>C Bladder Neck | 0 Open<br>3 Percutaneous<br>4 Percutaneous Endoscopic<br>7 Via Natural or Artificial Opening<br>8 Via Natural or Artificial Opening<br>   Endoscopic | Z No Device | X Diagnostic<br>Z No Qualifier |
| D Urethra | 0 Open<br>3 Percutaneous<br>4 Percutaneous Endoscopic<br>7 Via Natural or Artificial Opening<br>8 Via Natural or Artificial Opening<br>   Endoscopic<br>X External | Z No Device | X Diagnostic<br>Z No Qualifier |

**AHA:** 0TBB8ZZ - 2Q 2014, 8

**0** Medical and Surgical
**T** Urinary System
**C** Extirpation: Taking or cutting out solid matter from a body part

| Character 4<br>Body Part | Character 5<br>Approach | Character 6<br>Device | Character 7<br>Qualifier |
|---|---|---|---|
| 0 Kidney, Right<br>1 Kidney, Left<br>3 Kidney Pelvis, Right<br>4 Kidney Pelvis, Left<br>6 Ureter, Right<br>7 Ureter, Left<br>B Bladder<br>C Bladder Neck | 0 Open<br>3 Percutaneous<br>4 Percutaneous Endoscopic<br>7 Via Natural or Artificial Opening<br>8 Via Natural or Artificial Opening<br>   Endoscopic | Z No Device | Z No Qualifier |
| D Urethra | 0 Open<br>3 Percutaneous<br>4 Percutaneous Endoscopic<br>7 Via Natural or Artificial Opening<br>8 Via Natural or Artificial Opening<br>   Endoscopic<br>X External | Z No Device | Z No Qualifier |

**AHA:** 0TC68ZZ - 4Q 2013, 123

**0** Medical and Surgical
**T** Urinary System
**D** Extraction: Pulling or stripping out or off all or a portion of a body part by the use of force

| Character 4<br>Body Part | Character 5<br>Approach | Character 6<br>Device | Character 7<br>Qualifier |
|---|---|---|---|
| 0 Kidney, Right<br>1 Kidney, Left | 0 Open<br>3 Percutaneous<br>4 Percutaneous Endoscopic | Z No Device | Z No Qualifier |

**0** Medical and Surgical
**T** Urinary System
**F** Fragmentation: Breaking solid matter in a body part into pieces

| Character 4<br>Body Part | Character 5<br>Approach | Character 6<br>Device | Character 7<br>Qualifier |
|---|---|---|---|
| 3 Kidney Pelvis, Right<br>4 Kidney Pelvis, Left<br>6 Ureter, Right<br>7 Ureter, Left<br>B Bladder<br>C Bladder Neck<br>D Urethra  N C | 0 Open<br>3 Percutaneous<br>4 Percutaneous Endoscopic<br>7 Via Natural or Artificial Opening<br>8 Via Natural or Artificial Opening<br>   Endoscopic<br>X External | Z No Device | Z No Qualifier |

**AHA:** 0TF3XZZ - 4Q 2013, 122
N C 0TFDXZZ

**0** Medical and Surgical
**T** Urinary System
**H** Insertion: Putting in a nonbiological appliance that monitors, assists, performs, or prevents a physiological function but does not physically take the place of a body part

| Character 4<br>Body Part | Character 5<br>Approach | Character 6<br>Device | Character 7<br>Qualifier |
|---|---|---|---|
| 5 Kidney | 0 Open<br>3 Percutaneous<br>4 Percutaneous Endoscopic<br>7 Via Natural or Artificial Opening<br>8 Via Natural or Artificial Opening Endoscopic | 2 Monitoring Device<br>3 Infusion Device | Z No Qualifier |
| 9 Ureter | 0 Open<br>3 Percutaneous<br>4 Percutaneous Endoscopic<br>7 Via Natural or Artificial Opening<br>8 Via Natural or Artificial Opening Endoscopic | 2 Monitoring Device<br>3 Infusion Device<br>M Stimulator Lead | Z No Qualifier |
| B Bladder **N C** | 0 Open<br>3 Percutaneous<br>4 Percutaneous Endoscopic<br>7 Via Natural or Artificial Opening<br>8 Via Natural or Artificial Opening Endoscopic | 2 Monitoring Device<br>3 Infusion Device<br>L Artificial Sphincter<br>M Stimulator Lead | Z No Qualifier |
| C Bladder Neck | 0 Open<br>3 Percutaneous<br>4 Percutaneous Endoscopic<br>7 Via Natural or Artificial Opening<br>8 Via Natural or Artificial Opening Endoscopic | L Artificial Sphincter | Z No Qualifier |
| D Urethra | 0 Open<br>3 Percutaneous<br>4 Percutaneous Endoscopic<br>7 Via Natural or Artificial Opening<br>8 Via Natural or Artificial Opening Endoscopic<br>X External | 2 Monitoring Device<br>3 Infusion Device<br>L Artificial Sphincter | Z No Qualifier |

**N C** 0THB(0,3,4,7,8)MZ

**0** Medical and Surgical
**T** Urinary System
**J** Inspection: Visually and/or manually exploring a body part

| Character 4<br>Body Part | Character 5<br>Approach | Character 6<br>Device | Character 7<br>Qualifier |
|---|---|---|---|
| 5 Kidney<br>9 Ureter<br>B Bladder<br>D Urethra | 0 Open<br>3 Percutaneous<br>4 Percutaneous Endoscopic<br>7 Via Natural or Artificial Opening<br>8 Via Natural or Artificial Opening Endoscopic<br>X External | Z No Device | Z No Qualifier |

**0** Medical and Surgical
**T** Urinary System
**L** Occlusion: Completely closing an orifice or the lumen of a tubular body part

| Character 4 Body Part | Character 5 Approach | Character 6 Device | Character 7 Qualifier |
|---|---|---|---|
| 3 Kidney Pelvis, Right<br>4 Kidney Pelvis, Left<br>6 Ureter, Right<br>7 Ureter, Left<br>B Bladder<br>C Bladder Neck | 0 Open<br>3 Percutaneous<br>4 Percutaneous Endoscopic | C Extraluminal Device<br>D Intraluminal Device<br>Z No Device | Z No Qualifier |
| 3 Kidney Pelvis, Right<br>4 Kidney Pelvis, Left<br>6 Ureter, Right<br>7 Ureter, Left<br>B Bladder<br>C Bladder Neck | 7 Via Natural or Artificial Opening<br>8 Via Natural or Artificial Opening Endoscopic | D Intraluminal Device<br>Z No Device | Z No Qualifier |
| D Urethra | 0 Open<br>3 Percutaneous<br>4 Percutaneous Endoscopic<br>X External | C Extraluminal Device<br>D Intraluminal Device<br>Z No Device | Z No Qualifier |
| D Urethra | 7 Via Natural or Artificial Opening<br>8 Via Natural or Artificial Opening Endoscopic | D Intraluminal Device<br>Z No Device | Z No Qualifier |

**0** Medical and Surgical
**T** Urinary System
**M** Reattachment: Putting back in or on all or a portion of a separated body part to its normal location or other suitable location

| Character 4 Body Part | Character 5 Approach | Character 6 Device | Character 7 Qualifier |
|---|---|---|---|
| 0 Kidney, Right<br>1 Kidney, Left<br>2 Kidneys, Bilateral<br>3 Kidney Pelvis, Right<br>4 Kidney Pelvis, Left<br>6 Ureter, Right<br>7 Ureter, Left<br>8 Ureters, Bilateral<br>B Bladder<br>C Bladder Neck<br>D Urethra | 0 Open<br>4 Percutaneous Endoscopic | Z No Device | Z No Qualifier |

**0** Medical and Surgical
**T** Urinary System
**N** Release: Freeing a body part from an abnormal physical constraint by cutting or by the use of force

| Character 4 Body Part | Character 5 Approach | Character 6 Device | Character 7 Qualifier |
|---|---|---|---|
| 0 Kidney, Right<br>1 Kidney, Left<br>3 Kidney Pelvis, Right<br>4 Kidney Pelvis, Left<br>6 Ureter, Right<br>7 Ureter, Left<br>B Bladder<br>C Bladder Neck | 0 Open<br>3 Percutaneous<br>4 Percutaneous Endoscopic<br>7 Via Natural or Artificial Opening<br>8 Via Natural or Artificial Opening Endoscopic | Z No Device | Z No Qualifier |
| D Urethra | 0 Open<br>3 Percutaneous<br>4 Percutaneous Endoscopic<br>7 Via Natural or Artificial Opening<br>8 Via Natural or Artificial Opening Endoscopic<br>X External | Z No Device | Z No Qualifier |

| 0 | Medical and Surgical |
|---|---|
| T | Urinary System |
| P | Removal: Taking out or off a device from a body part |

| Character 4<br>Body Part | Character 5<br>Approach | Character 6<br>Device | Character 7<br>Qualifier |
|---|---|---|---|
| 5 Kidney | 0 Open<br>3 Percutaneous<br>4 Percutaneous Endoscopic<br>7 Via Natural or Artificial Opening<br>8 Via Natural or Artificial Opening Endoscopic | 0 Drainage Device<br>2 Monitoring Device<br>3 Infusion Device<br>7 Autologous Tissue Substitute<br>C Extraluminal Device<br>D Intraluminal Device<br>J Synthetic Substitute<br>K Nonautologous Tissue Substitute | Z No Qualifier |
| 5 Kidney | X External | 0 Drainage Device<br>2 Monitoring Device<br>3 Infusion Device<br>D Intraluminal Device | Z No Qualifier |
| 9 Ureter | 0 Open<br>3 Percutaneous<br>4 Percutaneous Endoscopic<br>7 Via Natural or Artificial Opening<br>8 Via Natural or Artificial Opening Endoscopic | 0 Drainage Device<br>2 Monitoring Device<br>3 Infusion Device<br>7 Autologous Tissue Substitute<br>C Extraluminal Device<br>D Intraluminal Device<br>J Synthetic Substitute<br>K Nonautologous Tissue Substitute<br>M Stimulator Lead | Z No Qualifier |
| 9 Ureter | X External | 0 Drainage Device<br>2 Monitoring Device<br>3 Infusion Device<br>D Intraluminal Device<br>M Stimulator Lead | Z No Qualifier |
| B Bladder  N C | 0 Open<br>3 Percutaneous<br>4 Percutaneous Endoscopic<br>7 Via Natural or Artificial Opening<br>8 Via Natural or Artificial Opening Endoscopic | 0 Drainage Device<br>2 Monitoring Device<br>3 Infusion Device<br>7 Autologous Tissue Substitute<br>C Extraluminal Device<br>D Intraluminal Device<br>J Synthetic Substitute<br>K Nonautologous Tissue Substitute<br>L Artificial Sphincter<br>M Stimulator Lead | Z No Qualifier |
| B Bladder | X External | 0 Drainage Device<br>2 Monitoring Device<br>3 Infusion Device<br>D Intraluminal Device<br>L Artificial Sphincter<br>M Stimulator Lead | Z No Qualifier |
| D Urethra | 0 Open<br>3 Percutaneous<br>4 Percutaneous Endoscopic<br>7 Via Natural or Artificial Opening<br>8 Via Natural or Artificial Opening Endoscopic | 0 Drainage Device<br>2 Monitoring Device<br>3 Infusion Device<br>7 Autologous Tissue Substitute<br>C Extraluminal Device<br>D Intraluminal Device<br>J Synthetic Substitute<br>K Nonautologous Tissue Substitute<br>L Artificial Sphincter | Z No Qualifier |
| D Urethra | X External | 0 Drainage Device<br>2 Monitoring Device<br>3 Infusion Device<br>D Intraluminal Device<br>L Artificial Sphincter | Z No Qualifier |

N C 0TPB(0,3,4,7,8)MZ

**0** Medical and Surgical
**T** Urinary System
**Q** Repair: Restoring, to the extent possible, a body part to its normal anatomic structure and function

| Character 4 Body Part | Character 5 Approach | Character 6 Device | Character 7 Qualifier |
|---|---|---|---|
| 0 Kidney, Right<br>1 Kidney, Left<br>3 Kidney Pelvis, Right<br>4 Kidney Pelvis, Left<br>6 Ureter, Right<br>7 Ureter, Left<br>B Bladder<br>C Bladder Neck | 0 Open<br>3 Percutaneous<br>4 Percutaneous Endoscopic<br>7 Via Natural or Artificial Opening<br>8 Via Natural or Artificial Opening Endoscopic | Z No Device | Z No Qualifier |
| D Urethra | 0 Open<br>3 Percutaneous<br>4 Percutaneous Endoscopic<br>7 Via Natural or Artificial Opening<br>8 Via Natural or Artificial Opening Endoscopic<br>X External | Z No Device | Z No Qualifier |

**0** Medical and Surgical
**T** Urinary System
**R** Replacement: Putting in or on biological or synthetic material that physically takes the place and/or function of all or a portion of a body part

| Character 4 Body Part | Character 5 Approach | Character 6 Device | Character 7 Qualifier |
|---|---|---|---|
| 3 Kidney Pelvis, Right<br>4 Kidney Pelvis, Left<br>6 Ureter, Right<br>7 Ureter, Left<br>B Bladder<br>C Bladder Neck | 0 Open<br>4 Percutaneous Endoscopic<br>7 Via Natural or Artificial Opening<br>8 Via Natural or Artificial Opening Endoscopic | 7 Autologous Tissue Substitute<br>J Synthetic Substitute<br>K Nonautologous Tissue Substitute | Z No Qualifier |
| D Urethra | 0 Open<br>4 Percutaneous Endoscopic<br>7 Via Natural or Artificial Opening<br>8 Via Natural or Artificial Opening Endoscopic<br>X External | 7 Autologous Tissue Substitute<br>J Synthetic Substitute<br>K Nonautologous Tissue Substitute | Z No Qualifier |

**0** Medical and Surgical
**T** Urinary System
**S** Reposition: Moving to its normal location, or other suitable location, all or a portion of a body part

| Character 4 Body Part | Character 5 Approach | Character 6 Device | Character 7 Qualifier |
|---|---|---|---|
| 0 Kidney, Right<br>1 Kidney, Left<br>2 Kidneys, Bilateral<br>3 Kidney Pelvis, Right<br>4 Kidney Pelvis, Left<br>6 Ureter, Right<br>7 Ureter, Left<br>8 Ureters, Bilateral<br>B Bladder<br>C Bladder Neck<br>D Urethra | 0 Open<br>4 Percutaneous Endoscopic | Z No Device | Z No Qualifier |

**0** Medical and Surgical
**T** Urinary System
**T** Resection: Cutting out or off, without replacement, all of a body part

| Character 4<br>Body Part | Character 5<br>Approach | Character 6<br>Device | Character 7<br>Qualifier |
|---|---|---|---|
| 0 Kidney, Right<br>1 Kidney, Left<br>2 Kidneys, Bilateral | 0 Open<br>4 Percutaneous Endoscopic | Z No Device | Z No Qualifier |
| 3 Kidney Pelvis, Right<br>4 Kidney Pelvis, Left<br>6 Ureter, Right<br>7 Ureter, Left<br>B Bladder<br>C Bladder Neck<br>D Urethra | 0 Open<br>4 Percutaneous Endoscopic<br>7 Via Natural or Artificial Opening<br>8 Via Natural or Artificial Opening<br>  Endoscopic | Z No Device | Z No Qualifier |

**0** Medical and Surgical
**T** Urinary System
**U** Supplement: Putting in or on biological or synthetic material that physically reinforces and/or augments the function of a portion of a body part

| Character 4<br>Body Part | Character 5<br>Approach | Character 6<br>Device | Character 7<br>Qualifier |
|---|---|---|---|
| 3 Kidney Pelvis, Right<br>4 Kidney Pelvis, Left<br>6 Ureter, Right<br>7 Ureter, Left<br>B Bladder<br>C Bladder Neck | 0 Open<br>4 Percutaneous Endoscopic<br>7 Via Natural or Artificial Opening<br>8 Via Natural or Artificial Opening<br>  Endoscopic | 7 Autologous Tissue Substitute<br>J Synthetic Substitute<br>K Nonautologous Tissue Substitute | Z No Qualifier |
| D Urethra | 0 Open<br>4 Percutaneous Endoscopic<br>7 Via Natural or Artificial Opening<br>8 Via Natural or Artificial Opening<br>  Endoscopic<br>X External | 7 Autologous Tissue Substitute<br>J Synthetic Substitute<br>K Nonautologous Tissue Substitute | Z No Qualifier |

**0** Medical and Surgical
**T** Urinary System
**V** Restriction: Partially closing an orifice or the lumen of a tubular body part

| Character 4<br>Body Part | Character 5<br>Approach | Character 6<br>Device | Character 7<br>Qualifier |
|---|---|---|---|
| 3 Kidney Pelvis, Right<br>4 Kidney Pelvis, Left<br>6 Ureter, Right<br>7 Ureter, Left<br>B Bladder<br>C Bladder Neck | 0 Open<br>3 Percutaneous<br>4 Percutaneous Endoscopic | C Extraluminal Device<br>D Intraluminal Device<br>Z No Device | Z No Qualifier |
| 3 Kidney Pelvis, Right<br>4 Kidney Pelvis, Left<br>6 Ureter, Right<br>7 Ureter, Left<br>B Bladder<br>C Bladder Neck | 7 Via Natural or Artificial Opening<br>8 Via Natural or Artificial Opening<br>  Endoscopic | D Intraluminal Device<br>Z No Device | Z No Qualifier |
| D Urethra | 0 Open<br>3 Percutaneous<br>4 Percutaneous Endoscopic | C Extraluminal Device<br>D Intraluminal Device<br>Z No Device | Z No Qualifier |
| D Urethra | 7 Via Natural or Artificial Opening<br>8 Via Natural or Artificial Opening<br>  Endoscopic | D Intraluminal Device<br>Z No Device | Z No Qualifier |
| D Urethra | X External | Z No Device | Z No Qualifier |

**0** Medical and Surgical
**T** Urinary System
**W** Revision: Correcting, to the extent possible, a portion of a malfunctioning device or the position of a displaced device

| Character 4<br>Body Part | Character 5<br>Approach | Character 6<br>Device | Character 7<br>Qualifier |
|---|---|---|---|
| 5 Kidney | 0 Open<br>3 Percutaneous<br>4 Percutaneous Endoscopic<br>7 Via Natural or Artificial Opening<br>8 Via Natural or Artificial Opening<br>   Endoscopic<br>X External | 0 Drainage Device<br>2 Monitoring Device<br>3 Infusion Device<br>7 Autologous Tissue Substitute<br>C Extraluminal Device<br>D Intraluminal Device<br>J Synthetic Substitute<br>K Nonautologous Tissue Substitute | Z No Qualifier |
| 9 Ureter | 0 Open<br>3 Percutaneous<br>4 Percutaneous Endoscopic<br>7 Via Natural or Artificial Opening<br>8 Via Natural or Artificial Opening<br>   Endoscopic<br>X External | 0 Drainage Device<br>2 Monitoring Device<br>3 Infusion Device<br>7 Autologous Tissue Substitute<br>C Extraluminal Device<br>D Intraluminal Device<br>J Synthetic Substitute<br>K Nonautologous Tissue Substitute<br>M Stimulator Lead | Z No Qualifier |
| B Bladder | 0 Open<br>3 Percutaneous<br>4 Percutaneous Endoscopic<br>7 Via Natural or Artificial Opening<br>8 Via Natural or Artificial Opening<br>   Endoscopic<br>X External | 0 Drainage Device<br>2 Monitoring Device<br>3 Infusion Device<br>7 Autologous Tissue Substitute<br>C Extraluminal Device<br>D Intraluminal Device<br>J Synthetic Substitute<br>K Nonautologous Tissue Substitute<br>L Artificial Sphincter<br>M Stimulator Lead | Z No Qualifier |
| D Urethra | 0 Open<br>3 Percutaneous<br>4 Percutaneous Endoscopic<br>7 Via Natural or Artificial Opening<br>8 Via Natural or Artificial Opening<br>   Endoscopic<br>X External | 0 Drainage Device<br>2 Monitoring Device<br>3 Infusion Device<br>7 Autologous Tissue Substitute<br>C Extraluminal Device<br>D Intraluminal Device<br>J Synthetic Substitute<br>K Nonautologous Tissue Substitute<br>L Artificial Sphincter | Z No Qualifier |

**0** Medical and Surgical
**T** Urinary System
**Y** Transplantation: Putting in or on all or a portion of a living body part taken from another individual or animal to physically take the place and/or function of all or a portion of a similar body part

| Character 4<br>Body Part | Character 5<br>Approach | Character 6<br>Device | Character 7<br>Qualifier |
|---|---|---|---|
| 0 Kidney, Right  **L C**<br>1 Kidney, Left  **L C** | 0 Open | Z No Device | 0 Allogeneic<br>1 Syngeneic<br>2 Zooplastic |

**L C** 0TY00Z(0,1,2), 0TY10Z(0,1,2)

# Female Reproductive System | 0U1-0UY

| **0** Medical and Surgical | | | |
|---|---|---|---|
| **U** Female Reproductive System | | | |
| **1** Bypass: Altering the route of passage of the contents of a tubular body part | | | |
| Character 4<br>Body Part | Character 5<br>Approach | Character 6<br>Device | Character 7<br>Qualifier |
| 5 Fallopian Tube, Right ♀<br>6 Fallopian Tube, Left ♀ | 0 Open<br>4 Percutaneous Endoscopic | 7 Autologous Tissue Substitute<br>J Synthetic Substitute<br>K Nonautologous Tissue Substitute<br>Z No Device | 5 Fallopian Tube, Right<br>6 Fallopian Tube, Left<br>9 Uterus |

| **0** Medical and Surgical | | | |
|---|---|---|---|
| **U** Female Reproductive System | | | |
| **2** Change: Taking out or off a device from a body part and putting back an identical or similar device in or on the same body part without cutting or puncturing the skin or a mucous membrane | | | |
| Character 4<br>Body Part | Character 5<br>Approach | Character 6<br>Device | Character 7<br>Qualifier |
| 3 Ovary ♀<br>8 Fallopian Tube ♀<br>M Vulva ♀ | X External | 0 Drainage Device<br>Y Other Device | Z No Qualifier |
| D Uterus and Cervix ♀ | X External | 0 Drainage Device<br>H Contraceptive Device<br>Y Other Device | Z No Qualifier |
| H Vagina and Cul-de-sac ♀ | X External | 0 Drainage Device<br>G Intraluminal Device, Pessary<br>Y Other Device | Z No Qualifier |

| **0** Medical and Surgical | | | |
|---|---|---|---|
| **U** Female Reproductive System | | | |
| **5** Destruction: Physical eradication of all or a portion of a body part by the direct use of energy, force, or a destructive agent | | | |
| Character 4<br>Body Part | Character 5<br>Approach | Character 6<br>Device | Character 7<br>Qualifier |
| 0 Ovary, Right ♀<br>1 Ovary, Left ♀<br>2 Ovaries, Bilateral ♀<br>4 Uterine Supporting Structure ♀ | 0 Open<br>3 Percutaneous<br>4 Percutaneous Endoscopic | Z No Device | Z No Qualifier |
| 5 Fallopian Tube, Right ♀<br>6 Fallopian Tube, Left ♀<br>7 Fallopian Tubes, Bilateral ♀ NC<br>9 Uterus ♀<br>B Endometrium ♀<br>C Cervix ♀<br>F Cul-de-sac ♀ | 0 Open<br>3 Percutaneous<br>4 Percutaneous Endoscopic<br>7 Via Natural or Artificial Opening<br>8 Via Natural or Artificial Opening Endoscopic | Z No Device | Z No Qualifier |
| G Vagina ♀<br>K Hymen ♀ | 0 Open<br>3 Percutaneous<br>4 Percutaneous Endoscopic<br>7 Via Natural or Artificial Opening<br>8 Via Natural or Artificial Opening Endoscopic<br>X External | Z No Device | Z No Qualifier |
| J Clitoris ♀<br>L Vestibular Gland ♀<br>M Vulva ♀ | 0 Open<br>X External | Z No Device | Z No Qualifier |

NC 0U57(0,3,4,7,8)ZZ

**0** Medical and Surgical
**U** Female Reproductive System
**7** Dilation: Expanding an orifice or the lumen of a tubular body part

| Character 4<br>Body Part | Character 5<br>Approach | Character 6<br>Device | Character 7<br>Qualifier |
|---|---|---|---|
| 5 Fallopian Tube, Right ♀<br>6 Fallopian Tube, Left ♀<br>7 Fallopian Tubes, Bilateral ♀<br>9 Uterus ♀<br>C Cervix ♀<br>G Vagina ♀ | 0 Open<br>3 Percutaneous<br>4 Percutaneous Endoscopic<br>7 Via Natural or Artificial Opening<br>8 Via Natural or Artificial Opening<br>   Endoscopic | D Intraluminal Device<br>Z No Device | Z No Qualifier |
| K Hymen ♀ | 0 Open<br>3 Percutaneous<br>4 Percutaneous Endoscopic<br>7 Via Natural or Artificial Opening<br>8 Via Natural or Artificial Opening<br>   Endoscopic<br>X External | D Intraluminal Device<br>Z No Device | Z No Qualifier |

**0** Medical and Surgical
**U** Female Reproductive System
**8** Division: Cutting into a body part, without draining fluids and/or gases from the body part, in order to separate or transect a body part

| Character 4<br>Body Part | Character 5<br>Approach | Character 6<br>Device | Character 7<br>Qualifier |
|---|---|---|---|
| 0 Ovary, Right ♀<br>1 Ovary, Left ♀<br>2 Ovaries, Bilateral ♀<br>4 Uterine Supporting Structure ♀ | 0 Open<br>3 Percutaneous<br>4 Percutaneous Endoscopic | Z No Device | Z No Qualifier |
| K Hymen ♀ | 7 Via Natural or Artificial Opening<br>8 Via Natural or Artificial Opening<br>   Endoscopic<br>X External | Z No Device | Z No Qualifier |

**0** Medical and Surgical
**U** Female Reproductive System
**9** Drainage: Taking or letting out fluids and/or gases from a body part

| Character 4<br>Body Part | Character 5<br>Approach | Character 6<br>Device | Character 7<br>Qualifier |
|---|---|---|---|
| 0 Ovary, Right ♀<br>1 Ovary, Left ♀<br>2 Ovaries, Bilateral ♀ | 0 Open<br>3 Percutaneous<br>4 Percutaneous Endoscopic | 0 Drainage Device | Z No Qualifier |
| 0 Ovary, Right ♀<br>1 Ovary, Left ♀<br>2 Ovaries, Bilateral ♀ | 0 Open<br>3 Percutaneous<br>4 Percutaneous Endoscopic | Z No Device | X Diagnostic<br>Z No Qualifier |
| 0 Ovary, Right ♀<br>1 Ovary, Left ♀<br>2 Ovaries, Bilateral ♀ | X External | Z No Device | Z No Qualifier |
| 4 Uterine Supporting Structure ♀ | 0 Open<br>3 Percutaneous<br>4 Percutaneous Endoscopic | 0 Drainage Device | Z No Qualifier |
| 4 Uterine Supporting Structure ♀ | 0 Open<br>3 Percutaneous<br>4 Percutaneous Endoscopic | Z No Device | X Diagnostic<br>Z No Qualifier |
| 5 Fallopian Tube, Right ♀<br>6 Fallopian Tube, Left ♀<br>7 Fallopian Tubes, Bilateral ♀<br>9 Uterus ♀<br>C Cervix ♀<br>F Cul-de-sac ♀ | 0 Open<br>3 Percutaneous<br>4 Percutaneous Endoscopic<br>7 Via Natural or Artificial Opening<br>8 Via Natural or Artificial Opening Endoscopic | 0 Drainage Device | Z No Qualifier |
| 5 Fallopian Tube, Right ♀<br>6 Fallopian Tube, Left ♀<br>7 Fallopian Tubes, Bilateral ♀<br>9 Uterus ♀<br>C Cervix ♀<br>F Cul-de-sac ♀ | 0 Open<br>3 Percutaneous<br>4 Percutaneous Endoscopic<br>7 Via Natural or Artificial Opening<br>8 Via Natural or Artificial Opening Endoscopic | Z No Device | X Diagnostic<br>Z No Qualifier |
| G Vagina ♀<br>K Hymen ♀ | 0 Open<br>3 Percutaneous<br>4 Percutaneous Endoscopic<br>7 Via Natural or Artificial Opening<br>8 Via Natural or Artificial Opening Endoscopic<br>X External | 0 Drainage Device | Z No Qualifier |
| G Vagina ♀<br>K Hymen ♀ | 0 Open<br>3 Percutaneous<br>4 Percutaneous Endoscopic<br>7 Via Natural or Artificial Opening<br>8 Via Natural or Artificial Opening Endoscopic<br>X External | Z No Device | X Diagnostic<br>Z No Qualifier |
| J Clitoris ♀<br>L Vestibular Gland ♀<br>M Vulva ♀ | 0 Open<br>X External | 0 Drainage Device | Z No Qualifier |
| J Clitoris ♀<br>L Vestibular Gland ♀<br>M Vulva ♀ | 0 Open<br>X External | Z No Device | X Diagnostic<br>Z No Qualifier |

**0** Medical and Surgical
**U** Female Reproductive System
**B** Excision: Cutting out or off, without replacement, a portion of a body part

| Character 4<br>Body Part | Character 5<br>Approach | Character 6<br>Device | Character 7<br>Qualifier |
|---|---|---|---|
| 0 Ovary, Right ♀<br>1 Ovary, Left ♀<br>2 Ovaries, Bilateral ♀<br>4 Uterine Supporting Structure ♀<br>5 Fallopian Tube, Right ♀<br>6 Fallopian Tube, Left ♀<br>7 Fallopian Tubes, Bilateral ♀<br>9 Uterus ♀<br>C Cervix ♀<br>F Cul-de-sac ♀ | 0 Open<br>3 Percutaneous<br>4 Percutaneous Endoscopic<br>7 Via Natural or Artificial Opening<br>8 Via Natural or Artificial Opening<br>  Endoscopic | Z No Device | X Diagnostic<br>Z No Qualifier |
| G Vagina ♀<br>K Hymen ♀ | 0 Open<br>3 Percutaneous<br>4 Percutaneous Endoscopic<br>7 Via Natural or Artificial Opening<br>8 Via Natural or Artificial Opening<br>  Endoscopic<br>X External | Z No Device | X Diagnostic<br>Z No Qualifier |
| J Clitoris ♀<br>L Vestibular Gland ♀<br>M Vulva ♀ | 0 Open<br>X External | Z No Device | X Diagnostic<br>Z No Qualifier |

**0** Medical and Surgical
**U** Female Reproductive System
**C** Extirpation: Taking or cutting out solid matter from a body part

| Character 4<br>Body Part | Character 5<br>Approach | Character 6<br>Device | Character 7<br>Qualifier |
|---|---|---|---|
| 0 Ovary, Right ♀<br>1 Ovary, Left ♀<br>2 Ovaries, Bilateral ♀<br>4 Uterine Supporting Structure ♀ | 0 Open<br>3 Percutaneous<br>4 Percutaneous Endoscopic | Z No Device | Z No Qualifier |
| 5 Fallopian Tube, Right ♀<br>6 Fallopian Tube, Left ♀<br>7 Fallopian Tubes, Bilateral ♀<br>9 Uterus ♀<br>B Endometrium ♀<br>C Cervix ♀<br>F Cul-de-sac ♀ | 0 Open<br>3 Percutaneous<br>4 Percutaneous Endoscopic<br>7 Via Natural or Artificial Opening<br>8 Via Natural or Artificial Opening<br>  Endoscopic | Z No Device | Z No Qualifier |
| G Vagina ♀<br>K Hymen ♀ | 0 Open<br>3 Percutaneous<br>4 Percutaneous Endoscopic<br>7 Via Natural or Artificial Opening<br>8 Via Natural or Artificial Opening<br>  Endoscopic<br>X External | Z No Device | Z No Qualifier |
| J Clitoris ♀<br>L Vestibular Gland ♀<br>M Vulva ♀ | 0 Open<br>X External | Z No Device | Z No Qualifier |

**AHA:** 0UC97ZZ - 2Q 2013, 38

**0** Medical and Surgical
**U** Female Reproductive System
**D** Extraction: Pulling or stripping out or off all or a portion of a body part by the use of force

| Character 4<br>Body Part | Character 5<br>Approach | Character 6<br>Device | Character 7<br>Qualifier |
|---|---|---|---|
| B Endometrium ♀ | 7 Via Natural or Artificial Opening<br>8 Via Natural or Artificial Opening<br>  Endoscopic | Z No Device | X Diagnostic<br>Z No Qualifier |
| N Ova ♀ | 0 Open<br>3 Percutaneous<br>4 Percutaneous Endoscopic | Z No Device | Z No Qualifier |

**0** Medical and Surgical
**U** Female Reproductive System
**F** Fragmentation: Breaking solid matter in a body part into pieces

| Character 4<br>Body Part | Character 5<br>Approach | Character 6<br>Device | Character 7<br>Qualifier |
|---|---|---|---|
| 5  Fallopian Tube, Right ♀ N C<br>6  Fallopian Tube, Left ♀ N C<br>7  Fallopian Tubes, Bilateral ♀ N C<br>9  Uterus ♀ N C | 0  Open<br>3  Percutaneous<br>4  Percutaneous Endoscopic<br>7  Via Natural or Artificial Opening<br>8  Via Natural or Artificial Opening<br>   Endoscopic<br>X  External | Z  No Device | Z  No Qualifier |

N C  0UF(5,6,7,9)XZZ

---

**0** Medical and Surgical
**U** Female Reproductive System
**H** Insertion: Putting in a nonbiological appliance that monitors, assists, performs, or prevents a physiological function but does not physically take the place of a body part

| Character 4<br>Body Part | Character 5<br>Approach | Character 6<br>Device | Character 7<br>Qualifier |
|---|---|---|---|
| 3  Ovary ♀ | 0  Open<br>3  Percutaneous<br>4  Percutaneous Endoscopic | 3  Infusion Device | Z  No Qualifier |
| 8  Fallopian Tube ♀<br>D  Uterus and Cervix ♀<br>H  Vagina and Cul-de-sac ♀ | 0  Open<br>3  Percutaneous<br>4  Percutaneous Endoscopic<br>7  Via Natural or Artificial Opening<br>8  Via Natural or Artificial Opening<br>   Endoscopic | 3  Infusion Device | Z  No Qualifier |
| 9  Uterus ♀ | 7  Via Natural or Artificial Opening<br>8  Via Natural or Artificial Opening<br>   Endoscopic | H  Contraceptive Device | Z  No Qualifier |
| C  Cervix ♀ | 0  Open<br>3  Percutaneous<br>4  Percutaneous Endoscopic | 1  Radioactive Element | Z  No Qualifier |
| C  Cervix ♀ | 7  Via Natural or Artificial Opening<br>8  Via Natural or Artificial Opening<br>   Endoscopic | 1  Radioactive Element<br>H  Contraceptive Device | Z  No Qualifier |
| F  Cul-de-sac ♀ | 7  Via Natural or Artificial Opening<br>8  Via Natural or Artificial Opening<br>   Endoscopic | G  Intraluminal Device, Pessary | Z  No Qualifier |
| G  Vagina ♀ | 0  Open<br>3  Percutaneous<br>4  Percutaneous Endoscopic<br>X  External | 1  Radioactive Element | Z  No Qualifier |
| G  Vagina ♀ | 7  Via Natural or Artificial Opening<br>8  Via Natural or Artificial Opening<br>   Endoscopic | 1  Radioactive Element<br>G  Intraluminal Device, Pessary | Z  No Qualifier |

**AHA:** 0UH97HZ - 2Q 2013, 34

---

**0** Medical and Surgical
**U** Female Reproductive System
**J** Inspection: Visually and/or manually exploring a body part

| Character 4<br>Body Part | Character 5<br>Approach | Character 6<br>Device | Character 7<br>Qualifier |
|---|---|---|---|
| 3  Ovary ♀ | 0  Open<br>3  Percutaneous<br>4  Percutaneous Endoscopic<br>X  External | Z  No Device | Z  No Qualifier |
| 8  Fallopian Tube ♀<br>D  Uterus and Cervix ♀<br>H  Vagina and Cul-de-sac ♀ | 0  Open<br>3  Percutaneous<br>4  Percutaneous Endoscopic<br>7  Via Natural or Artificial Opening<br>8  Via Natural or Artificial Opening<br>   Endoscopic<br>X  External | Z  No Device | Z  No Qualifier |
| M  Vulva ♀ | 0  Open<br>X  External | Z  No Device | Z  No Qualifier |

---

♂ Male          ♀ Female          N C Non-covered          L C Limited Coverage          **AHA** *AHA Coding Clinic*

**0** Medical and Surgical
**U** Female Reproductive System
**L** Occlusion: Completely closing an orifice or the lumen of a tubular body part

| Character 4<br>Body Part | Character 5<br>Approach | Character 6<br>Device | Character 7<br>Qualifier |
|---|---|---|---|
| 5 Fallopian Tube, Right ♀<br>6 Fallopian Tube, Left ♀<br>7 Fallopian Tubes, Bilateral ♀ NC | 0 Open<br>3 Percutaneous<br>4 Percutaneous Endoscopic | C Extraluminal Device<br>D Intraluminal Device<br>Z No Device | Z No Qualifier |
| 5 Fallopian Tube, Right ♀<br>6 Fallopian Tube, Left ♀<br>7 Fallopian Tubes, Bilateral ♀ NC | 7 Via Natural or Artificial Opening<br>8 Via Natural or Artificial Opening<br>Endoscopic | D Intraluminal Device<br>Z No Device | Z No Qualifier |
| F Cul-de-sac ♀<br>G Vagina ♀ | 7 Via Natural or Artificial Opening<br>8 Via Natural or Artificial Opening<br>Endoscopic | D Intraluminal Device<br>Z No Device | Z No Qualifier |

**NC** 0UL70(C,D,Z)Z, 0UL73(C,D,Z)Z, 0UL74(C,D,Z)Z, 0UL77(D,Z)Z, 0UL78(D,Z)Z

**0** Medical and Surgical
**U** Female Reproductive System
**M** Reattachment: Putting back in or on all or a portion of a separated body part to its normal location or other suitable location

| Character 4<br>Body Part | Character 5<br>Approach | Character 6<br>Device | Character 7<br>Qualifier |
|---|---|---|---|
| 0 Ovary, Right ♀<br>1 Ovary, Left ♀<br>2 Ovaries, Bilateral ♀<br>4 Uterine Supporting Structure ♀<br>5 Fallopian Tube, Right ♀<br>6 Fallopian Tube, Left ♀<br>7 Fallopian Tubes, Bilateral ♀<br>9 Uterus ♀<br>C Cervix ♀<br>F Cul-de-sac ♀<br>G Vagina ♀ | 0 Open<br>4 Percutaneous Endoscopic | Z No Device | Z No Qualifier |
| J Clitoris ♀<br>M Vulva ♀ | X External | Z No Device | Z No Qualifier |
| K Hymen ♀ | 0 Open<br>4 Percutaneous Endoscopic<br>X External | Z No Device | Z No Qualifier |

**0** Medical and Surgical
**U** Female Reproductive System
**N** Release: Freeing a body part from an abnormal physical constraint by cutting or by the use of force

| Character 4<br>Body Part | Character 5<br>Approach | Character 6<br>Device | Character 7<br>Qualifier |
|---|---|---|---|
| 0 Ovary, Right ♀<br>1 Ovary, Left ♀<br>2 Ovaries, Bilateral ♀<br>4 Uterine Supporting Structure ♀ | 0 Open<br>3 Percutaneous<br>4 Percutaneous Endoscopic | Z No Device | Z No Qualifier |
| 5 Fallopian Tube, Right ♀<br>6 Fallopian Tube, Left ♀<br>7 Fallopian Tubes, Bilateral ♀<br>9 Uterus ♀<br>C Cervix ♀<br>F Cul-de-sac ♀ | 0 Open<br>3 Percutaneous<br>4 Percutaneous Endoscopic<br>7 Via Natural or Artificial Opening<br>8 Via Natural or Artificial Opening<br>Endoscopic | Z No Device | Z No Qualifier |
| G Vagina ♀<br>K Hymen ♀ | 0 Open<br>3 Percutaneous<br>4 Percutaneous Endoscopic<br>7 Via Natural or Artificial Opening<br>8 Via Natural or Artificial Opening<br>Endoscopic<br>X External | Z No Device | Z No Qualifier |
| J Clitoris ♀<br>L Vestibular Gland ♀<br>M Vulva ♀ | 0 Open<br>X External | Z No Device | Z No Qualifier |

**0** Medical and Surgical
**U** Female Reproductive System
**P** Removal: Taking out or off a device from a body part

| Character 4<br>Body Part | Character 5<br>Approach | Character 6<br>Device | Character 7<br>Qualifier |
|---|---|---|---|
| 3 Ovary ♀ | 0 Open<br>3 Percutaneous<br>4 Percutaneous Endoscopic<br>X External | 0 Drainage Device<br>3 Infusion Device | Z No Qualifier |
| 8 Fallopian Tube ♀ | 0 Open<br>3 Percutaneous<br>4 Percutaneous Endoscopic<br>7 Via Natural or Artificial Opening<br>8 Via Natural or Artificial Opening<br>Endoscopic | 0 Drainage Device<br>3 Infusion Device<br>7 Autologous Tissue Substitute<br>C Extraluminal Device<br>D Intraluminal Device<br>J Synthetic Substitute<br>K Nonautologous Tissue Substitute | Z No Qualifier |
| 8 Fallopian Tube ♀ | X External | 0 Drainage Device<br>3 Infusion Device<br>D Intraluminal Device | Z No Qualifier |
| D Uterus and Cervix ♀ | 0 Open<br>3 Percutaneous<br>4 Percutaneous Endoscopic<br>7 Via Natural or Artificial Opening<br>8 Via Natural or Artificial Opening<br>Endoscopic | 0 Drainage Device<br>1 Radioactive Element<br>3 Infusion Device<br>7 Autologous Tissue Substitute<br>C Extraluminal Device<br>D Intraluminal Device<br>H Contraceptive Device<br>J Synthetic Substitute<br>K Nonautologous Tissue Substitute | Z No Qualifier |
| D Uterus and Cervix ♀ | X External | 0 Drainage Device<br>3 Infusion Device<br>D Intraluminal Device<br>H Contraceptive Device | Z No Qualifier |
| H Vagina and Cul-de-sac ♀ | 0 Open<br>3 Percutaneous<br>4 Percutaneous Endoscopic<br>7 Via Natural or Artificial Opening<br>8 Via Natural or Artificial Opening<br>Endoscopic | 0 Drainage Device<br>1 Radioactive Element<br>3 Infusion Device<br>7 Autologous Tissue Substitute<br>D Intraluminal Device<br>J Synthetic Substitute<br>K Nonautologous Tissue Substitute | Z No Qualifier |
| H Vagina and Cul-de-sac ♀ | X External | 0 Drainage Device<br>1 Radioactive Element<br>3 Infusion Device<br>D Intraluminal Device | Z No Qualifier |
| M Vulva ♀ | 0 Open | 0 Drainage Device<br>7 Autologous Tissue Substitute<br>J Synthetic Substitute<br>K Nonautologous Tissue Substitute | Z No Qualifier |
| M Vulva ♀ | X External | 0 Drainage Device | Z No Qualifier |

**0** Medical and Surgical
**U** Female Reproductive System
**Q** Repair: Restoring, to the extent possible, a body part to its normal anatomic structure and function

| Character 4<br>Body Part | Character 5<br>Approach | Character 6<br>Device | Character 7<br>Qualifier |
|---|---|---|---|
| 0 Ovary, Right ♀<br>1 Ovary, Left ♀<br>2 Ovaries, Bilateral ♀<br>4 Uterine Supporting Structure ♀ | 0 Open<br>3 Percutaneous<br>4 Percutaneous Endoscopic | Z No Device | Z No Qualifier |
| 5 Fallopian Tube, Right ♀<br>6 Fallopian Tube, Left ♀<br>7 Fallopian Tubes, Bilateral ♀<br>9 Uterus ♀<br>C Cervix ♀<br>F Cul-de-sac ♀ | 0 Open<br>3 Percutaneous<br>4 Percutaneous Endoscopic<br>7 Via Natural or Artificial Opening<br>8 Via Natural or Artificial Opening<br>   Endoscopic | Z No Device | Z No Qualifier |
| G Vagina ♀<br>K Hymen ♀ | 0 Open<br>3 Percutaneous<br>4 Percutaneous Endoscopic<br>7 Via Natural or Artificial Opening<br>8 Via Natural or Artificial Opening<br>   Endoscopic<br>X External | Z No Device | Z No Qualifier |
| J Clitoris ♀<br>L Vestibular Gland ♀<br>M Vulva ♀ | 0 Open<br>X External | Z No Device | Z No Qualifier |

**AHA:** 0UQJXZZ - 4Q 2013, 121

**0** Medical and Surgical
**U** Female Reproductive System
**S** Reposition: Moving to its normal location, or other suitable location, all or a portion of a body part

| Character 4<br>Body Part | Character 5<br>Approach | Character 6<br>Device | Character 7<br>Qualifier |
|---|---|---|---|
| 0 Ovary, Right ♀<br>1 Ovary, Left ♀<br>2 Ovaries, Bilateral ♀<br>4 Uterine Supporting Structure ♀<br>5 Fallopian Tube, Right ♀<br>6 Fallopian Tube, Left ♀<br>7 Fallopian Tubes, Bilateral ♀<br>C Cervix ♀<br>F Cul-de-sac ♀ | 0 Open<br>4 Percutaneous Endoscopic | Z No Device | Z No Qualifier |
| 9 Uterus ♀<br>G Vagina ♀ | 0 Open<br>4 Percutaneous Endoscopic<br>X External | Z No Device | Z No Qualifier |

**0 Medical and Surgical**
**U Female Reproductive System**
**T Resection: Cutting out or off, without replacement, all of a body part**

| Character 4<br>Body Part | Character 5<br>Approach | Character 6<br>Device | Character 7<br>Qualifier |
|---|---|---|---|
| 0 Ovary, Right ♀<br>1 Ovary, Left ♀<br>2 Ovaries, Bilateral ♀<br>5 Fallopian Tube, Right ♀<br>6 Fallopian Tube, Left ♀<br>7 Fallopian Tubes, Bilateral ♀<br>9 Uterus ♀ | 0 Open<br>4 Percutaneous Endoscopic<br>7 Via Natural or Artificial Opening<br>8 Via Natural or Artificial Opening Endoscopic<br>F Via Natural or Artificial Opening With Percutaneous Endoscopic Assistance | Z No Device | Z No Qualifier |
| 4 Uterine Supporting Structure ♀<br>C Cervix ♀<br>F Cul-de-sac ♀<br>G Vagina ♀ | 0 Open<br>4 Percutaneous Endoscopic<br>7 Via Natural or Artificial Opening<br>8 Via Natural or Artificial Opening Endoscopic | Z No Device | Z No Qualifier |
| J Clitoris ♀<br>L Vestibular Gland ♀<br>M Vulva ♀ | 0 Open<br>X External | Z No Device | Z No Qualifier |
| K Hymen ♀ | 0 Open<br>4 Percutaneous Endoscopic<br>7 Via Natural or Artificial Opening<br>8 Via Natural or Artificial Opening Endoscopic<br>X External | Z No Device | Z No Qualifier |

**AHA:** 0UT00ZZ - 1Q 2013, 24; 0UT90ZZ - 3Q 2013, 28; 0UTC0ZZ - 3Q 2013, 28

---

**0 Medical and Surgical**
**U Female Reproductive System**
**U Supplement: Putting in or on biological or synthetic material that physically reinforces and/or augments the function of a portion of a body part**

| Character 4<br>Body Part | Character 5<br>Approach | Character 6<br>Device | Character 7<br>Qualifier |
|---|---|---|---|
| 4 Uterine Supporting Structure ♀ | 0 Open<br>4 Percutaneous Endoscopic | 7 Autologous Tissue Substitute<br>J Synthetic Substitute<br>K Nonautologous Tissue Substitute | Z No Qualifier |
| 5 Fallopian Tube, Right ♀<br>6 Fallopian Tube, Left ♀<br>7 Fallopian Tubes, Bilateral ♀<br>F Cul-de-sac ♀ | 0 Open<br>4 Percutaneous Endoscopic<br>7 Via Natural or Artificial Opening<br>8 Via Natural or Artificial Opening Endoscopic | 7 Autologous Tissue Substitute<br>J Synthetic Substitute<br>K Nonautologous Tissue Substitute | Z No Qualifier |
| G Vagina ♀<br>K Hymen ♀ | 0 Open<br>4 Percutaneous Endoscopic<br>7 Via Natural or Artificial Opening<br>8 Via Natural or Artificial Opening Endoscopic<br>X External | 7 Autologous Tissue Substitute<br>J Synthetic Substitute<br>K Nonautologous Tissue Substitute | Z No Qualifier |
| J Clitoris ♀<br>M Vulva ♀ | 0 Open<br>X External | 7 Autologous Tissue Substitute<br>J Synthetic Substitute<br>K Nonautologous Tissue Substitute | Z No Qualifier |

---

**0 Medical and Surgical**
**U Female Reproductive System**
**V Restriction: Partially closing an orifice or the lumen of a tubular body part**

| Character 4<br>Body Part | Character 5<br>Approach | Character 6<br>Device | Character 7<br>Qualifier |
|---|---|---|---|
| C Cervix ♀ | 0 Open<br>3 Percutaneous<br>4 Percutaneous Endoscopic | C Extraluminal Device<br>D Intraluminal Device<br>Z No Device | Z No Qualifier |
| C Cervix ♀ | 7 Via Natural or Artificial Opening<br>8 Via Natural or Artificial Opening Endoscopic | D Intraluminal Device<br>Z No Device | Z No Qualifier |

---

♂ Male     ♀ Female     N C Non-covered     L C Limited Coverage     **AHA** *AHA Coding Clinic*

**0 Medical and Surgical**
**U Female Reproductive System**
**W Revision: Correcting, to the extent possible, a portion of a malfunctioning device or the position of a displaced device**

| Character 4<br>Body Part | Character 5<br>Approach | Character 6<br>Device | Character 7<br>Qualifier |
|---|---|---|---|
| 3 Ovary ♀ | 0 Open<br>3 Percutaneous<br>4 Percutaneous Endoscopic<br>X External | 0 Drainage Device<br>3 Infusion Device | Z No Qualifier |
| 8 Fallopian Tube ♀ | 0 Open<br>3 Percutaneous<br>4 Percutaneous Endoscopic<br>7 Via Natural or Artificial Opening<br>8 Via Natural or Artificial Opening<br>   Endoscopic<br>X External | 0 Drainage Device<br>3 Infusion Device<br>7 Autologous Tissue Substitute<br>C Extraluminal Device<br>D Intraluminal Device<br>J Synthetic Substitute<br>K Nonautologous Tissue Substitute | Z No Qualifier |
| D Uterus and Cervix ♀ | 0 Open<br>3 Percutaneous<br>4 Percutaneous Endoscopic<br>7 Via Natural or Artificial Opening<br>8 Via Natural or Artificial Opening<br>   Endoscopic | 0 Drainage Device<br>1 Radioactive Element<br>3 Infusion Device<br>7 Autologous Tissue Substitute<br>C Extraluminal Device<br>D Intraluminal Device<br>H Contraceptive Device<br>J Synthetic Substitute<br>K Nonautologous Tissue Substitute | Z No Qualifier |
| D Uterus and Cervix ♀ | X External | 0 Drainage Device<br>3 Infusion Device<br>7 Autologous Tissue Substitute<br>C Extraluminal Device<br>D Intraluminal Device<br>H Contraceptive Device<br>J Synthetic Substitute<br>K Nonautologous Tissue Substitute | Z No Qualifier |
| H Vagina and Cul-de-sac ♀ | 0 Open<br>3 Percutaneous<br>4 Percutaneous Endoscopic<br>7 Via Natural or Artificial Opening<br>8 Via Natural or Artificial Opening<br>   Endoscopic | 0 Drainage Device<br>1 Radioactive Element<br>3 Infusion Device<br>7 Autologous Tissue Substitute<br>D Intraluminal Device<br>J Synthetic Substitute<br>K Nonautologous Tissue Substitute | Z No Qualifier |
| H Vagina and Cul-de-sac ♀ | X External | 0 Drainage Device<br>3 Infusion Device<br>7 Autologous Tissue Substitute<br>D Intraluminal Device<br>J Synthetic Substitute<br>K Nonautologous Tissue Substitute | Z No Qualifier |
| M Vulva ♀ | 0 Open<br>X External | 0 Drainage Device<br>7 Autologous Tissue Substitute<br>J Synthetic Substitute<br>K Nonautologous Tissue Substitute | Z No Qualifier |

**0 Medical and Surgical**
**U Female Reproductive System**
**Y Transplantation: Putting in or on all or a portion of a living body part taken from another individual or animal to physically take the place and/or function of all or a portion of a similar body part**

| Character 4<br>Body Part | Character 5<br>Approach | Character 6<br>Device | Character 7<br>Qualifier |
|---|---|---|---|
| 0 Ovary, Right ♀<br>1 Ovary, Left ♀ | 0 Open | Z No Device | 0 Allogeneic<br>1 Syngeneic<br>2 Zooplastic |

# Male Reproductive System | 0V1-0VW

**0** Medical and Surgical
**V** Male Reproductive System
**1** Bypass: Altering the route of passage of the contents of a tubular body part

| Character 4 Body Part | Character 5 Approach | Character 6 Device | Character 7 Qualifier |
|---|---|---|---|
| N Vas Deferens, Right ♂<br>P Vas Deferens, Left ♂<br>Q Vas Deferens, Bilateral ♂ | 0 Open<br>4 Percutaneous Endoscopic | 7 Autologous Tissue Substitute<br>J Synthetic Substitute<br>K Nonautologous Tissue Substitute<br>Z No Device | J Epididymis, Right<br>K Epididymis, Left<br>N Vas Deferens, Right<br>P Vas Deferens, Left |

**0** Medical and Surgical
**V** Male Reproductive System
**2** Change: Taking out or off a device from a body part and putting back an identical or similar device in or on the same body part without cutting or puncturing the skin or a mucous membrane

| Character 4 Body Part | Character 5 Approach | Character 6 Device | Character 7 Qualifier |
|---|---|---|---|
| 4 Prostate and Seminal Vesicles ♂<br>8 Scrotum and Tunica Vaginalis ♂<br>D Testis ♂<br>M Epididymis and Spermatic Cord ♂<br>R Vas Deferens ♂<br>S Penis ♂ | X External | 0 Drainage Device<br>Y Other Device | Z No Qualifier |

**0** Medical and Surgical
**V** Male Reproductive System
**5** Destruction: Physical eradication of all or a portion of a body part by the direct use of energy, force, or a destructive agent

| Character 4 Body Part | Character 5 Approach | Character 6 Device | Character 7 Qualifier |
|---|---|---|---|
| 0 Prostate ♂ | 0 Open<br>3 Percutaneous<br>4 Percutaneous Endoscopic<br>7 Via Natural or Artificial Opening<br>8 Via Natural or Artificial Opening Endoscopic | Z No Device | Z No Qualifier |
| 1 Seminal Vesicle, Right ♂<br>2 Seminal Vesicle, Left ♂<br>3 Seminal Vesicles, Bilateral ♂<br>6 Tunica Vaginalis, Right ♂<br>7 Tunica Vaginalis, Left ♂<br>9 Testis, Right ♂<br>B Testis, Left ♂<br>C Testes, Bilateral ♂<br>F Spermatic Cord, Right ♂<br>G Spermatic Cord, Left ♂<br>H Spermatic Cords, Bilateral ♂<br>J Epididymis, Right ♂<br>K Epididymis, Left ♂<br>L Epididymis, Bilateral ♂<br>N Vas Deferens, Right ♂ NC<br>P Vas Deferens, Left ♂ NC<br>Q Vas Deferens, Bilateral ♂ NC | 0 Open<br>3 Percutaneous<br>4 Percutaneous Endoscopic | Z No Device | Z No Qualifier |
| 5 Scrotum ♂<br>S Penis ♂<br>T Prepuce ♂ | 0 Open<br>3 Percutaneous<br>4 Percutaneous Endoscopic<br>X External | Z No Device | Z No Qualifier |

NC 0V5N(0,3,4)ZZ, 0V5P(0,3,4)ZZ, 0V5Q(0,3,4)ZZ

**0** Medical and Surgical
**V** Male Reproductive System
**7** Dilation: Expanding an orifice or the lumen of a tubular body part

| Character 4 Body Part | Character 5 Approach | Character 6 Device | Character 7 Qualifier |
|---|---|---|---|
| N Vas Deferens, Right ♂<br>P Vas Deferens, Left ♂<br>Q Vas Deferens, Bilateral ♂ | 0 Open<br>3 Percutaneous<br>4 Percutaneous Endoscopic | D Intraluminal Device<br>Z No Device | Z No Qualifier |

---

♂ Male      ♀ Female      NC Non-covered      LC Limited Coverage      **AHA** *AHA Coding Clinic*

**0** Medical and Surgical
**V** Male Reproductive System
**9** Drainage: Taking or letting out fluids and/or gases from a body part

| Character 4<br>Body Part | Character 5<br>Approach | Character 6<br>Device | Character 7<br>Qualifier |
|---|---|---|---|
| 0 Prostate ♂ | 0 Open<br>3 Percutaneous<br>4 Percutaneous Endoscopic<br>7 Via Natural or Artificial Opening<br>8 Via Natural or Artificial Opening<br>　 Endoscopic | 0 Drainage Device | Z No Qualifier |
| 0 Prostate ♂ | 0 Open<br>3 Percutaneous<br>4 Percutaneous Endoscopic<br>7 Via Natural or Artificial Opening<br>8 Via Natural or Artificial Opening<br>　 Endoscopic | Z No Device | X Diagnostic<br>Z No Qualifier |
| 1 Seminal Vesicle, Right ♂<br>2 Seminal Vesicle, Left ♂<br>3 Seminal Vesicles, Bilateral ♂<br>6 Tunica Vaginalis, Right ♂<br>7 Tunica Vaginalis, Left ♂<br>9 Testis, Right ♂<br>B Testis, Left ♂<br>C Testes, Bilateral ♂<br>F Spermatic Cord, Right ♂<br>G Spermatic Cord, Left ♂<br>H Spermatic Cords, Bilateral ♂<br>J Epididymis, Right ♂<br>K Epididymis, Left ♂<br>L Epididymis, Bilateral ♂<br>N Vas Deferens, Right ♂<br>P Vas Deferens, Left ♂<br>Q Vas Deferens, Bilateral ♂ | 0 Open<br>3 Percutaneous<br>4 Percutaneous Endoscopic | 0 Drainage Device | Z No Qualifier |
| 1 Seminal Vesicle, Right ♂<br>2 Seminal Vesicle, Left ♂<br>3 Seminal Vesicles, Bilateral ♂<br>6 Tunica Vaginalis, Right ♂<br>7 Tunica Vaginalis, Left ♂<br>9 Testis, Right ♂<br>B Testis, Left ♂<br>C Testes, Bilateral ♂<br>F Spermatic Cord, Right ♂<br>G Spermatic Cord, Left ♂<br>H Spermatic Cords, Bilateral ♂<br>J Epididymis, Right ♂<br>K Epididymis, Left ♂<br>L Epididymis, Bilateral ♂<br>N Vas Deferens, Right ♂<br>P Vas Deferens, Left ♂<br>Q Vas Deferens, Bilateral ♂ | 0 Open<br>3 Percutaneous<br>4 Percutaneous Endoscopic | Z No Device | X Diagnostic<br>Z No Qualifier |
| 5 Scrotum ♂<br>S Penis ♂<br>T Prepuce ♂ | 0 Open<br>3 Percutaneous<br>4 Percutaneous Endoscopic<br>X External | 0 Drainage Device | Z No Qualifier |
| 5 Scrotum ♂<br>S Penis ♂<br>T Prepuce ♂ | 0 Open<br>3 Percutaneous<br>4 Percutaneous Endoscopic<br>X External | Z No Device | X Diagnostic<br>Z No Qualifier |

**0** Medical and Surgical
**V** Male Reproductive System
**B** Excision: Cutting out or off, without replacement, a portion of a body part

| Character 4<br>Body Part | Character 5<br>Approach | Character 6<br>Device | Character 7<br>Qualifier |
|---|---|---|---|
| 0 Prostate ♂ | 0 Open<br>3 Percutaneous<br>4 Percutaneous Endoscopic<br>7 Via Natural or Artificial Opening<br>8 Via Natural or Artificial Opening Endoscopic | Z No Device | X Diagnostic<br>Z No Qualifier |
| 1 Seminal Vesicle, Right ♂<br>2 Seminal Vesicle, Left ♂<br>3 Seminal Vesicles, Bilateral ♂<br>6 Tunica Vaginalis, Right ♂<br>7 Tunica Vaginalis, Left ♂<br>9 Testis, Right ♂<br>B Testis, Left ♂<br>C Testes, Bilateral ♂<br>F Spermatic Cord, Right ♂<br>G Spermatic Cord, Left ♂<br>H Spermatic Cords, Bilateral ♂<br>J Epididymis, Right ♂<br>K Epididymis, Left ♂<br>L Epididymis, Bilateral ♂<br>N Vas Deferens, Right ♂ **NC**<br>P Vas Deferens, Left ♂ **NC**<br>Q Vas Deferens, Bilateral ♂ **NC** | 0 Open<br>3 Percutaneous<br>4 Percutaneous Endoscopic | Z No Device | X Diagnostic<br>Z No Qualifier |
| 5 Scrotum ♂<br>S Penis ♂<br>T Prepuce ♂ | 0 Open<br>3 Percutaneous<br>4 Percutaneous Endoscopic<br>X External | Z No Device | X Diagnostic<br>Z No Qualifier |

**NC** 0VBN(0,3,4)ZZ, 0VBP(0,3,4)ZZ, 0VBQ(0,3,4)ZZ

**0** Medical and Surgical
**V** Male Reproductive System
**C** Extirpation: Taking or cutting out solid matter from a body part

| Character 4<br>Body Part | Character 5<br>Approach | Character 6<br>Device | Character 7<br>Qualifier |
|---|---|---|---|
| 0 Prostate ♂ | 0 Open<br>3 Percutaneous<br>4 Percutaneous Endoscopic<br>7 Via Natural or Artificial Opening<br>8 Via Natural or Artificial Opening Endoscopic | Z No Device | Z No Qualifier |
| 1 Seminal Vesicle, Right ♂<br>2 Seminal Vesicle, Left ♂<br>3 Seminal Vesicles, Bilateral ♂<br>6 Tunica Vaginalis, Right ♂<br>7 Tunica Vaginalis, Left ♂<br>9 Testis, Right ♂<br>B Testis, Left ♂<br>C Testes, Bilateral ♂<br>F Spermatic Cord, Right ♂<br>G Spermatic Cord, Left ♂<br>H Spermatic Cords, Bilateral ♂<br>J Epididymis, Right ♂<br>K Epididymis, Left ♂<br>L Epididymis, Bilateral ♂<br>N Vas Deferens, Right ♂<br>P Vas Deferens, Left ♂<br>Q Vas Deferens, Bilateral ♂ | 0 Open<br>3 Percutaneous<br>4 Percutaneous Endoscopic | Z No Device | Z No Qualifier |
| 5 Scrotum ♂<br>S Penis ♂<br>T Prepuce ♂ | 0 Open<br>3 Percutaneous<br>4 Percutaneous Endoscopic<br>X External | Z No Device | Z No Qualifier |

**0** Medical and Surgical
**V** Male Reproductive System
**H** Insertion: Putting in a nonbiological appliance that monitors, assists, performs, or prevents a physiological function but does not physically take the place of a body part

| Character 4 Body Part | Character 5 Approach | Character 6 Device | Character 7 Qualifier |
|---|---|---|---|
| 0  Prostate ♂ | 0  Open<br>3  Percutaneous<br>4  Percutaneous Endoscopic<br>7  Via Natural or Artificial Opening<br>8  Via Natural or Artificial Opening Endoscopic | 1  Radioactive Element | Z  No Qualifier |
| 4  Prostate and Seminal Vesicles ♂<br>8  Scrotum and Tunica Vaginalis ♂<br>D  Testis ♂<br>M  Epididymis and Spermatic Cord ♂<br>R  Vas Deferens ♂ | 0  Open<br>3  Percutaneous<br>4  Percutaneous Endoscopic<br>7  Via Natural or Artificial Opening<br>8  Via Natural or Artificial Opening Endoscopic | 3  Infusion Device | Z  No Qualifier |
| S  Penis ♂ | 0  Open<br>3  Percutaneous<br>4  Percutaneous Endoscopic<br>X  External | 3  Infusion Device | Z  No Qualifier |

**0** Medical and Surgical
**V** Male Reproductive System
**J** Inspection: Visually and/or manually exploring a body part

| Character 4 Body Part | Character 5 Approach | Character 6 Device | Character 7 Qualifier |
|---|---|---|---|
| 4  Prostate and Seminal Vesicles ♂<br>8  Scrotum and Tunica Vaginalis ♂<br>D  Testis ♂<br>M  Epididymis and Spermatic Cord ♂<br>R  Vas Deferens ♂<br>S  Penis ♂ | 0  Open<br>3  Percutaneous<br>4  Percutaneous Endoscopic<br>X  External | Z  No Device | Z  No Qualifier |

**0** Medical and Surgical
**V** Male Reproductive System
**L** Occlusion: Completely closing an orifice or the lumen of a tubular body part

| Character 4 Body Part | Character 5 Approach | Character 6 Device | Character 7 Qualifier |
|---|---|---|---|
| F  Spermatic Cord, Right ♂ NC<br>G  Spermatic Cord, Left ♂ NC<br>H  Spermatic Cords, Bilateral ♂ NC<br>N  Vas Deferens, Right ♂ NC<br>P  Vas Deferens, Left ♂ NC<br>Q  Vas Deferens, Bilateral ♂ NC | 0  Open<br>3  Percutaneous<br>4  Percutaneous Endoscopic | C  Extraluminal Device<br>D  Intraluminal Device<br>Z  No Device | Z  No Qualifier |

NC 0VLF0(C,D,Z)Z, 0VLF3(C,D,Z)Z, 0VLF4(C,D,Z)Z, 0VLG0(C,D,Z)Z, 0VLG3(C,D,Z)Z, 0VLG4(C,D,Z)Z, 0VLH0(C,D,Z)Z, 0VLH3(C,D,Z)Z, 0VLH4(C,D,Z)Z, 0VLN0(C,Z)Z, 0VLN3(C,Z)Z, 0VLN4(C,Z)Z, 0VLP0(C,Z)Z, 0VLP3(C,Z)Z, 0VLP4(C,Z)Z, 0VLQ0(C,Z)Z, 0VLQ3(C,Z)Z, 0VLQ4(C,Z)Z

**0** Medical and Surgical
**V** Male Reproductive System
**M** Reattachment: Putting back in or on all or a portion of a separated body part to its normal location or other suitable location

| Character 4 Body Part | Character 5 Approach | Character 6 Device | Character 7 Qualifier |
|---|---|---|---|
| 5  Scrotum ♂<br>S  Penis ♂ | X  External | Z  No Device | Z  No Qualifier |
| 6  Tunica Vaginalis, Right ♂<br>7  Tunica Vaginalis, Left ♂<br>9  Testis, Right ♂<br>B  Testis, Left ♂<br>C  Testes, Bilateral ♂<br>F  Spermatic Cord, Right ♂<br>G  Spermatic Cord, Left ♂<br>H  Spermatic Cords, Bilateral ♂ | 0  Open<br>4  Percutaneous Endoscopic | Z  No Device | Z  No Qualifier |

| **0** Medical and Surgical |
| **V** Male Reproductive System |
| **N** Release: Freeing a body part from an abnormal physical constraint by cutting or by the use of force |

| Character 4<br>Body Part | Character 5<br>Approach | Character 6<br>Device | Character 7<br>Qualifier |
|---|---|---|---|
| 0 Prostate ♂ | 0 Open<br>3 Percutaneous<br>4 Percutaneous Endoscopic<br>7 Via Natural or Artificial Opening<br>8 Via Natural or Artificial Opening Endoscopic | Z No Device | Z No Qualifier |
| 1 Seminal Vesicle, Right ♂<br>2 Seminal Vesicle, Left ♂<br>3 Seminal Vesicles, Bilateral ♂<br>6 Tunica Vaginalis, Right ♂<br>7 Tunica Vaginalis, Left ♂<br>9 Testis, Right ♂<br>B Testis, Left ♂<br>C Testes, Bilateral ♂<br>F Spermatic Cord, Right ♂<br>G Spermatic Cord, Left ♂<br>H Spermatic Cords, Bilateral ♂<br>J Epididymis, Right ♂<br>K Epididymis, Left ♂<br>L Epididymis, Bilateral ♂<br>N Vas Deferens, Right ♂<br>P Vas Deferens, Left ♂<br>Q Vas Deferens, Bilateral ♂ | 0 Open<br>3 Percutaneous<br>4 Percutaneous Endoscopic | Z No Device | Z No Qualifier |
| 5 Scrotum ♂<br>S Penis ♂<br>T Prepuce ♂ | 0 Open<br>3 Percutaneous<br>4 Percutaneous Endoscopic<br>X External | Z No Device | Z No Qualifier |

**0** Medical and Surgical
**V** Male Reproductive System
**P** Removal: Taking out or off a device from a body part

| Character 4<br>Body Part | Character 5<br>Approach | Character 6<br>Device | Character 7<br>Qualifier |
|---|---|---|---|
| 4 Prostate and Seminal Vesicles ♂ | 0 Open<br>3 Percutaneous<br>4 Percutaneous Endoscopic<br>7 Via Natural or Artificial Opening<br>8 Via Natural or Artificial Opening Endoscopic | 0 Drainage Device<br>1 Radioactive Element<br>3 Infusion Device<br>7 Autologous Tissue Substitute<br>J Synthetic Substitute<br>K Nonautologous Tissue Substitute | Z No Qualifier |
| 4 Prostate and Seminal Vesicles ♂ | X External | 0 Drainage Device<br>1 Radioactive Element<br>3 Infusion Device | Z No Qualifier |
| 8 Scrotum and Tunica Vaginalis ♂<br>D Testis ♂<br>S Penis ♂ | 0 Open<br>3 Percutaneous<br>4 Percutaneous Endoscopic<br>7 Via Natural or Artificial Opening<br>8 Via Natural or Artificial Opening Endoscopic | 0 Drainage Device<br>3 Infusion Device<br>7 Autologous Tissue Substitute<br>J Synthetic Substitute<br>K Nonautologous Tissue Substitute | Z No Qualifier |
| 8 Scrotum and Tunica Vaginalis ♂<br>D Testis ♂<br>S Penis ♂ | X External | 0 Drainage Device<br>3 Infusion Device | Z No Qualifier |
| M Epididymis and Spermatic Cord ♂ | 0 Open<br>3 Percutaneous<br>4 Percutaneous Endoscopic<br>7 Via Natural or Artificial Opening<br>8 Via Natural or Artificial Opening Endoscopic | 0 Drainage Device<br>3 Infusion Device<br>7 Autologous Tissue Substitute<br>C Extraluminal Device<br>J Synthetic Substitute<br>K Nonautologous Tissue Substitute | Z No Qualifier |
| M Epididymis and Spermatic Cord ♂ | X External | 0 Drainage Device<br>3 Infusion Device | Z No Qualifier |
| R Vas Deferens ♂ | 0 Open<br>3 Percutaneous<br>4 Percutaneous Endoscopic<br>7 Via Natural or Artificial Opening<br>8 Via Natural or Artificial Opening Endoscopic | 0 Drainage Device<br>3 Infusion Device<br>7 Autologous Tissue Substitute<br>C Extraluminal Device<br>D Intraluminal Device<br>J Synthetic Substitute<br>K Nonautologous Tissue Substitute | Z No Qualifier |
| R Vas Deferens ♂ | X External | 0 Drainage Device<br>3 Infusion Device<br>D Intraluminal Device | Z No Qualifier |

**0** Medical and Surgical
**V** Male Reproductive System
**Q** Repair: Restoring, to the extent possible, a body part to its normal anatomic structure and function

| Character 4<br>Body Part | Character 5<br>Approach | Character 6<br>Device | Character 7<br>Qualifier |
|---|---|---|---|
| 0 Prostate ♂ | 0 Open<br>3 Percutaneous<br>4 Percutaneous Endoscopic<br>7 Via Natural or Artificial Opening<br>8 Via Natural or Artificial Opening<br>   Endoscopic | Z No Device | Z No Qualifier |
| 1 Seminal Vesicle, Right ♂<br>2 Seminal Vesicle, Left ♂<br>3 Seminal Vesicles, Bilateral ♂<br>6 Tunica Vaginalis, Right ♂<br>7 Tunica Vaginalis, Left ♂<br>9 Testis, Right ♂<br>B Testis, Left ♂<br>C Testes, Bilateral ♂<br>F Spermatic Cord, Right ♂<br>G Spermatic Cord, Left ♂<br>H Spermatic Cords, Bilateral ♂<br>J Epididymis, Right ♂<br>K Epididymis, Left ♂<br>L Epididymis, Bilateral ♂<br>N Vas Deferens, Right ♂<br>P Vas Deferens, Left ♂<br>Q Vas Deferens, Bilateral ♂ | 0 Open<br>3 Percutaneous<br>4 Percutaneous Endoscopic | Z No Device | Z No Qualifier |
| 5 Scrotum ♂<br>S Penis ♂<br>T Prepuce ♂ | 0 Open<br>3 Percutaneous<br>4 Percutaneous Endoscopic<br>X External | Z No Device | Z No Qualifier |

**0** Medical and Surgical
**V** Male Reproductive System
**R** Replacement: Putting in or on biological or synthetic material that physically takes the place and/or function of all or a portion of a body part

| Character 4<br>Body Part | Character 5<br>Approach | Character 6<br>Device | Character 7<br>Qualifier |
|---|---|---|---|
| 9 Testis, Right ♂<br>B Testis, Left ♂<br>C Testes, Bilateral ♂ | 0 Open | J Synthetic Substitute | Z No Qualifier |

**0** Medical and Surgical
**V** Male Reproductive System
**S** Reposition: Moving to its normal location, or other suitable location, all or a portion of a body part

| Character 4<br>Body Part | Character 5<br>Approach | Character 6<br>Device | Character 7<br>Qualifier |
|---|---|---|---|
| 9 Testis, Right ♂<br>B Testis, Left ♂<br>C Testes, Bilateral ♂<br>F Spermatic Cord, Right ♂<br>G Spermatic Cord, Left ♂<br>H Spermatic Cords, Bilateral ♂ | 0 Open<br>3 Percutaneous<br>4 Percutaneous Endoscopic | Z No Device | Z No Qualifier |

**0** Medical and Surgical
**V** Male Reproductive System
**T** Resection: Cutting out or off, without replacement, all of a body part

| Character 4<br>Body Part | Character 5<br>Approach | Character 6<br>Device | Character 7<br>Qualifier |
|---|---|---|---|
| 0 Prostate ♂ | 0 Open<br>4 Percutaneous Endoscopic<br>7 Via Natural or Artificial Opening<br>8 Via Natural or Artificial Opening<br>   Endoscopic | Z No Device | Z No Qualifier |
| 1 Seminal Vesicle, Right ♂<br>2 Seminal Vesicle, Left ♂<br>3 Seminal Vesicles, Bilateral ♂<br>6 Tunica Vaginalis, Right ♂<br>7 Tunica Vaginalis, Left ♂<br>9 Testis, Right ♂<br>B Testis, Left ♂<br>C Testes, Bilateral ♂<br>F Spermatic Cord, Right ♂<br>G Spermatic Cord, Left ♂<br>H Spermatic Cords, Bilateral ♂<br>J Epididymis, Right ♂<br>K Epididymis, Left ♂<br>L Epididymis, Bilateral ♂<br>N Vas Deferens, Right ♂ NC<br>P Vas Deferens, Left ♂ NC<br>Q Vas Deferens, Bilateral ♂ NC | 0 Open<br>4 Percutaneous Endoscopic | Z No Device | Z No Qualifier |
| 5 Scrotum ♂<br>S Penis ♂<br>T Prepuce ♂ | 0 Open<br>4 Percutaneous Endoscopic<br>X External | Z No Device | Z No Qualifier |

NC 0VTN(0,4)ZZ, 0VTP(0,4)ZZ, 0VTQ(0,4)ZZ

**0** Medical and Surgical
**V** Male Reproductive System
**U** Supplement: Putting in or on biological or synthetic material that physically reinforces and/or augments the function of a portion of a body part

| Character 4<br>Body Part | Character 5<br>Approach | Character 6<br>Device | Character 7<br>Qualifier |
|---|---|---|---|
| 1 Seminal Vesicle, Right ♂<br>2 Seminal Vesicle, Left ♂<br>3 Seminal Vesicles, Bilateral ♂<br>6 Tunica Vaginalis, Right ♂<br>7 Tunica Vaginalis, Left ♂<br>F Spermatic Cord, Right ♂<br>G Spermatic Cord, Left ♂<br>H Spermatic Cords, Bilateral ♂<br>J Epididymis, Right ♂<br>K Epididymis, Left ♂<br>L Epididymis, Bilateral ♂<br>N Vas Deferens, Right ♂<br>P Vas Deferens, Left ♂<br>Q Vas Deferens, Bilateral ♂ | 0 Open<br>4 Percutaneous Endoscopic | 7 Autologous Tissue Substitute<br>J Synthetic Substitute<br>K Nonautologous Tissue Substitute | Z No Qualifier |
| 5 Scrotum ♂<br>S Penis ♂<br>T Prepuce ♂ | 0 Open<br>4 Percutaneous Endoscopic<br>X External | 7 Autologous Tissue Substitute<br>J Synthetic Substitute<br>K Nonautologous Tissue Substitute | Z No Qualifier |
| 9 Testis, Right ♂<br>B Testis, Left ♂<br>C Testes, Bilateral ♂ | 0 Open | 7 Autologous Tissue Substitute<br>J Synthetic Substitute<br>K Nonautologous Tissue Substitute | Z No Qualifier |

**0** Medical and Surgical
**V** Male Reproductive System
**W** Revision: Correcting, to the extent possible, a portion of a malfunctioning device or the position of a displaced device

| Character 4<br>Body Part | Character 5<br>Approach | Character 6<br>Device | Character 7<br>Qualifier |
|---|---|---|---|
| 4 Prostate and Seminal Vesicles ♂<br>8 Scrotum and Tunica Vaginalis ♂<br>D Testis ♂<br>S Penis ♂ | 0 Open<br>3 Percutaneous<br>4 Percutaneous Endoscopic<br>7 Via Natural or Artificial Opening<br>8 Via Natural or Artificial Opening<br>   Endoscopic<br>X External | 0 Drainage Device<br>3 Infusion Device<br>7 Autologous Tissue Substitute<br>J Synthetic Substitute<br>K Nonautologous Tissue Substitute | Z No Qualifier |
| M Epididymis and Spermatic Cord ♂ | 0 Open<br>3 Percutaneous<br>4 Percutaneous Endoscopic<br>7 Via Natural or Artificial Opening<br>8 Via Natural or Artificial Opening<br>   Endoscopic<br>X External | 0 Drainage Device<br>3 Infusion Device<br>7 Autologous Tissue Substitute<br>C Extraluminal Device<br>J Synthetic Substitute<br>K Nonautologous Tissue Substitute | Z No Qualifier |
| R Vas Deferens ♂ | 0 Open<br>3 Percutaneous<br>4 Percutaneous Endoscopic<br>7 Via Natural or Artificial Opening<br>8 Via Natural or Artificial Opening<br>   Endoscopic<br>X External | 0 Drainage Device<br>3 Infusion Device<br>7 Autologous Tissue Substitute<br>C Extraluminal Device<br>D Intraluminal Device<br>J Synthetic Substitute<br>K Nonautologous Tissue Substitute | Z No Qualifier |

# Anatomical Regions, General | 0W0-0WW

**0** Medical and Surgical
**W** Anatomical Regions, General
**0** Alteration: Modifying the anatomic structure of a body part without affecting the function of the body part

| Character 4<br>Body Part | Character 5<br>Approach | Character 6<br>Device | Character 7<br>Qualifier |
|---|---|---|---|
| 0 Head<br>2 Face<br>4 Upper Jaw<br>5 Lower Jaw<br>6 Neck<br>8 Chest Wall<br>F Abdominal Wall<br>K Upper Back<br>L Lower Back<br>M Perineum, Male ♂<br>N Perineum, Female ♀ | 0 Open<br>3 Percutaneous<br>4 Percutaneous Endoscopic | 7 Autologous Tissue Substitute<br>J Synthetic Substitute<br>K Nonautologous Tissue Substitute<br>Z No Device | Z No Qualifier |

**0** Medical and Surgical
**W** Anatomical Regions, General
**1** Bypass: Altering the route of passage of the contents of a tubular body part

| Character 4<br>Body Part | Character 5<br>Approach | Character 6<br>Device | Character 7<br>Qualifier |
|---|---|---|---|
| 1 Cranial Cavity | 0 Open | J Synthetic Substitute | 9 Pleural Cavity, Right<br>B Pleural Cavity, Left<br>G Peritoneal Cavity<br>J Pelvic Cavity |
| 9 Pleural Cavity, Right<br>B Pleural Cavity, Left<br>G Peritoneal Cavity<br>J Pelvic Cavity ♀ | 0 Open<br>4 Percutaneous Endoscopic | J Synthetic Substitute | 4 Cutaneous<br>9 Pleural Cavity, Right<br>B Pleural Cavity, Left<br>G Peritoneal Cavity<br>J Pelvic Cavity<br>Y Lower Vein |
| 9 Pleural Cavity, Right<br>B Pleural Cavity, Left<br>G Peritoneal Cavity<br>J Pelvic Cavity ♀ | 3 Percutaneous | J Synthetic Substitute | 4 Cutaneous |

**AHA:** 0W1G3J4 - 4Q 2013, 126; 0W1G4J4 - 4Q 2013, 127

---

**0 Medical and Surgical**
**W Anatomical Regions, General**
**2 Change: Taking out or off a device from a body part and putting back an identical or similar device in or on the same body part without cutting or puncturing the skin or a mucous membrane**

| Character 4 Body Part | Character 5 Approach | Character 6 Device | Character 7 Qualifier |
|---|---|---|---|
| 0  Head | X  External | 0  Drainage Device | Z  No Qualifier |
| 1  Cranial Cavity | | Y  Other Device | |
| 2  Face | | | |
| 4  Upper Jaw | | | |
| 5  Lower Jaw | | | |
| 6  Neck | | | |
| 8  Chest Wall | | | |
| 9  Pleural Cavity, Right | | | |
| B  Pleural Cavity, Left | | | |
| C  Mediastinum | | | |
| D  Pericardial Cavity | | | |
| F  Abdominal Wall | | | |
| G  Peritoneal Cavity | | | |
| H  Retroperitoneum | | | |
| J  Pelvic Cavity | | | |
| K  Upper Back | | | |
| L  Lower Back | | | |
| M  Perineum, Male | | | |
| N  Perineum, Female | | | |

**0 Medical and Surgical**
**W Anatomical Regions, General**
**3 Control: Stopping, or attempting to stop, postprocedural bleeding**

| Character 4 Body Part | Character 5 Approach | Character 6 Device | Character 7 Qualifier |
|---|---|---|---|
| 0  Head | 0  Open | Z  No Device | Z  No Qualifier |
| 1  Cranial Cavity | 3  Percutaneous | | |
| 2  Face | 4  Percutaneous Endoscopic | | |
| 4  Upper Jaw | | | |
| 5  Lower Jaw | | | |
| 6  Neck | | | |
| 8  Chest Wall | | | |
| 9  Pleural Cavity, Right | | | |
| B  Pleural Cavity, Left | | | |
| C  Mediastinum | | | |
| D  Pericardial Cavity | | | |
| F  Abdominal Wall | | | |
| G  Peritoneal Cavity | | | |
| H  Retroperitoneum | | | |
| J  Pelvic Cavity | | | |
| K  Upper Back | | | |
| L  Lower Back | | | |
| M  Perineum, Male | | | |
| N  Perineum, Female | | | |
| 3  Oral Cavity and Throat | 0  Open | Z  No Device | Z  No Qualifier |
| | 3  Percutaneous | | |
| | 4  Percutaneous Endoscopic | | |
| | 7  Via Natural or Artificial Opening | | |
| | 8  Via Natural or Artificial Opening Endoscopic | | |
| | X  External | | |
| P  Gastrointestinal Tract | 0  Open | Z  No Device | Z  No Qualifier |
| Q  Respiratory Tract | 3  Percutaneous | | |
| R  Genitourinary Tract | 4  Percutaneous Endoscopic | | |
| | 7  Via Natural or Artificial Opening | | |
| | 8  Via Natural or Artificial Opening Endoscopic | | |

**0** Medical and Surgical
**W** Anatomical Regions, General
**4** Creation: Making a new genital structure that does not take over the function of a body part

| Character 4<br>Body Part | Character 5<br>Approach | Character 6<br>Device | Character 7<br>Qualifier |
|---|---|---|---|
| M Perineum, Male ♂ N C | 0 Open | 7 Autologous Tissue Substitute<br>J Synthetic Substitute<br>K Nonautologous Tissue Substitute<br>Z No Device | 0 Vagina ♂ |
| N Perineum, Female ♀ N C | 0 Open | 7 Autologous Tissue Substitute<br>J Synthetic Substitute<br>K Nonautologous Tissue Substitute<br>Z No Device | 1 Penis ♀ |

N C 0W4M0(7,J,K,Z)0, 0W4N0(7,J,K,Z)1

**0** Medical and Surgical
**W** Anatomical Regions, General
**8** Division: Cutting into a body part, without draining fluids and/or gases from the body part, in order to separate or transect a body part

| Character 4<br>Body Part | Character 5<br>Approach | Character 6<br>Device | Character 7<br>Qualifier |
|---|---|---|---|
| N Perineum, Female ♀ | X External | Z No Device | Z No Qualifier |

**0** Medical and Surgical
**W** Anatomical Regions, General
**9** Drainage: Taking or letting out fluids and/or gases from a body part

| Character 4<br>Body Part | Character 5<br>Approach | Character 6<br>Device | Character 7<br>Qualifier |
|---|---|---|---|
| 0 Head<br>1 Cranial Cavity<br>2 Face<br>3 Oral Cavity and Throat<br>4 Upper Jaw<br>5 Lower Jaw<br>6 Neck<br>8 Chest Wall<br>9 Pleural Cavity, Right<br>B Pleural Cavity, Left<br>C Mediastinum<br>D Pericardial Cavity<br>F Abdominal Wall<br>G Peritoneal Cavity<br>H Retroperitoneum<br>J Pelvic Cavity<br>K Upper Back<br>L Lower Back<br>M Perineum, Male ♂<br>N Perineum, Female ♀ | 0 Open<br>3 Percutaneous<br>4 Percutaneous Endoscopic | 0 Drainage Device | Z No Qualifier |
| 0 Head<br>1 Cranial Cavity<br>2 Face<br>3 Oral Cavity and Throat<br>4 Upper Jaw<br>5 Lower Jaw<br>6 Neck<br>8 Chest Wall<br>9 Pleural Cavity, Right<br>B Pleural Cavity, Left<br>C Mediastinum<br>D Pericardial Cavity<br>F Abdominal Wall<br>G Peritoneal Cavity<br>H Retroperitoneum<br>J Pelvic Cavity<br>K Upper Back<br>L Lower Back<br>M Perineum, Male ♂<br>N Perineum, Female ♀ | 0 Open<br>3 Percutaneous<br>4 Percutaneous Endoscopic | Z No Device | X Diagnostic<br>Z No Qualifier |

**0** Medical and Surgical
**W** Anatomical Regions, General
**B** Excision: Cutting out or off, without replacement, a portion of a body part

| Character 4<br>Body Part | Character 5<br>Approach | Character 6<br>Device | Character 7<br>Qualifier |
|---|---|---|---|
| 0 Head<br>2 Face<br>4 Upper Jaw<br>5 Lower Jaw<br>8 Chest Wall<br>K Upper Back<br>L Lower Back<br>M Perineum, Male ♂<br>N Perineum, Female ♀ | 0 Open<br>3 Percutaneous<br>4 Percutaneous Endoscopic<br>X External | Z No Device | X Diagnostic<br>Z No Qualifier |
| 6 Neck<br>F Abdominal Wall | 0 Open<br>3 Percutaneous<br>4 Percutaneous Endoscopic | Z No Device | X Diagnostic<br>Z No Qualifier |
| 6 Neck<br>F Abdominal Wall | X External | Z No Device | 2 Stoma<br>X Diagnostic<br>Z No Qualifier |
| C Mediastinum<br>H Retroperitoneum | 0 Open<br>3 Percutaneous<br>4 Percutaneous Endoscopic | Z No Device | X Diagnostic<br>Z No Qualifier |

**AHA:** 0WBNXZZ - 4Q 2013, 120

---

**0** Medical and Surgical
**W** Anatomical Regions, General
**C** Extirpation: Taking or cutting out solid matter from a body part

| Character 4<br>Body Part | Character 5<br>Approach | Character 6<br>Device | Character 7<br>Qualifier |
|---|---|---|---|
| 1 Cranial Cavity<br>3 Oral Cavity and Throat<br>9 Pleural Cavity, Right<br>B Pleural Cavity, Left<br>C Mediastinum<br>D Pericardial Cavity<br>G Peritoneal Cavity<br>J Pelvic Cavity | 0 Open<br>3 Percutaneous<br>4 Percutaneous Endoscopic<br>X External | Z No Device | Z No Qualifier |
| P Gastrointestinal Tract<br>Q Respiratory Tract<br>R Genitourinary Tract | 0 Open<br>3 Percutaneous<br>4 Percutaneous Endoscopic<br>7 Via Natural or Artificial Opening<br>8 Via Natural or Artificial Opening<br>   Endoscopic<br>X External | Z No Device | Z No Qualifier |

---

**0** Medical and Surgical
**W** Anatomical Regions, General
**F** Fragmentation: Breaking solid matter in a body part into pieces

| Character 4<br>Body Part | Character 5<br>Approach | Character 6<br>Device | Character 7<br>Qualifier |
|---|---|---|---|
| 1 Cranial Cavity  NC<br>3 Oral Cavity and Throat  NC<br>9 Pleural Cavity, Right  NC<br>B Pleural Cavity, Left  NC<br>C Mediastinum  NC<br>D Pericardial Cavity<br>G Peritoneal Cavity  NC<br>J Pelvic Cavity  NC | 0 Open<br>3 Percutaneous<br>4 Percutaneous Endoscopic<br>X External | Z No Device | Z No Qualifier |
| P Gastrointestinal Tract  NC<br>Q Respiratory Tract  NC<br>R Genitourinary Tract | 0 Open<br>3 Percutaneous<br>4 Percutaneous Endoscopic<br>7 Via Natural or Artificial Opening<br>8 Via Natural or Artificial Opening<br>   Endoscopic<br>X External | Z No Device | Z No Qualifier |

NC 0WF(1,3,9,B,C,G,J,P,Q)XZZ

---

**0** Medical and Surgical
**W** Anatomical Regions, General
**H** Insertion: Putting in a nonbiological appliance that monitors, assists, performs, or prevents a physiological function but does not physically take the place of a body part

| Character 4<br>Body Part | Character 5<br>Approach | Character 6<br>Device | Character 7<br>Qualifier |
|---|---|---|---|
| 0 Head<br>1 Cranial Cavity<br>2 Face<br>3 Oral Cavity and Throat<br>4 Upper Jaw<br>5 Lower Jaw<br>6 Neck<br>8 Chest Wall<br>9 Pleural Cavity, Right<br>B Pleural Cavity, Left<br>C Mediastinum<br>D Pericardial Cavity<br>F Abdominal Wall<br>G Peritoneal Cavity<br>H Retroperitoneum<br>J Pelvic Cavity<br>K Upper Back<br>L Lower Back<br>M Perineum, Male ♂<br>N Perineum, Female ♀ | 0 Open<br>3 Percutaneous<br>4 Percutaneous Endoscopic | 1 Radioactive Element<br>3 Infusion Device<br>Y Other Device | Z No Qualifier |
| P Gastrointestinal Tract<br>Q Respiratory Tract<br>R Genitourinary Tract | 0 Open<br>3 Percutaneous<br>4 Percutaneous Endoscopic<br>7 Via Natural or Artificial Opening<br>8 Via Natural or Artificial Opening Endoscopic | 1 Radioactive Element<br>3 Infusion Device<br>Y Other Device | Z No Qualifier |

**0** Medical and Surgical
**W** Anatomical Regions, General
**J** Inspection: Visually and/or manually exploring a body part

| Character 4<br>Body Part | Character 5<br>Approach | Character 6<br>Device | Character 7<br>Qualifier |
|---|---|---|---|
| 0 Head<br>2 Face<br>3 Oral Cavity and Throat<br>4 Upper Jaw<br>5 Lower Jaw<br>6 Neck<br>8 Chest Wall<br>F Abdominal Wall<br>K Upper Back<br>L Lower Back<br>M Perineum, Male ♂<br>N Perineum, Female ♀ | 0 Open<br>3 Percutaneous<br>4 Percutaneous Endoscopic<br>X External | Z No Device | Z No Qualifier |
| 1 Cranial Cavity<br>9 Pleural Cavity, Right<br>B Pleural Cavity, Left<br>C Mediastinum<br>D Pericardial Cavity<br>G Peritoneal Cavity<br>H Retroperitoneum<br>J Pelvic Cavity | 0 Open<br>3 Percutaneous<br>4 Percutaneous Endoscopic | Z No Device | Z No Qualifier |
| P Gastrointestinal Tract<br>Q Respiratory Tract<br>R Genitourinary Tract | 0 Open<br>3 Percutaneous<br>4 Percutaneous Endoscopic<br>7 Via Natural or Artificial Opening<br>8 Via Natural or Artificial Opening Endoscopic | Z No Device | Z No Qualifier |

**AHA:** 0WJG4ZZ - 2Q 2013, 37

| **0** Medical and Surgical | | | |
| **W** Anatomical Regions, General | | | |
| **M** Reattachment: Putting back in or on all or a portion of a separated body part to its normal location or other suitable location | | | |

| Character 4<br>Body Part | Character 5<br>Approach | Character 6<br>Device | Character 7<br>Qualifier |
|---|---|---|---|
| 2 Face<br>4 Upper Jaw<br>5 Lower Jaw<br>6 Neck<br>8 Chest Wall<br>F Abdominal Wall<br>K Upper Back<br>L Lower Back<br>M Perineum, Male ♂<br>N Perineum, Female ♀ | 0 Open | Z No Device | Z No Qualifier |

| **0** Medical and Surgical | | | |
| **W** Anatomical Regions, General | | | |
| **P** Removal: Taking out or off a device from a body part | | | |

| Character 4<br>Body Part | Character 5<br>Approach | Character 6<br>Device | Character 7<br>Qualifier |
|---|---|---|---|
| 0 Head<br>2 Face<br>4 Upper Jaw<br>5 Lower Jaw<br>6 Neck<br>8 Chest Wall<br>C Mediastinum<br>F Abdominal Wall<br>K Upper Back<br>L Lower Back<br>M Perineum, Male ♂<br>N Perineum, Female ♀ | 0 Open<br>3 Percutaneous<br>4 Percutaneous Endoscopic<br>X External | 0 Drainage Device<br>1 Radioactive Element<br>3 Infusion Device<br>7 Autologous Tissue Substitute<br>J Synthetic Substitute<br>K Nonautologous Tissue Substitute<br>Y Other Device | Z No Qualifier |
| 1 Cranial Cavity<br>9 Pleural Cavity, Right<br>B Pleural Cavity, Left<br>G Peritoneal Cavity<br>J Pelvic Cavity | 0 Open<br>3 Percutaneous<br>4 Percutaneous Endoscopic | 0 Drainage Device<br>1 Radioactive Element<br>3 Infusion Device<br>J Synthetic Substitute<br>Y Other Device | Z No Qualifier |
| 1 Cranial Cavity<br>9 Pleural Cavity, Right<br>B Pleural Cavity, Left<br>G Peritoneal Cavity<br>J Pelvic Cavity | X External | 0 Drainage Device<br>1 Radioactive Element<br>3 Infusion Device | Z No Qualifier |
| D Pericardial Cavity<br>H Retroperitoneum | 0 Open<br>3 Percutaneous<br>4 Percutaneous Endoscopic | 0 Drainage Device<br>1 Radioactive Element<br>3 Infusion Device<br>Y Other Device | Z No Qualifier |
| D Pericardial Cavity<br>H Retroperitoneum | X External | 0 Drainage Device<br>1 Radioactive Element<br>3 Infusion Device | Z No Qualifier |
| P Gastrointestinal Tract<br>Q Respiratory Tract<br>R Genitourinary Tract | 0 Open<br>3 Percutaneous<br>4 Percutaneous Endoscopic<br>7 Via Natural or Artificial Opening<br>8 Via Natural or Artificial Opening Endoscopic<br>X External | 1 Radioactive Element<br>3 Infusion Device<br>Y Other Device | Z No Qualifier |

**0** Medical and Surgical
**W** Anatomical Regions, General
**Q** Repair: Restoring, to the extent possible, a body part to its normal anatomic structure and function

| Character 4<br>Body Part | Character 5<br>Approach | Character 6<br>Device | Character 7<br>Qualifier |
|---|---|---|---|
| 0 Head<br>2 Face<br>4 Upper Jaw<br>5 Lower Jaw<br>8 Chest Wall<br>K Upper Back<br>L Lower Back<br>M Perineum, Male ♂<br>N Perineum, Female ♀ | 0 Open<br>3 Percutaneous<br>4 Percutaneous Endoscopic<br>X External | Z No Device | Z No Qualifier |
| 6 Neck<br>F Abdominal Wall | 0 Open<br>3 Percutaneous<br>4 Percutaneous Endoscopic | Z No Device | Z No Qualifier |
| 6 Neck<br>F Abdominal Wall | X External | Z No Device | 2 Stoma<br>Z No Qualifier |
| C Mediastinum | 0 Open<br>3 Percutaneous<br>4 Percutaneous Endoscopic | Z No Device | Z No Qualifier |

**0** Medical and Surgical
**W** Anatomical Regions, General
**U** Supplement: Putting in or on biological or synthetic material that physically reinforces and/or augments the function of a portion of a body part

| Character 4<br>Body Part | Character 5<br>Approach | Character 6<br>Device | Character 7<br>Qualifier |
|---|---|---|---|
| 0 Head<br>2 Face<br>4 Upper Jaw<br>5 Lower Jaw<br>6 Neck<br>8 Chest Wall<br>C Mediastinum<br>F Abdominal Wall<br>K Upper Back<br>L Lower Back<br>M Perineum, Male ♂<br>N Perineum, Female ♀ | 0 Open<br>4 Percutaneous Endoscopic | 7 Autologous Tissue Substitute<br>J Synthetic Substitute<br>K Nonautologous Tissue Substitute | Z No Qualifier |

**0** Medical and Surgical
**W** Anatomical Regions, General
**W** Revision: Correcting, to the extent possible, a portion of a malfunctioning device or the position of a displaced device

| Character 4<br>Body Part | Character 5<br>Approach | Character 6<br>Device | Character 7<br>Qualifier |
|---|---|---|---|
| 0 Head<br>2 Face<br>4 Upper Jaw<br>5 Lower Jaw<br>6 Neck<br>8 Chest Wall<br>C Mediastinum<br>F Abdominal Wall<br>K Upper Back<br>L Lower Back<br>M Perineum, Male ♂<br>N Perineum, Female ♀ | 0 Open<br>3 Percutaneous<br>4 Percutaneous Endoscopic<br>X External | 0 Drainage Device<br>1 Radioactive Element<br>3 Infusion Device<br>7 Autologous Tissue Substitute<br>J Synthetic Substitute<br>K Nonautologous Tissue Substitute<br>Y Other Device | Z No Qualifier |
| 1 Cranial Cavity<br>9 Pleural Cavity, Right<br>B Pleural Cavity, Left<br>G Peritoneal Cavity<br>J Pelvic Cavity | 0 Open<br>3 Percutaneous<br>4 Percutaneous Endoscopic<br>X External | 0 Drainage Device<br>1 Radioactive Element<br>3 Infusion Device<br>J Synthetic Substitute<br>Y Other Device | Z No Qualifier |
| D Pericardial Cavity<br>H Retroperitoneum | 0 Open<br>3 Percutaneous<br>4 Percutaneous Endoscopic<br>X External | 0 Drainage Device<br>1 Radioactive Element<br>3 Infusion Device<br>Y Other Device | Z No Qualifier |
| P Gastrointestinal Tract<br>Q Respiratory Tract<br>R Genitourinary Tract | 0 Open<br>3 Percutaneous<br>4 Percutaneous Endoscopic<br>7 Via Natural or Artificial Opening<br>8 Via Natural or Artificial Opening Endoscopic<br>X External | 1 Radioactive Element<br>3 Infusion Device<br>Y Other Device | Z No Qualifier |

# Anatomical Regions, Upper Extremities | 0X0-0XX

**0** Medical and Surgical
**X** Anatomical Regions, Upper Extremities
**0** Alteration: Modifying the anatomic structure of a body part without affecting the function of the body part

| Character 4<br>Body Part | Character 5<br>Approach | Character 6<br>Device | Character 7<br>Qualifier |
|---|---|---|---|
| 2 Shoulder Region, Right<br>3 Shoulder Region, Left<br>4 Axilla, Right<br>5 Axilla, Left<br>6 Upper Extremity, Right<br>7 Upper Extremity, Left<br>8 Upper Arm, Right<br>9 Upper Arm, Left<br>B Elbow Region, Right<br>C Elbow Region, Left<br>D Lower Arm, Right<br>F Lower Arm, Left<br>G Wrist Region, Right<br>H Wrist Region, Left | 0 Open<br>3 Percutaneous<br>4 Percutaneous Endoscopic | 7 Autologous Tissue Substitute<br>J Synthetic Substitute<br>K Nonautologous Tissue Substitute<br>Z No Device | Z No Qualifier |

**0** Medical and Surgical
**X** Anatomical Regions, Upper Extremities
**2** Change: Taking out or off a device from a body part and putting back an identical or similar device in or on the same body part without cutting or puncturing the skin or a mucous membrane

| Character 4<br>Body Part | Character 5<br>Approach | Character 6<br>Device | Character 7<br>Qualifier |
|---|---|---|---|
| 6 Upper Extremity, Right<br>7 Upper Extremity, Left | X External | 0 Drainage Device<br>Y Other Device | Z No Qualifier |

**0** Medical and Surgical
**X** Anatomical Regions, Upper Extremities
**3** Control: Stopping, or attempting to stop, postprocedural bleeding

| Character 4<br>Body Part | Character 5<br>Approach | Character 6<br>Device | Character 7<br>Qualifier |
|---|---|---|---|
| 2 Shoulder Region, Right<br>3 Shoulder Region, Left<br>4 Axilla, Right<br>5 Axilla, Left<br>6 Upper Extremity, Right<br>7 Upper Extremity, Left<br>8 Upper Arm, Right<br>9 Upper Arm, Left<br>B Elbow Region, Right<br>C Elbow Region, Left<br>D Lower Arm, Right<br>F Lower Arm, Left<br>G Wrist Region, Right<br>H Wrist Region, Left<br>J Hand, Right<br>K Hand, Left | 0 Open<br>3 Percutaneous<br>4 Percutaneous Endoscopic | Z No Device | Z No Qualifier |

**0** Medical and Surgical
**X** Anatomical Regions, Upper Extremities
**6** Detachment: Cutting off all or a portion of the upper or lower extremities

| Character 4<br>Body Part | Character 5<br>Approach | Character 6<br>Device | Character 7<br>Qualifier |
|---|---|---|---|
| 0 Forequarter, Right<br>1 Forequarter, Left<br>2 Shoulder Region, Right<br>3 Shoulder Region, Left<br>B Elbow Region, Right<br>C Elbow Region, Left | 0 Open | Z No Device | Z No Qualifier |
| 8 Upper Arm, Right<br>9 Upper Arm, Left<br>D Lower Arm, Right<br>F Lower Arm, Left | 0 Open | Z No Device | 1 High<br>2 Mid<br>3 Low |
| J Hand, Right<br>K Hand, Left | 0 Open | Z No Device | 0 Complete<br>4 Complete 1st Ray<br>5 Complete 2nd Ray<br>6 Complete 3rd Ray<br>7 Complete 4th Ray<br>8 Complete 5th Ray<br>9 Partial 1st Ray<br>B Partial 2nd Ray<br>C Partial 3rd Ray<br>D Partial 4th Ray<br>F Partial 5th Ray |
| L Thumb, Right<br>M Thumb, Left<br>N Index Finger, Right<br>P Index Finger, Left<br>Q Middle Finger, Right<br>R Middle Finger, Left<br>S Ring Finger, Right<br>T Ring Finger, Left<br>V Little Finger, Right<br>W Little Finger, Left | 0 Open | Z No Device | 0 Complete<br>1 High<br>2 Mid<br>3 Low |

**0** Medical and Surgical
**X** Anatomical Regions, Upper Extremities
**9** Drainage: Taking or letting out fluids and/or gases from a body part

| Character 4<br>Body Part | Character 5<br>Approach | Character 6<br>Device | Character 7<br>Qualifier |
|---|---|---|---|
| 2 Shoulder Region, Right<br>3 Shoulder Region, Left<br>4 Axilla, Right<br>5 Axilla, Left<br>6 Upper Extremity, Right<br>7 Upper Extremity, Left<br>8 Upper Arm, Right<br>9 Upper Arm, Left<br>B Elbow Region, Right<br>C Elbow Region, Left<br>D Lower Arm, Right<br>F Lower Arm, Left<br>G Wrist Region, Right<br>H Wrist Region, Left<br>J Hand, Right<br>K Hand, Left | 0 Open<br>3 Percutaneous<br>4 Percutaneous Endoscopic | 0 Drainage Device | Z No Qualifier |
| 2 Shoulder Region, Right<br>3 Shoulder Region, Left<br>4 Axilla, Right<br>5 Axilla, Left<br>6 Upper Extremity, Right<br>7 Upper Extremity, Left<br>8 Upper Arm, Right<br>9 Upper Arm, Left<br>B Elbow Region, Right<br>C Elbow Region, Left<br>D Lower Arm, Right<br>F Lower Arm, Left<br>G Wrist Region, Right<br>H Wrist Region, Left<br>J Hand, Right<br>K Hand, Left | 0 Open<br>3 Percutaneous<br>4 Percutaneous Endoscopic | Z No Device | X Diagnostic<br>Z No Qualifier |

**0** Medical and Surgical
**X** Anatomical Regions, Upper Extremities
**B** Excision: Cutting out or off, without replacement, a portion of a body part

| Character 4<br>Body Part | Character 5<br>Approach | Character 6<br>Device | Character 7<br>Qualifier |
|---|---|---|---|
| 2 Shoulder Region, Right<br>3 Shoulder Region, Left<br>4 Axilla, Right<br>5 Axilla, Left<br>6 Upper Extremity, Right<br>7 Upper Extremity, Left<br>8 Upper Arm, Right<br>9 Upper Arm, Left<br>B Elbow Region, Right<br>C Elbow Region, Left<br>D Lower Arm, Right<br>F Lower Arm, Left<br>G Wrist Region, Right<br>H Wrist Region, Left<br>J Hand, Right<br>K Hand, Left | 0 Open<br>3 Percutaneous<br>4 Percutaneous Endoscopic | Z No Device | X Diagnostic<br>Z No Qualifier |

**0** Medical and Surgical
**X** Anatomical Regions, Upper Extremities
**H** Insertion: Putting in a nonbiological appliance that monitors, assists, performs, or prevents a physiological function but does not physically take the place of a body part

| Character 4<br>Body Part | Character 5<br>Approach | Character 6<br>Device | Character 7<br>Qualifier |
|---|---|---|---|
| 2 Shoulder Region, Right<br>3 Shoulder Region, Left<br>4 Axilla, Right<br>5 Axilla, Left<br>6 Upper Extremity, Right<br>7 Upper Extremity, Left<br>8 Upper Arm, Right<br>9 Upper Arm, Left<br>B Elbow Region, Right<br>C Elbow Region, Left<br>D Lower Arm, Right<br>F Lower Arm, Left<br>G Wrist Region, Right<br>H Wrist Region, Left<br>J Hand, Right<br>K Hand, Left | 0 Open<br>3 Percutaneous<br>4 Percutaneous Endoscopic | 1 Radioactive Element<br>3 Infusion Device<br>Y Other Device | Z No Qualifier |

**0** Medical and Surgical
**X** Anatomical Regions, Upper Extremities
**J** Inspection: Visually and/or manually exploring a body part

| Character 4<br>Body Part | Character 5<br>Approach | Character 6<br>Device | Character 7<br>Qualifier |
|---|---|---|---|
| 2 Shoulder Region, Right<br>3 Shoulder Region, Left<br>4 Axilla, Right<br>5 Axilla, Left<br>6 Upper Extremity, Right<br>7 Upper Extremity, Left<br>8 Upper Arm, Right<br>9 Upper Arm, Left<br>B Elbow Region, Right<br>C Elbow Region, Left<br>D Lower Arm, Right<br>F Lower Arm, Left<br>G Wrist Region, Right<br>H Wrist Region, Left<br>J Hand, Right<br>K Hand, Left | 0 Open<br>3 Percutaneous<br>4 Percutaneous Endoscopic<br>X External | Z No Device | Z No Qualifier |

**0** Medical and Surgical
**X** Anatomical Regions, Upper Extremities
**M** Reattachment: Putting back in or on all or a portion of a separated body part to its normal location or other suitable location

| Character 4<br>Body Part | Character 5<br>Approach | Character 6<br>Device | Character 7<br>Qualifier |
|---|---|---|---|
| 0 Forequarter, Right<br>1 Forequarter, Left<br>2 Shoulder Region, Right<br>3 Shoulder Region, Left<br>4 Axilla, Right<br>5 Axilla, Left<br>6 Upper Extremity, Right<br>7 Upper Extremity, Left<br>8 Upper Arm, Right<br>9 Upper Arm, Left<br>B Elbow Region, Right<br>C Elbow Region, Left<br>D Lower Arm, Right<br>F Lower Arm, Left<br>G Wrist Region, Right<br>H Wrist Region, Left<br>J Hand, Right<br>K Hand, Left<br>L Thumb, Right<br>M Thumb, Left<br>N Index Finger, Right<br>P Index Finger, Left<br>Q Middle Finger, Right<br>R Middle Finger, Left<br>S Ring Finger, Right<br>T Ring Finger, Left<br>V Little Finger, Right<br>W Little Finger, Left | 0 Open | Z No Device | Z No Qualifier |

**0** Medical and Surgical
**X** Anatomical Regions, Upper Extremities
**P** Removal: Taking out or off a device from a body part

| Character 4<br>Body Part | Character 5<br>Approach | Character 6<br>Device | Character 7<br>Qualifier |
|---|---|---|---|
| 6  Upper Extremity, Right<br>7  Upper Extremity, Left | 0  Open<br>3  Percutaneous<br>4  Percutaneous Endoscopic<br>X  External | 0  Drainage Device<br>1  Radioactive Element<br>3  Infusion Device<br>7  Autologous Tissue Substitute<br>J  Synthetic Substitute<br>K  Nonautologous Tissue Substitute<br>Y  Other Device | Z  No Qualifier |

**0** Medical and Surgical
**X** Anatomical Regions, Upper Extremities
**Q** Repair: Restoring, to the extent possible, a body part to its normal anatomic structure and function

| Character 4<br>Body Part | Character 5<br>Approach | Character 6<br>Device | Character 7<br>Qualifier |
|---|---|---|---|
| 2  Shoulder Region, Right<br>3  Shoulder Region, Left<br>4  Axilla, Right<br>5  Axilla, Left<br>6  Upper Extremity, Right<br>7  Upper Extremity, Left<br>8  Upper Arm, Right<br>9  Upper Arm, Left<br>B  Elbow Region, Right<br>C  Elbow Region, Left<br>D  Lower Arm, Right<br>F  Lower Arm, Left<br>G  Wrist Region, Right<br>H  Wrist Region, Left<br>J  Hand, Right<br>K  Hand, Left<br>L  Thumb, Right<br>M  Thumb, Left<br>N  Index Finger, Right<br>P  Index Finger, Left<br>Q  Middle Finger, Right<br>R  Middle Finger, Left<br>S  Ring Finger, Right<br>T  Ring Finger, Left<br>V  Little Finger, Right<br>W  Little Finger, Left | 0  Open<br>3  Percutaneous<br>4  Percutaneous Endoscopic<br>X  External | Z  No Device | Z  No Qualifier |

**0** Medical and Surgical
**X** Anatomical Regions, Upper Extremities
**R** Replacement: Putting in or on biological or synthetic material that physically takes the place and/or function of all or a portion of a body part

| Character 4<br>Body Part | Character 5<br>Approach | Character 6<br>Device | Character 7<br>Qualifier |
|---|---|---|---|
| L  Thumb, Right<br>M  Thumb, Left | 0  Open<br>4  Percutaneous Endoscopic | 7  Autologous Tissue Substitute | N  Toe, Right<br>P  Toe, Left |

**0** Medical and Surgical
**X** Anatomical Regions, Upper Extremities
**U** Supplement: Putting in or on biological or synthetic material that physically reinforces and/or augments the function of a portion of a body part

| Character 4<br>Body Part | Character 5<br>Approach | Character 6<br>Device | Character 7<br>Qualifier |
|---|---|---|---|
| 2 Shoulder Region, Right<br>3 Shoulder Region, Left<br>4 Axilla, Right<br>5 Axilla, Left<br>6 Upper Extremity, Right<br>7 Upper Extremity, Left<br>8 Upper Arm, Right<br>9 Upper Arm, Left<br>B Elbow Region, Right<br>C Elbow Region, Left<br>D Lower Arm, Right<br>F Lower Arm, Left<br>G Wrist Region, Right<br>H Wrist Region, Left<br>J Hand, Right<br>K Hand, Left<br>L Thumb, Right<br>M Thumb, Left<br>N Index Finger, Right<br>P Index Finger, Left<br>Q Middle Finger, Right<br>R Middle Finger, Left<br>S Ring Finger, Right<br>T Ring Finger, Left<br>V Little Finger, Right<br>W Little Finger, Left | 0 Open<br>4 Percutaneous Endoscopic | 7 Autologous Tissue Substitute<br>J Synthetic Substitute<br>K Nonautologous Tissue Substitute | Z No Qualifier |

**0** Medical and Surgical
**X** Anatomical Regions, Upper Extremities
**W** Revision: Correcting, to the extent possible, a portion of a malfunctioning device or the position of a displaced device

| Character 4<br>Body Part | Character 5<br>Approach | Character 6<br>Device | Character 7<br>Qualifier |
|---|---|---|---|
| 6 Upper Extremity, Right<br>7 Upper Extremity, Left | 0 Open<br>3 Percutaneous<br>4 Percutaneous Endoscopic<br>X External | 0 Drainage Device<br>3 Infusion Device<br>7 Autologous Tissue Substitute<br>J Synthetic Substitute<br>K Nonautologous Tissue Substitute<br>Y Other Device | Z No Qualifier |

**0** Medical and Surgical
**X** Anatomical Regions, Upper Extremities
**X** Transfer: Moving, without taking out, all or a portion of a body part to another location to take over the function of all or a portion of a body part

| Character 4<br>Body Part | Character 5<br>Approach | Character 6<br>Device | Character 7<br>Qualifier |
|---|---|---|---|
| N Index Finger, Right | 0 Open | Z No Device | L Thumb, Right |
| P Index Finger, Left | 0 Open | Z No Device | M Thumb, Left |

# Anatomical Regions, Lower Extremities | 0Y0-0YW

**0** Medical and Surgical
**Y** Anatomical Regions, Lower Extremities
**0** Alteration: Modifying the anatomic structure of a body part without affecting the function of the body part

| Character 4 Body Part | Character 5 Approach | Character 6 Device | Character 7 Qualifier |
|---|---|---|---|
| 0 Buttock, Right<br>1 Buttock, Left<br>9 Lower Extremity, Right<br>B Lower Extremity, Left<br>C Upper Leg, Right<br>D Upper Leg, Left<br>F Knee Region, Right<br>G Knee Region, Left<br>H Lower Leg, Right<br>J Lower Leg, Left<br>K Ankle Region, Right<br>L Ankle Region, Left | 0 Open<br>3 Percutaneous<br>4 Percutaneous Endoscopic | 7 Autologous Tissue Substitute<br>J Synthetic Substitute<br>K Nonautologous Tissue Substitute<br>Z No Device | Z No Qualifier |

**0** Medical and Surgical
**Y** Anatomical Regions, Lower Extremities
**2** Change: Taking out or off a device from a body part and putting back an identical or similar device in or on the same body part without cutting or puncturing the skin or a mucous membrane

| Character 4 Body Part | Character 5 Approach | Character 6 Device | Character 7 Qualifier |
|---|---|---|---|
| 9 Lower Extremity, Right<br>B Lower Extremity, Left | X External | 0 Drainage Device<br>Y Other Device | Z No Qualifier |

**0** Medical and Surgical
**Y** Anatomical Regions, Lower Extremities
**3** Control: Stopping, or attempting to stop, postprocedural bleeding

| Character 4 Body Part | Character 5 Approach | Character 6 Device | Character 7 Qualifier |
|---|---|---|---|
| 0 Buttock, Right<br>1 Buttock, Left<br>5 Inguinal Region, Right<br>6 Inguinal Region, Left<br>7 Femoral Region, Right<br>8 Femoral Region, Left<br>9 Lower Extremity, Right<br>B Lower Extremity, Left<br>C Upper Leg, Right<br>D Upper Leg, Left<br>F Knee Region, Right<br>G Knee Region, Left<br>H Lower Leg, Right<br>J Lower Leg, Left<br>K Ankle Region, Right<br>L Ankle Region, Left<br>M Foot, Right<br>N Foot, Left | 0 Open<br>3 Percutaneous<br>4 Percutaneous Endoscopic | Z No Device | Z No Qualifier |

**0** Medical and Surgical
**Y** Anatomical Regions, Lower Extremities
**6** Detachment: Cutting off all or a portion of the upper or lower extremities

| Character 4<br>Body Part | Character 5<br>Approach | Character 6<br>Device | Character 7<br>Qualifier |
|---|---|---|---|
| 2 Hindquarter, Right<br>3 Hindquarter, Left<br>4 Hindquarter, Bilateral<br>7 Femoral Region, Right<br>8 Femoral Region, Left<br>F Knee Region, Right<br>G Knee Region, Left | 0 Open | Z No Device | Z No Qualifier |
| C Upper Leg, Right<br>D Upper Leg, Left<br>H Lower Leg, Right<br>J Lower Leg, Left | 0 Open | Z No Device | 1 High<br>2 Mid<br>3 Low |
| M Foot, Right<br>N Foot, Left | 0 Open | Z No Device | 0 Complete<br>4 Complete 1st Ray<br>5 Complete 2nd Ray<br>6 Complete 3rd Ray<br>7 Complete 4th Ray<br>8 Complete 5th Ray<br>9 Partial 1st Ray<br>B Partial 2nd Ray<br>C Partial 3rd Ray<br>D Partial 4th Ray<br>F Partial 5th Ray |
| P 1st Toe, Right<br>Q 1st Toe, Left<br>R 2nd Toe, Right<br>S 2nd Toe, Left<br>T 3rd Toe, Right<br>U 3rd Toe, Left<br>V 4th Toe, Right<br>W 4th Toe, Left<br>X 5th Toe, Right<br>Y 5th Toe, Left | 0 Open | Z No Device | 0 Complete<br>1 High<br>2 Mid<br>3 Low |

**0** Medical and Surgical
**Y** Anatomical Regions, Lower Extremities
**9** Drainage: Taking or letting out fluids and/or gases from a body part

| Character 4<br>Body Part | Character 5<br>Approach | Character 6<br>Device | Character 7<br>Qualifier |
|---|---|---|---|
| 0 Buttock, Right<br>1 Buttock, Left<br>5 Inguinal Region, Right<br>6 Inguinal Region, Left<br>7 Femoral Region, Right<br>8 Femoral Region, Left<br>9 Lower Extremity, Right<br>B Lower Extremity, Left<br>C Upper Leg, Right<br>D Upper Leg, Left<br>F Knee Region, Right<br>G Knee Region, Left<br>H Lower Leg, Right<br>J Lower Leg, Left<br>K Ankle Region, Right<br>L Ankle Region, Left<br>M Foot, Right<br>N Foot, Left | 0 Open<br>3 Percutaneous<br>4 Percutaneous Endoscopic | 0 Drainage Device | Z No Qualifier |
| 0 Buttock, Right<br>1 Buttock, Left<br>5 Inguinal Region, Right<br>6 Inguinal Region, Left<br>7 Femoral Region, Right<br>8 Femoral Region, Left<br>9 Lower Extremity, Right<br>B Lower Extremity, Left<br>C Upper Leg, Right<br>D Upper Leg, Left<br>F Knee Region, Right<br>G Knee Region, Left<br>H Lower Leg, Right<br>J Lower Leg, Left<br>K Ankle Region, Right<br>L Ankle Region, Left<br>M Foot, Right<br>N Foot, Left | 0 Open<br>3 Percutaneous<br>4 Percutaneous Endoscopic | Z No Device | X Diagnostic<br>Z No Qualifier |

**0** Medical and Surgical
**Y** Anatomical Regions, Lower Extremities
**B** Excision: Cutting out or off, without replacement, a portion of a body part

| Character 4 Body Part | Character 5 Approach | Character 6 Device | Character 7 Qualifier |
|---|---|---|---|
| 0  Buttock, Right<br>1  Buttock, Left<br>5  Inguinal Region, Right<br>6  Inguinal Region, Left<br>7  Femoral Region, Right<br>8  Femoral Region, Left<br>9  Lower Extremity, Right<br>B  Lower Extremity, Left<br>C  Upper Leg, Right<br>D  Upper Leg, Left<br>F  Knee Region, Right<br>G  Knee Region, Left<br>H  Lower Leg, Right<br>J  Lower Leg, Left<br>K  Ankle Region, Right<br>L  Ankle Region, Left<br>M  Foot, Right<br>N  Foot, Left | 0  Open<br>3  Percutaneous<br>4  Percutaneous Endoscopic | Z  No Device | X  Diagnostic<br>Z  No Qualifier |

**0** Medical and Surgical
**Y** Anatomical Regions, Lower Extremities
**H** Insertion: Putting in a nonbiological appliance that monitors, assists, performs, or prevents a physiological function but does not physically take the place of a body part

| Character 4 Body Part | Character 5 Approach | Character 6 Device | Character 7 Qualifier |
|---|---|---|---|
| 0  Buttock, Right<br>1  Buttock, Left<br>5  Inguinal Region, Right<br>6  Inguinal Region, Left<br>7  Femoral Region, Right<br>8  Femoral Region, Left<br>9  Lower Extremity, Right<br>B  Lower Extremity, Left<br>C  Upper Leg, Right<br>D  Upper Leg, Left<br>F  Knee Region, Right<br>G  Knee Region, Left<br>H  Lower Leg, Right<br>J  Lower Leg, Left<br>K  Ankle Region, Right<br>L  Ankle Region, Left<br>M  Foot, Right<br>N  Foot, Left | 0  Open<br>3  Percutaneous<br>4  Percutaneous Endoscopic | 1  Radioactive Element<br>3  Infusion Device<br>Y  Other Device | Z  No Qualifier |

**0** Medical and Surgical
**Y** Anatomical Regions, Lower Extremities
**J** Inspection: Visually and/or manually exploring a body part

| Character 4 Body Part | Character 5 Approach | Character 6 Device | Character 7 Qualifier |
|---|---|---|---|
| 0  Buttock, Right<br>1  Buttock, Left<br>5  Inguinal Region, Right<br>6  Inguinal Region, Left<br>7  Femoral Region, Right<br>8  Femoral Region, Left<br>9  Lower Extremity, Right<br>A  Inguinal Region, Bilateral<br>B  Lower Extremity, Left<br>C  Upper Leg, Right<br>D  Upper Leg, Left<br>E  Femoral Region, Bilateral<br>F  Knee Region, Right<br>G  Knee Region, Left<br>H  Lower Leg, Right<br>J  Lower Leg, Left<br>K  Ankle Region, Right<br>L  Ankle Region, Left<br>M  Foot, Right<br>N  Foot, Left | 0  Open<br>3  Percutaneous<br>4  Percutaneous Endoscopic<br>X  External | Z  No Device | Z  No Qualifier |

**0** Medical and Surgical
**Y** Anatomical Regions, Lower Extremities
**M** Reattachment: Putting back in or on all or a portion of a separated body part to its normal location or other suitable location

| Character 4 Body Part | Character 5 Approach | Character 6 Device | Character 7 Qualifier |
|---|---|---|---|
| 0 Buttock, Right | 0 Open | Z No Device | Z No Qualifier |
| 1 Buttock, Left | | | |
| 2 Hindquarter, Right | | | |
| 3 Hindquarter, Left | | | |
| 4 Hindquarter, Bilateral | | | |
| 5 Inguinal Region, Right | | | |
| 6 Inguinal Region, Left | | | |
| 7 Femoral Region, Right | | | |
| 8 Femoral Region, Left | | | |
| 9 Lower Extremity, Right | | | |
| B Lower Extremity, Left | | | |
| C Upper Leg, Right | | | |
| D Upper Leg, Left | | | |
| F Knee Region, Right | | | |
| G Knee Region, Left | | | |
| H Lower Leg, Right | | | |
| J Lower Leg, Left | | | |
| K Ankle Region, Right | | | |
| L Ankle Region, Left | | | |
| M Foot, Right | | | |
| N Foot, Left | | | |
| P 1st Toe, Right | | | |
| Q 1st Toe, Left | | | |
| R 2nd Toe, Right | | | |
| S 2nd Toe, Left | | | |
| T 3rd Toe, Right | | | |
| U 3rd Toe, Left | | | |
| V 4th Toe, Right | | | |
| W 4th Toe, Left | | | |
| X 5th Toe, Right | | | |
| Y 5th Toe, Left | | | |

**0** Medical and Surgical
**Y** Anatomical Regions, Lower Extremities
**P** Removal: Taking out or off a device from a body part

| Character 4 Body Part | Character 5 Approach | Character 6 Device | Character 7 Qualifier |
|---|---|---|---|
| 9 Lower Extremity, Right | 0 Open | 0 Drainage Device | Z No Qualifier |
| B Lower Extremity, Left | 3 Percutaneous | 1 Radioactive Element | |
| | 4 Percutaneous Endoscopic | 3 Infusion Device | |
| | X External | 7 Autologous Tissue Substitute | |
| | | J Synthetic Substitute | |
| | | K Nonautologous Tissue Substitute | |
| | | Y Other Device | |

**0** Medical and Surgical
**Y** Anatomical Regions, Lower Extremities
**Q** Repair: Restoring, to the extent possible, a body part to its normal anatomic structure and function

| Character 4<br>Body Part | Character 5<br>Approach | Character 6<br>Device | Character 7<br>Qualifier |
|---|---|---|---|
| 0 Buttock, Right<br>1 Buttock, Left<br>5 Inguinal Region, Right<br>6 Inguinal Region, Left<br>7 Femoral Region, Right<br>8 Femoral Region, Left<br>9 Lower Extremity, Right<br>A Inguinal Region, Bilateral<br>B Lower Extremity, Left<br>C Upper Leg, Right<br>D Upper Leg, Left<br>E Femoral Region, Bilateral<br>F Knee Region, Right<br>G Knee Region, Left<br>H Lower Leg, Right<br>J Lower Leg, Left<br>K Ankle Region, Right<br>L Ankle Region, Left<br>M Foot, Right<br>N Foot, Left<br>P 1st Toe, Right<br>Q 1st Toe, Left<br>R 2nd Toe, Right<br>S 2nd Toe, Left<br>T 3rd Toe, Right<br>U 3rd Toe, Left<br>V 4th Toe, Right<br>W 4th Toe, Left<br>X 5th Toe, Right<br>Y 5th Toe, Left | 0 Open<br>3 Percutaneous<br>4 Percutaneous Endoscopic<br>X External | Z No Device | Z No Qualifier |

**0** Medical and Surgical
**Y** Anatomical Regions, Lower Extremities
**U** Supplement: Putting in or on biological or synthetic material that physically reinforces and/or augments the function of a portion of a body part

| Character 4<br>Body Part | Character 5<br>Approach | Character 6<br>Device | Character 7<br>Qualifier |
|---|---|---|---|
| 0 Buttock, Right<br>1 Buttock, Left<br>5 Inguinal Region, Right<br>6 Inguinal Region, Left<br>7 Femoral Region, Right<br>8 Femoral Region, Left<br>9 Lower Extremity, Right<br>A Inguinal Region, Bilateral<br>B Lower Extremity, Left<br>C Upper Leg, Right<br>D Upper Leg, Left<br>E Femoral Region, Bilateral<br>F Knee Region, Right<br>G Knee Region, Left<br>H Lower Leg, Right<br>J Lower Leg, Left<br>K Ankle Region, Right<br>L Ankle Region, Left<br>M Foot, Right<br>N Foot, Left<br>P 1st Toe, Right<br>Q 1st Toe, Left<br>R 2nd Toe, Right<br>S 2nd Toe, Left<br>T 3rd Toe, Right<br>U 3rd Toe, Left<br>V 4th Toe, Right<br>W 4th Toe, Left<br>X 5th Toe, Right<br>Y 5th Toe, Left | 0 Open<br>4 Percutaneous Endoscopic | 7 Autologous Tissue Substitute<br>J Synthetic Substitute<br>K Nonautologous Tissue Substitute | Z No Qualifier |

**0** Medical and Surgical
**Y** Anatomical Regions, Lower Extremities
**W** Revision: Correcting, to the extent possible, a portion of a malfunctioning device or the position of a displaced device

| Character 4<br>Body Part | Character 5<br>Approach | Character 6<br>Device | Character 7<br>Qualifier |
|---|---|---|---|
| 9 Lower Extremity, Right<br>B Lower Extremity, Left | 0 Open<br>3 Percutaneous<br>4 Percutaneous Endoscopic<br>X External | 0 Drainage Device<br>3 Infusion Device<br>7 Autologous Tissue Substitute<br>J Synthetic Substitute<br>K Nonautologous Tissue Substitute<br>Y Other Device | Z No Qualifier |

# Obstetrics | 102-10Y

| **1** Obstetrics **0** Pregnancy **2** Change: Taking out or off a device from a body part and putting back an identical or similar device in or on the same body part without cutting or puncturing the skin or a mucous membrane | | | |
|---|---|---|---|
| Character 4 Body Part | Character 5 Approach | Character 6 Device | Character 7 Qualifier |
| 0 Products of Conception ♀ | 7 Via Natural or Artificial Opening | 3 Monitoring Electrode Y Other Device | Z No Qualifier |

| **1** Obstetrics **0** Pregnancy **9** Drainage: Taking or letting out fluids and/or gases from a body part | | | |
|---|---|---|---|
| Character 4 Body Part | Character 5 Approach | Character 6 Device | Character 7 Qualifier |
| 0 Products of Conception ♀ | 0 Open 3 Percutaneous 4 Percutaneous Endoscopic 7 Via Natural or Artificial Opening 8 Via Natural or Artificial Opening Endoscopic | Z No Device | 9 Fetal Blood A Fetal Cerebrospinal Fluid B Fetal Fluid, Other C Amniotic Fluid, Therapeutic D Fluid, Other U Amniotic Fluid, Diagnostic |

**AHA:** 10907ZC - 2Q 2014, 10

| **1** Obstetrics **0** Pregnancy **A** Abortion: Artificially terminating a pregnancy | | | |
|---|---|---|---|
| Character 4 Body Part | Character 5 Approach | Character 6 Device | Character 7 Qualifier |
| 0 Products of Conception ♀ | 0 Open 3 Percutaneous 4 Percutaneous Endoscopic 8 Via Natural or Artificial Opening Endoscopic | Z No Device | Z No Qualifier |
| 0 Products of Conception ♀ | 7 Via Natural or Artificial Opening | Z No Device | 6 Vacuum W Laminaria X Abortifacient Z No Qualifier |

| **1** Obstetrics **0** Pregnancy **D** Extraction: Pulling or stripping out or off all or a portion of a body part by the use of force | | | |
|---|---|---|---|
| Character 4 Body Part | Character 5 Approach | Character 6 Device | Character 7 Qualifier |
| 0 Products of Conception ♀ | 0 Open | Z No Device | 0 Classical 1 Low Cervical 2 Extraperitoneal |
| 0 Products of Conception ♀ | 7 Via Natural or Artificial Opening | Z No Device | 3 Low Forceps 4 Mid Forceps 5 High Forceps 6 Vacuum 7 Internal Version 8 Other |
| 1 Products of Conception, Retained ♀ 2 Products of Conception, Ectopic ♀ | 7 Via Natural or Artificial Opening 8 Via Natural or Artificial Opening Endoscopic | Z No Device | Z No Qualifier |

**1 Obstetrics**
**0 Pregnancy**
**E Delivery:** Assisting the passage of the products of conception from the genital canal

| Character 4 Body Part | Character 5 Approach | Character 6 Device | Character 7 Qualifier |
|---|---|---|---|
| 0 Products of Conception ♀ | X External | Z No Device | Z No Qualifier |

**AHA:** 10E0XZZ - 2Q 2014, 9

**1 Obstetrics**
**0 Pregnancy**
**H Insertion:** Putting in a nonbiological appliance that monitors, assists, performs, or prevents a physiological function but does not physically take the place of a body part

| Character 4 Body Part | Character 5 Approach | Character 6 Device | Character 7 Qualifier |
|---|---|---|---|
| 0 Products of Conception ♀ | 0 Open<br>7 Via Natural or Artificial Opening | 3 Monitoring Electrode<br>Y Other Device | Z No Qualifier |

**AHA:** 10H07YZ - 2Q 2013, 36

**1 Obstetrics**
**0 Pregnancy**
**J Inspection:** Visually and/or manually exploring a body part

| Character 4 Body Part | Character 5 Approach | Character 6 Device | Character 7 Qualifier |
|---|---|---|---|
| 0 Products of Conception ♀<br>1 Products of Conception, Retained ♀<br>2 Products of Conception, Ectopic ♀ | 0 Open<br>3 Percutaneous<br>4 Percutaneous Endoscopic<br>7 Via Natural or Artificial Opening<br>8 Via Natural or Artificial Opening Endoscopic<br>X External | Z No Device | Z No Qualifier |

**1 Obstetrics**
**0 Pregnancy**
**P Removal:** Taking out or off a device from a body part, region or orifice

| Character 4 Body Part | Character 5 Approach | Character 6 Device | Character 7 Qualifier |
|---|---|---|---|
| 0 Products of Conception ♀ | 0 Open<br>7 Via Natural or Artificial Opening | 3 Monitoring Electrode<br>Y Other Device | Z No Qualifier |

**1 Obstetrics**
**0 Pregnancy**
**Q Repair:** Restoring, to the extent possible, a body part to its normal anatomic structure and function

| Character 4 Body Part | Character 5 Approach | Character 6 Device | Character 7 Qualifier |
|---|---|---|---|
| 0 Products of Conception ♀ | 0 Open<br>3 Percutaneous<br>4 Percutaneous Endoscopic<br>7 Via Natural or Artificial Opening<br>8 Via Natural or Artificial Opening Endoscopic | Y Other Device<br>Z No Device | E Nervous System<br>F Cardiovascular System<br>G Lymphatics and Hemic<br>H Eye<br>J Ear, Nose and Sinus<br>K Respiratory System<br>L Mouth and Throat<br>M Gastrointestinal System<br>N Hepatobiliary and Pancreas<br>P Endocrine System<br>Q Skin<br>R Musculoskeletal System<br>S Urinary System<br>T Female Reproductive System<br>V Male Reproductive System<br>Y Other Body System |

**1** Obstetrics
**0** Pregnancy
**S** Reposition: Moving to its normal location, or other suitable location, all or a portion of a body part

| Character 4<br>Body Part | Character 5<br>Approach | Character 6<br>Device | Character 7<br>Qualifier |
|---|---|---|---|
| 0 Products of Conception ♀ | 7 Via Natural or Artificial Opening<br>X External | Z No Device | Z No Qualifier |
| 2 Products of Conception, Ectopic ♀ | 0 Open<br>3 Percutaneous<br>4 Percutaneous Endoscopic<br>7 Via Natural or Artificial Opening<br>8 Via Natural or Artificial Opening<br>   Endoscopic | Z No Device | Z No Qualifier |

**1** Obstetrics
**0** Pregnancy
**T** Resection: Cutting out or off, without replacement, all of a body part

| Character 4<br>Body Part | Character 5<br>Approach | Character 6<br>Device | Character 7<br>Qualifier |
|---|---|---|---|
| 2 Products of Conception, Ectopic ♀ | 0 Open<br>3 Percutaneous<br>4 Percutaneous Endoscopic<br>7 Via Natural or Artificial Opening<br>8 Via Natural or Artificial Opening<br>   Endoscopic | Z No Device | Z No Qualifier |

**1** Obstetrics
**0** Pregnancy
**Y** Transplantation: Putting in or on all or a portion of a living body part taken from another individual or animal to physically take the place and/or function of all or a portion of a similar body part

| Character 4<br>Body Part | Character 5<br>Approach | Character 6<br>Device | Character 7<br>Qualifier |
|---|---|---|---|
| 0 Products of Conception ♀ | 3 Percutaneous<br>4 Percutaneous Endoscopic<br>7 Via Natural or Artificial Opening | Z No Device | E Nervous System<br>F Cardiovascular System<br>G Lymphatics and Hemic<br>H Eye<br>J Ear, Nose and Sinus<br>K Respiratory System<br>L Mouth and Throat<br>M Gastrointestinal System<br>N Hepatobiliary and Pancreas<br>P Endocrine System<br>Q Skin<br>R Musculoskeletal System<br>S Urinary System<br>T Female Reproductive System<br>V Male Reproductive System<br>Y Other Body System |

# Placement | 2W0-2Y5

**2** Placement
**W** Anatomical Regions
**0** Change: Taking out or off a device from a body part and putting back an identical or similar device in or on the same body part without cutting or puncturing the skin or a mucous membrane

| Character 4<br>Body Region | Character 5<br>Approach | Character 6<br>Device | Character 7<br>Qualifier |
|---|---|---|---|
| 0 Head<br>2 Neck<br>3 Abdominal Wall<br>4 Chest Wall<br>5 Back<br>6 Inguinal Region, Right<br>7 Inguinal Region, Left<br>8 Upper Extremity, Right<br>9 Upper Extremity, Left<br>A Upper Arm, Right<br>B Upper Arm, Left<br>C Lower Arm, Right<br>D Lower Arm, Left<br>E Hand, Right<br>F Hand, Left<br>G Thumb, Right<br>H Thumb, Left<br>J Finger, Right<br>K Finger, Left<br>L Lower Extremity, Right<br>M Lower Extremity, Left<br>N Upper Leg, Right<br>P Upper Leg, Left<br>Q Lower Leg, Right<br>R Lower Leg, Left<br>S Foot, Right<br>T Foot, Left<br>U Toe, Right<br>V Toe, Left | X External | 0 Traction Apparatus<br>1 Splint<br>2 Cast<br>3 Brace<br>4 Bandage<br>5 Packing Material<br>6 Pressure Dressing<br>7 Intermittent Pressure Device<br>Y Other Device | Z No Qualifier |
| 1 Face | X External | 0 Traction Apparatus<br>1 Splint<br>2 Cast<br>3 Brace<br>4 Bandage<br>5 Packing Material<br>6 Pressure Dressing<br>7 Intermittent Pressure Device<br>9 Wire<br>Y Other Device | Z No Qualifier |

**2** Placement
**W** Anatomical Regions
**1** Compression: Putting pressure on a body region

| Character 4<br>Body Region | Character 5<br>Approach | Character 6<br>Device | Character 7<br>Qualifier |
|---|---|---|---|
| 0 Head<br>1 Face<br>2 Neck<br>3 Abdominal Wall<br>4 Chest Wall<br>5 Back<br>6 Inguinal Region, Right<br>7 Inguinal Region, Left<br>8 Upper Extremity, Right<br>9 Upper Extremity, Left<br>A Upper Arm, Right<br>B Upper Arm, Left<br>C Lower Arm, Right<br>D Lower Arm, Left<br>E Hand, Right<br>F Hand, Left<br>G Thumb, Right<br>H Thumb, Left<br>J Finger, Right<br>K Finger, Left<br>L Lower Extremity, Right<br>M Lower Extremity, Left<br>N Upper Leg, Right<br>P Upper Leg, Left<br>Q Lower Leg, Right<br>R Lower Leg, Left<br>S Foot, Right<br>T Foot, Left<br>U Toe, Right<br>V Toe, Left | X External | 6 Pressure Dressing<br>7 Intermittent Pressure Device | Z No Qualifier |

**2** Placement
**W** Anatomical Regions
**2** Dressing: Putting material on a body region for protection

| Character 4 Body Region | Character 5 Approach | Character 6 Device | Character 7 Qualifier |
|---|---|---|---|
| 0 Head | X External | 4 Bandage | Z No Qualifier |
| 1 Face | | | |
| 2 Neck | | | |
| 3 Abdominal Wall | | | |
| 4 Chest Wall | | | |
| 5 Back | | | |
| 6 Inguinal Region, Right | | | |
| 7 Inguinal Region, Left | | | |
| 8 Upper Extremity, Right | | | |
| 9 Upper Extremity, Left | | | |
| A Upper Arm, Right | | | |
| B Upper Arm, Left | | | |
| C Lower Arm, Right | | | |
| D Lower Arm, Left | | | |
| E Hand, Right | | | |
| F Hand, Left | | | |
| G Thumb, Right | | | |
| H Thumb, Left | | | |
| J Finger, Right | | | |
| K Finger, Left | | | |
| L Lower Extremity, Right | | | |
| M Lower Extremity, Left | | | |
| N Upper Leg, Right | | | |
| P Upper Leg, Left | | | |
| Q Lower Leg, Right | | | |
| R Lower Leg, Left | | | |
| S Foot, Right | | | |
| T Foot, Left | | | |
| U Toe, Right | | | |
| V Toe, Left | | | |

**2** Placement
**W** Anatomical Regions
**3** Immobilization: Limiting or preventing motion of a body region

| Character 4 Body Region | Character 5 Approach | Character 6 Device | Character 7 Qualifier |
|---|---|---|---|
| 0 Head | X External | 1 Splint | Z No Qualifier |
| 2 Neck | | 2 Cast | |
| 3 Abdominal Wall | | 3 Brace | |
| 4 Chest Wall | | Y Other Device | |
| 5 Back | | | |
| 6 Inguinal Region, Right | | | |
| 7 Inguinal Region, Left | | | |
| 8 Upper Extremity, Right | | | |
| 9 Upper Extremity, Left | | | |
| A Upper Arm, Right | | | |
| B Upper Arm, Left | | | |
| C Lower Arm, Right | | | |
| D Lower Arm, Left | | | |
| E Hand, Right | | | |
| F Hand, Left | | | |
| G Thumb, Right | | | |
| H Thumb, Left | | | |
| J Finger, Right | | | |
| K Finger, Left | | | |
| L Lower Extremity, Right | | | |
| M Lower Extremity, Left | | | |
| N Upper Leg, Right | | | |
| P Upper Leg, Left | | | |
| Q Lower Leg, Right | | | |
| R Lower Leg, Left | | | |
| S Foot, Right | | | |
| T Foot, Left | | | |
| U Toe, Right | | | |
| V Toe, Left | | | |
| 1 Face | X External | 1 Splint | Z No Qualifier |
| | | 2 Cast | |
| | | 3 Brace | |
| | | 9 Wire | |
| | | Y Other Device | |

**2 Placement**
**W Anatomical Regions**
**4 Packing: Putting material in a body region or orifice**

| Character 4<br>Body Region | Character 5<br>Approach | Character 6<br>Device | Character 7<br>Qualifier |
|---|---|---|---|
| 0 Head<br>1 Face<br>2 Neck<br>3 Abdominal Wall<br>4 Chest Wall<br>5 Back<br>6 Inguinal Region, Right<br>7 Inguinal Region, Left<br>8 Upper Extremity, Right<br>9 Upper Extremity, Left<br>A Upper Arm, Right<br>B Upper Arm, Left<br>C Lower Arm, Right<br>D Lower Arm, Left<br>E Hand, Right<br>F Hand, Left<br>G Thumb, Right<br>H Thumb, Left<br>J Finger, Right<br>K Finger, Left<br>L Lower Extremity, Right<br>M Lower Extremity, Left<br>N Upper Leg, Right<br>P Upper Leg, Left<br>Q Lower Leg, Right<br>R Lower Leg, Left<br>S Foot, Right<br>T Foot, Left<br>U Toe, Right<br>V Toe, Left | X External | 5 Packing Material | Z No Qualifier |

**2 Placement**
**W Anatomical Regions**
**5 Removal: Taking out or off a device from a body part**

| Character 4<br>Body Region | Character 5<br>Approach | Character 6<br>Device | Character 7<br>Qualifier |
|---|---|---|---|
| 0 Head<br>2 Neck<br>3 Abdominal Wall<br>4 Chest Wall<br>5 Back<br>6 Inguinal Region, Right<br>7 Inguinal Region, Left<br>8 Upper Extremity, Right<br>9 Upper Extremity, Left<br>A Upper Arm, Right<br>B Upper Arm, Left<br>C Lower Arm, Right<br>D Lower Arm, Left<br>E Hand, Right<br>F Hand, Left<br>G Thumb, Right<br>H Thumb, Left<br>J Finger, Right<br>K Finger, Left<br>L Lower Extremity, Right<br>M Lower Extremity, Left<br>N Upper Leg, Right<br>P Upper Leg, Left<br>Q Lower Leg, Right<br>R Lower Leg, Left<br>S Foot, Right<br>T Foot, Left<br>U Toe, Right<br>V Toe, Left | X External | 0 Traction Apparatus<br>1 Splint<br>2 Cast<br>3 Brace<br>4 Bandage<br>5 Packing Material<br>6 Pressure Dressing<br>7 Intermittent Pressure Device<br>Y Other Device | Z No Qualifier |
| 1 Face | X External | 0 Traction Apparatus<br>1 Splint<br>2 Cast<br>3 Brace<br>4 Bandage<br>5 Packing Material<br>6 Pressure Dressing<br>7 Intermittent Pressure Device<br>9 Wire<br>Y Other Device | Z No Qualifier |

**2** Placement
**W** Anatomical Regions
**6** Traction: Exerting a pulling force on a body region in a distal direction

| Character 4<br>Body Region | Character 5<br>Approach | Character 6<br>Device | Character 7<br>Qualifier |
|---|---|---|---|
| 0 Head | X External | 0 Traction Apparatus | Z No Qualifier |
| 1 Face | | Z No Device | |
| 2 Neck | | | |
| 3 Abdominal Wall | | | |
| 4 Chest Wall | | | |
| 5 Back | | | |
| 6 Inguinal Region, Right | | | |
| 7 Inguinal Region, Left | | | |
| 8 Upper Extremity, Right | | | |
| 9 Upper Extremity, Left | | | |
| A Upper Arm, Right | | | |
| B Upper Arm, Left | | | |
| C Lower Arm, Right | | | |
| D Lower Arm, Left | | | |
| E Hand, Right | | | |
| F Hand, Left | | | |
| G Thumb, Right | | | |
| H Thumb, Left | | | |
| J Finger, Right | | | |
| K Finger, Left | | | |
| L Lower Extremity, Right | | | |
| M Lower Extremity, Left | | | |
| N Upper Leg, Right | | | |
| P Upper Leg, Left | | | |
| Q Lower Leg, Right | | | |
| R Lower Leg, Left | | | |
| S Foot, Right | | | |
| T Foot, Left | | | |
| U Toe, Right | | | |
| V Toe, Left | | | |

**AHA:** 2W60X0Z - 2Q 2013, 39

**2** Placement
**Y** Anatomical Orifices
**0** Change: Taking out or off a device from a body part and putting back an identical or similar device in or on the same body part without cutting or puncturing the skin or a mucous membrane

| Character 4<br>Body Region | Character 5<br>Approach | Character 6<br>Device | Character 7<br>Qualifier |
|---|---|---|---|
| 0 Mouth and Pharynx | X External | 5 Packing Material | Z No Qualifier |
| 1 Nasal | | | |
| 2 Ear | | | |
| 3 Anorectal | | | |
| 4 Female Genital Tract ♀ | | | |
| 5 Urethra | | | |

**2** Placement
**Y** Anatomical Orifices
**4** Packing: Putting material in a body region or orifice

| Character 4<br>Body Region | Character 5<br>Approach | Character 6<br>Device | Character 7<br>Qualifier |
|---|---|---|---|
| 0 Mouth and Pharynx | X External | 5 Packing Material | Z No Qualifier |
| 1 Nasal | | | |
| 2 Ear | | | |
| 3 Anorectal | | | |
| 4 Female Genital Tract ♀ | | | |
| 5 Urethra | | | |

**2** Placement
**Y** Anatomical Orifices
**5** Removal: Taking out or off a device from a body part

| Character 4<br>Body Region | Character 5<br>Approach | Character 6<br>Device | Character 7<br>Qualifier |
|---|---|---|---|
| 0 Mouth and Pharynx | X External | 5 Packing Material | Z No Qualifier |
| 1 Nasal | | | |
| 2 Ear | | | |
| 3 Anorectal | | | |
| 4 Female Genital Tract ♀ | | | |
| 5 Urethra | | | |

# Administration | 302-3E1

**3** Administration
**0** Circulatory
**2** Transfusion: Putting in blood or blood products

| Character 4<br>Body System / Region | Character 5<br>Approach | Character 6<br>Substance | Character 7<br>Qualifier |
|---|---|---|---|
| 3 Peripheral Vein<br>4 Central Vein | 0 Open<br>3 Percutaneous | A Stem Cells, Embryonic | Z No Qualifier |
| 3 Peripheral Vein<br>4 Central Vein | 0 Open<br>3 Percutaneous | G Bone Marrow<br>H Whole Blood<br>J Serum Albumin<br>K Frozen Plasma<br>L Fresh Plasma<br>M Plasma Cryoprecipitate<br>N Red Blood Cells<br>P Frozen Red Cells<br>Q White Cells<br>R Platelets<br>S Globulin<br>T Fibrinogen<br>V Antihemophilic Factors<br>W Factor IX<br>X Stem Cells, Cord Blood<br>Y Stem Cells, Hematopoietic | 0 Autologous<br>1 Nonautologous |
| 5 Peripheral Artery<br>6 Central Artery | 0 Open<br>3 Percutaneous | G Bone Marrow<br>H Whole Blood<br>J Serum Albumin<br>K Frozen Plasma<br>L Fresh Plasma<br>M Plasma Cryoprecipitate<br>N Red Blood Cells<br>P Frozen Red Cells<br>Q White Cells<br>R Platelets<br>S Globulin<br>T Fibrinogen<br>V Antihemophilic Factors<br>W Factor IX<br>X Stem Cells, Cord Blood<br>Y Stem Cells, Hematopoietic | 0 Autologous<br>1 Nonautologous |
| 7 Products of Conception, Circulatory ♀ | 3 Percutaneous<br>7 Via Natural or Artificial Opening | H Whole Blood<br>J Serum Albumin<br>K Frozen Plasma<br>L Fresh Plasma<br>M Plasma Cryoprecipitate<br>N Red Blood Cells<br>P Frozen Red Cells<br>Q White Cells<br>R Platelets<br>S Globulin<br>T Fibrinogen<br>V Antihemophilic Factors<br>W Factor IX | 1 Nonautologous |
| 8 Vein | 0 Open<br>3 Percutaneous | B 4-Factor Prothrombin Complex Concentrate | 1 Nonautologous |

**3** Administration
**C** Indwelling Device
**1** Irrigation: Putting in or on a cleansing substance

| Character 4<br>Body System / Region | Character 5<br>Approach | Character 6<br>Substance | Character 7<br>Qualifier |
|---|---|---|---|
| Z None | X External | 8 Irrigating Substance | Z No Qualifier |

**3 Administration**
**E Physiological Systems and Anatomical Regions**
**0 Introduction:** Putting in or on a therapeutic, diagnostic, nutritional, physiological, or prophylactic substance except blood or blood products

| Character 4<br>Body System / Region | Character 5<br>Approach | Character 6<br>Substance | Character 7<br>Qualifier |
|---|---|---|---|
| 0 Skin and Mucous Membranes | X External | 0 Antineoplastic | 5 Other Antineoplastic<br>M Monoclonal Antibody |
| 0 Skin and Mucous Membranes | X External | 2 Anti-infective | 8 Oxazolidinones<br>9 Other Anti-infective |
| 0 Skin and Mucous Membranes | X External | 3 Anti-inflammatory<br>4 Serum, Toxoid and Vaccine<br>B Local Anesthetic<br>K Other Diagnostic Substance<br>M Pigment<br>N Analgesics, Hypnotics, Sedatives<br>T Destructive Agent | Z No Qualifier |
| 0 Skin and Mucous Membranes | X External | G Other Therapeutic Substance | C Other Substance |
| 1 Subcutaneous Tissue | 0 Open | 2 Anti-infective | A Anti-Infective Envelope |
| 1 Subcutaneous Tissue | 3 Percutaneous | 0 Antineoplastic | 5 Other Antineoplastic<br>M Monoclonal Antibody |
| 1 Subcutaneous Tissue | 3 Percutaneous | 2 Anti-infective | 8 Oxazolidinones<br>9 Other Anti-infective<br>A Anti-Infective Envelope |
| 1 Subcutaneous Tissue | 3 Percutaneous | 3 Anti-inflammatory<br>4 Serum, Toxoid and Vaccine<br>6 Nutritional Substance<br>7 Electrolytic and Water Balance<br>Substance<br>B Local Anesthetic<br>H Radioactive Substance<br>K Other Diagnostic Substance<br>N Analgesics, Hypnotics, Sedatives<br>T Destructive Agent | Z No Qualifier |
| 1 Subcutaneous Tissue | 3 Percutaneous | G Other Therapeutic Substance | C Other Substance |
| 1 Subcutaneous Tissue | 3 Percutaneous | V Hormone | G Insulin<br>J Other Hormone |
| 2 Muscle | 3 Percutaneous | 0 Antineoplastic | 5 Other Antineoplastic<br>M Monoclonal Antibody |
| 2 Muscle | 3 Percutaneous | 2 Anti-infective | 8 Oxazolidinones<br>9 Other Anti-infective |
| 2 Muscle | 3 Percutaneous | 3 Anti-inflammatory<br>4 Serum, Toxoid and Vaccine<br>6 Nutritional Substance<br>7 Electrolytic and Water Balance<br>Substance<br>B Local Anesthetic<br>H Radioactive Substance<br>K Other Diagnostic Substance<br>N Analgesics, Hypnotics, Sedatives<br>T Destructive Agent | Z No Qualifier |
| 2 Muscle | 3 Percutaneous | G Other Therapeutic Substance | C Other Substance |
| 3 Peripheral Vein | 0 Open | 0 Antineoplastic | 2 High-dose Interleukin-2<br>3 Low-dose Interleukin-2<br>5 Other Antineoplastic<br>M Monoclonal Antibody<br>P Clofarabine |
| 3 Peripheral Vein | 0 Open | 1 Thrombolytic | 6 Recombinant Human-activated<br>Protein C<br>7 Other Thrombolytic |
| 3 Peripheral Vein | 0 Open | 2 Anti-infective | 8 Oxazolidinones<br>9 Other Anti-infective |

**3E0** continues on next page

**3** Administration – *continued*
**E** Physiological Systems and Anatomical Regions – *continued*
**0** Introduction: Putting in or on a therapeutic, diagnostic, nutritional, physiological, or prophylactic substance except blood or blood products – *continued*

| Character 4<br>Body System / Region | Character 5<br>Approach | Character 6<br>Substance | Character 7<br>Qualifier |
|---|---|---|---|
| 3 Peripheral Vein | 0 Open | 3 Anti-inflammatory<br>4 Serum, Toxoid and Vaccine<br>6 Nutritional Substance<br>7 Electrolytic and Water Balance<br>   Substance<br>F Intracirculatory Anesthetic<br>H Radioactive Substance<br>K Other Diagnostic Substance<br>N Analgesics, Hypnotics, Sedatives<br>P Platelet Inhibitor<br>R Antiarrhythmic<br>T Destructive Agent<br>X Vasopressor | Z No Qualifier |
| 3 Peripheral Vein | 0 Open | G Other Therapeutic Substance | C Other Substance<br>N Blood Brain Barrier Disruption |
| 3 Peripheral Vein | 0 Open | U Pancreatic Islet Cells | 0 Autologous<br>1 Nonautologous |
| 3 Peripheral Vein | 0 Open | V Hormone | G Insulin<br>H Human B-type Natriuretic Peptide<br>J Other Hormone |
| 3 Peripheral Vein | 0 Open | W Immunotherapeutic | K Immunostimulator<br>L Immunosuppressive |
| 3 Peripheral Vein | 3 Percutaneous | 0 Antineoplastic | 2 High-dose Interleukin-2<br>3 Low-dose Interleukin-2<br>5 Other Antineoplastic<br>M Monoclonal Antibody<br>P Clofarabine |
| 3 Peripheral Vein | 3 Percutaneous | 1 Thrombolytic | 6 Recombinant Human-activated<br>   Protein C<br>7 Other Thrombolytic |
| 3 Peripheral Vein | 3 Percutaneous | 2 Anti-infective | 8 Oxazolidinones<br>9 Other Anti-infective |
| 3 Peripheral Vein | 3 Percutaneous | 3 Anti-inflammatory<br>4 Serum, Toxoid and Vaccine<br>6 Nutritional Substance<br>7 Electrolytic and Water Balance<br>   Substance<br>F Intracirculatory Anesthetic<br>H Radioactive Substance<br>K Other Diagnostic Substance<br>N Analgesics, Hypnotics, Sedatives<br>P Platelet Inhibitor<br>R Antiarrhythmic<br>T Destructive Agent<br>X Vasopressor | Z No Qualifier |
| 3 Peripheral Vein | 3 Percutaneous | G Other Therapeutic Substance | C Other Substance<br>N Blood Brain Barrier Disruption<br>Q Glucarpidase |
| 3 Peripheral Vein | 3 Percutaneous | U Pancreatic Islet Cells | 0 Autologous<br>1 Nonautologous |
| 3 Peripheral Vein | 3 Percutaneous | V Hormone | G Insulin<br>H Human B-type Natriuretic Peptide<br>J Other Hormone |
| 3 Peripheral Vein | 3 Percutaneous | W Immunotherapeutic | K Immunostimulator<br>L Immunosuppressive |
| 4 Central Vein | 0 Open | 0 Antineoplastic | 2 High-dose Interleukin-2<br>3 Low-dose Interleukin-2<br>5 Other Antineoplastic<br>M Monoclonal Antibody<br>P Clofarabine |
| 4 Central Vein | 0 Open | 1 Thrombolytic | 6 Recombinant Human-activated<br>   Protein C<br>7 Other Thrombolytic |
| 4 Central Vein | 0 Open | 2 Anti-infective | 8 Oxazolidinones<br>9 Other Anti-infective |

**3E0** *continues on next page*

**3 Administration** – *continued*
**E Physiological Systems and Anatomical Regions** – *continued*
**0 Introduction: Putting in or on a therapeutic, diagnostic, nutritional, physiological, or prophylactic substance except blood or blood products** – *continued*

| Character 4<br>Body System / Region | Character 5<br>Approach | Character 6<br>Substance | Character 7<br>Qualifier |
|---|---|---|---|
| 4 Central Vein | 0 Open | 3 Anti-inflammatory<br>4 Serum, Toxoid and Vaccine<br>6 Nutritional Substance<br>7 Electrolytic and Water Balance Substance<br>F Intracirculatory Anesthetic<br>H Radioactive Substance<br>K Other Diagnostic Substance<br>N Analgesics, Hypnotics, Sedatives<br>P Platelet Inhibitor<br>R Antiarrhythmic<br>T Destructive Agent<br>X Vasopressor | Z No Qualifier |
| 4 Central Vein | 0 Open | G Other Therapeutic Substance | C Other Substance<br>N Blood Brain Barrier Disruption |
| 4 Central Vein | 0 Open | V Hormone | G Insulin<br>H Human B-type Natriuretic Peptide<br>J Other Hormone |
| 4 Central Vein | 0 Open | W Immunotherapeutic | K Immunostimulator<br>L Immunosuppressive |
| 4 Central Vein | 3 Percutaneous | 0 Antineoplastic | 2 High-dose Interleukin-2<br>3 Low-dose Interleukin-2<br>5 Other Antineoplastic<br>M Monoclonal Antibody<br>P Clofarabine |
| 4 Central Vein | 3 Percutaneous | 1 Thrombolytic | 6 Recombinant Human-activated Protein C<br>7 Other Thrombolytic |
| 4 Central Vein | 3 Percutaneous | 2 Anti-infective | 8 Oxazolidinones<br>9 Other Anti-infective |
| 4 Central Vein | 3 Percutaneous | 3 Anti-inflammatory<br>4 Serum, Toxoid and Vaccine<br>6 Nutritional Substance<br>7 Electrolytic and Water Balance Substance<br>F Intracirculatory Anesthetic<br>H Radioactive Substance<br>K Other Diagnostic Substance<br>N Analgesics, Hypnotics, Sedatives<br>P Platelet Inhibitor<br>R Antiarrhythmic<br>T Destructive Agent<br>X Vasopressor | Z No Qualifier |
| 4 Central Vein | 3 Percutaneous | G Other Therapeutic Substance | C Other Substance<br>N Blood Brain Barrier Disruption<br>Q Glucarpidase |
| 4 Central Vein | 3 Percutaneous | V Hormone | G Insulin<br>H Human B-type Natriuretic Peptide<br>J Other Hormone |
| 4 Central Vein | 3 Percutaneous | W Immunotherapeutic | K Immunostimulator<br>L Immunosuppressive |
| 5 Peripheral Artery<br>6 Central Artery | 0 Open<br>3 Percutaneous | 0 Antineoplastic | 2 High-dose Interleukin-2<br>3 Low-dose Interleukin-2<br>5 Other Antineoplastic<br>M Monoclonal Antibody<br>P Clofarabine |
| 5 Peripheral Artery<br>6 Central Artery | 0 Open<br>3 Percutaneous | 1 Thrombolytic | 6 Recombinant Human-activated Protein C<br>7 Other Thrombolytic |
| 5 Peripheral Artery<br>6 Central Artery | 0 Open<br>3 Percutaneous | 2 Anti-infective | 8 Oxazolidinones<br>9 Other Anti-infective |

**3E0** continues on next page

**3** Administration – *continued*
**E** Physiological Systems and Anatomical Regions – *continued*
**0** Introduction: Putting in or on a therapeutic, diagnostic, nutritional, physiological, or prophylactic substance except blood or blood products – *continued*

| Character 4<br>Body System / Region | Character 5<br>Approach | Character 6<br>Substance | Character 7<br>Qualifier |
|---|---|---|---|
| 5 Peripheral Artery<br>6 Central Artery | 0 Open<br>3 Percutaneous | 3 Anti-inflammatory<br>4 Serum, Toxoid and Vaccine<br>6 Nutritional Substance<br>7 Electrolytic and Water Balance<br>  Substance<br>F Intracirculatory Anesthetic<br>H Radioactive Substance<br>K Other Diagnostic Substance<br>N Analgesics, Hypnotics, Sedatives<br>P Platelet Inhibitor<br>R Antiarrhythmic<br>T Destructive Agent<br>X Vasopressor | Z No Qualifier |
| 5 Peripheral Artery<br>6 Central Artery | 0 Open<br>3 Percutaneous | G Other Therapeutic Substance | C Other Substance<br>N Blood Brain Barrier Disruption |
| 5 Peripheral Artery<br>6 Central Artery | 0 Open<br>3 Percutaneous | V Hormone | G Insulin<br>H Human B-type Natriuretic Peptide<br>J Other Hormone |
| 5 Peripheral Artery<br>6 Central Artery | 0 Open<br>3 Percutaneous | W Immunotherapeutic | K Immunostimulator<br>L Immunosuppressive |
| 7 Coronary Artery<br>8 Heart | 0 Open<br>3 Percutaneous | 1 Thrombolytic | 6 Recombinant Human-activated<br>  Protein C<br>7 Other Thrombolytic |
| 7 Coronary Artery<br>8 Heart | 0 Open<br>3 Percutaneous | G Other Therapeutic Substance | C Other Substance |
| 7 Coronary Artery<br>8 Heart | 0 Open<br>3 Percutaneous | K Other Diagnostic Substance<br>P Platelet Inhibitor | Z No Qualifier |
| 9 Nose | 3 Percutaneous<br>7 Via Natural or Artificial Opening<br>X External | 0 Antineoplastic | 5 Other Antineoplastic<br>M Monoclonal Antibody |
| 9 Nose | 3 Percutaneous<br>7 Via Natural or Artificial Opening<br>X External | 2 Anti-infective | 8 Oxazolidinones<br>9 Other Anti-infective |
| 9 Nose | 3 Percutaneous<br>7 Via Natural or Artificial Opening<br>X External | 3 Anti-inflammatory<br>4 Serum, Toxoid and Vaccine<br>B Local Anesthetic<br>H Radioactive Substance<br>K Other Diagnostic Substance<br>N Analgesics, Hypnotics, Sedatives<br>T Destructive Agent | Z No Qualifier |
| 9 Nose | 3 Percutaneous<br>7 Via Natural or Artificial Opening<br>X External | G Other Therapeutic Substance | C Other Substance |
| A Bone Marrow | 3 Percutaneous | 0 Antineoplastic | 5 Other Antineoplastic<br>M Monoclonal Antibody |
| A Bone Marrow | 3 Percutaneous | G Other Therapeutic Substance | C Other Substance |
| B Ear | 3 Percutaneous<br>7 Via Natural or Artificial Opening<br>X External | 0 Antineoplastic | 4 Liquid Brachytherapy Radioisotope<br>5 Other Antineoplastic<br>M Monoclonal Antibody |
| B Ear | 3 Percutaneous<br>7 Via Natural or Artificial Opening<br>X External | 2 Anti-infective | 8 Oxazolidinones<br>9 Other Anti-infective |
| B Ear | 3 Percutaneous<br>7 Via Natural or Artificial Opening<br>X External | 3 Anti-inflammatory<br>B Local Anesthetic<br>H Radioactive Substance<br>K Other Diagnostic Substance<br>N Analgesics, Hypnotics, Sedatives<br>T Destructive Agent | Z No Qualifier |
| B Ear | 3 Percutaneous<br>7 Via Natural or Artificial Opening<br>X External | G Other Therapeutic Substance | C Other Substance |
| C Eye | 3 Percutaneous<br>7 Via Natural or Artificial Opening<br>X External | 0 Antineoplastic | 4 Liquid Brachytherapy Radioisotope<br>5 Other Antineoplastic<br>M Monoclonal Antibody |

**3E0** *continues on next page*

| | | Character 4 Body System / Region | | Character 5 Approach | | Character 6 Substance | | Character 7 Qualifier |
|---|---|---|---|---|---|---|---|---|

**3** Administration – *continued*
**E** Physiological Systems and Anatomical Regions – *continued*
**0** Introduction: Putting in or on a therapeutic, diagnostic, nutritional, physiological, or prophylactic substance except blood or blood products – *continued*

| Character 4 Body System / Region | Character 5 Approach | Character 6 Substance | Character 7 Qualifier |
|---|---|---|---|
| C  Eye | 3  Percutaneous<br>7  Via Natural or Artificial Opening<br>X  External | 2  Anti-infective | 8  Oxazolidinones<br>9  Other Anti-infective |
| C  Eye | 3  Percutaneous<br>7  Via Natural or Artificial Opening<br>X  External | 3  Anti-inflammatory<br>B  Local Anesthetic<br>H  Radioactive Substance<br>K  Other Diagnostic Substance<br>M  Pigment<br>N  Analgesics, Hypnotics, Sedatives<br>T  Destructive Agent | Z  No Qualifier |
| C  Eye | 3  Percutaneous<br>7  Via Natural or Artificial Opening<br>X  External | G  Other Therapeutic Substance | C  Other Substance |
| C  Eye | 3  Percutaneous<br>7  Via Natural or Artificial Opening<br>X  External | S  Gas | F  Other Gas |
| D  Mouth and Pharynx | 3  Percutaneous<br>7  Via Natural or Artificial Opening<br>X  External | 0  Antineoplastic | 4  Liquid Brachytherapy Radioisotope<br>5  Other Antineoplastic<br>M  Monoclonal Antibody |
| D  Mouth and Pharynx | 3  Percutaneous<br>7  Via Natural or Artificial Opening<br>X  External | 2  Anti-infective | 8  Oxazolidinones<br>9  Other Anti-infective |
| D  Mouth and Pharynx | 3  Percutaneous<br>7  Via Natural or Artificial Opening<br>X  External | 3  Anti-inflammatory<br>4  Serum, Toxoid and Vaccine<br>6  Nutritional Substance<br>7  Electrolytic and Water Balance Substance<br>B  Local Anesthetic<br>H  Radioactive Substance<br>K  Other Diagnostic Substance<br>N  Analgesics, Hypnotics, Sedatives<br>R  Antiarrhythmic<br>T  Destructive Agent | Z  No Qualifier |
| D  Mouth and Pharynx | 3  Percutaneous<br>7  Via Natural or Artificial Opening<br>X  External | G  Other Therapeutic Substance | C  Other Substance |
| E  Products of Conception ♀<br>G  Upper GI<br>H  Lower GI<br>K  Genitourinary Tract<br>N  Male Reproductive ♂ | 3  Percutaneous<br>7  Via Natural or Artificial Opening<br>8  Via Natural or Artificial Opening Endoscopic | 0  Antineoplastic | 4  Liquid Brachytherapy Radioisotope<br>5  Other Antineoplastic<br>M  Monoclonal Antibody |
| E  Products of Conception ♀<br>G  Upper GI<br>H  Lower GI<br>K  Genitourinary Tract<br>N  Male Reproductive ♂ | 3  Percutaneous<br>7  Via Natural or Artificial Opening<br>8  Via Natural or Artificial Opening Endoscopic | 2  Anti-infective | 8  Oxazolidinones<br>9  Other Anti-infective |
| E  Products of Conception ♀<br>G  Upper GI<br>H  Lower GI<br>K  Genitourinary Tract<br>N  Male Reproductive ♂ | 3  Percutaneous<br>7  Via Natural or Artificial Opening<br>8  Via Natural or Artificial Opening Endoscopic | 3  Anti-inflammatory<br>6  Nutritional Substance<br>7  Electrolytic and Water Balance Substance<br>B  Local Anesthetic<br>H  Radioactive Substance<br>K  Other Diagnostic Substance<br>N  Analgesics, Hypnotics, Sedatives<br>T  Destructive Agent | Z  No Qualifier |
| E  Products of Conception ♀<br>G  Upper GI<br>H  Lower GI<br>K  Genitourinary Tract<br>N  Male Reproductive ♂ | 3  Percutaneous<br>7  Via Natural or Artificial Opening<br>8  Via Natural or Artificial Opening Endoscopic | G  Other Therapeutic Substance | C  Other Substance |
| E  Products of Conception ♀<br>G  Upper GI<br>H  Lower GI<br>K  Genitourinary Tract<br>N  Male Reproductive ♂ | 3  Percutaneous<br>7  Via Natural or Artificial Opening<br>8  Via Natural or Artificial Opening Endoscopic | S  Gas | F  Other Gas |
| F  Respiratory Tract | 3  Percutaneous | 0  Antineoplastic | 4  Liquid Brachytherapy Radioisotope<br>5  Other Antineoplastic<br>M  Monoclonal Antibody |

**3E0** *continues on next page*

Administration | 3E0–3E0

**3** Administration – *continued*
**E** Physiological Systems and Anatomical Regions – *continued*
**0** Introduction: Putting in or on a therapeutic, diagnostic, nutritional, physiological, or prophylactic substance except blood or blood products – *continued*

| Character 4<br>Body System / Region | Character 5<br>Approach | Character 6<br>Substance | Character 7<br>Qualifier |
|---|---|---|---|
| F Respiratory Tract | 3 Percutaneous | 2 Anti-infective | 8 Oxazolidinones<br>9 Other Anti-infective |
| F Respiratory Tract | 3 Percutaneous | 3 Anti-inflammatory<br>6 Nutritional Substance<br>7 Electrolytic and Water Balance<br>   Substance<br>B Local Anesthetic<br>H Radioactive Substance<br>K Other Diagnostic Substance<br>N Analgesics, Hypnotics, Sedatives<br>T Destructive Agent | Z No Qualifier |
| F Respiratory Tract | 3 Percutaneous | G Other Therapeutic Substance | C Other Substance |
| F Respiratory Tract | 3 Percutaneous | S Gas | D Nitric Oxide<br>F Other Gas |
| F Respiratory Tract | 7 Via Natural or Artificial Opening<br>8 Via Natural or Artificial Opening<br>   Endoscopic | 0 Antineoplastic | 4 Liquid Brachytherapy Radioisotope<br>5 Other Antineoplastic<br>M Monoclonal Antibody |
| F Respiratory Tract | 7 Via Natural or Artificial Opening<br>8 Via Natural or Artificial Opening<br>   Endoscopic | 2 Anti-infective | 8 Oxazolidinones<br>9 Other Anti-infective |
| F Respiratory Tract | 7 Via Natural or Artificial Opening<br>8 Via Natural or Artificial Opening<br>   Endoscopic | 3 Anti-inflammatory<br>6 Nutritional Substance<br>7 Electrolytic and Water Balance<br>   Substance<br>B Local Anesthetic<br>D Inhalation Anesthetic<br>H Radioactive Substance<br>K Other Diagnostic Substance<br>N Analgesics, Hypnotics, Sedatives<br>T Destructive Agent | Z No Qualifier |
| F Respiratory Tract | 7 Via Natural or Artificial Opening<br>8 Via Natural or Artificial Opening<br>   Endoscopic | G Other Therapeutic Substance | C Other Substance |
| F Respiratory Tract | 7 Via Natural or Artificial Opening<br>8 Via Natural or Artificial Opening<br>   Endoscopic | S Gas | D Nitric Oxide<br>F Other Gas |
| J Biliary and Pancreatic Tract | 3 Percutaneous<br>7 Via Natural or Artificial Opening<br>8 Via Natural or Artificial Opening<br>   Endoscopic | 0 Antineoplastic | 4 Liquid Brachytherapy Radioisotope<br>5 Other Antineoplastic<br>M Monoclonal Antibody |
| J Biliary and Pancreatic Tract | 3 Percutaneous<br>7 Via Natural or Artificial Opening<br>8 Via Natural or Artificial Opening<br>   Endoscopic | 2 Anti-infective | 8 Oxazolidinones<br>9 Other Anti-infective |
| J Biliary and Pancreatic Tract | 3 Percutaneous<br>7 Via Natural or Artificial Opening<br>8 Via Natural or Artificial Opening<br>   Endoscopic | 3 Anti-inflammatory<br>6 Nutritional Substance<br>7 Electrolytic and Water Balance<br>   Substance<br>B Local Anesthetic<br>H Radioactive Substance<br>K Other Diagnostic Substance<br>N Analgesics, Hypnotics, Sedatives<br>T Destructive Agent | Z No Qualifier |
| J Biliary and Pancreatic Tract | 3 Percutaneous<br>7 Via Natural or Artificial Opening<br>8 Via Natural or Artificial Opening<br>   Endoscopic | G Other Therapeutic Substance | C Other Substance |
| J Biliary and Pancreatic Tract | 3 Percutaneous<br>7 Via Natural or Artificial Opening<br>8 Via Natural or Artificial Opening<br>   Endoscopic | S Gas | F Other Gas |
| J Biliary and Pancreatic Tract | 3 Percutaneous<br>7 Via Natural or Artificial Opening<br>8 Via Natural or Artificial Opening<br>   Endoscopic | U Pancreatic Islet Cells | 0 Autologous<br>1 Nonautologous |
| L Pleural Cavity<br>M Peritoneal Cavity | 0 Open | 5 Adhesion Barrier | Z No Qualifier |

**3E0** *continues on next page*

**3 Administration** – *continued*
**E Physiological Systems and Anatomical Regions** – *continued*
**0 Introduction: Putting in or on a therapeutic, diagnostic, nutritional, physiological, or prophylactic substance except blood or blood products** – *continued*

| Character 4<br>Body System / Region | Character 5<br>Approach | Character 6<br>Substance | Character 7<br>Qualifier |
|---|---|---|---|
| L Pleural Cavity<br>M Peritoneal Cavity | 3 Percutaneous | 0 Antineoplastic | 4 Liquid Brachytherapy Radioisotope<br>5 Other Antineoplastic<br>M Monoclonal Antibody |
| L Pleural Cavity<br>M Peritoneal Cavity | 3 Percutaneous | 2 Anti-infective | 8 Oxazolidinones<br>9 Other Anti-infective |
| L Pleural Cavity<br>M Peritoneal Cavity | 3 Percutaneous | 3 Anti-inflammatory<br>6 Nutritional Substance<br>7 Electrolytic and Water Balance Substance<br>B Local Anesthetic<br>H Radioactive Substance<br>K Other Diagnostic Substance<br>N Analgesics, Hypnotics, Sedatives<br>T Destructive Agent | Z No Qualifier |
| L Pleural Cavity<br>M Peritoneal Cavity | 3 Percutaneous | G Other Therapeutic Substance | C Other Substance |
| L Pleural Cavity<br>M Peritoneal Cavity | 3 Percutaneous | S Gas | F Other Gas |
| L Pleural Cavity<br>M Peritoneal Cavity | 7 Via Natural or Artificial Opening | 0 Antineoplastic | 4 Liquid Brachytherapy Radioisotope<br>5 Other Antineoplastic<br>M Monoclonal Antibody |
| L Pleural Cavity<br>M Peritoneal Cavity | 7 Via Natural or Artificial Opening | S Gas | F Other Gas |
| P Female Reproductive ♀ | 0 Open | 5 Adhesion Barrier | Z No Qualifier |
| P Female Reproductive ♀ | 3 Percutaneous<br>7 Via Natural or Artificial Opening | 0 Antineoplastic | 4 Liquid Brachytherapy Radioisotope<br>5 Other Antineoplastic<br>M Monoclonal Antibody |
| P Female Reproductive ♀ | 3 Percutaneous<br>7 Via Natural or Artificial Opening | 2 Anti-infective | 8 Oxazolidinones<br>9 Other Anti-infective |
| P Female Reproductive ♀ | 3 Percutaneous<br>7 Via Natural or Artificial Opening | 3 Anti-inflammatory<br>6 Nutritional Substance<br>7 Electrolytic and Water Balance Substance<br>B Local Anesthetic<br>H Radioactive Substance<br>K Other Diagnostic Substance<br>L Sperm<br>N Analgesics, Hypnotics, Sedatives<br>T Destructive Agent | Z No Qualifier |
| P Female Reproductive ♀ | 3 Percutaneous<br>7 Via Natural or Artificial Opening | G Other Therapeutic Substance | C Other Substance |
| P Female Reproductive ♀ | 3 Percutaneous<br>7 Via Natural or Artificial Opening | Q Fertilized Ovum | 0 Autologous<br>1 Nonautologous |
| P Female Reproductive ♀ | 3 Percutaneous<br>7 Via Natural or Artificial Opening | S Gas | F Other Gas |
| P Female Reproductive ♀ | 8 Via Natural or Artificial Opening Endoscopic | 0 Antineoplastic | 4 Liquid Brachytherapy Radioisotope<br>5 Other Antineoplastic<br>M Monoclonal Antibody |
| P Female Reproductive ♀ | 8 Via Natural or Artificial Opening Endoscopic | 2 Anti-infective | 8 Oxazolidinones<br>9 Other Anti-infective |
| P Female Reproductive ♀ | 8 Via Natural or Artificial Opening Endoscopic | 3 Anti-inflammatory<br>6 Nutritional Substance<br>7 Electrolytic and Water Balance Substance<br>B Local Anesthetic<br>H Radioactive Substance<br>K Other Diagnostic Substance<br>N Analgesics, Hypnotics, Sedatives<br>T Destructive Agent | Z No Qualifier |
| P Female Reproductive ♀ | 8 Via Natural or Artificial Opening Endoscopic | G Other Therapeutic Substance | C Other Substance |

**3E0** *continues on next page*

♂ Male          ♀ Female          N C Non-covered          L C Limited Coverage          **AHA** *AHA Coding Clinic*

**3** Administration – *continued*
**E** Physiological Systems and Anatomical Regions – *continued*
**0** Introduction: Putting in or on a therapeutic, diagnostic, nutritional, physiological, or prophylactic substance except blood or blood products – *continued*

| Character 4<br>Body System / Region | Character 5<br>Approach | Character 6<br>Substance | Character 7<br>Qualifier |
|---|---|---|---|
| P Female Reproductive ♀ | 8 Via Natural or Artificial Opening Endoscopic | S Gas | F Other Gas |
| Q Cranial Cavity and Brain | 0 Open | A Stem Cells, Embryonic | Z No Qualifier |
| Q Cranial Cavity and Brain | 0 Open | E Stem Cells, Somatic | 0 Autologous<br>1 Nonautologous |
| Q Cranial Cavity and Brain | 3 Percutaneous | 0 Antineoplastic | 4 Liquid Brachytherapy Radioisotope<br>5 Other Antineoplastic<br>M Monoclonal Antibody |
| Q Cranial Cavity and Brain | 3 Percutaneous | 2 Anti-infective | 8 Oxazolidinones<br>9 Other Anti-infective |
| Q Cranial Cavity and Brain | 3 Percutaneous | 3 Anti-inflammatory<br>6 Nutritional Substance<br>7 Electrolytic and Water Balance Substance<br>A Stem Cells, Embryonic<br>B Local Anesthetic<br>H Radioactive Substance<br>K Other Diagnostic Substance<br>N Analgesics, Hypnotics, Sedatives<br>T Destructive Agent | Z No Qualifier |
| Q Cranial Cavity and Brain | 3 Percutaneous | E Stem Cells, Somatic | 0 Autologous<br>1 Nonautologous |
| Q Cranial Cavity and Brain | 3 Percutaneous | G Other Therapeutic Substance | C Other Substance |
| Q Cranial Cavity and Brain | 3 Percutaneous | S Gas | F Other Gas |
| Q Cranial Cavity and Brain | 7 Via Natural or Artificial Opening | 0 Antineoplastic | 4 Liquid Brachytherapy Radioisotope<br>5 Other Antineoplastic<br>M Monoclonal Antibody |
| Q Cranial Cavity and Brain | 7 Via Natural or Artificial Opening | S Gas | F Other Gas |
| R Spinal Canal | 0 Open | A Stem Cells, Embryonic | Z No Qualifier |
| R Spinal Canal | 0 Open | E Stem Cells, Somatic | 0 Autologous<br>1 Nonautologous |
| R Spinal Canal | 3 Percutaneous | 0 Antineoplastic | 2 High-dose Interleukin-2<br>3 Low-dose Interleukin-2<br>4 Liquid Brachytherapy Radioisotope<br>5 Other Antineoplastic<br>M Monoclonal Antibody |
| R Spinal Canal | 3 Percutaneous | 2 Anti-infective | 8 Oxazolidinones<br>9 Other Anti-infective |
| R Spinal Canal | 3 Percutaneous | 3 Anti-inflammatory<br>6 Nutritional Substance<br>7 Electrolytic and Water Balance Substance<br>A Stem Cells, Embryonic<br>B Local Anesthetic<br>C Regional Anesthetic<br>H Radioactive Substance<br>K Other Diagnostic Substance<br>N Analgesics, Hypnotics, Sedatives<br>T Destructive Agent | Z No Qualifier |
| R Spinal Canal | 3 Percutaneous | E Stem Cells, Somatic | 0 Autologous<br>1 Nonautologous |
| R Spinal Canal | 3 Percutaneous | G Other Therapeutic Substance | C Other Substance |
| R Spinal Canal | 3 Percutaneous | S Gas | F Other Gas |
| R Spinal Canal | 7 Via Natural or Artificial Opening | S Gas | F Other Gas |

**3E0** *continues on next page*

**3** Administration – *continued*
**E** Physiological Systems and Anatomical Regions – *continued*
**0** Introduction: Putting in or on a therapeutic, diagnostic, nutritional, physiological, or prophylactic substance except blood or blood products – *continued*

| Character 4<br>Body System / Region | Character 5<br>Approach | Character 6<br>Substance | Character 7<br>Qualifier |
|---|---|---|---|
| S Epidural Space | 3 Percutaneous | 0 Antineoplastic | 2 High-dose Interleukin-2<br>3 Low-dose Interleukin-2<br>4 Liquid Brachytherapy Radioisotope<br>5 Other Antineoplastic<br>M Monoclonal Antibody |
| S Epidural Space | 3 Percutaneous | 2 Anti-infective | 8 Oxazolidinones<br>9 Other Anti-infective |
| S Epidural Space | 3 Percutaneous | 3 Anti-inflammatory<br>6 Nutritional Substance<br>7 Electrolytic and Water Balance<br>   Substance<br>B Local Anesthetic<br>C Regional Anesthetic<br>H Radioactive Substance<br>K Other Diagnostic Substance<br>N Analgesics, Hypnotics, Sedatives<br>T Destructive Agent | Z No Qualifier |
| S Epidural Space | 3 Percutaneous | G Other Therapeutic Substance | C Other Substance |
| S Epidural Space | 3 Percutaneous | S Gas | F Other Gas |
| S Epidural Space | 7 Via Natural or Artificial Opening | S Gas | F Other Gas |
| T Peripheral Nerves and Plexi<br>X Cranial Nerves | 3 Percutaneous | 3 Anti-inflammatory<br>B Local Anesthetic<br>C Regional Anesthetic<br>T Destructive Agent | Z No Qualifier |
| T Peripheral Nerves and Plexi<br>X Cranial Nerves | 3 Percutaneous | G Other Therapeutic Substance | C Other Substance |
| U Joints | 0 Open | 2 Anti-infective | 8 Oxazolidinones<br>9 Other Anti-infective |
| U Joints | 0 Open | G Other Therapeutic Substance | B Recombinant Bone Morphogenetic<br>   Protein |
| U Joints | 3 Percutaneous | 0 Antineoplastic | 4 Liquid Brachytherapy Radioisotope<br>5 Other Antineoplastic<br>M Monoclonal Antibody |
| U Joints | 3 Percutaneous | 2 Anti-infective | 8 Oxazolidinones<br>9 Other Anti-infective |
| U Joints | 3 Percutaneous | 3 Anti-inflammatory<br>6 Nutritional Substance<br>7 Electrolytic and Water Balance<br>   Substance<br>B Local Anesthetic<br>H Radioactive Substance<br>K Other Diagnostic Substance<br>N Analgesics, Hypnotics, Sedatives<br>T Destructive Agent | Z No Qualifier |
| U Joints | 3 Percutaneous | G Other Therapeutic Substance | B Recombinant Bone Morphogenetic<br>   Protein<br>C Other Substance |
| U Joints | 3 Percutaneous | S Gas | F Other Gas |
| V Bones | 0 Open | G Other Therapeutic Substance | B Recombinant Bone Morphogenetic<br>   Protein |
| V Bones | 3 Percutaneous | 0 Antineoplastic | 5 Other Antineoplastic<br>M Monoclonal Antibody |
| V Bones | 3 Percutaneous | 2 Anti-infective | 8 Oxazolidinones<br>9 Other Anti-infective |

**3E0** *continues on next page*

**3** Administration – *continued*
**E** Physiological Systems and Anatomical Regions – *continued*
**0** Introduction: Putting in or on a therapeutic, diagnostic, nutritional, physiological, or prophylactic substance except blood or blood products – *continued*

| Character 4<br>Body System / Region | Character 5<br>Approach | Character 6<br>Substance | Character 7<br>Qualifier |
|---|---|---|---|
| V Bones | 3 Percutaneous | 3 Anti-inflammatory<br>6 Nutritional Substance<br>7 Electrolytic and Water Balance<br>   Substance<br>B Local Anesthetic<br>H Radioactive Substance<br>K Other Diagnostic Substance<br>N Analgesics, Hypnotics, Sedatives<br>T Destructive Agent | Z No Qualifier |
| V Bones | 3 Percutaneous | G Other Therapeutic Substance | B Recombinant Bone Morphogenetic<br>   Protein<br>C Other Substance |
| W Lymphatics | 3 Percutaneous | 0 Antineoplastic | 5 Other Antineoplastic<br>M Monoclonal Antibody |
| W Lymphatics | 3 Percutaneous | 2 Anti-infective | 8 Oxazolidinones<br>9 Other Anti-infective |
| W Lymphatics | 3 Percutaneous | 3 Anti-inflammatory<br>6 Nutritional Substance<br>7 Electrolytic and Water Balance<br>   Substance<br>B Local Anesthetic<br>H Radioactive Substance<br>K Other Diagnostic Substance<br>N Analgesics, Hypnotics, Sedatives<br>T Destructive Agent | Z No Qualifier |
| W Lymphatics | 3 Percutaneous | G Other Therapeutic Substance | C Other Substance |
| Y Pericardial Cavity | 3 Percutaneous | 0 Antineoplastic | 4 Liquid Brachytherapy Radioisotope<br>5 Other Antineoplastic<br>M Monoclonal Antibody |
| Y Pericardial Cavity | 3 Percutaneous | 2 Anti-infective | 8 Oxazolidinones<br>9 Other Anti-infective |
| Y Pericardial Cavity | 3 Percutaneous | 3 Anti-inflammatory<br>6 Nutritional Substance<br>7 Electrolytic and Water Balance<br>   Substance<br>B Local Anesthetic<br>H Radioactive Substance<br>K Other Diagnostic Substance<br>N Analgesics, Hypnotics, Sedatives<br>T Destructive Agent | Z No Qualifier |
| Y Pericardial Cavity | 3 Percutaneous | G Other Therapeutic Substance | C Other Substance |
| Y Pericardial Cavity | 3 Percutaneous | S Gas | F Other Gas |
| Y Pericardial Cavity | 7 Via Natural or Artificial Opening | 0 Antineoplastic | 4 Liquid Brachytherapy Radioisotope<br>5 Other Antineoplastic<br>M Monoclonal Antibody |
| Y Pericardial Cavity | 7 Via Natural or Artificial Opening | S Gas | F Other Gas |

**AHA:** 3E0G8TZ - 1Q 2013, 27; 3E03317 - 4Q 2013, 124; 3E0P7GC - 2Q 2014, 9; 3E013GC - 2Q 2014, 10

**3** Administration
**E** Physiological Systems and Anatomical Regions
**1** Irrigation: Putting in or on a cleansing substance

| Character 4 Body System / Region | Character 5 Approach | Character 6 Substance | Character 7 Qualifier |
|---|---|---|---|
| 0 Skin and Mucous Membranes<br>C Eye | 3 Percutaneous<br>X External | 8 Irrigating Substance | X Diagnostic<br>Z No Qualifier |
| 9 Nose<br>B Ear<br>F Respiratory Tract<br>G Upper GI<br>H Lower GI<br>J Biliary and Pancreatic Tract<br>K Genitourinary Tract<br>N Male Reproductive ♂<br>P Female Reproductive ♀ | 3 Percutaneous<br>7 Via Natural or Artificial Opening<br>8 Via Natural or Artificial Opening Endoscopic | 8 Irrigating Substance | X Diagnostic<br>Z No Qualifier |
| L Pleural Cavity<br>Q Cranial Cavity and Brain<br>R Spinal Canal<br>S Epidural Space<br>U Joints<br>Y Pericardial Cavity | 3 Percutaneous | 8 Irrigating Substance | X Diagnostic<br>Z No Qualifier |
| M Peritoneal Cavity | 3 Percutaneous | 8 Irrigating Substance | X Diagnostic<br>Z No Qualifier |
| M Peritoneal Cavity | 3 Percutaneous | 9 Dialysate | Z No Qualifier |

# Measurement and Monitoring | 4A0-4B0

| | | | |
|---|---|---|---|
| **4** Measurement and Monitoring | | | |
| **A** Physiological Systems | | | |
| **0** Measurement: Determining the level of a physiological or physical function at a point in time | | | |

| Character 4<br>Body System | Character 5<br>Approach | Character 6<br>Function / Device | Character 7<br>Qualifier |
|---|---|---|---|
| 0 Central Nervous | 0 Open | 2 Conductivity<br>4 Electrical Activity<br>B Pressure | Z No Qualifier |
| 0 Central Nervous | 3 Percutaneous | 4 Electrical Activity | Z No Qualifier |
| 0 Central Nervous | 3 Percutaneous | B Pressure<br>K Temperature<br>R Saturation | D Intracranial |
| 0 Central Nervous | 7 Via Natural or Artificial Opening | B Pressure<br>K Temperature<br>R Saturation | D Intracranial |
| 0 Central Nervous | X External | 2 Conductivity<br>4 Electrical Activity | Z No Qualifier |
| 1 Peripheral Nervous | 0 Open<br>3 Percutaneous<br>X External | 2 Conductivity | 9 Sensory<br>B Motor |
| 1 Peripheral Nervous | 0 Open<br>3 Percutaneous<br>X External | 4 Electrical Activity | Z No Qualifier |
| 2 Cardiac | 0 Open<br>3 Percutaneous | 4 Electrical Activity<br>9 Output<br>C Rate<br>F Rhythm<br>H Sound<br>P Action Currents | Z No Qualifier |
| 2 Cardiac | 0 Open<br>3 Percutaneous | N Sampling and Pressure | 6 Right Heart<br>7 Left Heart<br>8 Bilateral |
| 2 Cardiac | X External | 4 Electrical Activity | A Guidance<br>Z No Qualifier |
| 2 Cardiac | X External | 9 Output<br>C Rate<br>F Rhythm<br>H Sound<br>P Action Currents | Z No Qualifier |
| 2 Cardiac | X External | M Total Activity | 4 Stress |
| 3 Arterial | 0 Open<br>3 Percutaneous | 5 Flow<br>J Pulse | 1 Peripheral<br>3 Pulmonary<br>C Coronary |
| 3 Arterial | 0 Open<br>3 Percutaneous | B Pressure | 1 Peripheral<br>3 Pulmonary<br>C Coronary<br>F Other Thoracic |
| 3 Arterial | 0 Open<br>3 Percutaneous | H Sound<br>R Saturation | 1 Peripheral |
| 3 Arterial | X External | 5 Flow<br>B Pressure<br>H Sound<br>J Pulse<br>R Saturation | 1 Peripheral |
| 4 Venous | 0 Open<br>3 Percutaneous | 5 Flow<br>B Pressure<br>J Pulse | 0 Central<br>1 Peripheral<br>2 Portal<br>3 Pulmonary |
| 4 Venous | 0 Open<br>3 Percutaneous | R Saturation | 1 Peripheral |
| 4 Venous | X External | 5 Flow<br>B Pressure<br>J Pulse<br>R Saturation | 1 Peripheral |
| 5 Circulatory | X External | L Volume | Z No Qualifier |

**4A0** *continues on next page*

**4** Measurement and Monitoring – *continued*
**A** Physiological Systems – *continued*
**0** Measurement: Determining the level of a physiological or physical function at a point in time – *continued*

| Character 4<br>Body System | Character 5<br>Approach | Character 6<br>Function / Device | Character 7<br>Qualifier |
|---|---|---|---|
| 6 Lymphatic | 0 Open<br>3 Percutaneous | 5 Flow<br>B Pressure | Z No Qualifier |
| 7 Visual | X External | 0 Acuity<br>7 Mobility<br>B Pressure | Z No Qualifier |
| 8 Olfactory | X External | 0 Acuity | Z No Qualifier |
| 9 Respiratory | 7 Via Natural or Artificial Opening<br>8 Via Natural or Artificial Opening Endoscopic<br>X External | 1 Capacity<br>5 Flow<br>C Rate<br>D Resistance<br>L Volume<br>M Total Activity | Z No Qualifier |
| B Gastrointestinal | 7 Via Natural or Artificial Opening<br>8 Via Natural or Artificial Opening Endoscopic | 8 Motility<br>B Pressure<br>G Secretion | Z No Qualifier |
| C Biliary | 3 Percutaneous<br>4 Percutaneous Endoscopic<br>7 Via Natural or Artificial Opening<br>8 Via Natural or Artificial Opening Endoscopic | 5 Flow<br>B Pressure | Z No Qualifier |
| D Urinary | 7 Via Natural or Artificial Opening | 3 Contractility<br>5 Flow<br>B Pressure<br>D Resistance<br>L Volume | Z No Qualifier |
| F Musculoskeletal | 3 Percutaneous<br>X External | 3 Contractility | Z No Qualifier |
| H Products of Conception, Cardiac ♀ | 7 Via Natural or Artificial Opening<br>8 Via Natural or Artificial Opening Endoscopic<br>X External | 4 Electrical Activity<br>C Rate<br>F Rhythm<br>H Sound | Z No Qualifier |
| J Products of Conception, Nervous ♀ | 7 Via Natural or Artificial Opening<br>8 Via Natural or Artificial Opening Endoscopic<br>X External | 2 Conductivity<br>4 Electrical Activity<br>B Pressure | Z No Qualifier |
| Z None | 7 Via Natural or Artificial Opening | 6 Metabolism<br>K Temperature | Z No Qualifier |
| Z None | X External | 6 Metabolism<br>K Temperature<br>Q Sleep | Z No Qualifier |

**4** Measurement and Monitoring
**A** Physiological Systems
**1** Monitoring: Determining the level of a physiological or physical function repetitively over a period of time

| Character 4 Body System | Character 5 Approach | Character 6 Function / Device | Character 7 Qualifier |
|---|---|---|---|
| 0 Central Nervous | 0 Open | 2 Conductivity<br>B Pressure | Z No Qualifier |
| 0 Central Nervous | 0 Open | 4 Electrical Activity | G Intraoperative<br>Z No Qualifier |
| 0 Central Nervous | 3 Percutaneous | 4 Electrical Activity | G Intraoperative<br>Z No Qualifier |
| 0 Central Nervous | 3 Percutaneous | B Pressure<br>K Temperature<br>R Saturation | D Intracranial |
| 0 Central Nervous | 7 Via Natural or Artificial Opening | B Pressure<br>K Temperature<br>R Saturation | D Intracranial |
| 0 Central Nervous | X External | 2 Conductivity | Z No Qualifier |
| 0 Central Nervous | X External | 4 Electrical Activity | G Intraoperative<br>Z No Qualifier |
| 1 Peripheral Nervous | 0 Open<br>3 Percutaneous<br>X External | 2 Conductivity | 9 Sensory<br>B Motor |
| 1 Peripheral Nervous | 0 Open<br>3 Percutaneous<br>X External | 4 Electrical Activity | G Intraoperative<br>Z No Qualifier |
| 2 Cardiac | 0 Open<br>3 Percutaneous | 4 Electrical Activity<br>9 Output<br>C Rate<br>F Rhythm<br>H Sound | Z No Qualifier |
| 2 Cardiac | X External | 4 Electrical Activity | 5 Ambulatory<br>Z No Qualifier |
| 2 Cardiac | X External | 9 Output<br>C Rate<br>F Rhythm<br>H Sound | Z No Qualifier |
| 2 Cardiac | X External | M Total Activity | 4 Stress |
| 3 Arterial | 0 Open<br>3 Percutaneous | 5 Flow<br>B Pressure<br>J Pulse | 1 Peripheral<br>3 Pulmonary<br>C Coronary |
| 3 Arterial | 0 Open<br>3 Percutaneous | H Sound<br>R Saturation | 1 Peripheral |
| 3 Arterial | X External | 5 Flow<br>B Pressure<br>H Sound<br>J Pulse<br>R Saturation | 1 Peripheral |
| 4 Venous | 0 Open<br>3 Percutaneous | 5 Flow<br>B Pressure<br>J Pulse | 0 Central<br>1 Peripheral<br>2 Portal<br>3 Pulmonary |
| 4 Venous | 0 Open<br>3 Percutaneous | R Saturation | 0 Central<br>2 Portal<br>3 Pulmonary |
| 4 Venous | X External | 5 Flow<br>B Pressure<br>J Pulse | 1 Peripheral |
| 6 Lymphatic | 0 Open<br>3 Percutaneous | 5 Flow<br>B Pressure | Z No Qualifier |
| 9 Respiratory | 7 Via Natural or Artificial Opening<br>X External | 1 Capacity<br>5 Flow<br>C Rate<br>D Resistance<br>L Volume | Z No Qualifier |

**4A1** continues on next page

**4** Measurement and Monitoring – *continued*
**A** Physiological Systems – *continued*
**1** Monitoring: Determining the level of a physiological or physical function repetitively over a period of time – *continued*

| Character 4<br>Body System | Character 5<br>Approach | Character 6<br>Function / Device | Character 7<br>Qualifier |
|---|---|---|---|
| B Gastrointestinal | 7 Via Natural or Artificial Opening<br>8 Via Natural or Artificial Opening Endoscopic | 8 Motility<br>B Pressure<br>G Secretion | Z No Qualifier |
| D Urinary | 7 Via Natural or Artificial Opening | 3 Contractility<br>5 Flow<br>B Pressure<br>D Resistance<br>L Volume | Z No Qualifier |
| H Products of Conception, Cardiac ♀ | 7 Via Natural or Artificial Opening<br>8 Via Natural or Artificial Opening Endoscopic<br>X External | 4 Electrical Activity<br>C Rate<br>F Rhythm<br>H Sound | Z No Qualifier |
| J Products of Conception, Nervous ♀ | 7 Via Natural or Artificial Opening<br>8 Via Natural or Artificial Opening Endoscopic<br>X External | 2 Conductivity<br>4 Electrical Activity<br>B Pressure | Z No Qualifier |
| Z None | 7 Via Natural or Artificial Opening | K Temperature | Z No Qualifier |
| Z None | X External | K Temperature<br>Q Sleep | Z No Qualifier |

**4** Measurement and Monitoring
**B** Physiological Devices
**0** Measurement: Determining the level of a physiological or physical function at a point in time

| Character 4<br>Body System | Character 5<br>Approach | Character 6<br>Function / Device | Character 7<br>Qualifier |
|---|---|---|---|
| 0 Central Nervous<br>1 Peripheral Nervous<br>F Musculoskeletal | X External | V Stimulator | Z No Qualifier |
| 2 Cardiac | X External | S Pacemaker<br>T Defibrillator | Z No Qualifier |
| 9 Respiratory | X External | S Pacemaker | Z No Qualifier |

# Extracorporeal Assistance and Performance | 5A0-5A2

**5** Extracorporeal Assistance and Performance
**A** Physiological Systems
**0** Assistance: Taking over a portion of a physiological function by extracorporeal means

| Character 4<br>Body System | Character 5<br>Duration | Character 6<br>Function | Character 7<br>Qualifier |
|---|---|---|---|
| 2 Cardiac | 1 Intermittent<br>2 Continuous | 1 Output | 0 Balloon Pump<br>5 Pulsatile Compression<br>6 Other Pump<br>D Impeller Pump |
| 5 Circulatory | 1 Intermittent<br>2 Continuous | 2 Oxygenation | 1 Hyperbaric<br>C Supersaturated |
| 9 Respiratory | 3 Less than 24 Consecutive Hours<br>4 24-96 Consecutive Hours<br>5 Greater than 96 Consecutive Hours | 5 Ventilation | 7 Continuous Positive Airway Pressure<br>8 Intermittent Positive Airway Pressure<br>9 Continuous Negative Airway Pressure<br>B Intermittent Negative Airway Pressure<br>Z No Qualifier |

**AHA:** 5A02210 - 3Q 2013, 19

**5** Extracorporeal Assistance and Performance
**A** Physiological Systems
**1** Performance: Completely taking over a physiological function by extracorporeal means

| Character 4<br>Body System | Character 5<br>Duration | Character 6<br>Function | Character 7<br>Qualifier |
|---|---|---|---|
| 2 Cardiac | 0 Single | 1 Output | 2 Manual<br>4 Nonmechanical |
| 2 Cardiac | 1 Intermittent | 3 Pacing | Z No Qualifier |
| 2 Cardiac | 2 Continuous | 1 Output<br>3 Pacing | Z No Qualifier |
| 5 Circulatory | 2 Continuous | 2 Oxygenation | 3 Membrane |
| 9 Respiratory | 0 Single | 5 Ventilation | |
| 9 Respiratory | 3 Less than 24 Consecutive Hours<br>4 24-96 Consecutive Hours<br>5 Greater than 96 Consecutive Hours | 5 Ventilation | Z No Qualifier |
| C Biliary<br>D Urinary | 0 Single<br>6 Multiple | 0 Filtration | Z No Qualifier |

**AHA:** 5A1223Z - 3Q 2013, 19; 5A1221Z - 3Q 2013, 19, 1Q 2014, 11

**5** Extracorporeal Assistance and Performance
**A** Physiological Systems
**2** Restoration: Returning, or attempting to return, a physiological function to its original state by extracorporeal means

| Character 4<br>Body System | Character 5<br>Duration | Character 6<br>Function | Character 7<br>Qualifier |
|---|---|---|---|
| 2 Cardiac | 0 Single | 4 Rhythm | Z No Qualifier |

# Extracorporeal Therapies | 6A0-6A9

**6** Extracorporeal Therapies
**A** Physiological Systems
**0** Atmospheric Control: Extracorporeal control of atmospheric pressure and composition

| Character 4<br>Body System | Character 5<br>Duration | Character 6<br>Qualifier | Character 7<br>Qualifier |
|---|---|---|---|
| Z None | 0 Single<br>1 Multiple | Z No Qualifier | Z No Qualifier |

**6** Extracorporeal Therapies
**A** Physiological Systems
**1** Decompression: Extracorporeal elimination of undissolved gas from body fluids

| Character 4<br>Body System | Character 5<br>Duration | Character 6<br>Qualifier | Character 7<br>Qualifier |
|---|---|---|---|
| 5 Circulatory | 0 Single<br>1 Multiple | Z No Qualifier | Z No Qualifier |

**6** Extracorporeal Therapies
**A** Physiological Systems
**2** Electromagnetic Therapy: Extracorporeal treatment by electromagnetic rays

| Character 4<br>Body System | Character 5<br>Duration | Character 6<br>Qualifier | Character 7<br>Qualifier |
|---|---|---|---|
| 1 Urinary<br>2 Central Nervous | 0 Single<br>1 Multiple | Z No Qualifier | Z No Qualifier |

**6** Extracorporeal Therapies
**A** Physiological Systems
**3** Hyperthermia: Extracorporeal raising of body temperature

| Character 4<br>Body System | Character 5<br>Duration | Character 6<br>Qualifier | Character 7<br>Qualifier |
|---|---|---|---|
| Z None | 0 Single<br>1 Multiple | Z No Qualifier | Z No Qualifier |

**6 Extracorporeal Therapies**
**A Physiological Systems**
**4 Hypothermia: Extracorporeal lowering of body temperature**

| Character 4<br>Body System | Character 5<br>Duration | Character 6<br>Qualifier | Character 7<br>Qualifier |
|---|---|---|---|
| Z None | 0 Single<br>1 Multiple | Z No Qualifier | Z No Qualifier |

**6 Extracorporeal Therapies**
**A Physiological Systems**
**5 Pheresis: Extracorporeal separation of blood products**

| Character 4<br>Body System | Character 5<br>Duration | Character 6<br>Qualifier | Character 7<br>Qualifier |
|---|---|---|---|
| 5 Circulatory | 0 Single<br>1 Multiple | Z No Qualifier | 0 Erythrocytes<br>1 Leukocytes<br>2 Platelets<br>3 Plasma<br>T Stem Cells, Cord Blood<br>V Stem Cells, Hematopoietic |

**6 Extracorporeal Therapies**
**A Physiological Systems**
**6 Phototherapy: Extracorporeal treatment by light rays**

| Character 4<br>Body System | Character 5<br>Duration | Character 6<br>Qualifier | Character 7<br>Qualifier |
|---|---|---|---|
| 0 Skin<br>5 Circulatory | 0 Single<br>1 Multiple | Z No Qualifier | Z No Qualifier |

**6 Extracorporeal Therapies**
**A Physiological Systems**
**7 Ultrasound Therapy: Extracorporeal treatment by ultrasound**

| Character 4<br>Body System | Character 5<br>Duration | Character 6<br>Qualifier | Character 7<br>Qualifier |
|---|---|---|---|
| 5 Circulatory | 0 Single<br>1 Multiple | Z No Qualifier | 4 Head and Neck Vessels<br>5 Heart<br>6 Peripheral Vessels<br>7 Other Vessels<br>Z No Qualifier |

**6 Extracorporeal Therapies**
**A Physiological Systems**
**8 Ultraviolet Light Therapy: Extracorporeal treatment by ultraviolet light**

| Character 4<br>Body System | Character 5<br>Duration | Character 6<br>Qualifier | Character 7<br>Qualifier |
|---|---|---|---|
| 0 Skin | 0 Single<br>1 Multiple | Z No Qualifier | Z No Qualifier |

**6 Extracorporeal Therapies**
**A Physiological Systems**
**9 Shock Wave Therapy: Extracorporeal treatment by shock waves**

| Character 4<br>Body System | Character 5<br>Duration | Character 6<br>Qualifier | Character 7<br>Qualifier |
|---|---|---|---|
| 3 Musculoskeletal | 0 Single<br>1 Multiple | Z No Qualifier | Z No Qualifier |

# Osteopathic | 7W0

**7** Osteopathic
**W** Anatomical Regions
**0** Treatment: Manual treatment to eliminate or alleviate somatic dysfunction and related disorders

| Character 4<br>Body Region | Character 5<br>Approach | Character 6<br>Method | Character 7<br>Qualifier |
|---|---|---|---|
| 0 Head | X External | 0 Articulatory-Raising | Z None |
| 1 Cervical | | 1 Fascial Release | |
| 2 Thoracic | | 2 General Mobilization | |
| 3 Lumbar | | 3 High Velocity-Low Amplitude | |
| 4 Sacrum | | 4 Indirect | |
| 5 Pelvis | | 5 Low Velocity-High Amplitude | |
| 6 Lower Extremities | | 6 Lymphatic Pump | |
| 7 Upper Extremities | | 7 Muscle Energy-Isometric | |
| 8 Rib Cage | | 8 Muscle Energy-Isotonic | |
| 9 Abdomen | | 9 Other Method | |

# Other Procedures | 8C0-8E0

**8** Other Procedures
**C** Indwelling Device
**0** Other Procedures: Methodologies which attempt to remediate or cure a disorder or disease

| Character 4<br>Body Region | Character 5<br>Approach | Character 6<br>Method | Character 7<br>Qualifier |
|---|---|---|---|
| 1 Nervous System | X External | 6 Collection | J Cerebrospinal Fluid<br>L Other Fluid |
| 2 Circulatory System | X External | 6 Collection | K Blood<br>L Other Fluid |

**8** Other Procedures
**E** Physiological Systems and Anatomical Regions
**0** Other Procedures: Methodologies which attempt to remediate or cure a disorder or disease

| Character 4<br>Body Region | Character 5<br>Approach | Character 6<br>Method | Character 7<br>Qualifier |
|---|---|---|---|
| 1 Nervous System<br>U Female Reproductive System ♀ | X External | Y Other Method | 7 Examination |
| 2 Circulatory System | 3 Percutaneous | D Near Infrared Spectroscopy | Z No Qualifier |
| 9 Head and Neck Region<br>W Trunk Region | 0 Open<br>3 Percutaneous<br>4 Percutaneous Endoscopic<br>7 Via Natural or Artificial Opening<br>8 Via Natural or Artificial Opening<br>Endoscopic | C Robotic Assisted Procedure | Z No Qualifier |
| 9 Head and Neck Region<br>W Trunk Region | X External | B Computer Assisted Procedure | F With Fluoroscopy<br>G With Computerized Tomography<br>H With Magnetic Resonance Imaging<br>Z No Qualifier |
| 9 Head and Neck Region<br>W Trunk Region | X External | C Robotic Assisted Procedure | Z No Qualifier |
| 9 Head and Neck Region<br>W Trunk Region | X External | Y Other Method | 8 Suture Removal |
| H Integumentary System and Breast ♀ | 3 Percutaneous | 0 Acupuncture | 0 Anesthesia<br>Z No Qualifier |
| H Integumentary System and Breast ♀ | X External | 6 Collection | 2 Breast Milk |
| H Integumentary System and Breast ♀ | X External | Y Other Method | 9 Piercing |
| K Musculoskeletal System | X External | 1 Therapeutic Massage | Z No Qualifier |
| K Musculoskeletal System | X External | Y Other Method | 7 Examination |
| V Male Reproductive System ♂ | X External | 1 Therapeutic Massage | C Prostate<br>D Rectum |
| V Male Reproductive System ♂ | X External | 6 Collection | 3 Sperm |
| X Upper Extremity<br>Y Lower Extremity | 0 Open<br>3 Percutaneous<br>4 Percutaneous Endoscopic | C Robotic Assisted Procedure | Z No Qualifier |
| X Upper Extremity<br>Y Lower Extremity | X External | B Computer Assisted Procedure | F With Fluoroscopy<br>G With Computerized Tomography<br>H With Magnetic Resonance Imaging<br>Z No Qualifier |
| X Upper Extremity<br>Y Lower Extremity | X External | C Robotic Assisted Procedure | Z No Qualifier |
| X Upper Extremity<br>Y Lower Extremity | X External | Y Other Method | 8 Suture Removal |
| Z None | X External | Y Other Method | 1 In Vitro Fertilization<br>4 Yoga Therapy<br>5 Meditation<br>6 Isolation |

---

♂ Male    ♀ Female    **N C** Non-covered    **L C** Limited Coverage    **AHA** *AHA Coding Clinic*

# Chiropractic | 9WB

**9** Chiropractic
**W** Anatomical Regions
**B** Manipulation: Manual procedure that involves a directed thrust to move a joint past the physiological range of motion, without exceeding the anatomical limit

| Character 4 Body Region | Character 5 Approach | Character 6 Method | Character 7 Qualifier |
|---|---|---|---|
| 0 Head<br>1 Cervical<br>2 Thoracic<br>3 Lumbar<br>4 Sacrum<br>5 Pelvis<br>6 Lower Extremities<br>7 Upper Extremities<br>8 Rib Cage<br>9 Abdomen | X External | B Non-Manual<br>C Indirect Visceral<br>D Extra-Articular<br>F Direct Visceral<br>G Long Lever Specific Contact<br>H Short Lever Specific Contact<br>J Long and Short Lever Specific Contact<br>K Mechanically Assisted<br>L Other Method | Z None |

# Imaging | B00-BY4

**B** Imaging
**0** Central Nervous System
**0** Plain Radiography: Planar display of an image developed from the capture of external ionizing radiation on photographic or photoconductive plate

| Character 4 Body Part | Character 5 Contrast | Character 6 Qualifier | Character 7 Qualifier |
|---|---|---|---|
| B Spinal Cord | 0 High Osmolar<br>1 Low Osmolar<br>Y Other Contrast<br>Z None | Z None | Z None |

**B** Imaging
**0** Central Nervous System
**1** Fluoroscopy: Single plane or bi-plane real time display of an image developed from the capture of external ionizing radiation on a fluorescent screen. The image may also be stored by either digital or analog means

| Character 4 Body Part | Character 5 Contrast | Character 6 Qualifier | Character 7 Qualifier |
|---|---|---|---|
| B Spinal Cord | 0 High Osmolar<br>1 Low Osmolar<br>Y Other Contrast<br>Z None | Z None | Z None |

**B** Imaging
**0** Central Nervous System
**2** Computerized Tomography (CT Scan): Computer reformatted digital display of multiplanar images developed from the capture of multiple exposures of external ionizing radiation

| Character 4 Body Part | Character 5 Contrast | Character 6 Qualifier | Character 7 Qualifier |
|---|---|---|---|
| 0 Brain<br>7 Cisterna<br>8 Cerebral Ventricle(s)<br>9 Sella Turcica/Pituitary Gland<br>B Spinal Cord | 0 High Osmolar<br>1 Low Osmolar<br>Y Other Contrast | 0 Unenhanced and Enhanced<br>Z None | Z None |
| 0 Brain<br>7 Cisterna<br>8 Cerebral Ventricle(s)<br>9 Sella Turcica/Pituitary Gland<br>B Spinal Cord | Z None | Z None | Z None |

**B** Imaging
**0** Central Nervous System
**3** Magnetic Resonance Imaging (MRI): Computer reformatted digital display of multiplanar images developed from the capture of radiofrequency signals emitted by nuclei in a body site excited within a magnetic field

| Character 4<br>Body Part | Character 5<br>Contrast | Character 6<br>Qualifier | Character 7<br>Qualifier |
|---|---|---|---|
| 0 Brain<br>9 Sella Turcica/Pituitary Gland<br>B Spinal Cord<br>C Acoustic Nerves | Y Other Contrast | 0 Unenhanced and Enhanced<br>Z None | Z None |
| 0 Brain<br>9 Sella Turcica/Pituitary Gland<br>B Spinal Cord<br>C Acoustic Nerves | Z None | Z None | Z None |

**B** Imaging
**0** Central Nervous System
**4** Ultrasonography: Real time display of images of anatomy or flow information developed from the capture of reflected and attenuated high frequency sound waves

| Character 4<br>Body Part | Character 5<br>Contrast | Character 6<br>Qualifier | Character 7<br>Qualifier |
|---|---|---|---|
| 0 Brain<br>B Spinal Cord | Z None | Z None | Z None |

**B** Imaging
**2** Heart
**0** Plain Radiography: Planar display of an image developed from the capture of external ionizing radiation on photographic or photoconductive plate

| Character 4<br>Body Part | Character 5<br>Contrast | Character 6<br>Qualifier | Character 7<br>Qualifier |
|---|---|---|---|
| 0 Coronary Artery, Single<br>1 Coronary Arteries, Multiple<br>2 Coronary Artery Bypass Graft, Single<br>3 Coronary Artery Bypass Grafts,<br>   Multiple<br>4 Heart, Right<br>5 Heart, Left<br>6 Heart, Right and Left<br>7 Internal Mammary Bypass Graft, Right<br>8 Internal Mammary Bypass Graft, Left<br>F Bypass Graft, Other | 0 High Osmolar<br>1 Low Osmolar<br>Y Other Contrast | Z None | Z None |

**B** Imaging
**2** Heart
**1** Fluoroscopy: Single plane or bi-plane real time display of an image developed from the capture of external ionizing radiation on a fluorescent screen. The image may also be stored by either digital or analog means

| Character 4<br>Body Part | Character 5<br>Contrast | Character 6<br>Qualifier | Character 7<br>Qualifier |
|---|---|---|---|
| 0 Coronary Artery, Single<br>1 Coronary Arteries, Multiple<br>2 Coronary Artery Bypass Graft, Single<br>3 Coronary Artery Bypass Grafts,<br>   Multiple | 0 High Osmolar<br>1 Low Osmolar<br>Y Other Contrast | 1 Laser | 0 Intraoperative |
| 0 Coronary Artery, Single<br>1 Coronary Arteries, Multiple<br>2 Coronary Artery Bypass Graft, Single<br>3 Coronary Artery Bypass Grafts,<br>   Multiple | 0 High Osmolar<br>1 Low Osmolar<br>Y Other Contrast | Z None | Z None |
| 4 Heart, Right<br>5 Heart, Left<br>6 Heart, Right and Left<br>7 Internal Mammary Bypass Graft, Right<br>8 Internal Mammary Bypass Graft, Left<br>F Bypass Graft, Other | 0 High Osmolar<br>1 Low Osmolar<br>Y Other Contrast | Z None | Z None |

**B** Imaging
**2** Heart
**2** Computerized Tomography (CT Scan): Computer reformatted digital display of multiplanar images developed from the capture of multiple exposures of external ionizing radiation

| Character 4<br>Body Part | Character 5<br>Contrast | Character 6<br>Qualifier | Character 7<br>Qualifier |
|---|---|---|---|
| 1 Coronary Arteries, Multiple<br>3 Coronary Artery Bypass Grafts, Multiple<br>6 Heart, Right and Left | 0 High Osmolar<br>1 Low Osmolar<br>Y Other Contrast | 0 Unenhanced and Enhanced<br>Z None | Z None |
| 1 Coronary Arteries, Multiple<br>3 Coronary Artery Bypass Grafts, Multiple<br>6 Heart, Right and Left | Z None | 2 Intravascular Optical Coherence<br>Z None | Z None |

**B** Imaging
**2** Heart
**3** Magnetic Resonance Imaging (MRI): Computer reformatted digital display of multiplanar images developed from the capture of radiofrequency signals emitted by nuclei in a body site excited within a magnetic field

| Character 4<br>Body Part | Character 5<br>Contrast | Character 6<br>Qualifier | Character 7<br>Qualifier |
|---|---|---|---|
| 1 Coronary Arteries, Multiple<br>3 Coronary Artery Bypass Grafts, Multiple<br>6 Heart, Right and Left | Y Other Contrast | 0 Unenhanced and Enhanced<br>Z None | Z None |
| 1 Coronary Arteries, Multiple<br>3 Coronary Artery Bypass Grafts, Multiple<br>6 Heart, Right and Left | Z None | Z None | Z None |

**B** Imaging
**2** Heart
**4** Ultrasonography: Real time display of images of anatomy or flow information developed from the capture of reflected and attenuated high frequency sound waves

| Character 4<br>Body Part | Character 5<br>Contrast | Character 6<br>Qualifier | Character 7<br>Qualifier |
|---|---|---|---|
| 0 Coronary Artery, Single<br>1 Coronary Arteries, Multiple<br>4 Heart, Right<br>5 Heart, Left<br>6 Heart, Right and Left<br>B Heart with Aorta<br>C Pericardium<br>D Pediatric Heart | Y Other Contrast | Z None | Z None |
| 0 Coronary Artery, Single<br>1 Coronary Arteries, Multiple<br>4 Heart, Right<br>5 Heart, Left<br>6 Heart, Right and Left<br>B Heart with Aorta<br>C Pericardium<br>D Pediatric Heart | Z None | Z None | 3 Intravascular<br>4 Transesophageal<br>Z None |

**B** Imaging
**3** Upper Arteries
**0** Plain Radiography: Planar display of an image developed from the capture of external ionizing radiation on photographic or photoconductive plate

| Character 4<br>Body Part | Character 5<br>Contrast | Character 6<br>Qualifier | Character 7<br>Qualifier |
|---|---|---|---|
| 0 Thoracic Aorta | 0 High Osmolar | Z None | Z None |
| 1 Brachiocephalic-Subclavian Artery, Right | 1 Low Osmolar | | |
| 2 Subclavian Artery, Left | Y Other Contrast | | |
| 3 Common Carotid Artery, Right | Z None | | |
| 4 Common Carotid Artery, Left | | | |
| 5 Common Carotid Arteries, Bilateral | | | |
| 6 Internal Carotid Artery, Right | | | |
| 7 Internal Carotid Artery, Left | | | |
| 8 Internal Carotid Arteries, Bilateral | | | |
| 9 External Carotid Artery, Right | | | |
| B External Carotid Artery, Left | | | |
| C External Carotid Arteries, Bilateral | | | |
| D Vertebral Artery, Right | | | |
| F Vertebral Artery, Left | | | |
| G Vertebral Arteries, Bilateral | | | |
| H Upper Extremity Arteries, Right | | | |
| J Upper Extremity Arteries, Left | | | |
| K Upper Extremity Arteries, Bilateral | | | |
| L Intercostal and Bronchial Arteries | | | |
| M Spinal Arteries | | | |
| N Upper Arteries, Other | | | |
| P Thoraco-Abdominal Aorta | | | |
| Q Cervico-Cerebral Arch | | | |
| R Intracranial Arteries | | | |
| S Pulmonary Artery, Right | | | |
| T Pulmonary Artery, Left | | | |

**B** Imaging
**3** Upper Arteries
**1** Fluoroscopy: Single plane or bi-plane real time display of an image developed from the capture of external ionizing radiation on a fluorescent screen. The image may also be stored by either digital or analog means

| Character 4<br>Body Part | Character 5<br>Contrast | Character 6<br>Qualifier | Character 7<br>Qualifier |
|---|---|---|---|
| 0 Thoracic Aorta<br>1 Brachiocephalic-Subclavian Artery, Right<br>2 Subclavian Artery, Left<br>3 Common Carotid Artery, Right<br>4 Common Carotid Artery, Left<br>5 Common Carotid Arteries, Bilateral<br>6 Internal Carotid Artery, Right<br>7 Internal Carotid Artery, Left<br>8 Internal Carotid Arteries, Bilateral<br>9 External Carotid Artery, Right<br>B External Carotid Artery, Left<br>C External Carotid Arteries, Bilateral<br>D Vertebral Artery, Right<br>F Vertebral Artery, Left<br>G Vertebral Arteries, Bilateral<br>H Upper Extremity Arteries, Right<br>J Upper Extremity Arteries, Left<br>K Upper Extremity Arteries, Bilateral<br>L Intercostal and Bronchial Arteries<br>M Spinal Arteries<br>N Upper Arteries, Other<br>P Thoraco-Abdominal Aorta<br>Q Cervico-Cerebral Arch<br>R Intracranial Arteries<br>S Pulmonary Artery, Right<br>T Pulmonary Artery, Left | 0 High Osmolar<br>1 Low Osmolar<br>Y Other Contrast | 1 Laser | 0 Intraoperative |
| 0 Thoracic Aorta<br>1 Brachiocephalic-Subclavian Artery, Right<br>2 Subclavian Artery, Left<br>3 Common Carotid Artery, Right<br>4 Common Carotid Artery, Left<br>5 Common Carotid Arteries, Bilateral<br>6 Internal Carotid Artery, Right<br>7 Internal Carotid Artery, Left<br>8 Internal Carotid Arteries, Bilateral<br>9 External Carotid Artery, Right<br>B External Carotid Artery, Left<br>C External Carotid Arteries, Bilateral<br>D Vertebral Artery, Right<br>F Vertebral Artery, Left<br>G Vertebral Arteries, Bilateral<br>H Upper Extremity Arteries, Right<br>J Upper Extremity Arteries, Left<br>K Upper Extremity Arteries, Bilateral<br>L Intercostal and Bronchial Arteries<br>M Spinal Arteries<br>N Upper Arteries, Other<br>P Thoraco-Abdominal Aorta<br>Q Cervico-Cerebral Arch<br>R Intracranial Arteries<br>S Pulmonary Artery, Right<br>T Pulmonary Artery, Left | 0 High Osmolar<br>1 Low Osmolar<br>Y Other Contrast | Z None | Z None |
| 0 Thoracic Aorta<br>1 Brachiocephalic-Subclavian Artery, Right<br>2 Subclavian Artery, Left<br>3 Common Carotid Artery, Right<br>4 Common Carotid Artery, Left<br>5 Common Carotid Arteries, Bilateral<br>6 Internal Carotid Artery, Right<br>7 Internal Carotid Artery, Left<br>8 Internal Carotid Arteries, Bilateral<br>9 External Carotid Artery, Right<br>B External Carotid Artery, Left<br>C External Carotid Arteries, Bilateral<br>D Vertebral Artery, Right<br>F Vertebral Artery, Left<br>G Vertebral Arteries, Bilateral<br>H Upper Extremity Arteries, Right<br>J Upper Extremity Arteries, Left<br>K Upper Extremity Arteries, Bilateral<br>L Intercostal and Bronchial Arteries<br>M Spinal Arteries<br>N Upper Arteries, Other<br>P Thoraco-Abdominal Aorta<br>Q Cervico-Cerebral Arch<br>R Intracranial Arteries<br>S Pulmonary Artery, Right<br>T Pulmonary Artery, Left | Z None | Z None | Z None |

**B** Imaging
**3** Upper Arteries
**2** Computerized Tomography (CT Scan): Computer reformatted digital display of multiplanar images developed from the capture of multiple exposures of external ionizing radiation

| Character 4<br>Body Part | Character 5<br>Contrast | Character 6<br>Qualifier | Character 7<br>Qualifier |
|---|---|---|---|
| 0 Thoracic Aorta<br>5 Common Carotid Arteries, Bilateral<br>8 Internal Carotid Arteries, Bilateral<br>G Vertebral Arteries, Bilateral<br>R Intracranial Arteries<br>S Pulmonary Artery, Right<br>T Pulmonary Artery, Left | 0 High Osmolar<br>1 Low Osmolar<br>Y Other Contrast | Z None | Z None |
| 0 Thoracic Aorta<br>5 Common Carotid Arteries, Bilateral<br>8 Internal Carotid Arteries, Bilateral<br>G Vertebral Arteries, Bilateral<br>R Intracranial Arteries<br>S Pulmonary Artery, Right<br>T Pulmonary Artery, Left | Z None | 2 Intravascular Optical Coherence<br>Z None | Z None |

**B** Imaging
**3** Upper Arteries
**3** Magnetic Resonance Imaging (MRI): Computer reformatted digital display of multiplanar images developed from the capture of radiofrequency signals emitted by nuclei in a body site excited within a magnetic field

| Character 4<br>Body Part | Character 5<br>Contrast | Character 6<br>Qualifier | Character 7<br>Qualifier |
|---|---|---|---|
| 0 Thoracic Aorta<br>5 Common Carotid Arteries, Bilateral<br>8 Internal Carotid Arteries, Bilateral<br>G Vertebral Arteries, Bilateral<br>H Upper Extremity Arteries, Right<br>J Upper Extremity Arteries, Left<br>K Upper Extremity Arteries, Bilateral<br>M Spinal Arteries<br>Q Cervico-Cerebral Arch<br>R Intracranial Arteries | Y Other Contrast | 0 Unenhanced and Enhanced<br>Z None | Z None |
| 0 Thoracic Aorta<br>5 Common Carotid Arteries, Bilateral<br>8 Internal Carotid Arteries, Bilateral<br>G Vertebral Arteries, Bilateral<br>H Upper Extremity Arteries, Right<br>J Upper Extremity Arteries, Left<br>K Upper Extremity Arteries, Bilateral<br>M Spinal Arteries<br>Q Cervico-Cerebral Arch<br>R Intracranial Arteries | Z None | Z None | Z None |

**B** Imaging
**3** Upper Arteries
**4** Ultrasonography: Real time display of images of anatomy or flow information developed from the capture of reflected and attenuated high frequency sound waves

| Character 4<br>Body Part | Character 5<br>Contrast | Character 6<br>Qualifier | Character 7<br>Qualifier |
|---|---|---|---|
| 0 Thoracic Aorta<br>1 Brachiocephalic-Subclavian Artery, Right<br>2 Subclavian Artery, Left<br>3 Common Carotid Artery, Right<br>4 Common Carotid Artery, Left<br>5 Common Carotid Arteries, Bilateral<br>6 Internal Carotid Artery, Right<br>7 Internal Carotid Artery, Left<br>8 Internal Carotid Arteries, Bilateral<br>H Upper Extremity Arteries, Right<br>J Upper Extremity Arteries, Left<br>K Upper Extremity Arteries, Bilateral<br>R Intracranial Arteries<br>S Pulmonary Artery, Right<br>T Pulmonary Artery, Left<br>V Ophthalmic Arteries | Z None | Z None | 3 Intravascular<br>Z None |

---

♂ Male     ♀ Female     N C Non-covered     L C Limited Coverage     **AHA** *AHA Coding Clinic*

**B** Imaging
**4** Lower Arteries
**0** Plain Radiography: Planar display of an image developed from the capture of external ionizing radiation on photographic or photoconductive plate

| Character 4<br>Body Part | Character 5<br>Contrast | Character 6<br>Qualifier | Character 7<br>Qualifier |
|---|---|---|---|
| 0　Abdominal Aorta<br>2　Hepatic Artery<br>3　Splenic Arteries<br>4　Superior Mesenteric Artery<br>5　Inferior Mesenteric Artery<br>6　Renal Artery, Right<br>7　Renal Artery, Left<br>8　Renal Arteries, Bilateral<br>9　Lumbar Arteries<br>B　Intra-Abdominal Arteries, Other<br>C　Pelvic Arteries<br>D　Aorta and Bilateral Lower Extremity<br>　　Arteries<br>F　Lower Extremity Arteries, Right<br>G　Lower Extremity Arteries, Left<br>J　Lower Arteries, Other<br>M　Renal Artery Transplant | 0　High Osmolar<br>1　Low Osmolar<br>Y　Other Contrast | Z　None | Z　None |

**B** Imaging
**4** Lower Arteries
**1** Fluoroscopy: Single plane or bi-plane real time display of an image developed from the capture of external ionizing radiation on a fluorescent screen. The image may also be stored by either digital or analog means

| Character 4<br>Body Part | Character 5<br>Contrast | Character 6<br>Qualifier | Character 7<br>Qualifier |
|---|---|---|---|
| 0　Abdominal Aorta<br>2　Hepatic Artery<br>3　Splenic Arteries<br>4　Superior Mesenteric Artery<br>5　Inferior Mesenteric Artery<br>6　Renal Artery, Right<br>7　Renal Artery, Left<br>8　Renal Arteries, Bilateral<br>9　Lumbar Arteries<br>B　Intra-Abdominal Arteries, Other<br>C　Pelvic Arteries<br>D　Aorta and Bilateral Lower Extremity<br>　　Arteries<br>F　Lower Extremity Arteries, Right<br>G　Lower Extremity Arteries, Left<br>J　Lower Arteries, Other | 0　High Osmolar<br>1　Low Osmolar<br>Y　Other Contrast | 1　Laser | 0　Intraoperative |
| 0　Abdominal Aorta<br>2　Hepatic Artery<br>3　Splenic Arteries<br>4　Superior Mesenteric Artery<br>5　Inferior Mesenteric Artery<br>6　Renal Artery, Right<br>7　Renal Artery, Left<br>8　Renal Arteries, Bilateral<br>9　Lumbar Arteries<br>B　Intra-Abdominal Arteries, Other<br>C　Pelvic Arteries<br>D　Aorta and Bilateral Lower Extremity<br>　　Arteries<br>F　Lower Extremity Arteries, Right<br>G　Lower Extremity Arteries, Left<br>J　Lower Arteries, Other | 0　High Osmolar<br>1　Low Osmolar<br>Y　Other Contrast | Z　None | Z　None |
| 0　Abdominal Aorta<br>2　Hepatic Artery<br>3　Splenic Arteries<br>4　Superior Mesenteric Artery<br>5　Inferior Mesenteric Artery<br>6　Renal Artery, Right<br>7　Renal Artery, Left<br>8　Renal Arteries, Bilateral<br>9　Lumbar Arteries<br>B　Intra-Abdominal Arteries, Other<br>C　Pelvic Arteries<br>D　Aorta and Bilateral Lower Extremity<br>　　Arteries<br>F　Lower Extremity Arteries, Right<br>G　Lower Extremity Arteries, Left<br>J　Lower Arteries, Other | Z　None | Z　None | Z　None |

**B Imaging**
**4 Lower Arteries**
**2 Computerized Tomography (CT Scan):** Computer reformatted digital display of multiplanar images developed from the capture of multiple exposures of external ionizing radiation

| Character 4<br>Body Part | Character 5<br>Contrast | Character 6<br>Qualifier | Character 7<br>Qualifier |
|---|---|---|---|
| 0 Abdominal Aorta<br>1 Celiac Artery<br>4 Superior Mesenteric Artery<br>8 Renal Arteries, Bilateral<br>C Pelvic Arteries<br>F Lower Extremity Arteries, Right<br>G Lower Extremity Arteries, Left<br>H Lower Extremity Arteries, Bilateral<br>M Renal Artery Transplant | 0 High Osmolar<br>1 Low Osmolar<br>Y Other Contrast | Z None | Z None |
| 0 Abdominal Aorta<br>1 Celiac Artery<br>4 Superior Mesenteric Artery<br>8 Renal Arteries, Bilateral<br>C Pelvic Arteries<br>F Lower Extremity Arteries, Right<br>G Lower Extremity Arteries, Left<br>H Lower Extremity Arteries, Bilateral<br>M Renal Artery Transplant | Z None | 2 Intravascular Optical Coherence<br>Z None | Z None |

**B Imaging**
**4 Lower Arteries**
**3 Magnetic Resonance Imaging (MRI):** Computer reformatted digital display of multiplanar images developed from the capture of radiofrequency signals emitted by nuclei in a body site excited within a magnetic field

| Character 4<br>Body Part | Character 5<br>Contrast | Character 6<br>Qualifier | Character 7<br>Qualifier |
|---|---|---|---|
| 0 Abdominal Aorta<br>1 Celiac Artery<br>4 Superior Mesenteric Artery<br>8 Renal Arteries, Bilateral<br>C Pelvic Arteries<br>F Lower Extremity Arteries, Right<br>G Lower Extremity Arteries, Left<br>H Lower Extremity Arteries, Bilateral | Y Other Contrast | 0 Unenhanced and Enhanced<br>Z None | Z None |
| 0 Abdominal Aorta<br>1 Celiac Artery<br>4 Superior Mesenteric Artery<br>8 Renal Arteries, Bilateral<br>C Pelvic Arteries<br>F Lower Extremity Arteries, Right<br>G Lower Extremity Arteries, Left<br>H Lower Extremity Arteries, Bilateral | Z None | Z None | Z None |

**B Imaging**
**4 Lower Arteries**
**4 Ultrasonography:** Real time display of images of anatomy or flow information developed from the capture of reflected and attenuated high frequency sound waves

| Character 4<br>Body Part | Character 5<br>Contrast | Character 6<br>Qualifier | Character 7<br>Qualifier |
|---|---|---|---|
| 0 Abdominal Aorta<br>4 Superior Mesenteric Artery<br>5 Inferior Mesenteric Artery<br>6 Renal Artery, Right<br>7 Renal Artery, Left<br>8 Renal Arteries, Bilateral<br>B Intra-Abdominal Arteries, Other<br>F Lower Extremity Arteries, Right<br>G Lower Extremity Arteries, Left<br>H Lower Extremity Arteries, Bilateral<br>K Celiac and Mesenteric Arteries<br>L Femoral Artery<br>N Penile Arteries | Z None | Z None | 3 Intravascular<br>Z None |

**B** Imaging
**5** Veins
**0** Plain Radiography: Planar display of an image developed from the capture of external ionizing radiation on photographic or photoconductive plate

| Character 4<br>Body Part | Character 5<br>Contrast | Character 6<br>Qualifier | Character 7<br>Qualifier |
|---|---|---|---|
| 0 Epidural Veins | 0 High Osmolar | Z None | Z None |
| 1 Cerebral and Cerebellar Veins | 1 Low Osmolar | | |
| 2 Intracranial Sinuses | Y Other Contrast | | |
| 3 Jugular Veins, Right | | | |
| 4 Jugular Veins, Left | | | |
| 5 Jugular Veins, Bilateral | | | |
| 6 Subclavian Vein, Right | | | |
| 7 Subclavian Vein, Left | | | |
| 8 Superior Vena Cava | | | |
| 9 Inferior Vena Cava | | | |
| B Lower Extremity Veins, Right | | | |
| C Lower Extremity Veins, Left | | | |
| D Lower Extremity Veins, Bilateral | | | |
| F Pelvic (Iliac) Veins, Right | | | |
| G Pelvic (Iliac) Veins, Left | | | |
| H Pelvic (Iliac) Veins, Bilateral | | | |
| J Renal Vein, Right | | | |
| K Renal Vein, Left | | | |
| L Renal Veins, Bilateral | | | |
| M Upper Extremity Veins, Right | | | |
| N Upper Extremity Veins, Left | | | |
| P Upper Extremity Veins, Bilateral | | | |
| Q Pulmonary Vein, Right | | | |
| R Pulmonary Vein, Left | | | |
| S Pulmonary Veins, Bilateral | | | |
| T Portal and Splanchnic Veins | | | |
| V Veins, Other | | | |
| W Dialysis Shunt/Fistula | | | |

**B** Imaging
**5** Veins
**1** Fluoroscopy: Single plane or bi-plane real time display of an image developed from the capture of external ionizing radiation on a fluorescent screen. The image may also be stored by either digital or analog means

| Character 4<br>Body Part | Character 5<br>Contrast | Character 6<br>Qualifier | Character 7<br>Qualifier |
|---|---|---|---|
| 0 Epidural Veins | 0 High Osmolar | Z None | A Guidance |
| 1 Cerebral and Cerebellar Veins | 1 Low Osmolar | | Z None |
| 2 Intracranial Sinuses | Y Other Contrast | | |
| 3 Jugular Veins, Right | Z None | | |
| 4 Jugular Veins, Left | | | |
| 5 Jugular Veins, Bilateral | | | |
| 6 Subclavian Vein, Right | | | |
| 7 Subclavian Vein, Left | | | |
| 8 Superior Vena Cava | | | |
| 9 Inferior Vena Cava | | | |
| B Lower Extremity Veins, Right | | | |
| C Lower Extremity Veins, Left | | | |
| D Lower Extremity Veins, Bilateral | | | |
| F Pelvic (Iliac) Veins, Right | | | |
| G Pelvic (Iliac) Veins, Left | | | |
| H Pelvic (Iliac) Veins, Bilateral | | | |
| J Renal Vein, Right | | | |
| K Renal Vein, Left | | | |
| L Renal Veins, Bilateral | | | |
| M Upper Extremity Veins, Right | | | |
| N Upper Extremity Veins, Left | | | |
| P Upper Extremity Veins, Bilateral | | | |
| Q Pulmonary Vein, Right | | | |
| R Pulmonary Vein, Left | | | |
| S Pulmonary Veins, Bilateral | | | |
| T Portal and Splanchnic Veins | | | |
| V Veins, Other | | | |
| W Dialysis Shunt/Fistula | | | |

**B Imaging**
**5 Veins**
**2 Computerized Tomography (CT Scan):** Computer reformatted digital display of multiplanar images developed from the capture of multiple exposures of external ionizing radiation

| Character 4 Body Part | Character 5 Contrast | Character 6 Qualifier | Character 7 Qualifier |
|---|---|---|---|
| 2 Intracranial Sinuses | 0 High Osmolar | 0 Unenhanced and Enhanced | Z None |
| 8 Superior Vena Cava | 1 Low Osmolar | Z None | |
| 9 Inferior Vena Cava | Y Other Contrast | | |
| F Pelvic (Iliac) Veins, Right | | | |
| G Pelvic (Iliac) Veins, Left | | | |
| H Pelvic (Iliac) Veins, Bilateral | | | |
| J Renal Vein, Right | | | |
| K Renal Vein, Left | | | |
| L Renal Veins, Bilateral | | | |
| Q Pulmonary Vein, Right | | | |
| R Pulmonary Vein, Left | | | |
| S Pulmonary Veins, Bilateral | | | |
| T Portal and Splanchnic Veins | | | |
| 2 Intracranial Sinuses | Z None | 2 Intravascular Optical Coherence | Z None |
| 8 Superior Vena Cava | | Z None | |
| 9 Inferior Vena Cava | | | |
| F Pelvic (Iliac) Veins, Right | | | |
| G Pelvic (Iliac) Veins, Left | | | |
| H Pelvic (Iliac) Veins, Bilateral | | | |
| J Renal Vein, Right | | | |
| K Renal Vein, Left | | | |
| L Renal Veins, Bilateral | | | |
| Q Pulmonary Vein, Right | | | |
| R Pulmonary Vein, Left | | | |
| S Pulmonary Veins, Bilateral | | | |
| T Portal and Splanchnic Veins | | | |

**B Imaging**
**5 Veins**
**3 Magnetic Resonance Imaging (MRI):** Computer reformatted digital display of multiplanar images developed from the capture of radiofrequency signals emitted by nuclei in a body site excited within a magnetic field

| Character 4 Body Part | Character 5 Contrast | Character 6 Qualifier | Character 7 Qualifier |
|---|---|---|---|
| 1 Cerebral and Cerebellar Veins | Y Other Contrast | 0 Unenhanced and Enhanced | Z None |
| 2 Intracranial Sinuses | | Z None | |
| 5 Jugular Veins, Bilateral | | | |
| 8 Superior Vena Cava | | | |
| 9 Inferior Vena Cava | | | |
| B Lower Extremity Veins, Right | | | |
| C Lower Extremity Veins, Left | | | |
| D Lower Extremity Veins, Bilateral | | | |
| H Pelvic (Iliac) Veins, Bilateral | | | |
| L Renal Veins, Bilateral | | | |
| M Upper Extremity Veins, Right | | | |
| N Upper Extremity Veins, Left | | | |
| P Upper Extremity Veins, Bilateral | | | |
| S Pulmonary Veins, Bilateral | | | |
| T Portal and Splanchnic Veins | | | |
| V Veins, Other | | | |
| 1 Cerebral and Cerebellar Veins | Z None | Z None | Z None |
| 2 Intracranial Sinuses | | | |
| 5 Jugular Veins, Bilateral | | | |
| 8 Superior Vena Cava | | | |
| 9 Inferior Vena Cava | | | |
| B Lower Extremity Veins, Right | | | |
| C Lower Extremity Veins, Left | | | |
| D Lower Extremity Veins, Bilateral | | | |
| H Pelvic (Iliac) Veins, Bilateral | | | |
| L Renal Veins, Bilateral | | | |
| M Upper Extremity Veins, Right | | | |
| N Upper Extremity Veins, Left | | | |
| P Upper Extremity Veins, Bilateral | | | |
| S Pulmonary Veins, Bilateral | | | |
| T Portal and Splanchnic Veins | | | |
| V Veins, Other | | | |

**B** Imaging
**5** Veins
**4** Ultrasonography: Real time display of images of anatomy or flow information developed from the capture of reflected and attenuated high frequency sound waves

| Character 4<br>Body Part | Character 5<br>Contrast | Character 6<br>Qualifier | Character 7<br>Qualifier |
|---|---|---|---|
| 3 Jugular Veins, Right<br>4 Jugular Veins, Left<br>6 Subclavian Vein, Right<br>7 Subclavian Vein, Left<br>8 Superior Vena Cava<br>9 Inferior Vena Cava<br>B Lower Extremity Veins, Right<br>C Lower Extremity Veins, Left<br>D Lower Extremity Veins, Bilateral<br>J Renal Vein, Right<br>K Renal Vein, Left<br>L Renal Veins, Bilateral<br>M Upper Extremity Veins, Right<br>N Upper Extremity Veins, Left<br>P Upper Extremity Veins, Bilateral<br>T Portal and Splanchnic Veins | Z None | Z None | 3 Intravascular<br>A Guidance<br>Z None |

**B** Imaging
**7** Lymphatic System
**0** Plain Radiography: Planar display of an image developed from the capture of external ionizing radiation on photographic or photoconductive plate

| Character 4<br>Body Part | Character 5<br>Contrast | Character 6<br>Qualifier | Character 7<br>Qualifier |
|---|---|---|---|
| 0 Abdominal/Retroperitoneal<br>  Lymphatics, Unilateral<br>1 Abdominal/Retroperitoneal<br>  Lymphatics, Bilateral<br>4 Lymphatics, Head and Neck<br>5 Upper Extremity Lymphatics, Right<br>6 Upper Extremity Lymphatics, Left<br>7 Upper Extremity Lymphatics, Bilateral<br>8 Lower Extremity Lymphatics, Right<br>9 Lower Extremity Lymphatics, Left<br>B Lower Extremity Lymphatics, Bilateral<br>C Lymphatics, Pelvic | 0 High Osmolar<br>1 Low Osmolar<br>Y Other Contrast | Z None | Z None |

**B** Imaging
**8** Eye
**0** Plain Radiography: Planar display of an image developed from the capture of external ionizing radiation on photographic or photoconductive plate

| Character 4<br>Body Part | Character 5<br>Contrast | Character 6<br>Qualifier | Character 7<br>Qualifier |
|---|---|---|---|
| 0 Lacrimal Duct, Right<br>1 Lacrimal Duct, Left<br>2 Lacrimal Ducts, Bilateral | 0 High Osmolar<br>1 Low Osmolar<br>Y Other Contrast | Z None | Z None |
| 3 Optic Foramina, Right<br>4 Optic Foramina, Left<br>5 Eye, Right<br>6 Eye, Left<br>7 Eyes, Bilateral | Z None | Z None | Z None |

**B** Imaging
**8** Eye
**2** Computerized Tomography (CT Scan): Computer reformatted digital display of multiplanar images developed from the capture of multiple exposures of external ionizing radiation

| Character 4<br>Body Part | Character 5<br>Contrast | Character 6<br>Qualifier | Character 7<br>Qualifier |
|---|---|---|---|
| 5 Eye, Right<br>6 Eye, Left<br>7 Eyes, Bilateral | 0 High Osmolar<br>1 Low Osmolar<br>Y Other Contrast | 0 Unenhanced and Enhanced<br>Z None | Z None |
| 5 Eye, Right<br>6 Eye, Left<br>7 Eyes, Bilateral | Z None | Z None | Z None |

**B** Imaging
**8** Eye
**3** Magnetic Resonance Imaging (MRI): Computer reformatted digital display of multiplanar images developed from the capture of radiofrequency signals emitted by nuclei in a body site excited within a magnetic field

| Character 4<br>Body Part | Character 5<br>Contrast | Character 6<br>Qualifier | Character 7<br>Qualifier |
|---|---|---|---|
| 5 Eye, Right<br>6 Eye, Left<br>7 Eyes, Bilateral | Y Other Contrast | 0 Unenhanced and Enhanced<br>Z None | Z None |
| 5 Eye, Right<br>6 Eye, Left<br>7 Eyes, Bilateral | Z None | Z None | Z None |

**B** Imaging
**8** Eye
**4** Ultrasonography: Real time display of images of anatomy or flow information developed from the capture of reflected and attenuated high frequency sound waves

| Character 4<br>Body Part | Character 5<br>Contrast | Character 6<br>Qualifier | Character 7<br>Qualifier |
|---|---|---|---|
| 5 Eye, Right<br>6 Eye, Left<br>7 Eyes, Bilateral | Z None | Z None | Z None |

**B** Imaging
**9** Ear, Nose, Mouth and Throat
**0** Plain Radiography: Planar display of an image developed from the capture of external ionizing radiation on photographic or photoconductive plate

| Character 4<br>Body Part | Character 5<br>Contrast | Character 6<br>Qualifier | Character 7<br>Qualifier |
|---|---|---|---|
| 2 Paranasal Sinuses<br>F Nasopharynx/Oropharynx<br>H Mastoids | Z None | Z None | Z None |
| 4 Parotid Gland, Right<br>5 Parotid Gland, Left<br>6 Parotid Glands, Bilateral<br>7 Submandibular Gland, Right<br>8 Submandibular Gland, Left<br>9 Submandibular Glands, Bilateral<br>B Salivary Gland, Right<br>C Salivary Gland, Left<br>D Salivary Glands, Bilateral | 0 High Osmolar<br>1 Low Osmolar<br>Y Other Contrast | Z None | Z None |

**B** Imaging
**9** Ear, Nose, Mouth and Throat
**1** Fluoroscopy: Single plane or bi-plane real time display of an image developed from the capture of external ionizing radiation on a fluorescent screen. The image may also be stored by either digital or analog means

| Character 4<br>Body Part | Character 5<br>Contrast | Character 6<br>Qualifier | Character 7<br>Qualifier |
|---|---|---|---|
| G Pharynx and Epiglottis<br>J Larynx | Y Other Contrast<br>Z None | Z None | Z None |

**B** Imaging
**9** Ear, Nose, Mouth and Throat
**2** Computerized Tomography (CT Scan): Computer reformatted digital display of multiplanar images developed from the capture of multiple exposures of external ionizing radiation

| Character 4<br>Body Part | Character 5<br>Contrast | Character 6<br>Qualifier | Character 7<br>Qualifier |
|---|---|---|---|
| 0 Ear<br>2 Paranasal Sinuses<br>6 Parotid Glands, Bilateral<br>9 Submandibular Glands, Bilateral<br>D Salivary Glands, Bilateral<br>F Nasopharynx/Oropharynx<br>J Larynx | 0 High Osmolar<br>1 Low Osmolar<br>Y Other Contrast | 0 Unenhanced and Enhanced<br>Z None | Z None |
| 0 Ear<br>2 Paranasal Sinuses<br>6 Parotid Glands, Bilateral<br>9 Submandibular Glands, Bilateral<br>D Salivary Glands, Bilateral<br>F Nasopharynx/Oropharynx<br>J Larynx | Z None | Z None | Z None |

**B** Imaging
**9** Ear, Nose, Mouth and Throat
**3** Magnetic Resonance Imaging (MRI): Computer reformatted digital display of multiplanar images developed from the capture of radiofrequency signals emitted by nuclei in a body site excited within a magnetic field

| Character 4<br>Body Part | Character 5<br>Contrast | Character 6<br>Qualifier | Character 7<br>Qualifier |
|---|---|---|---|
| 0 Ear<br>2 Paranasal Sinuses<br>6 Parotid Glands, Bilateral<br>9 Submandibular Glands, Bilateral<br>D Salivary Glands, Bilateral<br>F Nasopharynx/Oropharynx<br>J Larynx | Y Other Contrast | 0 Unenhanced and Enhanced<br>Z None | Z None |
| 0 Ear<br>2 Paranasal Sinuses<br>6 Parotid Glands, Bilateral<br>9 Submandibular Glands, Bilateral<br>D Salivary Glands, Bilateral<br>F Nasopharynx/Oropharynx<br>J Larynx | Z None | Z None | Z None |

**B** Imaging
**B** Respiratory System
**0** Plain Radiography: Planar display of an image developed from the capture of external ionizing radiation on photographic or photoconductive plate

| Character 4<br>Body Part | Character 5<br>Contrast | Character 6<br>Qualifier | Character 7<br>Qualifier |
|---|---|---|---|
| 7 Tracheobronchial Tree, Right<br>8 Tracheobronchial Tree, Left<br>9 Tracheobronchial Trees, Bilateral | Y Other Contrast | Z None | Z None |
| D Upper Airways | Z None | Z None | Z None |

**B** Imaging
**B** Respiratory System
**1** Fluoroscopy: Single plane or bi-plane real time display of an image developed from the capture of external ionizing radiation on a fluorescent screen. The image may also be stored by either digital or analog means

| Character 4<br>Body Part | Character 5<br>Contrast | Character 6<br>Qualifier | Character 7<br>Qualifier |
|---|---|---|---|
| 2 Lung, Right<br>3 Lung, Left<br>4 Lungs, Bilateral<br>6 Diaphragm<br>C Mediastinum<br>D Upper Airways | Z None | Z None | Z None |
| 7 Tracheobronchial Tree, Right<br>8 Tracheobronchial Tree, Left<br>9 Tracheobronchial Trees, Bilateral | Y Other Contrast | Z None | Z None |

**B Imaging**
**B Respiratory System**
**2 Computerized Tomography (CT Scan): Computer reformatted digital display of multiplanar images developed from the capture of multiple exposures of external ionizing radiation**

| Character 4<br>Body Part | Character 5<br>Contrast | Character 6<br>Qualifier | Character 7<br>Qualifier |
|---|---|---|---|
| 4 Lungs, Bilateral<br>7 Tracheobronchial Tree, Right<br>8 Tracheobronchial Tree, Left<br>9 Tracheobronchial Trees, Bilateral<br>F Trachea/Airways | 0 High Osmolar<br>1 Low Osmolar<br>Y Other Contrast | 0 Unenhanced and Enhanced<br>Z None | Z None |
| 4 Lungs, Bilateral<br>7 Tracheobronchial Tree, Right<br>8 Tracheobronchial Tree, Left<br>9 Tracheobronchial Trees, Bilateral<br>F Trachea/Airways | Z None | Z None | Z None |

**B Imaging**
**B Respiratory System**
**3 Magnetic Resonance Imaging (MRI): Computer reformatted digital display of multiplanar images developed from the capture of radiofrequency signals emitted by nuclei in a body site excited within a magnetic field**

| Character 4<br>Body Part | Character 5<br>Contrast | Character 6<br>Qualifier | Character 7<br>Qualifier |
|---|---|---|---|
| G Lung Apices | Y Other Contrast | 0 Unenhanced and Enhanced<br>Z None | Z None |
| G Lung Apices | Z None | Z None | Z None |

**B Imaging**
**B Respiratory System**
**4 Ultrasonography: Real time display of images of anatomy or flow information developed from the capture of reflected and attenuated high frequency sound waves**

| Character 4<br>Body Part | Character 5<br>Contrast | Character 6<br>Qualifier | Character 7<br>Qualifier |
|---|---|---|---|
| B Pleura<br>C Mediastinum | Z None | Z None | Z None |

**B Imaging**
**D Gastrointestinal System**
**1 Fluoroscopy: Single plane or bi-plane real time display of an image developed from the capture of external ionizing radiation on a fluorescent screen. The image may also be stored by either digital or analog means**

| Character 4<br>Body Part | Character 5<br>Contrast | Character 6<br>Qualifier | Character 7<br>Qualifier |
|---|---|---|---|
| 1 Esophagus<br>2 Stomach<br>3 Small Bowel<br>4 Colon<br>5 Upper GI<br>6 Upper GI and Small Bowel<br>9 Duodenum<br>B Mouth/Oropharynx | Y Other Contrast<br>Z None | Z None | Z None |

**B Imaging**
**D Gastrointestinal System**
**2 Computerized Tomography (CT Scan): Computer reformatted digital display of multiplanar images developed from the capture of multiple exposures of external ionizing radiation**

| Character 4<br>Body Part | Character 5<br>Contrast | Character 6<br>Qualifier | Character 7<br>Qualifier |
|---|---|---|---|
| 4 Colon | 0 High Osmolar<br>1 Low Osmolar<br>Y Other Contrast | 0 Unenhanced and Enhanced<br>Z None | Z None |
| 4 Colon | Z None | Z None | Z None |

**B** Imaging
**D** Gastrointestinal System
**4** Ultrasonography: Real time display of images of anatomy or flow information developed from the capture of reflected and attenuated high frequency sound waves

| Character 4<br>Body Part | Character 5<br>Contrast | Character 6<br>Qualifier | Character 7<br>Qualifier |
|---|---|---|---|
| 1 Esophagus<br>2 Stomach<br>7 Gastrointestinal Tract<br>8 Appendix<br>9 Duodenum<br>C Rectum | Z None | Z None | Z None |

**B** Imaging
**F** Hepatobiliary System and Pancreas
**0** Plain Radiography: Planar display of an image developed from the capture of external ionizing radiation on photographic or photoconductive plate

| Character 4<br>Body Part | Character 5<br>Contrast | Character 6<br>Qualifier | Character 7<br>Qualifier |
|---|---|---|---|
| 0 Bile Ducts<br>3 Gallbladder and Bile Ducts<br>C Hepatobiliary System, All | 0 High Osmolar<br>1 Low Osmolar<br>Y Other Contrast | Z None | Z None |

**B** Imaging
**F** Hepatobiliary System and Pancreas
**1** Fluoroscopy: Single plane or bi-plane real time display of an image developed from the capture of external ionizing radiation on a fluorescent screen. The image may also be stored by either digital or analog means

| Character 4<br>Body Part | Character 5<br>Contrast | Character 6<br>Qualifier | Character 7<br>Qualifier |
|---|---|---|---|
| 0 Bile Ducts<br>1 Biliary and Pancreatic Ducts<br>2 Gallbladder<br>3 Gallbladder and Bile Ducts<br>4 Gallbladder, Bile Ducts and Pancreatic<br>  Ducts<br>8 Pancreatic Ducts | 0 High Osmolar<br>1 Low Osmolar<br>Y Other Contrast | Z None | Z None |

**B** Imaging
**F** Hepatobiliary System and Pancreas
**2** Computerized Tomography (CT Scan): Computer reformatted digital display of multiplanar images developed from the capture of multiple exposures of external ionizing radiation

| Character 4<br>Body Part | Character 5<br>Contrast | Character 6<br>Qualifier | Character 7<br>Qualifier |
|---|---|---|---|
| 5 Liver<br>6 Liver and Spleen<br>7 Pancreas<br>C Hepatobiliary System, All | 0 High Osmolar<br>1 Low Osmolar<br>Y Other Contrast | 0 Unenhanced and Enhanced<br>Z None | Z None |
| 5 Liver<br>6 Liver and Spleen<br>7 Pancreas<br>C Hepatobiliary System, All | Z None | Z None | Z None |

**B** Imaging
**F** Hepatobiliary System and Pancreas
**3** Magnetic Resonance Imaging (MRI): Computer reformatted digital display of multiplanar images developed from the capture of radiofrequency signals emitted by nuclei in a body site excited within a magnetic field

| Character 4<br>Body Part | Character 5<br>Contrast | Character 6<br>Qualifier | Character 7<br>Qualifier |
|---|---|---|---|
| 5 Liver<br>6 Liver and Spleen<br>7 Pancreas | Y Other Contrast | 0 Unenhanced and Enhanced<br>Z None | Z None |
| 5 Liver<br>6 Liver and Spleen<br>7 Pancreas | Z None | Z None | Z None |

**B Imaging**
**F Hepatobiliary System and Pancreas**
**4 Ultrasonography:** Real time display of images of anatomy or flow information developed from the capture of reflected and attenuated high frequency sound waves

| Character 4<br>Body Part | Character 5<br>Contrast | Character 6<br>Qualifier | Character 7<br>Qualifier |
|---|---|---|---|
| 0 Bile Ducts<br>2 Gallbladder<br>3 Gallbladder and Bile Ducts<br>5 Liver<br>6 Liver and Spleen<br>7 Pancreas<br>C Hepatobiliary System, All | Z None | Z None | Z None |

**B Imaging**
**G Endocrine System**
**2 Computerized Tomography (CT Scan):** Computer reformatted digital display of multiplanar images developed from the capture of multiple exposures of external ionizing radiation

| Character 4<br>Body Part | Character 5<br>Contrast | Character 6<br>Qualifier | Character 7<br>Qualifier |
|---|---|---|---|
| 2 Adrenal Glands, Bilateral<br>3 Parathyroid Glands<br>4 Thyroid Gland | 0 High Osmolar<br>1 Low Osmolar<br>Y Other Contrast | 0 Unenhanced and Enhanced<br>Z None | Z None |
| 2 Adrenal Glands, Bilateral<br>3 Parathyroid Glands<br>4 Thyroid Gland | Z None | Z None | Z None |

**B Imaging**
**G Endocrine System**
**3 Magnetic Resonance Imaging (MRI):** Computer reformatted digital display of multiplanar images developed from the capture of radiofrequency signals emitted by nuclei in a body site excited within a magnetic field

| Character 4<br>Body Part | Character 5<br>Contrast | Character 6<br>Qualifier | Character 7<br>Qualifier |
|---|---|---|---|
| 2 Adrenal Glands, Bilateral<br>3 Parathyroid Glands<br>4 Thyroid Gland | Y Other Contrast | 0 Unenhanced and Enhanced<br>Z None | Z None |
| 2 Adrenal Glands, Bilateral<br>3 Parathyroid Glands<br>4 Thyroid Gland | Z None | Z None | Z None |

**B Imaging**
**G Endocrine System**
**4 Ultrasonography:** Real time display of images of anatomy or flow information developed from the capture of reflected and attenuated high frequency sound waves

| Character 4<br>Body Part | Character 5<br>Contrast | Character 6<br>Qualifier | Character 7<br>Qualifier |
|---|---|---|---|
| 0 Adrenal Gland, Right<br>1 Adrenal Gland, Left<br>2 Adrenal Glands, Bilateral<br>3 Parathyroid Glands<br>4 Thyroid Gland | Z None | Z None | Z None |

**B Imaging**
**H Skin, Subcutaneous Tissue and Breast**
**0 Plain Radiography:** Planar display of an image developed from the capture of external ionizing radiation on photographic or photoconductive plate

| Character 4<br>Body Part | Character 5<br>Contrast | Character 6<br>Qualifier | Character 7<br>Qualifier |
|---|---|---|---|
| 0 Breast, Right<br>1 Breast, Left<br>2 Breasts, Bilateral | Z None | Z None | Z None |
| 3 Single Mammary Duct, Right<br>4 Single Mammary Duct, Left<br>5 Multiple Mammary Ducts, Right<br>6 Multiple Mammary Ducts, Left | 0 High Osmolar<br>1 Low Osmolar<br>Y Other Contrast<br>Z None | Z None | Z None |

**B** Imaging
**H** Skin, Subcutaneous Tissue and Breast
**3** Magnetic Resonance Imaging (MRI): Computer reformatted digital display of multiplanar images developed from the capture of radiofrequency signals emitted by nuclei in a body site excited within a magnetic field

| Character 4<br>Body Part | Character 5<br>Contrast | Character 6<br>Qualifier | Character 7<br>Qualifier |
|---|---|---|---|
| 0 Breast, Right<br>1 Breast, Left<br>2 Breasts, Bilateral<br>D Subcutaneous Tissue, Head/Neck<br>F Subcutaneous Tissue, Upper Extremity<br>G Subcutaneous Tissue, Thorax<br>H Subcutaneous Tissue, Abdomen and<br>　Pelvis<br>J Subcutaneous Tissue, Lower Extremity | Y Other Contrast | 0 Unenhanced and Enhanced<br>Z None | Z None |
| 0 Breast, Right<br>1 Breast, Left<br>2 Breasts, Bilateral<br>D Subcutaneous Tissue, Head/Neck<br>F Subcutaneous Tissue, Upper Extremity<br>G Subcutaneous Tissue, Thorax<br>H Subcutaneous Tissue, Abdomen and<br>　Pelvis<br>J Subcutaneous Tissue, Lower Extremity | Z None | Z None | Z None |

**B** Imaging
**H** Skin, Subcutaneous Tissue and Breast
**4** Ultrasonography: Real time display of images of anatomy or flow information developed from the capture of reflected and attenuated high frequency sound waves

| Character 4<br>Body Part | Character 5<br>Contrast | Character 6<br>Qualifier | Character 7<br>Qualifier |
|---|---|---|---|
| 0 Breast, Right<br>1 Breast, Left<br>2 Breasts, Bilateral<br>7 Extremity, Upper<br>8 Extremity, Lower<br>9 Abdominal Wall<br>B Chest Wall<br>C Head and Neck | Z None | Z None | Z None |

**B** Imaging
**L** Connective Tissue
**3** Magnetic Resonance Imaging (MRI): Computer reformatted digital display of multiplanar images developed from the capture of radiofrequency signals emitted by nuclei in a body site excited within a magnetic field

| Character 4<br>Body Part | Character 5<br>Contrast | Character 6<br>Qualifier | Character 7<br>Qualifier |
|---|---|---|---|
| 0 Connective Tissue, Upper Extremity<br>1 Connective Tissue, Lower Extremity<br>2 Tendons, Upper Extremity<br>3 Tendons, Lower Extremity | Y Other Contrast | 0 Unenhanced and Enhanced<br>Z None | Z None |
| 0 Connective Tissue, Upper Extremity<br>1 Connective Tissue, Lower Extremity<br>2 Tendons, Upper Extremity<br>3 Tendons, Lower Extremity | Z None | Z None | Z None |

**B** Imaging
**L** Connective Tissue
**4** Ultrasonography: Real time display of images of anatomy or flow information developed from the capture of reflected and attenuated high frequency sound waves

| Character 4<br>Body Part | Character 5<br>Contrast | Character 6<br>Qualifier | Character 7<br>Qualifier |
|---|---|---|---|
| 0 Connective Tissue, Upper Extremity<br>1 Connective Tissue, Lower Extremity<br>2 Tendons, Upper Extremity<br>3 Tendons, Lower Extremity | Z None | Z None | Z None |

**B** Imaging
**N** Skull and Facial Bones
**0** Plain Radiography: Planar display of an image developed from the capture of external ionizing radiation on photographic or photoconductive plate

| Character 4<br>Body Part | Character 5<br>Contrast | Character 6<br>Qualifier | Character 7<br>Qualifier |
|---|---|---|---|
| 0 Skull<br>1 Orbit, Right<br>2 Orbit, Left<br>3 Orbits, Bilateral<br>4 Nasal Bones<br>5 Facial Bones<br>6 Mandible<br>B Zygomatic Arch, Right<br>C Zygomatic Arch, Left<br>D Zygomatic Arches, Bilateral<br>G Tooth, Single<br>H Teeth, Multiple<br>J Teeth, All | Z None | Z None | Z None |
| 7 Temporomandibular Joint, Right<br>8 Temporomandibular Joint, Left<br>9 Temporomandibular Joints, Bilateral | 0 High Osmolar<br>1 Low Osmolar<br>Y Other Contrast<br>Z None | Z None | Z None |

**B** Imaging
**N** Skull and Facial Bones
**1** Fluoroscopy: Single plane or bi-plane real time display of an image developed from the capture of external ionizing radiation on a fluorescent screen. The image may also be stored by either digital or analog means

| Character 4<br>Body Part | Character 5<br>Contrast | Character 6<br>Qualifier | Character 7<br>Qualifier |
|---|---|---|---|
| 7 Temporomandibular Joint, Right<br>8 Temporomandibular Joint, Left<br>9 Temporomandibular Joints, Bilateral | 0 High Osmolar<br>1 Low Osmolar<br>Y Other Contrast<br>Z None | Z None | Z None |

**B** Imaging
**N** Skull and Facial Bones
**2** Computerized Tomography (CT Scan): Computer reformatted digital display of multiplanar images developed from the capture of multiple exposures of external ionizing radiation

| Character 4<br>Body Part | Character 5<br>Contrast | Character 6<br>Qualifier | Character 7<br>Qualifier |
|---|---|---|---|
| 0 Skull<br>3 Orbits, Bilateral<br>5 Facial Bones<br>6 Mandible<br>9 Temporomandibular Joints, Bilateral<br>F Temporal Bones | 0 High Osmolar<br>1 Low Osmolar<br>Y Other Contrast<br>Z None | Z None | Z None |

**B** Imaging
**N** Skull and Facial Bones
**3** Magnetic Resonance Imaging (MRI): Computer reformatted digital display of multiplanar images developed from the capture of radiofrequency signals emitted by nuclei in a body site excited within a magnetic field

| Character 4<br>Body Part | Character 5<br>Contrast | Character 6<br>Qualifier | Character 7<br>Qualifier |
|---|---|---|---|
| 9 Temporomandibular Joints, Bilateral | Y Other Contrast<br>Z None | Z None | Z None |

**B** Imaging
**P** Non-Axial Upper Bones
**0** Plain Radiography: Planar display of an image developed from the capture of external ionizing radiation on photographic or photoconductive plate

| Character 4<br>Body Part | Character 5<br>Contrast | Character 6<br>Qualifier | Character 7<br>Qualifier |
|---|---|---|---|
| 0 Sternoclavicular Joint, Right<br>1 Sternoclavicular Joint, Left<br>2 Sternoclavicular Joints, Bilateral<br>3 Acromioclavicular Joints, Bilateral<br>4 Clavicle, Right<br>5 Clavicle, Left<br>6 Scapula, Right<br>7 Scapula, Left<br>A Humerus, Right<br>B Humerus, Left<br>E Upper Arm, Right<br>F Upper Arm, Left<br>J Forearm, Right<br>K Forearm, Left<br>N Hand, Right<br>P Hand, Left<br>R Finger(s), Right<br>S Finger(s), Left<br>X Ribs, Right<br>Y Ribs, Left | Z None | Z None | Z None |
| 8 Shoulder, Right<br>9 Shoulder, Left<br>C Hand/Finger Joint, Right<br>D Hand/Finger Joint, Left<br>G Elbow, Right<br>H Elbow, Left<br>L Wrist, Right<br>M Wrist, Left | 0 High Osmolar<br>1 Low Osmolar<br>Y Other Contrast<br>Z None | Z None | Z None |

**B** Imaging
**P** Non-Axial Upper Bones
**1** Fluoroscopy: Single plane or bi-plane real time display of an image developed from the capture of external ionizing radiation on a fluorescent screen. The image may also be stored by either digital or analog means

| Character 4<br>Body Part | Character 5<br>Contrast | Character 6<br>Qualifier | Character 7<br>Qualifier |
|---|---|---|---|
| 0 Sternoclavicular Joint, Right<br>1 Sternoclavicular Joint, Left<br>2 Sternoclavicular Joints, Bilateral<br>3 Acromioclavicular Joints, Bilateral<br>4 Clavicle, Right<br>5 Clavicle, Left<br>6 Scapula, Right<br>7 Scapula, Left<br>A Humerus, Right<br>B Humerus, Left<br>E Upper Arm, Right<br>F Upper Arm, Left<br>J Forearm, Right<br>K Forearm, Left<br>N Hand, Right<br>P Hand, Left<br>R Finger(s), Right<br>S Finger(s), Left<br>X Ribs, Right<br>Y Ribs, Left | Z None | Z None | Z None |
| 8 Shoulder, Right<br>9 Shoulder, Left<br>L Wrist, Right<br>M Wrist, Left | 0 High Osmolar<br>1 Low Osmolar<br>Y Other Contrast<br>Z None | Z None | Z None |
| C Hand/Finger Joint, Right<br>D Hand/Finger Joint, Left<br>G Elbow, Right<br>H Elbow, Left | 0 High Osmolar<br>1 Low Osmolar<br>Y Other Contrast | Z None | Z None |

**B** Imaging
**P** Non-Axial Upper Bones
**2** Computerized Tomography (CT Scan): Computer reformatted digital display of multiplanar images developed from the capture of multiple exposures of external ionizing radiation

| Character 4<br>Body Part | Character 5<br>Contrast | Character 6<br>Qualifier | Character 7<br>Qualifier |
|---|---|---|---|
| 0 Sternoclavicular Joint, Right<br>1 Sternoclavicular Joint, Left<br>W Thorax | 0 High Osmolar<br>1 Low Osmolar<br>Y Other Contrast | Z None | Z None |
| 2 Sternoclavicular Joints, Bilateral<br>3 Acromioclavicular Joints, Bilateral<br>4 Clavicle, Right<br>5 Clavicle, Left<br>6 Scapula, Right<br>7 Scapula, Left<br>8 Shoulder, Right<br>9 Shoulder, Left<br>A Humerus, Right<br>B Humerus, Left<br>E Upper Arm, Right<br>F Upper Arm, Left<br>G Elbow, Right<br>H Elbow, Left<br>J Forearm, Right<br>K Forearm, Left<br>L Wrist, Right<br>M Wrist, Left<br>N Hand, Right<br>P Hand, Left<br>Q Hands and Wrists, Bilateral<br>R Finger(s), Right<br>S Finger(s), Left<br>T Upper Extremity, Right<br>U Upper Extremity, Left<br>V Upper Extremities, Bilateral<br>X Ribs, Right<br>Y Ribs, Left | 0 High Osmolar<br>1 Low Osmolar<br>Y Other Contrast<br>Z None | Z None | Z None |
| C Hand/Finger Joint, Right<br>D Hand/Finger Joint, Left | Z None | Z None | Z None |

**B** Imaging
**P** Non-Axial Upper Bones
**3** Magnetic Resonance Imaging (MRI): Computer reformatted digital display of multiplanar images developed from the capture of radiofrequency signals emitted by nuclei in a body site excited within a magnetic field

| Character 4<br>Body Part | Character 5<br>Contrast | Character 6<br>Qualifier | Character 7<br>Qualifier |
|---|---|---|---|
| 8 Shoulder, Right<br>9 Shoulder, Left<br>C Hand/Finger Joint, Right<br>D Hand/Finger Joint, Left<br>E Upper Arm, Right<br>F Upper Arm, Left<br>G Elbow, Right<br>H Elbow, Left<br>J Forearm, Right<br>K Forearm, Left<br>L Wrist, Right<br>M Wrist, Left | Y Other Contrast | 0 Unenhanced and Enhanced<br>Z None | Z None |
| 8 Shoulder, Right<br>9 Shoulder, Left<br>C Hand/Finger Joint, Right<br>D Hand/Finger Joint, Left<br>E Upper Arm, Right<br>F Upper Arm, Left<br>G Elbow, Right<br>H Elbow, Left<br>J Forearm, Right<br>K Forearm, Left<br>L Wrist, Right<br>M Wrist, Left | Z None | Z None | Z None |

**B** Imaging
**P** Non-Axial Upper Bones
**4** Ultrasonography: Real time display of images of anatomy or flow information developed from the capture of reflected and attenuated high frequency sound waves

| Character 4<br>Body Part | Character 5<br>Contrast | Character 6<br>Qualifier | Character 7<br>Qualifier |
|---|---|---|---|
| 8 Shoulder, Right<br>9 Shoulder, Left<br>G Elbow, Right<br>H Elbow, Left<br>L Wrist, Right<br>M Wrist, Left<br>N Hand, Right<br>P Hand, Left | Z None | Z None | 1 Densitometry<br>Z None |

**B** Imaging
**Q** Non-Axial Lower Bones
**0** Plain Radiography: Planar display of an image developed from the capture of external ionizing radiation on photographic or photoconductive plate

| Character 4<br>Body Part | Character 5<br>Contrast | Character 6<br>Qualifier | Character 7<br>Qualifier |
|---|---|---|---|
| 0 Hip, Right<br>1 Hip, Left | 0 High Osmolar<br>1 Low Osmolar<br>Y Other Contrast | Z None | Z None |
| 0 Hip, Right<br>1 Hip, Left | Z None | Z None | 1 Densitometry<br>Z None |
| 3 Femur, Right<br>4 Femur, Left | Z None | Z None | 1 Densitometry<br>Z None |
| 7 Knee, Right<br>8 Knee, Left<br>G Ankle, Right<br>H Ankle, Left | 0 High Osmolar<br>1 Low Osmolar<br>Y Other Contrast<br>Z None | Z None | Z None |
| D Lower Leg, Right<br>F Lower Leg, Left<br>J Calcaneus, Right<br>K Calcaneus, Left<br>L Foot, Right<br>M Foot, Left<br>P Toe(s), Right<br>Q Toe(s), Left<br>V Patella, Right<br>W Patella, Left | Z None | Z None | Z None |
| X Foot/Toe Joint, Right<br>Y Foot/Toe Joint, Left | 0 High Osmolar<br>1 Low Osmolar<br>Y Other Contrast | Z None | Z None |

**B** Imaging
**Q** Non-Axial Lower Bones
**1** Fluoroscopy: Single plane or bi-plane real time display of an image developed from the capture of external ionizing radiation on a fluorescent screen. The image may also be stored by either digital or analog means

| Character 4<br>Body Part | Character 5<br>Contrast | Character 6<br>Qualifier | Character 7<br>Qualifier |
|---|---|---|---|
| 0 Hip, Right<br>1 Hip, Left<br>7 Knee, Right<br>8 Knee, Left<br>G Ankle, Right<br>H Ankle, Left<br>X Foot/Toe Joint, Right<br>Y Foot/Toe Joint, Left | 0 High Osmolar<br>1 Low Osmolar<br>Y Other Contrast<br>Z None | Z None | Z None |
| 3 Femur, Right<br>4 Femur, Left<br>D Lower Leg, Right<br>F Lower Leg, Left<br>J Calcaneus, Right<br>K Calcaneus, Left<br>L Foot, Right<br>M Foot, Left<br>P Toe(s), Right<br>Q Toe(s), Left<br>V Patella, Right<br>W Patella, Left | Z None | Z None | Z None |

**B** Imaging
**Q** Non-Axial Lower Bones
**2** Computerized Tomography (CT Scan): Computer reformatted digital display of multiplanar images developed from the capture of multiple exposures of external ionizing radiation

| Character 4 Body Part | Character 5 Contrast | Character 6 Qualifier | Character 7 Qualifier |
|---|---|---|---|
| 0 Hip, Right | 0 High Osmolar | Z None | Z None |
| 1 Hip, Left | 1 Low Osmolar | | |
| 3 Femur, Right | Y Other Contrast | | |
| 4 Femur, Left | Z None | | |
| 7 Knee, Right | | | |
| 8 Knee, Left | | | |
| D Lower Leg, Right | | | |
| F Lower Leg, Left | | | |
| G Ankle, Right | | | |
| H Ankle, Left | | | |
| J Calcaneus, Right | | | |
| K Calcaneus, Left | | | |
| L Foot, Right | | | |
| M Foot, Left | | | |
| P Toe(s), Right | | | |
| Q Toe(s), Left | | | |
| R Lower Extremity, Right | | | |
| S Lower Extremity, Left | | | |
| V Patella, Right | | | |
| W Patella, Left | | | |
| X Foot/Toe Joint, Right | | | |
| Y Foot/Toe Joint, Left | | | |
| B Tibia/Fibula, Right | 0 High Osmolar | Z None | Z None |
| C Tibia/Fibula, Left | 1 Low Osmolar | | |
| | Y Other Contrast | | |

**B** Imaging
**Q** Non-Axial Lower Bones
**3** Magnetic Resonance Imaging (MRI): Computer reformatted digital display of multiplanar images developed from the capture of radiofrequency signals emitted by nuclei in a body site excited within a magnetic field

| Character 4 Body Part | Character 5 Contrast | Character 6 Qualifier | Character 7 Qualifier |
|---|---|---|---|
| 0 Hip, Right | Y Other Contrast | 0 Unenhanced and Enhanced | Z None |
| 1 Hip, Left | | Z None | |
| 3 Femur, Right | | | |
| 4 Femur, Left | | | |
| 7 Knee, Right | | | |
| 8 Knee, Left | | | |
| D Lower Leg, Right | | | |
| F Lower Leg, Left | | | |
| G Ankle, Right | | | |
| H Ankle, Left | | | |
| J Calcaneus, Right | | | |
| K Calcaneus, Left | | | |
| L Foot, Right | | | |
| M Foot, Left | | | |
| P Toe(s), Right | | | |
| Q Toe(s), Left | | | |
| V Patella, Right | | | |
| W Patella, Left | | | |
| 0 Hip, Right | Z None | Z None | Z None |
| 1 Hip, Left | | | |
| 3 Femur, Right | | | |
| 4 Femur, Left | | | |
| 7 Knee, Right | | | |
| 8 Knee, Left | | | |
| D Lower Leg, Right | | | |
| F Lower Leg, Left | | | |
| G Ankle, Right | | | |
| H Ankle, Left | | | |
| J Calcaneus, Right | | | |
| K Calcaneus, Left | | | |
| L Foot, Right | | | |
| M Foot, Left | | | |
| P Toe(s), Right | | | |
| Q Toe(s), Left | | | |
| V Patella, Right | | | |
| W Patella, Left | | | |

**B** Imaging
**Q** Non-Axial Lower Bones
**4** Ultrasonography: Real time display of images of anatomy or flow information developed from the capture of reflected and attenuated high frequency sound waves

| Character 4<br>Body Part | Character 5<br>Contrast | Character 6<br>Qualifier | Character 7<br>Qualifier |
|---|---|---|---|
| 0 Hip, Right<br>1 Hip, Left<br>2 Hips, Bilateral<br>7 Knee, Right<br>8 Knee, Left<br>9 Knees, Bilateral | Z None | Z None | Z None |

**B** Imaging
**R** Axial Skeleton, Except Skull and Facial Bones
**0** Plain Radiography: Planar display of an image developed from the capture of external ionizing radiation on photographic or photoconductive plate

| Character 4<br>Body Part | Character 5<br>Contrast | Character 6<br>Qualifier | Character 7<br>Qualifier |
|---|---|---|---|
| 0 Cervical Spine<br>7 Thoracic Spine<br>9 Lumbar Spine<br>G Whole Spine | Z None | Z None | 1 Densitometry<br>Z None |
| 1 Cervical Disc(s)<br>2 Thoracic Disc(s)<br>3 Lumbar Disc(s)<br>4 Cervical Facet Joint(s)<br>5 Thoracic Facet Joint(s)<br>6 Lumbar Facet Joint(s)<br>D Sacroiliac Joints | 0 High Osmolar<br>1 Low Osmolar<br>Y Other Contrast<br>Z None | Z None | Z None |
| 8 Thoracolumbar Joint<br>B Lumbosacral Joint<br>C Pelvis<br>F Sacrum and Coccyx<br>H Sternum | Z None | Z None | Z None |

**B** Imaging
**R** Axial Skeleton, Except Skull and Facial Bones
**1** Fluoroscopy: Single plane or bi-plane real time display of an image developed from the capture of external ionizing radiation on a fluorescent screen. The image may also be stored by either digital or analog means

| Character 4<br>Body Part | Character 5<br>Contrast | Character 6<br>Qualifier | Character 7<br>Qualifier |
|---|---|---|---|
| 0 Cervical Spine<br>1 Cervical Disc(s)<br>2 Thoracic Disc(s)<br>3 Lumbar Disc(s)<br>4 Cervical Facet Joint(s)<br>5 Thoracic Facet Joint(s)<br>6 Lumbar Facet Joint(s)<br>7 Thoracic Spine<br>8 Thoracolumbar Joint<br>9 Lumbar Spine<br>B Lumbosacral Joint<br>C Pelvis<br>D Sacroiliac Joints<br>F Sacrum and Coccyx<br>G Whole Spine<br>H Sternum | 0 High Osmolar<br>1 Low Osmolar<br>Y Other Contrast<br>Z None | Z None | Z None |

**B** Imaging
**R** Axial Skeleton, Except Skull and Facial Bones
**2** Computerized Tomography (CT Scan): Computer reformatted digital display of multiplanar images developed from the capture of multiple exposures of external ionizing radiation

| Character 4<br>Body Part | Character 5<br>Contrast | Character 6<br>Qualifier | Character 7<br>Qualifier |
|---|---|---|---|
| 0 Cervical Spine<br>7 Thoracic Spine<br>9 Lumbar Spine<br>C Pelvis<br>D Sacroiliac Joints<br>F Sacrum and Coccyx | 0 High Osmolar<br>1 Low Osmolar<br>Y Other Contrast<br>Z None | Z None | Z None |

**B** Imaging
**R** Axial Skeleton, Except Skull and Facial Bones
**3** Magnetic Resonance Imaging (MRI): Computer reformatted digital display of multiplanar images developed from the capture of radiofrequency signals emitted by nuclei in a body site excited within a magnetic field

| Character 4<br>Body Part | Character 5<br>Contrast | Character 6<br>Qualifier | Character 7<br>Qualifier |
|---|---|---|---|
| 0 Cervical Spine<br>1 Cervical Disc(s)<br>2 Thoracic Disc(s)<br>3 Lumbar Disc(s)<br>7 Thoracic Spine<br>9 Lumbar Spine<br>C Pelvis<br>F Sacrum and Coccyx | Y Other Contrast | 0 Unenhanced and Enhanced<br>Z None | Z None |
| 0 Cervical Spine<br>1 Cervical Disc(s)<br>2 Thoracic Disc(s)<br>3 Lumbar Disc(s)<br>7 Thoracic Spine<br>9 Lumbar Spine<br>C Pelvis<br>F Sacrum and Coccyx | Z None | Z None | Z None |

**B** Imaging
**R** Axial Skeleton, Except Skull and Facial Bones
**4** Ultrasonography: Real time display of images of anatomy or flow information developed from the capture of reflected and attenuated high frequency sound waves

| Character 4<br>Body Part | Character 5<br>Contrast | Character 6<br>Qualifier | Character 7<br>Qualifier |
|---|---|---|---|
| 0 Cervical Spine<br>7 Thoracic Spine<br>9 Lumbar Spine<br>F Sacrum and Coccyx | Z None | Z None | Z None |

**B** Imaging
**T** Urinary System
**0** Plain Radiography: Planar display of an image developed from the capture of external ionizing radiation on photographic or photoconductive plate

| Character 4<br>Body Part | Character 5<br>Contrast | Character 6<br>Qualifier | Character 7<br>Qualifier |
|---|---|---|---|
| 0 Bladder<br>1 Kidney, Right<br>2 Kidney, Left<br>3 Kidneys, Bilateral<br>4 Kidneys, Ureters and Bladder<br>5 Urethra<br>6 Ureter, Right<br>7 Ureter, Left<br>8 Ureters, Bilateral<br>B Bladder and Urethra<br>C Ileal Diversion Loop | 0 High Osmolar<br>1 Low Osmolar<br>Y Other Contrast<br>Z None | Z None | Z None |

**B** Imaging
**T** Urinary System
**1** Fluoroscopy: Single plane or bi-plane real time display of an image developed from the capture of external ionizing radiation on a fluorescent screen. The image may also be stored by either digital or analog means

| Character 4<br>Body Part | Character 5<br>Contrast | Character 6<br>Qualifier | Character 7<br>Qualifier |
|---|---|---|---|
| 0 Bladder<br>1 Kidney, Right<br>2 Kidney, Left<br>3 Kidneys, Bilateral<br>4 Kidneys, Ureters and Bladder<br>5 Urethra<br>6 Ureter, Right<br>7 Ureter, Left<br>B Bladder and Urethra<br>C Ileal Diversion Loop<br>D Kidney, Ureter and Bladder, Right<br>F Kidney, Ureter and Bladder, Left<br>G Ileal Loop, Ureters and Kidneys | 0 High Osmolar<br>1 Low Osmolar<br>Y Other Contrast<br>Z None | Z None | Z None |

**B** Imaging
**T** Urinary System
**2** Computerized Tomography (CT Scan): Computer reformatted digital display of multiplanar images developed from the capture of multiple exposures of external ionizing radiation

| Character 4<br>Body Part | Character 5<br>Contrast | Character 6<br>Qualifier | Character 7<br>Qualifier |
|---|---|---|---|
| 0 Bladder<br>1 Kidney, Right<br>2 Kidney, Left<br>3 Kidneys, Bilateral<br>9 Kidney Transplant | 0 High Osmolar<br>1 Low Osmolar<br>Y Other Contrast | 0 Unenhanced and Enhanced<br>Z None | Z None |
| 0 Bladder<br>1 Kidney, Right<br>2 Kidney, Left<br>3 Kidneys, Bilateral<br>9 Kidney Transplant | Z None | Z None | Z None |

**B** Imaging
**T** Urinary System
**3** Magnetic Resonance Imaging (MRI): Computer reformatted digital display of multiplanar images developed from the capture of radiofrequency signals emitted by nuclei in a body site excited within a magnetic field

| Character 4<br>Body Part | Character 5<br>Contrast | Character 6<br>Qualifier | Character 7<br>Qualifier |
|---|---|---|---|
| 0 Bladder<br>1 Kidney, Right<br>2 Kidney, Left<br>3 Kidneys, Bilateral<br>9 Kidney Transplant | Y Other Contrast | 0 Unenhanced and Enhanced<br>Z None | Z None |
| 0 Bladder<br>1 Kidney, Right<br>2 Kidney, Left<br>3 Kidneys, Bilateral<br>9 Kidney Transplant | Z None | Z None | Z None |

**B** Imaging
**T** Urinary System
**4** Ultrasonography: Real time display of images of anatomy or flow information developed from the capture of reflected and attenuated high frequency sound waves

| Character 4<br>Body Part | Character 5<br>Contrast | Character 6<br>Qualifier | Character 7<br>Qualifier |
|---|---|---|---|
| 0 Bladder<br>1 Kidney, Right<br>2 Kidney, Left<br>3 Kidneys, Bilateral<br>5 Urethra<br>6 Ureter, Right<br>7 Ureter, Left<br>8 Ureters, Bilateral<br>9 Kidney Transplant<br>J Kidneys and Bladder | Z None | Z None | Z None |

**B** Imaging
**U** Female Reproductive System
**0** Plain Radiography: Planar display of an image developed from the capture of external ionizing radiation on photographic or photoconductive plate

| Character 4<br>Body Part | Character 5<br>Contrast | Character 6<br>Qualifier | Character 7<br>Qualifier |
|---|---|---|---|
| 0 Fallopian Tube, Right ♀<br>1 Fallopian Tube, Left ♀<br>2 Fallopian Tubes, Bilateral ♀<br>6 Uterus ♀<br>8 Uterus and Fallopian Tubes ♀<br>9 Vagina ♀ | 0 High Osmolar<br>1 Low Osmolar<br>Y Other Contrast | Z None | Z None |

**B** Imaging
**U** Female Reproductive System
**1** Fluoroscopy: Single plane or bi-plane real time display of an image developed from the capture of external ionizing radiation on a fluorescent screen. The image may also be stored by either digital or analog means

| Character 4<br>Body Part | Character 5<br>Contrast | Character 6<br>Qualifier | Character 7<br>Qualifier |
|---|---|---|---|
| 0 Fallopian Tube, Right ♀<br>1 Fallopian Tube, Left ♀<br>2 Fallopian Tubes, Bilateral ♀<br>6 Uterus ♀<br>8 Uterus and Fallopian Tubes ♀<br>9 Vagina ♀ | 0 High Osmolar<br>1 Low Osmolar<br>Y Other Contrast<br>Z None | Z None | Z None |

**B** Imaging
**U** Female Reproductive System
**3** Magnetic Resonance Imaging (MRI): Computer reformatted digital display of multiplanar images developed from the capture of radiofrequency signals emitted by nuclei in a body site excited within a magnetic field

| Character 4<br>Body Part | Character 5<br>Contrast | Character 6<br>Qualifier | Character 7<br>Qualifier |
|---|---|---|---|
| 3 Ovary, Right ♀<br>4 Ovary, Left ♀<br>5 Ovaries, Bilateral ♀<br>6 Uterus ♀<br>9 Vagina ♀<br>B Pregnant Uterus ♀<br>C Uterus and Ovaries ♀ | Y Other Contrast | 0 Unenhanced and Enhanced<br>Z None | Z None |
| 3 Ovary, Right ♀<br>4 Ovary, Left ♀<br>5 Ovaries, Bilateral ♀<br>6 Uterus ♀<br>9 Vagina ♀<br>B Pregnant Uterus ♀<br>C Uterus and Ovaries ♀ | Z None | Z None | Z None |

**B** Imaging
**U** Female Reproductive System
**4** Ultrasonography: Real time display of images of anatomy or flow information developed from the capture of reflected and attenuated high frequency sound waves

| Character 4<br>Body Part | Character 5<br>Contrast | Character 6<br>Qualifier | Character 7<br>Qualifier |
|---|---|---|---|
| 0 Fallopian Tube, Right ♀<br>1 Fallopian Tube, Left ♀<br>2 Fallopian Tubes, Bilateral ♀<br>3 Ovary, Right ♀<br>4 Ovary, Left ♀<br>5 Ovaries, Bilateral ♀<br>6 Uterus ♀<br>C Uterus and Ovaries ♀ | Y Other Contrast<br>Z None | Z None | Z None |

**B** Imaging
**V** Male Reproductive System
**0** Plain Radiography: Planar display of an image developed from the capture of external ionizing radiation on photographic or photoconductive plate

| Character 4<br>Body Part | Character 5<br>Contrast | Character 6<br>Qualifier | Character 7<br>Qualifier |
|---|---|---|---|
| 0 Corpora Cavernosa ♂<br>1 Epididymis, Right ♂<br>2 Epididymis, Left ♂<br>3 Prostate ♂<br>5 Testicle, Right ♂<br>6 Testicle, Left ♂<br>8 Vasa Vasorum ♂ | 0 High Osmolar<br>1 Low Osmolar<br>Y Other Contrast | Z None | Z None |

♂ Male      ♀ Female      N C Non-covered      L C Limited Coverage      **AHA** *AHA Coding Clinic*

**B** Imaging
**V** Male Reproductive System
**1** Fluoroscopy: Single plane or bi-plane real time display of an image developed from the capture of external ionizing radiation on a fluorescent screen. The image may also be stored by either digital or analog means

| Character 4<br>Body Part | Character 5<br>Contrast | Character 6<br>Qualifier | Character 7<br>Qualifier |
|---|---|---|---|
| 0 Corpora Cavernosa ♂<br>8 Vasa Vasorum ♂ | 0 High Osmolar<br>1 Low Osmolar<br>Y Other Contrast<br>Z None | Z None | Z None |

**B** Imaging
**V** Male Reproductive System
**2** Computerized Tomography (CT Scan): Computer reformatted digital display of multiplanar images developed from the capture of multiple exposures of external ionizing radiation

| Character 4<br>Body Part | Character 5<br>Contrast | Character 6<br>Qualifier | Character 7<br>Qualifier |
|---|---|---|---|
| 3 Prostate ♂ | 0 High Osmolar<br>1 Low Osmolar<br>Y Other Contrast | 0 Unenhanced and Enhanced<br>Z None | Z None |
| 3 Prostate ♂ | Z None | Z None | Z None |

**B** Imaging
**V** Male Reproductive System
**3** Magnetic Resonance Imaging (MRI): Computer reformatted digital display of multiplanar images developed from the capture of radiofrequency signals emitted by nuclei in a body site excited within a magnetic field

| Character 4<br>Body Part | Character 5<br>Contrast | Character 6<br>Qualifier | Character 7<br>Qualifier |
|---|---|---|---|
| 0 Corpora Cavernosa ♂<br>3 Prostate ♂<br>4 Scrotum ♂<br>5 Testicle, Right ♂<br>6 Testicle, Left ♂<br>7 Testicles, Bilateral ♂ | Y Other Contrast | 0 Unenhanced and Enhanced<br>Z None | Z None |
| 0 Corpora Cavernosa ♂<br>3 Prostate ♂<br>4 Scrotum ♂<br>5 Testicle, Right ♂<br>6 Testicle, Left ♂<br>7 Testicles, Bilateral ♂ | Z None | Z None | Z None |

**B** Imaging
**V** Male Reproductive System
**4** Ultrasonography: Real time display of images of anatomy or flow information developed from the capture of reflected and attenuated high frequency sound waves

| Character 4<br>Body Part | Character 5<br>Contrast | Character 6<br>Qualifier | Character 7<br>Qualifier |
|---|---|---|---|
| 4 Scrotum ♂<br>9 Prostate and Seminal Vesicles ♂<br>B Penis ♂ | Z None | Z None | Z None |

**B** Imaging
**W** Anatomical Regions
**0** Plain Radiography: Planar display of an image developed from the capture of external ionizing radiation on photographic or photoconductive plate

| Character 4<br>Body Part | Character 5<br>Contrast | Character 6<br>Qualifier | Character 7<br>Qualifier |
|---|---|---|---|
| 0 Abdomen<br>1 Abdomen and Pelvis<br>3 Chest<br>B Long Bones, All<br>C Lower Extremity<br>J Upper Extremity<br>K Whole Body<br>L Whole Skeleton<br>M Whole Body, Infant | Z None | Z None | Z None |

**B** Imaging
**W** Anatomical Regions
**1** Fluoroscopy: Single plane or bi-plane real time display of an image developed from the capture of external ionizing radiation on a fluorescent screen. The image may also be stored by either digital or analog means

| Character 4<br>Body Part | Character 5<br>Contrast | Character 6<br>Qualifier | Character 7<br>Qualifier |
|---|---|---|---|
| 1 Abdomen and Pelvis<br>9 Head and Neck<br>C Lower Extremity<br>J Upper Extremity | 0 High Osmolar<br>1 Low Osmolar<br>Y Other Contrast<br>Z None | Z None | Z None |

**B** Imaging
**W** Anatomical Regions
**2** Computerized Tomography (CT Scan): Computer reformatted digital display of multiplanar images developed from the capture of multiple exposures of external ionizing radiation

| Character 4<br>Body Part | Character 5<br>Contrast | Character 6<br>Qualifier | Character 7<br>Qualifier |
|---|---|---|---|
| 0 Abdomen<br>1 Abdomen and Pelvis<br>4 Chest and Abdomen<br>5 Chest, Abdomen and Pelvis<br>8 Head<br>9 Head and Neck<br>F Neck<br>G Pelvic Region | 0 High Osmolar<br>1 Low Osmolar<br>Y Other Contrast | 0 Unenhanced and Enhanced<br>Z None | Z None |
| 0 Abdomen<br>1 Abdomen and Pelvis<br>4 Chest and Abdomen<br>5 Chest, Abdomen and Pelvis<br>8 Head<br>9 Head and Neck<br>F Neck<br>G Pelvic Region | Z None | Z None | Z None |

**B** Imaging
**W** Anatomical Regions
**3** Magnetic Resonance Imaging (MRI): Computer reformatted digital display of multiplanar images developed from the capture of radiofrequency signals emitted by nuclei in a body site excited within a magnetic field

| Character 4<br>Body Part | Character 5<br>Contrast | Character 6<br>Qualifier | Character 7<br>Qualifier |
|---|---|---|---|
| 0 Abdomen<br>8 Head<br>F Neck<br>G Pelvic Region<br>H Retroperitoneum<br>P Brachial Plexus | Y Other Contrast | 0 Unenhanced and Enhanced<br>Z None | Z None |
| 0 Abdomen<br>8 Head<br>F Neck<br>G Pelvic Region<br>H Retroperitoneum<br>P Brachial Plexus | Z None | Z None | Z None |
| 3 Chest | Y Other Contrast | 0 Unenhanced and Enhanced<br>Z None | Z None |

**B** Imaging
**W** Anatomical Regions
**4** Ultrasonography: Real time display of images of anatomy or flow information developed from the capture of reflected and attenuated high frequency sound waves

| Character 4<br>Body Part | Character 5<br>Contrast | Character 6<br>Qualifier | Character 7<br>Qualifier |
|---|---|---|---|
| 0 Abdomen<br>1 Abdomen and Pelvis<br>F Neck<br>G Pelvic Region | Z None | Z None | Z None |

**B** Imaging
**Y** Fetus and Obstetrical
**3** Magnetic Resonance Imaging (MRI): Computer reformatted digital display of multiplanar images developed from the capture of radiofrequency signals emitted by nuclei in a body site excited within a magnetic field

| Character 4 Body Part | Character 5 Contrast | Character 6 Qualifier | Character 7 Qualifier |
|---|---|---|---|
| 0 Fetal Head ♀<br>1 Fetal Heart ♀<br>2 Fetal Thorax ♀<br>3 Fetal Abdomen ♀<br>4 Fetal Spine ♀<br>5 Fetal Extremities ♀<br>6 Whole Fetus ♀ | Y Other Contrast | 0 Unenhanced and Enhanced<br>Z None | Z None |
| 0 Fetal Head ♀<br>1 Fetal Heart ♀<br>2 Fetal Thorax ♀<br>3 Fetal Abdomen ♀<br>4 Fetal Spine ♀<br>5 Fetal Extremities ♀<br>6 Whole Fetus ♀ | Z None | Z None | Z None |

**B** Imaging
**Y** Fetus and Obstetrical
**4** Ultrasonography: Real time display of images of anatomy or flow information developed from the capture of reflected and attenuated high frequency sound waves

| Character 4 Body Part | Character 5 Contrast | Character 6 Qualifier | Character 7 Qualifier |
|---|---|---|---|
| 7 Fetal Umbilical Cord ♀<br>8 Placenta ♀<br>9 First Trimester, Single Fetus ♀<br>B First Trimester, Multiple Gestation ♀<br>C Second Trimester, Single Fetus ♀<br>D Second Trimester, Multiple Gestation ♀<br>F Third Trimester, Single Fetus ♀<br>G Third Trimester, Multiple Gestation ♀ | Z None | Z None | Z None |

# Nuclear Medicine | C01-CW7

**C** Nuclear Medicine
**0** Central Nervous System
**1** Planar Nuclear Medicine Imaging: Introduction of radioactive materials into the body for single plane display of images developed from the capture of radioactive emissions

| Character 4<br>Body Part | Character 5<br>Radionuclide | Character 6<br>Qualifier | Character 7<br>Qualifier |
|---|---|---|---|
| 0 Brain | 1 Technetium 99m (Tc-99m)<br>Y Other Radionuclide | Z None | Z None |
| 5 Cerebrospinal Fluid | D Indium 111 (In-111)<br>Y Other Radionuclide | Z None | Z None |
| Y Central Nervous System | Y Other Radionuclide | Z None | Z None |

**C** Nuclear Medicine
**0** Central Nervous System
**2** Tomographic (Tomo) Nuclear Medicine Imaging: Introduction of radioactive materials into the body for three dimensional display of images developed from the capture of radioactive emissions

| Character 4<br>Body Part | Character 5<br>Radionuclide | Character 6<br>Qualifier | Character 7<br>Qualifier |
|---|---|---|---|
| 0 Brain | 1 Technetium 99m (Tc-99m)<br>F Iodine 123 (I-123)<br>S Thallium 201 (Tl-201)<br>Y Other Radionuclide | Z None | Z None |
| 5 Cerebrospinal Fluid | D Indium 111 (In-111)<br>Y Other Radionuclide | Z None | Z None |
| Y Central Nervous System | Y Other Radionuclide | Z None | Z None |

**C** Nuclear Medicine
**0** Central Nervous System
**3** Positron Emission Tomographic (PET) Imaging: Introduction of radioactive materials into the body for three dimensional display of images developed from the simultaneous capture, 180 degrees apart, of radioactive emissions

| Character 4<br>Body Part | Character 5<br>Radionuclide | Character 6<br>Qualifier | Character 7<br>Qualifier |
|---|---|---|---|
| 0 Brain | B Carbon 11 (C-11)<br>K Fluorine 18 (F-18)<br>M Oxygen 15 (O-15)<br>Y Other Radionuclide | Z None | Z None |
| Y Central Nervous System | Y Other Radionuclide | Z None | Z None |

**C** Nuclear Medicine
**0** Central Nervous System
**5** Nonimaging Nuclear Medicine Probe: Introduction of radioactive materials into the body for the study of distribution and fate of certain substances by the detection of radioactive emissions; or, alternatively, measurement of absorption of radioactive emissions from an external source

| Character 4<br>Body Part | Character 5<br>Radionuclide | Character 6<br>Qualifier | Character 7<br>Qualifier |
|---|---|---|---|
| 0 Brain | V Xenon 133 (Xe-133)<br>Y Other Radionuclide | Z None | Z None |
| Y Central Nervous System | Y Other Radionuclide | Z None | Z None |

**C Nuclear Medicine**
**2 Heart**
**1 Planar Nuclear Medicine Imaging:** Introduction of radioactive materials into the body for single plane display of images developed from the capture of radioactive emissions

| Character 4<br>Body Part | Character 5<br>Radionuclide | Character 6<br>Qualifier | Character 7<br>Qualifier |
|---|---|---|---|
| 6 Heart, Right and Left | 1 Technetium 99m (Tc-99m)<br>Y Other Radionuclide | Z None | Z None |
| G Myocardium | 1 Technetium 99m (Tc-99m)<br>D Indium 111 (In-111)<br>S Thallium 201 (Tl-201)<br>Y Other Radionuclide<br>Z None | Z None | Z None |
| Y Heart | Y Other Radionuclide | Z None | Z None |

**C Nuclear Medicine**
**2 Heart**
**2 Tomographic (Tomo) Nuclear Medicine Imaging:** Introduction of radioactive materials into the body for three dimensional display of images developed from the capture of radioactive emissions

| Character 4<br>Body Part | Character 5<br>Radionuclide | Character 6<br>Qualifier | Character 7<br>Qualifier |
|---|---|---|---|
| 6 Heart, Right and Left | 1 Technetium 99m (Tc-99m)<br>Y Other Radionuclide | Z None | Z None |
| G Myocardium | 1 Technetium 99m (Tc-99m)<br>D Indium 111 (In-111)<br>K Fluorine 18 (F-18)<br>S Thallium 201 (Tl-201)<br>Y Other Radionuclide<br>Z None | Z None | Z None |
| Y Heart | Y Other Radionuclide | Z None | Z None |

**C Nuclear Medicine**
**2 Heart**
**3 Positron Emission Tomographic (PET) Imaging:** Introduction of radioactive materials into the body for three dimensional display of images developed from the simultaneous capture, 180 degrees apart, of radioactive emissions

| Character 4<br>Body Part | Character 5<br>Radionuclide | Character 6<br>Qualifier | Character 7<br>Qualifier |
|---|---|---|---|
| G Myocardium | K Fluorine 18 (F-18)<br>M Oxygen 15 (O-15)<br>Q Rubidium 82 (Rb-82)<br>R Nitrogen 13 (N-13)<br>Y Other Radionuclide | Z None | Z None |
| Y Heart | Y Other Radionuclide | Z None | Z None |

**C Nuclear Medicine**
**2 Heart**
**5 Nonimaging Nuclear Medicine Probe:** Introduction of radioactive materials into the body for the study of distribution and fate of certain substances by the detection of radioactive emissions; or, alternatively, measurement of absorption of radioactive emissions from an external source

| Character 4<br>Body Part | Character 5<br>Radionuclide | Character 6<br>Qualifier | Character 7<br>Qualifier |
|---|---|---|---|
| 6 Heart, Right and Left | 1 Technetium 99m (Tc-99m)<br>Y Other Radionuclide | Z None | Z None |
| Y Heart | Y Other Radionuclide | Z None | Z None |

**C Nuclear Medicine**
**5 Veins**
**1 Planar Nuclear Medicine Imaging: Introduction of radioactive materials into the body for single plane display of images developed from the capture of radioactive emissions**

| Character 4<br>Body Part | Character 5<br>Radionuclide | Character 6<br>Qualifier | Character 7<br>Qualifier |
|---|---|---|---|
| B Lower Extremity Veins, Right<br>C Lower Extremity Veins, Left<br>D Lower Extremity Veins, Bilateral<br>N Upper Extremity Veins, Right<br>P Upper Extremity Veins, Left<br>Q Upper Extremity Veins, Bilateral<br>R Central Veins | 1 Technetium 99m (Tc-99m)<br>Y Other Radionuclide | Z None | Z None |
| Y Veins | Y Other Radionuclide | Z None | Z None |

**C Nuclear Medicine**
**7 Lymphatic and Hematologic System**
**1 Planar Nuclear Medicine Imaging: Introduction of radioactive materials into the body for single plane display of images developed from the capture of radioactive emissions**

| Character 4<br>Body Part | Character 5<br>Radionuclide | Character 6<br>Qualifier | Character 7<br>Qualifier |
|---|---|---|---|
| 0 Bone Marrow | 1 Technetium 99m (Tc-99m)<br>D Indium 111 (In-111)<br>Y Other Radionuclide | Z None | Z None |
| 2 Spleen<br>5 Lymphatics, Head and Neck<br>D Lymphatics, Pelvic<br>J Lymphatics, Head<br>K Lymphatics, Neck<br>L Lymphatics, Upper Chest<br>M Lymphatics, Trunk<br>N Lymphatics, Upper Extremity<br>P Lymphatics, Lower Extremity | 1 Technetium 99m (Tc-99m)<br>Y Other Radionuclide | Z None | Z None |
| 3 Blood | D Indium 111 (In-111)<br>Y Other Radionuclide | Z None | Z None |
| Y Lymphatic and Hematologic System | Y Other Radionuclide | Z None | Z None |

**C Nuclear Medicine**
**7 Lymphatic and Hematologic System**
**2 Tomographic (Tomo) Nuclear Medicine Imaging: Introduction of radioactive materials into the body for three dimensional display of images developed from the capture of radioactive emissions**

| Character 4<br>Body Part | Character 5<br>Radionuclide | Character 6<br>Qualifier | Character 7<br>Qualifier |
|---|---|---|---|
| 2 Spleen | 1 Technetium 99m (Tc-99m)<br>Y Other Radionuclide | Z None | Z None |
| Y Lymphatic and Hematologic System | Y Other Radionuclide | Z None | Z None |

**C Nuclear Medicine**
**7 Lymphatic and Hematologic System**
**5 Nonimaging Nuclear Medicine Probe: Introduction of radioactive materials into the body for the study of distribution and fate of certain substances by the detection of radioactive emissions; or, alternatively, measurement of absorption of radioactive emissions from an external source**

| Character 4<br>Body Part | Character 5<br>Radionuclide | Character 6<br>Qualifier | Character 7<br>Qualifier |
|---|---|---|---|
| 5 Lymphatics, Head and Neck<br>D Lymphatics, Pelvic<br>J Lymphatics, Head<br>K Lymphatics, Neck<br>L Lymphatics, Upper Chest<br>M Lymphatics, Trunk<br>N Lymphatics, Upper Extremity<br>P Lymphatics, Lower Extremity | 1 Technetium 99m (Tc-99m)<br>Y Other Radionuclide | Z None | Z None |
| Y Lymphatic and Hematologic System | Y Other Radionuclide | Z None | Z None |

**C** Nuclear Medicine
**7** Lymphatic and Hematologic System
**6** Nonimaging Nuclear Medicine Assay: Introduction of radioactive materials into the body for the study of body fluids and blood elements, by the detection of radioactive emissions

| Character 4<br>Body Part | Character 5<br>Radionuclide | Character 6<br>Qualifier | Character 7<br>Qualifier |
|---|---|---|---|
| 3  Blood | 1  Technetium 99m (Tc-99m)<br>7  Cobalt 58 (Co-58)<br>C  Cobalt 57 (Co-57)<br>D  Indium 111 (In-111)<br>H  Iodine 125 (I-125)<br>W  Chromium (Cr-51)<br>Y  Other Radionuclide | Z  None | Z  None |
| Y  Lymphatic and Hematologic System | Y  Other Radionuclide | Z  None | Z  None |

**C** Nuclear Medicine
**8** Eye
**1** Planar Nuclear Medicine Imaging: Introduction of radioactive materials into the body for single plane display of images developed from the capture of radioactive emissions

| Character 4<br>Body Part | Character 5<br>Radionuclide | Character 6<br>Qualifier | Character 7<br>Qualifier |
|---|---|---|---|
| 9  Lacrimal Ducts, Bilateral | 1  Technetium 99m (Tc-99m)<br>Y  Other Radionuclide | Z  None | Z  None |
| Y  Eye | Y  Other Radionuclide | Z  None | Z  None |

**C** Nuclear Medicine
**9** Ear, Nose, Mouth and Throat
**1** Planar Nuclear Medicine Imaging: Introduction of radioactive materials into the body for single plane display of images developed from the capture of radioactive emissions

| Character 4<br>Body Part | Character 5<br>Radionuclide | Character 6<br>Qualifier | Character 7<br>Qualifier |
|---|---|---|---|
| B  Salivary Glands, Bilateral | 1  Technetium 99m (Tc-99m)<br>Y  Other Radionuclide | Z  None | Z  None |
| Y  Ear, Nose, Mouth and Throat | Y  Other Radionuclide | Z  None | Z  None |

**C** Nuclear Medicine
**B** Respiratory System
**1** Planar Nuclear Medicine Imaging: Introduction of radioactive materials into the body for single plane display of images developed from the capture of radioactive emissions

| Character 4<br>Body Part | Character 5<br>Radionuclide | Character 6<br>Qualifier | Character 7<br>Qualifier |
|---|---|---|---|
| 2  Lungs and Bronchi | 1  Technetium 99m (Tc-99m)<br>9  Krypton (Kr-81m)<br>T  Xenon 127 (Xe-127)<br>V  Xenon 133 (Xe-133)<br>Y  Other Radionuclide | Z  None | Z  None |
| Y  Respiratory System | Y  Other Radionuclide | Z  None | Z  None |

**C** Nuclear Medicine
**B** Respiratory System
**2** Tomographic (Tomo) Nuclear Medicine Imaging: Introduction of radioactive materials into the body for three dimensional display of images developed from the capture of radioactive emissions

| Character 4<br>Body Part | Character 5<br>Radionuclide | Character 6<br>Qualifier | Character 7<br>Qualifier |
|---|---|---|---|
| 2  Lungs and Bronchi | 1  Technetium 99m (Tc-99m)<br>9  Krypton (Kr-81m)<br>Y  Other Radionuclide | Z  None | Z  None |
| Y  Respiratory System | Y  Other Radionuclide | Z  None | Z  None |

**C** Nuclear Medicine
**B** Respiratory System
**3** Positron Emission Tomographic (PET) Imaging: Introduction of radioactive materials into the body for three dimensional display of images developed from the simultaneous capture, 180 degrees apart, of radioactive emissions

| Character 4<br>Body Part | Character 5<br>Radionuclide | Character 6<br>Qualifier | Character 7<br>Qualifier |
|---|---|---|---|
| 2 Lungs and Bronchi | K Fluorine 18 (F-18)<br>Y Other Radionuclide | Z None | Z None |
| Y Respiratory System | Y Other Radionuclide | Z None | Z None |

**C** Nuclear Medicine
**D** Gastrointestinal System
**1** Planar Nuclear Medicine Imaging: Introduction of radioactive materials into the body for single plane display of images developed from the capture of radioactive emissions

| Character 4<br>Body Part | Character 5<br>Radionuclide | Character 6<br>Qualifier | Character 7<br>Qualifier |
|---|---|---|---|
| 5 Upper Gastrointestinal Tract<br>7 Gastrointestinal Tract | 1 Technetium 99m (Tc-99m)<br>D Indium 111 (In-111)<br>Y Other Radionuclide | Z None | Z None |
| Y Digestive System | Y Other Radionuclide | Z None | Z None |

**C** Nuclear Medicine
**D** Gastrointestinal System
**2** Tomographic (Tomo) Nuclear Medicine Imaging: Introduction of radioactive materials into the body for three dimensional display of images developed from the capture of radioactive emissions

| Character 4<br>Body Part | Character 5<br>Radionuclide | Character 6<br>Qualifier | Character 7<br>Qualifier |
|---|---|---|---|
| 7 Gastrointestinal Tract | 1 Technetium 99m (Tc-99m)<br>D Indium 111 (In-111)<br>Y Other Radionuclide | Z None | Z None |
| Y Digestive System | Y Other Radionuclide | Z None | Z None |

**C** Nuclear Medicine
**F** Hepatobiliary System and Pancreas
**1** Planar Nuclear Medicine Imaging: Introduction of radioactive materials into the body for single plane display of images developed from the capture of radioactive emissions

| Character 4<br>Body Part | Character 5<br>Radionuclide | Character 6<br>Qualifier | Character 7<br>Qualifier |
|---|---|---|---|
| 4 Gallbladder<br>5 Liver<br>6 Liver and Spleen<br>C Hepatobiliary System, All | 1 Technetium 99m (Tc-99m)<br>Y Other Radionuclide | Z None | Z None |
| Y Hepatobiliary System and Pancreas | Y Other Radionuclide | Z None | Z None |

**C** Nuclear Medicine
**F** Hepatobiliary System and Pancreas
**2** Tomographic (Tomo) Nuclear Medicine Imaging: Introduction of radioactive materials into the body for three dimensional display of images developed from the capture of radioactive emissions

| Character 4<br>Body Part | Character 5<br>Radionuclide | Character 6<br>Qualifier | Character 7<br>Qualifier |
|---|---|---|---|
| 4 Gallbladder<br>5 Liver<br>6 Liver and Spleen | 1 Technetium 99m (Tc-99m)<br>Y Other Radionuclide | Z None | Z None |
| Y Hepatobiliary System and Pancreas | Y Other Radionuclide | Z None | Z None |

---

♂ Male          ♀ Female          N C Non-covered          L C Limited Coverage          **AHA** AHA Coding Clinic

**C** Nuclear Medicine
**G** Endocrine System
**1** Planar Nuclear Medicine Imaging: Introduction of radioactive materials into the body for single plane display of images developed from the capture of radioactive emissions

| Character 4 Body Part | Character 5 Radionuclide | Character 6 Qualifier | Character 7 Qualifier |
|---|---|---|---|
| 1 Parathyroid Glands | 1 Technetium 99m (Tc-99m) <br> S Thallium 201 (Tl-201) <br> Y Other Radionuclide | Z None | Z None |
| 2 Thyroid Gland | 1 Technetium 99m (Tc-99m) <br> F Iodine 123 (I-123) <br> G Iodine 131 (I-131) <br> Y Other Radionuclide | Z None | Z None |
| 4 Adrenal Glands, Bilateral | G Iodine 131 (I-131) <br> Y Other Radionuclide | Z None | Z None |
| Y Endocrine System | Y Other Radionuclide | Z None | Z None |

**C** Nuclear Medicine
**G** Endocrine System
**2** Tomographic (Tomo) Nuclear Medicine Imaging: Introduction of radioactive materials into the body for three dimensional display of images developed from the capture of radioactive emissions

| Character 4 Body Part | Character 5 Radionuclide | Character 6 Qualifier | Character 7 Qualifier |
|---|---|---|---|
| 1 Parathyroid Glands | 1 Technetium 99m (Tc-99m) <br> S Thallium 201 (Tl-201) <br> Y Other Radionuclide | Z None | Z None |
| Y Endocrine System | Y Other Radionuclide | Z None | Z None |

**C** Nuclear Medicine
**G** Endocrine System
**4** Nonimaging Nuclear Medicine Uptake: Introduction of radioactive materials into the body for measurements of organ function, from the detection of radioactive emissions

| Character 4 Body Part | Character 5 Radionuclide | Character 6 Qualifier | Character 7 Qualifier |
|---|---|---|---|
| 2 Thyroid Gland | 1 Technetium 99m (Tc-99m) <br> F Iodine 123 (I-123) <br> G Iodine 131 (I-131) <br> Y Other Radionuclide | Z None | Z None |
| Y Endocrine System | Y Other Radionuclide | Z None | Z None |

**C** Nuclear Medicine
**H** Skin, Subcutaneous Tissue and Breast
**1** Planar Nuclear Medicine Imaging: Introduction of radioactive materials into the body for single plane display of images developed from the capture of radioactive emissions

| Character 4 Body Part | Character 5 Radionuclide | Character 6 Qualifier | Character 7 Qualifier |
|---|---|---|---|
| 0 Breast, Right <br> 1 Breast, Left <br> 2 Breasts, Bilateral | 1 Technetium 99m (Tc-99m) <br> S Thallium 201 (Tl-201) <br> Y Other Radionuclide | Z None | Z None |
| Y Skin, Subcutaneous Tissue and Breast | Y Other Radionuclide | Z None | Z None |

**C** Nuclear Medicine
**H** Skin, Subcutaneous Tissue and Breast
**2** Tomographic (Tomo) Nuclear Medicine Imaging: Introduction of radioactive materials into the body for three dimensional display of images developed from the capture of radioactive emissions

| Character 4 Body Part | Character 5 Radionuclide | Character 6 Qualifier | Character 7 Qualifier |
|---|---|---|---|
| 0 Breast, Right <br> 1 Breast, Left <br> 2 Breasts, Bilateral | 1 Technetium 99m (Tc-99m) <br> S Thallium 201 (Tl-201) <br> Y Other Radionuclide | Z None | Z None |
| Y Skin, Subcutaneous Tissue and Breast | Y Other Radionuclide | Z None | Z None |

**C** Nuclear Medicine
**P** Musculoskeletal System
**1** Planar Nuclear Medicine Imaging: Introduction of radioactive materials into the body for single plane display of images developed from the capture of radioactive emissions

| Character 4 Body Part | Character 5 Radionuclide | Character 6 Qualifier | Character 7 Qualifier |
|---|---|---|---|
| 1 Skull<br>4 Thorax<br>5 Spine<br>6 Pelvis<br>7 Spine and Pelvis<br>8 Upper Extremity, Right<br>9 Upper Extremity, Left<br>B Upper Extremities, Bilateral<br>C Lower Extremity, Right<br>D Lower Extremity, Left<br>F Lower Extremities, Bilateral<br>Z Musculoskeletal System, All | 1 Technetium 99m (Tc-99m)<br>Y Other Radionuclide | Z None | Z None |
| Y Musculoskeletal System, Other | Y Other Radionuclide | Z None | Z None |

**C** Nuclear Medicine
**P** Musculoskeletal System
**2** Tomographic (Tomo) Nuclear Medicine Imaging: Introduction of radioactive materials into the body for three dimensional display of images developed from the capture of radioactive emissions

| Character 4 Body Part | Character 5 Radionuclide | Character 6 Qualifier | Character 7 Qualifier |
|---|---|---|---|
| 1 Skull<br>2 Cervical Spine<br>3 Skull and Cervical Spine<br>4 Thorax<br>6 Pelvis<br>7 Spine and Pelvis<br>8 Upper Extremity, Right<br>9 Upper Extremity, Left<br>B Upper Extremities, Bilateral<br>C Lower Extremity, Right<br>D Lower Extremity, Left<br>F Lower Extremities, Bilateral<br>G Thoracic Spine<br>H Lumbar Spine<br>J Thoracolumbar Spine | 1 Technetium 99m (Tc-99m)<br>Y Other Radionuclide | Z None | Z None |
| Y Musculoskeletal System, Other | Y Other Radionuclide | Z None | Z None |

**C** Nuclear Medicine
**P** Musculoskeletal System
**5** Nonimaging Nuclear Medicine Probe: Introduction of radioactive materials into the body for the study of distribution and fate of certain substances by the detection of radioactive emissions; or, alternatively, measurement of absorption of radioactive emissions from an external source

| Character 4 Body Part | Character 5 Radionuclide | Character 6 Qualifier | Character 7 Qualifier |
|---|---|---|---|
| 5 Spine<br>N Upper Extremities<br>P Lower Extremities | Z None | Z None | Z None |
| Y Musculoskeletal System, Other | Y Other Radionuclide | Z None | Z None |

**C** Nuclear Medicine
**T** Urinary System
**1** Planar Nuclear Medicine Imaging: Introduction of radioactive materials into the body for single plane display of images developed from the capture of radioactive emissions

| Character 4 Body Part | Character 5 Radionuclide | Character 6 Qualifier | Character 7 Qualifier |
|---|---|---|---|
| 3 Kidneys, Ureters and Bladder | 1 Technetium 99m (Tc-99m)<br>F Iodine 123 (I-123)<br>G Iodine 131 (I-131)<br>Y Other Radionuclide | Z None | Z None |
| H Bladder and Ureters | 1 Technetium 99m (Tc-99m)<br>Y Other Radionuclide | Z None | Z None |
| Y Urinary System | Y Other Radionuclide | Z None | Z None |

**C** Nuclear Medicine
**T** Urinary System
**2** Tomographic (Tomo) Nuclear Medicine Imaging: Introduction of radioactive materials into the body for three dimensional display of images developed from the capture of radioactive emissions

| Character 4<br>Body Part | Character 5<br>Radionuclide | Character 6<br>Qualifier | Character 7<br>Qualifier |
|---|---|---|---|
| 3 Kidneys, Ureters and Bladder | 1 Technetium 99m (Tc-99m)<br>Y Other Radionuclide | Z None | Z None |
| Y Urinary System | Y Other Radionuclide | Z None | Z None |

**C** Nuclear Medicine
**T** Urinary System
**6** Nonimaging Nuclear Medicine Assay: Introduction of radioactive materials into the body for the study of body fluids and blood elements, by the detection of radioactive emissions

| Character 4<br>Body Part | Character 5<br>Radionuclide | Character 6<br>Qualifier | Character 7<br>Qualifier |
|---|---|---|---|
| 3 Kidneys, Ureters and Bladder | 1 Technetium 99m (Tc-99m)<br>F Iodine 123 (I-123)<br>G Iodine 131 (I-131)<br>H Iodine 125 (I-125)<br>Y Other Radionuclide | Z None | Z None |
| Y Urinary System | Y Other Radionuclide | Z None | Z None |

**C** Nuclear Medicine
**V** Male Reproductive System
**1** Planar Nuclear Medicine Imaging: Introduction of radioactive materials into the body for single plane display of images developed from the capture of radioactive emissions

| Character 4<br>Body Part | Character 5<br>Radionuclide | Character 6<br>Qualifier | Character 7<br>Qualifier |
|---|---|---|---|
| 9 Testicles, Bilateral ♂ | 1 Technetium 99m (Tc-99m)<br>Y Other Radionuclide | Z None | Z None |
| Y Male Reproductive System ♂ | Y Other Radionuclide | Z None | Z None |

**C** Nuclear Medicine
**W** Anatomical Regions
**1** Planar Nuclear Medicine Imaging: Introduction of radioactive materials into the body for single plane display of images developed from the capture of radioactive emissions

| Character 4<br>Body Part | Character 5<br>Radionuclide | Character 6<br>Qualifier | Character 7<br>Qualifier |
|---|---|---|---|
| 0 Abdomen<br>1 Abdomen and Pelvis<br>4 Chest and Abdomen<br>6 Chest and Neck<br>B Head and Neck<br>D Lower Extremity<br>J Pelvic Region<br>M Upper Extremity<br>N Whole Body | 1 Technetium 99m (Tc-99m)<br>D Indium 111 (In-111)<br>F Iodine 123 (I-123)<br>G Iodine 131 (I-131)<br>L Gallium 67 (Ga-67)<br>S Thallium 201 (Tl-201)<br>Y Other Radionuclide | Z None | Z None |
| 3 Chest | 1 Technetium 99m (Tc-99m)<br>D Indium 111 (In-111)<br>F Iodine 123 (I-123)<br>G Iodine 131 (I-131)<br>K Fluorine 18 (F-18)<br>L Gallium 67 (Ga-67)<br>S Thallium 201 (Tl-201)<br>Y Other Radionuclide | Z None | Z None |
| Y Anatomical Regions, Multiple | Y Other Radionuclide | Z None | Z None |
| Z Anatomical Region, Other | Z None | Z None | Z None |

**C** Nuclear Medicine
**W** Anatomical Regions
**2** Tomographic (Tomo) Nuclear Medicine Imaging: Introduction of radioactive materials into the body for three dimensional display of images developed from the capture of radioactive emissions

| Character 4<br>Body Part | Character 5<br>Radionuclide | Character 6<br>Qualifier | Character 7<br>Qualifier |
|---|---|---|---|
| 0 Abdomen<br>1 Abdomen and Pelvis<br>3 Chest<br>4 Chest and Abdomen<br>6 Chest and Neck<br>B Head and Neck<br>D Lower Extremity<br>J Pelvic Region<br>M Upper Extremity | 1 Technetium 99m (Tc-99m)<br>D Indium 111 (In-111)<br>F Iodine 123 (I-123)<br>G Iodine 131 (I-131)<br>K Fluorine 18 (F-18)<br>L Gallium 67 (Ga-67)<br>S Thallium 201 (Tl-201)<br>Y Other Radionuclide | Z None | Z None |
| Y Anatomical Regions, Multiple | Y Other Radionuclide | Z None | Z None |

**C** Nuclear Medicine
**W** Anatomical Regions
**3** Positron Emission Tomographic (PET) Imaging: Introduction of radioactive materials into the body for three dimensional display of images developed from the simultaneous capture, 180 degrees apart, of radioactive emissions

| Character 4<br>Body Part | Character 5<br>Radionuclide | Character 6<br>Qualifier | Character 7<br>Qualifier |
|---|---|---|---|
| N Whole Body | Y Other Radionuclide | Z None | Z None |

**C** Nuclear Medicine
**W** Anatomical Regions
**5** Nonimaging Nuclear Medicine Probe: Introduction of radioactive materials into the body for the study of distribution and fate of certain substances by the detection of radioactive emissions; or, alternatively, measurement of absorption of radioactive emissions from an external source

| Character 4<br>Body Part | Character 5<br>Radionuclide | Character 6<br>Qualifier | Character 7<br>Qualifier |
|---|---|---|---|
| 0 Abdomen<br>1 Abdomen and Pelvis<br>3 Chest<br>4 Chest and Abdomen<br>6 Chest and Neck<br>B Head and Neck<br>D Lower Extremity<br>J Pelvic Region<br>M Upper Extremity | 1 Technetium 99m (Tc-99m)<br>D Indium 111 (In-111)<br>Y Other Radionuclide | Z None | Z None |

**C** Nuclear Medicine
**W** Anatomical Regions
**7** Systemic Nuclear Medicine Therapy: Introduction of unsealed radioactive materials into the body for treatment

| Character 4<br>Body Part | Character 5<br>Radionuclide | Character 6<br>Qualifier | Character 7<br>Qualifier |
|---|---|---|---|
| 0 Abdomen<br>3 Chest | N Phosphorus 32 (P-32)<br>Y Other Radionuclide | Z None | Z None |
| G Thyroid | G Iodine 131 (I-131)<br>Y Other Radionuclide | Z None | Z None |
| N Whole Body | 8 Samarium 153 (Sm-153)<br>G Iodine 131 (I-131)<br>N Phosphorus 32 (P-32)<br>P Strontium 89 (Sr-89)<br>Y Other Radionuclide | Z None | Z None |
| Y Anatomical Regions, Multiple | Y Other Radionuclide | Z None | Z None |

# Radiation Therapy | D00-DWY

**D** Radiation Therapy
**0** Central and Peripheral Nervous System
**0** Beam Radiation

| Character 4<br>Treatment Site | Character 5<br>Modality Qualifier | Character 6<br>Isotope | Character 7<br>Qualifier |
|---|---|---|---|
| 0 Brain<br>1 Brain Stem<br>6 Spinal Cord<br>7 Peripheral Nerve | 0 Photons <1 MeV<br>1 Photons 1 - 10 MeV<br>2 Photons >10 MeV<br>4 Heavy Particles (Protons,Ions)<br>5 Neutrons<br>6 Neutron Capture | Z None | Z None |
| 0 Brain<br>1 Brain Stem<br>6 Spinal Cord<br>7 Peripheral Nerve | 3 Electrons | Z None | 0 Intraoperative<br>Z None |

**D** Radiation Therapy
**0** Central and Peripheral Nervous System
**1** Brachytherapy

| Character 4<br>Treatment Site | Character 5<br>Modality Qualifier | Character 6<br>Isotope | Character 7<br>Qualifier |
|---|---|---|---|
| 0 Brain<br>1 Brain Stem<br>6 Spinal Cord<br>7 Peripheral Nerve | 9 High Dose Rate (HDR)<br>B Low Dose Rate (LDR) | 7 Cesium 137 (Cs-137)<br>8 Iridium 192 (Ir-192)<br>9 Iodine 125 (I-125)<br>B Palladium 103 (Pd-103)<br>C Californium 252 (Cf-252)<br>Y Other Isotope | Z None |

**D** Radiation Therapy
**0** Central and Peripheral Nervous System
**2** Stereotactic Radiosurgery

| Character 4<br>Treatment Site | Character 5<br>Modality Qualifier | Character 6<br>Isotope | Character 7<br>Qualifier |
|---|---|---|---|
| 0 Brain<br>1 Brain Stem<br>6 Spinal Cord<br>7 Peripheral Nerve | D Stereotactic Other Photon<br>   Radiosurgery<br>H Stereotactic Particulate Radiosurgery<br>J Stereotactic Gamma Beam<br>   Radiosurgery | Z None | Z None |

**D** Radiation Therapy
**0** Central and Peripheral Nervous System
**Y** Other Radiation

| Character 4<br>Treatment Site | Character 5<br>Modality Qualifier | Character 6<br>Isotope | Character 7<br>Qualifier |
|---|---|---|---|
| 0 Brain<br>1 Brain Stem<br>6 Spinal Cord<br>7 Peripheral Nerve | 7 Contact Radiation<br>8 Hyperthermia<br>F Plaque Radiation<br>K Laser Interstitial Thermal Therapy | Z None | Z None |

**D Radiation Therapy**
**7 Lymphatic and Hematologic System**
**0 Beam Radiation**

| Character 4 Treatment Site | Character 5 Modality Qualifier | Character 6 Isotope | Character 7 Qualifier |
|---|---|---|---|
| 0 Bone Marrow<br>1 Thymus<br>2 Spleen<br>3 Lymphatics, Neck<br>4 Lymphatics, Axillary<br>5 Lymphatics, Thorax<br>6 Lymphatics, Abdomen<br>7 Lymphatics, Pelvis<br>8 Lymphatics, Inguinal | 0 Photons <1 MeV<br>1 Photons 1 - 10 MeV<br>2 Photons >10 MeV<br>4 Heavy Particles (Protons,Ions)<br>5 Neutrons<br>6 Neutron Capture | Z None | Z None |
| 0 Bone Marrow<br>1 Thymus<br>2 Spleen<br>3 Lymphatics, Neck<br>4 Lymphatics, Axillary<br>5 Lymphatics, Thorax<br>6 Lymphatics, Abdomen<br>7 Lymphatics, Pelvis<br>8 Lymphatics, Inguinal | 3 Electrons | Z None | 0 Intraoperative<br>Z None |

**D Radiation Therapy**
**7 Lymphatic and Hematologic System**
**1 Brachytherapy**

| Character 4 Treatment Site | Character 5 Modality Qualifier | Character 6 Isotope | Character 7 Qualifier |
|---|---|---|---|
| 0 Bone Marrow<br>1 Thymus<br>2 Spleen<br>3 Lymphatics, Neck<br>4 Lymphatics, Axillary<br>5 Lymphatics, Thorax<br>6 Lymphatics, Abdomen<br>7 Lymphatics, Pelvis<br>8 Lymphatics, Inguinal | 9 High Dose Rate (HDR)<br>B Low Dose Rate (LDR) | 7 Cesium 137 (Cs-137)<br>8 Iridium 192 (Ir-192)<br>9 Iodine 125 (I-125)<br>B Palladium 103 (Pd-103)<br>C Californium 252 (Cf-252)<br>Y Other Isotope | Z None |

**D Radiation Therapy**
**7 Lymphatic and Hematologic System**
**2 Stereotactic Radiosurgery**

| Character 4 Treatment Site | Character 5 Modality Qualifier | Character 6 Isotope | Character 7 Qualifier |
|---|---|---|---|
| 0 Bone Marrow<br>1 Thymus<br>2 Spleen<br>3 Lymphatics, Neck<br>4 Lymphatics, Axillary<br>5 Lymphatics, Thorax<br>6 Lymphatics, Abdomen<br>7 Lymphatics, Pelvis<br>8 Lymphatics, Inguinal | D Stereotactic Other Photon Radiosurgery<br>H Stereotactic Particulate Radiosurgery<br>J Stereotactic Gamma Beam Radiosurgery | Z None | Z None |

**D Radiation Therapy**
**7 Lymphatic and Hematologic System**
**Y Other Radiation**

| Character 4 Treatment Site | Character 5 Modality Qualifier | Character 6 Isotope | Character 7 Qualifier |
|---|---|---|---|
| 0 Bone Marrow<br>1 Thymus<br>2 Spleen<br>3 Lymphatics, Neck<br>4 Lymphatics, Axillary<br>5 Lymphatics, Thorax<br>6 Lymphatics, Abdomen<br>7 Lymphatics, Pelvis<br>8 Lymphatics, Inguinal | 8 Hyperthermia<br>F Plaque Radiation | Z None | Z None |

**D Radiation Therapy**
**8 Eye**
**0 Beam Radiation**

| Character 4<br>Treatment Site | Character 5<br>Modality Qualifier | Character 6<br>Isotope | Character 7<br>Qualifier |
|---|---|---|---|
| 0 Eye | 0 Photons <1 MeV<br>1 Photons 1 - 10 MeV<br>2 Photons >10 MeV<br>4 Heavy Particles (Protons,Ions)<br>5 Neutrons<br>6 Neutron Capture | Z None | Z None |
| 0 Eye | 3 Electrons | Z None | 0 Intraoperative<br>Z None |

**D Radiation Therapy**
**8 Eye**
**1 Brachytherapy**

| Character 4<br>Treatment Site | Character 5<br>Modality Qualifier | Character 6<br>Isotope | Character 7<br>Qualifier |
|---|---|---|---|
| 0 Eye | 9 High Dose Rate (HDR)<br>B Low Dose Rate (LDR) | 7 Cesium 137 (Cs-137)<br>8 Iridium 192 (Ir-192)<br>9 Iodine 125 (I-125)<br>B Palladium 103 (Pd-103)<br>C Californium 252 (Cf-252)<br>Y Other Isotope | Z None |

**D Radiation Therapy**
**8 Eye**
**2 Stereotactic Radiosurgery**

| Character 4<br>Treatment Site | Character 5<br>Modality Qualifier | Character 6<br>Isotope | Character 7<br>Qualifier |
|---|---|---|---|
| 0 Eye | D Stereotactic Other Photon<br>Radiosurgery<br>H Stereotactic Particulate Radiosurgery<br>J Stereotactic Gamma Beam<br>Radiosurgery | Z None | Z None |

**D Radiation Therapy**
**8 Eye**
**Y Other Radiation**

| Character 4<br>Treatment Site | Character 5<br>Modality Qualifier | Character 6<br>Isotope | Character 7<br>Qualifier |
|---|---|---|---|
| 0 Eye | 7 Contact Radiation<br>8 Hyperthermia<br>F Plaque Radiation | Z None | Z None |

**D Radiation Therapy**
**9 Ear, Nose, Mouth and Throat**
**0 Beam Radiation**

| Character 4<br>Treatment Site | Character 5<br>Modality Qualifier | Character 6<br>Isotope | Character 7<br>Qualifier |
|---|---|---|---|
| 0 Ear<br>1 Nose<br>3 Hypopharynx<br>4 Mouth<br>5 Tongue<br>6 Salivary Glands<br>7 Sinuses<br>8 Hard Palate<br>9 Soft Palate<br>B Larynx<br>D Nasopharynx<br>F Oropharynx | 0 Photons <1 MeV<br>1 Photons 1 - 10 MeV<br>2 Photons >10 MeV<br>4 Heavy Particles (Protons,Ions)<br>5 Neutrons<br>6 Neutron Capture | Z None | Z None |
| 0 Ear<br>1 Nose<br>3 Hypopharynx<br>4 Mouth<br>5 Tongue<br>6 Salivary Glands<br>7 Sinuses<br>8 Hard Palate<br>9 Soft Palate<br>B Larynx<br>D Nasopharynx<br>F Oropharynx | 3 Electrons | Z None | 0 Intraoperative<br>Z None |

**D Radiation Therapy**
**9 Ear, Nose, Mouth and Throat**
**1 Brachytherapy**

| Character 4<br>Treatment Site | Character 5<br>Modality Qualifier | Character 6<br>Isotope | Character 7<br>Qualifier |
|---|---|---|---|
| 0 Ear<br>1 Nose<br>3 Hypopharynx<br>4 Mouth<br>5 Tongue<br>6 Salivary Glands<br>7 Sinuses<br>8 Hard Palate<br>9 Soft Palate<br>B Larynx<br>D Nasopharynx<br>F Oropharynx | 9 High Dose Rate (HDR)<br>B Low Dose Rate (LDR) | 7 Cesium 137 (Cs-137)<br>8 Iridium 192 (Ir-192)<br>9 Iodine 125 (I-125)<br>B Palladium 103 (Pd-103)<br>C Californium 252 (Cf-252)<br>Y Other Isotope | Z None |

**D Radiation Therapy**
**9 Ear, Nose, Mouth and Throat**
**2 Stereotactic Radiosurgery**

| Character 4<br>Treatment Site | Character 5<br>Modality Qualifier | Character 6<br>Isotope | Character 7<br>Qualifier |
|---|---|---|---|
| 0 Ear<br>1 Nose<br>4 Mouth<br>5 Tongue<br>6 Salivary Glands<br>7 Sinuses<br>8 Hard Palate<br>9 Soft Palate<br>B Larynx<br>C Pharynx<br>D Nasopharynx | D Stereotactic Other Photon<br>   Radiosurgery<br>H Stereotactic Particulate Radiosurgery<br>J Stereotactic Gamma Beam<br>   Radiosurgery | Z None | Z None |

**D Radiation Therapy**
**9 Ear, Nose, Mouth and Throat**
**Y Other Radiation**

| Character 4<br>Treatment Site | Character 5<br>Modality Qualifier | Character 6<br>Isotope | Character 7<br>Qualifier |
|---|---|---|---|
| 0 Ear<br>1 Nose<br>5 Tongue<br>6 Salivary Glands<br>7 Sinuses<br>8 Hard Palate<br>9 Soft Palate | 7 Contact Radiation<br>8 Hyperthermia<br>F Plaque Radiation | Z None | Z None |
| 3 Hypopharynx<br>F Oropharynx | 7 Contact Radiation<br>8 Hyperthermia | Z None | Z None |
| 4 Mouth<br>B Larynx<br>D Nasopharynx | 7 Contact Radiation<br>8 Hyperthermia<br>C Intraoperative Radiation Therapy<br>  (IORT)<br>F Plaque Radiation | Z None | Z None |
| C Pharynx | C Intraoperative Radiation Therapy<br>  (IORT)<br>F Plaque Radiation | Z None | Z None |

**D Radiation Therapy**
**B Respiratory System**
**0 Beam Radiation**

| Character 4<br>Treatment Site | Character 5<br>Modality Qualifier | Character 6<br>Isotope | Character 7<br>Qualifier |
|---|---|---|---|
| 0 Trachea<br>1 Bronchus<br>2 Lung<br>5 Pleura<br>6 Mediastinum<br>7 Chest Wall<br>8 Diaphragm | 0 Photons <1 MeV<br>1 Photons 1 - 10 MeV<br>2 Photons >10 MeV<br>4 Heavy Particles (Protons,Ions)<br>5 Neutrons<br>6 Neutron Capture | Z None | Z None |
| 0 Trachea<br>1 Bronchus<br>2 Lung<br>5 Pleura<br>6 Mediastinum<br>7 Chest Wall<br>8 Diaphragm | 3 Electrons | Z None | 0 Intraoperative<br>Z None |

**D Radiation Therapy**
**B Respiratory System**
**1 Brachytherapy**

| Character 4<br>Treatment Site | Character 5<br>Modality Qualifier | Character 6<br>Isotope | Character 7<br>Qualifier |
|---|---|---|---|
| 0 Trachea<br>1 Bronchus<br>2 Lung<br>5 Pleura<br>6 Mediastinum<br>7 Chest Wall<br>8 Diaphragm | 9 High Dose Rate (HDR)<br>B Low Dose Rate (LDR) | 7 Cesium 137 (Cs-137)<br>8 Iridium 192 (Ir-192)<br>9 Iodine 125 (I-125)<br>B Palladium 103 (Pd-103)<br>C Californium 252 (Cf-252)<br>Y Other Isotope | Z None |

**D Radiation Therapy**
**B Respiratory System**
**2 Stereotactic Radiosurgery**

| Character 4<br>Treatment Site | Character 5<br>Modality Qualifier | Character 6<br>Isotope | Character 7<br>Qualifier |
|---|---|---|---|
| 0 Trachea<br>1 Bronchus<br>2 Lung<br>5 Pleura<br>6 Mediastinum<br>7 Chest Wall<br>8 Diaphragm | D Stereotactic Other Photon<br>   Radiosurgery<br>H Stereotactic Particulate Radiosurgery<br>J Stereotactic Gamma Beam<br>   Radiosurgery | Z None | Z None |

**D Radiation Therapy**
**B Respiratory System**
**Y Other Radiation**

| Character 4<br>Treatment Site | Character 5<br>Modality Qualifier | Character 6<br>Isotope | Character 7<br>Qualifier |
|---|---|---|---|
| 0 Trachea<br>1 Bronchus<br>2 Lung<br>5 Pleura<br>6 Mediastinum<br>7 Chest Wall<br>8 Diaphragm | 7 Contact Radiation<br>8 Hyperthermia<br>F Plaque Radiation<br>K Laser Interstitial Thermal Therapy | Z None | Z None |

**D Radiation Therapy**
**D Gastrointestinal System**
**0 Beam Radiation**

| Character 4<br>Treatment Site | Character 5<br>Modality Qualifier | Character 6<br>Isotope | Character 7<br>Qualifier |
|---|---|---|---|
| 0 Esophagus<br>1 Stomach<br>2 Duodenum<br>3 Jejunum<br>4 Ileum<br>5 Colon<br>7 Rectum | 0 Photons <1 MeV<br>1 Photons 1 - 10 MeV<br>2 Photons >10 MeV<br>4 Heavy Particles (Protons,Ions)<br>5 Neutrons<br>6 Neutron Capture | Z None | Z None |
| 0 Esophagus<br>1 Stomach<br>2 Duodenum<br>3 Jejunum<br>4 Ileum<br>5 Colon<br>7 Rectum | 3 Electrons | Z None | 0 Intraoperative<br>Z None |

**D Radiation Therapy**
**D Gastrointestinal System**
**1 Brachytherapy**

| Character 4<br>Treatment Site | Character 5<br>Modality Qualifier | Character 6<br>Isotope | Character 7<br>Qualifier |
|---|---|---|---|
| 0 Esophagus<br>1 Stomach<br>2 Duodenum<br>3 Jejunum<br>4 Ileum<br>5 Colon<br>7 Rectum | 9 High Dose Rate (HDR)<br>B Low Dose Rate (LDR) | 7 Cesium 137 (Cs-137)<br>8 Iridium 192 (Ir-192)<br>9 Iodine 125 (I-125)<br>B Palladium 103 (Pd-103)<br>C Californium 252 (Cf-252)<br>Y Other Isotope | Z None |

**D** Radiation Therapy
**D** Gastrointestinal System
**2** Stereotactic Radiosurgery

| Character 4 Treatment Site | Character 5 Modality Qualifier | Character 6 Isotope | Character 7 Qualifier |
|---|---|---|---|
| 0 Esophagus<br>1 Stomach<br>2 Duodenum<br>3 Jejunum<br>4 Ileum<br>5 Colon<br>7 Rectum | D Stereotactic Other Photon<br>   Radiosurgery<br>H Stereotactic Particulate Radiosurgery<br>J Stereotactic Gamma Beam<br>   Radiosurgery | Z None | Z None |

**D** Radiation Therapy
**D** Gastrointestinal System
**Y** Other Radiation

| Character 4 Treatment Site | Character 5 Modality Qualifier | Character 6 Isotope | Character 7 Qualifier |
|---|---|---|---|
| 0 Esophagus | 7 Contact Radiation<br>8 Hyperthermia<br>F Plaque Radiation<br>K Laser Interstitial Thermal Therapy | Z None | Z None |
| 1 Stomach<br>2 Duodenum<br>3 Jejunum<br>4 Ileum<br>5 Colon<br>7 Rectum | 7 Contact Radiation<br>8 Hyperthermia<br>C Intraoperative Radiation Therapy<br>   (IORT)<br>F Plaque Radiation<br>K Laser Interstitial Thermal Therapy | Z None | Z None |
| 8 Anus | C Intraoperative Radiation Therapy<br>   (IORT)<br>F Plaque Radiation<br>K Laser Interstitial Thermal Therapy | Z None | Z None |

**D** Radiation Therapy
**F** Hepatobiliary System and Pancreas
**0** Beam Radiation

| Character 4 Treatment Site | Character 5 Modality Qualifier | Character 6 Isotope | Character 7 Qualifier |
|---|---|---|---|
| 0 Liver<br>1 Gallbladder<br>2 Bile Ducts<br>3 Pancreas | 0 Photons <1 MeV<br>1 Photons 1 - 10 MeV<br>2 Photons >10 MeV<br>4 Heavy Particles (Protons,Ions)<br>5 Neutrons<br>6 Neutron Capture | Z None | Z None |
| 0 Liver<br>1 Gallbladder<br>2 Bile Ducts<br>3 Pancreas | 3 Electrons | Z None | 0 Intraoperative<br>Z None |

**D** Radiation Therapy
**F** Hepatobiliary System and Pancreas
**1** Brachytherapy

| Character 4 Treatment Site | Character 5 Modality Qualifier | Character 6 Isotope | Character 7 Qualifier |
|---|---|---|---|
| 0 Liver<br>1 Gallbladder<br>2 Bile Ducts<br>3 Pancreas | 9 High Dose Rate (HDR)<br>B Low Dose Rate (LDR) | 7 Cesium 137 (Cs-137)<br>8 Iridium 192 (Ir-192)<br>9 Iodine 125 (I-125)<br>B Palladium 103 (Pd-103)<br>C Californium 252 (Cf-252)<br>Y Other Isotope | Z None |

**D** Radiation Therapy
**F** Hepatobiliary System and Pancreas
**2** Stereotactic Radiosurgery

| Character 4<br>Treatment Site | Character 5<br>Modality Qualifier | Character 6<br>Isotope | Character 7<br>Qualifier |
|---|---|---|---|
| 0 Liver<br>1 Gallbladder<br>2 Bile Ducts<br>3 Pancreas | D Stereotactic Other Photon<br>Radiosurgery<br>H Stereotactic Particulate Radiosurgery<br>J Stereotactic Gamma Beam<br>Radiosurgery | Z None | Z None |

**D** Radiation Therapy
**F** Hepatobiliary System and Pancreas
**Y** Other Radiation

| Character 4<br>Treatment Site | Character 5<br>Modality Qualifier | Character 6<br>Isotope | Character 7<br>Qualifier |
|---|---|---|---|
| 0 Liver<br>1 Gallbladder<br>2 Bile Ducts<br>3 Pancreas | 7 Contact Radiation<br>8 Hyperthermia<br>C Intraoperative Radiation Therapy<br>(IORT)<br>F Plaque Radiation<br>K Laser Interstitial Thermal Therapy | Z None | Z None |

**D** Radiation Therapy
**G** Endocrine System
**0** Beam Radiation

| Character 4<br>Treatment Site | Character 5<br>Modality Qualifier | Character 6<br>Isotope | Character 7<br>Qualifier |
|---|---|---|---|
| 0 Pituitary Gland<br>1 Pineal Body<br>2 Adrenal Glands<br>4 Parathyroid Glands<br>5 Thyroid | 0 Photons <1 MeV<br>1 Photons 1 - 10 MeV<br>2 Photons >10 MeV<br>5 Neutrons<br>6 Neutron Capture | Z None | Z None |
| 0 Pituitary Gland<br>1 Pineal Body<br>2 Adrenal Glands<br>4 Parathyroid Glands<br>5 Thyroid | 3 Electrons | Z None | 0 Intraoperative<br>Z None |

**D** Radiation Therapy
**G** Endocrine System
**1** Brachytherapy

| Character 4<br>Treatment Site | Character 5<br>Modality Qualifier | Character 6<br>Isotope | Character 7<br>Qualifier |
|---|---|---|---|
| 0 Pituitary Gland<br>1 Pineal Body<br>2 Adrenal Glands<br>4 Parathyroid Glands<br>5 Thyroid | 9 High Dose Rate (HDR)<br>B Low Dose Rate (LDR) | 7 Cesium 137 (Cs-137)<br>8 Iridium 192 (Ir-192)<br>9 Iodine 125 (I-125)<br>B Palladium 103 (Pd-103)<br>C Californium 252 (Cf-252)<br>Y Other Isotope | Z None |

**D** Radiation Therapy
**G** Endocrine System
**2** Stereotactic Radiosurgery

| Character 4<br>Treatment Site | Character 5<br>Modality Qualifier | Character 6<br>Isotope | Character 7<br>Qualifier |
|---|---|---|---|
| 0 Pituitary Gland<br>1 Pineal Body<br>2 Adrenal Glands<br>4 Parathyroid Glands<br>5 Thyroid | D Stereotactic Other Photon<br>Radiosurgery<br>H Stereotactic Particulate Radiosurgery<br>J Stereotactic Gamma Beam<br>Radiosurgery | Z None | Z None |

**D** Radiation Therapy
**G** Endocrine System
**Y** Other Radiation

| Character 4<br>Treatment Site | Character 5<br>Modality Qualifier | Character 6<br>Isotope | Character 7<br>Qualifier |
|---|---|---|---|
| 0  Pituitary Gland<br>1  Pineal Body<br>2  Adrenal Glands<br>4  Parathyroid Glands<br>5  Thyroid | 7  Contact Radiation<br>8  Hyperthermia<br>F  Plaque Radiation<br>K  Laser Interstitial Thermal Therapy | Z  None | Z  None |

**D** Radiation Therapy
**H** Skin
**0** Beam Radiation

| Character 4<br>Treatment Site | Character 5<br>Modality Qualifier | Character 6<br>Isotope | Character 7<br>Qualifier |
|---|---|---|---|
| 2  Skin, Face<br>3  Skin, Neck<br>4  Skin, Arm<br>6  Skin, Chest<br>7  Skin, Back<br>8  Skin, Abdomen<br>9  Skin, Buttock<br>B  Skin, Leg | 0  Photons <1 MeV<br>1  Photons 1 - 10 MeV<br>2  Photons >10 MeV<br>4  Heavy Particles (Protons,Ions)<br>5  Neutrons<br>6  Neutron Capture | Z  None | Z  None |
| 2  Skin, Face<br>3  Skin, Neck<br>4  Skin, Arm<br>6  Skin, Chest<br>7  Skin, Back<br>8  Skin, Abdomen<br>9  Skin, Buttock<br>B  Skin, Leg | 3  Electrons | Z  None | 0  Intraoperative<br>Z  None |

**D** Radiation Therapy
**H** Skin
**Y** Other Radiation

| Character 4<br>Treatment Site | Character 5<br>Modality Qualifier | Character 6<br>Isotope | Character 7<br>Qualifier |
|---|---|---|---|
| 2  Skin, Face<br>3  Skin, Neck<br>4  Skin, Arm<br>6  Skin, Chest<br>7  Skin, Back<br>8  Skin, Abdomen<br>9  Skin, Buttock<br>B  Skin, Leg | 7  Contact Radiation<br>8  Hyperthermia<br>F  Plaque Radiation | Z  None | Z  None |
| 5  Skin, Hand<br>C  Skin, Foot | F  Plaque Radiation | Z  None | Z  None |

**D** Radiation Therapy
**M** Breast
**0** Beam Radiation

| Character 4<br>Treatment Site | Character 5<br>Modality Qualifier | Character 6<br>Isotope | Character 7<br>Qualifier |
|---|---|---|---|
| 0  Breast, Left<br>1  Breast, Right | 0  Photons <1 MeV<br>1  Photons 1 - 10 MeV<br>2  Photons >10 MeV<br>4  Heavy Particles (Protons,Ions)<br>5  Neutrons<br>6  Neutron Capture | Z  None | Z  None |
| 0  Breast, Left<br>1  Breast, Right | 3  Electrons | Z  None | 0  Intraoperative<br>Z  None |

**D  Radiation Therapy**
**M  Breast**
**1  Brachytherapy**

| Character 4 Treatment Site | Character 5 Modality Qualifier | Character 6 Isotope | Character 7 Qualifier |
|---|---|---|---|
| 0  Breast, Left<br>1  Breast, Right | 9  High Dose Rate (HDR)<br>B  Low Dose Rate (LDR) | 7  Cesium 137 (Cs-137)<br>8  Iridium 192 (Ir-192)<br>9  Iodine 125 (I-125)<br>B  Palladium 103 (Pd-103)<br>C  Californium 252 (Cf-252)<br>Y  Other Isotope | Z  None |

**D  Radiation Therapy**
**M  Breast**
**2  Stereotactic Radiosurgery**

| Character 4 Treatment Site | Character 5 Modality Qualifier | Character 6 Isotope | Character 7 Qualifier |
|---|---|---|---|
| 0  Breast, Left<br>1  Breast, Right | D  Stereotactic Other Photon Radiosurgery<br>H  Stereotactic Particulate Radiosurgery<br>J  Stereotactic Gamma Beam Radiosurgery | Z  None | Z  None |

**D  Radiation Therapy**
**M  Breast**
**Y  Other Radiation**

| Character 4 Treatment Site | Character 5 Modality Qualifier | Character 6 Isotope | Character 7 Qualifier |
|---|---|---|---|
| 0  Breast, Left<br>1  Breast, Right | 7  Contact Radiation<br>8  Hyperthermia<br>F  Plaque Radiation<br>K  Laser Interstitial Thermal Therapy | Z  None | Z  None |

**D  Radiation Therapy**
**P  Musculoskeletal System**
**0  Beam Radiation**

| Character 4 Treatment Site | Character 5 Modality Qualifier | Character 6 Isotope | Character 7 Qualifier |
|---|---|---|---|
| 0  Skull<br>2  Maxilla<br>3  Mandible<br>4  Sternum<br>5  Rib(s)<br>6  Humerus<br>7  Radius/Ulna<br>8  Pelvic Bones<br>9  Femur<br>B  Tibia/Fibula<br>C  Other Bone | 0  Photons <1 MeV<br>1  Photons 1 - 10 MeV<br>2  Photons >10 MeV<br>4  Heavy Particles (Protons,Ions)<br>5  Neutrons<br>6  Neutron Capture | Z  None | Z  None |
| 0  Skull<br>2  Maxilla<br>3  Mandible<br>4  Sternum<br>5  Rib(s)<br>6  Humerus<br>7  Radius/Ulna<br>8  Pelvic Bones<br>9  Femur<br>B  Tibia/Fibula<br>C  Other Bone | 3  Electrons | Z  None | 0  Intraoperative<br>Z  None |

**D** Radiation Therapy
**P** Musculoskeletal System
**Y** Other Radiation

| Character 4 Treatment Site | Character 5 Modality Qualifier | Character 6 Isotope | Character 7 Qualifier |
|---|---|---|---|
| 0 Skull | 7 Contact Radiation | Z None | Z None |
| 2 Maxilla | 8 Hyperthermia | | |
| 3 Mandible | F Plaque Radiation | | |
| 4 Sternum | | | |
| 5 Rib(s) | | | |
| 6 Humerus | | | |
| 7 Radius/Ulna | | | |
| 8 Pelvic Bones | | | |
| 9 Femur | | | |
| B Tibia/Fibula | | | |
| C Other Bone | | | |

**D** Radiation Therapy
**T** Urinary System
**0** Beam Radiation

| Character 4 Treatment Site | Character 5 Modality Qualifier | Character 6 Isotope | Character 7 Qualifier |
|---|---|---|---|
| 0 Kidney | 0 Photons <1 MeV | Z None | Z None |
| 1 Ureter | 1 Photons 1 - 10 MeV | | |
| 2 Bladder | 2 Photons >10 MeV | | |
| 3 Urethra | 4 Heavy Particles (Protons,Ions) | | |
| | 5 Neutrons | | |
| | 6 Neutron Capture | | |
| 0 Kidney | 3 Electrons | Z None | 0 Intraoperative |
| 1 Ureter | | | Z None |
| 2 Bladder | | | |
| 3 Urethra | | | |

**D** Radiation Therapy
**T** Urinary System
**1** Brachytherapy

| Character 4 Treatment Site | Character 5 Modality Qualifier | Character 6 Isotope | Character 7 Qualifier |
|---|---|---|---|
| 0 Kidney | 9 High Dose Rate (HDR) | 7 Cesium 137 (Cs-137) | Z None |
| 1 Ureter | B Low Dose Rate (LDR) | 8 Iridium 192 (Ir-192) | |
| 2 Bladder | | 9 Iodine 125 (I-125) | |
| 3 Urethra | | B Palladium 103 (Pd-103) | |
| | | C Californium 252 (Cf-252) | |
| | | Y Other Isotope | |

**D** Radiation Therapy
**T** Urinary System
**2** Stereotactic Radiosurgery

| Character 4 Treatment Site | Character 5 Modality Qualifier | Character 6 Isotope | Character 7 Qualifier |
|---|---|---|---|
| 0 Kidney | D Stereotactic Other Photon Radiosurgery | Z None | Z None |
| 1 Ureter | H Stereotactic Particulate Radiosurgery | | |
| 2 Bladder | J Stereotactic Gamma Beam Radiosurgery | | |
| 3 Urethra | | | |

**D  Radiation Therapy**
**T  Urinary System**
**Y  Other Radiation**

| Character 4<br>Treatment Site | Character 5<br>Modality Qualifier | Character 6<br>Isotope | Character 7<br>Qualifier |
|---|---|---|---|
| 0  Kidney<br>1  Ureter<br>2  Bladder<br>3  Urethra | 7  Contact Radiation<br>8  Hyperthermia<br>C  Intraoperative Radiation Therapy<br>   (IORT)<br>F  Plaque Radiation | Z  None | Z  None |

**D  Radiation Therapy**
**U  Female Reproductive System**
**0  Beam Radiation**

| Character 4<br>Treatment Site | Character 5<br>Modality Qualifier | Character 6<br>Isotope | Character 7<br>Qualifier |
|---|---|---|---|
| 0  Ovary ♀<br>1  Cervix ♀<br>2  Uterus ♀ | 0  Photons <1 MeV<br>1  Photons 1 - 10 MeV<br>2  Photons >10 MeV<br>4  Heavy Particles (Protons,Ions)<br>5  Neutrons<br>6  Neutron Capture | Z  None | Z  None |
| 0  Ovary ♀<br>1  Cervix ♀<br>2  Uterus ♀ | 3  Electrons | Z  None | 0  Intraoperative<br>Z  None |

**D  Radiation Therapy**
**U  Female Reproductive System**
**1  Brachytherapy**

| Character 4<br>Treatment Site | Character 5<br>Modality Qualifier | Character 6<br>Isotope | Character 7<br>Qualifier |
|---|---|---|---|
| 0  Ovary ♀<br>1  Cervix ♀<br>2  Uterus ♀ | 9  High Dose Rate (HDR)<br>B  Low Dose Rate (LDR) | 7  Cesium 137 (Cs-137)<br>8  Iridium 192 (Ir-192)<br>9  Iodine 125 (I-125)<br>B  Palladium 103 (Pd-103)<br>C  Californium 252 (Cf-252)<br>Y  Other Isotope | Z  None |

**D  Radiation Therapy**
**U  Female Reproductive System**
**2  Stereotactic Radiosurgery**

| Character 4<br>Treatment Site | Character 5<br>Modality Qualifier | Character 6<br>Isotope | Character 7<br>Qualifier |
|---|---|---|---|
| 0  Ovary ♀<br>1  Cervix ♀<br>2  Uterus ♀ | D  Stereotactic Other Photon<br>   Radiosurgery<br>H  Stereotactic Particulate Radiosurgery<br>J  Stereotactic Gamma Beam<br>   Radiosurgery | Z  None | Z  None |

**D  Radiation Therapy**
**U  Female Reproductive System**
**Y  Other Radiation**

| Character 4<br>Treatment Site | Character 5<br>Modality Qualifier | Character 6<br>Isotope | Character 7<br>Qualifier |
|---|---|---|---|
| 0  Ovary ♀<br>1  Cervix ♀<br>2  Uterus ♀ | 7  Contact Radiation<br>8  Hyperthermia<br>C  Intraoperative Radiation Therapy<br>   (IORT)<br>F  Plaque Radiation | Z  None | Z  None |

**D Radiation Therapy**
**V Male Reproductive System**
**0 Beam Radiation**

| Character 4<br>Treatment Site | Character 5<br>Modality Qualifier | Character 6<br>Isotope | Character 7<br>Qualifier |
|---|---|---|---|
| 0 Prostate ♂<br>1 Testis ♂ | 0 Photons <1 MeV<br>1 Photons 1 - 10 MeV<br>2 Photons >10 MeV<br>4 Heavy Particles (Protons,Ions)<br>5 Neutrons<br>6 Neutron Capture | Z None | Z None |
| 0 Prostate ♂<br>1 Testis ♂ | 3 Electrons | Z None | 0 Intraoperative<br>Z None |

**D Radiation Therapy**
**V Male Reproductive System**
**1 Brachytherapy**

| Character 4<br>Treatment Site | Character 5<br>Modality Qualifier | Character 6<br>Isotope | Character 7<br>Qualifier |
|---|---|---|---|
| 0 Prostate ♂<br>1 Testis ♂ | 9 High Dose Rate (HDR)<br>B Low Dose Rate (LDR) | 7 Cesium 137 (Cs-137)<br>8 Iridium 192 (Ir-192)<br>9 Iodine 125 (I-125)<br>B Palladium 103 (Pd-103)<br>C Californium 252 (Cf-252)<br>Y Other Isotope | Z None |

**D Radiation Therapy**
**V Male Reproductive System**
**2 Stereotactic Radiosurgery**

| Character 4<br>Treatment Site | Character 5<br>Modality Qualifier | Character 6<br>Isotope | Character 7<br>Qualifier |
|---|---|---|---|
| 0 Prostate ♂<br>1 Testis ♂ | D Stereotactic Other Photon<br>  Radiosurgery<br>H Stereotactic Particulate Radiosurgery<br>J Stereotactic Gamma Beam<br>  Radiosurgery | Z None | Z None |

**D Radiation Therapy**
**V Male Reproductive System**
**Y Other Radiation**

| Character 4<br>Treatment Site | Character 5<br>Modality Qualifier | Character 6<br>Isotope | Character 7<br>Qualifier |
|---|---|---|---|
| 0 Prostate ♂ | 7 Contact Radiation<br>8 Hyperthermia<br>C Intraoperative Radiation Therapy<br>  (IORT)<br>F Plaque Radiation<br>K Laser Interstitial Thermal Therapy | Z None | Z None |
| 1 Testis ♂ | 7 Contact Radiation<br>8 Hyperthermia<br>F Plaque Radiation | Z None | Z None |

**D Radiation Therapy**
**W Anatomical Regions**
**0 Beam Radiation**

| Character 4<br>Treatment Site | Character 5<br>Modality Qualifier | Character 6<br>Isotope | Character 7<br>Qualifier |
|---|---|---|---|
| 1 Head and Neck<br>2 Chest<br>3 Abdomen<br>4 Hemibody<br>5 Whole Body<br>6 Pelvic Region | 0 Photons <1 MeV<br>1 Photons 1 - 10 MeV<br>2 Photons >10 MeV<br>4 Heavy Particles (Protons,Ions)<br>5 Neutrons<br>6 Neutron Capture | Z None | Z None |
| 1 Head and Neck<br>2 Chest<br>3 Abdomen<br>4 Hemibody<br>5 Whole Body<br>6 Pelvic Region | 3 Electrons | Z None | 0 Intraoperative<br>Z None |

**D Radiation Therapy**
**W Anatomical Regions**
**1 Brachytherapy**

| Character 4<br>Treatment Site | Character 5<br>Modality Qualifier | Character 6<br>Isotope | Character 7<br>Qualifier |
|---|---|---|---|
| 1 Head and Neck<br>2 Chest<br>3 Abdomen<br>6 Pelvic Region | 9 High Dose Rate (HDR)<br>B Low Dose Rate (LDR) | 7 Cesium 137 (Cs-137)<br>8 Iridium 192 (Ir-192)<br>9 Iodine 125 (I-125)<br>B Palladium 103 (Pd-103)<br>C Californium 252 (Cf-252)<br>Y Other Isotope | Z None |

**D Radiation Therapy**
**W Anatomical Regions**
**2 Stereotactic Radiosurgery**

| Character 4<br>Treatment Site | Character 5<br>Modality Qualifier | Character 6<br>Isotope | Character 7<br>Qualifier |
|---|---|---|---|
| 1 Head and Neck<br>2 Chest<br>3 Abdomen<br>6 Pelvic Region | D Stereotactic Other Photon<br>Radiosurgery<br>H Stereotactic Particulate Radiosurgery<br>J Stereotactic Gamma Beam<br>Radiosurgery | Z None | Z None |

**D Radiation Therapy**
**W Anatomical Regions**
**Y Other Radiation**

| Character 4<br>Treatment Site | Character 5<br>Modality Qualifier | Character 6<br>Isotope | Character 7<br>Qualifier |
|---|---|---|---|
| 1 Head and Neck<br>2 Chest<br>3 Abdomen<br>4 Hemibody<br>6 Pelvic Region | 7 Contact Radiation<br>8 Hyperthermia<br>F Plaque Radiation | Z None | Z None |
| 5 Whole Body | 7 Contact Radiation<br>8 Hyperthermia<br>F Plaque Radiation | Z None | Z None |
| 5 Whole Body | G Isotope Administration | D Iodine 131 (I-131)<br>F Phosphorus 32 (P-32)<br>G Strontium 89 (Sr-89)<br>H Strontium 90 (Sr-90)<br>Y Other Isotope | Z None |

# Physical Rehabilitation and Diagnostic Audiology | F00-F15

**F** Physical Rehabilitation and Diagnostic Audiology
**0** Rehabilitation
**0** Speech Assessment: Measurement of speech and related functions

| Character 4<br>Body System / Region | Character 5<br>Type Qualifier | Character 6<br>Equipment | Character 7<br>Qualifier |
|---|---|---|---|
| 3 Neurological System - Whole Body | G Communicative/Cognitive Integration Skills | K Audiovisual<br>M Augmentative / Alternative Communication<br>P Computer<br>Y Other Equipment<br>Z None | Z None |
| Z None | 0 Filtered Speech<br>3 Staggered Spondaic Word<br>Q Performance Intensity Phonetically Balanced Speech Discrimination<br>R Brief Tone Stimuli<br>S Distorted Speech<br>T Dichotic Stimuli<br>V Temporal Ordering of Stimuli<br>W Masking Patterns | 1 Audiometer<br>2 Sound Field / Booth<br>K Audiovisual<br>Z None | Z None |
| Z None | 1 Speech Threshold<br>2 Speech/Word Recognition | 1 Audiometer<br>2 Sound Field / Booth<br>9 Cochlear Implant<br>K Audiovisual<br>Z None | Z None |
| Z None | 4 Sensorineural Acuity Level | 1 Audiometer<br>2 Sound Field / Booth<br>Z None | Z None |
| Z None | 5 Synthetic Sentence Identification | 1 Audiometer<br>2 Sound Field / Booth<br>9 Cochlear Implant<br>K Audiovisual | Z None |
| Z None | 6 Speech and/or Language Screening<br>7 Nonspoken Language<br>8 Receptive/Expressive Language<br>C Aphasia<br>G Communicative/Cognitive Integration Skills<br>L Augmentative/Alternative Communication System | K Audiovisual<br>M Augmentative / Alternative Communication<br>P Computer<br>Y Other Equipment<br>Z None | Z None |
| Z None | 9 Articulation/Phonology | K Audiovisual<br>P Computer<br>Q Speech Analysis<br>Y Other Equipment<br>Z None | Z None |
| Z None | B Motor Speech | K Audiovisual<br>N Biosensory Feedback<br>P Computer<br>Q Speech Analysis<br>T Aerodynamic Function<br>Y Other Equipment<br>Z None | Z None |
| Z None | D Fluency | K Audiovisual<br>N Biosensory Feedback<br>P Computer<br>Q Speech Analysis<br>S Voice Analysis<br>T Aerodynamic Function<br>Y Other Equipment<br>Z None | Z None |
| Z None | F Voice | K Audiovisual<br>N Biosensory Feedback<br>P Computer<br>S Voice Analysis<br>T Aerodynamic Function<br>Y Other Equipment<br>Z None | Z None |
| Z None | H Bedside Swallowing and Oral Function<br>P Oral Peripheral Mechanism | Y Other Equipment<br>Z None | Z None |
| Z None | J Instrumental Swallowing and Oral Function | T Aerodynamic Function<br>W Swallowing<br>Y Other Equipment | Z None |
| Z None | K Orofacial Myofunctional | K Audiovisual<br>P Computer<br>Y Other Equipment<br>Z None | Z None |

**F00** *continues on next page*

**F** Physical Rehabilitation and Diagnostic Audiology – *continued*
**0** Rehabilitation – *continued*
**0** Speech Assessment: Measurement of speech and related functions – *continued*

| Character 4 Body System / Region | Character 5 Type Qualifier | Character 6 Equipment | Character 7 Qualifier |
|---|---|---|---|
| Z None | M Voice Prosthetic | K Audiovisual<br>P Computer<br>S Voice Analysis<br>V Speech Prosthesis<br>Y Other Equipment<br>Z None | Z None |
| Z None | N Non-invasive Instrumental Status | N Biosensory Feedback<br>P Computer<br>Q Speech Analysis<br>S Voice Analysis<br>T Aerodynamic Function<br>Y Other Equipment | Z None |
| Z None | X Other Specified Central Auditory Processing | Z None | Z None |

♂ Male          ♀ Female          N C Non-covered          L C Limited Coverage          **AHA** *AHA Coding Clinic*

**F Physical Rehabilitation and Diagnostic Audiology**
**0 Rehabilitation**
**1 Motor and/or Nerve Function Assessment: Measurement of motor, nerve, and related functions**

| Character 4<br>Body System / Region | Character 5<br>Type Qualifier | Character 6<br>Equipment | Character 7<br>Qualifier |
|---|---|---|---|
| 0 Neurological System - Head and Neck<br>1 Neurological System - Upper Back /<br>Upper Extremity<br>2 Neurological System - Lower Back /<br>Lower Extremity<br>3 Neurological System - Whole Body | 0 Muscle Performance | E Orthosis<br>F Assistive, Adaptive, Supportive or<br>Protective<br>U Prosthesis<br>Y Other Equipment<br>Z None | Z None |
| 0 Neurological System - Head and Neck<br>1 Neurological System - Upper Back /<br>Upper Extremity<br>2 Neurological System - Lower Back /<br>Lower Extremity<br>3 Neurological System - Whole Body | 1 Integumentary Integrity<br>3 Coordination/Dexterity<br>4 Motor Function<br>G Reflex Integrity | Z None | Z None |
| 0 Neurological System - Head and Neck<br>1 Neurological System - Upper Back /<br>Upper Extremity<br>2 Neurological System - Lower Back /<br>Lower Extremity<br>3 Neurological System - Whole Body | 5 Range of Motion and Joint Integrity<br>6 Sensory<br>Awareness/Processing/Integrity | Y Other Equipment<br>Z None | Z None |
| D Integumentary System - Head and<br>Neck<br>F Integumentary System - Upper Back /<br>Upper Extremity<br>G Integumentary System - Lower Back /<br>Lower Extremity<br>H Integumentary System - Whole Body<br>J Musculoskeletal System - Head and<br>Neck<br>K Musculoskeletal System - Upper Back<br>/ Upper Extremity<br>L Musculoskeletal System - Lower Back<br>/ Lower Extremity<br>M Musculoskeletal System - Whole Body | 0 Muscle Performance | E Orthosis<br>F Assistive, Adaptive, Supportive or<br>Protective<br>U Prosthesis<br>Y Other Equipment<br>Z None | Z None |
| D Integumentary System - Head and<br>Neck<br>F Integumentary System - Upper Back /<br>Upper Extremity<br>G Integumentary System - Lower Back /<br>Lower Extremity<br>H Integumentary System - Whole Body<br>J Musculoskeletal System - Head and<br>Neck<br>K Musculoskeletal System - Upper Back<br>/ Upper Extremity<br>L Musculoskeletal System - Lower Back<br>/ Lower Extremity<br>M Musculoskeletal System - Whole Body | 1 Integumentary Integrity | Z None | Z None |
| D Integumentary System - Head and<br>Neck<br>F Integumentary System - Upper Back /<br>Upper Extremity<br>G Integumentary System - Lower Back /<br>Lower Extremity<br>H Integumentary System - Whole Body<br>J Musculoskeletal System - Head and<br>Neck<br>K Musculoskeletal System - Upper Back<br>/ Upper Extremity<br>L Musculoskeletal System - Lower Back<br>/ Lower Extremity<br>M Musculoskeletal System - Whole Body | 5 Range of Motion and Joint Integrity<br>6 Sensory<br>Awareness/Processing/Integrity | Y Other Equipment<br>Z None | Z None |
| N Genitourinary System | 0 Muscle Performance | E Orthosis<br>F Assistive, Adaptive, Supportive or<br>Protective<br>U Prosthesis<br>Y Other Equipment<br>Z None | Z None |
| Z None | 2 Visual Motor Integration | K Audiovisual<br>M Augmentative / Alternative<br>Communication<br>N Biosensory Feedback<br>P Computer<br>Q Speech Analysis<br>S Voice Analysis<br>Y Other Equipment<br>Z None | Z None |
| Z None | 7 Facial Nerve Function | 7 Electrophysiologic | Z None |

**F01** *continues on next page*

**F** Physical Rehabilitation and Diagnostic Audiology – *continued*
**0** Rehabilitation – *continued*
**1** Motor and/or Nerve Function Assessment: Measurement of motor, nerve, and related functions – *continued*

| Character 4 Body System / Region | Character 5 Type Qualifier | Character 6 Equipment | Character 7 Qualifier |
|---|---|---|---|
| Z None | 9 Somatosensory Evoked Potentials | J Somatosensory | Z None |
| Z None | B Bed Mobility<br>C Transfer<br>F Wheelchair Mobility | E Orthosis<br>F Assistive, Adaptive, Supportive or Protective<br>U Prosthesis<br>Z None | Z None |
| Z None | D Gait and/or Balance | E Orthosis<br>F Assistive, Adaptive, Supportive or Protective<br>U Prosthesis<br>Y Other Equipment<br>Z None | Z None |

**F** Physical Rehabilitation and Diagnostic Audiology
**0** Rehabilitation
**2** Activities of Daily Living Assessment: Measurement of functional level for activities of daily living

| Character 4<br>Body System / Region | Character 5<br>Type Qualifier | Character 6<br>Equipment | Character 7<br>Qualifier |
|---|---|---|---|
| 0 Neurological System - Head and Neck | 9 Cranial Nerve Integrity<br>D Neuromotor Development | Y Other Equipment<br>Z None | Z None |
| 1 Neurological System - Upper Back /<br>Upper Extremity<br>2 Neurological System - Lower Back /<br>Lower Extremity<br>3 Neurological System - Whole Body | D Neuromotor Development | Y Other Equipment<br>Z None | Z None |
| 4 Circulatory System - Head and Neck<br>5 Circulatory System - Upper Back /<br>Upper Extremity<br>6 Circulatory System - Lower Back /<br>Lower Extremity<br>8 Respiratory System - Head and Neck<br>9 Respiratory System - Upper Back /<br>Upper Extremity<br>B Respiratory System - Lower Back /<br>Lower Extremity | G Ventilation, Respiration and<br>Circulation | C Mechanical<br>G Aerobic Endurance and Conditioning<br>Y Other Equipment<br>Z None | Z None |
| 7 Circulatory System - Whole Body<br>C Respiratory System - Whole Body | 7 Aerobic Capacity and Endurance | E Orthosis<br>G Aerobic Endurance and Conditioning<br>U Prosthesis<br>Y Other Equipment<br>Z None | Z None |
| 7 Circulatory System - Whole Body<br>C Respiratory System - Whole Body | G Ventilation, Respiration and<br>Circulation | C Mechanical<br>G Aerobic Endurance and Conditioning<br>Y Other Equipment<br>Z None | Z None |
| Z None | 0 Bathing/Showering<br>1 Dressing<br>3 Grooming/Personal Hygiene<br>4 Home Management | E Orthosis<br>F Assistive, Adaptive, Supportive or<br>Protective<br>U Prosthesis<br>Z None | Z None |
| Z None | 2 Feeding/Eating<br>8 Anthropometric Characteristics<br>F Pain | Y Other Equipment<br>Z None | Z None |
| Z None | 5 Perceptual Processing | K Audiovisual<br>M Augmentative / Alternative<br>Communication<br>N Biosensory Feedback<br>P Computer<br>Q Speech Analysis<br>S Voice Analysis<br>Y Other Equipment<br>Z None | Z None |
| Z None | 6 Psychosocial Skills | Z None | Z None |
| Z None | B Environmental, Home and Work<br>Barriers<br>C Ergonomics and Body Mechanics | E Orthosis<br>F Assistive, Adaptive, Supportive or<br>Protective<br>U Prosthesis<br>Y Other Equipment<br>Z None | Z None |
| Z None | H Vocational Activities and Functional<br>Community or Work Reintegration<br>Skills | E Orthosis<br>F Assistive, Adaptive, Supportive or<br>Protective<br>G Aerobic Endurance and Conditioning<br>U Prosthesis<br>Y Other Equipment<br>Z None | Z None |

| | | | |
|---|---|---|---|
| **F** Physical Rehabilitation and Diagnostic Audiology | | | |
| **0** Rehabilitation | | | |
| **6** Speech Treatment: Application of techniques to improve, augment, or compensate for speech and related functional impairment | | | |
| Character 4 Body System / Region | Character 5 Type Qualifier | Character 6 Equipment | Character 7 Qualifier |
| 3 Neurological System - Whole Body | 6 Communicative/Cognitive Integration Skills | K Audiovisual<br>M Augmentative / Alternative Communication<br>P Computer<br>Y Other Equipment<br>Z None | Z None |
| Z None | 0 Nonspoken Language<br>3 Aphasia<br>6 Communicative/Cognitive Integration Skills | K Audiovisual<br>M Augmentative / Alternative Communication<br>P Computer<br>Y Other Equipment<br>Z None | Z None |
| Z None | 1 Speech-Language Pathology and Related Disorders Counseling<br>2 Speech-Language Pathology and Related Disorders Prevention | K Audiovisual<br>Z None | Z None |
| Z None | 4 Articulation/Phonology | K Audiovisual<br>P Computer<br>Q Speech Analysis<br>T Aerodynamic Function<br>Y Other Equipment<br>Z None | Z None |
| Z None | 5 Aural Rehabilitation | K Audiovisual<br>L Assistive Listening<br>M Augmentative / Alternative Communication<br>N Biosensory Feedback<br>P Computer<br>Q Speech Analysis<br>S Voice Analysis<br>Y Other Equipment<br>Z None | Z None |
| Z None | 7 Fluency | 4 Electroacoustic Immitance / Acoustic Reflex<br>K Audiovisual<br>N Biosensory Feedback<br>Q Speech Analysis<br>S Voice Analysis<br>T Aerodynamic Function<br>Y Other Equipment<br>Z None | Z None |
| Z None | 8 Motor Speech | K Audiovisual<br>N Biosensory Feedback<br>P Computer<br>Q Speech Analysis<br>S Voice Analysis<br>T Aerodynamic Function<br>Y Other Equipment<br>Z None | Z None |
| Z None | 9 Orofacial Myofunctional | K Audiovisual<br>P Computer<br>Y Other Equipment<br>Z None | Z None |
| Z None | B Receptive/Expressive Language | K Audiovisual<br>L Assistive Listening<br>M Augmentative / Alternative Communication<br>P Computer<br>Y Other Equipment<br>Z None | Z None |
| Z None | C Voice | K Audiovisual<br>N Biosensory Feedback<br>P Computer<br>S Voice Analysis<br>T Aerodynamic Function<br>V Speech Prosthesis<br>Y Other Equipment<br>Z None | Z None |
| Z None | D Swallowing Dysfunction | M Augmentative / Alternative Communication<br>T Aerodynamic Function<br>V Speech Prosthesis<br>Y Other Equipment<br>Z None | Z None |

**F** Physical Rehabilitation and Diagnostic Audiology
**0** Rehabilitation
**7** Motor Treatment: Exercise or activities to increase or facilitate motor function

| Character 4<br>Body System / Region | Character 5<br>Type Qualifier | Character 6<br>Equipment | Character 7<br>Qualifier |
|---|---|---|---|
| 0 Neurological System - Head and Neck<br>1 Neurological System - Upper Back /<br>   Upper Extremity<br>2 Neurological System - Lower Back /<br>   Lower Extremity<br>3 Neurological System - Whole Body<br>D Integumentary System - Head and<br>   Neck<br>F Integumentary System - Upper Back /<br>   Upper Extremity<br>G Integumentary System - Lower Back /<br>   Lower Extremity<br>H Integumentary System - Whole Body<br>J Musculoskeletal System - Head and<br>   Neck<br>K Musculoskeletal System - Upper Back<br>   / Upper Extremity<br>L Musculoskeletal System - Lower Back<br>   / Lower Extremity<br>M Musculoskeletal System - Whole Body | 0 Range of Motion and Joint Mobility<br>1 Muscle Performance<br>2 Coordination/Dexterity<br>3 Motor Function | E Orthosis<br>F Assistive, Adaptive, Supportive or<br>   Protective<br>U Prosthesis<br>Y Other Equipment<br>Z None | Z None |
| 0 Neurological System - Head and Neck<br>1 Neurological System - Upper Back /<br>   Upper Extremity<br>2 Neurological System - Lower Back /<br>   Lower Extremity<br>3 Neurological System - Whole Body<br>D Integumentary System - Head and<br>   Neck<br>F Integumentary System - Upper Back /<br>   Upper Extremity<br>G Integumentary System - Lower Back /<br>   Lower Extremity<br>H Integumentary System - Whole Body<br>J Musculoskeletal System - Head and<br>   Neck<br>K Musculoskeletal System - Upper Back<br>   / Upper Extremity<br>L Musculoskeletal System - Lower Back<br>   / Lower Extremity<br>M Musculoskeletal System - Whole Body | 6 Therapeutic Exercise | B Physical Agents<br>C Mechanical<br>D Electrotherapeutic<br>E Orthosis<br>F Assistive, Adaptive, Supportive or<br>   Protective<br>G Aerobic Endurance and Conditioning<br>H Mechanical or Electromechanical<br>U Prosthesis<br>Y Other Equipment<br>Z None | Z None |
| 0 Neurological System - Head and Neck<br>1 Neurological System - Upper Back /<br>   Upper Extremity<br>2 Neurological System - Lower Back /<br>   Lower Extremity<br>3 Neurological System - Whole Body<br>D Integumentary System - Head and<br>   Neck<br>F Integumentary System - Upper Back /<br>   Upper Extremity<br>G Integumentary System - Lower Back /<br>   Lower Extremity<br>H Integumentary System - Whole Body<br>J Musculoskeletal System - Head and<br>   Neck<br>K Musculoskeletal System - Upper Back<br>   / Upper Extremity<br>L Musculoskeletal System - Lower Back<br>   / Lower Extremity<br>M Musculoskeletal System - Whole Body | 7 Manual Therapy Techniques | Z None | Z None |
| 4 Circulatory System - Head and Neck<br>5 Circulatory System - Upper Back /<br>   Upper Extremity<br>6 Circulatory System - Lower Back /<br>   Lower Extremity<br>7 Circulatory System - Whole Body<br>8 Respiratory System - Head and Neck<br>9 Respiratory System - Upper Back /<br>   Upper Extremity<br>B Respiratory System - Lower Back /<br>   Lower Extremity<br>C Respiratory System - Whole Body | 6 Therapeutic Exercise | B Physical Agents<br>C Mechanical<br>D Electrotherapeutic<br>E Orthosis<br>F Assistive, Adaptive, Supportive or<br>   Protective<br>G Aerobic Endurance and Conditioning<br>H Mechanical or Electromechanical<br>U Prosthesis<br>Y Other Equipment<br>Z None | Z None |
| N Genitourinary System | 1 Muscle Performance | E Orthosis<br>F Assistive, Adaptive, Supportive or<br>   Protective<br>U Prosthesis<br>Y Other Equipment<br>Z None | Z None |

**F07** continues on next page

**F** Physical Rehabilitation and Diagnostic Audiology – *continued*
**0** Rehabilitation – *continued*
**7** Motor Treatment: Exercise or activities to increase or facilitate motor function – *continued*

| Character 4 Body System / Region | Character 5 Type Qualifier | Character 6 Equipment | Character 7 Qualifier |
|---|---|---|---|
| N Genitourinary System | 6 Therapeutic Exercise | B Physical Agents<br>C Mechanical<br>D Electrotherapeutic<br>E Orthosis<br>F Assistive, Adaptive, Supportive or Protective<br>G Aerobic Endurance and Conditioning<br>H Mechanical or Electromechanical<br>U Prosthesis<br>Y Other Equipment<br>Z None | Z None |
| Z None | 4 Wheelchair Mobility | D Electrotherapeutic<br>E Orthosis<br>F Assistive, Adaptive, Supportive or Protective<br>U Prosthesis<br>Y Other Equipment<br>Z None | Z None |
| Z None | 5 Bed Mobility | C Mechanical<br>E Orthosis<br>F Assistive, Adaptive, Supportive or Protective<br>U Prosthesis<br>Y Other Equipment<br>Z None | Z None |
| Z None | 8 Transfer Training | C Mechanical<br>D Electrotherapeutic<br>E Orthosis<br>F Assistive, Adaptive, Supportive or Protective<br>U Prosthesis<br>Y Other Equipment<br>Z None | Z None |
| Z None | 9 Gait Training/Functional Ambulation | C Mechanical<br>D Electrotherapeutic<br>E Orthosis<br>F Assistive, Adaptive, Supportive or Protective<br>G Aerobic Endurance and Conditioning<br>U Prosthesis<br>Y Other Equipment<br>Z None | Z None |

**F** Physical Rehabilitation and Diagnostic Audiology
**0** Rehabilitation
**8** Activities of Daily Living Treatment: Exercise or activities to facilitate functional competence for activities of daily living

| Character 4<br>Body System / Region | Character 5<br>Type Qualifier | Character 6<br>Equipment | Character 7<br>Qualifier |
|---|---|---|---|
| D Integumentary System - Head and Neck<br>F Integumentary System - Upper Back / Upper Extremity<br>G Integumentary System - Lower Back / Lower Extremity<br>H Integumentary System - Whole Body<br>J Musculoskeletal System - Head and Neck<br>K Musculoskeletal System - Upper Back / Upper Extremity<br>L Musculoskeletal System - Lower Back / Lower Extremity<br>M Musculoskeletal System - Whole Body | 5 Wound Management | B Physical Agents<br>C Mechanical<br>D Electrotherapeutic<br>E Orthosis<br>F Assistive, Adaptive, Supportive or Protective<br>U Prosthesis<br>Y Other Equipment<br>Z None | Z None |
| Z None | 0 Bathing/Showering Techniques<br>1 Dressing Techniques<br>2 Grooming/Personal Hygiene | E Orthosis<br>F Assistive, Adaptive, Supportive or Protective<br>U Prosthesis<br>Y Other Equipment<br>Z None | Z None |
| Z None | 3 Feeding/Eating | C Mechanical<br>D Electrotherapeutic<br>E Orthosis<br>F Assistive, Adaptive, Supportive or Protective<br>U Prosthesis<br>Y Other Equipment<br>Z None | Z None |
| Z None | 4 Home Management | D Electrotherapeutic<br>E Orthosis<br>F Assistive, Adaptive, Supportive or Protective<br>U Prosthesis<br>Y Other Equipment<br>Z None | Z None |
| Z None | 6 Psychosocial Skills | Z None | Z None |
| Z None | 7 Vocational Activities and Functional Community or Work Reintegration Skills | B Physical Agents<br>C Mechanical<br>D Electrotherapeutic<br>E Orthosis<br>F Assistive, Adaptive, Supportive or Protective<br>G Aerobic Endurance and Conditioning<br>U Prosthesis<br>Y Other Equipment<br>Z None | Z None |

**F** Physical Rehabilitation and Diagnostic Audiology
**0** Rehabilitation
**9** Hearing Treatment: Application of techniques to improve, augment, or compensate for hearing and related functional impairment

| Character 4<br>Body System / Region | Character 5<br>Type Qualifier | Character 6<br>Equipment | Character 7<br>Qualifier |
|---|---|---|---|
| Z None | 0 Hearing and Related Disorders Counseling<br>1 Hearing and Related Disorders Prevention | K Audiovisual<br>Z None | Z None |
| Z None | 2 Auditory Processing | K Audiovisual<br>L Assistive Listening<br>P Computer<br>Y Other Equipment<br>Z None | Z None |
| Z None | 3 Cerumen Management | X Cerumen Management<br>Z None | Z None |

**F Physical Rehabilitation and Diagnostic Audiology**
**0 Rehabilitation**
**B Cochlear Implant Treatment:** Application of techniques to improve the communication abilities of individuals with cochlear implant

| Character 4<br>Body System / Region | Character 5<br>Type Qualifier | Character 6<br>Equipment | Character 7<br>Qualifier |
|---|---|---|---|
| Z None | 0 Cochlear Implant Rehabilitation | 1 Audiometer<br>2 Sound Field / Booth<br>9 Cochlear Implant<br>K Audiovisual<br>P Computer<br>Y Other Equipment | Z None |

**F Physical Rehabilitation and Diagnostic Audiology**
**0 Rehabilitation**
**C Vestibular Treatment:** Application of techniques to improve, augment, or compensate for vestibular and related functional impairment

| Character 4<br>Body System / Region | Character 5<br>Type Qualifier | Character 6<br>Equipment | Character 7<br>Qualifier |
|---|---|---|---|
| 3 Neurological System - Whole Body<br>H Integumentary System - Whole Body<br>M Musculoskeletal System - Whole Body | 3 Postural Control | E Orthosis<br>F Assistive, Adaptive, Supportive or<br>   Protective<br>U Prosthesis<br>Y Other Equipment<br>Z None | Z None |
| Z None | 0 Vestibular | 8 Vestibular / Balance<br>Z None | Z None |
| Z None | 1 Perceptual Processing<br>2 Visual Motor Integration | K Audiovisual<br>L Assistive Listening<br>N Biosensory Feedback<br>P Computer<br>Q Speech Analysis<br>S Voice Analysis<br>T Aerodynamic Function<br>Y Other Equipment<br>Z None | Z None |

**F Physical Rehabilitation and Diagnostic Audiology**
**0 Rehabilitation**
**D Device Fitting:** Fitting of a device designed to facilitate or support achievement of a higher level of function

| Character 4<br>Body System / Region | Character 5<br>Type Qualifier | Character 6<br>Equipment | Character 7<br>Qualifier |
|---|---|---|---|
| Z None | 0 Tinnitus Masker | 5 Hearing Aid Selection / Fitting / Test<br>Z None | Z None |
| Z None | 1 Monaural Hearing Aid<br>2 Binaural Hearing Aid<br>5 Assistive Listening Device | 1 Audiometer<br>2 Sound Field / Booth<br>5 Hearing Aid Selection / Fitting / Test<br>K Audiovisual<br>L Assistive Listening<br>Z None | Z None |
| Z None | 3 Augmentative/Alternative<br>   Communication System | M Augmentative / Alternative<br>   Communication | Z None |
| Z None | 4 Voice Prosthetic | S Voice Analysis<br>V Speech Prosthesis | Z None |
| Z None | 6 Dynamic Orthosis<br>7 Static Orthosis<br>8 Prosthesis<br>9 Assistive, Adaptive, Supportive or<br>   Protective Devices | E Orthosis<br>F Assistive, Adaptive, Supportive or<br>   Protective<br>U Prosthesis<br>Z None | Z None |

**F** Physical Rehabilitation and Diagnostic Audiology
**0** Rehabilitation
**F** Caregiver Training: Training in activities to support patient's optimal level of function

| Character 4<br>Body System / Region | Character 5<br>Type Qualifier | Character 6<br>Equipment | Character 7<br>Qualifier |
|---|---|---|---|
| Z None | 0 Bathing/Showering Technique<br>1 Dressing<br>2 Feeding and Eating<br>3 Grooming/Personal Hygiene<br>4 Bed Mobility<br>5 Transfer<br>6 Wheelchair Mobility<br>7 Therapeutic Exercise<br>8 Airway Clearance Techniques<br>9 Wound Management<br>B Vocational Activities and Functional Community or Work Reintegration Skills<br>C Gait Training/Functional Ambulation<br>D Application, Proper Use and Care of Devices<br>F Application, Proper Use and Care of Orthoses<br>G Application, Proper Use and Care of Prosthesis<br>H Home Management | E Orthosis<br>F Assistive, Adaptive, Supportive or Protective<br>U Prosthesis<br>Z None | Z None |
| Z None | J Communication Skills | K Audiovisual<br>L Assistive Listening<br>M Augmentative / Alternative Communication<br>P Computer<br>Z None | Z None |

| F Physical Rehabilitation and Diagnostic Audiology |
| --- |
| 1 Diagnostic Audiology |
| 3 Hearing Assessment: Measurement of hearing and related functions |

| Character 4<br>Body System / Region | Character 5<br>Type Qualifier | Character 6<br>Equipment | Character 7<br>Qualifier |
| --- | --- | --- | --- |
| Z None | 0 Hearing Screening | 0 Occupational Hearing<br>1 Audiometer<br>2 Sound Field / Booth<br>3 Tympanometer<br>8 Vestibular / Balance<br>9 Cochlear Implant<br>Z None | Z None |
| Z None | 1 Pure Tone Audiometry, Air<br>2 Pure Tone Audiometry, Air and Bone | 0 Occupational Hearing<br>1 Audiometer<br>2 Sound Field / Booth<br>Z None | Z None |
| Z None | 3 Bekesy Audiometry<br>6 Visual Reinforcement Audiometry<br>9 Short Increment Sensitivity Index<br>B Stenger<br>C Pure Tone Stenger | 1 Audiometer<br>2 Sound Field / Booth<br>Z None | Z None |
| Z None | 4 Conditioned Play Audiometry<br>5 Select Picture Audiometry | 1 Audiometer<br>2 Sound Field / Booth<br>K Audiovisual<br>Z None | Z None |
| Z None | 7 Alternate Binaural or Monaural<br>Loudness Balance | 1 Audiometer<br>K Audiovisual<br>Z None | Z None |
| Z None | 8 Tone Decay<br>D Tympanometry<br>F Eustachian Tube Function<br>G Acoustic Reflex Patterns<br>H Acoustic Reflex Threshold<br>J Acoustic Reflex Decay | 3 Tympanometer<br>4 Electroacoustic Immitance / Acoustic Reflex<br>Z None | Z None |
| Z None | K Electrocochleography<br>L Auditory Evoked Potentials | 7 Electrophysiologic<br>Z None | Z None |
| Z None | M Evoked Otoacoustic Emissions, Screening<br>N Evoked Otoacoustic Emissions, Diagnostic | 6 Otoacoustic Emission (OAE)<br>Z None | Z None |
| Z None | P Aural Rehabilitation Status | 1 Audiometer<br>2 Sound Field / Booth<br>4 Electroacoustic Immitance / Acoustic Reflex<br>9 Cochlear Implant<br>K Audiovisual<br>L Assistive Listening<br>P Computer<br>Z None | Z None |
| Z None | Q Auditory Processing | K Audiovisual<br>P Computer<br>Y Other Equipment<br>Z None | Z None |

**Physical Rehabilitation and Diagnostic Audiology | F14–F15**

**F** Physical Rehabilitation and Diagnostic Audiology
**1** Diagnostic Audiology
**4** Hearing Aid Assessment: Measurement of the appropriateness and/or effectiveness of a hearing device

| Character 4<br>Body System / Region | Character 5<br>Type Qualifier | Character 6<br>Equipment | Character 7<br>Qualifier |
|---|---|---|---|
| Z None | 0 Cochlear Implant | 1 Audiometer<br>2 Sound Field / Booth<br>3 Tympanometer<br>4 Electroacoustic Immitance / Acoustic Reflex<br>5 Hearing Aid Selection / Fitting / Test<br>7 Electrophysiologic<br>9 Cochlear Implant<br>K Audiovisual<br>L Assistive Listening<br>P Computer<br>Y Other Equipment<br>Z None | Z None |
| Z None | 1 Ear Canal Probe Microphone<br>6 Binaural Electroacoustic Hearing Aid Check<br>8 Monaural Electroacoustic Hearing Aid Check | 5 Hearing Aid Selection / Fitting / Test<br>Z None | Z None |
| Z None | 2 Monaural Hearing Aid<br>3 Binaural Hearing Aid | 1 Audiometer<br>2 Sound Field / Booth<br>3 Tympanometer<br>4 Electroacoustic Immitance / Acoustic Reflex<br>5 Hearing Aid Selection / Fitting / Test<br>K Audiovisual<br>L Assistive Listening<br>P Computer<br>Z None | Z None |
| Z None | 4 Assistive Listening System/Device Selection | 1 Audiometer<br>2 Sound Field / Booth<br>3 Tympanometer<br>4 Electroacoustic Immitance / Acoustic Reflex<br>K Audiovisual<br>L Assistive Listening<br>Z None | Z None |
| Z None | 5 Sensory Aids | 1 Audiometer<br>2 Sound Field / Booth<br>3 Tympanometer<br>4 Electroacoustic Immitance / Acoustic Reflex<br>5 Hearing Aid Selection / Fitting / Test<br>K Audiovisual<br>L Assistive Listening<br>Z None | Z None |
| Z None | 7 Ear Protector Attentuation | 0 Occupational Hearing<br>Z None | Z None |

**F** Physical Rehabilitation and Diagnostic Audiology
**1** Diagnostic Audiology
**5** Vestibular Assessment: Measurement of the vestibular system and related functions

| Character 4<br>Body System / Region | Character 5<br>Type Qualifier | Character 6<br>Equipment | Character 7<br>Qualifier |
|---|---|---|---|
| Z None | 0 Bithermal, Binaural Caloric Irrigation<br>1 Bithermal, Monaural Caloric Irrigation<br>2 Unithermal Binaural Screen<br>3 Oscillating Tracking<br>4 Sinusoidal Vertical Axis Rotational<br>5 Dix-Hallpike Dynamic<br>6 Computerized Dynamic Posturography | 8 Vestibular / Balance<br>Z None | Z None |
| Z None | 7 Tinnitus Masker | 5 Hearing Aid Selection / Fitting / Test<br>Z None | Z None |

# Mental Health | GZ1-GZJ

**G** Mental Health
**Z** None
**1** Psychological Tests: The administration and interpretation of standardized psychological tests and measurement instruments for the assessment of psychological function

| Character 4<br>Qualifier | Character 5<br>Qualifier | Character 6<br>Qualifier | Character 7<br>Qualifier |
|---|---|---|---|
| 0 Developmental<br>1 Personality and Behavioral<br>2 Intellectual and Psychoeducational<br>3 Neuropsychological<br>4 Neurobehavioral and Cognitive Status | Z None | Z None | Z None |

**G** Mental Health
**Z** None
**2** Crisis Intervention: Treatment of a traumatized, acutely disturbed or distressed individual for the purpose of short-term stabilization

| Character 4<br>Qualifier | Character 5<br>Qualifier | Character 6<br>Qualifier | Character 7<br>Qualifier |
|---|---|---|---|
| Z None | Z None | Z None | Z None |

**G** Mental Health
**Z** None
**3** Medication Management: Monitoring and adjusting the use of medications for the treatment of a mental health disorder

| Character 4<br>Qualifier | Character 5<br>Qualifier | Character 6<br>Qualifier | Character 7<br>Qualifier |
|---|---|---|---|
| Z None | Z None | Z None | Z None |

**G** Mental Health
**Z** None
**5** Individual Psychotherapy: Treatment of an individual with a mental health disorder by behavioral, cognitive, psychoanalytic, psychodynamic or psychophysiological means to improve functioning or well-being

| Character 4<br>Qualifier | Character 5<br>Qualifier | Character 6<br>Qualifier | Character 7<br>Qualifier |
|---|---|---|---|
| 0 Interactive<br>1 Behavioral<br>2 Cognitive<br>3 Interpersonal<br>4 Psychoanalysis<br>5 Psychodynamic<br>6 Supportive<br>8 Cognitive-Behavioral<br>9 Psychophysiological | Z None | Z None | Z None |

**G** Mental Health
**Z** None
**6** Counseling: The application of psychological methods to treat an individual with normal developmental issues and psychological problems in order to increase function, improve well-being, alleviate distress, maladjustment or resolve crises

| Character 4<br>Qualifier | Character 5<br>Qualifier | Character 6<br>Qualifier | Character 7<br>Qualifier |
|---|---|---|---|
| 0 Educational<br>1 Vocational<br>3 Other Counseling | Z None | Z None | Z None |

**G** Mental Health
**Z** None
**7** Family Psychotherapy: Treatment that includes one or more family members of an individual with a mental health disorder by behavioral, cognitive, psychoanalytic, psychodynamic or psychophysiological means to improve functioning or well-being

| Character 4<br>Qualifier | Character 5<br>Qualifier | Character 6<br>Qualifier | Character 7<br>Qualifier |
|---|---|---|---|
| 2 Other Family Psychotherapy | Z None | Z None | Z None |

♂ Male          ♀ Female          **N C** Non-covered          **L C** Limited Coverage          **AHA** *AHA Coding Clinic*

**G** Mental Health
**Z** None
**B** Electroconvulsive Therapy: The application of controlled electrical voltages to treat a mental health disorder

| Character 4<br>Qualifier | Character 5<br>Qualifier | Character 6<br>Qualifier | Character 7<br>Qualifier |
|---|---|---|---|
| 0 Unilateral-Single Seizure<br>1 Unilateral-Multiple Seizure<br>2 Bilateral-Single Seizure<br>3 Bilateral-Multiple Seizure<br>4 Other Electroconvulsive Therapy | Z None | Z None | Z None |

**G** Mental Health
**Z** None
**C** Biofeedback: Provision of information from the monitoring and regulating of physiological processes in conjunction with cognitive-behavioral techniques to improve patient functioning or well-being

| Character 4<br>Qualifier | Character 5<br>Qualifier | Character 6<br>Qualifier | Character 7<br>Qualifier |
|---|---|---|---|
| 9 Other Biofeedback | Z None | Z None | Z None |

**G** Mental Health
**Z** None
**F** Hypnosis: Induction of a state of heightened suggestibility by auditory, visual and tactile techniques to elicit an emotional or behavioral response

| Character 4<br>Qualifier | Character 5<br>Qualifier | Character 6<br>Qualifier | Character 7<br>Qualifier |
|---|---|---|---|
| Z None | Z None | Z None | Z None |

**G** Mental Health
**Z** None
**G** Narcosynthesis: Administration of intravenous barbiturates in order to release suppressed or repressed thoughts

| Character 4<br>Qualifier | Character 5<br>Qualifier | Character 6<br>Qualifier | Character 7<br>Qualifier |
|---|---|---|---|
| Z None | Z None | Z None | Z None |

**G** Mental Health
**Z** None
**H** Group Psychotherapy: Treatment of two or more individuals with a mental health disorder by behavioral, cognitive, psychoanalytic, psychodynamic or psychophysiological means to improve functioning or well-being

| Character 4<br>Qualifier | Character 5<br>Qualifier | Character 6<br>Qualifier | Character 7<br>Qualifier |
|---|---|---|---|
| Z None | Z None | Z None | Z None |

**G** Mental Health
**Z** None
**J** Light Therapy: Application of specialized light treatments to improve functioning or well-being

| Character 4<br>Qualifier | Character 5<br>Qualifier | Character 6<br>Qualifier | Character 7<br>Qualifier |
|---|---|---|---|
| Z None | Z None | Z None | Z None |

# Substance Abuse Treatment | HZ2-HZ9

**H** Substance Abuse Treatment
**Z** None
**2** Detoxification Services: Detoxification from alcohol and/or drugs

| Character 4 Qualifier | Character 5 Qualifier | Character 6 Qualifier | Character 7 Qualifier |
|---|---|---|---|
| Z None | Z None | Z None | Z None |

**H** Substance Abuse Treatment
**Z** None
**3** Individual Counseling: The application of psychological methods to treat an individual with addictive behavior

| Character 4 Qualifier | Character 5 Qualifier | Character 6 Qualifier | Character 7 Qualifier |
|---|---|---|---|
| 0 Cognitive | Z None | Z None | Z None |
| 1 Behavioral | | | |
| 2 Cognitive-Behavioral | | | |
| 3 12-Step | | | |
| 4 Interpersonal | | | |
| 5 Vocational | | | |
| 6 Psychoeducation | | | |
| 7 Motivational Enhancement | | | |
| 8 Confrontational | | | |
| 9 Continuing Care | | | |
| B Spiritual | | | |
| C Pre/Post-Test Infectious Disease | | | |

**H** Substance Abuse Treatment
**Z** None
**4** Group Counseling: The application of psychological methods to treat two or more individuals with addictive behavior

| Character 4 Qualifier | Character 5 Qualifier | Character 6 Qualifier | Character 7 Qualifier |
|---|---|---|---|
| 0 Cognitive | Z None | Z None | Z None |
| 1 Behavioral | | | |
| 2 Cognitive-Behavioral | | | |
| 3 12-Step | | | |
| 4 Interpersonal | | | |
| 5 Vocational | | | |
| 6 Psychoeducation | | | |
| 7 Motivational Enhancement | | | |
| 8 Confrontational | | | |
| 9 Continuing Care | | | |
| B Spiritual | | | |
| C Pre/Post-Test Infectious Disease | | | |

**H** Substance Abuse Treatment
**Z** None
**5** Individual Psychotherapy: Treatment of an individual with addictive behavior by behavioral, cognitive, psychoanalytic, psychodynamic or psychophysiological means

| Character 4 Qualifier | Character 5 Qualifier | Character 6 Qualifier | Character 7 Qualifier |
|---|---|---|---|
| 0 Cognitive | Z None | Z None | Z None |
| 1 Behavioral | | | |
| 2 Cognitive-Behavioral | | | |
| 3 12-Step | | | |
| 4 Interpersonal | | | |
| 5 Interactive | | | |
| 6 Psychoeducation | | | |
| 7 Motivational Enhancement | | | |
| 8 Confrontational | | | |
| 9 Supportive | | | |
| B Psychoanalysis | | | |
| C Psychodynamic | | | |
| D Psychophysiological | | | |

**H** Substance Abuse Treatment
**Z** None
**6** Family Counseling: The application of psychological methods that includes one or more family members to treat an individual with addictive behavior

| Character 4<br>Qualifier | Character 5<br>Qualifier | Character 6<br>Qualifier | Character 7<br>Qualifier |
|---|---|---|---|
| 3 Other Family Counseling | Z None | Z None | Z None |

**H** Substance Abuse Treatment
**Z** None
**8** Medication Management: Monitoring and adjusting the use of replacement medications for the treatment of addiction

| Character 4<br>Qualifier | Character 5<br>Qualifier | Character 6<br>Qualifier | Character 7<br>Qualifier |
|---|---|---|---|
| 0 Nicotine Replacement<br>1 Methadone Maintenance<br>2 Levo-alpha-acetyl-methadol (LAAM)<br>3 Antabuse<br>4 Naltrexone<br>5 Naloxone<br>6 Clonidine<br>7 Bupropion<br>8 Psychiatric Medication<br>9 Other Replacement Medication | Z None | Z None | Z None |

**H** Substance Abuse Treatment
**Z** None
**9** Pharmacotherapy: The use of replacement medications for the treatment of addiction

| Character 4<br>Qualifier | Character 5<br>Qualifier | Character 6<br>Qualifier | Character 7<br>Qualifier |
|---|---|---|---|
| 0 Nicotine Replacement<br>1 Methadone Maintenance<br>2 Levo-alpha-acetyl-methadol (LAAM)<br>3 Antabuse<br>4 Naltrexone<br>5 Naloxone<br>6 Clonidine<br>7 Bupropion<br>8 Psychiatric Medication<br>9 Other Replacement Medication | Z None | Z None | Z None |

# APPENDIX A:

## Definitions

### Section 0 – Medical and Surgical
### Character 3: Operation

| | |
|---|---|
| **Alteration** | **Definition:** Modifying the anatomic structure of a body part without affecting the function of the body part |
| | **Explanation:** Principal purpose is to improve appearance |
| | **Includes/Examples:** Face lift, breast augmentation |
| **Bypass** | **Definition:** Altering the route of passage of the contents of a tubular body part |
| | **Explanation:** Rerouting contents of a body part to a downstream area of the normal route, to a similar route and body part, or to an abnormal route and dissimilar body part. Includes one or more anastomoses, with or without the use of a device |
| | **Includes/Examples:** Coronary artery bypass, colostomy formation |
| **Change** | **Definition:** Taking out or off a device from a body part and putting back an identical or similar device in or on the same body part without cutting or puncturing the skin or a mucous membrane |
| | **Explanation:** All CHANGE procedures are coded using the approach EXTERNAL |
| | **Includes/Examples:** Urinary catheter change, gastrostomy tube change |
| **Control** | **Definition:** Stopping, or attempting to stop, postprocedural bleeding |
| | **Explanation:** The site of the bleeding is coded as an anatomical region and not to a specific body part |
| | **Includes/Examples:** Control of post-prostatectomy hemorrhage, control of post-tonsillectomy hemorrhage |
| **Creation** | **Definition:** Making a new genital structure that does not take over the function of a body part |
| | **Explanation:** Used only for sex change operations |
| | **Includes/Examples:** Creation of vagina in a male, creation of penis in a female |
| **Destruction** | **Definition:** Physical eradication of all or a portion of a body part by the direct use of energy, force, or a destructive agent |
| | **Explanation:** None of the body part is physically taken out |
| | **Includes/Examples:** Fulguration of rectal polyp, cautery of skin lesion |
| **Detachment** | **Definition:** Cutting off all or a portion of the upper or lower extremities |
| | **Explanation:** The body part value is the site of the detachment, with a qualifier if applicable to further specify the level where the extremity was detached |
| | **Includes/Examples:** Below knee amputation, disarticulation of shoulder |
| **Dilation** | **Definition:** Expanding an orifice or the lumen of a tubular body part |
| | **Explanation:** The orifice can be a natural orifice or an artificially created orifice. Accomplished by stretching a tubular body part using intraluminal pressure or by cutting part of the orifice or wall of the tubular body part |
| | **Includes/Examples:** Percutaneous transluminal angioplasty, pyloromyotomy |
| **Division** | **Definition:** Cutting into a body part, without draining fluids and/or gases from the body part, in order to separate or transect a body part |
| | **Explanation:** All or a portion of the body part is separated into two or more portions |
| | **Includes/Examples:** Spinal cordotomy, osteotomy |
| **Drainage** | **Definition:** Taking or letting out fluids and/or gases from a body part |
| | **Explanation:** The qualifier DIAGNOSTIC is used to identify drainage procedures that are biopsies |
| | **Includes/Examples:** Thoracentesis, incision and drainage |
| **Excision** | **Definition:** Cutting out or off, without replacement, a portion of a body part |
| | **Explanation:** The qualifier DIAGNOSTIC is used to identify excision procedures that are biopsies |
| | **Includes/Examples:** Partial nephrectomy, liver biopsy |

| | |
|---|---|
| **Extirpation** | **Definition:** Taking or cutting out solid matter from a body part |
| | **Explanation:** The solid matter may be an abnormal byproduct of a biological function or a foreign body; it may be embedded in a body part or in the lumen of a tubular body part. The solid matter may or may not have been previously broken into pieces |
| | **Includes/Examples:** Thrombectomy, choledocholithotomy, endarterectomy |
| **Extraction** | **Definition:** Pulling or stripping out or off all or a portion of a body part by the use of force |
| | **Explanation:** The qualifier DIAGNOSTIC is used to identify extraction procedures that are biopsies |
| | **Includes/Examples:** Dilation and curettage, vein stripping |
| **Fragmentation** | **Definition:** Breaking solid matter in a body part into pieces |
| | **Explanation:** Physical force (e.g., manual, ultrasonic) applied directly or indirectly is used to break the solid matter into pieces. The solid matter may be an abnormal byproduct of a biological function or a foreign body. The pieces of solid matter are not taken out |
| | **Includes/Examples:** Extracorporeal shockwave lithotripsy, transurethral lithotripsy |
| **Fusion** | **Definition:** Joining together portions of an articular body part rendering the articular body part immobile |
| | **Explanation:** The body part is joined together by fixation device, bone graft, or other means |
| | **Includes/Examples:** Spinal fusion, ankle arthrodesis |
| **Insertion** | **Definition:** Putting in a nonbiological appliance that monitors, assists, performs, or prevents a physiological function but does not physically take the place of a body part |
| | **Includes/Examples:** Insertion of radioactive implant, insertion of central venous catheter |
| **Inspection** | **Definition:** Visually and/or manually exploring a body part |
| | **Explanation:** Visual exploration may be performed with or without optical instrumentation. Manual exploration may be performed directly or through intervening body layers |
| | **Includes/Examples:** Diagnostic arthroscopy, exploratory laparotomy |
| **Map** | **Definition:** Locating the route of passage of electrical impulses and/or locating functional areas in a body part |
| | **Explanation:** Applicable only to the cardiac conduction mechanism and the central nervous system |
| | **Includes/Examples:** Cardiac mapping, cortical mapping |
| **Occlusion** | **Definition:** Completely closing an orifice or the lumen of a tubular body part |
| | **Explanation:** The orifice can be a natural orifice or an artificially created orifice |
| | **Includes/Examples:** Fallopian tube ligation, ligation of inferior vena cava |
| **Reattachment** | **Definition:** Putting back in or on all or a portion of a separated body part to its normal location or other suitable location |
| | **Explanation:** Vascular circulation and nervous pathways may or may not be reestablished |
| | **Includes/Examples:** Reattachment of hand, reattachment of avulsed kidney |
| **Release** | **Definition:** Freeing a body part from an abnormal physical constraint by cutting or by use of force |
| | **Explanation:** Some of the restraining tissue may be taken out but none of the body part is taken out |
| | **Includes/Examples:** Adhesiolysis, carpal tunnel release |
| **Removal** | **Definition:** Taking out or off a device from a body part |
| | **Explanation:** If a device is taken out and a similar device put in without cutting or puncturing the skin or mucous membrane, the procedure is coded to the root operation CHANGE. Otherwise, the procedure for taking out a device is coded to the root operation REMOVAL |
| | **Includes/Examples:** Drainage tube removal, cardiac pacemaker removal |

| | |
|---|---|
| **Repair** | **Definition:** Restoring, to the extent possible, a body part to its normal anatomic structure and function<br><br>**Explanation:** Used only when the method to accomplish the repair is not one of the other root operations<br><br>**Includes/Examples:** Colostomy takedown, suture of laceration |
| **Replacement** | **Definition:** Putting in or on biological or synthetic material that physically takes the place and/or function of all or a portion of a body part<br><br>**Explanation:** The body part may have been taken out or replaced, or may be taken out, physically eradicated, or rendered nonfunctional during the Replacement procedure. A Removal procedure is coded for taking out the device used in a previous replacement procedure<br><br>**Includes/Examples:** Total hip replacement, bone graft, free skin graft |
| **Reposition** | **Definition:** Moving to its normal location, or other suitable location, all or a portion of a body part<br><br>**Explanation:** The body part is moved to a new location from an abnormal location, or from a normal location where it is not functioning correctly. The body part may or may not be cut out or off to be moved to the new location<br><br>**Includes/Examples:** Reposition of undescended testicle, fracture reduction |
| **Resection** | **Definition:** Cutting out or off, without replacement, all of a body part<br><br>**Includes/Examples:** Total nephrectomy, total lobectomy of lung |
| **Restriction** | **Definition:** Partially closing an orifice or the lumen of a tubular body part<br><br>**Explanation:** The orifice can be a natural orifice or an artificially created orifice<br><br>**Includes/Examples:** Esophagogastric fundoplication, cervical cerclage |
| **Revision** | **Definition:** Correcting, to the extent possible, a portion of a malfunctioning device or the position of a displaced device<br><br>**Explanation:** Revision can include correcting a malfunctioning or displaced device by taking out or putting in components of the device, such as a screw or pin<br><br>**Includes/Examples:** Adjustment of position of pacemaker lead, recementing of hip prosthesis |
| **Supplement** | **Definition:** Putting in or on biological or synthetic material that physically reinforces and/or augments the function of a portion of a body part<br><br>**Explanation:** The biological material is non-living, or is living and from the same individual. The body part may have been previously replaced, and the Supplement procedure is performed to physically reinforce and/or augment the function of the replaced body part<br><br>**Includes/Examples:** Herniorrhaphy using mesh, free nerve graft, mitral valve ring annuloplasty, put a new acetabular liner in a previous hip replacement |
| **Transfer** | **Definition:** Moving, without taking out, all or a portion of a body part to another location to take over the function of all or a portion of a body part<br><br>**Explanation:** The body part transferred remains connected to its vascular and nervous supply<br><br>**Includes/Examples:** Tendon transfer, skin pedicle flap transfer |
| **Transplantation** | **Definition:** Putting in or on all or a portion of a living body part taken from another individual or animal to physically take the place and/or function of all or a portion of a similar body part<br><br>**Explanation:** The native body part may or may not be taken out, and the transplanted body part may take over all or a portion of its function<br><br>**Includes/Examples:** Kidney transplant, heart transplant |

# Section 0 – Medical and Surgical
*Character 4: Body Part Definitions*

| Body Part | Definition |
|---|---|
| 1st Toe, Left<br>1st Toe, Right | **Includes:** Hallux |
| Abdomen Muscle, Left<br>Abdomen Muscle, Right | **Includes:** External oblique muscle<br>Internal oblique muscle<br>Pyramidalis muscle<br>Rectus abdominis muscle<br>Transversus abdominis muscle |
| Abdominal Aorta | **Includes:** Inferior phrenic artery<br>Lumbar artery<br>Median sacral artery<br>Middle suprarenal artery<br>Ovarian artery<br>Testicular artery |

| Body Part | Definition |
|---|---|
| Abdominal Sympathetic Nerve | **Includes:**<br>Abdominal aortic plexus<br>Auerbach's (myenteric) plexus<br>Celiac (solar) plexus<br>Celiac ganglion<br>Gastric plexus<br>Hepatic plexus<br>Inferior hypogastric plexus<br>Inferior mesenteric ganglion<br>Inferior mesenteric plexus<br>Meissner's (submucous) plexus<br>Myenteric (Auerbach's) plexus<br>Pancreatic plexus<br>Pelvic splanchnic nerve<br>Renal plexus<br>Solar (celiac) plexus<br>Splenic plexus<br>Submucous (Meissner's) plexus<br>Superior hypogastric plexus<br>Superior mesenteric ganglion<br>Superior mesenteric plexus<br>Suprarenal plexus |
| Abducens Nerve | **Includes:** Sixth cranial nerve |
| Accessory Nerve | **Includes:** Eleventh cranial nerve |
| Acoustic Nerve | **Includes:**<br>Cochlear nerve<br>Eighth cranial nerve<br>Scarpa's (vestibular) ganglion<br>Spiral ganglion<br>Vestibular (Scarpa's) ganglion<br>Vestibular nerve<br>Vestibulocochlear nerve |
| Adenoids | **Includes:**<br>Pharyngeal tonsil |
| Adrenal Gland<br>Adrenal Gland, Left<br>Adrenal Gland, Right<br>Adrenal Glands, Bilateral | **Includes:**<br>Suprarenal gland |
| Ampulla of Vater | **Includes:**<br>Duodenal ampulla<br>Hepatopancreatic ampulla |
| Anal Sphincter | **Includes:**<br>External anal sphincter<br>Internal anal sphincter |
| Ankle Bursa and Ligament, Left<br>Ankle Bursa and Ligament, Right | **Includes:**<br>Calcaneofibular ligament<br>Deltoid ligament<br>Ligament of the lateral malleolus<br>Talofibular ligament |
| Ankle Joint, Left<br>Ankle Joint, Right | **Includes:**<br>Inferior tibiofibular joint<br>Talocrural joint |
| Anterior Chamber, Left<br>Anterior Chamber, Right | **Includes:**<br>Aqueous humour |
| Anterior Tibial Artery, Left<br>Anterior Tibial Artery, Right | **Includes:**<br>Anterior lateral malleolar artery<br>Anterior medial malleolar artery<br>Anterior tibial recurrent artery<br>Dorsalis pedis artery<br>Posterior tibial recurrent artery |
| Anus | **Includes:**<br>Anal orifice |
| Aortic Valve | **Includes:**<br>Aortic annulus |
| Appendix | **Includes:** Vermiform appendix |
| Ascending Colon | **Includes:** Hepatic flexure |
| Atrial Septum | **Includes:** Interatrial septum |
| Atrium, Left | **Includes:**<br>Atrium pulmonale<br>Left auricular appendix |
| Atrium, Right | **Includes:**<br>Atrium dextrum cordis<br>Right auricular appendix<br>Sinus venosus |

| Body Part | Definition |
|---|---|
| Auditory Ossicle, Left<br>Auditory Ossicle, Right | Includes:<br>Incus<br>Malleus<br>Ossicular chain<br>Stapes |
| Axillary Artery, Left<br>Axillary Artery, Right | Includes:<br>Anterior circumflex humeral artery<br>Lateral thoracic artery<br>Posterior circumflex humeral artery<br>Subscapular artery<br>Superior thoracic artery<br>Thoracoacromial artery |
| Azygos Vein | Includes:<br>Right ascending lumbar vein<br>Right subcostal vein |
| Basal Ganglia | Includes:<br>Basal nuclei<br>Claustrum<br>Corpus striatum<br>Globus pallidus<br>Substantia nigra<br>Subthalamic nucleus |
| Basilic Vein, Left<br>Basilic Vein, Right | Includes:<br>Median antebrachial vein<br>Median cubital vein |
| Bladder | Includes: Trigone of bladder |
| Brachial Artery, Left<br>Brachial Artery, Right | Includes:<br>Inferior ulnar collateral artery<br>Profunda brachii<br>Superior ulnar collateral artery |
| Brachial Plexus | Includes:<br>Axillary nerve<br>Dorsal scapular nerve<br>First intercostal nerve<br>Long thoracic nerve<br>Musculocutaneous nerve<br>Subclavius nerve<br>Suprascapular nerve |
| Brachial Vein, Left<br>Brachial Vein, Right | Includes:<br>Radial vein<br>Ulnar vein |
| Brain | Includes:<br>Cerebrum<br>Corpus callosum<br>Encephalon |
| Breast, Bilateral<br>Breast, Left<br>Breast, Right | Includes:<br>Mammary duct<br>Mammary gland |
| Buccal Mucosa | Includes:<br>Buccal gland<br>Molar gland<br>Palatine gland |
| Carotid Bodies, Bilateral<br>Carotid Body, Left<br>Carotid Body, Right | Includes: Carotid glomus |
| Carpal Joint, Left<br>Carpal Joint, Right | Includes:<br>Intercarpal joint<br>Midcarpal joint |
| Carpal, Left<br>Carpal, Right | Includes:<br>Capitate bone<br>Hamate bone<br>Lunate bone<br>Pisiform bone<br>Scaphoid bone<br>Trapezium bone<br>Trapezoid bone<br>Triquetral bone |
| Celiac Artery | Includes: Celiac trunk |
| Cephalic Vein, Left<br>Cephalic Vein, Right | Includes: Accessory cephalic vein |
| Cerebellum | Includes: Culmen |
| Cerebral Hemisphere | Includes:<br>Frontal lobe<br>Occipital lobe<br>Parietal lobe<br>Temporal lobe |

| Body Part | Definition |
|---|---|
| Cerebral Meninges | Includes:<br>Arachnoid mater<br>Leptomeninges<br>Pia mater |
| Cerebral Ventricle | Includes:<br>Aqueduct of Sylvius<br>Cerebral aqueduct (Sylvius)<br>Choroid plexus<br>Ependyma<br>Foramen of Monro (intraventricular)<br>Fourth ventricle<br>Interventricular foramen (Monro)<br>Left lateral ventricle<br>Right lateral ventricle<br>Third ventricle |
| Cervical Nerve | Includes:<br>Greater occipital nerve<br>Spinal nerve, cervical<br>Suboccipital nerve<br>Third occipital nerve |
| Cervical Plexus | Includes:<br>Ansa cervicalis<br>Cutaneous (transverse) cervical nerve<br>Great auricular nerve<br>Lesser occipital nerve<br>Supraclavicular nerve<br>Transverse (cutaneous) cervical nerve |
| Cervical Vertebra | Includes:<br>Spinous process<br>Vertebral arch<br>Vertebral foramen<br>Vertebral lamina<br>Vertebral pedicle |
| Cervical Vertebral Joint | Includes:<br>Atlantoaxial joint<br>Cervical facet joint |
| Cervical Vertebral Joints, 2 or more | Includes: Cervical facet joint |
| Cervicothoracic Vertebral Joint | Includes: Cervicothoracic facet joint |
| Cisterna Chyli | Includes:<br>Intestinal lymphatic trunk<br>Lumbar lymphatic trunk |
| Coccygeal Glomus | Includes:<br>Coccygeal body |
| Colic Vein | Includes:<br>Ileocolic vein<br>Left colic vein<br>Middle colic vein<br>Right colic vein |
| Conduction Mechanism | Includes:<br>Atrioventricular node<br>Bundle of His<br>Bundle of Kent<br>Sinoatrial node |
| Conjunctiva, Left<br>Conjunctiva, Right | Includes: Plica semilunaris |
| Dura Mater | Includes:<br>Cranial dura mater<br>Dentate ligament<br>Diaphragma sellae<br>Falx cerebri<br>Spinal dura mater<br>Tentorium cerebelli |
| Elbow Bursa and Ligament, Left<br>Elbow Bursa and Ligament, Right | Includes:<br>Annular ligament<br>Olecranon bursa<br>Radial collateral ligament<br>Ulnar collateral ligament |
| Elbow Joint, Left<br>Elbow Joint, Right | Includes:<br>Distal humerus, involving joint<br>Humeroradial joint<br>Humeroulnar joint<br>Proximal radioulnar joint |
| Epidural Space | Includes:<br>Cranial epidural space<br>Extradural space<br>Spinal epidural space |
| Epiglottis | Includes: Glossoepiglottic fold |

| Body Part | Definition |
|---|---|
| Esophagogastric Junction | **Includes:**<br>Cardia<br>Cardioesophageal junction<br>Gastroesophageal (GE) junction |
| Esophagus, Lower | **Includes:** Abdominal esophagus |
| Esophagus, Middle | **Includes:** Thoracic esophagus |
| Esophagus, Upper | **Includes:** Cervical esophagus |
| Ethmoid Bone, Left<br>Ethmoid Bone, Right | **Includes:** Cribriform plate |
| Ethmoid Sinus, Left<br>Ethmoid Sinus, Right | **Includes:** Ethmoidal air cell |
| Eustachian Tube, Left<br>Eustachian Tube, Right | **Includes:**<br>Auditory tube<br>Pharyngotympanic tube |
| External Auditory Canal, Left<br>External Auditory Canal, Right | **Includes:** External auditory meatus |
| External Carotid Artery, Left<br>External Carotid Artery, Right | **Includes:**<br>Ascending pharyngeal artery<br>Internal maxillary artery<br>Lingual artery<br>Maxillary artery<br>Occipital artery<br>Posterior auricular artery<br>Superior thyroid artery |
| External Ear, Bilateral<br>External Ear, Left<br>External Ear, Right | **Includes:**<br>Antihelix<br>Antitragus<br>Auricle<br>Earlobe<br>Helix<br>Pinna<br>Tragus |
| External Iliac Artery, Left<br>External Iliac Artery, Right | **Includes:**<br>Deep circumflex iliac artery<br>Inferior epigastric artery |
| External Jugular Vein, Left<br>External Jugular Vein, Right | **Includes:** Posterior auricular vein |
| Extraocular Muscle, Left<br>Extraocular Muscle, Right | **Includes:**<br>Inferior oblique muscle<br>Inferior rectus muscle<br>Lateral rectus muscle<br>Medial rectus muscle<br>Superior oblique muscle<br>Superior rectus muscle |
| Eye, Left<br>Eye, Rigt | **Includes:**<br>Ciliary body<br>Posterior chamber |
| Face Artery | **Includes:**<br>Angular artery<br>Ascending palatine artery<br>External maxillary artery<br>Facial artery<br>Inferior labial artery<br>Submental artery<br>Superior labial artery |
| Face Vein, Left<br>Face Vein, Right | **Includes:**<br>Angular vein<br>Anterior facial vein<br>Common facial vein<br>Deep facial vein<br>Frontal vein<br>Posterior facial (retromandibular) vein<br>Supraorbital vein |

| Body Part | Definition |
|---|---|
| Facial Muscle | **Includes:**<br>Buccinator muscle<br>Corrugator supercilii muscle<br>Depressor anguli oris muscle<br>Depressor labii inferioris muscle<br>Depressor septi nasi muscle<br>Depressor supercilii muscle<br>Levator anguli oris muscle<br>Levator labii superioris alaeque nasi muscle<br>Levator labii superioris muscle<br>Mentalis muscle<br>Nasalis muscle<br>Occipitofrontalis muscle<br>Orbicularis oris muscle<br>Procerus muscle<br>Risorius muscle<br>Zygomaticus muscle |
| Facial Nerve | **Includes:**<br>Chorda tympani<br>Geniculate ganglion<br>Greater superficial petrosal nerve<br>Nerve to the stapedius<br>Parotid plexus<br>Posterior auricular nerve<br>Seventh cranial nerve<br>Submandibular ganglion |
| Fallopian Tube, Left<br>Fallopian Tube, Right | **Includes:**<br>Oviduct<br>Salpinx<br>Uterine tube |
| Femoral Artery, Left<br>Femoral Artery, Right | **Includes:**<br>Circumflex iliac artery<br>Deep femoral artery<br>Descending genicular artery<br>External pudendal artery<br>Superficial epigastric artery |
| Femoral Nerve | **Includes:**<br>Anterior crural nerve<br>Saphenous nerve |
| Femoral Shaft, Left<br>Femoral Shaft, Right | **Includes:** Body of femur |
| Femoral Vein, Left<br>Femoral Vein, Right | **Includes:**<br>Deep femoral (profunda femoris) vein<br>Popliteal vein<br>Profunda femoris (deep femoral) vein |
| Fibula, Left<br>Fibula, Right | **Includes:**<br>Body of fibula<br>Head of fibula<br>Lateral malleolus |
| Finger Nail | **Includes:**<br>Nail bed<br>Nail plate |
| Finger Phalangeal Joint, Left<br>Finger Phalangeal Joint, Right | **Includes:** Interphalangeal (IP) joint |
| Foot Artery, Left<br>Foot Artery, Right | **Includes:**<br>Arcuate artery<br>Dorsal metatarsal artery<br>Lateral plantar artery<br>Lateral tarsal artery<br>Medial plantar artery |
| Foot Bursa and Ligament, Left<br>Foot Bursa and Ligament, Right | **Includes:**<br>Calcaneocuboid ligament<br>Cuneonavicular ligament<br>Intercuneiform ligament<br>Interphalangeal ligament<br>Metatarsal ligament<br>Metatarsophalangeal ligament<br>Subtalar ligament<br>Talocalcaneal ligament<br>Talocalcaneonavicular ligament<br>Tarsometatarsal ligament |
| Foot Muscle, Left<br>Foot Muscle, Right | **Includes:**<br>Abductor hallucis muscle<br>Adductor hallucis muscle<br>Extensor digitorum brevis muscle<br>Extensor hallucis brevis muscle<br>Flexor digitorum brevis muscle<br>Flexor hallucis brevis muscle<br>Quadratus plantae muscle |

| Body Part | Definition |
|-----------|------------|
| Foot Vein, Left<br>Foot Vein, Right | **Includes:**<br>Common digital vein<br>Dorsal metatarsal vein<br>Dorsal venous arch<br>Plantar digital vein<br>Plantar metatarsal vein<br>Plantar venous arch |
| Frontal Bone, Left<br>Frontal Bone, Right | **Includes:**<br>Zygomatic process of frontal bone |
| Gastric Artery | **Includes:**<br>Left gastric artery<br>Right gastric artery |
| Glenoid Cavity, Left<br>Glenoid Cavity, Right | **Includes:**<br>Glenoid fossa (of scapula) |
| Glomus Jugulare | **Includes:** Jugular body |
| Glossopharyngeal Nerve | **Includes:**<br>Carotid sinus nerve<br>Ninth cranial nerve<br>Tympanic nerve |
| Greater Omentum | **Includes:**<br>Gastrocolic ligament<br>Gastrocolic omentum<br>Gastrophrenic ligament<br>Gastrosplenic ligament |
| Greater Saphenous Vein, Left<br>Greater Saphenous Vein, Right | **Includes:**<br>External pudendal vein<br>Great saphenous vein<br>Superficial circumflex iliac vein<br>Superficial epigastric vein |
| Hand Artery, Left<br>Hand Artery, Right | **Includes:**<br>Deep palmar arch<br>Princeps pollicis artery<br>Radialis indicis<br>Superficial palmar arch |
| Hand Bursa and Ligament, Left<br>Hand Bursa and Ligament, Right | **Includes:** Carpometacarpal ligament<br>Intercarpal ligament<br>Interphalangeal ligament<br>Lunotriquetral ligament<br>Metacarpal ligament<br>Metacarpophalangeal ligament<br>Pisohamate ligament<br>Pisometacarpal ligament<br>Scapholunate ligament<br>Scaphotrapezium ligament |
| Hand Muscle, Left<br>Hand Muscle, Right | **Includes:**<br>Hypothenar muscle<br>Palmar interosseous muscle<br>Thenar muscle |
| Hand Vein, Left<br>Hand Vein, Right | **Includes:**<br>Dorsal metacarpal vein<br>Palmar (volar) digital vein<br>Palmar (volar) metacarpal vein<br>Superficial palmar venous arch<br>Volar (palmar) digital vein<br>Volar (palmar) metacarpal vein |
| Head and Neck Bursa and Ligament | **Includes:**<br>Alar ligament of axis<br>Cervical interspinous ligament<br>Cervical intertransverse ligament<br>Cervical ligamentum flavum<br>Lateral temporomandibular ligament<br>Sphenomandibular ligament<br>Stylomandibular ligament<br>Transverse ligament of atlas |
| Head and Neck Sympathetic Nerve | **Includes:**<br>Cavernous plexus<br>Cervical ganglion<br>Ciliary ganglion<br>Internal carotid plexus<br>Otic ganglion<br>Pterygopalatine (sphenopalatine) ganglion<br>Sphenopalatine (pterygopalatine) ganglion<br>Stellate ganglion<br>Submandibular ganglion<br>Submaxillary ganglion |

| Body Part | Definition |
|-----------|------------|
| Head Muscle | **Includes:**<br>Auricularis muscle<br>Masseter muscle<br>Pterygoid muscle<br>Splenius capitis muscle<br>Temporalis muscle<br>Temporoparietalis muscle |
| Heart, Left | **Includes:**<br>Left coronary sulcus<br>Obtuse margin |
| Heart, Right | **Includes:** Right coronary sulcus |
| Hemiazygos Vein | **Includes:**<br>Left ascending lumbar vein<br>Left subcostal vein |
| Hepatic Artery | **Includes:**<br>Common hepatic artery<br>Gastroduodenal artery<br>Hepatic artery proper |
| Hip Bursa and Ligament, Left<br>Hip Bursa and Ligament, Right | **Includes:**<br>Iliofemoral ligament<br>Ischiofemoral ligament<br>Pubofemoral ligament<br>Transverse acetabular ligament<br>Trochanteric bursa |
| Hip Joint, Left<br>Hip Joint, Right | **Includes:**<br>Acetabulofemoral joint |
| Hip Muscle, Left<br>Hip Muscle, Right | **Includes:**<br>Gemellus muscle<br>Gluteus maximus muscle<br>Gluteus medius muscle<br>Gluteus minimus muscle<br>Iliacus muscle<br>Obturator muscle<br>Piriformis muscle<br>Psoas muscle<br>Quadratus femoris muscle<br>Tensor fasciae latae muscle |
| Humeral Head, Left<br>Humeral Head, Right | **Includes:**<br>Greater tuberosity<br>Lesser tuberosity<br>Neck of humerus (anatomical)(surgical) |
| Humeral Shaft, Left<br>Humeral Shaft, Right | **Includes:**<br>Distal humerus<br>Humerus, distal<br>Lateral epicondyle of humerus<br>Medial epicondyle of humerus |
| Hypogastric Vein, Left<br>Hypogastric Vein, Right | **Includes:**<br>Gluteal vein<br>Internal iliac vein<br>Internal pudendal vein<br>Lateral sacral vein<br>Middle hemorrhoidal vein<br>Obturator vein<br>Uterine vein<br>Vaginal vein<br>Vesical vein |
| Hypoglossal Nerve | **Includes:** Twelfth cranial nerve |
| Hypothalamus | **Includes:** Mammillary body |
| Inferior Mesenteric Artery | **Includes:**<br>Sigmoid artery<br>Superior rectal artery |
| Inferior Mesenteric Vein | **Includes:**<br>Sigmoid vein<br>Superior rectal vein |
| Inferior Vena Cava | **Includes:**<br>Postcava<br>Right inferior phrenic vein<br>Right ovarian vein<br>Right second lumbar vein<br>Right suprarenal vein<br>Right testicular vein |
| Inguinal Region, Bilateral<br>Inguinal Region, Left<br>Inguinal Region, Right | **Includes:**<br>Inguinal canal<br>Inguinal triangle |

| Body Part | Definition |
|---|---|
| Inner Ear, Left<br>Inner Ear, Right | Includes:<br>Bony labyrinth<br>Bony vestibule<br>Cochlea<br>Round window<br>Semicircular canal |
| Innominate Artery | Includes:<br>Brachiocephalic artery<br>Brachiocephalic trunk |
| Innominate Vein, Left<br>Innominate Vein, Right | Includes:<br>Brachiocephalic vein<br>Inferior thyroid vein |
| Internal Carotid Artery, Left<br>Internal Carotid Artery, Right | Includes:<br>Caroticotympanic artery<br>Carotid sinus<br>Ophthalmic artery |
| Internal Iliac Artery, Left<br>Internal Iliac Artery, Right | Includes:<br>Deferential artery<br>Hypogastric artery<br>Iliolumbar artery<br>Inferior gluteal artery<br>Inferior vesical artery<br>Internal pudendal artery<br>Lateral sacral artery<br>Middle rectal artery<br>Obturator artery<br>Superior gluteal artery<br>Umbilical artery<br>Uterine artery<br>Vaginal artery |
| Internal Mammary Artery, Left<br>Internal Mammary Artery, Right | Includes:<br>Anterior intercostal artery<br>Internal thoracic artery<br>Musculophrenic artery<br>Pericardiophrenic artery<br>Superior epigastric artery |
| Intracranial Artery | Includes:<br>Anterior cerebral artery<br>Anterior choroidal artery<br>Anterior communicating artery<br>Basilar artery<br>Circle of Willis<br>Middle cerebral artery<br>Posterior cerebral artery<br>Posterior communicating artery<br>Posterior inferior cerebellar artery (PICA) |
| Intracranial Vein | Includes:<br>Anterior cerebral vein<br>Basal (internal) cerebral vein<br>Dural venous sinus<br>Great cerebral vein<br>Inferior cerebellar vein<br>Inferior cerebral vein<br>Internal (basal) cerebral vein<br>Middle cerebral vein<br>Ophthalmic vein<br>Superior cerebellar vein<br>Superior cerebral vein |
| Jejunum | Includes: Duodenojejunal flexure |
| Kidney | Includes:<br>Renal calyx<br>Renal capsule<br>Renal cortex<br>Renal segment |
| Kidney Pelvis, Left<br>Kidney Pelvis, Right | Includes:<br>Ureteropelvic junction (UPJ) |
| Kidney, Left<br>Kidney, Right<br>Kidneys, Bilateral | Includes:<br>Renal calyx<br>Renal capsule<br>Renal cortex<br>Renal segment |
| Knee Bursa and Ligament, Left<br>Knee Bursa and Ligament, Right | Includes:<br>Anterior cruciate ligament (ACL)<br>Lateral collateral ligament (LCL)<br>Ligament of head of fibula<br>Medial collateral ligament (MCL)<br>Patellar ligament<br>Popliteal ligament<br>Posterior cruciate ligament (PCL)<br>Prepatellar bursa |

| Body Part | Definition |
|---|---|
| Knee Joint, Left<br>Knee Joint, Right | Includes:<br>Femoropatellar joint<br>Femorotibial joint<br>Lateral meniscus<br>Medial meniscus<br>Patellofemoral joint<br>Tibiofemoral joint |
| Knee Joint, Femoral Surface, Left<br>Knee Joint, Femoral Surface, Right | Includes:<br>Femoropatellar joint<br>Patellofemoral joint |
| Knee Joint, Tibial Surface, Left<br>Knee Joint, Tibial Surface, Right | Includes:<br>Femorotibial joint<br>Tibiofemoral joint |
| Knee Tendon, Left<br>Knee Tendon, Right | Includes:<br>Patellar tendon |
| Lacrimal Duct, Left<br>Lacrimal Duct, Right | Includes:<br>Lacrimal canaliculus<br>Lacrimal punctum<br>Lacrimal sac<br>Nasolacrimal duct |
| Larynx | Includes:<br>Aryepiglottic fold<br>Arytenoid cartilage<br>Corniculate cartilage<br>Cricoid cartilage<br>Cuneiform cartilage<br>False vocal cord<br>Glottis<br>Rima glottidis<br>Thyroid cartilage<br>Ventricular fold |
| Lens, Left<br>Lens, Right | Includes:<br>Zonule of Zinn |
| Lesser Omentum | Includes:<br>Gastrohepatic omentum<br>Hepatogastric ligament |
| Lesser Saphenous Vein, Left<br>Lesser Saphenous Vein, Right | Includes:<br>Small saphenous vein |
| Liver | Includes: Quadrate lobe |
| Lower Arm and Wrist Muscle, Left<br>Lower Arm and Wrist Muscle, Right | Includes:<br>Anatomical snuffbox<br>Brachioradialis muscle<br>Extensor carpi radialis muscle<br>Extensor carpi ulnaris muscle<br>Flexor carpi radialis muscle<br>Flexor carpi ulnaris muscle<br>Flexor pollicis longus muscle<br>Palmaris longus muscle<br>Pronator quadratus muscle<br>Pronator teres muscle |
| Lower Eyelid, Left<br>Lower Eyelid, Right | Includes:<br>Inferior tarsal plate<br>Medial canthus |
| Lower Femur, Left<br>Lower Femur, Right | Includes:<br>Lateral condyle of femur<br>Lateral epicondyle of femur<br>Medial condyle of femur<br>Medial epicondyle of femur |
| Lower Leg Muscle, Left<br>Lower Leg Muscle, Right | Includes:<br>Extensor digitorum longus muscle<br>Extensor hallucis longus muscle<br>Fibularis brevis muscle<br>Fibularis longus muscle<br>Flexor digitorum longus muscle<br>Flexor hallucis longus muscle<br>Gastrocnemius muscle<br>Peroneus brevis muscle<br>Peroneus longus muscle<br>Popliteus muscle<br>Soleus muscle<br>Tibialis anterior muscle<br>Tibialis posterior muscle |
| Lower Leg Tendon, Left<br>Lower Leg Tendon, Right | Includes:<br>Achilles tendon |
| Lower Lip | Includes:<br>Frenulum labii inferioris<br>Labial gland<br>Vermilion border |

| Body Part | Definition |
|---|---|
| Lumbar Nerve | **Includes:**<br>Lumbosacral trunk<br>Spinal nerve, lumbar<br>Superior clunic (cluneal) nerve |
| Lumbar Plexus | **Includes:**<br>Accessory obturator nerve<br>Genitofemoral nerve<br>Iliohypogastric nerve<br>Ilioinguinal nerve<br>Lateral femoral cutaneous nerve<br>Obturator nerve<br>Superior gluteal nerve |
| Lumbar Spinal Cord | **Includes:**<br>Cauda equina<br>Conus medullaris |
| Lumbar Sympathetic Nerve | **Includes:**<br>Lumbar ganglion<br>Lumbar splanchnic nerve |
| Lumbar Vertebra | **Includes:**<br>Spinous process<br>Vertebral arch<br>Vertebral foramen<br>Vertebral lamina<br>Vertebral pedicle |
| Lumbar Vertebral Joint | **Includes:**<br>Lumbar facet joint |
| Lumbosacral Joint | **Includes:** Lumbosacral facet joint |
| Lymphatic, Aortic | **Includes:**<br>Celiac lymph node<br>Gastric lymph node<br>Hepatic lymph node<br>Lumbar lymph node<br>Pancreaticosplenic lymph node<br>Paraaortic lymph node<br>Retroperitoneal lymph node |
| Lymphatic, Head | **Includes:**<br>Buccinator lymph node<br>Infraauricular lymph node<br>Infraparotid lymph node<br>Parotid lymph node<br>Preauricular lymph node<br>Submandibular lymph node<br>Submaxillary lymph node<br>Submental lymph node<br>Subparotid lymph node<br>Suprahyoid lymph node |
| Lymphatic, Left Axillary | **Includes:**<br>Anterior (pectoral) lymph node<br>Apical (subclavicular) lymph node<br>Brachial (lateral) lymph node<br>Central axillary lymph node<br>Lateral (brachial) lymph node<br>Pectoral (anterior) lymph node<br>Posterior (subscapular) lymph node<br>Subclavicular (apical) lymph node<br>Subscapular (posterior) lymph node |
| Lymphatic, Left Lower Extremity | **Includes:**<br>Femoral lymph node<br>Popliteal lymph node |
| Lymphatic, Left Neck | **Includes:**<br>Cervical lymph node<br>Jugular lymph node<br>Mastoid (postauricular) lymph node<br>Occipital lymph node<br>Postauricular (mastoid) lymph node<br>Retropharyngeal lymph node<br>Supraclavicular (Virchow's) lymph node<br>Virchow's (supraclavicular) lymph node |
| Lymphatic, Left Upper Extremity | **Includes:**<br>Cubital lymph node<br>Deltopectoral (infraclavicular) lymph node<br>Epitrochlear lymph node<br>Infraclavicular (deltopectoral) lymph node<br>Supratrochlear lymph node |
| Lymphatic, Mesenteric | **Includes:**<br>Inferior mesenteric lymph node<br>Pararectal lymph node<br>Superior mesenteric lymph node |
| Lymphatic, Pelvis | **Includes:**<br>Common iliac (subaortic) lymph node<br>Gluteal lymph node<br>Iliac lymph node<br>Inferior epigastric lymph node<br>Obturator lymph node<br>Sacral lymph node<br>Subaortic (common iliac) lymph node<br>Suprainguinal lymph node |
| Lymphatic, Right Axillary | **Includes:**<br>Anterior (pectoral) lymph node<br>Apical (subclavicular) lymph node<br>Brachial (lateral) lymph node<br>Central axillary lymph node<br>Lateral (brachial) lymph node<br>Pectoral (anterior) lymph node<br>Posterior (subscapular) lymph node<br>Subclavicular (apical) lymph node<br>Subscapular (posterior) lymph node |
| Lymphatic, Right Lower Extremity | **Includes:**<br>Femoral lymph node<br>Popliteal lymph node |
| Lymphatic, Right Neck | **Includes:**<br>Cervical lymph node<br>Jugular lymph node<br>Mastoid (postauricular) lymph node<br>Occipital lymph node<br>Postauricular (mastoid) lymph node<br>Retropharyngeal lymph node<br>Right jugular trunk<br>Right lymphatic duct<br>Right subclavian trunk<br>Supraclavicular (Virchow's) lymph node<br>Virchow's (supraclavicular) lymph node |
| Lymphatic, Right Upper Extremity | **Includes:**<br>Cubital lymph node<br>Deltopectoral (infraclavicular) lymph node<br>Epitrochlear lymph node<br>Infraclavicular (deltopectoral) lymph node<br>Supratrochlear lymph node |
| Lymphatic, Thorax | **Includes:**<br>Intercostal lymph node<br>Mediastinal lymph node<br>Parasternal lymph node<br>Paratracheal lymph node<br>Tracheobronchial lymph node |
| Mandible, Left<br>Mandible, Right | **Includes:**<br>Alveolar process of mandible<br>Condyloid process<br>Mandibular notch<br>Mental foramen |
| Mastoid Sinus, Left<br>Mastoid Sinus, Right | **Includes:**<br>Mastoid air cells |
| Maxilla, Left<br>Maxilla, Right | **Includes:**<br>Alveolar process of maxilla |
| Maxillary Sinus, Left<br>Maxillary Sinus, Right | **Includes:**<br>Antrum of Highmore |
| Median Nerve | **Includes:**<br>Anterior interosseous nerve<br>Palmar cutaneous nerve |
| Medulla Oblongata | **Includes:** Myelencephalon |
| Mesentery | **Includes:**<br>Mesoappendix<br>Mesocolon |
| Metacarpocarpal Joint, Left<br>Metacarpocarpal Joint, Right | **Includes:**<br>Carpometacarpal (CMC) joint |
| Metatarsal-Phalangeal Joint, Left<br>Metatarsal-Phalangeal Joint, Right | **Includes:**<br>Metatarsophalangeal (MTP) joint |
| Metatarsal-Tarsal Joint, Left<br>Metatarsal-Tarsal Joint, Right | **Includes:**<br>Tarsometatarsal joint |
| Middle Ear, Left<br>Middle Ear, Right | **Includes:**<br>Oval window<br>Tympanic cavity |
| Minor Salivary Gland | **Includes:** Anterior lingual gland |
| Mitral Valve | **Includes:**<br>Bicuspid valve<br>Left atrioventricular valve<br>Mitral annulus |

| Body Part | Definition |
|-----------|------------|
| Nasal Bone | **Includes:** Vomer of nasal septum |
| Nasal Septum | **Includes:**<br>Quadrangular cartilage<br>Septal cartilage<br>Vomer bone |
| Nasal Turbinate | **Includes:**<br>Inferior turbinate<br>Middle turbinate<br>Nasal concha<br>Superior turbinate |
| Nasopharynx | **Includes:**<br>Choana<br>Fossa of Rosenmuller<br>Pharyngeal recess<br>Rhinopharynx |
| Neck Muscle, Left<br>Neck Muscle, Right | **Includes:**<br>Anterior vertebral muscle<br>Arytenoid muscle<br>Cricothyroid muscle<br>Infrahyoid muscle<br>Levator scapulae muscle<br>Platysma muscle<br>Scalene muscle<br>Splenius cervicis muscle<br>Sternocleidomastoid muscle<br>Suprahyoid muscle<br>Thyroarytenoid muscle |
| Nipple, Left<br>Nipple, Right | **Includes:**<br>Areola |
| Nose | **Includes:**<br>Columella<br>External naris<br>Greater alar cartilage<br>Internal naris<br>Lateral nasal cartilage<br>Lesser alar cartilage<br>Nasal cavity<br>Nostril |
| Occipital Bone, Left<br>Occipital Bone, Right | **Includes:**<br>Foramen magnum |
| Oculomotor Nerve | **Includes:** Third cranial nerve |
| Olfactory Nerve | **Includes:**<br>First cranial nerve<br>Olfactory bulb |
| Optic Nerve | **Includes:**<br>Optic chiasma<br>Second cranial nerve |
| Orbit, Left<br>Orbit, Right | **Includes:**<br>Bony orbit<br>Orbital portion of ethmoid bone<br>Orbital portion of frontal bone<br>Orbital portion of lacrimal bone<br>Orbital portion of maxilla<br>Orbital portion of palatine bone<br>Orbital portion of sphenoid bone<br>Orbital portion of zygomatic bone |
| Pancreatic Duct | **Includes:** Duct of Wirsung |
| Pancreatic Duct, Accessory | **Includes:** Duct of Santorini |
| Parotid Duct, Left<br>Parotid Duct, Right | **Includes:**<br>Stensen's duct |
| Pelvic Bone, Left<br>Pelvic Bone, Right | **Includes:**<br>Iliac crest<br>Ilium<br>Ischium<br>Pubis |
| Pelvic Cavity | **Includes:** Retropubic space |
| Penis | **Includes:**<br>Corpus cavernosum<br>Corpus spongiosum |
| Perineum Muscle | **Includes:**<br>Bulbospongiosus muscle<br>Cremaster muscle<br>Deep transverse perineal muscle<br>Ischiocavernosus muscle<br>Superficial transverse perineal muscle |
| Peritoneum | **Includes:** Epiploic foramen |

| Body Part | Definition |
|-----------|------------|
| Peroneal Artery, Left<br>Peroneal Artery, Right | **Includes:**<br>Fibular artery |
| Peroneal Nerve | **Includes:**<br>Common fibular nerve<br>Common peroneal nerve<br>External popliteal nerve<br>Lateral sural cutaneous nerve |
| Pharynx | **Includes:**<br>Hypopharynx<br>Laryngopharynx<br>Oropharynx<br>Piriform recess (sinus) |
| Phrenic Nerve | **Includes:** Accessory phrenic nerve |
| Pituitary Gland | **Includes:**<br>Adenohypophysis<br>Hypophysis<br>Neurohypophysis |
| Pons | **Includes:**<br>Apneustic center<br>Basis pontis<br>Locus ceruleus<br>Pneumotaxic center<br>Pontine tegmentum<br>Superior olivary nucleus |
| Popliteal Artery, Left<br>Popliteal Artery, Right | **Includes:**<br>Inferior genicular artery<br>Middle genicular artery<br>Superior genicular artery<br>Sural artery |
| Portal Vein | **Includes:** Hepatic portal vein |
| Prepuce | **Includes:**<br>Foreskin<br>Glans penis |
| Pudendal Nerve | **Includes:**<br>Posterior labial nerve<br>Posterior scrotal nerve |
| Pulmonary Artery, Left | **Includes:**<br>Arterial canal (duct)<br>Botallo's duct<br>Pulmoaortic canal |
| Pulmonary Valve | **Includes:**<br>Pulmonary annulus<br>Pulmonic valve |
| Pulmonary Vein, Left | **Includes:**<br>Left inferior pulmonary vein<br>Left superior pulmonary vein |
| Pulmonary Vein, Right | **Includes:**<br>Right inferior pulmonary vein<br>Right superior pulmonary vein |
| Radial Artery, Left<br>Radial Artery, Right | **Includes:**<br>Radial recurrent artery |
| Radial Nerve | **Includes:**<br>Dorsal digital nerve<br>Musculospiral nerve<br>Palmar cutaneous nerve<br>Posterior interosseous nerve |
| Radius, Left<br>Radius, Right | **Includes:**<br>Ulnar notch |
| Rectum | **Includes:** Anorectal junction |
| Renal Artery, Left<br>Renal Artery, Right | **Includes:**<br>Inferior suprarenal artery<br>Renal segmental artery |
| Renal Vein, Left | **Includes:**<br>Left inferior phrenic vein<br>Left ovarian vein<br>Left second lumbar vein<br>Left suprarenal vein<br>Left testicular vein |
| Retina, Left<br>Retina, Right | **Includes:**<br>Fovea<br>Macula<br>Optic disc |
| Retroperitoneum | **Includes:** Retroperitoneal space |
| Sacral Nerve | **Includes:** Spinal nerve, sacral |

| Body Part | Definition |
|---|---|
| Sacral Plexus | **Includes:**<br>Inferior gluteal nerve<br>Posterior femoral cutaneous nerve<br>Pudendal nerve |
| Sacral Sympathetic Nerve | **Includes:**<br>Ganglion impar (ganglion of Walther)<br>Pelvic splanchnic nerve<br>Sacral ganglion<br>Sacral splanchnic nerve |
| Sacrococcygeal Joint | **Includes:** Sacrococcygeal symphysis |
| Scapula, Left<br>Scapula, Right | **Includes:**<br>Acromion (process)<br>Coracoid process |
| Sciatic Nerve | **Includes:** Ischiatic nerve |
| Shoulder Bursa and Ligament, Left<br>Shoulder Bursa and Ligament, Right | **Includes:**<br>Acromioclavicular ligament<br>Coracoacromial ligament<br>Coracoclavicular ligament<br>Coracohumeral ligament<br>Costoclavicular ligament<br>Glenohumeral ligament<br>Glenoid ligament (labrum)<br>Interclavicular ligament<br>Sternoclavicular ligament<br>Subacromial bursa<br>Transverse humeral ligament<br>Transverse scapular ligament |
| Shoulder Joint, Left<br>Shoulder Joint, Right | **Includes:**<br>Glenohumeral joint |
| Shoulder Muscle, Left<br>Shoulder Muscle, Right | **Includes:**<br>Deltoid muscle<br>Infraspinatus muscle<br>Subscapularis muscle<br>Supraspinatus muscle<br>Teres major muscle<br>Teres minor muscle |
| Sigmoid Colon | **Includes:**<br>Rectosigmoid junction<br>Sigmoid flexure |
| Skin | **Includes:**<br>Dermis<br>Epidermis<br>Sebaceous gland<br>Sweat gland |
| Sphenoid Bone, Left<br>Sphenoid Bone, Right | **Includes:**<br>Greater wing<br>Lesser wing<br>Optic foramen<br>Pterygoid process<br>Sella turcica |
| Spinal Canal | **Includes:** Vertebral canal |
| Spinal Meninges | **Includes:**<br>Arachnoid mater<br>Denticulate ligament<br>Leptomeninges<br>Pia mater |
| Spleen | **Includes:** Accessory spleen |
| Splenic Artery | **Includes:**<br>Left gastroepiploic artery<br>Pancreatic artery<br>Short gastric artery |
| Splenic Vein | **Includes:**<br>Left gastroepiploic vein<br>Pancreatic vein |
| Sternum | **Includes:**<br>Manubrium<br>Suprasternal notch<br>Xiphoid process |
| Stomach, Pylorus | **Includes:**<br>Pyloric antrum<br>Pyloric canal<br>Pyloric sphincter |
| Subarachnoid Space | **Includes:**<br>Cranial subarachnoid space<br>Spinal subarachnoid space |

| Body Part | Definition |
|---|---|
| Subclavian Artery, Left<br>Subclavian Artery, Right | **Includes:**<br>Costocervical trunk<br>Dorsal scapular artery<br>Internal thoracic artery |
| Subcutaneous Tissue and Fascia, Anterior Neck | **Includes:**<br>Deep cervical fascia<br>Pretracheal fascia |
| Subcutaneous Tissue and Fascia, Chest | **Includes:** Pectoral fascia |
| Subcutaneous Tissue and Fascia, Face | **Includes:**<br>Masseteric fascia<br>Orbital fascia |
| Subcutaneous Tissue and Fascia, Right Foot<br>Subcutaneous Tissue and Fascia, Left Foot | **Includes:**<br>Plantar fascia (aponeurosis) |
| Subcutaneous Tissue and Fascia, Right Hand<br>Subcutaneous Tissue and Fascia, Left Hand | **Includes:**<br>Palmar fascia (aponeurosis) |
| Subcutaneous Tissue and Fascia, Right Lower Arm<br>Subcutaneous Tissue and Fascia, Left Lower Arm | **Includes:**<br>Antebrachial fascia<br>Bicipital aponeurosis |
| Subcutaneous Tissue and Fascia, Posterior Neck | **Includes:**<br>Prevertebral fascia |
| Subcutaneous Tissue and Fascia, Scalp | **Includes:** Galea aponeurotica |
| Subcutaneous Tissue and Fascia, Trunk | **Includes:**<br>External oblique aponeurosis<br>Transversalis fascia |
| Subcutaneous Tissue and Fascia, Right Upper Arm<br>Subcutaneous Tissue and Fascia, Left Upper Arm | **Includes:**<br>Axillary fascia<br>Deltoid fascia<br>Infraspinatus fascia<br>Subscapular aponeurosis<br>Supraspinatus fascia |
| Subcutaneous Tissue and Fascia, Right Upper Leg<br>Subcutaneous Tissue and Fascia, Left Upper Leg | **Includes:**<br>Crural fascia<br>Fascia lata<br>Iliac fascia<br>Iliotibial tract (band) |
| Subdural Space | **Includes:**<br>Cranial subdural space<br>Spinal subdural space |
| Submaxillary Gland, Left<br>Submaxillary Gland, Right | **Includes:**<br>Submandibular gland |
| Superior Mesenteric Artery | **Includes:**<br>Ileal artery<br>Ileocolic artery<br>Inferior pancreaticoduodenal artery<br>Jejunal artery |
| Superior Mesenteric Vein | **Includes:** Right gastroepiploic vein |
| Superior Vena Cava | **Includes:** Precava |
| Tarsal Joint, Left<br>Tarsal Joint, Right | **Includes:**<br>Calcaneocuboid joint<br>Cuboideonavicular joint<br>Cuneonavicular joint<br>Intercuneiform joint<br>Subtalar (talocalcaneal) joint<br>Talocalcaneal (subtalar) joint<br>Talocalcaneonavicular joint |
| Tarsal, Left<br>Tarsal, Right | **Includes:**<br>Calcaneus<br>Cuboid bone<br>Intermediate cuneiform bone<br>Lateral cuneiform bone<br>Medial cuneiform bone<br>Navicular bone<br>Talus bone |
| Temporal Artery, Left<br>Temporal Artery, Right | **Includes:**<br>Middle temporal artery<br>Superficial temporal artery<br>Transverse facial artery |
| Temporal Bone, Left<br>Temporal Bone, Right | **Includes:**<br>Mastoid process<br>Petrous part of temoporal bone<br>Tympanic part of temoporal bone<br>Zygomatic process of temporal bone |

| Body Part | Definition |
|---|---|
| Thalamus | Includes:<br>Epithalamus<br>Geniculate nucleus<br>Metathalamus<br>Pulvinar |
| Thoracic Aorta | Includes:<br>Aortic arch<br>Aortic intercostal artery<br>Ascending aorta<br>Bronchial artery<br>Esophageal artery<br>Subcostal artery |
| Thoracic Duct | Includes:<br>Left jugular trunk<br>Left subclavian trunk |
| Thoracic Nerve | Includes:<br>Intercostal nerve<br>Intercostobrachial nerve<br>Spinal nerve, thoracic<br>Subcostal nerve |
| Thoracic Sympathetic Nerve | Includes:<br>Cardiac plexus<br>Esophageal plexus<br>Greater splanchnic nerve<br>Inferior cardiac nerve<br>Least splanchnic nerve<br>Lesser splanchnic nerve<br>Middle cardiac nerve<br>Pulmonary plexus<br>Superior cardiac nerve<br>Thoracic aortic plexus<br>Thoracic ganglion |
| Thoracic Vertebra | Includes:<br>Spinous process<br>Vertebral arch<br>Vertebral foramen<br>Vertebral lamina<br>Vertebral pedicle |
| Thoracic Vertebral Joint | Includes:<br>Costotransverse joint<br>Costovertebral joint<br>Thoracic facet joint |
| Thoracolumbar Vertebral Joint | Includes: Thoracolumbar facet joint |
| Thorax Bursa and Ligament, Left<br>Thorax Bursa and Ligament, Right | Includes:<br>Costotransverse ligament<br>Costoxiphoid ligament<br>Sternocostal ligament |
| Thorax Muscle, Left<br>Thorax Muscle, Right | Includes:<br>Intercostal muscle<br>Levatores costarum muscle<br>Pectoralis major muscle<br>Pectoralis minor muscle<br>Serratus anterior muscle<br>Subclavius muscle<br>Subcostal muscle<br>Transverse thoracis muscle |
| Thymus | Includes: Thymus gland |
| Thyroid Artery, Left<br>Thyroid Artery, Right | Includes:<br>Cricothyroid artery<br>Hyoid artery<br>Sternocleidomastoid artery<br>Superior laryngeal artery<br>Superior thyroid artery<br>Thyrocervical trunk |
| Tibia, Left<br>Tibia, Right | Includes:<br>Lateral condyle of tibia<br>Medial condyle of tibia<br>Medial malleolus |
| Tibial Nerve | Includes:<br>Lateral plantar nerve<br>Medial plantar nerve<br>Medial popliteal nerve<br>Medial sural cutaneous nerve |
| Toe Nail | Includes:<br>Nail bed<br>Nail plate |
| Toe Phalangeal Joint, Left<br>Toe Phalangeal Joint, Right | Includes:<br>Interphalangeal (IP) joint |

| Body Part | Definition |
|---|---|
| Tongue | Includes:<br>Frenulum linguae<br>Lingual tonsil |
| Tongue, Palate, Pharynx Muscle | Includes:<br>Chondroglossus muscle<br>Genioglossus muscle<br>Hyoglossus muscle<br>Inferior longitudinal muscle<br>Levator veli palatini muscle<br>Palatoglossal muscle<br>Palatopharyngeal muscle<br>Pharyngeal constrictor muscle<br>Salpingopharyngeus muscle<br>Styloglossus muscle<br>Stylopharyngeus muscle<br>Superior longitudinal muscle<br>Tensor veli palatini muscle |
| Tonsils | Includes: Palatine tonsil |
| Transverse Colon | Includes: Splenic flexure |
| Tricuspid Valve | Includes:<br>Right atrioventricular valve<br>Tricuspid annulus |
| Trigeminal Nerve | Includes:<br>Fifth cranial nerve<br>Gasserian ganglion<br>Mandibular nerve<br>Maxillary nerve<br>Ophthalmic nerve<br>Trifacial nerve |
| Trochlear Nerve | Includes: Fourth cranial nerve |
| Trunk Bursa and Ligament, Left<br>Trunk Bursa and Ligament, Right | Includes:<br>Iliolumbar ligament<br>Interspinous ligament<br>Intertransverse ligament<br>Ligamentum flavum<br>Pubic ligament<br>Sacrococcygeal ligament<br>Sacroiliac ligament<br>Sacrospinous ligament<br>Sacrotuberous ligament<br>Supraspinous ligament |
| Trunk Muscle, Left<br>Trunk Muscle, Right | Includes:<br>Coccygeus muscle<br>Erector spinae muscle<br>Interspinalis muscle<br>Intertransversarius muscle<br>Latissimus dorsi muscle<br>Levator ani muscle<br>Quadratus lumborum muscle<br>Rhomboid major muscle<br>Rhomboid minor muscle<br>Serratus posterior muscle<br>Transversospinalis muscle<br>Trapezius muscle |
| Tympanic Membrane, Left<br>Tympanic Membrane, Right | Includes:<br>Pars flaccida |
| Ulna, Left<br>Ulna, Right | Includes:<br>Olecranon process<br>Radial notch |
| Ulnar Artery, Left<br>Ulnar Artery, Right | Includes:<br>Anterior ulnar recurrent artery<br>Common interosseous artery<br>Posterior ulnar recurrent artery |
| Ulnar Nerve | Includes: Cubital nerve |
| Upper Arm Muscle, Left<br>Upper Arm Muscle, Right | Includes:<br>Biceps brachii muscle<br>Brachialis muscle<br>Coracobrachialis muscle<br>Triceps brachii muscle |
| Upper Eyelid, Left<br>Upper Eyelid, Right | Includes:<br>Lateral canthus<br>Levator palpebrae superioris muscle<br>Orbicularis oculi muscle<br>Superior tarsal plate |
| Upper Femur, Left<br>Upper Femur, Right | Includes:<br>Femoral head<br>Greater trochanter<br>Lesser trochanter<br>Neck of femur |

| Body Part | Definition |
|---|---|
| Upper Leg Muscle, Left<br>Upper Leg Muscle, Right | **Includes:**<br>Adductor brevis muscle<br>Adductor longus muscle<br>Adductor magnus muscle<br>Biceps femoris muscle<br>Gracilis muscle<br>Pectineus muscle<br>Quadriceps (femoris)<br>Rectus femoris muscle<br>Sartorius muscle<br>Semimembranosus muscle<br>Semitendinosus muscle<br>Vastus intermedius muscle<br>Vastus lateralis muscle<br>Vastus medialis muscle |
| Upper Lip | **Includes:**<br>Frenulum labii superioris<br>Labial gland<br>Vermilion border |
| Ureter<br>Ureter, Left<br>Ureter, Right<br>Ureters, Bilateral | **Includes:**<br>Ureteral orifice<br>Ureterovesical orifice |
| Urethra | **Includes:**<br>Bulbourethral (Cowper's) gland<br>Cowper's (bulbourethral) gland<br>External urethral sphincter<br>Internal urethral sphincter<br>Membranous urethra<br>Penile urethra<br>Prostatic urethra |
| Uterine Supporting Structure | **Includes:**<br>Broad ligament<br>Infundibulopelvic ligament<br>Ovarian ligament<br>Round ligament of uterus |
| Uterus | **Includes:**<br>Fundus uteri<br>Myometrium<br>Perimetrium<br>Uterine cornu |
| Uvula | **Includes:** Palatine uvula |
| Vagus Nerve | **Includes:**<br>Anterior vagal trunk<br>Pharyngeal plexus<br>Pneumogastric nerve<br>Posterior vagal trunk<br>Pulmonary plexus<br>Recurrent laryngeal nerve<br>Superior laryngeal nerve<br>Tenth cranial nerve |
| Vas Deferens<br>Vas Deferens, Bilateral<br>Vas Deferens, Left<br>Vas Deferens, Right | **Includes:**<br>Ductus deferens<br>Ejaculatory duct |
| Ventricle, Right | **Includes:** Conus arteriosus |
| Ventricular Septum | **Includes:** Interventricular septum |
| Vertebral Artery, Left<br>Vertebral Artery, Right | **Includes:** Anterior spinal artery<br>Posterior spinal artery |
| Vertebral Vein, Left<br>Vertebral Vein, Right | **Includes:**<br>Deep cervical vein<br>Suboccipital venous plexus |
| Vestibular Gland | **Includes:**<br>Bartholin's (greater vestibular) gland<br>Greater vestibular (Bartholin's) gland<br>Paraurethral (Skene's) gland<br>Skene's (paraurethral) gland |
| Vitreous, Left<br>Vitreous, Right | **Includes:**<br>Vitreous body |
| Vocal Cord, Left<br>Vocal Cord, Right | **Includes:**<br>Vocal fold |
| Vulva | **Includes:**<br>Labia majora<br>Labia minora |

| Body Part | Definition |
|---|---|
| Wrist Bursa and Ligament, Left<br>Wrist Bursa and Ligament, Right | **Includes:**<br>Palmar ulnocarpal ligament<br>Radial collateral carpal ligament<br>Radiocarpal ligament<br>Radioulnar ligament<br>Ulnar collateral carpal ligament |
| Wrist Joint, Left<br>Wrist Joint, Right | **Includes:**<br>Distal radioulnar joint<br>Radiocarpal joint |

## Section 0 – Medical and Surgical
*Character 5: Approach*

| External | **Definition:** Procedures performed directly on the skin or mucous membrane and procedures performed indirectly by the application of external force through the skin or mucous membrane |
|---|---|
| Open | **Definition:** Cutting through the skin or mucous membrane and any other body layers necessary to expose the site of the procedure |
| Percutaneous | **Definition:** Entry, by puncture or minor incision, of instrumentation through the skin or mucous membrane and any other body layers necessary to reach the site of the procedure |
| Percutaneous Endoscopic | **Definition:** Entry, by puncture or minor incision, of instrumentation through the skin or mucous membrane and any other body layers necessary to reach and visualize the site of the procedure |
| Via Natural or Artificial Opening | **Definition:** Entry of instrumentation through a natural or artificial external opening to reach the site of the procedure |
| Via Natural or Artificial Opening Endoscopic | **Definition:** Entry of instrumentation through a natural or artificial external opening to reach and visualize the site of the procedure |
| Via Natural or Artificial Opening With Percutaneous Endoscopic Assistance | **Definition:** Entry of instrumentation through a natural or artificial external opening and entry, by puncture or minor incision, of instrumentation through the skin or mucous membrane and any other body layers necessary to aid in the performance of the procedure |

## Section 0 – Medical and Surgical
*Character 6: Device*

| Artificial Sphincter in Gastrointestinal System | **Includes:**<br>Artificial anal sphincter (AAS)<br>Artificial bowel sphincter (neosphincter) |
|---|---|
| Artificial Sphincter in Urinary System | **Includes:**<br>AMS 800® Urinary Control System<br>Artificial urinary sphincter (AUS) |
| Autologous Arterial Tissue in Heart and Great Vessels | **Includes:**<br>Autologous artery graft |
| Autologous Arterial Tissue in Lower Arteries | **Includes:**<br>Autologous artery graft |
| Autologous Arterial Tissue in Lower Veins | **Includes:**<br>Autologous artery graft |
| Autologous Arterial Tissue in Upper Arteries | **Includes:**<br>Autologous artery graft |
| Autologous Arterial Tissue in Upper Veins | **Includes:**<br>Autologous artery graft |
| Autologous Tissue Substitute | **Includes:**<br>Autograft<br>Cultured epidermal cell autograft<br>Epicel® cultured epidermal autograft |
| Autologous Venous Tissue in Heart and Great Vessels | **Includes:**<br>Autologous vein graft |
| Autologous Venous Tissue in Lower Arteries | **Includes:**<br>Autologous vein graft |
| Autologous Venous Tissue in Lower Veins | **Includes:**<br>Autologous vein graft |
| Autologous Venous Tissue in Upper Arteries | **Includes:**<br>Autologous vein graft |
| Autologous Venous Tissue in Upper Veins | **Includes:**<br>Autologous vein graft |
| Bone Growth Stimulator in Head and Facial Bones | **Includes:**<br>Electrical bone growth stimulator (EBGS)<br>Ultrasonic osteogenic stimulator<br>Ultrasound bone healing system |
| Bone Growth Stimulator in Lower Bones | **Includes:**<br>Electrical bone growth stimulator (EBGS)<br>Ultrasonic osteogenic stimulator<br>Ultrasound bone healing system |

| | |
|---|---|
| **Bone Growth Stimulator in Upper Bones** | **Includes:**<br>Electrical bone growth stimulator (EBGS)<br>Ultrasonic osteogenic stimulator<br>Ultrasound bone healing system |
| **Cardiac Lead in Heart and Great Vessels** | **Includes:**<br>Cardiac contractility modulation lead |
| **Cardiac Lead, Defibrillator for Insertion in Heart and Great Vessels** | **Includes:**<br>ACUITY™ Steerable Lead<br>Attain Ability® lead<br>Attain StarFix® (OTW) lead<br>Cardiac resynchronization therapy (CRT) lead<br>Corox (OTW) Bipolar Lead<br>Durata® Defibrillation Lead<br>ENDOTAK RELIANCE® (G) Defibrillation Lead |
| **Cardiac Lead, Pacemaker for Insertion in Heart and Great Vessels** | **Includes:**<br>ACUITY™ Steerable Lead<br>Attain Ability® lead<br>Attain StarFix® (OTW) lead<br>Cardiac resynchronization therapy (CRT) lead<br>Corox (OTW) Bipolar Lead |
| **Cardiac Resynchronization Defibrillator Pulse Generator for Insertion in Subcutaneous Tissue and Fascia** | **Includes:**<br>COGNIS® CRT-D<br>Concerto II CRT-D<br>Consulta CRT-D<br>CONTAK RENEWAL® 3 RF (HE) CRT-D<br>LIVIAN™ CRT-D<br>Maximo II DR CRT-D<br>Ovatio™ CRT-D<br>Protecta XT CRT-D<br>Viva (XT)(S) |
| **Cardiac Resynchronization Pacemaker Pulse Generator for Insertion in Subcutaneous Tissue and Fascia** | **Includes:**<br>Consulta CRT-P<br>Stratos LV<br>Synchra CRT-P |
| **Contraceptive Device in Female Reproductive System** | **Includes:**<br>Intrauterine Device (IUD) |
| **Contraceptive Device in Subcutaneous Tissue and Fascia** | **Includes:**<br>Subdermal progesterone implant |
| **Contractility Modulation Device for Insertion in Subcutaneous Tissue and Fascia** | **Includes:**<br>Optimizer™ III implantable pulse generator |
| **Defibrillator Generator for Insertion in Subcutaneous Tissue and Fascia** | **Includes:**<br>Evera (XT)(S)(DR/VR)<br>Implantable cardioverter-defibrillator (ICD)<br>Maximo II DR (VR)<br>Protecta XT DR (XT VR)<br>Secura (DR) (VR)<br>Virtuoso (II) (DR) (VR) |
| **Diaphragmatic Pacemaker Lead in Respiratory System** | **Includes:**<br>Phrenic nerve stimulator lead |
| **Drainage Device** | **Includes:**<br>Cystostomy tube<br>Foley catheter<br>Percutaneous nephrostomy catheter<br>Thoracostomy tube |
| **Epiretinal Visual Prosthesis in Eye** | **Includes:** Epiretinal visual prosthesis |
| **External Fixation Device in Head and Facial Bones** | **Includes:**<br>External fixator |
| **External Fixation Device in Lower Bones** | **Includes:** External fixator |
| **External Fixation Device in Lower Joints** | **Includes:** External fixator |
| **External Fixation Device in Upper Bones** | **Includes:** External fixator |
| **External Fixation Device in Upper Joints** | **Includes:** External fixator |
| **External Fixation Device, Hybrid for Insertion in Upper Bones** | **Includes:**<br>Delta frame external fixator<br>Sheffield hybrid external fixator |
| **External Fixation Device, Hybrid for Insertion in Lower Bones** | **Includes:**<br>Delta frame external fixator<br>Sheffield hybrid external fixator |
| **External Fixation Device, Hybrid for Reposition in Lower Bones** | **Includes:**<br>Delta frame external fixator<br>Sheffield hybrid external fixator |
| **External Fixation Device, Hybrid for Reposition in Upper Bones** | **Includes:**<br>Delta frame external fixator<br>Sheffield hybrid external fixator |
| **External Fixation Device, Limb Lengthening for Insertion in Lower Bones** | **Includes:**<br>Ilizarov-Vecklich device |
| **External Fixation Device, Limb Lengthening for Insertion in Upper Bones** | **Includes:**<br>Ilizarov-Vecklich device |

| | |
|---|---|
| **External Fixation Device, Monoplanar for Insertion in Lower Bones** | **Includes:**<br>Uniplanar external fixator |
| **External Fixation Device, Monoplanar for Insertion in Upper Bones** | **Includes:**<br>Uniplanar external fixator |
| **External Fixation Device, Monoplanar for Reposition in Lower Bones** | **Includes:**<br>Uniplanar external fixator |
| **External Fixation Device, Monoplanar for Reposition in Upper Bones** | **Includes:**<br>Uniplanar external fixator |
| **External Fixation Device, Ring for Insertion in Upper Bones** | **Includes:**<br>Ilizarov external fixator<br>Sheffield ring external fixator |
| **External Fixation Device, Ring for Reposition in Upper Bones** | **Includes:**<br>Ilizarov external fixator<br>Sheffield ring external fixator |
| **External Fixation Device, Ring for Insertion in Lower Bones** | **Includes:**<br>Ilizarov external fixator<br>Sheffield ring external fixator |
| **External Fixation Device, Ring for Reposition in Lower Bones** | **Includes:**<br>Ilizarov external fixator<br>Sheffield ring external fixator |
| **External Heart Assist System in Heart and Great Vessels** | **Includes:**<br>Biventricular external heart assist system<br>BVS 5000 Ventricular Assist Device<br>Centrimag® Blood Pump<br>TandemHeart® System<br>Thoratec Paracorporeal Ventricular Assist Device |
| **Extraluminal Device** | **Includes:**<br>LAP-BAND® Adjustable Gastric Banding System<br>REALIZE® Adjustable Gastric Band<br>TigerPaw® system for closure of left atrial appendage |
| **Feeding Device in Gastrointestinal System** | **Includes:**<br>Percutaneous endoscopic gastrojejunostomy (PEG/J) tube<br>Percutaneous endoscopic gastrostomy (PEG) tube |
| **Hearing Device in Ear, Nose, Sinus** | **Includes:**<br>Esteem® implantable hearing system |
| **Hearing Device, Bone Conduction for Insertion in Ear, Nose, Sinus** | **Includes:**<br>Bone anchored hearing device |
| **Hearing Device in Head and Facial Bones** | **Includes:**<br>Bone anchored hearing device |
| **Hearing Device, Multiple Channel Cochlear Prosthesis for Insertion in Ear, Nose, Sinus** | **Includes:**<br>Cochlear implant (CI), multiple channel (electrode) |
| **Hearing Device, Single Channel Cochlear Prosthesis for Insertion in Ear, Nose, Sinus** | **Includes:**<br>Cochlear implant (CI), single channel (electrode) |
| **Implantable Heart Assist System in Heart and Great Vessels** | **Includes:**<br>Berlin Heart Ventricular Assist Device<br>DeBakey Left Ventricular Assist Device<br>DuraHeart Left Ventricular Assist System<br>HeartMate II® Left Ventricular Assist Device (LVAD)<br>HeartMate XVE® Left Ventricular Assist Device (LVAD)<br>MicroMed HeartAssist<br>Novacor Left Ventricular Assist Device<br>Thoratec IVAD (Implantable Ventricular Assist Device) |
| **Infusion Device** | **Includes:**<br>Ascenda Intrathecal Catheter<br>InDura, intrathecal catheter (1P) (spinal)<br>Non-tunneled central venous catheter<br>Peripherally inserted central catheter (PICC)<br>Tunneled spinal (intrathecal) catheter |
| **Infusion Device, Pump in Subcutaneous Tissue and Fascia** | **Includes:**<br>Implantable drug infusion pump (anti-spasmodic) (chemotherapy)(pain)<br>Injection reservoir, pump<br>Pump reservoir<br>Subcutaneous injection reservoir, pump<br>SynchroMed pump |
| **Interbody Fusion Device in Lower Joints** | **Includes:**<br>Axial Lumbar Interbody Fusion System<br>AxiaLIF® System<br>CoRoent® XL<br>Direct Lateral Interbody Fusion (DLIF) device<br>EXtreme Lateral Interbody Fusion (XLIF) device<br>Interbody fusion (spine) cage<br>XLIF® System |
| **Interbody Fusion Device in Upper Joints** | **Includes:**<br>BAK/C® Interbody Cervical Fusion System<br>Interbody fusion (spine) cage |

| | | | |
|---|---|---|---|
| **Internal Fixation Device in Head and Facial Bones** | **Includes:**<br>Bone screw (interlocking)(lag)(pedicle)(recessed)<br>Kirschner wire (K-wire)<br>Neutralization plate | **Intraluminal Device, Bioactive in Upper Arteries** | **Includes:**<br>Bioactive embolization coil(s)<br>Micrus CERECYTE Microcoil |
| **Internal Fixation Device in Lower Bones** | **Includes:**<br>Bone screw (interlocking)(lag)(pedicle)(recessed)<br>Clamp and rod internal fixation system (CRIF)<br>Kirschner wire (K-wire)<br>Neutralization plate | **Intraluminal Device, Drug-eluting in Heart and Great Vessels** | **Includes:**<br>CYPHER® Stent<br>Endeavor® (III)(IV) (Sprint) Zotarolimus-eluting Coronary Stent System<br>Everolimus-eluting coronary stent<br>Paclitaxel-eluting coronary stent<br>Sirolimus-eluting coronary stent<br>TAXUS® Liberté® Paclitaxel-eluting Coronary Stent System<br>XIENCE Everolimus Eluting Coronary Stent System<br>Zotarolimus-eluting coronary stent |
| **Internal Fixation Device in Lower Joints** | **Includes:**<br>Fusion screw (compression)(lag)(locking)<br>Joint fixation plate<br>Kirschner wire (K-wire) | | |
| **Internal Fixation Device in Upper Bones** | **Includes:**<br>Bone screw (interlocking)(lag)(pedicle)(recessed)<br>Clamp and rod internal fixation system (CRIF)<br>Kirschner wire (K-wire)<br>Neutralization plate | **Intraluminal Device, Drug-eluting in Upper Arteries** | **Includes:**<br>Paclitaxel-eluting peripheral stent<br>Zilver® PTX® (paclitaxel) Drug-Eluting Peripheral Stent |
| **Internal Fixation Device in Upper Joints** | **Includes:**<br>Fusion screw (compression)(lag)(locking)<br>Joint fixation plate<br>Kirschner wire (K-wire) | **Intraluminal Device, Drug-eluting in Lower Arteries** | **Includes:**<br>Paclitaxel-eluting peripheral stent<br>Zilver® PTX® (paclitaxel) Drug-Eluting Peripheral Stent |
| **Internal Fixation Device, Intramedullary in Upper Bones** | **Includes:**<br>Intramedullary (IM) rod (nail)<br>Intramedullary skeletal kinetic distractor (ISKD)<br>Kuntscher nail | **Intraluminal Device, Endobronchial Valve in Respiratory System** | **Includes:**<br>Spiration IBV™ Valve System |
| **Internal Fixation Device, Intramedullary in Lower Bones** | **Includes:**<br>Intramedullary (IM) rod (nail)<br>Intramedullary skeletal kinetic distractor (ISKD)<br>Kuntscher nail | **Intraluminal Device, Endotracheal Airway in Respiratory System** | **Includes:**<br>Endotracheal tube (cuffed)(double-lumen) |
| | | **Intraluminal Device, Pessary in Female Reproductive System** | **Includes:**<br>Pessary ring<br>Vaginal pessary |
| **Internal Fixation Device, Rigid Plate for Insertion in Upper Bones** | **Includes:**<br>Titanium Sternal Fixation System (TSFS) | **Liner in Lower Joints** | **Includes:**<br>Hip (joint) liner<br>Joint liner (insert)<br>Knee (implant) insert |
| **Internal Fixation Device, Rigid Plate for Reposition in Upper Bones** | **Includes:**<br>Titanium Sternal Fixation System (TSFS) | | |
| **Intraluminal Device** | **Includes:**<br>Absolute Pro Vascular (OTW) Self-Expanding Stent System<br>Acculink (RX) Carotid Stent System<br>AneuRx® AAA Advantage®<br>Assurant (Cobalt) stent<br>Carotid WALLSTENT® Monorail® Endoprothesis<br>CoAxia NeuroFlo catheter<br>Colonic Z-Stent®<br>Complete (SE) stent<br>Driver stent (RX) (OTW)<br>E-Luminexx™ (Biliary)(Vascular) Stent<br>Embolization coil(s)<br>Endurant® Endovascular Stent Graft<br>Express® (LD) Premounted Stent System<br>Express® Biliary SD Monorail® Premounted Stent System<br>Express® SD Renal Monorail® Premounted Stent System<br>FLAIR® Endovascular Stent Graft<br>Formula™ Balloon-Expandable Renal Stent System<br>Herculink (RX) Elite Renal Stent System<br>LifeStent® (Flexstar)(XL) Vascular Stent System<br>Micro-Driver stent (RX) (OTW)<br>MULTI-LINK (VISION) (MINI-VISION) (ULTRA) Coronary Stent System<br>Omnilink Elite Vascular Balloon Expandable Stent System<br>Pipeline™ Embolization device (PED)<br>Protégé® RX Carotid Stent System<br>Stent, intraluminal (cardiovascular) (gastrointestinal) (hepatobiliary) (urinary)<br>Talent® Converter<br>Talent® Occluder<br>Talent® Stent Graft (abdominal)(thoracic)<br>Therapeutic occlusion coil(s)<br>Ultraflex™ Precision Colonic Stent System<br>Valiant Thoracic Stent Graft<br>WALLSTENT® Endoprothesis<br>Xact Carotid Stent System<br>Zenith Flex® AAA Endovascular Graft<br>Zenith® Renu™ AAA Ancillary Graft<br>Zenith TX2® TAA Endovascular Graft | **Monitoring Device** | **Includes:**<br>Blood glucose monitoring system<br>Cardiac event recorder<br>Continuous Glucose Monitoring (CGM) device<br>Implantable glucose monitoring device<br>Loop recorder, implantable<br>Reveal (DX)(XT) |
| | | **Monitoring Device, Hemodynamic for Insertion in Subcutaneous Tissue and Fascia** | **Includes:**<br>Implantable hemodynamic monitor (IHM)<br>Implantable hemodynamic monitoring system (IHMS) |
| | | **Monitoring Device, Pressure Sensor for Insertion in Heart and Great Vessels** | **Includes:**<br>CardioMEMS® pressure sensor<br>EndoSure® sensor |
| | | **Neurostimulator Lead in Central Nervous System** | **Includes:**<br>Cortical strip neurostimulator lead<br>DBS lead<br>Deep brain neurostimulator lead<br>RNS System lead<br>Spinal cord neurostimulator lead |
| | | **Neurostimulator Lead in Peripheral Nervous System** | **Includes:**<br>InterStim® Therapy lead |
| | | **Neurostimulator Generator in Head and Facial Bones** | **Includes:**<br>RNS system neurostimulator generator |
| | | **Nonautologous Tissue Substitute** | **Includes:**<br>Acellular Hydrated Dermis<br>Bone bank bone graft<br>Tissue bank graft |
| | | **Pacemaker, Dual Chamber for Insertion in Subcutaneous Tissue and Fascia** | **Includes:**<br>Advisa (MRI)<br>EnRhythm<br>Kappa<br>Revo MRI™ SureScan® pacemaker<br>Two lead pacemaker<br>Versa |
| | | **Pacemaker, Single Chamber for Insertion in Subcutaneous Tissue and Fascia** | **Includes:**<br>Single lead pacemaker (atrium)(ventricle) |
| | | **Pacemaker, Single Chamber Rate Responsive for Insertion in Subcutaneous Tissue and Fascia** | **Includes:**<br>Single lead rate responsive pacemaker (atrium)(ventricle) |
| | | **Radioactive Element** | **Includes:**<br>Brachytherapy seeds |
| | | **Resurfacing Device in Lower Joints** | **Includes:**<br>CONSERVE® PLUS Total Resurfacing Hip System<br>Cormet Hip Resurfacing System |
| **Intraluminal Device, Airway in Ear, Nose, Sinus** | **Includes:**<br>Nasopharyngeal airway (NPA) | **Spacer in Lower Joints** | **Includes:**<br>Joint spacer (antibiotic) |
| **Intraluminal Device, Airway in Gastrointestinal System** | **Includes:**<br>Esophageal obturator airway (EOA) | **Spacer in Upper Joints** | **Includes:**<br>Joint spacer (antibiotic) |
| **Intraluminal Device, Airway in Mouth and Throat** | **Includes:**<br>Guedel airway<br>Oropharyngeal airway (OPA) | | |

| | |
|---|---|
| Spinal Stabilization Device, Facet Replacement for Insertion in Upper Joints | Includes:<br>Facet replacement spinal stabilization device |
| Spinal Stabilization Device, Facet Replacement for Insertion in Lower Joints | Includes:<br>Facet replacement spinal stabilization device |
| Spinal Stabilization Device, Interspinous Process for Insertion in Upper Joints | Includes:<br>Interspinous process spinal stabilization device<br>X-STOP® Spacer |
| Spinal Stabilization Device, Interspinous Process for Insertion in Lower Joints | Includes:<br>Interspinous process spinal stabilization device<br>X-STOP® Spacer |
| Spinal Stabilization Device, Pedicle-Based for Insertion in Upper Joints | Includes:<br>Dynesys® Dynamic Stabilization System<br>Pedicle-based dynamic stabilization device |
| Spinal Stabilization Device, Pedicle-Based for Insertion in Lower Joints | Includes:<br>Dynesys® Dynamic Stabilization System<br>Pedicle-based dynamic stabilization device |
| Stimulator Generator in Subcutaneous Tissue and Fascia | Includes:<br>Baroreflex Activation Therapy® (BAT®)<br>Diaphragmatic pacemaker generator<br>Mark IV Breathing Pacemaker System<br>Phrenic nerve stimulator generator<br>Rheos® System Device |
| Stimulator Generator, Multiple Array for Insertion in Subcutaneous Tissue and Fascia | Includes:<br>Activa PC neurostimulator<br>Enterra gastric neurostimulator<br>Neurostimulator generator, multiple channel<br>PrimeAdvanced neurostimulator (SureScan) (MRI Safe) |
| Stimulator Generator, Multiple Array Rechargeable for Insertion in Subcutaneous Tissue and Fascia | Includes:<br>Activa SC neurostimulator<br>Neurostimulator generator, multiple channel rechargeable<br>RestoreAdvanced neurostimulator (SureScan) (MRI Safe)<br>RestoreSensor neurostimulator (SureScan) (MRI Safe)<br>RestoreUltra neurostimulator (SureScan) (MRI Safe) |
| Stimulator Generator, Single Array for Insertion in Subcutaneous Tissue and Fascia | Includes:<br>Activa SC neurostimulator<br>InterStim® Therapy neurostimulator<br>Itrel (3)(4) neurostimulator<br>Neurostimulator generator, single channel |
| Stimulator Generator, Single Array Rechargeable for Insertion in Subcutaneous Tissue and Fascia | Includes:<br>Neurostimulator generator, single channel rechargeable |
| Stimulator Lead in Gastrointestinal System | Includes:<br>Gastric electrical stimulation (GES) lead<br>Gastric pacemaker lead |
| Stimulator Lead in Muscles | Includes:<br>Electrical muscle stimulation (EMS) lead<br>Electronic muscle stimulator lead<br>Neuromuscular electrical stimulation (NEMS) lead |
| Stimulator Lead in Upper Arteries | Includes:<br>Baroreflex Activation Therapy® (BAT®)<br>Carotid (artery) sinus (baroreceptor) lead<br>Rheos® System lead |
| Stimulator Lead in Urinary System | Includes:<br>Sacral nerve modulation (SNM) lead<br>Sacral neuromodulation lead<br>Urinary incontinence stimulator lead |

| | |
|---|---|
| Synthetic Substitute | Includes:<br>AbioCor® Total Replacement Heart<br>AMPLATZER® Muscular VSD Occluder<br>Annuloplasty ring<br>Bard® Composix® (E/X)(LP) mesh<br>Bard® Composix® Kugel® patch<br>Bard® Dulex™ mesh<br>Bard® Ventralex™ Hernia Patch<br>BRYAN® Cervical Disc System<br>Ex-PRESS™ mini glaucoma shunt<br>Flexible Composite Mesh<br>GORE® DUALMESH®<br>Holter valve ventricular shunt<br>MitraClip valve repair system<br>Nitinol framed polymer mesh<br>Open Pivot (mechanical) valve<br>Open Pivot Aortic Valve Graft (AVG)<br>Partially absorbable mesh<br>PHYSIOMESH™ Flexible Composite Mesh<br>Polymethylmethacrylate (PMMA)<br>Polypropylene mesh<br>PRESTIGE® Cervical Disc<br>PROCEED™ Ventral Patch<br>Prodisc-C<br>Prodisc-L<br>PROLENE Polypropylene Hernia System (PHS)<br>Rebound HRD® (Hernia Repair Device)<br>SynCardia Total Artificial Heart<br>Total artificial (replacement) heart<br>ULTRAPRO Hernia System (UHS)<br>ULTRAPRO Partially Absorbable Lightweight Mesh<br>ULTRAPRO Plug<br>Ventrio™ Hernia Patch<br>Zimmer® NexGen® LPS Mobile Bearing Knee<br>Zimmer® NexGen® LPS-Flex Mobile Knee |
| Synthetic Substitute, Ceramic for Replacement in Lower Joints | Includes:<br>Novation® Ceramic AHS® (Articulation Hip System) |
| Synthetic Substitute, Ceramic on Polyethylene for Replacement in Lower Joints | Includes:<br>Oxidized zirconium ceramic hip bearing surface |
| Synthetic Substitute, Intraocular Telescope for Replacement in Eye | Includes:<br>Implantable Miniature Telescope™ (IMT) |
| Synthetic Substitute, Metal for Replacement in Lower Joints | Includes:<br>Cobalt/chromium head and socket |
| Synthetic Substitute, Metal on Polyethylene for Replacement in Lower Joints | Includes:<br>Cobalt/chromium head and polyethylene socket |
| Synthetic Substitute, Polyethylene for Replacement in Lower Joints | Includes:<br>Polyethylene socket |
| Synthetic Substitute, Reverse Ball and Socket for Replacement in Upper Joints | Includes:<br>Delta III Reverse shoulder prosthesis<br>Reverse® Shoulder Prosthesis |
| Tissue Expander in Skin and Breast | Includes:<br>Tissue expander (inflatable)(injectable) |
| Tissue Expander in Subcutaneous Tissue and Fascia | Includes:<br>Tissue expander (inflatable)(injectable) |
| Tracheostomy Device in Respiratory System | Includes:<br>Tracheostomy tube |
| Vascular Access Device in Subcutaneous Tissue and Fascia | Includes:<br>Tunneled central venous catheter<br>Vectra® Vascular Access Graft |
| Vascular Access Device, Reservoir in Subcutaneous Tissue and Fascia | Includes:<br>Implanted (venous)(access) port<br>Injection reservoir, port<br>Subcutaneous injection reservoir, port |
| Zooplastic Tissue in Heart and Great Vessels | Includes:<br>3f (Aortic) Bioprosthesis valve<br>Bovine pericardial valve<br>Bovine pericardium graft<br>Contegra Pulmonary Valved Conduit<br>CoreValve transcatheter aortic valve<br>Epic™ Stented Tissue Valve (aortic)<br>Freestyle (Stentless) Aortic Root Bioprosthesis<br>Hancock Bioprosthesis (aortic) (mitral) valve<br>Hancock Bioprosthetic Valved Conduit<br>Mosaic Bioprosthesis (aortic) (mitral) valve<br>Melody® transcatheter pulmonary valve<br>Mitroflow® Aortic Pericardial Heart Valve<br>Porcine (bioprosthetic) valve<br>SAPIEN transcatheter aortic valve<br>SJM Biocor® Stented Valve System<br>Stented tissue valve<br>Trifecta™ Valve (aortic)<br>Xenograft |

## Section 1 – Obstetrics
*Character 3: Operation*

| Abortion | **Definition:** Artificially terminating a pregnancy |
|---|---|
| Change | **Definition:** Taking out or off a device from a body part and putting back an identical or similar device in or on the same body part without cutting or puncturing the skin or a mucous membrane |
| | **Explanation:** All CHANGE procedures are coded using the approach EXTERNAL |
| Delivery | **Definition:** Assisting the passage of the products of conception from the genital canal |
| Drainage | **Definition:** Taking or letting out fluids and/or gases from a body part |
| | **Explanation:** The qualifier DIAGNOSTIC is used to identify drainage procedures that are biopsies |
| Extraction | **Definition:** Pulling or stripping out or off all or a portion of a body part by the use of force |
| | **Explanation:** The qualifier DIAGNOSTIC is used to identify extraction procedures that are biopsies |
| Insertion | **Definition:** Putting in a nonbiological appliance that monitors, assists, performs, or prevents a physiological function but does not physically take the place of a body part |
| Inspection | **Definition:** Visually and/or manually exploring a body part |
| | **Explanation:** Visual exploration may be performed with or without optical instrumentation. Manual exploration may be performed directly or through intervening body layers |
| Removal | **Definition:** Taking out or off a device from a body part, region or orifice |
| | **Explanation:** If a device is taken out and a similar device put in without cutting or puncturing the skin or mucous membrane, the procedure is coded to the root operation CHANGE. Otherwise, the procedure for taking out a device is coded to the root operation REMOVAL |
| Repair | **Definition:** Restoring, to the extent possible, a body part to its normal anatomic structure and function |
| | **Explanation:** Used only when the method to accomplish the repair is not one of the other root operations |
| Reposition | **Definition:** Moving to its normal location or other suitable location all or a portion of a body part |
| | **Explanation:** The body part is moved to a new location from an abnormal location, or from a normal location where it is not functioning correctly. The body part may or may not be cut out or off to be moved to the new location |
| Resection | **Definition:** Cutting out or off, without replacement, all of a body part |
| Transplantation | **Definition:** Putting in or on all or a portion of a living body part taken from another individual or animal to physically take the place and/or function of all or a portion of a similar body part |
| | **Explanation:** The native body part may or may not be taken out, and the transplanted body part may take over all or a portion of its function |

## Section 1 – Obstetrics
*Character 5: Approach*

| External | **Definition:** Procedures performed directly on the skin or mucous membrane and procedures performed indirectly by the application of external force through the skin or mucous membrane |
|---|---|
| Open | **Definition:** Cutting through the skin or mucous membrane and any other body layers necessary to expose the site of the procedure |
| Percutaneous | **Definition:** Entry, by puncture or minor incision, of instrumentation through the skin or mucous membrane and any other body layers necessary to reach the site of the procedure |
| Percutaneous Endoscopic | **Definition:** Entry, by puncture or minor incision, of instrumentation through the skin or mucous membrane and any other body layers necessary to reach and visualize the site of the procedure |
| Via Natural or Artificial Opening | **Definition:** Entry of instrumentation through a natural or artificial external opening to reach the site of the procedure |
| Via Natural or Artificial Opening Endoscopic | **Definition:** Entry of instrumentation through a natural or artificial external opening to reach and visualize the site of the procedure |

## Section 2 – Placement
*Character 3: Operation*

| Change | **Definition:** Taking out or off a device from a body part and putting back an identical or similar device in or on the same body part without cutting or puncturing the skin or a mucous membrane |
|---|---|
| Compression | **Definition:** Putting pressure on a body region |
| Dressing | **Definition:** Putting material on a body region for protection |
| Immobilization | **Definition:** Limiting or preventing motion of a body region |
| Packing | **Definition:** Putting material in a body region or orifice |
| Removal | **Definition:** Taking out or off a device from a body part |
| Traction | **Definition:** Exerting a pulling force on a body region in a distal direction |

## Section 2 – Placement
*Character 5: Approach*

| External | **Definition:** Procedures performed directly on the skin or mucous membrane and procedures performed indirectly by the application of external force through the skin or mucous membrane |
|---|---|

## Section 3 – Administration
*Character 3: Operation*

| Introduction | **Definition:** Putting in or on a therapeutic, diagnostic, nutritional, physiological, or prophylactic substance except blood or blood products |
|---|---|
| Irrigation | **Definition:** Putting in or on a cleansing substance |
| Transfusion | **Definition:** Putting in blood or blood products |

## Section 3 – Administration
*Character 5: Approach*

| External | **Definition:** Procedures performed directly on the skin or mucous membrane and procedures performed indirectly by the application of external force through the skin or mucous membrane |
|---|---|
| Open | **Definition:** Cutting through the skin or mucous membrane and any other body layers necessary to expose the site of the procedure |
| Percutaneous | **Definition:** Entry, by puncture or minor incision, of instrumentation through the skin or mucous membrane and any other body layers necessary to reach the site of the procedure |
| Via Natural or Artificial Opening | **Definition:** Entry of instrumentation through a natural or artificial external opening to reach the site of the procedure |
| Via Natural or Artificial Opening Endoscopic | **Definition:** Entry of instrumentation through a natural or artificial external opening to reach and visualize the site of the procedure |

## Section 3 – Administration
*Character 6: Substance*

| 4-Factor Prothrombin Complex Concentrate | Kcentra |
|---|---|
| Adhesion Barrier | Seprafilm |
| Anti-Infective Envelope | AIGISRx Antibacterial envelope Antimircrobial envelope |
| Clofarabine | Clolar |
| Glucarpidase | Voraxaze |
| Human B-type Natriuretic Peptide | Nesiritide |
| Other Thrombolytic | Tissue Plasminogen Activator (tPA)(r-tPA) |
| Oxazolidinones | Zyvox |
| Recombinant Bone Morphogenetic Protein | Bone morphogenetic protein 2 (BMP 2) rhBMP-2 |

## Section 4 – Measurement and Monitoring
*Character 3: Operation*

| Measurement | **Definition:** Determining the level of a physiological or physical function at a point in time |
|---|---|
| Monitoring | **Definition:** Determining the level of a physiological or physical function repetitively over a period of time |

## Section 4 – Measurement and Monitoring
*Character 5: Approach Definitions*

| External | **Definition:** Procedures performed directly on the skin or mucous membrane and procedures performed indirectly by the application of external force through the skin or mucous membrane |
|---|---|
| Open | **Definition:** Cutting through the skin or mucous membrane and any other body layers necessary to expose the site of the procedure |
| Percutaneous | **Definition:** Entry, by puncture or minor incision, of instrumentation through the skin or mucous membrane and any other body layers necessary to reach the site of the procedure |

| Percutaneous Endo-scopic | Definition: Entry, by puncture or minor incision, of instrumentation through the skin or mucous membrane and any other body layers necessary to reach and visualize the site of the procedure |
|---|---|
| Via Natural or Artificial Opening | Definition: Entry of instrumentation through a natural or artificial external opening to reach the site of the procedure |
| Via Natural or Artificial Opening Endoscopic | Definition: Entry of instrumentation through a natural or artificial external opening to reach and visualize the site of the procedure |

## Section 5 – Extracorporeal Assistance and Performance
*Character 3: Operation*

| Assistance | Definition: Taking over a portion of a physiological function by extracorporeal means |
|---|---|
| Performance | Definition: Completely taking over a physiological function by extracorporeal means |
| Restoration | Definition: Returning, or attempting to return, a physiological function to its original state by extracorporeal means. |

## Section 6 – Extracorporeal Therapies
*Character 3: Operation*

| Atmospheric Control | Definition: Extracorporeal control of atmospheric pressure and composition |
|---|---|
| Decompression | Definition: Extracorporeal elimination of undissolved gas from body fluids |
| Electromagnetic Therapy | Definition: Extracorporeal treatment by electromagnetic rays |
| Hyperthermia | Definition: Extracorporeal raising of body temperature |
| Hypothermia | Definition: Extracorporeal lowering of body temperature |
| Pheresis | Definition: Extracorporeal separation of blood products |
| Phototherapy | Definition: Extracorporeal treatment by light rays |
| Shock Wave Therapy | Definition: Extracorporeal treatment by shock waves |
| Ultrasound Therapy | Definition: Extracorporeal treatment by ultrasound |
| Ultraviolet Light Therapy | Definition: Extracorporeal treatment by ultraviolet light |

## Section 7 – Osteopathic
*Character 3: Operation*

| Treatment | Definition: Manual treatment to eliminate or alleviate somatic dysfunction and related disorders |
|---|---|

*Character 5: Approach*

| External | Definition: Procedures performed directly on the skin or mucous membrane and procedures performed indirectly by the application of external force through the skin or mucous membrane |
|---|---|

## Section 8 – Other Procedures
*Character 3: Operation*

| Other Procedures | Definition: Methodologies which attempt to remediate or cure a disorder or disease |
|---|---|

## Section 8 – Other Procedures
*Character 5: Approach*

| External | Definition: Procedures performed directly on the skin or mucous membrane and procedures performed indirectly by the application of external force through the skin or mucous membrane |
|---|---|
| Percutaneous | Definition: Entry, by puncture or minor incision, of instrumentation through the skin or mucous membrane and any other body layers necessary to reach the site of the procedure |
| Percutaneous Endoscopic | Definition: Entry, by puncture or minor incision, of instrumentation through the skin or mucous membrane and any other body layers necessary to reach and visualize the site of the procedure |
| Via Natural or Artificial Opening | Definition: Entry of instrumentation through a natural or artificial external opening to reach the site of the procedure |
| Via Natural or Artificial Opening Endoscopic | Definition: Entry of instrumentation through a natural or artificial external opening to reach and visualize the site of the procedure |

## Section 9 – Chiropractic
*Character 3: Operation*

| Manipulation | Definition: Manual procedure that involves a directed thrust to move a joint past the physiological range of motion, without exceeding the anatomical limit |
|---|---|

## Section 9 – Chiropractic
*Character 5: Approach*

| External | Definition: Procedures performed directly on the skin or mucous membrane and procedures performed indirectly by the application of external force through the skin or mucous membrane |
|---|---|

## Section B – Imaging
*Character 3: Type*

| Computerized Tomography (CT Scan) | Definition: Computer reformatted digital display of multiplanar images developed from the capture of multiple exposures of external ionizing radiation |
|---|---|
| Fluoroscopy | Definition: Single plane or bi-plane real time display of an image developed from the capture of external ionizing radiation on a fluorescent screen. The image may also be stored by either digital or analog means |
| Magnetic Resonance Imaging (MRI) | Definition: Computer reformatted digital display of multiplanar images developed from the capture of radiofrequency signals emitted by nuclei in a body site excited within a magnetic field |
| Plain Radiography | Definition: Planar display of an image developed from the capture of external ionizing radiation on photographic or photoconductive plate |
| Ultrasonography | Definition: Real time display of images of anatomy or flow information developed from the capture of reflected and attenuated high frequency sound waves |

## Section C – Nuclear Medicine
*Character 3: Type*

| Nonimaging Nuclear Medicine Assay | Definition: Introduction of radioactive materials into the body for the study of body fluids and blood elements, by the detection of radioactive emissions |
|---|---|
| Nonimaging Nuclear Medicine Probe | Definition: Introduction of radioactive materials into the body for the study of distribution and fate of certain substances by the detection of radioactive emissions; or, alternatively, measurement of absorption of radioactive emissions from an external source |
| Nonimaging Nuclear Medicine Uptake | Definition: Introduction of radioactive materials into the body for measurements of organ function, from the detection of radioactive emissions |
| Planar Nuclear Medicine Imaging | Definition: Introduction of radioactive materials into the body for single plane display of images developed from the capture of radioactive emissions |
| Positron Emission Tomographic (PET) Imaging | Definition: Introduction of radioactive materials into the body for three dimensional display of images developed from the simultaneous capture, 180 degrees apart, of radioactive emissions |
| Systemic Nuclear Medicine Therapy | Definition: Introduction of unsealed radioactive materials into the body for treatment |
| Tomographic (Tomo) Nuclear Medicine Imaging | Definition: Introduction of radioactive materials into the body for three dimensional display of images developed from the capture of radioactive emissions |

## Section F – Physical Rehabilitation and Diagnostic Audiology
*Character 3: Type*

| Activities of Daily Living Assessment | Definition: Measurement of functional level for activities of daily living |
|---|---|
| Activities of Daily Living Treatment | Definition: Exercise or activities to facilitate functional competence for activities of daily living |
| Caregiver Training | Definition: Training in activities to support patient's optimal level of function |
| Cochlear Implant Treatment | Definition: Application of techniques to improve the communication abilities of individuals with cochlear implant |
| Device Fitting | Definition: Fitting of a device designed to facilitate or support achievement of a higher level of function |
| Hearing Aid Assessment | Definition: Measurement of the appropriateness and/or effectiveness of a hearing device |
| Hearing Assessment | Definition: Measurement of hearing and related functions |
| Hearing Treatment | Definition: Application of techniques to improve, augment, or compensate for hearing and related functional impairment |
| Motor and/or Nerve Function Assessment | Definition: Measurement of motor, nerve, and related functions |
| Motor Treatment | Definition: Exercise or activities to increase or facilitate motor function |
| Speech Assessment | Definition: Measurement of speech and related functions |
| Speech Treatment | Definition: Application of techniques to improve, augment, or compensate for speech and related functional impairment |
| Vestibular Assessment | Definition: Measurement of the vestibular system and related functions |
| Vestibular Treatment | Definition: Application of techniques to improve, augment, or compensate for vestibular and related functional impairment |

## Section F – Physical Rehabilitation and Diagnostic Audiology
*Character 5: Type Qualifier*

| | |
|---|---|
| **Acoustic Reflex Decay** | **Definition:** Measures reduction in size/strength of acoustic reflex over time<br><br>**Includes/Examples:** Includes site of lesion test |
| **Acoustic Reflex Patterns** | **Definition:** Defines site of lesion based upon presence/absence of acoustic reflexes with ipsilateral vs. contralateral stimulation |
| **Acoustic Reflex Threshold** | **Definition:** Determines minimal intensity that acoustic reflex occurs with ipsilateral and/or contralateral stimulation |
| **Aerobic Capacity and Endurance** | **Definition:** Measures autonomic responses to positional changes; perceived exertion, dyspnea or angina during activity; performance during exercise protocols; standard vital signs; and blood gas analysis or oxygen consumption |
| **Alternate Binaural or Monaural Loudness Balance** | **Definition:** Determines auditory stimulus parameter that yields the same objective sensation<br><br>**Includes/Examples:** Sound intensities that yield same loudness perception |
| **Anthropometric Characteristics** | **Definition:** Measures edema, body fat composition, height, weight, length and girth |
| **Aphasia** (Assessment) | **Definition:** Measures expressive and receptive speech and language function including reading and writing |
| **Aphasia** (Treatment) | **Definition:** Applying techniques to improve, augment, or compensate for receptive/expressive language impairments |
| **Articulation** (Assessment)<br><br>**Phonology** (Assessment) | **Definition:** Measures speech production |
| **Articulation** (Treatment)<br><br>**Phonology** (Treatment) | **Definition:** Applying techniques to correct, improve, or compensate for speech productive impairment |
| **Assistive Listening Device** | **Definition:** Assists in use of effective and appropriate assistive listening device/system |
| **Assistive Listening System Device Selection** | **Definition:** Measures the effectiveness and appropriateness of assistive listening systems/devices |
| **Assistive, Adaptive, Supportive or Protective Devices** | **Explanation:** Devices to facilitate or support achievement of a higher level of function in wheelchair mobility; bed mobility; transfer or ambulation ability; bath and showering ability; dressing; grooming; personal hygiene; play or leisure |
| **Auditory Evoked Potentials** | **Definition:** Measures electric responses produced by the VIIIth cranial nerve and brainstem following auditory stimulation |
| **Auditory Processing** (Assessment) | **Definition:** Evaluates ability to receive and process auditory information and comprehension of spoken language |
| **Auditory Processing** (Treatment) | **Definition:** Applying techniques to improve the receiving and processing of auditory information and comprehension of spoken language |
| **Augmentative / Alternative Communication System** (Assessment) | **Definition:** Determines the appropriateness of aids, techniques, symbols, and/or strategies to augment or replace speech and enhance communication<br><br>**Includes/Examples:** Includes the use of telephones, writing equipment, emergency equipment, and TDD |
| **Augmentative / Alternative Communication System** (Treatment) | **Includes/Examples:** Includes augmentative communication devices and aids |
| **Aural Rehabilitation** | **Definition:** Applying techniques to improve the communication abilities associated with hearing loss |
| **Aural Rehabilitation Status** | **Definition:** Measures impact of a hearing loss including evaluation of receptive and expressive communication skills |
| **Bathing/Showering** | **Includes/Examples:** Includes obtaining and using supplies; soaping, rinsing, and drying body parts; maintaining bathing position; and transferring to and from bathing positions |
| **Bathing Techniques**<br><br>**Showering Techniques** | **Definition:** Activities to facilitate obtaining and using supplies, soaping, rinsing and drying body parts, maintaining bathing position, and transferring to and from bathing positions |
| **Bed Mobility** (Assessment) | **Definition:** Transitional movement within bed |
| **Bed Mobility** (Treatment) | **Definition:** Exercise or activities to facilitate transitional movements within bed |
| **Bedside Swallowing and Oral Function** | **Includes/Examples:** Bedside swallowing includes assessment of sucking, masticating, coughing, and swallowing. Oral function includes assessment of musculature for controlled movements, structures and functions to determine coordination and phonation |
| **Bekesy Audiometry** | **Definition:** Uses an instrument that provides a choice of discrete or continuously varying pure tones; choice of pulsed or continuous signal |
| **Binaural Electroacoustic Hearing Aid Check** | **Definition:** Determines mechanical and electroacoustic function of bilateral hearing aids using hearing aid test box |

| | |
|---|---|
| **Binaural Hearing Aid** (Assessment) | **Definition:** Measures the candidacy, effectiveness, and appropriateness of a hearing aids<br><br>**Explanation:** Measures bilateral fit |
| **Binaural Hearing Aid** (Treatment) | **Explanation:** Assists in achieving maximum understanding and performance |
| **Bithermal, Binaural Caloric Irrigation** | **Definition:** Measures the rhythmic eye movements stimulated by changing the temperature of the vestibular system |
| **Bithermal, Monaural Caloric Irrigation** | **Definition:** Measures the rhythmic eye movements stimulated by changing the temperature of the vestibular system in one ear |
| **Brief Tone Stimuli** | **Definition:** Measures specific central auditory process |
| **Cerumen Management** | **Definition:** Includes examination of external auditory canal and tympanic membrane and removal of cerumen from external ear canal |
| **Cochlear Implant** | **Definition:** Measures candidacy for cochlear implant |
| **Cochlear Implant Rehabilitation** | **Definition:** Applying techniques to improve the communication abilities of individuals with cochlear implant; includes programming the device, providing patients/families with information |
| **Communicative / Cognitive Integration Skills** (Assessment) | **Definition:** Measures ability to use higher cortical functions<br><br>**Includes/Examples:** Includes orientation, recognition, attention span, initiation and termination of activity, memory, sequencing, categorizing, concept formation, spatial operations, judgment, problem solving, generalization and pragmatic communication |
| **Communicative / Cognitive Integration Skills** (Treatment) | **Definition:** Activities to facilitate the use of higher cortical functions<br><br>**Includes/Examples:** Includes level of arousal, orientation, recognition, attention span, initiation and termination of activity, memory sequencing, judgment and problem solving, learning and generalization, and pragmatic communication |
| **Computerized Dynamic Posturography** | **Definition:** Measures the status of the peripheral and central vestibular system and the sensory/motor component of balance; evaluates the efficacy of vestibular rehabilitation |
| **Conditioned Play Audiometry** | **Definition:** Behavioral measures using nonspeech and speech stimuli to obtain frequency-specific and ear-specific information on auditory status from the patient<br><br>**Explanation:** Obtains speech reception threshold by having patient point to pictures of spondaic words |
| **Coordination** (Assessment)<br><br>**Dexterity** (Assessment) | **Definition:** Measures large and small muscle groups for controlled goal-directed movements<br><br>**Explanation:** Dexterity includes object manipulation |
| **Coordination** (Treatment)<br><br>**Dexterity** (Treatment) | **Definition:** Exercise or activities to facilitate gross coordination and fine coordination |
| **Cranial Nerve Integrity** | **Definition:** Measures cranial nerve sensory and motor functions, including tastes, smell and facial expression |
| **Dichotic Stimuli** | **Definition:** Measures specific central auditory process |
| **Distorted Speech** | **Definition:** Measures specific central auditory process |
| **Dix-Hallpike Dynamic** | **Definition:** Measures nystagmus following Dix-Hallpike maneuver |
| **Dressing** | **Includes/Examples:** Includes selecting clothing and accessories, obtaining clothing from storage, dressing and, fastening and adjusting clothing and shoes, and applying and removing personal devices, prosthesis or orthosis |
| **Dressing Techniques** | **Definition:** Activities to facilitate selecting clothing and accessories, dressing and undressing, adjusting clothing and shoes, applying and removing devices, prostheses or orthoses |
| **Dynamic Orthosis** | **Includes/Examples:** Includes customized and prefabricated splints, inhibitory casts, spinal and other braces, and protective devices; allows motion through transfer of movement from other body parts or by use of outside forces |
| **Ear Canal Probe Microphone** | **Definition:** Real ear measures |
| **Ear Protector Attentuation** | **Definition:** Measures ear protector fit and effectiveness |
| **Electrocochleography** | **Definition:** Measures the VIIIth cranial nerve action potential |
| **Environmental Barriers**<br><br>**Home Barriers**<br><br>**Work Barriers** | **Definition:** Measures current and potential barriers to optimal function, including safety hazards, access problems and home or office design |
| **Ergonomics and Body Mechanics** | **Definition:** Ergonomic measurement of job tasks, work hardening or work conditioning needs; functional capacity; and body mechanics |
| **Eustachian Tube Function** | **Definition:** Measures eustachian tube function and patency of eustachian tube |
| **Evoked Otoacoustic Emissions, Diagnostic** | **Definition:** Measures auditory evoked potentials in a diagnostic format |
| **Evoked Otoacoustic Emissions, Screening** | **Definition:** Measures auditory evoked potentials in a screening format |

|  |  |
|---|---|
| Facial Nerve Function | **Definition:** Measures electrical activity of the VIIth cranial nerve (facial nerve) |
| Feeding (Assessment)<br>Eating (Assessment) | **Includes/Examples:** Includes setting up food, selecting and using utensils and tableware, bringing food or drink to mouth, cleaning face, hands, and clothing, and management of alternative methods of nourishment |
| Feeding (Treatment)<br>Eating (Treatment) | **Definition:** Exercise or activities to facilitate setting up food, selecting and using utensils and tableware, bringing food or drink to mouth, cleaning face, hands, and clothing, and management of alternative methods of nourishment |
| Filtered Speech | **Definition:** Uses high or low pass filtered speech stimuli to assess central auditory processing disorders, site of lesion testing |
| Fluency (Assessment) | **Definition:** Measures speech fluency or stuttering |
| Fluency (Treatment) | **Definition:** Applying techniques to improve and augment fluent speech |
| Gait<br>Balance | **Definition:** Measures biomechanical, arthrokinematic and other spatial and temporal characteristics of gait and balance |
| Gait Training<br>Functional Ambulation | **Definition:** Exercise or activities to facilitate ambulation on a variety of surfaces and in a variety of environments |
| Grooming (Assessment)<br>Personal Hygiene (Assessment) | **Includes/Examples:** Includes ability to obtain and use supplies in a sequential fashion, general grooming, oral hygiene, toilet hygiene, personal care devices, including care for artificial airways |
| Grooming (Treatment)<br>Personal Hygiene (Treatment) | **Definition:** Activities to facilitate obtaining and using supplies in a sequential fashion: general grooming, oral hygiene, toilet hygiene, cleaning body, and personal care devices, including artificial airways |
| Hearing and Related Disorders Counseling | **Definition:** Provides patients/families/caregivers with information, support, referrals to facilitate recovery from a communication disorder<br>**Includes/Examples:** Includes strategies for psychosocial adjustment to hearing loss for clients and families/caregivers |
| Hearing and Related Disorders Prevention | **Definition:** Provides patients/families/caregivers with information and support to prevent communication disorders |
| Hearing Screening | **Definition:** Pass/refer measures designed to identify need for further audiologic assessment |
| Home Management (Assessment) | **Definition:** Obtaining and maintaining personal and household possessions and environment<br>**Includes/Examples:** Includes clothing care, cleaning, meal preparation and cleanup, shopping, money management, household maintenance, safety procedures, and childcare/parenting |
| Home Management (Treatment) | **Definition:** Activities to facilitate obtaining and maintaining personal household possessions and environment<br>**Includes/Examples:** Includes clothing care, cleaning, meal preparation and clean-up, shopping, money management, household maintenance, safety procedures, childcare/parenting |
| Instrumental Swallowing and Oral Function | **Definition:** Measures swallowing function using instrumental diagnostic procedures<br>**Explanation:** Methods include videofluoroscopy, ultrasound, manometry, endoscopy |
| Integumentary Integrity | **Includes/Examples:** Includes burns, skin conditions, ecchymosis, bleeding, blisters, scar tissue, wounds and other traumas, tissue mobility, turgor and texture |
| Manual Therapy Techniques | **Definition:** Techniques in which the therapist uses his/her hands to administer skilled movements<br>**Includes/Examples:** Includes connective tissue massage, joint mobilization and manipulation, manual lymph drainage, manual traction, soft tissue mobilization and manipulation |
| Masking Patterns | **Definition:** Measures central auditory processing status |
| Monaural Electroacoustic Hearing Aid Check | **Definition:** Determines mechanical and electroacoustic function of one hearing aid using hearing aid test box |
| Monaural Hearing Aid (Assessment) | **Definition:** Measures the candidacy, effectiveness, and appropriateness of a hearing aid<br>**Explanation:** Measures unilateral fit |
| Monaural Hearing Aid (Treatment) | **Explanation:** Assists in achieving maximum understanding and performance |
| Motor Function (Assessment) | **Definition:** Measures the body's functional and versatile movement patterns<br>**Includes/Examples:** Includes motor assessment scales, analysis of head, trunk and limb movement, and assessment of motor learning |
| Motor Function (Treatment) | **Definition:** Exercise or activities to facilitate crossing midline, laterality, bilateral integration, praxis, neuromuscular relaxation, inhibition, facilitation, motor function and motor learning |
| Motor Speech (Assessment) | **Definition:** Measures neurological motor aspects of speech production |
| Motor Speech (Treatment) | **Definition:** Applying techniques to improve and augment the impaired neurological motor aspects of speech production |
| Muscle Performance (Assessment) | **Definition:** Measures muscle strength, power and endurance using manual testing, dynamometry or computer-assisted electromechanical muscle test; functional muscle strength, power and endurance; muscle pain, tone, or soreness; or pelvic-floor musculature<br>**Explanation:** Muscle endurance refers to the ability to contract a muscle repeatedly over time |
| Muscle Performance (Treatment) | **Definition:** Exercise or activities to increase the capacity of a muscle to do work in terms of strength, power, and/or endurance<br>**Explanation:** Muscle strength is the force exerted to overcome resistance in one maximal effort. Muscle power is work produced per unit of time, or the product of strength and speed. Muscle endurance is the ability to contract a muscle repeatedly over time |
| Neuromotor Development | **Definition:** Measures motor development, righting and equilibrium reactions, and reflex and equilibrium reactions |
| Neurophysiologic Intraoperative | **Definition:** Monitors neural status during surgery |
| Non-invasive Instrumental Status | **Definition:** Instrumental measures of oral, nasal, vocal, and velopharyngeal functions as they pertain to speech production |
| Nonspoken Language (Assessment) | **Definition:** Measures nonspoken language (print, sign, symbols) for communication |
| Nonspoken Language (Treatment) | **Definition:** Applying techniques that improve, augment, or compensate spoken communication |
| Oral Peripheral Mechanism | **Definition:** Structural measures of face, jaw, lips, tongue, teeth, hard and soft palate, pharynx as related to speech production |
| Orofacial Myofunctional (Assessment) | **Definition:** Measures orofacial myofunctional patterns for speech and related functions |
| Orofacial Myofunctional (Treatment) | **Definition:** Applying techniques to improve, alter, or augment impaired orofacial myofunctional patterns and related speech production errors |
| Oscillating Tracking | **Definition:** Measures ability to visually track |
| Pain | **Definition:** Measures muscle soreness, pain and soreness with joint movement, and pain perception<br>**Includes/Examples:** Includes questionnaires, graphs, symptom magnification scales or visual analog scales |
| Perceptual Processing (Assessment) | **Definition:** Measures stereognosis, kinesthesia, body schema, right-left discrimination, form constancy, position in space, visual closure, figure-ground, depth perception, spatial relations and topographical orientation |
| Perceptual Processing (Treatment) | **Definition:** Exercise and activities to facilitate perceptual processing<br>**Explanation:** Includes stereognosis, kinesthesia, body schema, right-left discrimination, form constancy, position in space, visual closure, figure-ground, depth perception, spatial relations, and topographical orientation<br>**Includes/Examples:** Includes stereognosis, kinesthesia, body schema, right-left discrimination, form constancy, position in space, visual closure, figure-ground, depth perception, spatial relations, and topographical orientation |
| Performance Intensity Phonetically Balanced Speech Discrimination | **Definition:** Measures word recognition over varying intensity levels |
| Postural Control | **Definition:** Exercise or activities to increase postural alignment and control |
| Prosthesis | **Explanation:** Artificial substitutes for missing body parts that augment performance or function |
| Psychosocial Skills (Assessment) | **Definition:** The ability to interact in society and to process emotions<br>**Includes/Examples:** Includes psychological (values, interests, self-concept); social (role performance, social conduct, interpersonal skills, self expression); self-management (coping skills, time management, self-control) |
| Psychosocial Skills (Treatment) | **Definition:** The ability to interact in society and to process emotions<br>**Includes/Examples:** Includes psychological (values, interests, self-concept); social (role performance, social conduct, interpersonal skills, self expression); self-management (coping skills, time management, self-control) |
| Pure Tone Audiometry, Air | **Definition:** Air-conduction pure tone threshold measures with appropriate masking |
| Pure Tone Audiometry, Air and Bone | **Definition:** Air-conduction and bone-conduction pure tone threshold measures with appropriate masking |
| Pure Tone Stenger | **Definition:** Measures unilateral nonorganic hearing loss based on simultaneous presentation of pure tones of differing volume |

| | |
|---|---|
| **Range of Motion and Joint Integrity** | **Definition:** Measures quantity, quality, grade, and classification of joint movement and/or mobility |
| | **Explanation:** Range of Motion is the space, distance or angle through which movement occurs at a joint or series of joints. Joint integrity is the conformance of joints to expected anatomic, biomechanical and kinematic norms |
| **Range of Motion and Joint Mobility** | **Definition:** Exercise or activities to increase muscle length and joint mobility |
| **Receptive Language** (Assessment)<br><br>**Expressive Language** (Assessment) | **Definition:** Measures receptive and expressive language |
| **Receptive Language** (Treatment)<br><br>**Expressive Language** (Treatment) | **Definition:** Applying techniques to improve and augment receptive/expressive language |
| **Reflex Integrity** | **Definition:** Measures the presence, absence, or exaggeration of developmentally appropriate, pathologic or normal reflexes |
| **Select Picture Audiometry** | **Definition:** Establishes hearing threshold levels for speech using pictures |
| **Sensorineural Acuity Level** | **Definition:** Measures sensorineural acuity masking presented via bone conduction |
| **Sensory Aids** | **Definition:** Determines the appropriateness of a sensory prosthetic device, other than a hearing aid or assistive listening system/device |
| **Sensory Awareness**<br><br>**Sensory Processing**<br><br>**Sensory Integrity** | **Includes/Examples:** Includes light touch, pressure, temperature, pain, sharp/dull, proprioception, vestibular, visual, auditory, gustatory, and olfactory |
| **Short Increment Sensitivity Index** | **Definition:** Measures the ear's ability to detect small intensity changes; site of lesion test requiring a behavioral response |
| **Sinusoidal Vertical Axis Rotational** | **Definition:** Measures nystagmus following rotation |
| **Somatosensory Evoked Potentials** | **Definition:** Measures neural activity from sites throughout the body |
| **Speech Recognition**<br><br>**Word Recognition** | **Definition:** Measures ability to repeat/identify single syllable words; scores given as a percentage; includes word recognition/speech discrimination |
| **Speech Screening**<br><br>**Language Screening** | **Definition:** Identifies need for further speech and/or language evaluation |
| **Speech Threshold** | **Definition:** Measures minimal intensity needed to repeat spondaic words |
| **Speech-Language Pathology and Related Disorders Counseling** | **Definition:** Provides patients/families with information, support, referrals to facilitate recovery from a communication disorder |
| **Speech-Language Pathology and Related Disorders Prevention** | **Definition:** Applying techniques to avoid or minimize onset and/or development of a communication disorder |
| **Staggered Spondaic Word** | **Definition:** Measures central auditory processing site of lesion based upon dichotic presentation of spondaic words |
| **Static Orthosis** | **Includes/Examples:** Includes customized and prefabricated splints, inhibitory casts, spinal and other braces, and protective devices; has no moving parts, maintains joint(s) in desired position. |
| **Stenger** | **Definition:** Measures unilateral nonorganic hearing loss based on simultaneous presentation of signals of differing volume |
| **Swallowing Dysfunction** | **Definition:** Activities to improve swallowing function in coordination with respiratory function |
| | **Includes/Examples:** Includes function and coordination of sucking, mastication, coughing, swallowing |
| **Synthetic Sentence Identification** | **Definition:** Measures central auditory dysfunction using identification of third order approximations of sentences and competing messages |
| **Temporal Ordering of Stimuli** | **Definition:** Measures specific central auditory process |
| **Therapeutic Exercise** | **Definition:** Exercise or activities to facilitate sensory awareness, sensory processing, sensory integration, balance training, conditioning, reconditioning |
| | **Includes/Examples:** Includes developmental activities, breathing exercises, aerobic endurance activities, aquatic exercises, stretching and ventilatory muscle training |
| **Tinnitus Masker** (Assessment) | **Definition:** Determines candidacy for tinnitus masker |
| **Tinnitus Masker** (Treatment) | **Explanation:** Used to verify physical fit, acoustic appropriateness, and benefit; assists in achieving maximum benefit |

| | |
|---|---|
| **Tone Decay** | **Definition:** Measures decrease in hearing sensitivity to a tone; site of lesion test requiring a behavioral response |
| **Transfer** | **Definition:** Transitional movement from one surface to another |
| **Transfer Training** | **Definition:** Exercise or activities to facilitate movement from one surface to another |
| **Tympanometry** | **Definition:** Measures the integrity of the middle ear; measures ease at which sound flows through the tympanic membrane while air pressure against the membrane is varied |
| **Unithermal Binaural Screen** | **Definition:** Measures the rhythmic eye movements stimulated by changing the temperature of the vestibular system in both ears using warm water, screening format |
| **Ventilation, Respiration, and Circulation** | **Definition:** Measures ventilatory muscle strength, power and endurance, pulmonary function and ventilatory mechanics |
| | **Includes/Examples:** Includes ability to clear airway, activities that aggravate or relieve edema, pain, dyspnea or other symptoms, chest wall mobility, cardiopulmonary response to performance of ADL and IAD, cough and sputum, standard vital signs |
| **Vestibular** | **Definition:** Applying techniques to compensate for balance disorders; includes habituation, exercise therapy, and balance retraining |
| **Visual Motor Integration** (Assessment) | **Definition:** Coordinating the interaction of information from the eyes with body movement during activity |
| **Visual Motor Integration** (Treatment) | **Definition:** Exercise or activities to facilitate coordinating the interaction of information from eyes with body movement during activity |
| **Visual Reinforcement Audiometry** | **Definition:** Behavioral measures using nonspeech and speech stimuli to obtain frequency/ear-specific information on auditory status |
| | **Includes/Examples:** Includes a conditioned response of looking toward a visual reinforcer (e.g., lights, animated toy) every time auditory stimuli are heard |
| **Vocational Activities and Functional Community or Work Reintegration Skills** (Assessment) | **Definition:** Measures environmental, home, work (job/school/play) barriers that keep patients from functioning optimally in their environment |
| | **Includes/Examples:** Includes assessment of vocational skill and interests, environment of work (job/school/play), injury potential and injury prevention or reduction, ergonomic stressors, transportation skills, and ability to access and use community resources |
| **Vocational Activities and Functional Community or Work Reintegration Skills** (Treatment) | **Definition:** Activities to facilitate vocational exploration, body mechanics training, job acquisition, and environmental or work (job/school/play) task adaptation |
| | **Includes/Examples:** Includes injury prevention and reduction, ergonomic stressor reduction, job coaching and simulation, work hardening and conditioning, driving training, transportation skills, and use of community resources |
| **Voice** (Assessment) | **Definition:** Measures vocal structure, function and production |
| **Voice** (Treatment) | **Definition:** Applying techniques to improve voice and vocal function |
| **Voice Prosthetic** (Assessment) | **Definition:** Determines the appropriateness of voice prosthetic/adaptive device to enhance or facilitate communication |
| **Voice Prosthetic** (Treatment) | **Includes/Examples:** Includes electrolarynx, and other assistive, adaptive, supportive devices |
| **Wheelchair Mobility** (Assessment) | **Definition:** Measures fit and functional abilities within wheelchair in a variety of environments |
| **Wheelchair Mobility** (Treatment) | **Definition:** Management, maintenance and controlled operation of a wheelchair, scooter or other device, in and on a variety of surfaces and environments |
| **Wound Management** | **Includes/Examples:** Includes non-selective and selective debridement (enzymes, autolysis, sharp debridement), dressings (wound coverings, hydrogel, vacuum-assisted closure), topical agents, etc. |

## Section G – Mental Health
### Character 3: Type

| | |
|---|---|
| **Biofeedback** | **Definition:** Provision of information from the monitoring and regulating of physiological processes in conjunction with cognitive-behavioral techniques to improve patient functioning or well-being |
| | **Includes/Examples:** Includes EEG, blood pressure, skin temperature or peripheral blood flow, ECG, electrooculogram, EMG, respirometry or capnometry, GSR/EDR, perineometry to monitor/regulate bowel/bladder activity, electrogastrogram to monitor/regulate gastric motility |
| **Counseling** | **Definition:** The application of psychological methods to treat an individual with normal developmental issues and psychological problems in order to increase function, improve well-being, alleviate distress, maladjustment or resolve crises |
| **Crisis Intervention** | **Definition:** Treatment of a traumatized, acutely disturbed or distressed individual for the purpose of short-term stabilization |
| | **Includes/Examples:** Includes defusing, debriefing, counseling, psychotherapy and/or coordination of care with other providers or agencies |

| Electroconvulsive Therapy | **Definition:** The application of controlled electrical voltages to treat a mental health disorder |
|---|---|
| | **Includes/Examples:** Includes appropriate sedation and other preparation of the individual |
| Family Psychotherapy | **Definition:** Treatment that includes one or more family members of an individual with a mental health disorder by behavioral, cognitive, psychoanalytic, psychodynamic or psychophysiological means to improve functioning or well-being |
| | **Explanation:** Remediation of emotional or behavioral problems presented by one or more family members in cases where psychotherapy with more than one family member is indicated |
| Group Psychotherapy | **Definition:** Treatment of two or more individuals with a mental health disorder by behavioral, cognitive, psychoanalytic, psychodynamic or psychophysiological means to improve functioning or well-being |
| Hypnosis | **Definition:** Induction of a state of heightened suggestibility by auditory, visual and tactile techniques to elicit an emotional or behavioral response |
| Individual Psychotherapy | **Definition:** Treatment of an individual with a mental health disorder by behavioral, cognitive, psychoanalytic, psychodynamic or psychophysiological means to improve functioning or well-being |
| Light Therapy | **Definition:** Application of specialized light treatments to improve functioning or well-being |
| Medication Management | **Definition:** Monitoring and adjusting the use of medications for the treatment of a mental health disorder |
| Narcosynthesis | **Definition:** Administration of intravenous barbiturates in order to release suppressed or repressed thoughts |
| Psychological Tests | **Definition:** The administration and interpretation of standardized psychological tests and measurement instruments for the assessment of psychological function |

## Section G – Mental Health
### Character 4: Qualifier

| Behavioral | **Definition:** Primarily to modify behavior |
|---|---|
| | **Includes/Examples:** Includes modeling and role playing, positive reinforcement of target behaviors, response cost, and training of self-management skills |
| Cognitive | **Definition:** Primarily to correct cognitive distortions and errors |
| Cognitive-Behavioral | **Definition:** Combining cognitive and behavioral treatment strategies to improve functioning |
| | **Explanation:** Maladaptive responses are examined to determine how cognitions relate to behavior patterns in response to an event. Uses learning principles and information-processing models |
| Developmental | **Definition:** Age-normed developmental status of cognitive, social and adaptive behavior skills |
| Intellectual and Psychoeducational | **Definition:** Intellectual abilities, academic achievement and learning capabilities (including behaviors and emotional factors affecting learning) |
| Interactive | **Definition:** Uses primarily physical aids and other forms of non-oral interaction with a patient who is physically, psychologically or developmentally unable to use ordinary language for communication |
| | **Includes/Examples:** Includes the use of toys in symbolic play |
| Interpersonal | **Definition:** Helps an individual make changes in interpersonal behaviors to reduce psychological dysfunction |
| | **Includes/Examples:** Includes exploratory techniques, encouragement of affective expression, clarification of patient statements, analysis of communication patterns, use of therapy relationship and behavior change techniques |
| Neurobehavioral Status Cognitive Status | **Definition:** Includes neurobehavioral status exam, interview(s), and observation for the clinical assessment of thinking, reasoning and judgment, acquired knowledge, attention, memory, visual spatial abilities, language functions, and planning |
| Neuropsychological | **Definition:** Thinking, reasoning and judgment, acquired knowledge, attention, memory, visual spatial abilities, language functions, planning |
| Personality and Behavioral | **Definition:** Mood, emotion, behavior, social functioning, psychopathological conditions, personality traits and characteristics |
| Psychoanalysis | **Definition:** Methods of obtaining a detailed account of past and present mental and emotional experiences to determine the source and eliminate or diminish the undesirable effects of unconscious conflicts |
| | **Explanation:** Accomplished by making the individual aware of their existence, origin, and inappropriate expression in emotions and behavior |
| Psychodynamic | **Definition:** Exploration of past and present emotional experiences to understand motives and drives using insight-oriented techniques to reduce the undesirable effects of internal conflicts on emotions and behavior |
| | **Explanation:** Techniques include empathetic listening, clarifying self-defeating behavior patterns, and exploring adaptive alternatives |

| Psychophysiological | **Definition:** Monitoring and alteration of physiological processes to help the individual associate physiological reactions combined with cognitive and behavioral strategies to gain improved control of these processes to help the individual cope more effectively |
|---|---|
| Supportive | **Definition:** Formation of therapeutic relationship primarily for providing emotional support to prevent further deterioration in functioning during periods of particular stress |
| | **Explanation:** Often used in conjunction with other therapeutic approaches |
| Vocational | **Definition:** Exploration of vocational interests, aptitudes and required adaptive behavior skills to develop and carry out a plan for achieving a successful vocational placement |
| | **Includes/Examples:** Includes enhancing work related adjustment and/or pursuing viable options in training education or preparation |

## Section H – Substance Abuse Treatment
### Character 3: Type

| Detoxification Services | **Definition:** Detoxification from alcohol and/or drugs |
|---|---|
| | **Explanation:** Not a treatment modality, but helps the patient stabilize physically and psychologically until the body becomes free of drugs and the effects of alcohol |
| Family Counseling | **Definition:** The application of psychological methods that includes one or more family members to treat an individual with addictive behavior |
| | **Explanation:** Provides support and education for family members of addicted individuals. Family member participation is seen as a critical area of substance abuse treatment |
| Group Counseling | **Definition:** The application of psychological methods to treat two or more individuals with addictive behavior |
| | **Explanation:** Provides structured group counseling sessions and healing power through the connection with others |
| Individual Counseling | **Definition:** The application of psychological methods to treat an individual with addictive behavior |
| | **Explanation:** Comprised of several different techniques, which apply various strategies to address drug addiction |
| Individual Psychotherapy | **Definition:** Treatment of an individual with addictive behavior by behavioral, cognitive, psychoanalytic, psychodynamic or psychophysiological means |
| Medication Management | **Definition:** Monitoring and adjusting the use of replacement medications for the treatment of addiction |
| Pharmacotherapy | **Definition:** The use of replacement medications for the treatment of addiction |

## APPENDIX B:
### Body Part Key

| Abdominal aortic plexus | **Use:** Abdominal Sympathetic Nerve |
|---|---|
| Abdominal esophagus | **Use:** Esophagus, Lower |
| Abductor hallucis muscle | **Use:** Foot Muscle, Right Foot Muscle, Left |
| Accessory cephalic vein | **Use:** Cephalic Vein, Right Cephalic Vein, Left |
| Accessory obturator nerve | **Use:** Lumbar Plexus |
| Accessory phrenic nerve | **Use:** Phrenic Nerve |
| Accessory spleen | **Use:** Spleen |
| Acetabulofemoral joint | **Use:** Hip Joint, Right Hip Joint, Left |
| Achilles tendon | **Use:** Lower Leg Tendon, Right Lower Leg Tendon, Left |
| Acromioclavicular ligament | **Use:** Shoulder Bursa and Ligament, Right Shoulder Bursa and Ligament, Left |
| Acromion (process) | **Use:** Scapula, Right Scapula, Left |

| | |
|---|---|
| Adductor brevis muscle | Use:<br>Upper Leg Muscle, Right<br>Upper Leg Muscle, Left |
| Adductor hallucis muscle | Use:<br>Foot Muscle, Right<br>Foot Muscle, Left |
| Adductor longus muscle<br>Adductor magnus muscle | Use:<br>Upper Leg Muscle, Right<br>Upper Leg Muscle, Left |
| Adenohypophysis | Use:<br>Pituitary Gland |
| Alar ligament of axis | Use:<br>Head and Neck Bursa and Ligament |
| Alveolar process of mandible | Use:<br>Mandible, Right<br>Mandible, Left |
| Alveolar process of maxilla | Use:<br>Maxilla, Right<br>Maxilla, Left |
| Anal orifice | Use:<br>Anus |
| Anatomical snuffbox | Use:<br>Lower Arm and Wrist Muscle, Right<br>Lower Arm and Wrist Muscle, Left |
| Angular artery | Use:<br>Face Artery |
| Angular vein | Use:<br>Face Vein, Right<br>Face Vein, Left |
| Annular ligament | Use:<br>Elbow Bursa and Ligament, Right<br>Elbow Bursa and Ligament, Left |
| Anorectal junction | Use:<br>Rectum |
| Ansa cervicalis | Use:<br>Cervical Plexus |
| Antebrachial fascia | Use:<br>Subcutaneous Tissue and Fascia, Right Lower Arm<br>Subcutaneous Tissue and Fascia, Left Lower Arm |
| Anterior (pectoral) lymph node | Use:<br>Lymphatic, Right Axillary<br>Lymphatic, Left Axillary |
| Anterior cerebral artery | Use:<br>Intracranial Artery |
| Anterior cerebral vein | Use:<br>Intracranial Vein |
| Anterior choroidal artery | Use:<br>Intracranial Artery |
| Anterior circumflex humeral artery | Use:<br>Axillary Artery, Right<br>Axillary Artery, Left |
| Anterior communicating artery | Use:<br>Intracranial Artery |
| Anterior cruciate ligament (ACL) | Use:<br>Knee Bursa and Ligament, Right<br>Knee Bursa and Ligament, Left |
| Anterior crural nerve | Use:<br>Femoral Nerve |
| Anterior facial vein | Use:<br>Face Vein, Right<br>Face Vein, Left |
| Anterior intercostal artery | Use:<br>Internal Mammary Artery, Right<br>Internal Mammary Artery, Left |
| Anterior interosseous nerve | Use:<br>Median Nerve |
| Anterior lateral malleolar artery | Use:<br>Anterior Tibial Artery, Right<br>Anterior Tibial Artery, Left |
| Anterior lingual gland | Use:<br>Minor Salivary Gland |
| Anterior medial malleolar artery | Use:<br>Anterior Tibial Artery, Right<br>Anterior Tibial Artery, Left |

| | |
|---|---|
| Anterior spinal artery | Use:<br>Vertebral Artery, Right<br>Vertebral Artery, Left |
| Anterior tibial recurrent artery | Use:<br>Anterior Tibial Artery, Right<br>Anterior Tibial Artery, Left |
| Anterior ulnar recurrent artery | Use:<br>Ulnar Artery, Right<br>Ulnar Artery, Left |
| Anterior vagal trunk | Use:<br>Vagus Nerve |
| Anterior vertebral muscle | Use:<br>Neck Muscle, Right<br>Neck Muscle, Left |
| Antihelix<br>Antitragus | Use:<br>External Ear, Right<br>External Ear, Left<br>External Ear, Bilateral |
| Antrum of Highmore | Use:<br>Maxillary Sinus, Right<br>Maxillary Sinus, Left |
| Aortic annulus | Use:<br>Aortic Valve |
| Aortic arch<br>Aortic intercostal artery | Use:<br>Thoracic Aorta |
| Apical (subclavicular) lymph node | Use:<br>Lymphatic, Right Axillary<br>Lymphatic, Left Axillary |
| Apneustic center | Use:<br>Pons |
| Aqueduct of Sylvius | Use:<br>Cerebral Ventricle |
| Aqueous humour | Use:<br>Anterior Chamber, Right<br>Anterior Chamber, Left |
| Arachnoid mater | Use:<br>Cerebral Meninges<br>Spinal Meninges |
| Arcuate artery | Use:<br>Foot Artery, Right<br>Foot Artery, Left |
| Areola | Use:<br>Nipple, Right<br>Nipple, Left |
| Arterial canal (duct) | Use:<br>Pulmonary Artery, Left |
| Aryepiglottic fold<br>Arytenoid cartilage | Use:<br>Larynx |
| Arytenoid muscle | Use:<br>Neck Muscle, Right<br>Neck Muscle, Left |
| Ascending aorta | Use:<br>Thoracic Aorta |
| Ascending palatine artery | Use:<br>Face Artery |
| Ascending pharyngeal artery | Use:<br>External Carotid Artery, Right<br>External Carotid Artery, Left |
| Atlantoaxial joint | Use:<br>Cervical Vertebral Joint |
| Atrioventricular node | Use:<br>Conduction Mechanism |
| Atrium dextrum cordis | Use:<br>Atrium, Right |
| Atrium pulmonale | Use:<br>Atrium, Left |
| Auditory tube | Use:<br>Eustachian Tube, Right<br>Eustachian Tube, Left |
| Auerbach's (myenteric) plexus | Use:<br>Abdominal Sympathetic Nerve |
| Auricle | Use:<br>External Ear, Right<br>External Ear, Left<br>External Ear, Bilateral |

| | | | |
|---|---|---|---|
| **Auricularis muscle** | Use:<br>Head Muscle | **Bundle of His**<br>**Bundle of Kent** | Use:<br>Conduction Mechanism |
| **Axillary fascia** | Use:<br>Subcutaneous Tissue and Fascia, Right Upper Arm<br>Subcutaneous Tissue and Fascia, Left Upper Arm | **Calcaneocuboid joint** | Use:<br>Tarsal Joint, Right<br>Tarsal Joint, Left |
| **Axillary nerve** | Use:<br>Brachial Plexus | **Calcaneocuboid ligament** | Use:<br>Foot Bursa and Ligament, Right<br>Foot Bursa and Ligament, Left |
| **Bartholin's (greater vestibular) gland** | Use:<br>Vestibular Gland | **Calcaneofibular ligament** | Use:<br>Ankle Bursa and Ligament, Right<br>Ankle Bursa and Ligament, Left |
| **Basal (internal) cerebral vein** | Use:<br>Intracranial Vein | **Calcaneus** | Use:<br>Tarsal, Right<br>Tarsal, Left |
| **Basal nuclei** | Use:<br>Basal Ganglia | **Capitate bone** | Use:<br>Carpal, Right<br>Carpal, Left |
| **Basilar artery** | Use:<br>Intracranial Artery | **Cardia** | Use:<br>Esophagogastric Junction |
| **Basis pontis** | Use:<br>Pons | **Cardiac plexus** | Use:<br>Thoracic Sympathetic Nerve |
| **Biceps brachii muscle** | Use:<br>Upper Arm Muscle, Right<br>Upper Arm Muscle, Left | **Cardioesophageal junction** | Use:<br>Esophagogastric Junction |
| **Biceps femoris muscle** | Use:<br>Upper Leg Muscle, Right<br>Upper Leg Muscle, Left | **Caroticotympanic artery** | Use:<br>Internal Carotid Artery, Right<br>Internal Carotid Artery, Left |
| **Bicipital aponeurosis** | Use:<br>Subcutaneous Tissue and Fascia, Right Lower Arm<br>Subcutaneous Tissue and Fascia, Left Lower Arm | **Carotid glomus** | Use:<br>Carotid Body, Left<br>Carotid Body, Right<br>Carotid Bodies, Bilateral |
| **Bicuspid valve** | Use:<br>Mitral Valve | **Carotid sinus** | Use:<br>Internal Carotid Artery, Right<br>Internal Carotid Artery, Left |
| **Body of femur** | Use:<br>Femoral Shaft, Right<br>Femoral Shaft, Left | **Carotid sinus nerve** | Use:<br>Glossopharyngeal Nerve |
| **Body of fibula** | Use:<br>Fibula, Right<br>Fibula, Left | **Carpometacarpal (CMC) joint** | Use:<br>Metacarpocarpal Joint, Right<br>Metacarpocarpal Joint, Left |
| **Bony labyrinth** | Use:<br>Inner Ear, Right<br>Inner Ear, Left | **Carpometacarpal ligament** | Use:<br>Hand Bursa and Ligament, Right<br>Hand Bursa and Ligament, Left |
| **Bony orbit** | Use:<br>Orbit, Right<br>Orbit, Left | **Cauda equina** | Use:<br>Lumbar Spinal Cord |
| **Bony vestibule** | Use:<br>Inner Ear, Right<br>Inner Ear, Left | **Cavernous plexus** | Use:<br>Head and Neck Sympathetic Nerve |
| **Botallo's duct** | Use:<br>Pulmonary Artery, Left | **Celiac (solar) plexus**<br>**Celiac ganglion** | Use:<br>Abdominal Sympathetic Nerve |
| **Brachial (lateral) lymph node** | Use:<br>Lymphatic, Right Axillary<br>Lymphatic, Left Axillary | **Celiac lymph node** | Use:<br>Lymphatic, Aortic |
| **Brachialis muscle** | Use:<br>Upper Arm Muscle, Right<br>Upper Arm Muscle, Left | **Celiac trunk** | Use:<br>Celiac Artery |
| **Brachiocephalic artery**<br>**Brachiocephalic trunk** | Use:<br>Innominate Artery | **Central axillary lymph node** | Use:<br>Lymphatic, Right Axillary<br>Lymphatic, Left Axillary |
| **Brachiocephalic vein** | Use:<br>Innominate Vein, Right<br>Innominate Vein, Left | **Cerebral aqueduct (Sylvius)** | Use:<br>Cerebral Ventricle |
| **Brachioradialis muscle** | Use:<br>Lower Arm and Wrist Muscle, Right<br>Lower Arm and Wrist Muscle, Left | **Cerebrum** | Use:<br>Brain |
| **Broad ligament** | Use:<br>Uterine Supporting Structure | **Cervical esophagus** | Use:<br>Esophagus, Upper |
| **Bronchial artery** | Use:<br>Thoracic Aorta | **Cervical facet joint** | Use:<br>Cervical Vertebral Joint<br>Cervical Vertebral Joints, 2 or more |
| **Buccal gland** | Use:<br>Buccal Mucosa | **Cervical ganglion** | Use:<br>Head and Neck Sympathetic Nerve |
| **Buccinator lymph node** | Use:<br>Lymphatic, Head | **Cervical interspinous ligament**<br>**Cervical intertransverse ligament**<br>**Cervical ligamentum flavum** | Use:<br>Head and Neck Bursa and Ligament |
| **Buccinator muscle** | Use:<br>Facial Muscle | **Cervical lymph node** | Use:<br>Lymphatic, Right Neck<br>Lymphatic, Left Neck |
| **Bulbospongiosus muscle** | Use:<br>Perineum Muscle | **Cervicothoracic facet joint** | Use:<br>Cervicothoracic Vertebral Joint |
| **Bulbourethral (Cowper's) gland** | Use:<br>Urethra | | |

| | |
|---|---|
| Choana | Use:<br>Nasopharynx |
| Chondroglossus muscle | Use:<br>Tongue, Palate, Pharynx Muscle |
| Chorda tympani | Use:<br>Facial Nerve |
| Choroid plexus | Use:<br>Cerebral Ventricle |
| Ciliary body | Use:<br>Eye, Right<br>Eye, Left |
| Ciliary ganglion | Use:<br>Head and Neck Sympathetic Nerve |
| Circle of Willis | Use:<br>Intracranial Artery |
| Circumflex iliac artery | Use:<br>Femoral Artery, Right<br>Femoral Artery, Left |
| Claustrum | Use:<br>Basal Ganglia |
| Coccygeal body | Use:<br>Coccygeal Glomus |
| Coccygeus muscle | Use:<br>Trunk Muscle, Right<br>Trunk Muscle, Left |
| Cochlea | Use:<br>Inner Ear, Right<br>Inner Ear, Left |
| Cochlear nerve | Use:<br>Acoustic Nerve |
| Columella | Use:<br>Nose |
| Common digital vein | Use:<br>Foot Vein, Right<br>Foot Vein, Left |
| Common facial vein | Use:<br>Face Vein, Right<br>Face Vein, Left |
| Common fibular nerve | Use:<br>Peroneal Nerve |
| Common hepatic artery | Use:<br>Hepatic Artery |
| Common iliac (subaortic) lymph node | Use:<br>Lymphatic, Pelvis |
| Common interosseous artery | Use:<br>Ulnar Artery, Right<br>Ulnar Artery, Left |
| Common peroneal nerve | Use:<br>Peroneal Nerve |
| Condyloid process | Use:<br>Mandible, Right<br>Mandible, Left |
| Conus arteriosus | Use:<br>Ventricle, Right |
| Conus medullaris | Use:<br>Lumbar Spinal Cord |
| Coracoacromial ligament | Use:<br>Shoulder Bursa and Ligament, Right<br>Shoulder Bursa and Ligament, Left |
| Coracobrachialis muscle | Use:<br>Upper Arm Muscle, Right<br>Upper Arm Muscle, Left |
| Coracoclavicular ligament<br>Coracohumeral ligament | Use:<br>Shoulder Bursa and Ligament, Right<br>Shoulder Bursa and Ligament, Left |
| Coracoid process | Use:<br>Scapula, Right<br>Scapula, Left |
| Corniculate cartilage | Use:<br>Larynx |
| Corpus callosum | Use:<br>Brain |
| Corpus cavernosum<br>Corpus spongiosum | Use:<br>Penis |
| Corpus striatum | Use:<br>Basal Ganglia |
| Corrugator supercilii muscle | Use:<br>Facial Muscle |
| Costocervical trunk | Use:<br>Subclavian Artery, Right<br>Subclavian Artery, Left |
| Costoclavicular ligament | Use:<br>Shoulder Bursa and Ligament, Right<br>Shoulder Bursa and Ligament, Left |
| Costotransverse joint | Use:<br>Thoracic Vertebral Joint<br>Thoracic Vertebral Joints, 2 to 7<br>Thoracic Vertebral Joints, 8 or more |
| Costotransverse ligament | Use:<br>Thorax Bursa and Ligament, Right<br>Thorax Bursa and Ligament, Left |
| Costovertebral joint | Use:<br>Thoracic Vertebral Joint<br>Thoracic Vertebral Joints, 2 to 7<br>Thoracic Vertebral Joints, 8 or more |
| Costoxiphoid ligament | Use:<br>Thorax Bursa and Ligament, Right<br>Thorax Bursa and Ligament, Left |
| Cowper's (bulbourethral) gland | Use:<br>Urethra |
| Cranial dura mater | Use:<br>Dura Mater |
| Cranial epidural space | Use:<br>Epidural Space |
| Cranial subarachnoid space | Use:<br>Subarachnoid Space |
| Cranial subdural space | Use:<br>Subdural Space |
| Cremaster muscle | Use:<br>Perineum Muscle |
| Cribriform plate | Use:<br>Ethmoid Bone, Right<br>Ethmoid Bone, Left |
| Cricoid cartilage | Use:<br>Larynx |
| Cricothyroid artery | Use:<br>Thyroid Artery, Right<br>Thyroid Artery, Left |
| Cricothyroid muscle | Use:<br>Neck Muscle, Right<br>Neck Muscle, Left |
| Crural fascia | Use:<br>Subcutaneous Tissue and Fascia, Right Upper Leg<br>Subcutaneous Tissue and Fascia, Left Upper Leg |
| Cubital lymph node | Use:<br>Lymphatic, Right Upper Extremity<br>Lymphatic, Left Upper Extremity |
| Cubital nerve | Use:<br>Ulnar Nerve |
| Cuboid bone | Use:<br>Tarsal, Right<br>Tarsal, Left |
| Cuboideonavicular joint | Use:<br>Tarsal Joint, Right<br>Tarsal Joint, Left |
| Culmen | Use:<br>Cerebellum |
| Cuneiform cartilage | Use:<br>Larynx |
| Cuneonavicular joint | Use:<br>Tarsal Joint, Right<br>Tarsal Joint, Left |
| Cuneonavicular ligament | Use:<br>Foot Bursa and Ligament, Right<br>Foot Bursa and Ligament, Left |
| Cutaneous (transverse) cervical nerve | Use:<br>Cervical Plexus |
| Deep cervical fascia | Use:<br>Subcutaneous Tissue and Fascia, Anterior Neck |

| | | | |
|---|---|---|---|
| Deep cervical vein | Use:<br>Vertebral Vein, Right<br>Vertebral Vein, Left | Dorsal venous arch | Use:<br>Foot Vein, Right<br>Foot Vein, Left |
| Deep circumflex iliac artery | Use:<br>External Iliac Artery, Right<br>External Iliac Artery, Left | Dorsalis pedis artery | Use:<br>Anterior Tibial Artery, Right<br>Anterior Tibial Artery, Left |
| Deep facial vein | Use:<br>Face Vein, Right<br>Face Vein, Left | Duct of Santorini | Use:<br>Pancreatic Duct, Accessory |
| Deep femoral (profunda femoris) vein | Use:<br>Femoral Vein, Right<br>Femoral Vein, Left | Duct of Wirsung | Use:<br>Pancreatic Duct |
| Deep femoral artery | Use:<br>Femoral Artery, Right<br>Femoral Artery, Left | Ductus deferens | Use:<br>Vas Deferens, Right<br>Vas Deferens, Left<br>Vas Deferens, Bilateral<br>Vas Deferens |
| Deep palmar arch | Use:<br>Hand Artery, Right<br>Hand Artery, Left | Duodenal ampulla | Use:<br>Ampulla of Vater |
| Deep transverse perineal muscle | Use:<br>Perineum Muscle | Duodenojejunal flexure | Use:<br>Jejunum |
| Deferential artery | Use:<br>Internal Iliac Artery, Right<br>Internal Iliac Artery, Left | Dural venous sinus | Use:<br>Intracranial Vein |
| Deltoid fascia | Use:<br>Subcutaneous Tissue and Fascia, Right Upper Arm<br>Subcutaneous Tissue and Fascia, Left Upper Arm | Earlobe | Use:<br>External Ear, Right<br>External Ear, Left<br>External Ear, Bilateral |
| Deltoid ligament | Use:<br>Ankle Bursa and Ligament, Right<br>Ankle Bursa and Ligament, Left | Eighth cranial nerve | Use:<br>Acoustic Nerve |
| Deltoid muscle | Use:<br>Shoulder Muscle, Right<br>Shoulder Muscle, Left | Ejaculatory duct | Use:<br>Vas Deferens, Right<br>Vas Deferens, Left<br>Vas Deferens, Bilateral<br>Vas Deferens |
| Deltopectoral (infraclavicular) lymph node | Use:<br>Lymphatic, Right Upper Extremity<br>Lymphatic, Left Upper Extremity | Eleventh cranial nerve | Use:<br>Accessory Nerve |
| Dentate ligament | Use:<br>Dura Mater | Encephalon | Use:<br>Brain |
| Denticulate ligament | Use:<br>Spinal meninges | Ependyma | Use:<br>Cerebral Ventricle |
| Depressor anguli oris muscle<br>Depressor labii inferioris muscle<br>Depressor septi nasi muscle<br>Depressor supercilii muscle | Use:<br>Facial Muscle | Epidermis | Use:<br>Skin |
| | | Epiploic foramen | Use:<br>Peritoneum |
| Dermis | Use:<br>Skin | Epithalamus | Use:<br>Thalamus |
| Descending genicular artery | Use:<br>Femoral Artery, Right<br>Femoral Artery, Left | Epitrochlear lymph node | Use:<br>Lymphatic, Right Upper Extremity<br>Lymphatic, Left Upper Extremity |
| Diaphragma sellae | Use:<br>Dura Mater | Erector spinae muscle | Use:<br>Trunk Muscle, Right<br>Trunk Muscle, Left |
| Distal humerus | Use:<br>Humeral Shaft, Right<br>Humeral Shaft, Left | Esophageal artery | Use:<br>Thoracic Aorta |
| Distal humerus, involving joint | Use:<br>Elbow Joint, Right<br>Elbow Joint, Left | Esophageal plexus | Use:<br>Thoracic Sympathetic Nerve |
| Distal radioulnar joint | Use:<br>Wrist Joint, Right<br>Wrist Joint, Left | Ethmoidal air cell | Use:<br>Ethmoid Sinus, Right<br>Ethmoid Sinus, Left |
| Dorsal digital nerve | Use:<br>Radial Nerve | Extensor carpi radialis muscle<br>Extensor carpi ulnaris muscle | Use:<br>Lower Arm and Wrist Muscle, Right<br>Lower Arm and Wrist Muscle, Left |
| Dorsal metacarpal vein | Use:<br>Hand Vein, Right<br>Hand Vein, Left | Extensor digitorum brevis muscle | Use:<br>Foot Muscle, Right<br>Foot Muscle, Left |
| Dorsal metatarsal artery | Use:<br>Foot Artery, Right<br>Foot Artery, Left | Extensor digitorum longus muscle | Use:<br>Lower Leg Muscle, Right<br>Lower Leg Muscle, Left |
| Dorsal metatarsal vein | Use:<br>Foot Vein, Right<br>Foot Vein, Left | Extensor hallucis brevis muscle | Use:<br>Foot Muscle, Right<br>Foot Muscle, Left |
| Dorsal scapular artery | Use:<br>Subclavian Artery, Right<br>Subclavian Artery, Left | Extensor hallucis longus muscle | Use:<br>Lower Leg Muscle, Right<br>Lower Leg Muscle, Left |
| Dorsal scapular nerve | Use:<br>Brachial Plexus | External anal sphincter | Use:<br>Anal Sphincter |

| | |
|---|---|
| External auditory meatus | Use:<br>External Auditory Canal, Right<br>External Auditory Canal, Left |
| External maxillary artery | Use:<br>Face Artery |
| External naris | Use:<br>Nose |
| External oblique aponeurosis | Use:<br>Subcutaneous Tissue and Fascia, Trunk |
| External oblique muscle | Use:<br>Abdomen Muscle, Right<br>Abdomen Muscle, Left |
| External popliteal nerve | Use:<br>Peroneal Nerve |
| External pudendal artery | Use:<br>Femoral Artery, Right<br>Femoral Artery, Left |
| External pudendal vein | Use:<br>Greater Saphenous Vein, Right<br>Greater Saphenous Vein, Left |
| External urethral sphincter | Use:<br>Urethra |
| Extradural space | Use:<br>Epidural Space |
| Facial artery | Use:<br>Face Artery |
| False vocal cord | Use:<br>Larynx |
| Falx cerebri | Use:<br>Dura Mater |
| Fascia lata | Use:<br>Subcutaneous Tissue and Fascia, Right Upper Leg<br>Subcutaneous Tissue and Fascia, Left Upper Leg |
| Femoral head | Use:<br>Upper Femur, Right<br>Upper Femur, Left |
| Femoral lymph node | Use:<br>Lymphatic, Right Lower Extremity<br>Lymphatic, Left Lower Extremity |
| Femoropatellar joint | Use:<br>Knee Joint, Right<br>Knee Joint, Left<br>Knee Joint, Femoral Surface, Right<br>Knee Joint, Femoral Surface, Left |
| Femorotibial joint | Use:<br>Knee Joint, Right<br>Knee Joint, Left<br>Knee Joint, Tibial Surface, Right<br>Knee Joint, Tibial Surface, Left |
| Fibular artery | Use:<br>Peroneal Artery, Right<br>Peroneal Artery, Left |
| Fibularis brevis muscle<br>Fibularis longus muscle | Use:<br>Lower Leg Muscle, Right<br>Lower Leg Muscle, Left |
| Fifth cranial nerve | Use:<br>Trigeminal Nerve |
| First cranial nerve | Use:<br>Olfactory Nerve |
| First intercostal nerve | Use:<br>Brachial Plexus |
| Flexor carpi radialis muscle<br>Flexor carpi ulnaris muscle | Use:<br>Lower Arm and Wrist Muscle, Right<br>Lower Arm and Wrist Muscle, Left |
| Flexor digitorum brevis muscle | Use:<br>Foot Muscle, Right<br>Foot Muscle, Left |
| Flexor digitorum longus muscle | Use:<br>Lower Leg Muscle, Right<br>Lower Leg Muscle, Left |
| Flexor hallucis brevis muscle | Use:<br>Foot Muscle, Right<br>Foot Muscle, Left |

| | |
|---|---|
| Flexor hallucis longus muscle | Use:<br>Lower Leg Muscle, Right<br>Lower Leg Muscle, Left |
| Flexor pollicis longus muscle | Use:<br>Lower Arm and Wrist Muscle, Right<br>Lower Arm and Wrist Muscle, Left |
| Foramen magnum | Use:<br>Occipital Bone, Right<br>Occipital Bone, Left |
| Foramen of Monro (intraventricular) | Use:<br>Cerebral Ventricle |
| Foreskin | Use:<br>Prepuce |
| Fossa of Rosenmuller | Use:<br>Nasopharynx |
| Fourth cranial nerve | Use:<br>Trochlear Nerve |
| Fourth ventricle | Use:<br>Cerebral Ventricle |
| Fovea | Use:<br>Retina, Right<br>Retina, Left |
| Frenulum labii inferioris | Use:<br>Lower Lip |
| Frenulum labii superioris | Use:<br>Upper Lip |
| Frenulum linguae | Use:<br>Tongue |
| Frontal lobe | Use:<br>Cerebral Hemisphere |
| Frontal vein | Use:<br>Face Vein, Right<br>Face Vein, Left |
| Fundus uteri | Use:<br>Uterus |
| Galea aponeurotica | Use:<br>Subcutaneous Tissue and Fascia, Scalp |
| Ganglion impar (ganglion of Walther) | Use:<br>Sacral Sympathetic Nerve |
| Gasserian ganglion | Use:<br>Trigeminal Nerve |
| Gastric lymph node | Use:<br>Lymphatic, Aortic |
| Gastric plexus | Use:<br>Abdominal Sympathetic Nerve |
| Gastrocnemius muscle | Use:<br>Lower Leg Muscle, Right<br>Lower Leg Muscle, Left |
| Gastrocolic ligament<br>Gastrocolic omentum | Use:<br>Greater Omentum |
| Gastroduodenal artery | Use:<br>Hepatic Artery |
| Gastroesophageal (GE) junction | Use:<br>Esophagogastric Junction |
| Gastrohepatic omentum | Use:<br>Lesser Omentum |
| Gastrophrenic ligament<br>Gastrosplenic ligament | Use:<br>Greater Omentum |
| Gemellus muscle | Use:<br>Hip Muscle, Right<br>Hip Muscle, Left |
| Geniculate ganglion | Use:<br>Facial Nerve |
| Geniculate nucleus | Use:<br>Thalamus |
| Genioglossus muscle | Use:<br>Tongue, Palate, Pharynx Muscle |
| Genitofemoral nerve | Use:<br>Lumbar Plexus |
| Glans penis | Use:<br>Prepuce |

| | |
|---|---|
| Glenohumeral joint | Use:<br>Shoulder Joint, Right<br>Shoulder Joint, Left |
| Glenohumeral ligament | Use:<br>Shoulder Bursa and Ligament, Right<br>Shoulder Bursa and Ligament, Left |
| Glenoid fossa (of scapula) | Use:<br>Glenoid Cavity, Right<br>Glenoid Cavity, Left |
| Glenoid ligament (labrum) | Use:<br>Shoulder Bursa and Ligament, Right<br>Shoulder Bursa and Ligament, Left |
| Globus pallidus | Use:<br>Basal Ganglia |
| Glossoepiglottic fold | Use:<br>Epiglottis |
| Glottis | Use:<br>Larynx |
| Gluteal lymph node | Use:<br>Lymphatic, Pelvis |
| Gluteal vein | Use:<br>Hypogastric Vein, Right<br>Hypogastric Vein, Left |
| Gluteus maximus muscle<br>Gluteus medius muscle<br>Gluteus minimus muscle | Use:<br>Hip Muscle, Right<br>Hip Muscle, Left |
| Gracilis muscle | Use:<br>Upper Leg Muscle, Right<br>Upper Leg Muscle, Left |
| Great auricular nerve | Use:<br>Cervical Plexus |
| Great cerebral vein | Use:<br>Intracranial Vein |
| Great saphenous vein | Use:<br>Greater Saphenous Vein, Right<br>Greater Saphenous Vein, Left |
| Greater alar cartilage | Use:<br>Nose |
| Greater occipital nerve | Use:<br>Cervical Nerve |
| Greater splanchnic nerve | Use:<br>Thoracic Sympathetic Nerve |
| Greater superficial petrosal nerve | Use:<br>Facial Nerve |
| Greater trochanter | Use:<br>Upper Femur, Right<br>Upper Femur, Left |
| Greater tuberosity | Use:<br>Humeral Head, Right<br>Humeral Head, Left |
| Greater vestibular (Bartholin's) gland | Use:<br>Vestibular Gland |
| Greater wing | Use:<br>Sphenoid Bone, Right<br>Sphenoid Bone, Left |
| Hallux | Use:<br>1st Toe, Right<br>1st Toe, Left |
| Hamate bone | Use:<br>Carpal, Right<br>Carpal, Left |
| Head of fibula | Use:<br>Fibula, Right<br>Fibula, Left |
| Helix | Use:<br>External Ear, Right<br>External Ear, Left<br>External Ear, Bilateral |
| Hepatic artery proper | Use:<br>Hepatic Artery |
| Hepatic flexure | Use:<br>Ascending Colon |
| Hepatic lymph node | Use:<br>Lymphatic, Aortic |

| | |
|---|---|
| Hepatic plexus | Use:<br>Abdominal Sympathetic Nerve |
| Hepatic portal vein | Use:<br>Portal Vein |
| Hepatogastric ligament | Use:<br>Lesser Omentum |
| Hepatopancreatic ampulla | Use:<br>Ampulla of Vater |
| Humeroradial joint<br>Humeroulnar joint | Use:<br>Elbow Joint, Right<br>Elbow Joint, Left |
| Humerus, distal | Use:<br>Humeral Shaft, Right<br>Humeral Shaft, Left |
| Hyoglossus muscle | Use:<br>Tongue, Palate, Pharynx Muscle |
| Hyoid artery | Use:<br>Thyroid Artery, Right<br>Thyroid Artery, Left |
| Hypogastric artery | Use:<br>Internal Iliac Artery, Right<br>Internal Iliac Artery, Left |
| Hypopharynx | Use:<br>Pharynx |
| Hypophysis | Use:<br>Pituitary Gland |
| Hypothenar muscle | Use:<br>Hand Muscle, Right<br>Hand Muscle, Left |
| Ileal artery<br>Ileocolic artery | Use:<br>Superior Mesenteric Artery |
| Ileocolic vein | Use:<br>Colic Vein |
| Iliac crest | Use:<br>Pelvic Bone, Right<br>Pelvic Bone, Left |
| Iliac fascia | Use:<br>Subcutaneous Tissue and Fascia, Right Upper Leg<br>Subcutaneous Tissue and Fascia, Left Upper Leg |
| Iliac lymph node | Use:<br>Lymphatic, Pelvis |
| Iliacus muscle | Use:<br>Hip Muscle, Right<br>Hip Muscle, Left |
| Iliofemoral ligament | Use:<br>Hip Bursa and Ligament, Right<br>Hip Bursa and Ligament, Left |
| Iliohypogastric nerve<br>Ilioinguinal nerve | Use:<br>Lumbar Plexus |
| Iliolumbar artery | Use:<br>Internal Iliac Artery, Right<br>Internal Iliac Artery, Left |
| Iliolumbar ligament | Use:<br>Trunk Bursa and Ligament, Right<br>Trunk Bursa and Ligament, Left |
| Iliotibial tract (band) | Use:<br>Subcutaneous Tissue and Fascia, Right Upper Leg<br>Subcutaneous Tissue and Fascia, Left Upper Leg |
| Ilium | Use:<br>Pelvic Bone, Right<br>Pelvic Bone, Left |
| Incus | Use:<br>Auditory Ossicle, Right<br>Auditory Ossicle, Left |
| Inferior cardiac nerve | Use:<br>Thoracic Sympathetic Nerve |
| Inferior cerebellar vein<br>Inferior cerebral vein | Use:<br>Intracranial Vein |
| Inferior epigastric artery | Use:<br>External Iliac Artery, Right<br>External Iliac Artery, Left |
| Inferior epigastric lymph node | Use:<br>Lymphatic, Pelvis |

| | | | |
|---|---|---|---|
| **Inferior genicular artery** | Use:<br>Popliteal Artery, Right<br>Popliteal Artery, Left | **Intercarpal joint** | Use:<br>Carpal Joint, Right<br>Carpal Joint, Left |
| **Inferior gluteal artery** | Use:<br>Internal Iliac Artery, Right<br>Internal Iliac Artery, Left | **Intercarpal ligament** | Use:<br>Hand Bursa and Ligament, Right<br>Hand Bursa and Ligament, Left |
| **Inferior gluteal nerve** | Use:<br>Sacral Plexus | **Interclavicular ligament** | Use:<br>Shoulder Bursa and Ligament, Right<br>Shoulder Bursa and Ligament, Left |
| **Inferior hypogastric plexus** | Use:<br>Abdominal Sympathetic Nerve | **Intercostal lymph node** | Use:<br>Lymphatic, Thorax |
| **Inferior labial artery** | Use:<br>Face Artery | **Intercostal muscle** | Use:<br>Thorax Muscle, Right<br>Thorax Muscle, Left |
| **Inferior longitudinal muscle** | Use:<br>Tongue, Palate, Pharynx Muscle | **Intercostal nerve**<br>**Intercostobrachial nerve** | Use:<br>Thoracic Nerve |
| **Inferior mesenteric ganglion** | Use:<br>Abdominal Sympathetic Nerve | **Intercuneiform joint** | Use:<br>Tarsal Joint, Right<br>Tarsal Joint, Left |
| **Inferior mesenteric lymph node** | Use:<br>Lymphatic, Mesenteric | **Intercuneiform ligament** | Use:<br>Foot Bursa and Ligament, Right<br>Foot Bursa and Ligament, Left |
| **Inferior mesenteric plexus** | Use:<br>Abdominal Sympathetic Nerve | **Intermediate cuneiform bone** | Use:<br>Tarsal, Right<br>Tarsal, Left |
| **Inferior oblique muscle** | Use:<br>Extraocular Muscle, Right<br>Extraocular Muscle, Left | **Internal (basal) cerebral vein** | Use:<br>Intracranial Vein |
| **Inferior pancreaticoduodenal artery** | Use:<br>Superior Mesenteric Artery | **Internal anal sphincter** | Use:<br>Anal Sphincter |
| **Inferior phrenic artery** | Use:<br>Abdominal Aorta | **Internal carotid plexus** | Use:<br>Head and Neck Sympathetic Nerve |
| **Inferior rectus muscle** | Use:<br>Extraocular Muscle, Right<br>Extraocular Muscle, Left | **Internal iliac vein** | Use:<br>Hypogastric Vein, Right<br>Hypogastric Vein, Left |
| **Inferior suprarenal artery** | Use:<br>Renal Artery, Right<br>Renal Artery, Left | **Internal maxillary artery** | Use:<br>External Carotid Artery, Right<br>External Carotid Artery, Left |
| **Inferior tarsal plate** | Use:<br>Lower Eyelid, Right<br>Lower Eyelid, Left | **Internal naris** | Use:<br>Nose |
| **Inferior thyroid vein** | Use:<br>Innominate Vein, Right<br>Innominate Vein, Left | **Internal oblique muscle** | Use:<br>Abdomen Muscle, Right<br>Abdomen Muscle, Left |
| **Inferior tibiofibular joint** | Use:<br>Ankle Joint, Right<br>Ankle Joint, Left | **Internal pudendal artery** | Use:<br>Internal Iliac Artery, Right<br>Internal Iliac Artery, Left |
| **Inferior turbinate** | Use:<br>Nasal Turbinate | **Internal pudendal vein** | Use:<br>Hypogastric Vein, Right<br>Hypogastric Vein, Left |
| **Inferior ulnar collateral artery** | Use:<br>Brachial Artery, Right<br>Brachial Artery, Left | **Internal thoracic artery** | Use:<br>Internal Mammary Artery, Right<br>Internal Mammary Artery, Left<br>Subclavian Artery, Right<br>Subclavian Artery, Left |
| **Inferior vesical artery** | Use:<br>Internal Iliac Artery, Right<br>Internal Iliac Artery, Left | **Internal urethral sphincter** | Use:<br>Urethra |
| **Infraauricular lymph node** | Use:<br>Lymphatic, Head | **Interphalangeal (IP) joint** | Use:<br>Finger Phalangeal Joint, Right<br>Finger Phalangeal Joint, Left<br>Toe Phalangeal Joint, Right<br>Toe Phalangeal Joint, Left |
| **Infraclavicular (deltopectoral) lymph node** | Use:<br>Lymphatic, Right Upper Extremity<br>Lymphatic, Left Upper Extremity | **Interphalangeal ligament** | Use:<br>Hand Bursa and Ligament, Right<br>Hand Bursa and Ligament, Left<br>Foot Bursa and Ligament, Right<br>Foot Bursa and Ligament, Left |
| **Infrahyoid muscle** | Use:<br>Neck Muscle, Right<br>Neck Muscle, Left | | |
| **Infraparotid lymph node** | Use:<br>Lymphatic, Head | **Interspinalis muscle** | Use:<br>Trunk Muscle, Right<br>Trunk Muscle, Left |
| **Infraspinatus fascia** | Use:<br>Subcutaneous Tissue and Fascia, Right Upper Arm<br>Subcutaneous Tissue and Fascia, Left Upper Arm | **Interspinous ligament** | Use:<br>Trunk Bursa and Ligament, Right<br>Trunk Bursa and Ligament, Left |
| **Infraspinatus muscle** | Use:<br>Shoulder Muscle, Right<br>Shoulder Muscle, Left | **Intertransversarius muscle** | Use:<br>Trunk Muscle, Right<br>Trunk Muscle, Left |
| **Infundibulopelvic ligament** | Use:<br>Uterine Supporting Structure | | |
| **Inguinal canal**<br>**Inguinal triangle** | Use:<br>Inguinal Region, Right<br>Inguinal Region, Left<br>Inguinal Region, Bilateral | | |
| **Interatrial septum** | Use:<br>Atrial Septum | | |

| | |
|---|---|
| Intertransverse ligament | **Use:**<br>Trunk Bursa and Ligament, Right<br>Trunk Bursa and Ligament, Left |
| Interventricular foramen (Monro) | **Use:**<br>Cerebral Ventricle |
| Interventricular septum | **Use:**<br>Ventricular Septum |
| Intestinal lymphatic trunk | **Use:**<br>Cisterna Chyli |
| Ischiatic nerve | **Use:**<br>Sciatic Nerve |
| Ischiocavernosus muscle | **Use:**<br>Perineum Muscle |
| Ischiofemoral ligament | **Use:**<br>Hip Bursa and Ligament, Right<br>Hip Bursa and Ligament, Left |
| Ischium | **Use:**<br>Pelvic Bone, Right<br>Pelvic Bone, Left |
| Jejunal artery | **Use:**<br>Superior Mesenteric Artery |
| Jugular body | **Use:**<br>Glomus Jugulare |
| Jugular lymph node | **Use:**<br>Lymphatic, Right Neck<br>Lymphatic, Left Neck |
| Labia majora<br>Labia minora | **Use:**<br>Vulva |
| Labial gland | **Use:**<br>Upper Lip<br>Lower Lip |
| Lacrimal canaliculus<br>Lacrimal punctum<br>Lacrimal sac | **Use:**<br>Lacrimal Duct, Right<br>Lacrimal Duct, Left |
| Laryngopharynx | **Use:**<br>Pharynx |
| Lateral (brachial) lymph node | **Use:**<br>Lymphatic, Right Axillary<br>Lymphatic, Left Axillary |
| Lateral canthus | **Use:**<br>Upper Eyelid, Right<br>Upper Eyelid, Left |
| Lateral collateral ligament (LCL) | **Use:**<br>Knee Bursa and Ligament, Right<br>Knee Bursa and Ligament, Left |
| Lateral condyle of femur | **Use:**<br>Lower Femur, Right<br>Lower Femur, Left |
| Lateral condyle of tibia | **Use:**<br>Tibia, Right<br>Tibia, Left |
| Lateral cuneiform bone | **Use:**<br>Tarsal, Right<br>Tarsal, Left |
| Lateral epicondyle of femur | **Use:**<br>Lower Femur, Right<br>Lower Femur, Left |
| Lateral epicondyle of humerus | **Use:**<br>Humeral Shaft, Right<br>Humeral Shaft, Left |
| Lateral femoral cutaneous nerve | **Use:**<br>Lumbar Plexus |
| Lateral malleolus | **Use:**<br>Fibula, Right<br>Fibula, Left |
| Lateral meniscus | **Use:**<br>Knee Joint, Right<br>Knee Joint, Left |
| Lateral nasal cartilage | **Use:**<br>Nose |
| Lateral plantar artery | **Use:**<br>Foot Artery, Right<br>Foot Artery, Left |
| Lateral plantar nerve | **Use:**<br>Tibial Nerve |

| | |
|---|---|
| Lateral rectus muscle | **Use:**<br>Extraocular Muscle, Right<br>Extraocular Muscle, Left |
| Lateral sacral artery | **Use:**<br>Internal Iliac Artery, Right<br>Internal Iliac Artery, Left |
| Lateral sacral vein | **Use:**<br>Hypogastric Vein, Right<br>Hypogastric Vein, Left |
| Lateral sural cutaneous nerve | **Use:**<br>Peroneal Nerve |
| Lateral tarsal artery | **Use:**<br>Foot Artery, Right<br>Foot Artery, Left |
| Lateral temporomandibular ligament | **Use:**<br>Head and Neck Bursa and Ligament |
| Lateral thoracic artery | **Use:**<br>Axillary Artery, Right<br>Axillary Artery, Left |
| Latissimus dorsi muscle | **Use:**<br>Trunk Muscle, Right<br>Trunk Muscle, Left |
| Least splanchnic nerve | **Use:**<br>Thoracic Sympathetic Nerve |
| Left ascending lumbar vein | **Use:**<br>Hemiazygos Vein |
| Left atrioventricular valve | **Use:**<br>Mitral Valve |
| Left auricular appendix | **Use:**<br>Atrium, Left |
| Left colic vein | **Use:**<br>Colic Vein |
| Left coronary sulcus | **Use:**<br>Heart, Left |
| Left gastric artery | **Use:**<br>Gastric Artery |
| Left gastroepiploic artery | **Use:**<br>Splenic Artery |
| Left gastroepiploic vein | **Use:**<br>Splenic Vein |
| Left inferior phrenic vein | **Use:**<br>Renal Vein, Left |
| Left inferior pulmonary vein | **Use:**<br>Pulmonary Vein, Left |
| Left jugular trunk | **Use:**<br>Thoracic Duct |
| Left lateral ventricle | **Use:**<br>Cerebral Ventricle |
| Left ovarian vein<br>Left second lumbar vein | **Use:**<br>Renal Vein, Left |
| Left subclavian trunk | **Use:**<br>Thoracic Duct |
| Left subcostal vein | **Use:**<br>Hemiazygos Vein |
| Left superior pulmonary vein | **Use:**<br>Pulmonary Vein, Left |
| Left suprarenal vein<br>Left testicular vein | **Use:**<br>Renal Vein, Left |
| Leptomeninges | **Use:**<br>Cerebral Meninges<br>Spinal Meninges |
| Lesser alar cartilage | **Use:**<br>Nose |
| Lesser occipital nerve | **Use:**<br>Cervical Plexus |
| Lesser splanchnic nerve | **Use:**<br>Thoracic Sympathetic Nerve |
| Lesser trochanter | **Use:**<br>Upper Femur, Right<br>Upper Femur, Left |
| Lesser tuberosity | **Use:**<br>Humeral Head, Right<br>Humeral Head, Left |

| | |
|---|---|
| **Lesser wing** | **Use:**<br>Sphenoid Bone, Right<br>Sphenoid Bone, Left |
| **Levator anguli oris muscle** | **Use:**<br>Facial Muscle |
| **Levator ani muscle** | **Use:**<br>Trunk Muscle, Right<br>Trunk Muscle, Left |
| **Levator labii superioris alaeque nasi muscle**<br>**Levator labii superioris muscle** | **Use:**<br>Facial Muscle |
| **Levator palpebrae superioris muscle** | **Use:**<br>Upper Eyelid, Right<br>Upper Eyelid, Left |
| **Levator scapulae muscle** | **Use:**<br>Neck Muscle, Right<br>Neck Muscle, Left |
| **Levator veli palatini muscle** | **Use:**<br>Tongue, Palate, Pharynx Muscle |
| **Levatores costarum muscle** | **Use:**<br>Thorax Muscle, Right<br>Thorax Muscle, Left |
| **Ligament of head of fibula** | **Use:**<br>Knee Bursa and Ligament, Right<br>Knee Bursa and Ligament, Left |
| **Ligament of the lateral malleolus** | **Use:**<br>Ankle Bursa and Ligament, Right<br>Ankle Bursa and Ligament, Left |
| **Ligamentum flavum** | **Use:**<br>Trunk Bursa and Ligament, Right<br>Trunk Bursa and Ligament, Left |
| **Lingual artery** | **Use:**<br>External Carotid Artery, Right<br>External Carotid Artery, Left |
| **Lingual tonsil** | **Use:**<br>Tongue |
| **Locus ceruleus** | **Use:**<br>Pons |
| **Long thoracic nerve** | **Use:**<br>Brachial Plexus |
| **Lumbar artery** | **Use:**<br>Abdominal Aorta |
| **Lumbar facet joint** | **Use:**<br>Lumbar Vertebral Joint<br>Lumbar Vertebral Joints, 2 or more |
| **Lumbar ganglion** | **Use:**<br>Lumbar Sympathetic Nerve |
| **Lumbar lymph node** | **Use:**<br>Lymphatic, Aortic |
| **Lumbar lymphatic trunk** | **Use:**<br>Cisterna Chyli |
| **Lumbar splanchnic nerve** | **Use:**<br>Lumbar Sympathetic Nerve |
| **Lumbosacral facet joint** | **Use:**<br>Lumbosacral Joint |
| **Lumbosacral trunk** | **Use:**<br>Lumbar Nerve |
| **Lunate bone** | **Use:**<br>Carpal, Right<br>Carpal, Left |
| **Lunotriquetral ligament** | **Use:**<br>Hand Bursa and Ligament, Right<br>Hand Bursa and Ligament, Left |
| **Macula** | **Use:**<br>Retina, Right<br>Retina, Left |
| **Malleus** | **Use:**<br>Auditory Ossicle, Right<br>Auditory Ossicle, Left |
| **Mammary duct**<br>**Mammary gland** | **Use:**<br>Breast, Right<br>Breast, Left<br>Breast, Bilateral |
| **Mammillary body** | **Use:**<br>Hypothalamus |

| | |
|---|---|
| **Mandibular nerve** | **Use:**<br>Trigeminal Nerve |
| **Mandibular notch** | **Use:**<br>Mandible, Right<br>Mandible, Left |
| **Manubrium** | **Use:**<br>Sternum |
| **Masseter muscle** | **Use:**<br>Head Muscle |
| **Masseteric fascia** | **Use:**<br>Subcutaneous Tissue and Fascia, Face |
| **Mastoid (postauricular) lymph node** | **Use:**<br>Lymphatic, Right Neck<br>Lymphatic, Left Neck |
| **Mastoid air cells** | **Use:**<br>Mastoid Sinus, Right<br>Mastoid Sinus, Left |
| **Mastoid process** | **Use:**<br>Temporal Bone, Right<br>Temporal Bone, Left |
| **Maxillary artery** | **Use:**<br>External Carotid Artery, Right<br>External Carotid Artery, Left |
| **Maxillary nerve** | **Use:**<br>Trigeminal Nerve |
| **Medial canthus** | **Use:**<br>Lower Eyelid, Right<br>Lower Eyelid, Left |
| **Medial collateral ligament (MCL)** | **Use:**<br>Knee Bursa and Ligament, Right<br>Knee Bursa and Ligament, Left |
| **Medial condyle of femur** | **Use:**<br>Lower Femur, Right<br>Lower Femur, Left |
| **Medial condyle of tibia** | **Use:**<br>Tibia, Right<br>Tibia, Left |
| **Medial cuneiform bone** | **Use:**<br>Tarsal, Right<br>Tarsal, Left |
| **Medial epicondyle of femur** | **Use:**<br>Lower Femur, Right<br>Lower Femur, Left |
| **Medial epicondyle of humerus** | **Use:**<br>Humeral Shaft, Right<br>Humeral Shaft, Left |
| **Medial malleolus** | **Use:**<br>Tibia, Right<br>Tibia, Left |
| **Medial meniscus** | **Use:**<br>Knee Joint, Right<br>Knee Joint, Left |
| **Medial plantar artery** | **Use:**<br>Foot Artery, Right<br>Foot Artery, Left |
| **Medial plantar nerve**<br>**Medial popliteal nerve** | **Use:**<br>Tibial Nerve |
| **Medial rectus muscle** | **Use:**<br>Extraocular Muscle, Right<br>Extraocular Muscle, Left |
| **Medial sural cutaneous nerve** | **Use:**<br>Tibial Nerve |
| **Median antebrachial vein**<br>**Median cubital vein** | **Use:**<br>Basilic Vein, Right<br>Basilic Vein, Left |
| **Median sacral artery** | **Use:**<br>Abdominal Aorta |
| **Mediastinal lymph node** | **Use:**<br>Lymphatic, Thorax |
| **Meissner's (submucous) plexus** | **Use:**<br>Abdominal Sympathetic Nerve |
| **Membranous urethra** | **Use:**<br>Urethra |

| | |
|---|---|
| Mental foramen | **Use:**<br>Mandible, Right<br>Mandible, Left |
| Mentalis muscle | **Use:**<br>Facial Muscle |
| Mesoappendix<br>Mesocolon | **Use:**<br>Mesentery |
| Metacarpal ligament<br>Metacarpophalangeal ligament | **Use:**<br>Hand Bursa and Ligament, Right<br>Hand Bursa and Ligament, Left |
| Metatarsal ligament | **Use:**<br>Foot Bursa and Ligament, Right<br>Foot Bursa and Ligament, Left |
| Metatarsophalangeal (MTP) joint | **Use:**<br>Metatarsal-Phalangeal Joint, Right<br>Metatarsal-Phalangeal Joint, Left |
| Metatarsophalangeal ligament | **Use:**<br>Foot Bursa and Ligament, Right<br>Foot Bursa and Ligament, Left |
| Metathalamus | **Use:**<br>Thalamus |
| Midcarpal joint | **Use:**<br>Carpal Joint, Right<br>Carpal Joint, Left |
| Middle cardiac nerve | **Use:**<br>Thoracic Sympathetic Nerve |
| Middle cerebral artery | **Use:**<br>Intracranial Artery |
| Middle cerebral vein | **Use:**<br>Intracranial Vein |
| Middle colic vein | **Use:**<br>Colic Vein |
| Middle genicular artery | **Use:**<br>Popliteal Artery, Right<br>Popliteal Artery, Left |
| Middle hemorrhoidal vein | **Use:**<br>Hypogastric Vein, Right<br>Hypogastric Vein, Left |
| Middle rectal artery | **Use:**<br>Internal Iliac Artery, Right<br>Internal Iliac Artery, Left |
| Middle suprarenal artery | **Use:**<br>Abdominal Aorta |
| Middle temporal artery | **Use:**<br>Temporal Artery, Right<br>Temporal Artery, Left |
| Middle turbinate | **Use:**<br>Nasal Turbinate |
| Mitral annulus | **Use:**<br>Mitral Valve |
| Molar gland | **Use:**<br>Buccal Mucosa |
| Musculocutaneous nerve | **Use:**<br>Brachial Plexus |
| Musculophrenic artery | **Use:**<br>Internal Mammary Artery, Right<br>Internal Mammary Artery, Left |
| Musculospiral nerve | **Use:**<br>Radial Nerve |
| Myelencephalon | **Use:**<br>Medulla Oblongata |
| Myenteric (Auerbach's) plexus | **Use:**<br>Abdominal Sympathetic Nerve |
| Myometrium | **Use:**<br>Uterus |
| Nail bed<br>Nail plate | **Use:**<br>Finger Nail<br>Toe Nail |
| Nasal cavity | **Use:**<br>Nose |
| Nasal concha | **Use:**<br>Nasal Turbinate |
| Nasalis muscle | **Use:**<br>Facial Muscle |

| | |
|---|---|
| Nasolacrimal duct | **Use:**<br>Lacrimal Duct, Right<br>Lacrimal Duct, Left |
| Navicular bone | **Use:**<br>Tarsal, Right<br>Tarsal, Left |
| Neck of femur | **Use:**<br>Upper Femur, Right<br>Upper Femur, Left |
| Neck of humerus (anatomical)<br>(surgical) | **Use:**<br>Humeral Head, Right<br>Humeral Head, Left |
| Nerve to the stapedius | **Use:**<br>Facial Nerve |
| Neurohypophysis | **Use:**<br>Pituitary Gland |
| Ninth cranial nerve | **Use:**<br>Glossopharyngeal Nerve |
| Nostril | **Use:**<br>Nose |
| Obturator artery | **Use:**<br>Internal Iliac Artery, Right<br>Internal Iliac Artery, Left |
| Obturator lymph node | **Use:**<br>Lymphatic, Pelvis |
| Obturator muscle | **Use:**<br>Hip Muscle, Right<br>Hip Muscle, Left |
| Obturator nerve | **Use:**<br>Lumbar Plexus |
| Obturator vein | **Use:**<br>Hypogastric Vein, Right<br>Hypogastric Vein, Left |
| Obtuse margin | **Use:**<br>Heart, Left |
| Occipital artery | **Use:**<br>External Carotid Artery, Right<br>External Carotid Artery, Left |
| Occipital lobe | **Use:**<br>Cerebral Hemisphere |
| Occipital lymph node | **Use:**<br>Lymphatic, Right Neck<br>Lymphatic, Left Neck |
| Occipitofrontalis muscle | **Use:**<br>Facial Muscle |
| Olecranon bursa | **Use:**<br>Elbow Bursa and Ligament, Right<br>Elbow Bursa and Ligament, Left |
| Olecranon process | **Use:**<br>Ulna, Right<br>Ulna, Left |
| Olfactory bulb | **Use:**<br>Olfactory Nerve |
| Ophthalmic artery | **Use:**<br>Internal Carotid Artery, Right<br>Internal Carotid Artery, Left |
| Ophthalmic nerve | **Use:**<br>Trigeminal Nerve |
| Ophthalmic vein | **Use:**<br>Intracranial Vein |
| Optic chiasma | **Use:**<br>Optic Nerve |
| Optic disc | **Use:**<br>Retina, Right<br>Retina, Left |
| Optic foramen | **Use:**<br>Sphenoid Bone, Right<br>Sphenoid Bone, Left |
| Orbicularis oculi muscle | **Use:**<br>Upper Eyelid, Right<br>Upper Eyelid, Left |
| Orbicularis oris muscle | **Use:**<br>Facial Muscle |

| | |
|---|---|
| Orbital fascia | Use:<br>Subcutaneous Tissue and Fascia, Face |
| Orbital portion of ethmoid bone<br>Orbital portion of frontal bone<br>Orbital portion of lacrimal bone<br>Orbital portion of maxilla<br>Orbital portion of palatine bone<br>Orbital portion of sphenoid bone<br>Orbital portion of zygomatic bone | Use:<br>Orbit, Right<br>Orbit, Left |
| Oropharynx | Use:<br>Pharynx |
| Ossicular chain | Use:<br>Auditory Ossicle, Right<br>Auditory Ossicle, Left |
| Otic ganglion | Use:<br>Head and Neck Sympathetic Nerve |
| Oval window | Use:<br>Middle Ear, Right<br>Middle Ear, Left |
| Ovarian artery | Use:<br>Abdominal Aorta |
| Ovarian ligament | Use:<br>Uterine Supporting Structure |
| Oviduct | Use:<br>Fallopian Tube, Right<br>Fallopian Tube, Left |
| Palatine gland | Use:<br>Buccal Mucosa |
| Palatine tonsil | Use:<br>Tonsils |
| Palatine uvula | Use:<br>Uvula |
| Palatoglossal muscle<br>Palatopharyngeal muscle | Use:<br>Tongue, Palate, Pharynx Muscle |
| Palmar (volar) digital vein<br>Palmar (volar) metacarpal vein | Use:<br>Hand Vein, Right<br>Hand Vein, Left |
| Palmar cutaneous nerve | Use:<br>Median Nerve<br>Radial Nerve |
| Palmar fascia (aponeurosis) | Use:<br>Subcutaneous Tissue and Fascia, Right Hand<br>Subcutaneous Tissue and Fascia, Left Hand |
| Palmar interosseous muscle | Use:<br>Hand Muscle, Right<br>Hand Muscle, Left |
| Palmar ulnocarpal ligament | Use:<br>Wrist Bursa and Ligament, Right<br>Wrist Bursa and Ligament, Left |
| Palmaris longus muscle | Use:<br>Lower Arm and Wrist Muscle, Right<br>Lower Arm and Wrist Muscle, Left |
| Pancreatic artery | Use:<br>Splenic Artery |
| Pancreatic plexus | Use:<br>Abdominal Sympathetic Nerve |
| Pancreatic vein | Use:<br>Splenic Vein |
| Pancreaticosplenic lymph node<br>Paraaortic lymph node | Use:<br>Lymphatic, Aortic |
| Pararectal lymph node | Use:<br>Lymphatic, Mesenteric |
| Parasternal lymph node<br>Paratracheal lymph node | Use:<br>Lymphatic, Thorax |
| Paraurethral (Skene's) gland | Use:<br>Vestibular Gland |
| Parietal lobe | Use:<br>Cerebral Hemisphere |
| Parotid lymph node | Use:<br>Lymphatic, Head |

| | |
|---|---|
| Parotid plexus | Use:<br>Facial Nerve |
| Pars flaccida | Use:<br>Tympanic Membrane, Right<br>Tympanic Membrane, Left |
| Patellar ligament | Use:<br>Knee Bursa and Ligament, Right<br>Knee Bursa and Ligament, Left |
| Patellar tendon | Use:<br>Knee Tendon, Right<br>Knee Tendon, Left |
| Patellofemoral joint | Use:<br>Knee Joint, Right<br>Knee Joint, Left<br>Knee Joint, Femoral Surface, Right<br>Knee Joint, Femoral Surface, Left |
| Pectineus muscle | Use:<br>Upper Leg Muscle, Right<br>Upper Leg Muscle, Left |
| Pectoral (anterior) lymph node | Use:<br>Lymphatic, Right Axillary<br>Lymphatic, Left Axillary |
| Pectoral fascia | Use:<br>Subcutaneous Tissue and Fascia, Chest |
| Pectoralis major muscle<br>Pectoralis minor muscle | Use:<br>Thorax Muscle, Right<br>Thorax Muscle, Left |
| Pelvic splanchnic nerve | Use:<br>Abdominal Sympathetic Nerve<br>Sacral Sympathetic Nerve |
| Penile urethra | Use:<br>Urethra |
| Pericardiophrenic artery | Use:<br>Internal Mammary Artery, Right<br>Internal Mammary Artery, Left |
| Perimetrium | Use:<br>Uterus |
| Peroneus brevis muscle<br>Peroneus longus muscle | Use:<br>Lower Leg Muscle, Right<br>Lower Leg Muscle, Left |
| Petrous part of temporal bone | Use:<br>Temporal Bone, Right<br>Temporal Bone, Left |
| Pharyngeal constrictor muscle | Use:<br>Tongue, Palate, Pharynx Muscle |
| Pharyngeal plexus | Use:<br>Vagus Nerve |
| Pharyngeal recess | Use:<br>Nasopharynx |
| Pharyngeal tonsil | Use:<br>Adenoids |
| Pharyngotympanic tube | Use:<br>Eustachian Tube, Right<br>Eustachian Tube, Left |
| Pia mater | Use:<br>Cerebral Meninges<br>Spinal Meninges |
| Pinna | Use:<br>External Ear, Right<br>External Ear, Left<br>External Ear, Bilateral |
| Piriform recess (sinus) | Use:<br>Pharynx |
| Piriformis muscle | Use:<br>Hip Muscle, Right<br>Hip Muscle, Left |
| Pisiform bone | Use:<br>Carpal, Right<br>Carpal, Left |
| Pisohamate ligament<br>Pisometacarpal ligament | Use:<br>Hand Bursa and Ligament, Right<br>Hand Bursa and Ligament, Left |
| Plantar digital vein | Use:<br>Foot Vein, Right<br>Foot Vein, Left |

| | | | |
|---|---|---|---|
| Plantar fascia (aponeurosis) | Use:<br>Subcutaneous Tissue and Fascia, Right Foot<br>Subcutaneous Tissue and Fascia, Left Foot | Posterior ulnar recurrent artery | Use:<br>Ulnar Artery, Right<br>Ulnar Artery, Left |
| Plantar metatarsal vein<br>Plantar venous arch | Use:<br>Foot Vein, Right<br>Foot Vein, Left | Posterior vagal trunk | Use:<br>Vagus Nerve |
| Platysma muscle | Use:<br>Neck Muscle, Right<br>Neck Muscle, Left | Preauricular lymph node | Use:<br>Lymphatic, Head |
| Plica semilunaris | Use:<br>Conjunctiva, Right<br>Conjunctiva, Left | Precava | Use:<br>Superior Vena Cava |
| Pneumogastric nerve | Use:<br>Vagus Nerve | Prepatellar bursa | Use:<br>Knee Bursa and Ligament, Right<br>Knee Bursa and Ligament, Left |
| Pneumotaxic center<br>Pontine tegmentum | Use:<br>Pons | Pretracheal fascia | Use:<br>Subcutaneous Tissue and Fascia, Anterior Neck |
| Popliteal ligament | Use:<br>Knee Bursa and Ligament, Right<br>Knee Bursa and Ligament, Left | Prevertebral fascia | Use:<br>Subcutaneous Tissue and Fascia, Posterior Neck |
| Popliteal lymph node | Use:<br>Lymphatic, Right Lower Extremity<br>Lymphatic, Left Lower Extremity | Princeps pollicis artery | Use:<br>Hand Artery, Right<br>Hand Artery, Left |
| Popliteal vein | Use:<br>Femoral Vein, Right<br>Femoral Vein, Left | Procerus muscle | Use:<br>Facial Muscle |
| Popliteus muscle | Use:<br>Lower Leg Muscle, Right<br>Lower Leg Muscle, Left | Profunda brachii | Use:<br>Brachial Artery, Right<br>Brachial Artery, Left |
| Postauricular (mastoid) lymph node | Use:<br>Lymphatic, Right Neck<br>Lymphatic, Left Neck | Profunda femoris (deep femoral) vein | Use:<br>Femoral Vein, Right<br>Femoral Vein, Left |
| Postcava | Use:<br>Inferior Vena Cava | Pronator quadratus muscle<br>Pronator teres muscle | Use:<br>Lower Arm and Wrist Muscle, Right<br>Lower Arm and Wrist Muscle, Left |
| Posterior (subscapular) lymph node | Use:<br>Lymphatic, Right Axillary<br>Lymphatic, Left Axillary | Prostatic urethra | Use:<br>Urethra |
| Posterior auricular artery | Use:<br>External Carotid Artery, Right<br>External Carotid Artery, Left | Proximal radioulnar joint | Use:<br>Elbow Joint, Right<br>Elbow Joint, Left |
| Posterior auricular nerve | Use:<br>Facial Nerve | Psoas muscle | Use:<br>Hip Muscle, Right<br>Hip Muscle, Left |
| Posterior auricular vein | Use:<br>External Jugular Vein, Right<br>External Jugular Vein, Left | Pterygoid muscle | Use:<br>Head Muscle |
| Posterior cerebral artery | Use:<br>Intracranial Artery | Pterygoid process | Use:<br>Sphenoid Bone, Right<br>Sphenoid Bone, Left |
| Posterior chamber | Use:<br>Eye, Right<br>Eye, Left | Pterygopalatine (sphenopala-tine) ganglion | Use:<br>Head and Neck Sympathetic Nerve |
| Posterior circumflex humeral artery | Use:<br>Axillary Artery, Right<br>Axillary Artery, Left | Pubic ligament | Use:<br>Trunk Bursa and Ligament, Right<br>Trunk Bursa and Ligament, Left |
| Posterior communicating artery | Use:<br>Intracranial Artery | Pubis | Use:<br>Pelvic Bone, Right<br>Pelvic Bone, Left |
| Posterior cruciate ligament (PCL) | Use:<br>Knee Bursa and Ligament, Right<br>Knee Bursa and Ligament, Left | Pubofemoral ligament | Use:<br>Hip Bursa and Ligament, Right<br>Hip Bursa and Ligament, Left |
| Posterior facial (retromandibu-lar) vein | Use:<br>Face Vein, Right<br>Face Vein, Left | Pudendal nerve | Use:<br>Sacral Plexus |
| Posterior femoral cutaneous nerve | Use:<br>Sacral Plexus | Pulmoaortic canal | Use:<br>Pulmonary Artery, Left |
| Posterior inferior cerebellar artery (PICA) | Use:<br>Intracranial Artery | Pulmonary annulus | Use:<br>Pulmonary Valve |
| Posterior interosseous nerve | Use:<br>Radial Nerve | Pulmonary plexus | Use:<br>Vagus Nerve<br>Thoracic Sympathetic Nerve |
| Posterior labial nerve<br>Posterior scrotal nerve | Use:<br>Pudendal Nerve | Pulmonic valve | Use:<br>Pulmonary Valve |
| Posterior spinal artery | Use:<br>Vertebral Artery, Right<br>Vertebral Artery, Left | Pulvinar | Use:<br>Thalamus |
| | | Pyloric antrum<br>Pyloric canal<br>Pyloric sphincter | Use:<br>Stomach, Pylorus |
| Posterior tibial recurrent artery | Use:<br>Anterior Tibial Artery, Right<br>Anterior Tibial Artery, Left | Pyramidalis muscle | Use:<br>Abdomen Muscle, Right<br>Abdomen Muscle, Left |

| | |
|---|---|
| Quadrangular cartilage | Use:<br>Nasal Septum |
| Quadrate lobe | Use:<br>Liver |
| Quadratus femoris muscle | Use:<br>Hip Muscle, Right<br>Hip Muscle, Left |
| Quadratus lumborum muscle | Use:<br>Trunk Muscle, Right<br>Trunk Muscle, Left |
| Quadratus plantae muscle | Use:<br>Foot Muscle, Right<br>Foot Muscle, Left |
| Quadriceps (femoris) | Use:<br>Upper Leg Muscle, Right<br>Upper Leg Muscle, Left |
| Radial collateral carpal ligament | Use:<br>Wrist Bursa and Ligament, Right<br>Wrist Bursa and Ligament, Left |
| Radial collateral ligament | Use:<br>Elbow Bursa and Ligament, Right<br>Elbow Bursa and Ligament, Left |
| Radial notch | Use:<br>Ulna, Right<br>Ulna, Left |
| Radial recurrent artery | Use:<br>Radial Artery, Right<br>Radial Artery, Left |
| Radial vein | Use:<br>Brachial Vein, Right<br>Brachial Vein, Left |
| Radialis indicis | Use:<br>Hand Artery, Right<br>Hand Artery, Left |
| Radiocarpal joint | Use:<br>Wrist Joint, Right<br>Wrist Joint, Left |
| Radiocarpal ligament<br>Radioulnar ligament | Use:<br>Wrist Bursa and Ligament, Right<br>Wrist Bursa and Ligament, Left |
| Rectosigmoid junction | Use:<br>Sigmoid Colon |
| Rectus abdominis muscle | Use:<br>Abdomen Muscle, Right<br>Abdomen Muscle, Left |
| Rectus femoris muscle | Use:<br>Upper Leg Muscle, Right<br>Upper Leg Muscle, Left |
| Recurrent laryngeal nerve | Use:<br>Vagus Nerve |
| Renal calyx<br>Renal capsule<br>Renal cortex | Use:<br>Kidney<br>Kidney, Right<br>Kidney, Left<br>Kidneys, Bilateral |
| Renal plexus | Use:<br>Abdominal Sympathetic Nerve |
| Renal segment | Use:<br>Kidney<br>Kidney, Right<br>Kidney, Left<br>Kidneys, Bilateral |
| Renal segmental artery | Use:<br>Renal Artery, Right<br>Renal Artery, Left |
| Retroperitoneal lymph node | Use:<br>Lymphatic, Aortic |
| Retroperitoneal space | Use:<br>Retroperitoneum |
| Retropharyngeal lymph node | Use:<br>Lymphatic, Right Neck<br>Lymphatic, Left Neck |
| Retropubic space | Use:<br>Pelvic Cavity |
| Rhinopharynx | Use:<br>Nasopharynx |

| | |
|---|---|
| Rhomboid major muscle<br>Rhomboid minor muscle | Use:<br>Trunk Muscle, Right<br>Trunk Muscle, Left |
| Right ascending lumbar vein | Use:<br>Azygos Vein |
| Right atrioventricular valve | Use:<br>Tricuspid Valve |
| Right auricular appendix | Use:<br>Atrium, Right |
| Right colic vein | Use:<br>Colic Vein |
| Right coronary sulcus | Use:<br>Heart, Right |
| Right gastric artery | Use:<br>Gastric Artery |
| Right gastroepiploic vein | Use:<br>Superior Mesenteric Vein |
| Right inferior phrenic vein | Use:<br>Inferior Vena Cava |
| Right inferior pulmonary vein | Use:<br>Pulmonary Vein, Right |
| Right jugular trunk | Use:<br>Lymphatic, Right Neck |
| Right lateral ventricle | Use:<br>Cerebral Ventricle |
| Right lymphatic duct | Use:<br>Lymphatic, Right Neck |
| Right ovarian vein<br>Right second lumbar vein | Use:<br>Inferior Vena Cava |
| Right subclavian trunk | Use:<br>Lymphatic, Right Neck |
| Right subcostal vein | Use:<br>Azygos Vein |
| Right superior pulmonary vein | Use:<br>Pulmonary Vein, Right |
| Right suprarenal vein<br>Right testicular vein | Use:<br>Inferior Vena Cava |
| Rima glottidis | Use:<br>Larynx |
| Risorius muscle | Use:<br>Facial Muscle |
| Round ligament of uterus | Use:<br>Uterine Supporting Structure |
| Round window | Use:<br>Inner Ear, Right<br>Inner Ear, Left |
| Sacral ganglion | Use:<br>Sacral Sympathetic Nerve |
| Sacral lymph node | Use:<br>Lymphatic, Pelvis |
| Sacral splanchnic nerve | Use:<br>Sacral Sympathetic Nerve |
| Sacrococcygeal ligament | Use:<br>Trunk Bursa and Ligament, Right<br>Trunk Bursa and Ligament, Left |
| Sacrococcygeal symphysis | Use:<br>Sacrococcygeal Joint |
| Sacroiliac ligament<br>Sacrospinous ligament<br>Sacrotuberous ligament | Use:<br>Trunk Bursa and Ligament, Right<br>Trunk Bursa and Ligament, Left |
| Salpingopharyngeus muscle | Use:<br>Tongue, Palate, Pharynx Muscle |
| Salpinx | Use:<br>Fallopian Tube, Right<br>Fallopian Tube, Left |
| Saphenous nerve | Use:<br>Femoral Nerve |
| Sartorius muscle | Use:<br>Upper Leg Muscle, Right<br>Upper Leg Muscle, Left |
| Scalene muscle | Use:<br>Neck Muscle, Right<br>Neck Muscle, Left |

| | |
|---|---|
| Scaphoid bone | Use:<br>Carpal, Right<br>Carpal, Left |
| Scapholunate ligament<br>Scaphotrapezium ligament | Use:<br>Hand Bursa and Ligament, Right<br>Hand Bursa and Ligament, Left |
| Scarpa's (vestibular) ganglion | Use:<br>Acoustic Nerve |
| Sebaceous gland | Use:<br>Skin |
| Second cranial nerve | Use:<br>Optic Nerve |
| Sella turcica | Use:<br>Sphenoid Bone, Right<br>Sphenoid Bone, Left |
| Semicircular canal | Use:<br>Inner Ear, Right<br>Inner Ear, Left |
| Semimembranosus muscle<br>Semitendinosus muscle | Use:<br>Upper Leg Muscle, Right<br>Upper Leg Muscle, Left |
| Septal cartilage | Use:<br>Nasal Septum |
| Serratus anterior muscle | Use:<br>Thorax Muscle, Right<br>Thorax Muscle, Left |
| Serratus posterior muscle | Use:<br>Trunk Muscle, Right<br>Trunk Muscle, Left |
| Seventh cranial nerve | Use:<br>Facial Nerve |
| Short gastric artery | Use:<br>Splenic Artery |
| Sigmoid artery | Use:<br>Inferior Mesenteric Artery |
| Sigmoid flexure | Use:<br>Sigmoid Colon |
| Sigmoid vein | Use:<br>Inferior Mesenteric Vein |
| Sinoatrial node | Use:<br>Conduction Mechanism |
| Sinus venosus | Use:<br>Atrium, Right |
| Sixth cranial nerve | Use:<br>Abducens Nerve |
| Skene's (paraurethral) gland | Use:<br>Vestibular Gland |
| Small saphenous vein | Use:<br>Lesser Saphenous Vein, Right<br>Lesser Saphenous Vein, Left |
| Solar (celiac) plexus | Use:<br>Abdominal Sympathetic Nerve |
| Soleus muscle | Use:<br>Lower Leg Muscle, Right<br>Lower Leg Muscle, Left |
| Sphenomandibular ligament | Use:<br>Head and Neck Bursa and Ligament |
| Sphenopalatine (pterygopala-<br>tine) ganglion | Use:<br>Head and Neck Sympathetic Nerve |
| Spinal dura mater | Use:<br>Dura Mater |
| Spinal epidural space | Use:<br>Epidural Space |
| Spinal nerve, cervical | Use:<br>Cervical Nerve |
| Spinal nerve, lumbar | Use:<br>Lumbar Nerve |
| Spinal nerve, sacral | Use:<br>Sacral Nerve |
| Spinal nerve, thoracic | Use:<br>Thoracic Nerve |
| Spinal subarachnoid space | Use:<br>Subarachnoid Space |
| Spinal subdural space | Use:<br>Subdural Space |
| Spinous process | Use:<br>Cervical Vertebra<br>Thoracic Vertebra<br>Lumbar Vertebra |
| Spiral ganglion | Use:<br>Acoustic Nerve |
| Splenic flexure | Use:<br>Transverse Colon |
| Splenic plexus | Use:<br>Abdominal Sympathetic Nerve |
| Splenius capitis muscle | Use:<br>Head Muscle |
| Splenius cervicis muscle | Use:<br>Neck Muscle, Right<br>Neck Muscle, Left |
| Stapes | Use:<br>Auditory Ossicle, Right<br>Auditory Ossicle, Left |
| Stellate ganglion | Use:<br>Head and Neck Sympathetic Nerve |
| Stensen's duct | Use:<br>Parotid Duct, Right<br>Parotid Duct, Left |
| Sternoclavicular ligament | Use:<br>Shoulder Bursa and Ligament, Right<br>Shoulder Bursa and Ligament, Left |
| Sternocleidomastoid artery | Use:<br>Thyroid Artery, Right<br>Thyroid Artery, Left |
| Sternocleidomastoid muscle | Use:<br>Neck Muscle, Right<br>Neck Muscle, Left |
| Sternocostal ligament | Use:<br>Thorax Bursa and Ligament, Right<br>Thorax Bursa and Ligament, Left |
| Styloglossus muscle | Use:<br>Tongue, Palate, Pharynx Muscle |
| Stylomandibular ligament | Use:<br>Head and Neck Bursa and Ligament |
| Stylopharyngeus muscle | Use:<br>Tongue, Palate, Pharynx Muscle |
| Subacromial bursa | Use:<br>Shoulder Bursa and Ligament, Right<br>Shoulder Bursa and Ligament, Left |
| Subaortic (common iliac)<br>lymph node | Use:<br>Lymphatic, Pelvis |
| Subclavicular (apical) lymph<br>node | Use:<br>Lymphatic, Right Axillary<br>Lymphatic, Left Axillary |
| Subclavius muscle | Use:<br>Thorax Muscle, Right<br>Thorax Muscle, Left |
| Subclavius nerve | Use:<br>Brachial Plexus |
| Subcostal artery | Use:<br>Thoracic Aorta |
| Subcostal muscle | Use:<br>Thorax Muscle. Right<br>Thorax Muscle, Left |
| Subcostal nerve | Use:<br>Thoracic Nerve |
| Submandibular ganglion | Use:<br>Facial Nerve<br>Head and Neck Sympathetic Nerve |
| Submandibular gland | Use:<br>Submaxillary Gland, Right<br>Submaxillary Gland, Left |
| Submandibular lymph node | Use:<br>Lymphatic, Head |
| Submaxillary ganglion | Use:<br>Head and Neck Sympathetic Nerve |

| | |
|---|---|
| Submaxillary lymph node | Use:<br>Lymphatic, Head |
| Submental artery | Use:<br>Face Artery |
| Submental lymph node | Use:<br>Lymphatic, Head |
| Submucous (Meissner's) plexus | Use:<br>Abdominal Sympathetic Nerve |
| Suboccipital nerve | Use:<br>Cervical Nerve |
| Suboccipital venous plexus | Use:<br>Vertebral Vein, Right<br>Vertebral Vein, Left |
| Subparotid lymph node | Use:<br>Lymphatic, Head |
| Subscapular (posterior) lymph node | Use:<br>Lymphatic, Right Axillary<br>Lymphatic, Left Axillary |
| Subscapular aponeurosis | Use:<br>Subcutaneous Tissue and Fascia, Right Upper Arm<br>Subcutaneous Tissue and Fascia, Left Upper Arm |
| Subscapular artery | Use:<br>Axillary Artery, Right<br>Axillary Artery, Left |
| Subscapularis muscle | Use:<br>Shoulder Muscle, Right<br>Shoulder Muscle, Left |
| Substantia nigra | Use:<br>Basal Ganglia |
| Subtalar (talocalcaneal) joint | Use:<br>Tarsal Joint, Right<br>Tarsal Joint, Left |
| Subtalar ligament | Use:<br>Foot Bursa and Ligament, Right<br>Foot Bursa and Ligament, Left |
| Subthalamic nucleus | Use:<br>Basal Ganglia |
| Superficial circumflex iliac vein | Use:<br>Greater Saphenous Vein, Right<br>Greater Saphenous Vein, Left |
| Superficial epigastric artery | Use:<br>Femoral Artery, Right<br>Femoral Artery, Left |
| Superficial epigastric vein | Use:<br>Greater Saphenous Vein, Right<br>Greater Saphenous Vein, Left |
| Superficial palmar arch | Use:<br>Hand Artery, Right<br>Hand Artery, Left |
| Superficial palmar venous arch | Use:<br>Hand Vein, Right<br>Hand Vein, Left |
| Superficial temporal artery | Use:<br>Temporal Artery, Right<br>Temporal Artery, Left |
| Superficial transverse perineal muscle | Use:<br>Perineum Muscle |
| Superior cardiac nerve | Use:<br>Thoracic Sympathetic Nerve |
| Superior cerebellar vein<br>Superior cerebral vein | Use:<br>Intracranial Vein |
| Superior clunic (cluneal) nerve | Use:<br>Lumbar Nerve |
| Superior epigastric artery | Use:<br>Internal Mammary Artery, Right<br>Internal Mammary Artery, Left |
| Superior genicular artery | Use:<br>Popliteal Artery, Right<br>Popliteal Artery, Left |
| Superior gluteal artery | Use:<br>Internal Iliac Artery, Right<br>Internal Iliac Artery, Left |
| Superior gluteal nerve | Use:<br>Lumbar Plexus |
| Superior hypogastric plexus | Use:<br>Abdominal Sympathetic Nerve |
| Superior labial artery | Use:<br>Face Artery |
| Superior laryngeal artery | Use:<br>Thyroid Artery, Right<br>Thyroid Artery, Left |
| Superior laryngeal nerve | Use:<br>Vagus Nerve |
| Superior longitudinal muscle | Use:<br>Tongue, Palate, Pharynx Muscle |
| Superior mesenteric ganglion | Use:<br>Abdominal Sympathetic Nerve |
| Superior mesenteric lymph node | Use:<br>Lymphatic, Mesenteric |
| Superior mesenteric plexus | Use:<br>Abdominal Sympathetic Nerve |
| Superior oblique muscle | Use:<br>Extraocular Muscle, Right<br>Extraocular Muscle, Left |
| Superior olivary nucleus | Use:<br>Pons |
| Superior rectal artery | Use:<br>Inferior Mesenteric Artery |
| Superior rectal vein | Use:<br>Inferior Mesenteric Vein |
| Superior rectus muscle | Use:<br>Extraocular Muscle, Right<br>Extraocular Muscle, Left |
| Superior tarsal plate | Use:<br>Upper Eyelid, Right<br>Upper Eyelid, Left |
| Superior thoracic artery | Use:<br>Axillary Artery, Right<br>Axillary Artery, Left |
| Superior thyroid artery | Use:<br>External Carotid Artery, Right<br>External Carotid Artery, Left<br>Thyroid Artery, Right<br>Thyroid Artery, Left |
| Superior turbinate | Use:<br>Nasal Turbinate |
| Superior ulnar collateral artery | Use:<br>Brachial Artery, Right<br>Brachial Artery, Left |
| Supraclavicular (Virchow's) lymph node | Use:<br>Lymphatic, Right Neck<br>Lymphatic, Left Neck |
| Supraclavicular nerve | Use:<br>Cervical Plexus |
| Suprahyoid lymph node | Use:<br>Lymphatic, Head |
| Suprahyoid muscle | Use:<br>Neck Muscle, Right<br>Neck Muscle, Left |
| Suprainguinal lymph node | Use:<br>Lymphatic, Pelvis |
| Supraorbital vein | Use:<br>Face Vein, Right<br>Face Vein, Left |
| Suprarenal gland | Use:<br>Adrenal Gland, Left<br>Adrenal Gland, Right<br>Adrenal Glands, Bilateral<br>Adrenal Gland |
| Suprarenal plexus | Use:<br>Abdominal Sympathetic Nerve |
| Suprascapular nerve | Use:<br>Brachial Plexus |
| Supraspinatus fascia | Use:<br>Subcutaneous Tissue and Fascia, Right Upper Arm<br>Subcutaneous Tissue and Fascia, Left Upper Arm |
| Supraspinatus muscle | Use:<br>Shoulder Muscle, Right<br>Shoulder Muscle, Left |

|  |  |
|------|-----|
| Supraspinous ligament | **Use:**<br>Trunk Bursa and Ligament, Right<br>Trunk Bursa and Ligament, Left |
| Suprasternal notch | **Use:**<br>Sternum |
| Supratrochlear lymph node | **Use:**<br>Lymphatic, Right Upper Extremity<br>Lymphatic, Left Upper Extremity |
| Sural artery | **Use:**<br>Popliteal Artery, Right<br>Popliteal Artery, Left |
| Sweat gland | **Use:**<br>Skin |
| Talocalcaneal (subtalar) joint | **Use:**<br>Tarsal Joint, Right<br>Tarsal Joint, Left |
| Talocalcaneal ligament | **Use:**<br>Foot Bursa and Ligament, Right<br>Foot Bursa and Ligament, Left |
| Talocalcaneonavicular joint | **Use:**<br>Tarsal Joint, Right<br>Tarsal Joint, Left |
| Talocalcaneonavicular ligament | **Use:**<br>Foot Bursa and Ligament, Right<br>Foot Bursa and Ligament, Left |
| Talocrural joint | **Use:**<br>Ankle Joint, Right<br>Ankle Joint, Left |
| Talofibular ligament | **Use:**<br>Ankle Bursa and Ligament, Right<br>Ankle Bursa and Ligament, Left |
| Talus bone | **Use:**<br>Tarsal, Right<br>Tarsal, Left |
| Tarsometatarsal joint | **Use:**<br>Metatarsal-Tarsal Joint, Right<br>Metatarsal-Tarsal Joint, Left |
| Tarsometatarsal ligament | **Use:**<br>Foot Bursa and Ligament, Right<br>Foot Bursa and Ligament, Left |
| Temporal lobe | **Use:**<br>Cerebral Hemisphere |
| Temporalis muscle<br>Temporoparietalis muscle | **Use:**<br>Head Muscle |
| Tensor fasciae latae muscle | **Use:**<br>Hip Muscle, Right<br>Hip Muscle, Left |
| Tensor veli palatini muscle | **Use:**<br>Tongue, Palate, Pharynx Muscle |
| Tenth cranial nerve | **Use:**<br>Vagus Nerve |
| Tentorium cerebelli | **Use:**<br>Dura Mater |
| Teres major muscle<br>Teres minor muscle | **Use:**<br>Shoulder Muscle, Right<br>Shoulder Muscle, Left |
| Testicular artery | **Use:**<br>Abdominal Aorta |
| Thenar muscle | **Use:**<br>Hand Muscle, Right<br>Hand Muscle, Left |
| Third cranial nerve | **Use:**<br>Oculomotor Nerve |
| Third occipital nerve | **Use:**<br>Cervical Nerve |
| Third ventricle | **Use:**<br>Cerebral Ventricle |
| Thoracic aortic plexus | **Use:**<br>Thoracic Sympathetic Nerve |
| Thoracic esophagus | **Use:**<br>Esophagus, Middle |
| Thoracic facet joint | **Use:**<br>Thoracic Vertebral Joint<br>Thoracic Vertebral Joints, 2 to 7<br>Thoracic Vertebral Joints, 8 or more |

|  |  |
|------|-----|
| Thoracic ganglion | **Use:**<br>Thoracic Sympathetic Nerve |
| Thoracoacromial artery | **Use:**<br>Axillary Artery, Right<br>Axillary Artery, Left |
| Thoracolumbar facet joint | **Use:**<br>Thoracolumbar Vertebral Joint |
| Thymus gland | **Use:**<br>Thymus |
| Thyroarytenoid muscle | **Use:**<br>Neck Muscle, Right<br>Neck Muscle, Left |
| Thyrocervical trunk | **Use:**<br>Thyroid Artery, Right<br>Thyroid Artery, Left |
| Thyroid cartilage | **Use:**<br>Larynx |
| Tibialis anterior muscle<br>Tibialis posterior muscle | **Use:**<br>Lower Leg Muscle, Right<br>Lower Leg Muscle, Left |
| Tibiofemoral joint | **Use:**<br>Knee Joint, Right<br>Knee Joint, Left<br>Knee Joint, Tibial Surface, Right<br>Knee Joint, Tibial Surface, Left |
| Tracheobronchial lymph node | **Use:**<br>Lymphatic, Thorax |
| Tragus | **Use:**<br>External Ear, Right<br>External Ear, Left<br>External Ear, Bilateral |
| Transversalis fascia | **Use:**<br>Subcutaneous Tissue and Fascia, Trunk |
| Transverse (cutaneous) cervical nerve | **Use:**<br>Cervical Plexus |
| Transverse acetabular ligament | **Use:**<br>Hip Bursa and Ligament, Right<br>Hip Bursa and Ligament, Left |
| Transverse facial artery | **Use:**<br>Temporal Artery, Right<br>Temporal Artery, Left |
| Transverse humeral ligament | **Use:**<br>Shoulder Bursa and Ligament, Right<br>Shoulder Bursa and Ligament, Left |
| Transverse ligament of atlas | **Use:**<br>Head and Neck Bursa and Ligament |
| Transverse scapular ligament | **Use:**<br>Shoulder Bursa and Ligament, Right<br>Shoulder Bursa and Ligament, Left |
| Transverse thoracis muscle | **Use:**<br>Thorax Muscle, Right<br>Thorax Muscle, Left |
| Transversospinalis muscle | **Use:**<br>Trunk Muscle, Right<br>Trunk Muscle, Left |
| Transversus abdominis muscle | **Use:**<br>Abdomen Muscle, Right<br>Abdomen Muscle, Left |
| Trapezium bone | **Use:**<br>Carpal, Right<br>Carpal, Left |
| Trapezius muscle | **Use:**<br>Trunk Muscle, Right<br>Trunk Muscle, Left |
| Trapezoid bone | **Use:**<br>Carpal, Right<br>Carpal, Left |
| Triceps brachii muscle | **Use:**<br>Upper Arm Muscle, Right<br>Upper Arm Muscle, Left |
| Tricuspid annulus | **Use:**<br>Tricuspid Valve |
| Trifacial nerve | **Use:**<br>Trigeminal Nerve |

| | |
|---|---|
| Trigone of bladder | Use:<br>Bladder |
| Triquetral bone | Use:<br>Carpal, Right<br>Carpal, Left |
| Trochanteric bursa | Use:<br>Hip Bursa and Ligament, Right<br>Hip Bursa and Ligament, Left |
| Twelfth cranial nerve | Use:<br>Hypoglossal Nerve |
| Tympanic cavity | Use:<br>Middle Ear, Right<br>Middle Ear, Left |
| Tympanic nerve | Use:<br>Glossopharyngeal Nerve |
| Tympanic part of temoporal bone | Use:<br>Temporal Bone, Right<br>Temporal Bone, Left |
| Ulnar collateral carpal ligament | Use:<br>Wrist Bursa and Ligament, Right<br>Wrist Bursa and Ligament, Left |
| Ulnar collateral ligament | Use:<br>Elbow Bursa and Ligament, Right<br>Elbow Bursa and Ligament, Left |
| Ulnar notch | Use:<br>Radius, Right<br>Radius, Left |
| Ulnar vein | Use:<br>Brachial Vein, Right<br>Brachial Vein, Left |
| Umbilical artery | Use:<br>Internal Iliac Artery, Right<br>Internal Iliac Artery, Left |
| Ureteral orifice | Use:<br>Ureter<br>Ureter, Right<br>Ureter, Left<br>Ureters, Bilateral |
| Ureteropelvic junction (UPJ) | Use:<br>Kidney Pelvis, Right<br>Kidney Pelvis, Left |
| Ureterovesical orifice | Use:<br>Ureter<br>Ureter, Right<br>Ureter, Left<br>Ureters, Bilateral |
| Uterine artery | Use:<br>Internal Iliac Artery, Right<br>Internal Iliac Artery, Left |
| Uterine cornu | Use:<br>Uterus |
| Uterine tube | Use:<br>Fallopian Tube, Right<br>Fallopian Tube, Left |
| Uterine vein | Use:<br>Hypogastric Vein, Right<br>Hypogastric Vein, Left |
| Vaginal artery | Use:<br>Internal Iliac Artery, Right<br>Internal Iliac Artery, Left |
| Vaginal vein | Use:<br>Hypogastric Vein, Right<br>Hypogastric Vein, Left |
| Vastus intermedius muscle<br>Vastus lateralis muscle<br>Vastus medialis muscle | Use:<br>Upper Leg Muscle, Right<br>Upper Leg Muscle, Left |
| Ventricular fold | Use:<br>Larynx |
| Vermiform appendix | Use:<br>Appendix |
| Vermilion border | Use:<br>Upper Lip<br>Lower Lip |

| | |
|---|---|
| Vertebral arch | Use:<br>Cervical Vertebra<br>Thoracic Vertebra<br>Lumbar Vertebra |
| Vertebral canal | Use:<br>Spinal Canal |
| Vertebral foramen<br>Vertebral lamina<br>Vertebral pedicle | Use:<br>Cervical Vertebra<br>Thoracic Vertebra<br>Lumbar Vertebra |
| Vesical vein | Use:<br>Hypogastric Vein, Right<br>Hypogastric Vein, Left |
| Vestibular (Scarpa's) ganglion<br>Vestibular nerve<br>Vestibulocochlear nerve | Use:<br>Acoustic Nerve |
| Virchow's (supraclavicular) lymph node | Use:<br>Lymphatic, Right Neck<br>Lymphatic, Left Neck |
| Vitreous body | Use:<br>Vitreous, Right<br>Vitreous, Left |
| Vocal fold | Use:<br>Vocal Cord, Right<br>Vocal Cord, Left |
| Volar (palmar) digital vein<br>Volar (palmar) metacarpal vein | Use:<br>Hand Vein, Right<br>Hand Vein, Left |
| Vomer bone | Use:<br>Nasal Septum |
| Vomer of nasal septum | Use:<br>Nasal Bone |
| Xiphoid process | Use:<br>Sternum |
| Zonule of Zinn | Use:<br>Lens, Right<br>Lens, Left |
| Zygomatic process of frontal bone | Use:<br>Frontal Bone, Right<br>Frontal Bone, Left |
| Zygomatic process of temporal bone | Use:<br>Temporal Bone, Right<br>Temporal Bone, Left |
| Zygomaticus muscle | Use:<br>Facial Muscle |

## APPENDIX C: Device Key

| | |
|---|---|
| 3f (Aortic) Bioprosthesis valve | Use:<br>Zooplastic Tissue in Heart and Great Vessels |
| AbioCor® Total Replacement Heart | Use:<br>Synthetic Substitute |
| Acellular Hydrated Dermis | Use:<br>Nonautologous Tissue Substitute |
| Activa PC neurostimulator | Use:<br>Stimulator Generator, Multiple Array for Insertion in Subcutaneous Tissue and Fascia |
| Activa RC neurostimulator | Use:<br>Stimulator Generator, Multiple Array Rechargeable for Insertion in Subcutaneous Tissue and Fascia |
| Activa SC neurostimulator | Use:<br>Stimulator Generator, Single Array for Insertion in Subcutaneous Tissue and Fascia |
| ACUITY™ Steerable Lead | Use:<br>Cardiac Lead, Pacemaker for Insertion in Heart and Great Vessels<br>Cardiac Lead, Defibrillator for Insertion in Heart and Great Vessels |
| AMPLATZER® Muscular VSD Occluder | Use:<br>Synthetic Substitute |
| AMS 800® Urinary Control System | Use:<br>Artificial Sphincter in Urinary System |
| AneuRx® AAA Advantage® | Use:<br>Intraluminal Device |
| Annuloplasty ring | Use:<br>Synthetic Substitute |

|  |  |
|---|---|
| Artificial anal sphincter (AAS) | Use:<br>Artificial Sphincter in Gastrointestinal System |
| Artificial bowel sphincter (neosphincter) | Use:<br>Artificial Sphincter in Gastrointestinal System |
| Artificial urinary sphincter (AUS) | Use:<br>Artificial Sphincter in Urinary System |
| Assurant (Cobalt) stent | Use:<br>Intraluminal Device |
| Attain Ability® Lead | Use:<br>Cardiac Lead, Pacemaker for Insertion in Heart and Great Vessels<br>Cardiac Lead, Defibrillator for Insertion in Heart and Great Vessels |
| Attain StarFix® (OTW) Lead | Use:<br>Cardiac Lead, Pacemaker for Insertion in Heart and Great Vessels<br>Cardiac Lead, Defibrillator for Insertion in Heart and Great Vessels |
| Autograft | Use:<br>Autologous Tissue Substitute |
| Autologous artery graft | Use:<br>Autologous Arterial Tissue in Heart and Great Vessels<br>Autologous Arterial Tissue in Upper Arteries<br>Autologous Arterial Tissue in Lower Arteries<br>Autologous Arterial Tissue in Upper Veins<br>Autologous Arterial Tissue in Lower Veins |
| Autologous vein graft | Use:<br>Autologous Venous Tissue in Heart and Great Vessels<br>Autologous Venous Tissue in Upper Arteries<br>Autologous Venous Tissue in Lower Arteries<br>Autologous Venous Tissue in Upper Veins<br>Autologous Venous Tissue in Lower Veins |
| Axial Lumbar Interbody Fusion System | Use:<br>Interbody Fusion Device in Lower Joints |
| AxiaLIF® System | Use:<br>Interbody Fusion Device in Lower Joints |
| BAK/C® Interbody Cervical Fusion System | Use:<br>Interbody Fusion Device in Upper Joints |
| Bard® Composix® (E/X)(LP) mesh | Use:<br>Synthetic Substitute |
| Bard® Composix® Kugel® patch | Use:<br>Synthetic Substitute |
| Bard® Dulex™ mesh | Use:<br>Synthetic Substitute |
| Bard® Ventralex™ Hernia Patch | Use:<br>Synthetic Substitute |
| Baroreflex Activation Therapy® (BAT®) | Use:<br>Stimulator Lead in Upper Arteries<br>Cardiac Rhythm Related Device in Subcutaneous Tissue and Fascia |
| Berlin Heart Ventricular Assist Device | Use:<br>Implantable Heart Assist System in Heart and Great Vessels |
| Bioactive embolization coil(s) | Use:<br>Intraluminal Device, Bioactive in Upper Arteries |
| Biventricular external heart assist system | Use:<br>External Heart Assist System in Heart and Great Vessels |
| Blood glucose monitoring system | Use:<br>Monitoring Device |
| Bone anchored hearing device | Use:<br>Hearing Device, Bone Conduction for Insertion in Ear, Nose, Sinus<br>Hearing Device in Head and Facial Bones |
| Bone bank bone graft | Use:<br>Nonautologous Tissue Substitute |
| Bone screw (interlocking)(lag) (pedicle)(recessed) | Use:<br>Internal Fixation Device in Head and Facial Bones<br>Internal Fixation Device in Upper Bones<br>Internal Fixation Device in Lower Bones |
| Bovine pericardial valve | Use:<br>Zooplastic Tissue in Heart and Great Vessels |
| Bovine pericardium graft | Use:<br>Zooplastic Tissue in Heart and Great Vessels |
| Brachytherapy seeds | Use:<br>Radioactive Element |
| BRYAN® Cervical Disc System | Use:<br>Synthetic Substitute |
| BVS 5000 Ventricular Assist Device | Use:<br>External Heart Assist System in Heart and Great Vessels |
| Cardiac contractility modulation lead | Use:<br>Cardiac Lead in Heart and Great Vessels |
| Cardiac event recorder | Use:<br>Monitoring Device |
| Cardiac resynchronization therapy (CRT) lead | Use:<br>Cardiac Lead, Pacemaker for Insertion in Heart and Great Vessels<br>Cardiac Lead, Defibrillator for Insertion in Heart and Great Vessels |
| CardioMEMS® pressure sensor | Use:<br>Monitoring Device, Pressure Sensor for Insertion in Heart and Great Vessels |
| Carotid (artery) sinus (baroreceptor) lead | Use:<br>Stimulator Lead in Upper Arteries |
| Carotid WALLSTENT® Monorail® Endoprosthesis | Use:<br>Intraluminal Device |
| Centrimag® Blood Pump | Use:<br>Intraluminal Device |
| Clamp and rod internal fixation system (CRIF) | Use:<br>Internal Fixation Device in Upper Bones<br>Internal Fixation Device in Lower Bones |
| CoAxia NeuroFlo catheter | Use:<br>Intraluminal Device |
| Cobalt/chromium head and polyethylene socket | Use:<br>Synthetic Substitute, Metal on Polyethylene for Replacement in Lower Joints |
| Cobalt/chromium head and socket | Use:<br>Synthetic Substitute, Metal for Replacement in Lower Joints |
| Cochlear implant (CI), multiple channel (electrode) | Use:<br>Hearing Device, Multiple Channel Cochlear Prosthesis for Insertion in Ear, Nose, Sinus |
| Cochlear implant (CI), single channel (electrode) | Use:<br>Hearing Device, Single Channel Cochlear Prosthesis for Insertion in Ear, Nose, Sinus |
| COGNIS® CRT-D | Use:<br>Cardiac Resynchronization Defibrillator Pulse Generator for Insertion in Subcutaneous Tissue and Fascia |
| Colonic Z-Stent® | Use:<br>Intraluminal Device |
| Complete (SE) stent | Use:<br>Intraluminal Device |
| Concerto II CRT-D | Use:<br>Cardiac Resynchronization Defibrillator Pulse Generator for Insertion in Subcutaneous Tissue and Fascia |
| CONSERVE® PLUS Total Resurfacing Hip System | Use:<br>Resurfacing Device in Lower Joints |
| Consulta CRT-D | Use:<br>Cardiac Resynchronization Defibrillator Pulse Generator for Insertion in Subcutaneous Tissue and Fascia |
| Consulta CRT-P | Use:<br>Cardiac Resynchronization Pacemaker Pulse Generator for Insertion in Subcutaneous Tissue and Fascia |
| CONTAK RENEWAL® 3 RF (HE) CRT-D | Use:<br>Cardiac Resynchronization Defibrillator Pulse Generator for Insertion in Subcutaneous Tissue and Fascia |
| Contegra Pulmonary Valved Conduit | Use:<br>Zooplastic Tissue in Heart and Great Vessels |
| Continuous Glucose Monitoring (CGM) device | Use:<br>Monitoring Device |
| CoreValve Transcatheter Aortic Valve | Use:<br>Zooplastic Tissue in Heart and Great Vessels |
| Cormet Hip Resurfacing System | Use:<br>Resurfacing Device in Lower Joints |
| CoRoent® XL | Use:<br>Interbody Fusion Device in Lower Joints |
| Corox OTW (Bipolar) Lead | Use:<br>Cardiac Lead, Pacemaker for Insertion in Heart and Great Vessels<br>Cardiac Lead, Defibrillator for Insertion in Heart and Great Vessels |
| Cortical strip neurostimulator lead | Use:<br>Neurostimulator Lead in Central Nervous System |
| Cultured epidermal cell autograft | Use:<br>Autologous Tissue Substitute |
| CYPHER® Stent | Use:<br>Intraluminal Device, Drug-eluting in Heart and Great Vessels |
| Cystostomy tube | Use:<br>Drainage Device |
| DBS lead | Use:<br>Neurostimulator Lead in Central Nervous System |

| | |
|---|---|
| **DeBakey Left Ventricular Assist Device** | **Use:**<br>Implantable Heart Assist System in Heart and Great Vessels |
| **Deep Brain Neurostimulator Lead** | **Use:**<br>Neurostimulator Lead in Central Nervous System |
| **Delta Frame External Fixator** | **Use:**<br>External Fixation Device, Hybrid for Insertion in Upper Bones<br>External Fixation Device, Hybrid for Reposition in Upper Bones<br>External Fixation Device, Hybrid for Insertion in Lower Bones<br>External Fixation Device, Hybrid for Reposition in Lower Bones |
| **Delta III Reverse shoulder prosthesis** | **Use:**<br>Synthetic Substitute, Reverse Ball and Socket for Replacement in Upper Joints |
| **Diaphragmatic Pacemaker Generator** | **Use:**<br>Stimulator Generator in Subcutaneous Tissue and Fascia |
| **Direct Lateral Interbody Fusion (DLIF) device** | **Use:**<br>Interbody Fusion Device in Lower Joints |
| **Driver stent (RX) (OTW)** | **Use:**<br>Intraluminal Device |
| **DuraHeart Left Ventricular Assist System** | **Use:**<br>Implantable Heart Assist System in Heart and Great Vessels |
| **Durata® Defibrillation Lead** | **Use:**<br>Cardiac Lead, Defibrillator for Insertion in Heart and Great Vessels |
| **Dynesys® Dynamic Stabilization System** | **Use:**<br>Spinal Stabilization Device, Pedicle-Based for Insertion in Upper Joints<br>Spinal Stabilization Device, Pedicle-Based for Insertion in Lower Joints |
| **E-Luminexx™ (Biliary)(Vascular) Stent** | **Use:**<br>Intraluminal Device |
| **Electrical bone growth stimulator (EBGS)** | **Use:**<br>Bone Growth Stimulator in Head and Facial Bones<br>Bone Growth Stimulator in Upper Bones<br>Bone Growth Stimulator in Lower Bones |
| **Electrical muscle stimulation (EMS) lead** | **Use:**<br>Stimulator Lead in Muscles |
| **Electronic muscle stimulator lead** | **Use:**<br>Stimulator Lead in Muscles |
| **Embolization coil(s)** | **Use:**<br>Intraluminal Device |
| **Endeavor® (III)(IV) (Sprint) Zotarolimus-eluting Coronary Stent System** | **Use:**<br>Intraluminal Device, Drug-eluting in Heart and Great Vessels |
| **EndoSure® sensor** | **Use:**<br>Monitoring Device, Pressure Sensor for Insertion in Heart and Great Vessels |
| **ENDOTAK RELIANCE® (G) Defibrillation Lead** | **Use:**<br>Cardiac Lead, Defibrillator for Insertion in Heart and Great Vessels |
| **Endotracheal tube (cuffed) (double-lumen)** | **Use:**<br>Intraluminal Device, Endotracheal Airway in Respiratory System |
| **Endurant® Endovascular Stent Graft** | **Use:**<br>Intraluminal Device |
| **EnRhythm** | **Use:**<br>Pacemaker, Dual Chamber for Insertion in Subcutaneous Tissue and Fascia |
| **Enterra gastric neurostimulator** | **Use:**<br>Stimulator Generator, Multiple Array for Insertion in Subcutaneous Tissue and Fascia |
| **Epicel® cultured epidermal autograft** | **Use:**<br>Autologous Tissue Substitute |
| **Epic™ Stented Tissue Valve (aortic)** | **Use:**<br>Zooplastic Tissue in Heart and Great Vessels |
| **Epiretinal visual prosthesis** | **Use:**<br>Epiretinal Visual Prosthesis in Eye |
| **Esophageal obturator airway (EOA)** | **Use:**<br>Intraluminal Device, Airway in Gastrointestinal System |
| **Esteem® implantable hearing system** | **Use:**<br>Hearing Device in Ear, Nose, Sinus |
| **Everolimus-eluting coronary stent** | **Use:**<br>Intraluminal Device, Drug-eluting in Heart and Great Vessels |
| **Ex-PRESS™ mini glaucoma shunt** | **Use:**<br>Synthetic Substitute |
| **Express® (LD) Premounted Stent System** | **Use:**<br>Intraluminal Device |
| **Express® Biliary SD Monorail® Premounted Stent System** | **Use:**<br>Intraluminal Device |
| **Express® SD Renal Monorail® Premounted Stent System** | **Use:**<br>Intraluminal Device |
| **External fixator** | **Use:**<br>External Fixation Device in Head and Facial Bones<br>External Fixation Device in Upper Bones<br>External Fixation Device in Lower Bones<br>External Fixation Device in Upper Joints<br>External Fixation Device in Lower Joints |
| **EXtreme Lateral Interbody Fusion (XLIF) device** | **Use:**<br>Interbody Fusion Device in Lower Joints |
| **Facet replacement spinal stabilization device** | **Use:**<br>Spinal Stabilization Device, Facet Replacement for Insertion in Upper Joints<br>Spinal Stabilization Device, Facet Replacement for Insertion in Lower Joints |
| **FLAIR® Endovascular Stent Graft** | **Use:**<br>Synthetic Substitute |
| **Flexible Composite Mesh** | **Use:**<br>Synthetic Substitute |
| **Foley catheter** | **Use:**<br>Drainage Device |
| **Formula™ Balloon-Expandable Renal Stent System** | **Use:**<br>Intraluminal Device |
| **Freestyle (Stentless) Aortic Root Bioprosthesis** | **Use:**<br>Zooplastic Tissue in Heart and Great Vessels |
| **Fusion screw (compression) (lag)(locking)** | **Use:**<br>Internal Fixation Device in Upper Joints<br>Internal Fixation Device in Lower Joints |
| **Gastric electrical stimulation (GES) lead** | **Use:**<br>Stimulator Lead in Gastrointestinal System |
| **Gastric pacemaker lead** | **Use:**<br>Stimulator Lead in Gastrointestinal System |
| **GORE® DUALMESH®** | **Use:**<br>Synthetic Substitute |
| **Guedel airway** | **Use:**<br>Intraluminal Device, Airway in Mouth and Throat |
| **Hancock Bioprosthesis (aortic) (mitral) valve** | **Use:**<br>Zooplastic Tissue in Heart and Great Vessels |
| **Hancock Bioprosthetic Valved Conduit** | **Use:**<br>Zooplastic Tissue in Heart and Great Vessels |
| **HeartMate II® Left Ventricular Assist Device (LVAD)** | **Use:**<br>Implantable Heart Assist System in Heart and Great Vessels |
| **HeartMate XVE® Left Ventricular Assist Device (LVAD)** | **Use:**<br>Implantable Heart Assist System in Heart and Great Vessels |
| **Hip (joint) liner** | **Use:**<br>Liner in Lower Joints |
| **Holter valve ventricular shunt** | **Use:**<br>Synthetic Substitute |
| **Ilizarov external fixator** | **Use:**<br>External Fixation Device, Ring for Insertion in Upper Bones<br>External Fixation Device, Ring for Reposition in Upper Bones<br>External Fixation Device, Ring for Insertion in Lower Bones<br>External Fixation Device, Ring for Reposition in Lower Bones |
| **Ilizarov-Vecklich device** | **Use:**<br>External Fixation Device, Limb Lengthening for Insertion in Upper Bones<br>External Fixation Device, Limb Lengthening for Insertion in Lower Bones |
| **Impella® (2.5)(5.0)(LD) cardiac assist device** | **Use:**<br>Intraluminal Device |
| **Implantable cardioverter-defibrillator (ICD)** | **Use:**<br>Defibrillator Generator for Insertion in Subcutaneous Tissue and Fascia |
| **Implantable drug infusion pump (anti-spasmodic) (chemotherapy) (pain)** | **Use:**<br>Infusion Device, Pump in Subcutaneous Tissue and Fascia |
| **Implantable glucose monitoring device** | **Use:**<br>Monitoring Device |
| **Implantable hemodynamic monitor (IHM)** | **Use:**<br>Monitoring Device, Hemodynamic for Insertion in Subcutaneous Tissue and Fascia |
| **Implantable hemodynamic monitoring system (IHMS)** | **Use:**<br>Monitoring Device, Hemodynamic for Insertion in Subcutaneous Tissue and Fascia |
| **Implantable Miniature Telescope™ (IMT)** | **Use:**<br>Synthetic Substitute, Intraocular Telescope for Replacement in Eye |
| **Implanted (venous)(access) port** | **Use:**<br>Vascular Access Device, Reservoir in Subcutaneous Tissue and Fascia |

| | |
|---|---|
| InDura, intrathecal catheter (1P) (spinal) | **Use:** Infusion Device |
| Injection reservoir, port | **Use:** Vascular Access Device, Reservoir in Subcutaneous Tissue and Fascia |
| Injection reservoir, pump | **Use:** Infusion Device, Pump in Subcutaneous Tissue and Fascia |
| Interbody fusion (spine) cage | **Use:** Interbody Fusion Device in Upper Joints<br>Interbody Fusion Device in Lower Joints |
| Interspinous process spinal stabilization device | **Use:** Spinal Stabilization Device, Interspinous Process for Insertion in Upper Joints<br>Spinal Stabilization Device, Interspinous Process for Insertion in Lower Joints |
| InterStim® Therapy lead | **Use:** Neurostimulator Lead in Peripheral Nervous System |
| InterStim® Therapy neurostimulator | **Use:** Stimulator Generator Single Array for Insertion in Subcutaneous Tissue and Fascia |
| Intramedullary (IM) rod (nail) | **Use:** Internal Fixation Device, Intramedullary in Upper Bones<br>Internal Fixation Device, Intramedullary in Lower Bones |
| Intramedullary skeletal kinetic distractor (ISKD) | **Use:** Internal Fixation Device, Intramedullary in Upper Bones<br>Internal Fixation Device, Intramedullary in Lower Bones |
| Intrauterine Device (IUD) | **Use:** Contraceptive Device in Female Reproductive System |
| Itrel (3)(4) neurostimulator | **Use:** Stimulator Generator, Single Array for Insertion in Subcutaneous Tissue and Fascia |
| Joint fixation plate | **Use:** Internal Fixation Device in Upper Joints<br>Internal Fixation Device in Lower Joints |
| Joint liner (insert) | **Use:** Liner in Lower Joints |
| Joint spacer (antibiotic) | **Use:** Spacer in Upper Joints<br>Spacer in Lower Joints |
| Kappa | **Use:** Pacemaker, Dual Chamber for Insertion in Subcutaneous Tissue and Fascia |
| Kinetra® neurostimulator | **Use:** Stimulator Generator, Multiple Array for Insertion in Subcutaneous Tissue and Fascia |
| Kirschner wire (K-wire) | **Use:** Internal Fixation Device in Head and Facial Bones<br>Internal Fixation Device in Upper Bones<br>Internal Fixation Device in Lower Bones<br>Internal Fixation Device in Upper Joints<br>Internal Fixation Device in Lower Joints |
| Knee (implant) insert | **Use:** Liner in Lower Joints |
| Kuntscher nail | **Use:** Internal Fixation Device, Intramedullary in Upper Bones<br>Internal Fixation Device, Intramedullary in Lower Bones |
| LAP-BAND® Adjustable Gastric Banding System | **Use:** Extraluminal Device |
| LifeStent® (Flexstar)(XL) Vascular Stent System | **Use:** Intraluminal Device |
| LIVIAN™ CRT-D | **Use:** Cardiac Resynchronization Defibrillator Pulse Generator for Insertion in Subcutaneous Tissue and Fascia |
| Loop recorder, implantable | **Use:** Monitoring Device |
| Mark IV Breathing Pacemaker System | **Use:** Stimulator Generator in Subcutaneous Tissue and Fascia |
| Maximo II DR (VR) | **Use:** Defibrillator Generator for Insertion in Subcutaneous Tissue and Fascia |
| Maximo II DR CRT-D | **Use:** Cardiac Resynchronization Defibrillator Pulse Generator for Insertion in Subcutaneous Tissue and Fascia |
| Melody® transcatheter pulmonary valve | **Use:** Zooplastic Tissue in Heart and Great Vessels |
| Micro-Driver stent (RX) (OTW) | **Use:** Intraluminal Device |

| | |
|---|---|
| MicroMed HeartAssist | **Use:** Implantable Heart Assist System in Heart and Great Vessels |
| Micrus CERECYTE Microcoil | **Use:** Intraluminal Device, Bioactive in Upper Arteries |
| MitraClip valve repair system | **Use:** Synthetic Substitute |
| Mitroflow® Aortic Pericardial Heart Valve | **Use:** Zooplastic Tissue in Heart and Great Vessels |
| Nasopharyngeal airway (NPA) | **Use:** Intraluminal Device, Airway in Ear, Nose, Sinus |
| Neuromuscular electrical stimulation (NEMS) lead | **Use:** Stimulator Lead in Muscles |
| Neurostimulator generator, multiple channel | **Use:** Stimulator Generator, Multiple Array for Insertion in Subcutaneous Tissue and Fascia |
| Neurostimulator generator, multiple channel rechargeable | **Use:** Stimulator Generator, Multiple Array Rechargeable for Insertion in Subcutaneous Tissue and Fascia |
| Neurostimulator generator, single channel | **Use:** Stimulator Generator, Single Array for Insertion in Subcutaneous Tissue and Fascia |
| Neurostimulator generator, single channel rechargeable | **Use:** Stimulator Generator, Single Array Rechargeable for Insertion in Subcutaneous Tissue and Fascia |
| Neutralization plate | **Use:** Internal Fixation Device in Head and Facial Bones<br>Internal Fixation Device in Upper Bones<br>Internal Fixation Device in Lower Bones |
| Nitinol framed polymer mesh | **Use:** Synthetic Substitute |
| Non-tunneled central venous catheter | **Use:** Infusion Device |
| Novacor Left Ventricular Assist Device | **Use:** Implantable Heart Assist System in Heart and Great Vessels |
| Novation® Ceramic AHS® (Articulation Hip System) | **Use:** Synthetic Substitute, Ceramic for Replacement in Lower Joints |
| Optimizer™ III implantable pulse generator | **Use:** Contractility Modulation Device for Insertion in Subcutaneous Tissue and Fascia |
| Oropharyngeal airway (OPA) | **Use:** Intraluminal Device, Airway in Mouth and Throat |
| Ovatio™ CRT-D | **Use:** Cardiac Resynchronization Defibrillator Pulse Generator for Insertion in Subcutaneous Tissue and Fascia |
| Oxidized zirconium ceramic hip bearing surface | **Use:** Synthetic Substitute, Ceramic on Polyethylene for Replacement in Lower Joints |
| Paclitaxel-eluting coronary stent | **Use:** Intraluminal Device, Drug-eluting in Heart and Great Vessels |
| Paclitaxel-eluting peripheral stent | **Use:** Intraluminal Device, Drug-eluting in Upper Arteries<br>Intraluminal Device, Drug-eluting in Lower Arteries |
| Partially absorbable mesh | **Use:** Synthetic Substitute |
| Pedicle-based dynamic stabilization device | **Use:** Spinal Stabilization Device, Pedicle-Based for Insertion in Upper Joints<br>Spinal Stabilization Device, Pedicle-Based for Insertion in Lower Joints |
| Percutaneous endoscopic gastrojejunostomy (PEG/J) tube | **Use:** Feeding Device in Gastrointestinal System |
| Percutaneous endoscopic gastrostomy (PEG) tube | **Use:** Feeding Device in Gastrointestinal System |
| Percutaneous nephrostomy catheter | **Use:** Drainage Device |
| Peripherally inserted central catheter (PICC) | **Use:** Infusion Device |
| Pessary ring | **Use:** Intraluminal Device, Pessary in Female Reproductive System |
| Phrenic nerve stimulator generator | **Use:** Stimulator Generator in Subcutaneous Tissue and Fascia |
| Phrenic nerve stimulator lead | **Use:** Diaphragmatic Pacemaker Lead in Respiratory System |
| PHYSIOMESH™ Flexible Composite Mesh | **Use:** Synthetic Substitute |

|  |  |
|---|---|
| Pipeline™ Embolization device (PED) | Use: Intraluminal Device |
| Polyethylene socket | Use: Synthetic Substitute, Polyethylene for Replacement in Lower Joints |
| Polymethylmethacrylate (PMMA) | Use: Synthetic Substitute |
| Polypropylene mesh | Use: Synthetic Substitute |
| Porcine (bioprosthetic) valve | Use: Zooplastic Tissue in Heart and Great Vessels |
| PRESTIGE® Cervical Disc | Use: Synthetic Substitute |
| PrimeAdvanced Neurostimulator | Use: Stimulator Generator, Multiple Array for Insertion in Subcutaneous Tissue and Fascia |
| PROCEED™ Ventral Patch | Use: Synthetic Substitute |
| Prodisc-C | Use: Synthetic Substitute |
| Prodisc-L | Use: Synthetic Substitute |
| PROLENE Polypropylene Hernia System (PHS) | Use: Synthetic Substitute |
| Protecta XT CRT-D | Use: Cardiac Resynchronization Defibrillator Pulse Generator for Insertion in Subcutaneous Tissue and Fascia |
| Protecta XT DR (XT VR) | Use: Defibrillator Generator for Insertion in Subcutaneous Tissue and Fascia |
| Protégé® RX Carotid Stent System | Use: Intraluminal Device |
| Pump reservoir | Use: Infusion Device, Pump in Subcutaneous Tissue and Fascia |
| REALIZE® Adjustable Gastric Band | Use: Extraluminal Device |
| Rebound HRD® (Hernia Repair Device) | Use: Synthetic Substitute |
| RestoreAdvanced neurostimulator | Use: Stimulator Generator, Multiple Array Rechargeable for Insertion in Subcutaneous Tissue and Fascia |
| RestoreSensor neurostimulator | Use: Stimulator Generator, Multiple Array Rechargeable for Insertion in Subcutaneous Tissue and Fascia |
| RestoreUltra neurostimulator | Use: Stimulator Generator, Multiple Array Rechargeable for Insertion in Subcutaneous Tissue and Fascia |
| Reveal (DX)(XT) | Use: Monitoring Device |
| Reverse® Shoulder Prosthesis | Use: Synthetic Substitute, Reverse Ball and Socket for Replacement in Upper Joints |
| Revo MRI™ SureScan® pacemaker | Use: Pacemaker, Dual Chamber for Insertion in Subcutaneous Tissue and Fascia |
| Rheos® System device | Use: Cardiac Rhythm Related Device in Subcutaneous Tissue and Fascia |
| Rheos® System lead | Use: Stimulator Lead in Upper Arteries |
| RNS System lead | Use: Neurostimulator Lead in Central Nervous System |
| RNS system neurostimulator generator | Use: Neurostimulator Generator in Head and Facial Bones |
| Sacral nerve modulation (SNM) lead | Use: Stimulator Lead in Urinary System |
| Sacral neuromodulation lead | Use: Stimulator Lead in Urinary System |
| SAPIEN transcatheter aortic valve | Use: Zooplastic Tissue in Heart and Great Vessels |
| Secura (DR) (VR) | Use: Defibrillator Generator for Insertion in Subcutaneous Tissue and Fascia |
| Sheffield hybrid external fixator | Use: External Fixation Device, Hybrid for Insertion in Upper Bones External Fixation Device, Hybrid for Reposition in Upper Bones External Fixation Device, Hybrid for Insertion in Lower Bones External Fixation Device, Hybrid for Reposition in Lower Bones |
| Sheffield ring external fixator | Use: External Fixation Device, Ring for Insertion in Upper Bones External Fixation Device, Ring for Reposition in Upper Bones External Fixation Device, Ring for Insertion in Lower Bones External Fixation Device, Ring for Reposition in Lower Bones |
| Single lead pacemaker (atrium) (ventricle) | Use: Pacemaker, Single Chamber for Insertion in Subcutaneous Tissue and Fascia |
| Single lead rate responsive pacemaker (atrium)(ventricle) | Use: Pacemaker, Single Chamber Rate Responsive for Insertion in Subcutaneous Tissue and Fascia |
| Sirolimus-eluting coronary stent | Use: Intraluminal Device, Drug-eluting in Heart and Great Vessels |
| SJM Biocor® Stented Valve System | Use: Zooplastic Tissue in Heart and Great Vessels |
| Soletra® single-channel neurostimulator | Use: Stimulator Generator, Single Array for Insertion in Subcutaneous Tissue and Fascia |
| Spinal cord neurostimulator lead | Use: Neurostimulator Lead in Central Nervous System |
| Spiration IBV™ Valve System | Use: Intraluminal Device, Endobronchial Valve in Respiratory System |
| Stent (angioplasty)(emboliza- tion) | Use: Intraluminal Device |
| Stented tissue valve | Use: Zooplastic Tissue in Heart and Great Vessels |
| Stratos LV | Use: Cardiac Resynchronization Pacemaker Pulse Generator for Insertion in Subcutaneous Tissue and Fascia |
| Subcutaneous injection reservoir, port | Use: Vascular Access Device, Reservoir in Subcutaneous Tissue and Fascia |
| Subcutaneous injection reservoir, pump | Use: Infusion Device, Pump in Subcutaneous Tissue and Fascia |
| Subdermal progesterone implant | Use: Contraceptive Device in Subcutaneous Tissue and Fascia |
| SynCardia Total Artificial Heart | Use: Synthetic Substitute |
| Synchra CRT-P | Use: Cardiac Resynchronization Pacemaker Pulse Generator for Insertion in Subcutaneous Tissue and Fascia |
| Talent® Converter | Use: Intraluminal Device |
| Talent® Occluder | Use: Intraluminal Device |
| Talent® Stent Graft (abdominal) (thoracic) | Use: Intraluminal Device |
| TandemHeart® System | Use: Intraluminal Device |
| TAXUS® Liberté® Paclitaxel- eluting Coronary Stent System | Use: Intraluminal Device, Drug-eluting in Heart and Great Vessels |
| Therapeutic occlusion coil(s) | Use: Intraluminal Device |
| Thoracostomy tube | Use: Drainage Device |
| Thoratec IVAD (Implantable Ventricular Assist Device) | Use: Implantable Heart Assist System in Heart and Great Vessels |
| Thoratec Paracorporeal Ventricular Assist Device | Use: External Heart Assist System in Heart and Great Vessels |
| TigerPaw® system for closure of left atrial appendage | Use: Extraluminal Device |
| Tissue bank graft | Use: Nonautologous Tissue Substitute |
| Tissue expander (inflatable) (injectable) | Use: Tissue Expander in Skin and Breast Tissue Expander in Subcutaneous Tissue and Fascia |
| Titanium Sternal Fixation System (TSFS) | Use: Internal Fixation Device, Rigid Plate for Insertion in Upper Bones Internal Fixation Device, Rigid Plate for Reposition in Upper Bones |
| Total artificial (replacement) heart | Use: Synthetic Substitute |
| Tracheostomy tube | Use: Tracheostomy Device in Respiratory System |

| | |
|---|---|
| Trifecta™ Valve (aortic) | Use:<br>Zooplastic Tissue in Heart and Great Vessels |
| Tunneled central venous catheter | Use:<br>Vascular Access Device in Subcutaneous Tissue and Fascia |
| Tunneled spinal (intrathecal) catheter | Use:<br>Infusion Device |
| Two lead pacemaker | Use:<br>Pacemaker, Dual Chamber for Insertion in Subcutaneous Tissue and Fascia |
| Ultraflex™ Precision Colonic Stent System | Use:<br>Intraluminal Device |
| ULTRAPRO Hernia System (UHS) | Use:<br>Synthetic Substitute |
| ULTRAPRO Partially Absorbable Lightweight Mesh | Use:<br>Synthetic Substitute |
| ULTRAPRO Plug | Use:<br>Synthetic Substitute |
| Ultrasonic osteogenic stimulator | Use:<br>Bone Growth Stimulator in Head and Facial Bones<br>Bone Growth Stimulator in Upper Bones<br>Bone Growth Stimulator in Lower Bones |
| Ultrasound bone healing system | Use:<br>Bone Growth Stimulator in Head and Facial Bones<br>Bone Growth Stimulator in Upper Bones<br>Bone Growth Stimulator in Lower Bones |
| Uniplanar external fixator | Use:<br>External Fixation Device, Monoplanar for Insertion in Upper Bones<br>External Fixation Device, Monoplanar for Reposition in Upper Bones<br>External Fixation Device, Monoplanar for Insertion in Lower Bones<br>External Fixation Device, Monoplanar for Reposition in Lower Bones |
| Urinary incontinence stimulator lead | Use:<br>Stimulator Lead in Urinary System |
| Vaginal pessary | Use:<br>Intraluminal Device, Pessary in Female Reproductive System |
| Valiant Thoracic Stent Graft | Use:<br>Synthetic Substitute |
| Vectra® Vascular Access Graft | Use:<br>Vascular Access Device in Subcutaneous Tissue and Fascia |
| Ventrio™ Hernia Patch | Use:<br>Synthetic Substitute |
| Versa | Use:<br>Pacemaker, Dual Chamber for Insertion in Subcutaneous Tissue and Fascia |
| Virtuoso (II) (DR) (VR) | Use:<br>Defibrillator Generator for Insertion in Subcutaneous Tissue and Fascia |
| WALLSTENT® Endoprosthesis | Use:<br>Intraluminal Device |
| X-STOP® Spacer | Use:<br>Spinal Stabilization Device, Interspinous Process for Insertion in Upper Joints<br>Spinal Stabilization Device, Interspinous Process for Insertion in Lower Joints |
| Xenograft | Use:<br>Zooplastic Tissue in Heart and Great Vessels |
| XIENCE V Everolimus Eluting Coronary Stent System | Use:<br>Intraluminal Device, Drug-eluting in Heart and Great Vessels |
| XLIF® System | Use:<br>Interbody Fusion Device in Lower Joints |
| Zenith Flex® AAA Endovascular Graft | Use:<br>Intraluminal Device |
| Zenith TX2® TAA Endovascular Graft | Use:<br>Intraluminal Device |
| Zenith® Renu™ AAA Ancillary Graft | Use:<br>Intraluminal Device |
| Zilver® PTX® (paclitaxel) Drug-Eluting Peripheral Stent | Use:<br>Intraluminal Device, Drug-eluting in Upper Arteries<br>Intraluminal Device, Drug-eluting in Lower Arteries |
| Zimmer® NexGen® LPS Mobile Bearing Knee | Use:<br>Synthetic Substitute |
| Zimmer® NexGen® LPS-Flex Mobile Knee | Use:<br>Synthetic Substitute |
| Zotarolimus-eluting coronary stent | Use:<br>Intraluminal Device, Drug-eluting in Heart and Great Vessels |

# APPENDIX D:
## Comparison of Medical and Surgical Root Operations

### Procedures that take out or eliminate all or a portion of a body part

| Operation | Action | Target | Clarification | Example |
|---|---|---|---|---|
| Excision | Cutting out or off | Portion of a body part | Without replacing body part | Sigmoid polypectomy |
| Resection | Cutting out or off | All of a body part | Without replacing body part | Total nephrectomy |
| Extraction | Pulling out or off by physical force | All or a portion of a body part | Without replacing body part | Toenail extraction |
| Destruction | Eradicating | All or a portion of a body part | Without taking out or replacing body part | Rectal polyp fulguration |
| Detachment | Cutting off | All or a portion of an extremity | Without replacing extremity | Below knee amputation |

### Procedures that involve putting in or on, putting back, or moving living body parts

| Operation | Action | Target | Clarification | Example |
|---|---|---|---|---|
| Transplantation | Putting in or on | All or a portion of a living body part from other individual or animal | Physically takes the place and/or function of all or a portion of a body part | Heart transplant |
| Reattachment | Putting back in or on | All or a portion of a separated body part | Put in its normal or other suitable location | Finger reattachment |
| Reposition | Moving | All or a portion of a body part | Put in its normal or other suitable location. Body part may or may not be cut out or off | Reposition undescended testicle |
| Transfer | Moving | All or a portion of a body part | Without taking out body part; assumes function of similar body part and remains connected to its vascular and nervous supply | Tendon transfer |

### Procedures that take out or eliminate solid matter, fluids, or gases from a body part

| Operation | Action | Target | Clarification | Example |
|---|---|---|---|---|
| Drainage | Taking or letting out | Fluids and/or gases from a body part | Without taking out any of the body part | Incision and drainage |
| Extirpation | Taking or cutting out | Solid matter in a body part | Without taking out any of the body part | Thrombectomy |
| Fragmentation | Breaking down | Solid matter in a body part | Without taking out any of the body part or any solid matter | Lithotripsy of gallstones |

### Procedures that only involve examination of body parts and regions

| Operation | Action | Target | Clarification | Example |
|---|---|---|---|---|
| Inspection | Visual and/or manual exploration | A body part | Performed with or without optical instrumentation, directly or through body layers | Diagnostic arthroscopy |
| Map | Locating | Route of passage of electrical impulses or functional areas in a body part | Applicable only to cardiac conduction mechanism and central nervous system | Cardiac mapping |

## Procedures that alter the diameter/route of a tubular body part

| Operation | Action | Target | Clarification | Example |
|---|---|---|---|---|
| Bypass | Altering the route of passage | Contents of tubular body part | May include use of living tissue, non-living biological material or synthetic material which does not take the place of the body part | Gastrojejunal bypass |
| Dilation | Expanding | Orifice or lumen of tubular body part | By application of intraluminal pressure or by cutting the wall or orifice | Coronary artery dilation |
| Occlusion | Completely closing | Orifice or lumen of tubular body part | N/A | Fallopian tube ligation |
| Restriction | Partially closing | Orifice or lumen of tubular body part | N/A | Cervical cerclage |

## Procedures that always involve devices

| Operation | Action | Target | Clarification | Example |
|---|---|---|---|---|
| Insertion | Putting in | Device in or on a body part | Does not physically take the place of a body part | Pacemaker insertion |
| Replacement | Putting in or on | Biological or synthetic material; or living tissue taken from same individual | Physically takes the place of all or a portion of a body part | Total hip replacement |
| Supplement | Putting in or on | Biological or synthetic material; or living tissue taken from same individual | Physically reinforces or augments a body part | Herniorrhaphy using mesh |
| Removal | Taking out or off | Device from a body part | N/A | Cardiac pacemaker removal |
| Change | Taking out or off and putting back | Identical or similar device in or on a body part | Without cutting or puncturing skin or mucous membrane | Drainage tube change |
| Revision | Correcting | Malfunctioning or displaced device in or on a body part | To the extent possible | Hip prosthesis adjustment |

## Procedures that involve cutting and separation only

| Operation | Action | Target | Clarification | Example |
|---|---|---|---|---|
| Division | Separating | A body part | Without taking out any of the body part | Osteotomy |
| Release | Freeing | A body part | Eliminating abnormal constraint without taking out any of the body part | Peritoneal adhesiolysis |

## Procedures involving other repairs

| Operation | Action | Target | Clarification | Example |
|---|---|---|---|---|
| Control | Stopping or attempting to stop | Postprocedural bleeding | Limited to anatomic regions and extremities | Control of postprostatectomy bleeding |
| Repair | Restoring | A body part to its normal structure | To the extent possible | Suture of laceration |

## Procedures with other objectives

| Operation | Action | Target | Clarification | Example |
|---|---|---|---|---|
| Alteration | Modifying | Anatomic structure of a body part | Without affecting function of body part, performed for cosmetic purposes | Face lift |
| Creation | Making | New genital structure | Does not physically take the place of a body part, used for sex change operations | Artificial vagina creation |
| Fusion | Joining together | An articular body part | Rendering body part immobile | Spinal fusion |

## Components of the Medical and Surgical Approach Definition

| Access Location | Method | Type of Instrumentation | Approach | Example |
|---|---|---|---|---|
| Skin or Mucous Membrane | Open | N/A | Open | Abdominal hysterectomy |
| Skin or Mucous Membrane | Instrumental | Without Visualization | Percutaneous | Needle biopsy of liver |
| Skin or Mucous Membrane | Instrumental | With Visualization | Percutaneous Endoscopic | Arthroscopy |
| Orifice | Instrumental | Without Visualization | Via Natural or Artificial Opening | Endotracheal tube insertion |
| Orifice | Instrumental | With Visualization | Via Natural or Artificial Opening Endoscopic | Sigmoidoscopy |
| Skin or Mucous Membrane | Open | With Visualization | Via Natural or Artificial Opening with Percutaneous Endoscopic Assistance | Laparoscopic-assisted vaginal hysterectomy |
| Skin or Mucous Membrane | N/A | N/A | External | Closed fracture reduction |

## APPENDIX F:

### Device Aggregation Table

| Specific Device | for Operation | in Body System | General Device |
|---|---|---|---|
| Autologous Arterial Tissue | All applicable | Heart and Great Vessels Lower Arteries Lower Veins Upper Arteries Upper Veins | 7 Autologous Tissue Substitute |
| Autologous Venous Tissue | All applicable | Heart and Great Vessels Lower Arteries Lower Veins Upper Arteries Upper Veins | 7 Autologous Tissue Substitute |
| Cardiac Lead, Defibrillator | Insertion | Heart and Great Vessels | M Cardiac Lead |
| Cardiac Lead, Pacemaker | Insertion | Heart and Great Vessels | M Cardiac Lead |
| Cardiac Resynchronization Defibrillator Pulse Generator | Insertion | Subcutaneous Tissue and Fascia | P Cardiac Rhythm Related Device |
| Cardiac Resynchronization Pacemaker Pulse Generator | Insertion | Subcutaneous Tissue and Fascia | P Cardiac Rhythm Related Device |
| Contractility Modulation Device | Insertion | Subcutaneous Tissue and Fascia | P Cardiac Rhythm Related Device |
| Defibrillator Generator | Insertion | Subcutaneous Tissue and Fascia | P Cardiac Rhythm Related Device |
| Epiretinal Visual Prosthesis | All applicable | Eye | J Synthetic Substitute |
| External Fixation Device, Hybrid | Insertion | Lower Bones Upper Bones | 5 External Fixation Device |
| External Fixation Device, Hybrid | Reposition | Lower Bones Upper Bones | 5 External Fixation Device |
| External Fixation Device, Limb Lengthening | Insertion | Lower Bones Upper Bones | 5 External Fixation Device |
| External Fixation Device, Monoplanar | Insertion | Lower Bones Upper Bones | 5 External Fixation Device |
| External Fixation Device, Monoplanar | Reposition | Lower Bones Upper Bones | 5 External Fixation Device |
| External Fixation Device, Ring | Insertion | Lower Bones Upper Bones | 5 External Fixation Device |
| External Fixation Device, Ring | Reposition | Lower Bones Upper Bones | 5 External Fixation Device |
| Hearing Device, Bone Conduction | Insertion | Ear, Nose, Sinus | S Hearing Device |
| Hearing Device, Multiple Channel Cochlear Prosthesis | Insertion | Ear, Nose, Sinus | S Hearing Device |
| Hearing Device, Single Channel Cochlear Prosthesis | Insertion | Ear, Nose, Sinus | S Hearing Device |
| Internal Fixation Device, Intramedullary | All applicable | Lower Bones Upper Bones | 4 Internal Fixation Device |
| Internal Fixation Device, Rigid Plate | Insertion | Upper Bones | 4 Internal Fixation Device |

| Specific Device | for Operation | in Body System | General Device |
|---|---|---|---|
| Internal Fixation Device, Rigid Plate | Reposition | Upper Bones | 4 Internal Fixation Device |
| Intraluminal Device, Pessary | All applicable | Female Reproductive System | D Intraluminal Device |
| Intraluminal Device, Airway | All applicable | Ear, Nose, Sinus Gastrointestinal System Mouth and Throat | D Intraluminal Device |
| Intraluminal Device, Bioactive | All applicable | Upper Arteries | D Intraluminal Device |
| Intraluminal Device, Drug-eluting | All applicable | Heart and Great Vessels Lower Arteries Upper Arteries | D Intraluminal Device |
| Intraluminal Device, Endobronchial Valve | All applicable | Respiratory System | D Intraluminal Device |
| Intraluminal Device, Endotracheal Airway | All applicable | Respiratory System | D Intraluminal Device |
| Intraluminal Device, Radioactive | All applicable | Heart and Great Vessels | D Intraluminal Device |
| Monitoring Device, Hemodynamic | Insertion | Subcutaneous Tissue and Fascia | 2 Monitoring Device |
| Monitoring Device, Pressure Sensor | Insertion | Heart and Great Vessels | 2 Monitoring Device |
| Pacemaker, Dual Chamber | Insertion | Subcutaneous Tissue and Fascia | P Cardiac Rhythm Related Device |
| Pacemaker, Single Chamber | Insertion | Subcutaneous Tissue and Fascia | P Cardiac Rhythm Related Device |
| Pacemaker, Single Chamber Rate Responsive | Insertion | Subcutaneous Tissue and Fascia | P Cardiac Rhythm Related Device |

| Specific Device | for Operation | in Body System | General Device |
|---|---|---|---|
| Spinal Stabilization Device, Facet Replacement | Insertion | Lower Joints Upper Joints | 4 Internal Fixation Device |
| Spinal Stabilization Device, Interspinous Process | Insertion | Lower Joints Upper Joints | 4 Internal Fixation Device |
| Spinal Stabilization Device, Pedicle-Based | Insertion | Lower Joints Upper Joints | 4 Internal Fixation Device |
| Stimulator Generator, Multiple Array | Insertion | Subcutaneous Tissue and Fascia | M Stimulator Generator |
| Stimulator Generator, Multiple Array Rechargeable | Insertion | Subcutaneous Tissue and Fascia | M Stimulator Generator |
| Stimulator Generator, Single Array | Insertion | Subcutaneous Tissue and Fascia | M Stimulator Generator |
| Stimulator Generator, Single Array Rechargeable | Insertion | Subcutaneous Tissue and Fascia | M Stimulator Generator |
| Synthetic Substitute, Ceramic | Replacement | Lower Joints | J Synthetic Substitute |
| Synthetic Substitute, Ceramic on Polyethylene | Replacement | Lower Joints | J Synthetic Substitute |
| Synthetic Substitute, Intraocular Telescope | Replacement | Eye | J Synthetic Substitute |
| Synthetic Substitute, Metal | Replacement | Lower Joints | J Synthetic Substitute |
| Synthetic Substitute, Metal on Polyethylene | Replacement | Lower Joints | J Synthetic Substitute |
| Synthetic Substitute, Polyethylene | Replacement | Lower Joints | J Synthetic Substitute |
| Synthetic Substitute, Reverse Ball and Socket | Replacement | Upper Joints | J Synthetic Substitute |

## APPENDIX G:
### Coding Practice Quiz Answers

### Section 0 – Medical and Surgical

| Procedure | Code |
|---|---|
| 1. | 0HB2XZZ |
| 2. | 0UB14ZZ |
| 3. | 0TB03ZX |
| 4. | 0DB68ZX |
| 5. | 0FB20ZZ |
| 6. | 0CB1XZZ |
| 7. | 0FBG0ZZ |
| 8. | 0KBS3ZX |
| 9. | 0DBN8ZZ |
| 10. | 0LBN0ZZ |
| 11. | 0DTH0ZZ |
| 12. | 0GT00ZZ |
| 13. | 0TT10ZZ |
| 14. | 07T60ZZ |
| 15. | 0UT9FZZ |
| 16. | 0HTT0ZZ |
| 17. | 02TD0ZZ |
| 18. | 0VT00ZZ |
| 19. | 0FT44ZZ |
| 20. | 09TQ4ZZ, 09TR4ZZ |
| 21. | 0X6B0ZZ |
| 22. | 0Y6H0Z1 |
| 23. | 0X6K0Z8 |
| 24. | 0Y620ZZ |
| 25. | 0X6L0Z3 |
| 26. | 0X6J0Z0 |
| 27. | 0Y6N0Z9 |
| 28. | 0X680Z2 |
| 29. | 0Y6W0Z1 |
| 30. | 0Y6C0Z3 |
| 31. | 0H5GXZZ |
| 32. | 0C5T3ZZ |
| 33. | 02583ZZ |
| 34. | 095KXZZ |
| 35. | 0V508ZZ |
| 36. | 065Y3ZZ |
| 37. | 0U524ZZ |
| 38. | 085G3ZZ |
| 39. | 0B5P422 |
| 40. | 06H03DZ |
| 41. | 0CDWXZ2, 0CDXXZ2 |
| 42. | 0HDQXZZ |
| 43. | 08DJ3ZZ |
| 44. | 0UDN4ZZ |
| 45. | 0HDMXZZ |
| 46. | 0JD80ZZ |
| 47. | 0UDB8ZX |
| 48. | 0JDF3ZZ |
| 49. | 09D77ZZ |
| 50. | 06DY3ZZ |
| 51. | 0T9B70Z |
| 52. | 0D90XZZ |
| 53. | 0W9G3ZZ |
| 54. | 0U914ZZ |
| 55. | 0F9100Z |
| 56. | 0S9C00Z |
| 57. | 0W9B3ZZ |
| 58. | 059C3ZZ |
| 59. | 0W9930Z |
| 60. | 099V4ZZ |
| 61. | 0TF6XZZ, 0TF7XZZ |
| 62. | 0FF98ZZ |
| 63. | 02FN0ZZ |
| 64. | 0TFB8ZZ |
| 65. | 0UF68ZZ |
| 66. | 0L8V3ZZ |
| 67. | 02883ZZ |
| 68. | 0P8N0ZZ |
| 69. | 0D848ZZ |
| 70. | 018R3ZZ |
| 71. | 0TN60ZZ |
| 72. | 0HNDXZZ |
| 73. | 0CN7XZZ |
| 74. | 0MN14ZZ |
| 75. | 02NG0ZZ |
| 76. | 0LNP3ZZ |
| 77. | 0DNW4ZZ |
| 78. | 0RNJXZZ |
| 79. | 01NG0ZZ |
| 80. | 0UN14ZZ, 0UN64ZZ |
| 81. | 0FY00Z0 |
| 82. | 02YA0Z2 |
| 83. | 0BYK0Z0 |
| 84. | 0DYE0Z0 |
| 85. | 0FYG0Z0, 0TY10Z0 |
| 86. | 0HM0XZZ |
| 87. | 09M0XZZ |
| 88. | 0KMT0ZZ |
| 89. | 0CMXXZ1 |
| 90. | 0XMK0ZZ |
| 91. | 0LX70ZZ |
| 92. | 01X64Z5 |
| 93. | 0JXM0ZC |
| 94. | 0XXP0ZM |
| 95. | 0JX43ZZ |
| 96. | 00XK4ZM |
| 97. | 0LXP4ZZ |
| 98. | 0HX0XZZ |
| 99. | 0KXK0Z6, 0KXL0Z6 |
| 100. | 0HX6XZZ |

| Procedure | Code | Procedure | Code | Procedure | Code | Procedure | Code |
|-----------|------|-----------|------|-----------|------|-----------|------|
| 101. | 0QSG0ZZ | 151. | 0SRC0JZ | 201. | 0RJJ4ZZ | 6. | 2W44X5Z |
| 102. | 0DS64ZZ | 152. | 0HRV076 | 202. | 09JY4ZZ | 7. | 2W27X4Z |
| 103. | 0MSP4ZZ | 153. | 0LRS0KZ | 203. | 0FJ00ZZ | 8. | 2Y50X5Z |
| 104. | 01S40ZZ | 154. | 02RG08Z | 204. | 0TJB8ZZ | 9. | 2W18X7Z |
| 105. | 0QS634Z | 155. | 08RJ3JZ | 205. | 0DJD8ZZ | 10. | 2W0PX6Z |
| 106. | 0UVC7ZZ | 156. | 08C8XZZ | 206. | 0W3R8ZZ | | |
| 107. | 02VR0CZ | 157. | 03C83ZZ | 207. | 0X3F0ZZ | | |
| 108. | 07VK3DZ | 158. | 0DC68ZZ | 208. | 0W3H0ZZ | **Section 3 – Administration** | |
| 109. | 03VG0CZ | 159. | 0HCGXZZ | 209. | 0W3C0ZZ | Procedure | Code |
| 110. | 08VX7DZ | 160. | 0TCB8ZZ | 210. | 0Y3F4ZZ | 1. | 3E1M39Z |
| | | | | | | 2. | 3E0P7LZ |
| 111. | 06L33ZZ | 161. | 09CKXZZ | 211. | 01Q60ZZ | 3. | 3E0436Z |
| 112. | 03LL3DZ | 162. | 0DCV4ZZ | 212. | 0DQ90ZZ | 4. | 3E0G8GC |
| 113. | 0UL74CZ | 163. | 08CX0ZZ | 213. | 0WQN0ZZ | 5. | 3E1U38Z |
| 114. | 03L80ZZ | 164. | 0UCG7ZZ or 0UCGXZZ | 214. | 0LQ30ZZ | 6. | 3E0S33Z |
| 115. | 03LG3DZ | 165. | 03CH0ZZ | 215. | 0WQF0ZZ | 7. | 30263V1 |
| 116. | 0F798ZZ | 166. | 02UF0JZ | 216. | 00K83ZZ | 8. | 3E0P3Q1 |
| 117. | 02703DZ, 02703ZZ | 167. | 0YU64JZ | 217. | 02K83ZZ | 9. | 30243G0 |
| 118. | 0T7C8ZZ | 168. | 01U547Z | 218. | 00K00ZZ | 10. | 3E0102A |
| 119. | 047L0ZZ | 169. | 0SUS09Z, 0SPB09Z | 219. | 00K74ZZ | | |
| 120. | 0D717ZZ | 170. | 0UUG0JZ | 220. | 02K80ZZ | **Section 4 - Measurement and Monitoring** | |
| | | | | | | Procedure | Code |
| 121. | 03773ZZ | 171. | 02UA0JZ | 221. | 0RGP04Z | 1. | 4A02XM4 |
| 122. | 087X7DZ | 172. | 0WUF0JZ | 222. | 0SG10AJ | 2. | 4A0C85Z |
| 123. | 0U778ZZ | 173. | 0LU207Z | 223. | 0RGQ0KZ | 3. | 4A023N8 |
| 124. | 0B718ZZ | 174. | 08U9X7Z | 224. | 0SG507Z | 4. | 4A04XJ1 |
| 125. | 0T778DZ | 175. | 0SUR0BZ | 225. | 0SGQ34Z | 5. | 4A12X45 |
| 126. | 0D160ZA | 176. | 0S2YX0Z | 226. | 0W020ZZ | 6. | 4A09XCZ |
| 127. | 031S0JG | 177. | 0B21XFZ | 227. | 0H0V0JZ | 7. | 4A1H7CZ |
| 128. | 0B113F4 | 178. | 0W2BX0Z | 228. | 090K07Z | 8. | 4A07X7Z |
| 129. | 02103D4 | 179. | 0020X0Z | 229. | 0W0F0ZZ | 9. | 4A1239Z |
| 130. | 041L0KL | 180. | 0T2BX0Z | 230. | 0J0L3ZZ, 0J0M3ZZ | 10. | 4A08X0Z |
| | | | | 231. | 0W4N0K1 | | |
| 131. | 00160J6 | 181. | 01PY0MZ | 232. | 0W4M0J0 | **Section 5 – Extracorporeal Assistance and Performance** | |
| 132. | 0D1L0Z4 | 182. | 02PYX2Z | | | Procedure | Code |
| 133. | 0T170ZC | 183. | 0FPG00Z | **Section 1 – Obstetrics** | | 1. | 5A1935Z |
| 134. | 02100Z9 | 184. | 0BP1XFZ | Procedure | Code | 2. | 5A1C00Z |
| 135. | 0W190JG | 185. | 0DP6XUZ | 1. | 10A07ZW | 3. | 5A2204Z |
| 136. | 0JH80DZ | 186. | 0UPH71Z | 2. | 10E0XZZ | 4. | 5A09358 |
| 137. | 02H73JZ | 187. | 0QPN04Z | 3. | 10A07ZX | 5. | 5A1D60Z |
| 138. | 0JH606Z | 188. | 0TP98DZ | 4. | 10J07ZZ | 6. | 5A02210 |
| 139. | 05HM33Z | 189. | 0DP6X0Z | 5. | 10D00Z2 | 7. | 5A1223Z |
| 140. | 09HE06Z | 190. | 0PPJX5Z | 6. | 10903ZA | 8. | 5A15223 |
| | | | | 7. | 10Y04ZS | 9. | 5A1945Z |
| 141. | 02HV32Z | 191. | 02WYX2Z | 8. | 10Q00ZK | 10. | 5A02115 |
| 142. | 0BH081Z | 192. | 0SW90JZ | 9. | 10T24ZZ | | |
| 143. | 0JHT3VZ | 193. | 02WA3MZ | 10. | 10P073Z | **Section 6 – Extracorporeal Therapies** | |
| 144. | 0QHY0MZ | 194. | 0QWH04Z | | | Procedure | Code |
| 145. | 0VH081Z | 195. | 0JWT0WZ | **Section 2 – Placement** | | 1. | 6A550Z2 |
| 146. | 0HRDX73 | 196. | 0WJ90ZZ | Procedure | Code | 2. | 6A801ZZ |
| 147. | 0QR70KZ | 197. | 0CJS8ZZ | 1. | 2Y42X5Z | 3. | 6A4Z0ZZ |
| 148. | 08R83KZ | 198. | 0SJD0ZZ | 2. | 2W6MX0Z | 4. | 6A650ZZ |
| 149. | 0HRV0JZ | 199. | 0UJD8ZZ | 3. | 2W5AX1Z | 5. | 6A930ZZ |
| 150. | 04R00JZ | 200. | 0DJD7ZZ | 4. | 2W32X3Z | 6. | 6A0Z1ZZ |
| | | | | 5. | 2Y04X5Z | 7. | 6A221ZZ |

| Procedure | Code |
|-----------|--------|
| 8. | 6A750ZZ |
| 9. | 6A551Z3 |
| 10. | 6A210ZZ |

## Section 7 – Osteopathic

| Procedure | Code |
|-----------|--------|
| 1. | 7W06X8Z |
| 2. | 7W00X5Z |
| 3. | 7W07X6Z |
| 4. | 7W04X4Z |
| 5. | 7W01X0Z |

## Section 8 – Other Procedures

| Procedure | Code |
|-----------|--------|
| 1. | 8E023DZ |
| 2. | 8E09XBG |
| 3. | 8E0WXY8 |
| 4. | 8E0ZXY6 |
| 5. | 8E0W0CZ |

## Section 9 – Chiropractics

| Procedure | Code |
|-----------|--------|
| 1. | 9WB3XGZ |
| 2. | 9WB9XCZ |
| 3. | 9WB6XDZ |
| 4. | 9WB4XJZ |
| 5. | 9WB0XKZ |

## Section B – Imaging

| Procedure | Code |
|-----------|--------|
| 1. | BW21ZZZ |
| 2. | B342ZZ3 |
| 3. | B5181ZA |
| 4. | BF43ZZZ |
| 5. | B2151ZZ |
| 6. | BD11YZZ |
| 7. | BP0JZZZ |
| 8. | BY4DZZZ |
| 9. | BB240ZZ |
| 10. | B41G1ZZ |

## Section C – Nuclear Medicine

| Procedure | Code |
|-----------|--------|
| 1. | C226YZZ |
| 2. | CT631ZZ |
| 3. | CP151ZZ |
| 4. | CH22SZZ |
| 5. | C23GQZZ |
| 6. | CW1BLZZ |
| 7. | C050VZZ |
| 8. | CD15YZZ |
| 9. | C030BZZ |
| 10. | C763HZZ |

## Section D – Radiation Therapy

| Procedure | Code |
|-----------|--------|
| 1. | D8Y0FZZ |
| 2. | D0011ZZ |
| 3. | DDY5CZZ |
| 4. | DV109BZ |
| 5. | DM013ZZ |
| 6. | DWY68ZZ |
| 7. | D9Y57ZZ |
| 8. | DF034ZZ |
| 9. | D016B9Z |
| 10. | DWY5GFZ |

## Section F – Physical Rehabilitation and Diagnostic Audiology

| Procedure | Code |
|-----------|--------|
| 1. | F13Z31Z |
| 2. | F0DZ8UZ |
| 3. | F07L0ZZ |
| 4. | F00ZHYZ |
| 5. | F0FZ8ZZ |
| 6. | F0DZ7EZ |
| 7. | F02ZFZZ |
| 8. | F0FZJMZ |
| 9. | F07M6ZZ |
| 10. | F09Z2KZ |

## Section G – Mental Health

| Procedure | Code |
|-----------|--------|
| 1. | GZ58ZZZ |
| 2. | GZGZZZZ |
| 3. | GZJZZZZ |
| 4. | GZB1ZZZ |
| 5. | GZ2ZZZZ |
| 6. | GZ13ZZZ |
| 7. | GZFZZZZ |
| 8. | GZ10ZZZ |
| 9. | GZ61ZZZ |
| 10. | GZ72ZZZ |

## Section H – Substance Abuse Treatment

| Procedure | Code |
|-----------|--------|
| 1. | HZ94ZZZ |
| 2. | HZ63ZZZ |
| 3. | HZ81ZZZ |
| 4. | HZ54ZZZ |
| 5. | HZ2ZZZZ |
| 6. | HZ47ZZZ |
| 7. | HZ53ZZZ |
| 8. | HZ3CZZZ |
| 9. | HZ5CZZZ |
| 10. | HZ42ZZZ |